# Clinical Nursing Skills and Techniques

**To Rebecca and Chip**
whose mother I am proud to be
Anne G. Perry

**To Ruth**
a very good friend
Patricia A. Potter

# Clinical Nursing Skills and Techniques

**ANNE G. PERRY, RN, MSN, ANP**

Associate Professor, School of Nursing, and
Coordinator of Critical Care Education, The University Hospital,
St. Louis University, St. Louis, Missouri
Doctoral Candidate, Southern Illinois University at Edwardsville, Edwardsville, Illinois

**PATRICIA A. POTTER, RN, MSN**

Director of Nursing Practice
Barnes Hospital, St. Louis, Missouri

**SECOND EDITION**

*With 757 Illustrations*

**The C. V. Mosby Company**

ST. LOUIS • BALTIMORE • PHILADELPHIA • TORONTO 1990

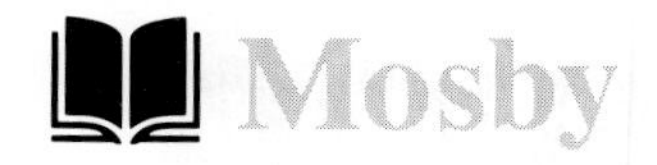

Editor: Nancy L. Coon
Developmental editor: Susan R. Epstein
Project manager: Carol Sullivan Wiseman
Production editor: Florence Achenbach
Design: Gail Morey Hudson
Photographer: Patrick Watson
Illustrator: Vicki Friedman



Printed in the United States of America

The C.V. Mosby Company
11830 Westline Industrial Drive, St. Louis, Missouri, 63146

**Library of Congress Cataloging in publication data**

Clinical nursing skills and techniques Anne G. Perry,
Patricia A. Potter.—2nd ed.
p. cm.
Includes bibliographical references.
ISBN 0-8016-5493-9
1. Nursing—Handbooks, manuals, etc. 2. Medicine, Clinical—Handbooks, manuals, etc. I. Perry, Anne Griffin. II. Potter,
[DNLM: 1. Nursing Care—handbooks. WY 39 C6413]
RT51.C65 1990
610.73—dc20
DNLM/DLC
for Library of Congress 89-13387
CIP

C/VH/VH 9 8 7 6 5 4 3

# CONTRIBUTORS

**PAMELA J. BECKER, RN, MSN**

Pulmonary Clinical Nurse Specialist
Barnes Hospital
St. Louis, Missouri

**CAROL BRANCH, RN, MSN**

St. Louis, Missouri

**LYNDAL GUENTHER BRAND, RN, BSN, MSN**

Director of Education
St. Louis Regional Medical Center
St. Louis, Missouri

**RITA H. CANFIELD, RN, MSN**

Instructor, School of Nursing
Southern Illinois University-Edwardsville
Edwardsville, Illinois

**PATRICIA DETTENMEIER, RN, MSN**

Clinical Nurse Specialist
Department of Pulmonology
St. Louis University Medical Center
St. Louis, Missouri

**MARY V. DYER, RN, MSN**

Oncology Clinical Nurse Specialist
South Florida Comprehensive Cancer Center Network
Salick Health Care, Inc.
Atlantis, Florida

**PATRICIA GELDBACH, RN, MA**

Assistant Director, Operating Room Department
St. Luke's Hospital
Chesterfield, Missouri

**EILEEN GIMPER, RN, PhD**

Associate Professor of Nursing
Duquesne University
Pittsburgh, Pennsylvania

**PAULA BRENNAN GOLDBERG, RN, MS, MSN**

Oncology Clinical Nurse Specialist
Barnes Hospital
St. Louis, Missouri

**PAT HANICK, RN, BSN**

Enterostomal Therapy Nurse Specialist
Barnes Hospital
St. Louis, Missouri

**SHIRLEY JOHNSON, RN, BSN**

Director, Medical Nursing
Barnes Hospital
St. Louis, Missouri

**JILL FELDMAN MALEN, RN, NS, MS**

Pulmonary/Thoracic Clinical Nurse Specialist
Barnes Hospital
St. Louis, Missouri

**ELIZABETH MEINERS MANTYCH, RN, MSN**

Nursing Instructor
Southern Illinois University-Edwardsville
Edwardsville, Illinois

**MARY MERCER, RN, MSN**

Clinical Nurse Specialist
Cardiac Rehabilitation
St. John's Mercy Medical Center
St. Louis, Missouri

**KATHLEEN DESKA PAGANA, RN, PhD**

Assistant Professor of Nursing
Lycoming College
Williamsport, Pennsylvania

**JUDITH A. ROOS, RN, MSN**

Nursing Education Coordinator, Staff Development
The University Hospital
St. Louis, Missouri

**JANICE J. RUMFELT, RNC, MSN**

Assistant Professor, School of Nursing
Southern Illinois University-Edwardsville
Edwardsville, Illinois

**JOANN SHEW, RN, MSN(R)**

Psychiatric Mental Health Clinical Nurse Specialist
St. John's Mercy Medical Center
St. Louis, Missouri

**MARLENE MARI SMITH, RN, BSN, MED**

Instructor, St. Louis Regional Medical Center and Clinics
St. Louis, Missouri

**MARGARET M. TIMM, BSN, MS**

Executive Director, Valley Home Health Inc.
Charleroi, Pennsylvania

**LAUREL A. WIERSEMA, RN, MSN**

Surgical Clinical Nurse Specialist
Barnes Hospital
St. Louis, Missouri

**PAMELA J. WILLIAMS, RN, MSN**

Surgical Intensive Care Nurse
Veterans Administration Medical Center
St. Louis, Missouri

# PREFACE

CLINICAL NURSING SKILLS AND TECHNIQUES has been developed to address the need for a back-to-basics approach to nursing practice. With so much emphasis on psychosocial aspects of nursing and specialization in today's curricula, it is possible that the profession has unwittingly lost sight of fundamental knowledge and skills the nurse must possess to effectively deliver quality health care to clients. Readers will find no conceptual material here—no theories, no classical frameworks characteristic of fundamentals texts—just procedures students will be required to competently demonstrate in their course work and that nurses will be expected to implement in their daily practice. And yet this text is not simply a "how-to" manual. Rather, the intent is to stimulate readers to think, to anticipate, and to formulate ideas based on sound, current nursing principle and within the nursing process framework.

The vast majority of readers will be exposed to this material in a first-semester or first-year fundamentals or skills course; however, because this text goes far beyond basic knowledge and skills, it can be of benefit throughout the students' course work either as a supplemental or as a reference text and can extend into the nurse's practice.

*Clinical Nursing Skills and Techniques* can also serve as a useful guide for entry-level practitioners who may need to refamiliarize themselves with various skills as they embark on nursing careers in many avenues of health care.

## ORGANIZATION

### Unit Format

CLINICAL NURSING SKILLS AND TECHNIQUES contains 47 chapters logically organized by broad subject matter, in 14 units. Unit I lays the groundwork for the rest of the text, with chapters on admitting, transfer and discharge, recording and reporting, and communication. Unit II covers skills of safety and comfort. Unit III presents hygiene skills. Unit IV provides detailed skills concerning vital signs and physical assessment. Unit V includes five oxygen-related chapters. Unit VI examines skills a nurse needs to administer a wide variety of medications. Unit VII deals with fluids, featuring timely chapters on vascular access devices and blood therapy. Unit VIII presents nutrition-related skills. Unit IX describes skills concerned with elimination. Unit X deals with posture, mobility, and ambulation, including a chapter on orthopedic measures. Unit XI describes skills needed for infection control. Unit XII focuses on care of the surgical client and intraoperative care. Unit XIII takes a look at skills related to dressings, binders and bandages, hot and cold therapy, and wound care and irrigation. The text concludes with a unit on special procedures, including specimen collection, diagnostic procedures, and postmortem care.

### Chapter Format

Each chapter begins with learning objectives, key terms, a list of the skills in the chapter, and an overview. The overview provides a general discussion of content, helpful guidelines to follow while performing all skills, and prerequisite knowledge and skills that should be mastered before performing the skills in the chapter. Helpful cross-references are provided for quick access to information in other chapters.

### Skills Format

Each skill begins with an introduction that includes the various purposes for the procedure. Procedures in each chapter are presented in a consistent, easy-to-follow two-column format, which provides the steps of the procedure and the rationale for each step. Steps of the procedure are presented according to the five steps of the nursing process.

Three additional features are included in each skill. Subordinate to *Evaluation* are *Expected Outcomes,* which help students determine the effect of the skill, and *Unexpected Outcomes,* which identify potential problems that may result. Second, *Recording and Reporting Guidelines* assists readers in developing charting skills. Third, *Follow-up Activities* are outlined, which include such ongoing care as monitoring vital signs and exercises.

Each skill concludes with a listing of special, teaching, and home care considerations as appropriate. This section provides information relating to clients with special conditions that may contraindicate performing all or part of the procedure, age-specific concerns, helpful tips, or alerts concerning complications that may result. Teaching considerations assist the nurse to ensure that client teaching is comprehensive and effective. Home care considerations include guidelines for adapting procedures for the home setting, assessment of the home environment as it relates to the clients' health care needs, and appropriate teaching and follow-up care.

## SPECIAL FEATURES

Much care and research has gone into special learning features. What has been included is a result of astute comments and suggestions from instructors, practicing nurses, and students in a wide variety of programs and settings. Learner-directed objectives are provided at the beginning of each chapter. The focus is on specific content within the chapter. Instructors are encouraged to add to the list as necessary. Key terms have also been provided. They represent common terminology discussed within the chapter. Definitions are also found in the glossary at the end of the book. Prerequisite knowledge and skills provide a frame of reference for students to test what they already know or to refer to other chapters before proceeding.

The inclusion of many illustrations and photographs, often shown in a series for a particular skill and placed in proximity to steps being described, will also aid students as they master techniques.

Performance checklists for each skill are found in the Instructor's Manual that accompanies this text. The uses of this important evaluative tool are twofold. The instructor may indicate to the students whether they successfully completed each step and may write comments in the space provided should the student need further instructions or guidance. If not employed as evaluative tools, students may request checklists from their instructors for self-evaluation purposes.

The versatility and adaptability of *Clinical Nursing Skills and Techniques* are boundless. It is a valuable learning tool for students and entry-level practitioners, providing the know-how to perform safely and efficiently and to still address the challenges of a rapidly changing profession.

## ACKNOWLEDGMENTS

A textbook such as this would not be possible without the diligent efforts of many people. To guide us in our writing, we depended on and are grateful to the many reviewers who lent their knowledge and expertise in a wide variety of areas.

The contributions of many individuals at the The C.V. Mosby Company were combined to make this textbook a reality. The authors especially wish to thank:

Alison Miller, vice-president. Her belief in this project provided much of the motivation behind this work. She has remained a close friend and confidante.

Nancy L. Coon, editor. Her committment to this project never wavered. Her demands for excellence were equally matched with encouragement, support, and good humor.

Suzi Epstein, developmental editor. Her support and encouragement proved valuable throughout this project.

Bess Arends, a special person who always has the ability to instill confidence and support when it is most needed.

Special effort was taken to ensure a high-quality illustration program. Thanks go out to:

Vicki M. Friedman and Marcy H. Hartstein, surgical illustrators. Their artistic contributions have made the textbook visually appealing.

Patrick Watson, photographer, a talented artist whose photographs make each chapter unique.

Anne G. Perry
Patricia A. Potter

# CONTENTS

SKILL 46-2 *Assisting with Bone Marrrow Aspiration,* 992


---

Teaching Considerations and Home Care Considerations written and/or reviewed by Eileen Gimper and Margaret M. Timm.

# UNIT I

# SUPPORTING THE CLIENT THROUGH THE HEALTH CARE SYSTEM

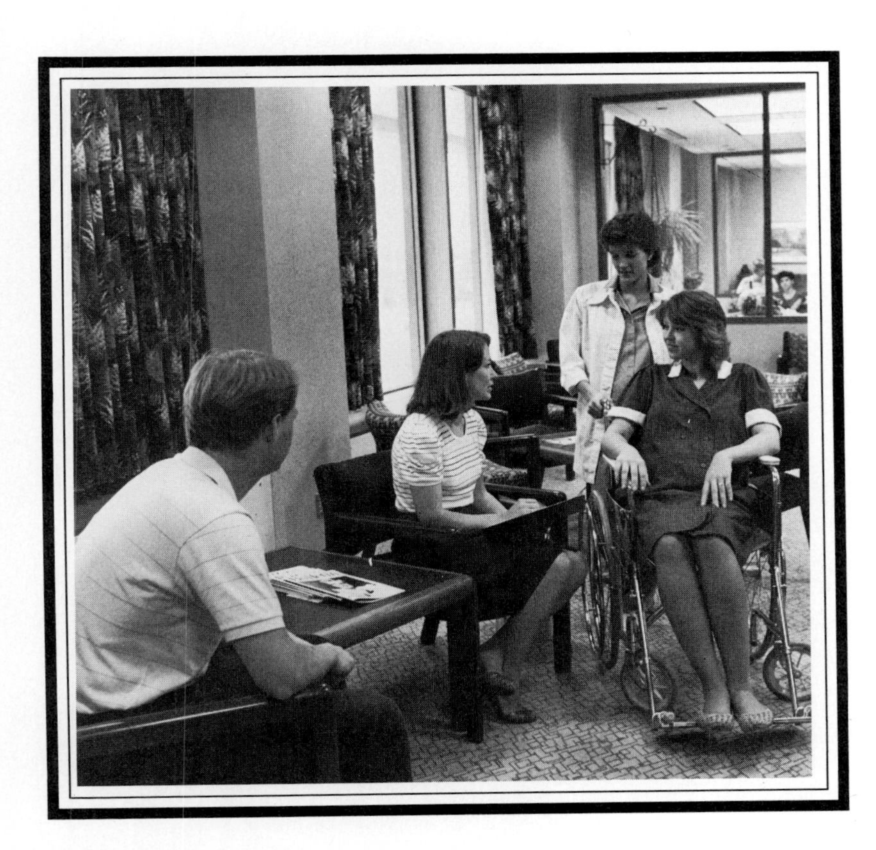

*When a client enters the health care delivery system, a variety of experiences can cause significant emotional and physical stress. The period of time spent within a health care facility often disrupts living routines, family relationships, or family financial planning. Various health care personnel responsible for the client's care at admission often repeatedly ask the same questions, causing a client to feel simply like a number walking through a maze of health care services. Laboratory tests and diagnostic examinations can cause physical discomforts that heighten the client's anxieties.*

# 1

# ADMITTING, TRANSFER, AND DISCHARGE

### OBJECTIVES

*Mastery of content in this chapter will enable the nurse to:*

- Define key terms.
- Perform the following skills: admit a client to an agency; admit a client to a nursing division; make a health care referral; transfer a client to a nursing division; transfer a client to a different agency; discharge a client.
- Describe methods for maintaining continuity of a client's care during admission, transfer, or discharge.
- Identify the purposes of health care referrals.
- Explain the importance of including the client's family in the admission, transfer, or discharge process.
- Describe the roles of various health professionals in discharge planning.

### KEY TERMS

*Discharge planning*
*Extended care facility*
*Nursing home*
*Patient's Bill of Rights*

### SKILLS

**1-1** Admitting Clients to a Health Care Agency
**1-2** Admitting Clients to a Nursing Division
**1-3** Making Referrals for Health Care Services
**1-4** Transferring Clients to a Different Nursing Division
**1-5** Transferring Clients to a Different Agency
**1-6** Discharging Clients from a Health Care Agency

Once the client is in a health care setting, it may be necessary to use the services of different health care specialties. Transfer from one health care service to another or referral for a special service causes further disruption as a client becomes confused over what expectations each health care provider holds.

Discharge planning is a process that facilitates the client's transition from a health care agency to the most independent level of care, whether that be home or another agency. However, discharge from an agency can be stressful if a client feels unprepared to resume normal activities or unable to adapt therapeutic regimens to living at home. A client must know what to expect before discharge. Without the necessary equipment and professional resources to care for continuing health problems, the client risks loss of any rehabilitation gains made before discharge. Failure to understand restrictions or implications of health problems may cause a client to develop complications after leaving the health care setting. Poor discharge planning ignores the client's needs within the home and increases the chance of the client reentering the health care system prematurely. An emphasis in current health care is to anticipate the client's discharge needs before the client enters the health care system.

The nurse plays a key role in coordinating the client's care from admission to eventual discharge. To separate the processes of admission and discharge is a critical error. The nurse identifies clients' learning needs, anticipates physical deficits that impose implications for resuming normal activities, assesses needs for family support, and assists in having health care resources made available in the home setting as needed. Ultimately the client and family should be prepared to understand the implications of health alterations and the responsibilities for continued care in the home.

### GUIDELINES

1. Identify as early as possible those clients who require discharge planning to foster continuity of care throughout their stay in the health care setting.
2. Include the client and family in planning early for all moves through the health care system.
3. Consider the client's past experiences in health care settings.

4. Communicate and document a plan of care to all health care personnel assuming the client's care.
5. Assist other health care personnel in assessing appropriate resources needed as clients move through the health care system.

### PREREQUISITE KNOWLEDGE

1. Therapeutic communication techniques (Chapter 3).
2. Process for collecting a nursing history.
3. Principles of medical asepsis.
4. Process for writing a nursing care plan.
5. Methods of reporting and recording (Chapter 2).
6. Teaching and learning principles.

### PREREQUISITE SKILLS

1. Methods for maintaining a safe environment (Chapter 4).
2. Physical assessment (Chapter 13).
3. Assessment of vital signs (Chapter 12).
4. Basic handwashing techniques (Chapter 37).
5. Methods for collecting specimens (Chapter 45).
6. Correct physical transfer techniques (Chapter 33).
7. Skills appropriate to client's teaching needs:
   a. Dressing changes (Chapter 41).
   b. Assessing a pulse (Chapter 12).
   c. Administering medications (Chapters 19 and 21).

### *THE PATIENT'S BILL OF RIGHTS*

1. The patient has the right to considerate and respectful care.
2. The patient has the right to obtain from his physician complete current information concerning his diagnosis, treatment and prognosis in terms the patient can be reasonably expected to understand.
3. The patient has the right to receive from his physician information necessary to give informed consent prior to the start of any procedure and/or treatment. . . . Where medically significant alternatives for care of treatment exist, or when the patient requests information concerning medical alternatives, the patient has the right to such information (and) to know the name of the person responsible for the procedures and/or treatment.
4. The patient has the right to refuse treatment to the extent permitted by law, and to be informed of the medical consequences of his action.
5. The patient has the right to every consideration of his privacy concerning his own medical care program.
6. The patient has the right to expect that all communications and records pertaining to his care should be treated as confidential.
7. The patient has the right to expect that within its capacity a hospital must make reasonable response to the request of a patient for services.
8. The patient has the right to obtain information as to any relationship of his hospital to other health care and educational institutions insofar as his care is concerned (and) any professional relationships among individuals, by name, who are treating him.
9. The patient has the right to be advised if the hospital proposes to engage in or perform human experimentation affecting his care or treatment (and) has the right to refuse to participate.
10. The patient has the right to expect reasonable continuity of care.
11. The patient has the right to examine and receive an explanation of his bill regardless of source of payment.
12. The patient has the right to know what hospital rules and regulations apply to his conduct as a patient.



## *SKILL 1-1* *Admitting Clients to a Health Care Agency*

Whether a client is entering a hospital, a nursing home, or a rehabilitation center, it is essential that as much information as possible be gathered so that the client ultimately receives the required care. Likewise the nurse considers the emotional influence the admission process has on the client so as to provide therapeutic support. Inclusion of available friends or family members into the admission process improves the likelihood of their support during the client's experience within a health care setting.

Each institution follows a different set of policies and procedures for admitting a client. Responsibilities can be understood when the nurse becomes familiarized with those policies and procedures.

A client's condition determines how extensive the admitting procedure will be. For example, the client entering a hospital through the emergency room may not be in a condition to tolerate the procedures that take place in an admitting office. Family members provide pertinent information for the hospital's records while the client is transported directly to the nursing division. In contrast, an elderly client who can no longer attend to daily chores but who is still independent enough to perform some self-care will undergo extensive screening before being accepted as a resident of a nursing home.

Admitting officers, secretaries, and technicians are the personnel primarily involved with the procedures for the initial admission of clients into an agency. Nurses and social workers are extensively involved with assessing the appropriateness of a client's placement into extended care and nursing home facilities.

There is considerable anxiety for the client about what the admission process will be like. It is important for all personnel to treat the client courteously and professionally. If one person shows an uncaring attitude, the client may assume that all personnel are unprofessional. By making the client and family feel welcome, the nursing personnel accomplish the first step in establishing a therapeutic rapport.

### Purposes

1. Begin acquiring information necessary to plan individualized care and discharge planning.
2. Minimize anxiety or misconceptions held by the client or family members.
3. Provide client and family members information that enhances their understanding of expectations of health care providers.
4. Ensure client comfort and safety.
5. Preserve the client's legal rights as a health care recipient.

## *Procedure 1-1*

| Steps | Rationale |
|---|---|
| **Implementation** | |
| 1. Maintain professional relationship with client. | |
| a. Welcome and escort client and family to interviewing area. | Courteous welcome helps relieve anxiety of anticipating first encounter with agency personnel. Interviewing area provides privacy for client. |
| 2. Provide for client's safety. | |
| a. Acquire identifying information including client's full legal name, age, birth date, address, next of kin, physician, religion, previous admissions. | Ensures correct legal identification of client. |
| b. Apply identification band (ID) to client's wrist containing following information: client's full legal name, hospital/agency number, physician, birth date. Be sure band is secure. | Serves to officially identify client when therapies or procedures are performed, e.g., medication administration, surgical procedures, or x-ray examinations. |
| 3. Provide for client's legal rights. | |
| a. Instruct client or legal guardian to read general consent form for treatment. Assess client's understanding of consent form. Request client or family member to sign form if there is agreement to be admitted for treatment. | Gives agency right to perform routine procedures and therapies, select room placement, and provide required nursing care. |
| 4. Orient client and family to health care agency. | |
| a. Provide any brochures describing purpose of agency, organization, and policies or rules that affect person's conduct as client. | American Hospital Association's "Patient's Bill of Rights" cites client's right to have access to this information (see box). |
| 5. Assess client's needs. | |
| a. Assign client's room on basis of client's condition, health care needs, and personal preferences. | Ensures that clients requiring frequent observation and therapy are close to central nursing station. Consideration of client's personal preferences during room selection minimizes client's anxiety and prevents conflict with other clients. Room environment can provide sensory stimulation for sensorially deprived clients. |
| 6. Prepare client for routine diagnostic testing. | |
| a. Instruct client on method for collecting urine specimen (Chapter 46). Technicians in admitting office collect routine blood specimens, chest x-ray, and electrocardiogram. | Serves to screen clients for presence of common physical alterations. |
| 7. Provide for continuity of care. | |
| a. Notify nursing division of client's admission: name, assigned room and bed, admitting physician, diagnosis, pertinent information related to client's condition (e.g., intravenous line infusing, need for oxygen). | Allows nursing personnel to prepare room and obtain necessary equipment for client's arrival. When client is admitted from emergency room, nursing division receives full report of client's condition so that personnel in nursing unit can prepare adequately for arrival and begin treatment immediately. |
| b. Transport client and family members to nursing division using escort. (Client's condition determines if ambulation or use of wheelchair or stretcher is appropriate.) | Member of hospital staff should accompany client to assigned room to ensure client's safe arrival. |

| Steps | Rationale |
|---|---|
| c. In nursing division introduce client and family to nurse assuming client's care. | Gives client sense of personalization during admission process. |
| d. Share pertinent observations about client's behavior with nursing staff, e.g., anxiety or fear, or level of knowledge regarding need for health care. | Promotes continuity of care so that nursing staff can assist client in coping with new environment and procedures. |

### Special Considerations

- When client is admitted in serious or unstable condition, family may be source for admitting information.
- Clients who wish to remain anonymous may be admitted under assumed name. Clients who are victims of crime may enter with assumed name to prevent their assailant from locating them. Clients admitted to emergency room unconscious may not be identified until family members arrive.
- Print on band must always be legible; illegible bands are replaced immediately.
- For consent form to be valid client or guardian must be mentally and physically competent, be a legal adult, give voluntary consent, understand risks and benefits of treatment, and have opportunity to ask questions.
- In some institutions nurses choose a client's room assignment. Otherwise, admitting personnel should confer with nursing staff. Confused, disoriented, or verbally abusive clients should be placed in private rooms to prevent disruption of roommate's sleep or rest. Clients who are highly susceptible to infection or who are infectious often require private rooms or consideration regarding the condition of a roommate. Clients who smoke should be separated from nonsmokers and clients using oxygen. Clients who will be restricted to bed for prolonged periods or who are isolated benefit from having a window for sensory stimulation.
- The following are risk criteria that may be used in screening clients who may need early assistance with discharge planning: clients over 72 years old and living alone, clients under 18 years old and suspected of being abused or neglected, out-of-town clients who must remain in town temporarily, clients who have no relatives, chronically ill clients being rehospitalized, clients with a condition likely to cause increasing impairment, clients with terminal illness, clients in need of special equipment at home, and adult clients unable to care for themselves.

### Teaching Considerations

- Clients admitted the morning of a surgical procedure or treatment are called *same day admissions.* They receive basic instructions regarding the purpose of surgery or treatment, preparatory procedures, and postsurgical or treatment care. Admission forms, consent forms, diagnostic tests, and teaching may be completed before the actual day of surgery. Often family members are offered instructional booklets pertaining to the client's surgery or treatment.

## *SKILL 1-2 Admitting Clients to a Nursing Division*

The nurse plays an active role in coordinating the admission process to a nursing division. As is the case with the initial admission process, a client's condition will influence the extent and type of admission activities. When a critically ill client reaches a hospital's nursing division, it becomes necessary for the client to undergo extensive examination and treatment procedures almost immediately. There is often little time for the nurse to orient the client and family to the division or learn of their fears or concerns. When a client enters a hospital for elective treatment, the nurse has time to prepare the client psychologically for hospitalization. The client will often undergo diagnostic studies, but the process is less urgent than that for an emergency admission.

The health care setting also influences the types of activities a client will undergo during admission. In a nursing home the nurse thoroughly assesses the client's ability to perform activities of daily living, whereas in a clinic the initial interview may focus on the client's current symptoms and previous health problems. In a hospital setting, the nurse collects a nursing history (Fig. 1-1) to identify relevant health problems and begin the formation of an individualized plan of care.

### Purposes

1. Identify presence of any acute signs or symptoms of health problems.
2. Initiate the nursing process relative to care of the client's health care needs.
3. Orient client and family to the health care setting.
4. Provide for client comfort and safety.
5. Provide client and family information pertinent to the type of care the client will receive.
6. Identify at an early stage the client's need for discharge planning.

**Barnes Hospital**

NURSES ADMISSION NOTE C-2

Date 4/18 Time 2:30pm Informant patient Age 41

T 37⁸ P 84 R 18 B/P 150/88 Ht. 5'10" Wt. 158 lb.

Chief Complaint and History of Present Illness:

Had experienced symptoms of weight loss, despite an increased appetite. Tests in physicians' office diagnosed Diabetes. Admitted for control

ADDRESSOGRAPH

| Type of previous illness/surgery | Date | Type of previous illness/surgery | Date |
|---|---|---|---|
| Appendectomy | 1985 | | |
| Fractured Ⓡ arm | 1978 | | |
| | | | |

Has received blood products in the past: ☐ Yes ☐ No If yes, List dates________ Reactions: ☐ Yes ☐ No

Allergies: ________

| Medication Name | Dose/Frequency | Time of Last Dose | Name | Dose/Frequency | Time of Last Dose |
|---|---|---|---|---|---|
| | | | | | |
| | | | | | |
| | | | | | |
| | | | | | |
| | | | | | |
| | | | | | |

Patient Provided: ☒ Admission Kit ☒ I.D. Band ☒ Sensitivity/Allergy Band

Patient Instructed: ☒ Valuables Policy ☒ Waiver signed ☒ Smoking/Visitor policy ☒ Nurses Call/Emergency/TV/Phone ☒ Chaplain availability ☐ Patient rights *(Psych. only)* SIGNATURE: T. Eelian RN

**DIRECTIONS: Circle those that apply. Comment on those circled if needed.**

**Sensory**

*Sensory Alteration*

- EYES: (Decreased acuity) (Blurred vision) Photophobia Discharge Prosthesis
  EARS: Tinnitus Discharge Hard of hearing (R or L)
  NOSE: (Congestion) Obstruction Discharge Epistaxis
  THROAT: Sore throat Hoarseness TOUCH: Reduced/absent tactile perception
  ASSIST DEVICES/MEASURES: (Glasses) Contacts Hearing aid Tracheostomy
  Comments: Glasses for reading. Has noticed blurred vision for last 2 weeks

**Skin/Mucous Membrane**

*Impaired Skin Integrity*
*Alt. in mucous membranes*

- Poor hygiene Poor turgor Diaphoretic Bruises Scars Erythema Petechiae Rash (Itching) Jaundice Wound *(describe)* Pale/dry membranes Coated tongue Stomatitis Carious teeth Halitosis
  Comments: Skin dry, flaky, warm to touch

**Respiratory**

*Ineffective airway clearance*
*Ineffective breathing patterns*
*Impaired gas exchange*

- Cough Hemoptysis Dyspnea Orthopnea Cyanosis Restlessness Home 02 L/min
  Use of accessory muscles Pursed lip breathing Pain with breathing
  Smoker *(packs/day ___ years ___)* (Lung sounds *(describe)*)
  Comments: Clear bilaterally

**Circulatory**

*Decreased cardiac output*
*Alt. periph. tissue perfusion*
*Alt. fluid volume*

- Fatigue Chest pain Palpitations Syncope Numbness Tingling Edema
  Weak/absent peripheral pulse (Capillary refill *(describe)*) (Extremities *(describe color/temperature)*)
  Comments: Refill good in fingers and toes. — Feet warm, dorsalis pedis pulses 3+ bilaterally

**Nutrition**

*Alt. in nutrition*

- Diet: Regular at home, Physician informed him 1800 ADA to be ordered
  Dysphagia Heartburn Nausea Vomiting (Appetite increase) decrease Decreased taste
  Weight gain/loss 15 lbs. Difficulty chewing Dentures - lower/upper
  Comments: Lost weight over course of 2 months

*Continued.*

***Fig. 1-1*** Nurses admission note.

Courtesy Barnes Hospital, St. Louis.

**Elimination**

*Alt. in bowel elimination*
*Alt. in urinary elimination*

- BOWEL: (Constipation) Diarrhea Incontinence Melena Tarry stools Ostomy
  Abd. pain/cramps/gas Hemorrhoids Last BM 4/16 Usual pattern *(describe)*
  Medications/Enemas MOM (rarely) (Bowel Sounds) *(describe)*
  Comments: occasional constipation, noted more when travelling. Bowel sounds active, all 4 quadrants
  URINARY: (Frequency) Urgency Incontinence (Polyuria) Dysuria Hematuria
  (Nocturia) x2 Anuria Retention Urinary appliance
  Comments: Noted Symptoms over last 3 months

**Activity/Exercise Alteration**

*Impaired physical mobility*
*Self care deficit*
*Activity intolerance*

- Self Care *(describe limitations to eat/bathe/dress/toilet/ambulate)* Fatigue Purposeful movement limited/absent
  Decreased strength Altered weight bearing Limited ROM Abnormal gait Impaired coordination
  Exercise routine Runs 1 mile 3x/week Assist devices used
  Comments: Very active, plays on softball team Very independent

**Comfort**

*Alteration in comfort*
*Alteration in sleep pattern*

- Pain *(describe character and patient behaviors)* Restlessness (Sleep pattern) *(Describe)* 10:30 pm to 7:00 am
  Pain control/sleeping aids used None
  Comments: Awakens due to nocturia

**Immune Function**

*Potential for infection*

- Fever in last 48° Lymphadenopathy Transplant history Chemotherapy *(date)*
  Radiation therapy *(date)* Venous access device
  Comments: Normal findings

**Sexuality/ Reproductive**

*Alt. in sexual function/ response*

- Vaginal/urethral discharge Pap smear LMP Mammogram
  Knowledge of self breast exam/(testicular exam) Change in relationship with partner
  Limitation imposed by disease/therapy
  Comments: Describes self as having good sexual relationship w/wife

**Neuro/Cerebral Function**

*Alt. in thought process*
*Alt. in communication*
*Potential for violence*

- (Alert) Oriented x 3 Memory impairment Impaired attention span (H/A) Dizziness
  Inappropriate behavior Inaccurate interpretation of environment Difficulty expressing self verbally
  Numbness Impaired judgement/perception
  Comments: Notices H/A at work, usually following Stressful day

**Cognitive Response**

*Lack of knowledge*

- Foreign language Poor understanding Inexperience with therapy (Requests information)
  Comments: Very receptive to questions, states "I want to learn how to take care of myself"

**Emotional Response**

*Alt. in coping mechanism*
*Alt. in self concept*

- VERBALIZES: Fear of therapy or surgery Loss of control Inability to cope Poor self-esteem
  Identifies stressors *(describe)* (Anxious) Angry Crying Irritable Inappropriate affect Low mood
  Comments: Expresses concern regarding hospitalization affecting work Schedule

**Social System**

*Alt. in support system*

- (Employed)/unemployed Lives: 2 floor home
  In nursing home/other Support person wife - Anne
  Ability to assist after discharge wife very supportive
  Home environment affecting self-care No problems
  Comments: Had a brother who was diagnosed to have diabetes

**Values/Beliefs**

*Value/belief conflict*

- Expresses attitudes/beliefs re: Hospitalization/Implications of care
  Inappropriate perceptions of illness *(patient/family)*
  Patient preference for spiritual assistance Catholic
  Comments:

**Health Management Pattern**

*Alt. in health maintenance*
*Potential for injury*

- Last physical 4/11 Alcohol use 4-5 drinks/week Drug Use none
  Noncompliance with therapies (Lack of knowledge) *(describe)* Needs equipment/finances/resources
  Comments: Unfamiliar with insulin and administration techniques

**Referrals**

- (Dietitian) Social service (Nurse specialist) AT/OT/PT Pastoral care Speech therapy

**Nurse Signature** T. Eolian RN

140996 Rev. 9/87

***Fig. 1-1, cont'd.*** Nurses admission note.

## *Procedure 1-2*

| Steps | Rationale |
|---|---|
| **Nursing Diagnosis** | |
| 1. Cluster data from observations, physical measurements, and nursing history to reveal actual or potential nursing diagnoses. | Any diagnosis may be identified on basis of client's unique health care problems. |
| **Planning** | |
| 1. Wash hands. | Reduces spread of microorganisms. |
| 2. Prepare assigned room with necessary equipment and personal care items: a. Bedpan/urinal b. Wash basin c. Bath towel and washcloth d. Toiletry items (e.g., soap, toothpaste, hand lotion) e. Tissue paper f. Water pitcher and drinking glass g. Kidney or emesis basin h. Thermometer i. Sphygmomanometer | Promotes client's comfort by preventing unnecessary delays during care delivery. Clients often prefer to bring personal care items from home into health agency. |
| 3. Prepare client's bed by adjusting it to lowest horizontal position. Turn down top sheet and spread. | Makes getting into bed easier and safer for client. If client is to be transferred to bed from stretcher, bed should be placed in high position. |
| **Implementation** | |
| 1. Greet client and family cordially. Introduce yourself by name and job title; state that you are responsible for client's care. | Reduces anxiety client may feel regarding admission. Knowing which nurse is responsible for care expedites requests client may have. |
| 2. Escort client and family members to assigned room. Introduce them to roommate if semiprivate room is assigned. | Orientation begins with introduction to roommate. |
| 3. Assess client's general appearance, noting signs or symptoms of physical distress. | If client is experiencing acute physical problems, nurse will postpone routine admission procedures until client's immediate needs are met. |
| 4. Assess client's and family members' psychological status by noting nonverbal behaviors and verbal responses to greetings and explanations. | Client's level of anxiety influences ability to adapt to health care environment. |
| 5. Check physician's orders for any treatment measures that should be initiated immediately. | Delay in initiation of therapies can cause worsening of client's condition. |
| 6. Orient client to nursing division. | |
| a. Introduce staff members who enter room. Always introduce client by last name. | Promotes client's ability to recognize care givers. |
| b. Explain who head nurse or charge nurse of division is and role in solving problems. | Provides means for client to communicate any problems. |
| c. Explain visiting hours and their purpose. | Family members' willingness to observe visiting hour policy ensures client will receive adequate rest. |
| d. Discuss smoking policy. | |
| e. Demonstrate how to use equipment in room, e.g., bed, overbed table, lighting. | Client's safety depends on understanding correct use of equipment. |
| f. Show client how to use nurse call light. | Ensures client knows how to call for assistance. |
| g. Escort client to bathroom (if able to ambulate). | |
| h. Explain hours for mealtime and nourishments. | |
| i. Describe services available, e.g., chaplain visitation, gift shop, activity therapy. | Offers client options for making decisions. |
| 7. Assess client's vital signs (Chapter 12). | Provides baseline measurement to compare future findings. Determines alterations from normal expected range. |
| 8. Obtain nursing history to include the following assessment categories: a. Client's perceptions of illness. b. Past medical history. c. Presenting signs and symptoms. d. Risk factors for illness. | Provides data necessary to develop individualized plan of care based upon client's identified health problems. |

| Steps | Rationale |
|---|---|
| e. History of allergies (nurse provides client with allergy band, similar in size to ID band, that lists foods, drugs, or substances to which client is allergic). | Allergy band alerts nurses to substances to which client is allergic. Prevents accidental administration of substances when client is confused or nonresponsive. |
| f. Medication history (if medications are brought to agency, nurse instructs client to take drugs home, otherwise medications are stored in division for safekeeping). | Therapeutic drug administration depends on correct dosages, proper timing of dosages, and avoidance of drug incompatibilities. Some agencies allow clients to self-administer drugs. See agency policy. |
| g. Alterations in activities of daily living. | Identifying client and family needs helps planning for eventual discharge from agency. |
| h. Family resources and support. | |
| i. Potential risk factors affecting discharge planning. | Allows nurse to refer client to necessary support services early to plan for discharge. |
| j. Client's knowledge of health problems and implications for long-term care. | Allows nurse to plan for necessary instruction to prepare client for eventual discharge. |
| 9. Conduct physical assessment of appropriate body systems (Chapter 13). | Provides objective data for identifying client's health problems. |
| 10. Instruct client on proper technique to acquire urine specimen (Chapter 45). Label specimen and attach requisition. | Urinalysis is basic test to screen for renal and metabolic problems, fluid and electrolyte alterations, and lower urinary tract alterations. |
| 11. If not obtained in admitting, explain to client that technicians will be obtaining blood specimens and performing electrocardiogram (ECG) and chest x-ray (Chapter 46). | Complete blood count (CBC) is routine test used to screen for anemias. Blood typing and cross-match is necessary for clients who require surgery or who are expected to receive blood transfusions. ECG screens for conduction defects of heart. X-ray screens for preexisting lung disease. |
| 12. Inform client about procedures or treatments that are scheduled for next shift or day, e.g., visit by physician, additional x-rays, diet restrictions. | Client has right to be informed of any scheduled procedures or treatments. Being able to anticipate planned therapies minimizes anxiety. |
| 13. Give client opportunity to ask questions about procedures or therapies. | Provides opportunity to clarify any misconceptions. |
| 14. Collect any valuables in client's possession. Complete a valuables listing sheet and have client sign. Place valuables and listing sheet in available safe. | Accurate inventory and lockup of client's valuables prevent loss during hospitalization. |
| 15. Allow client and family time together to spend alone if desired. (Anxious or fearful clients may prefer opportunity to converse.) | Admission procedure can be stressful and fatiguing. Allows time for client and family to make decisions or share concerns before visitation ends. |
| 16. Be sure call light is within reach, bed is in low position, and side rails are raised. | Provides for client's safety. |
| 17. Wash hands. | Reduces spread of microorganisms. |

## Recording and Reporting

| Steps | Rationale |
|---|---|
| 1. Record history and assessment findings on appropriate forms (see Fig. 1-1). | Prompt and thorough documentation prevents deletion of data. Client's condition may require immediate medical intervention. |
| 2. Notify physician of client's admission and report any unusual findings. | |
| 3. Begin to develop nursing care plan in nurses' notes, Kardex, or forms used by nursing staff. | Provides for continuity of individualized care. |

## Follow-up Activities

| Steps | Rationale |
|---|---|
| 1. Review physician orders and initiate all ordered interventions, e.g., diet, medications administration, preparation for diagnostic tests. | Delay in initiating therapies may complicate client's health problems. |
| 2. Return to client's room to allow client to ask questions. | Multiple activities that occur during admission may leave client confused or anxious. |

## Special Considerations

- Clients admitted to hospital room after surgery or from emergency room may require special equipment. Unit aides or nursing assistants often prepare the following room equipment:
  Intravenous (IV) pole
  Suction equipment
  Oxygen wall regulator and tubing
  Overhead frame with trapeze
- Client should be informed that a different nurse will provide care on each shift. (Explain time frame for day, evening, and night shifts.) When primary care is method of care delivery, primary nurse coordinates nursing activities throughout the hospital stay.

- Each client's condition is confidential. Do not tell one client another client's diagnosis.
- Examples of conditions that dictate temporary postponement of admitting procedure are respiratory distress, acute pain, vital sign alterations, loss of consciousness, hemorrhaging.
- Clients unable to use bedside equipment or call light will require more frequent monitoring by nurse.
- Label front of client's medical record with list of allergies.
- Nature of client's illness determines number and type of diagnostic tests obtained at admission.

### Teaching Considerations

- Teaching can occur during the admission process. A nurse can provide information regarding physical assessment findings, planned diagnostic procedures, or hospital routines. A formal teaching plan should not begin until assessment is completed and a care plan is developed.

## *SKILL 1-3 Making Referrals for Health Care Services*

Often a client requires the services of various departments within an agency, such as dietary, social work, or physical therapy. The nurse may be first to recognize the client's need. For example, a client may have had a poor appetite for several days and reveals to the nurse a dislike for many of the food choices on the menu. A referral to a dietitian could result in identifying food preferences that are appropriate to the client's diet. In many agencies a physician's order is necessary for a referral, especially when therapies are planned, for example, physical or occupational therapy. Whatever type of referral is made, it is essential that the nurse collaborate with members of other disciplines so that the individualized needs of the client are met.

### Purposes

1. Provide expert services the nurse or physician cannot provide.
2. Improve continuity of health care throughout a client's convalescence.
3. Adequately prepare a client for discharge.

## *Procedure 1-3*

| Steps | Rationale |
| --- | --- |
| **Assessment** | |
| 1. Assess client's current and posthospital needs for services from other hospital departments. | Other health professionals specialize in skills and knowledge that afford clients services the nurse often cannot offer. |
| a. Dietary—recognize factors such as client's repeated intolerance to diet, weight loss, or verbalized discontent with food choices. Client may express poor understanding of newly prescribed diet or diet restrictions. | Registered dietitian can determine nutrient and food source requirements based on client's physical condition. Dietitian has educational aides available to teach about diets. |
| b. Social work—assess client's need for counseling for major crises, e.g., terminal illness, loss of body part, family problems; need for relocation after discharge to nursing home or extended care facility; financial resources to cover medical costs; equipment for home health care; transport home after discharge. | Social worker is qualified to conduct regular counseling sessions with clients needing assistance to cope with life crises. Social workers are also knowledgeable of many community resources to help client with health care problems. |
| c. Physical therapy—assess client's need for regular exercise and mobility training after injury, surgery, or as result of chronic illness. Consider length of client's potential rehabilitation period. | Physical therapist is licensed to assist in examination and treatment of physically disabled or handicapped persons. Therapist assists in rehabilitating clients and restoring normal function. |
| d. Occupational therapy—assess client's need to learn new vocational skills or techniques to perform activities of daily living after a disability resulting from injury or illness. | Occupational therapists train clients to adapt to physical handicaps by learning new vocational skills or activities of daily living. |
| e. Speech therapy—assess client's ability to communicate, which has been altered as result of surgery, injury, or illness. | Speech therapist is trained to assist client with disorders affecting normal oral communication. |
| f. Home health services—assess client's need for intermittent skilled nursing care and physical or speech therapy after discharge. | Home health nurses provide a follow-up visit, as well as regular and frequent nursing services, e.g., administration of injections, wound care, ostomy care, that can help shorten a client's length of stay within a hospital. |

| Steps | Rationale |
|---|---|
| **Nursing Diagnosis** | |
| 1. Cluster data to reveal actual or potential nursing diagnoses: | A client's need for referral to health care services may result from any number of diagnoses. |
| a. Impaired adjustment: related to disability that causes life change. | If client is unable to modify behavior as a result of change in health status, social service may prove beneficial. |
| b. Impaired physical mobility: related to musculoskeletal impairment. | Limitation in independent physical movement may necessitate physical therapy or occupational therapy referral. |
| c. Altered nutrition—less than or more than body requirements: related to altered dietary intake. | For clients experiencing insufficient or excessive intake of nutrients, a dietitian is an appropriate referral. |
| d. Impaired verbal communication: related to injury to speech center. | If client is unable to speak or speech is impaired physically, a speech therapist may become a referral. |
| **Planning** | |
| 1. Develop individualized goals for client: | |
| a. Client's participation in referral process. | Client must be involved in decision-making process. |
| 2. Confer with client's physician regarding client's need for referral. | Physician's order is often needed for referral. Physician is knowledgeable of factors related to client's condition that may contraindicate or require specific therapies. |
| 3. Inquire as to client's desire to participate in referral. Allow client to ask questions about purpose of referral. | Allows client right to refuse any proposed treatment measure. |
| **Implementation** | |
| 1. Obtain necessary order for referral and communicate with appropriate department client's specific health care needs that will influence therapies. (When order is not needed nurse may confer directly with health care provider.) | Department accepting referral will require basic information about client before visits begin. Information related to nursing care needs may influence type of therapy referral service provides. |
| 2. Explain to client that therapist from another department will be visiting. | Client has right to know of proposed treatment measures. |
| 3. Consult with referral service about nursing implications related to prescribed treatments, e.g., exercises, diet restrictions, communication techniques. | Therapies initiated by referral service may pose implications for type and extent of care the nurse delivers. |
| **Evaluation** | |
| 1. Determine extent to which client's needs are met by referral service, e.g., has client's dietary intake improved or has weight gain occurred? Is client's range of motion (ROM) or motor strength improving? Is client learning alternative communication techniques? | Nurse is in best position to judge efficacy of care and coordinate all available resources. Continuing problems may indicate need for different referral or adjustment in nursing care plan. |
| 2. Determine client's satisfaction with referral. | Client may dislike therapist or disagree with need for referral, interfering with success of treatment plan. |
| ***Expected outcomes*** | |
| 1. Client is following treatment plan developed by referral therapist. | Therapist's objectives of care are being followed. |
| ***Unexpected outcomes*** | |
| 1. Client is unwilling or unable to follow treatment plan of referral service. | Client's health problem may become more complicated and thus interfere with ability to follow plan. Client may lack motivation or interest in plan. |
| **Recording and Reporting** | |
| 1. Record information regarding type of referral and frequency of visits in Kardex and nurses' notes. (Each therapist records client's progress with therapy in medical record.) | Provides continuity of care. Nurses can plan activities around therapist's visits. |

### Special Considerations

- Availability of services varies by size and type of health care agency. Often nurse must attempt to meet client's needs independently.
- Dietitian's functions include performing complete diet history, measuring caloric intakes, recommending nutritional supplements, e.g., tube feedings, diet education.
- Social worker is not a psychologist or psychiatrist. If clients have serious emotional problems, psychiatric referral is necessary.
- Physical therapists may plan special exercise programs, assist clients in learning crutch walking or how to use wheelchair, use special heat or cold therapies for musculoskeletal disorders. Examples of activities occupational therapists may plan are teaching stroke clients how to dress or use eating utensils, teaching amputee how to use artificial arm, teaching spinal cord–injured client how to use facilities in kitchen at home.
- Conditions in which clients may benefit from speech referrals include laryngectomies, cleft palate, stroke (cerebrovascular accident), hearing loss.
- Physician is legally responsible for informing client about treatments.
- In many agencies multidisciplinary team conferences provide excellent opportunity for discussing client's needs and making referrals.
- Nurse specialists offer consultation on complex nursing care problems and can provide client education.

## SKILL 1-4 Transferring Clients to a Different Nursing Division

It may become necessary for a client to move or transfer to another room on a nursing division, to another division within an agency, or to a division within a different agency. When a client simply changes a room in a division, it is usually for the purpose of locating the client closer to the central nursing station for more frequent observation, changing room accommodations to private or semiprivate, separating incompatible clients, or acquiring roommates who are compatible, for example, clients of the same age. A transfer to another room requires the nurse to move all supplies, equipment, and the client's personal belongings; to transport the client to the new room; and to make sure the staff in the admitting and other departments know about the room change. Transfers to different divisions require considerably more preparation. Nursing personnel in the sending division coordinate activities with personnel in the receiving division. It is important for nurses in receiving divisions to acquire complete information about the client's medical needs and nursing care so that continuity of care is not sacrificed.

### Purpose

1. Locate client in a division that provides special care or care suited to the client's needs, for example, from an intensive care unit to a general nursing division or from a self-care floor in a nursing home to a hospice unit.

## Procedure 1-4

| Steps | Rationale |
|---|---|
| **Assessment** | |
| 1. Determine reason for transfer alone or in collaboration with client's physician, e.g., change in client's condition, availability of specialty trained nursing staff. | Ensures that client has access to best resources and facilities within health care agency. |
| 2. Assess client's current physical condition. | Determines client's stability for transfer and need for any supportive equipment before move. |
| 3. Assess method for transport. | Ensures client's safety during transport. |
| **Nursing Diagnosis** | |
| 1. Cluster data from observations, physical measurements, and nursing history to reveal actual or potential nursing diagnoses. | Any diagnosis may be identified on basis of client's unique health care problems. |
| **Planning** | |
| 1. Develop individualized goals for client: | |
| a. Maintain client's physical well-being during transport to division. | Client's condition can change while being transported. |
| b. Promote continuity of the client's care in receiving division. | Receiving staff should be able to continue client's care without interruption. |
| c. Safely transport the client's personal belongings. | Items can easily be misplaced during transfer. |

| Steps | Rationale |
|---|---|
| 2. Obtain transfer orders from sending physician. Order should include receiving physician's name. | Receiving physician assumes legal responsibility for client's care. (Agencies differ as to content and form of orders.) |
| 3. Explain to client and family division and room to which client is being transferred, purpose of transfer, type of nursing division receiving client, manner in which client's needs will be communicated to new division, time transfer will occur, assurance family will be notified. Information desk will inform visitors of room change. | Client may experience fear or anxiety about moving to new division with different nursing personnel. Anxiety also commonly occurs over fear family members will not locate client. Client has right to be informed of transfer and can refuse to move. |
| 4. Determine if receiving unit is prepared to accept client. | Transfer should occur smoothly to prevent delays in moving client to new room. |
| 5. Obtain equipment required for transfer: a. IV pole b. Oxygen c. Wheelchair d. Stretcher | Ensures safe and efficient transport of client. |

## Implementation

| Steps | Rationale |
|---|---|
| 1. Provide nurse in receiving unit verbal phone report of client's current condition; major therapies being received, e.g., oxygen, intravenous fluids; pending treatments or procedures ordered for day; special nursing care needs, e.g., need for air mattress, need for time to discuss body image changes. | Continuity of care is maintained by conveying pertinent nursing care information to receiving division. |
| 2. Gather client's personal belongings: clothing in closet, drawers, and suitcase; cosmetic items; books, magazines, cards, flowers; glasses, dentures, hearing aid. Complete clothing and valuables list if agency policy requires it. | Avoids loss of articles in transfer. |
| 3. Gather reusable equipment and supplies at bedside: a. Bedpan/urinal b. Washbasin c. Water pitcher d. Kidney or emesis basin | Prevents exchange charge being billed to client. |
| 4. Be sure all documentation including care plan, is completed and current in client's medical record. | Accurate information is necessary for receiving division to resume client's care without error or delay. |
| 5. Collect medical record, Kardex, medication tickets and forms, and medications. | Medical record accompanies client to any division within agency. |
| 6. Assist client in transferring to wheelchair or stretcher (Chapter 33). | Transfer technique prevents accidental falls and avoids excess exertion. |
| 7. Chart time of transfer, receiving division, and method of transport. | Nurse from sending division is responsible for transport and should document procedure while in own division. |
| 8. Transport client, supplies, belongings, and records to receiving division. | Nurse responsible for client's care must ensure client's safety during transfer. |
| 9. Announce client's arrival at central nursing station and introduce client to nurse assuming care. | Orientation to new division's personnel conveys feeling of concern for client's welfare. |
| 10. Deposit records, forms, Kardex, and medications at desk area. | Records and medications are usually stored at central nursing station. |
| 11. Transport client to new room and assist in transfer to bed. | Transfer is complete once client is safely in bed. |
| 12. Ask receiving nurse for any further questions regarding client's condition or care. | Receiving nurse may observe client's behavior, physical signs, or condition of equipment that requires clarification. |
| 13. Sending nurse makes sure agency departments are notified of client's transfer. | In order to provide necessary support services (e.g., dietary and pharmacy) agency departments must be able to locate client. |

## Evaluation

| Steps | Rationale |
|---|---|
| 1. Receiving nurse measures client's vital signs and conducts general evaluation of client's condition. | Evaluates client's tolerance of transfer and confirms or disputes information gathered from sending division's report and medical report. |

### *Expected outcomes*

| Steps | Rationale |
|---|---|
| 1. Client's vital signs are stable compared to normal baseline values. 2. There are no physical signs or symptoms demonstrating change in client's condition. | Physical and emotional stress of transfer has not created change in client's condition. |

| Steps | Rationale |
|---|---|
| ***Unexpected outcomes*** | |
| 1. Client's vital signs change significantly from previous baseline values, e.g., pulse is tachycardic or bradycardic, blood pressure hypo- or hypertensive. | During transfer physical changes developed to cause an alteration in vital signs. Anxiety and pain may alter vital signs (Chapter 12). |
| 2. Physical assessment reveals change in client's condition. | Client's condition can change as a result of the stress of transfer itself or lack of available supplies and treatment modalities during transfer. |
| **Recording and Reporting** | |
| 1. Receiving nurse documents client's arrival in nurses' notes by recording date and time of arrival, method of transport, client's condition, and care provided. | Receiving nurse is legally responsible for immediately documenting client's arrival and any care administered. |
| **Follow-up Activities** | |
| 1. Receiving nurse cordially greets client, introduces self, and explains policies unique to new nursing division. | Orientation to new environment minimizes client's psychologic discomfort. |
| 2. Receiving nurse assists client in storing and organizing personal care items and unstored valuables. | Client may experience concern over potential loss of items during transfer. |
| 3. Receiving nurse reviews client's record and implements any ordered treatments or procedures. | Ensures continuity of care between nursing divisions. |

## Special Considerations

- Clients who can ambulate with little or no assistance can use a wheelchair. Clients restricted to bed should be transferred by stretcher.
- Special equipment, e.g., portable oxygen tanks, suction devices, and cardiac monitoring equipment, can be used in transport of a client.
- For clients who are highly anxious, a verbal report to receiving division made from phone in client's room can allay anxiety. (Only done when client's condition is stable or recovering).
- Orderlies may assist, but registered nurse should always accompany client in transport.
- Assessment priorities depend on client's condition, e.g., client transferred to nursing division after surgery requires assessment of surgical site and dressings. Client transferred to hospice unit may require assessment of pain and related symptoms.

## Teaching Considerations

- At time of transfer the client may be overly anxious or their condition may make teaching inappropriate. Give client information required to understand reason for transfer. It may be possible to instruct family members on more details, particularly if the transfer is a result of a serious change in the client's condition.

# *SKILL 1-5 Transferring Clients to a Different Agency*

When clients transfer to a new agency, their nursing care should continue as before. However, policies and procedures of the new agency may change the methods for care delivery. The client expects care to continue smoothly without changes or interruptions in therapy that may hinder progress toward recovery.

Because there is minimal opportunity for members of both nursing staffs to communicate, it is essential that the client's plan of care be documented thoroughly in medical records and transfer forms. In some institutions the nursing Kardex is not a permanent part of the medical record; therefore, the nurses' notes should provide a comprehensive review of the client's current nursing care needs.

## Purposes

1. Locate a client within an agency providing similar services closer to the client's home.
2. Locate a client within an agency that provides different health care services, such as rehabilitation.

## *Procedure 1-5*

| Steps | Rationale |
|---|---|
| **Assessment** | |
| 1. Assess reason for client's transfer in collaboration with physician, e.g., change in condition, resources available at agency, client or family preferences regarding client's location. | Client should have access to agency with best resources to meet health care needs. |
| 2. Assess client's physical condition and determine vehicle for transport. | Determines if client is stable for transfer. Client's safety is best assured by using a vehicle equipped with life support equipment. |
| 3. Assess method of transport to transferring vehicle, e.g., wheelchair or stretcher. | Ensures client's safety. |
| **Nursing Diagnosis** | |
| 1. Cluster data from observations, physical measurements, and nursing history to reveal actual or potential nursing diagnoses. | Any diagnosis may be identified on basis of client's unique health care problems. |
| **Planning** | |
| 1. Develop individualized goals for client: | |
| a. Maintain client's physical well-being during transfer to agency. | Client may be transported over long distances and require use of life support equipment. |
| b. Promote continuity of client's care in new agency. | New agency policies can make it difficult for client's care to be resumed as it was previously. |
| c. Protect client's belongings during transport. | |
| 2. Arrange for client's transport to agency by chosen vehicle. | Transfer should occur without delays so client has access to all needed resources at all times. |
| 3. Obtain a transfer order from sending physician. Order should include name of receiving agency, physician, and client's stability for transfer. | Client's physician is legally responsible for releasing client from medical care and arranging for receiving physician. Transfer will be temporarily postponed if client is considered unstable. Client has legal right to refuse transfer against medical advice. |
| 4. Explain to client or family purpose of transfer, location of agency, time for transfer, method for communicating client's needs to agency personnel, procedures for actual transport to agency. | Explanation of transfer procedures minimize client's anxiety. |
| 5. Obtain special equipment needed for transport, e.g., IV pole, oxygen. | Ensures safe and efficient transport of client. |
| **Implementation** | |
| 1. Make sure documentation in client's record is complete and accurate. | Accurate information is necessary for receiving agency to resume client's care. |
| 2. Obtain from client release form giving permission to have copy of medical record made for receiving agency. | Medical personnel from receiving agency rely upon client's medical record as primary resource in resuming client's care plan. Information in client's record is confidential and its use requires client's signed release. |
| 3. Complete nursing care transfer form according to agency policy. | Form provides summary of client's pertinent nursing care needs to ensure continuity of care. |
| 4. Gather client's personal care items, clothing, and valuables. Secure in suitcase or container. | Articles can easily be lost in transfer. |
| 5. Anticipate problems client may develop just before or during transfer. Perform necessary nursing therapies. | Ensures client's comfort and safety in transport. |
| 6. Assist in transferring client to stretcher or wheelchair using proper body mechanics. | Client transported to outside agency is more easily moved by stretcher into transport vehicle. Transfer technique prevents accidental falls or injury to client and nurse. |
| 7. Perform final assessment of client's physical stability, i.e., check vital signs, check for clear airway, inspect patency of intravenous lines, note client's level of consciousness. | Minimizes risk of client developing complications during transfer. |
| 8. Accompany client to transport vehicle. | Ensures medically qualified personnel are in attendance until client leaves agency. |

### Special Considerations

- Multidisciplinary conference can be useful in selecting best agency for a transfer.
- Clients who are relatively stable may be transported in van or car. Clients requiring more physical monitoring should transfer in well-equipped ambulance. Emergency transfers over long distances may occur by helicopter.
- Some institutions may require an order for certain members of the staff to accompany client during transfer.
- Agency policies dictate what portion of a client's medical record is copied, because record is property of agency.
- Routine nursing care measures are not as important to record on transfer form as individualized therapies. Nurse may ask client to assist in providing information.
- Measures nurse may implement just before transfer include suctioning of airway, changing soiled dressing, administering prescribed medications, bathing incontinent client, emptying drainage collection devices.
- In many states, a nurse or therapist from the receiving agency visits client before transfer to conduct a personal assessment of client. This facilitates treatment and reduces client anxiety.

## *SKILL 1-6* *Discharging Clients From a Health Care Agency*

Successful discharge planning is a coordinated, interdisciplinary process that ensures that all clients have a plan for continuing care after they leave the hospital (The American Hospital Association [AHA], 1983). Reimbursement pressures have resulted in shorter hospital stays for clients. Unfortunately, an "average" client who is hospitalized only a few days with no complications, is often unprepared to resume a normal life-style at home. It is common for health team members to direct more attention to the discharge needs of the severely debilitated client who will require continued health care in the home or an extended care facility.

In 1985, the Society for Hospital Social Work Directors of the AHA described four levels of outcomes for clients at discharge:

1. Client and family understanding of the diagnosis, anticipated level of function, discharge medications, and anticipated medical follow-up.
2. Specialized instruction or training so that the client or family can provide post-hospital care.
3. Coordination of community support systems that enable the client to return home.
4. Relocation of the client or transfer to another health care facility and coordination of support systems.

Typically nurses are actively involved in assisting clients with the first and second outcomes, whereas social workers manage the third and fourth. However in many institutions a nurse may be the one individual to coordinate the efforts of all health team members in meeting each of the outcomes. If the client's need for discharge planning is identified early during a hospital stay, there is a greater likelihood for mutual goal setting with the client and family and a realistic discharge plan.

Documentation of a client's discharge plan is important so that health team members work toward the same outcomes. The Joint Commission on Accreditation of Health Care Organizations (JCAHO) has adopted standards to address timely and smooth discharge planning for all clients (Nash, 1988). The standards focus on the importance of hospital-wide policies and procedures and documentation systems.

Frequently clients require skilled nursing care after discharge. The nature of the client's condition, the type of therapies required, and the availability of family or friends in the home help determine the need for home health care services. A nurse from a home health care agency may receive a referral to make visits in the client's home to provide skilled care. Third-party payers only reimburse for skilled nursing services such as wound and dressing care, administration of intravenous fluids, and health teaching for ostomy care and injection administration. Nurses in the agency caring for the client play an important role in determining the need for a home health care nurse. If a family member is capable of learning certain skills, a home health care nurse may need to make only a few home visits to be sure the skills are performed correctly.

### Purposes

1. Reduce client anxiety over leaving the health care agency.
2. Determine need and make referrals for home health care or extended care services.
3. Ensure client ability to perform self-care after discharge.
4. Provide family members with knowledge and skills needed to administer care to the client in a home setting.
5. Assist client and family in preparing the home environment for the client's discharge.

## Procedure 1-6

| Step | Rationale |
|---|---|
| **Assessment** | |
| 1. From time of admission assess client's health care needs for discharge, using nursing history, care plan, and ongoing assessments of physical abilities and cognitive function. | Plan for discharge begins at admission and continues throughout course of client's stay in agency. |
| 2. Assess client's and family members' need for health teaching related to therapies to administer at home; restrictions resulting from health alterations; complications to observe for. | Client's and family's understanding of health care needs will improve likelihood of client's ability to achieve self-care at home. Inclusion of family member in teaching sessions provides client with available resource when home. |
| 3. Assess with client and family any environmental factors within home setting that might interfere with self-care activities, e.g., size of rooms, doorway clearances, steps, bathroom facilities. (A home health care nurse may be available on referral to assist with assessment.) | Environmental barriers may pose risks to client's safety as a result of limitation created by client's illness or need for certain therapies. |
| 4. Collaborate with physician and other disciplines (e.g., physical therapy) in assessing need for referral for skilled home health care services or an extended care facility. | Clients eligible for home health care are confined to home as result of illness, are under physician's care, and require skilled nursing care on intermittent basis. A multidisciplinary assessment ensures a comprehensive discharge plan. |
| 5. Assess client's acceptance of health problems and related restrictions. | Client's acceptance of health status can affect willingness to adhere to therapies and restrictions after discharge. |
| 6. Consult other health team members about client's needs after discharge, e.g., dietitian, social worker, home health care nurse. (see Skill 1-3). | Members of all health care disciplines should collaborate to determine client's needs and functional abilities. |
| **Nursing Diagnosis** | |
| 1. Cluster data to reveal actual or potential nursing diagnoses: | |
| a. Self-care deficit: related to physical or cognitive impairment. | Client may be physically unable to care for self or not have family members present or educated to care for client. |
| b. Knowledge deficit regarding self-care activities: related to unfamiliarity with restrictions. | Client and family members have not been properly instructed on client's health care needs and procedures to follow. |
| c. Potential for injury: related to environmental barriers. | Physical restrictions place client at risk in home setting unless nurse can instruct on ways to change home environment or on way to cope with existing barriers. |
| d. Anxiety: related to impending discharge. | Client may be apprehensive about returning to home environment or feel helpless over change in health status. |
| e. Impaired home maintenance management: related to physical impairment, inadequate family support. | Poses implications for referral of client to home health care or community resources. |
| **Planning** | |
| 1. Develop individualized goals for client's discharge: | |
| a. Client will understand health care problems and related implications. | Client and family teaching will better prepare client to care for individual needs. |
| b. Client will be able to care for individual needs. | Planned discussion periods will give client opportunity to ask questions, clarify information. |
| c. Client's home environment will be safe. | Family members can make changes in advance of client's arrival to make home environment safer. A home health care nurse may be able to assess client's home environment. |
| d. Health care resources in the home are available. | Early referral to home health care services will allow those nurses to assess client's needs more thoroughly. |
| 2. Ask client and family members for suggestions on ways to prepare for discharge. | Client, as part of discharge planning team, may be able to identify additional need for support or resources that nurse's assessment did not reveal. |
| **Implementation** | |
| ***Preparation before day of discharge*** | |
| 1. Suggest methods for altering physical arrangement of home environment to meet client's needs. | Client's level of independence and ability to retain function can be maintained within environment conducive to safety. Advanced preparation is often needed before client actually returns home. |

| Step | Rationale |
|---|---|
| 2. Provide client and family with information about community health care resources. | Communities often offer services client or family cannot provide. |
| 3. Conduct teaching sessions with client and family as soon as possible during hospitalization, e.g., signs and symptoms of complications; skills: injections, wound care, transfer techniques, colostomy care; information regarding medications, diet, exercise; restrictions imposed by illness or surgery. | Gives client and family opportunities to practice new skills, ask questions, and obtain necessary feedback from nurse to ensure learning has occurred. |
| 4. Complete any referral forms indicating client's health care needs and functional abilities. | Continuity of health care is ensured through communication of individualized plan of care to all health team members. |
| ***Day of discharge*** | |
| 1. Let client and family ask questions or discuss issues related to home health care. | Allows for final clarification of information previously discussed. Helps relieve client's anxiety. |
| 2. Check physician's discharge orders for prescriptions, change in treatments, or need for special appliances. (Orders should be written as early as possible.) | Discharge is authorized only by physician. Early check of orders permits nurse to attend to any last minute treatments or procedures well in advance of client's actual discharge. |
| 3. Determine if client or family member has arranged for client's transport home. | Client's condition at discharge will determine method for transport. |
| 4. Offer assistance as client dresses and packs all personal belongings. Provide privacy as needed. | Promotes client's comfort. |
| 5. Make final check of all closets and drawers to be sure all of client's belongings have been removed. | Prevents loss of client's personal items. |
| 6. Obtain copy of valuables list signed by client and have security or appropriate administrator deliver valuables to client. | Client's signature on list will verify receipt of items. |
| 7. Be sure all valuables are accounted for. | Removes nursing of liability for any losses. |
| 8. Provide client with any prescriptions or medications ordered by physician. Review dosage of drug, schedule for administration, precautions, and other pertinent information with client and family member. | Review of drug information provides feedback to determine client's success in learning about medications. |
| 9. Contact agency's business office to determine if client needs to finalize arrangements for payment of bill. Arrange for client or family member to visit office. | Source of concern for many clients is whether agency has accepted insurance or other payment forms. |
| 10. Acquire utility cart to move client's belongings. Obtain wheelchair for clients unable to ambulate. Clients leaving by ambulance will be transported on ambulance stretchers. | Provides for safe transport of client. |
| 11. Use proper body mechanics and transfer techniques in assisting client to wheelchair or stretcher. | Prevents injury to nurse and client. |
| 12. Escort client to entrance of agency where source of transportation is waiting. | Agency policy requires escort to ensure client's safe exit. |
| 13. Lock wheelchair wheels. Assist client in transferring into automobile or transport vehicle. Help family member place personal belongings in vehicle. | Agency's liability ends once client is safely in vehicle. |
| 14. Return to division and notify admitting or appropriate department of time of client's discharge. | Allows agency to prepare for admission of next client. |
| **Evaluation (optional)** | |
| 1. Confer with home health care nurses or client about client's progress in home. | Maintains continuity of care. Communicates sense of concern to client. |
| ***Expected outcomes*** | |
| 1. Client is able to perform self-care at home or receives necessary assistance from home health care nurse. | Client has adapted to home environment with limitations posed by illness. |
| ***Unexpected outcomes*** | |
| 1. Client continues to have health problems affecting life-style. | Reassessment of client's health problems requires more appropriate plan of care. |
| **Recording and Reporting** | |
| 1. Complete documentation of client's discharge on discharge summary form (Fig. 1-2). In many institutions client receives signed copy of form. | Discharge summary is essential for documenting client's status at time client leaves health care agency. Signed copy demonstrates plan was communicated to and agreed to by client. |
| 2. Complete documentation of status of client's health problems at time of discharge. | Allows final evaluation of client's plan of care. |

**Barnes Hospital**

PATIENT DISCHARGE SUMMARY

C-16

Addressograph Plate

Date 10/17/88 Time 1030

**MEANS:** ☐ Ambulatory ☒ Wheelchair ☐ Stretcher

**METHODS:** ☒ M.D. order ☐ AMA with release ☐ AMA without release

Afebrile 24 hours? ☒ Yes ☐ No TPR $36^{8}$-72-16 B/P 124/72

☐ Physician notified of irregularities

**DISCHARGED TO:** ☐ Home ☐ Nursing Home ☒ Home with Home Health Care ☐ Other

If discharged to Nursing Home or other facility/service:

Name ______ Address/Phone ______

☐ Release of Information form signed ☐ Chart copied ☐ Transfer form completed ☐ Transportation Arranged

**DISCHARGE CONSIDERATIONS:**

☐ Valuables from cashier ☒ NA

☐ PTA meds returned ☒ NA

☐ Scripts given ☒ NA

DISCHARGE INSTRUCTIONS

**FOR PROBLEMS OR FOLLOW-UP:**

Physician Dr. Stan Jones Phone 362-5000 Appt. 10/24/86

Other: ______

Activity: To remain in bed with Ⓛ foot elevated on two pillows. May be up only to go to the bathroom.

Diet: To follow 1800 calorie ADA diet as instructed by the dietitian. For questions about diet, call the dietitian (Sue Marlin) 362-3184.

Medications: To take usual dosage of 30 units NPH insulin and 8 units of regular insulin every morning before breakfast.

Wound Care: Change dressings to Ⓛ foot daily using moistened fine mesh gauze with dry 4x4 gauze and wrap dressings with 4 kling gauze.

Teaching Materials Given: Copy of "Controlling Your Diabetes" and "Diabetic Menu Planning."

Special Instructions: Call doctor for increased pain, redness, swelling or drainage from Ⓛ foot wound. Barnes Home Health nurses will be visiting daily to change dressing to Ⓛ foot.

**My discharge instructions have been explained and a copy has been given to me.**

Patient/Significant Other *John Owens* Relation HUSBAND

Nurse *B. Rand, RN*

***Fig. 1-2*** Discharge summary form.

Courtesy Barnes Hospital, St. Louis.

| Step | Rationale |
|---|---|
| **Follow-up Activities** | |
| 1. Notify housekeeping of need to clean client's room. | Room must be thoroughly prepared before new client's admission. |

## Special Considerations

- Potential areas to assess in planning for home care will include diet management; proper, safe administration of medications; exercise limitations; wound care; risks associated with health alterations; signs and symptoms of common complications.
- Examples of environmental barriers include lack of running water, stairs, throw rugs, furniture placement, lighting, bathroom facilities. Clients most at risk for problems in home environment include those with sensory alterations, mobility restrictions, energy limitation, financial restrictions.
- Clients being discharged to nursing home are often fearful of new environment and potential loss of independence.
- Client must require skilled nursing care to be eligible for third-party payment (Medicare or insurance). Examples of skilled care include administration of injections, changing dressings, colostomy care, tracheostomy care, administration of IVs, rehabilitative care, indwelling catheter care, teaching of injections, nasogastric diet, inhalation therapy, diabetic care, care of bedridden client.
- Examples of methods for changing home environment: clients with ambulation restrictions benefit from handrails along staircase, elimination of throw rugs, removal of footstools and clutter on floors. Clients with visual alterations may benefit from better illumination of stairwells, elimination of throw rugs. Clients with mobility restrictions may benefit from grab bars or handrails installed around toilets and bathtub, chairs and beds set at heights to ease bending at waist or knees, and low-set cabinets for easy access to items.
- Examples of community resources: hospital equipment companies and rental agencies, Meals-on-Wheels program (delivery of hot meals to home), day-care centers for elderly, emergency call-for-help telephone services, community clinics.
- Some hospitals provide limited supplies of dressings, syringes, or appliances such as crutches and canes.
- Family members should accept valuables if client is confused, seriously weakened, or comatose.
- In some agencies there are nurses whose primary responsibility is to evaluate client's adjustment after discharge. This may involve direct contact with client and family.

## Teaching Considerations

- Before client leaves agency, nurse should provide for return demonstration of any skills taught.
- Clients who have short stays in health care agency may not receive teaching until day of discharge.
- Some prescriptions cannot be anticipated. Day of discharge may be only opportunity to teach client about medications. Some agencies have brochures or cards that provide specific information about individual drugs.

## Home Care Considerations

- The AHA (1983) recommends consideration of the following factors in planning for care at home:
  a. Desire of client.
  b. Desire and capability of family to assume responsibility and to understand and follow treatment plan.
  c. Capabilities of resources in community for home health care services.
  d. Physical environment of home.
  e. Financial resources to provide adequate food and health care expenses.
- Hospital discharge planners may be social workers or registered nurses working independently of the nurses who provide care to the client in the hospital. The discharge planner is not usually the case finder; the staff nurse will likely recommend the client for home care services. Therefore, the discharge planner should obtain as much information as possible from the staff nurse regarding condition of the client and anticipated needs before developing a discharge plan.
- The ideal discharge planning situation occurs when the discharge planner is assigned to specified clinical units within the hospital, thereby encouraging the staff nurse and discharge planner to jointly communicate and develop the discharge plan for the client.
- Home health care nurses require detailed information about the home environment, such as support systems and social and economic considerations that may modify and shape care, to develop complete and accurate care plans for the client. Without such information, the home health care nurse may need to assess the situation too quickly to develop a clear plan of care.
- Assess availability and skill of the primary care giver, such as spouse or neighbor: assess time available, ability, willingness, emotional and physical stamina, and knowledge to give care.
- Assess attitude of immediate family members: ability to adjust to demands of client care; impact of care demands on their lives, including noise levels and preparations of special diets; and potential ongoing nature of the client's needs. Family members who are not properly prepared for their role as caregivers may be overwhelmed by the client's needs, which can lead to neglect or unnecessary hospital readmissions.
- Assess additional resources including friends or neighbors who are available to help.
- Evaluate emergency preparations: call bell or phone rigged up within client's reach; appropriate written protocol.
- The hospital discharge planner has an obligation to warn insurance payors when they appear to be making payment decisions that adversely affect treatment needs of the client. Discharge planners must offer clients the option of paying privately for care when payors stop payment. Providers must provide, in writing, reasonable notice of the option to pay privately when payors stop payment.

## Referring the Client to Home Health Care

- Referral to a home health care agency may be made by the following:
  a. Hospital discharge planner.
  b. Client's physician through the office staff.
  c. Client or family.

d. Public health or community nurse.
e. Nurse in private practice.
f. Other health care workers.
g. Social service personnel. However, a physician's order must be obtained for the home health care agency to render care to the client.

- Assess referral for appropriateness of client admission to the home health care agency based on the following admission criteria:
  a. Client is confined to place of residence (homebound).
  b. Client is under care of a physician.
  c. Client needs part-time or intermittent skilled nursing services.
  d. Reasonable expectation exists that the client's medical, nursing, and social needs can be adequately met by the home health care agency in client's place of residence.
  l. Home health care services are necessary and reasonable for treatment of client's illness or injury.
- Obtain as much information as possible about the client before the nurse visits the client in the home setting; a visit to the client and family during hospitalization, if possible, permits the development of a more comprehensive plan of care.
- Document client intake information on the referral form for home health care admission to service.
- Review information in conjunction with established home health care agency admission criteria.
- Inform client or family member and client's physician as to the decision to accept or not accept the client for admission to the home health care agency.

## BIBLIOGRAPHY

American Hospital Association: Introduction to discharge planning for hospitals, Chicago, 1983, American Hospital Publishing Inc.

Bowen BJ: Use of combined admissions form ends repeated patient questioning, Hospitals 55:63, 1981.

Bridge P and Carlson RA: Preadmission assessment of the elderly, Can Nurse 79:27, 1983.

Cunningham LS: Early assessment for discharge planning: adopting a high-risk screening program, QRB 10:561, 1984.

Drew L, Biordi D, Gillies D: How discharge planners and home health nurses view their patients, Nursing Management 19(4):66, 1988.

Eggland ET, Nurses' guide to home health care, Nursing '87, 17(10):75, 1987.

Federal Register, 53:116, June 16, 1988.

Feuer L: Discharge planning: home caregivers need your support, too, Nursing Management 18(4):58, 1987.

Harvey BL: Your patient's discharge plan—does it include homecare referral? Nursing '81 11:48, 1981.

Kozier B and Erb G: Concepts and issues in nursing practice. In Germino B, ed. Home Health Care, Reading, Maine, 1988, Addison-Wesley Publishing Co.

Nash TB: What's new about the new discharge planning standards? Discharge Planning Update 8(5):1, 1988.

Pilcher M: Postdischarge care: how to follow up, Nursing '86 16(8):50, 1986.

Potter P and Perry A: Fundamentals of nursing, ed 2, St. Louis, 1989, The CV Mosby Co.

Reichelt PA and Newcomb J: Organizational factors in discharge planning, J Nurs Adm 10:36, 1980.

Reifsnider E and Damron B: When you hand over a patient for home care, RN 49(1):17, 1986.

Rossen S: Adapting discharge planning to prospective pricing, Hospitals 58:71, 1984.

Smallegan M: Decision making for nursing home admission: a preliminary study, J Gerontol Nurs 7:280, 1981.

Vivens S and Wookfork C: Nursing home admissions made more rational, Geriatr Nurs 4:361, 1983.

Weinberger B: Discharge planning the sooner, the better, Nursing '89 19(2):75, 1989.

Wells M: Discharge planning, Nursing '83 13(11):45, 1983.

# 2

# REPORTING AND RECORDING

### OBJECTIVES

*Mastery of content in this chapter will enable the nurse to:*

- Define key terms.
- Describe guidelines for effectively communicating via reporting and recording.
- Give a change-of-shift report to a nursing team.
- Explain how to verify telephone reports.
- Describe guidelines to use in completing an incident report.
- Identify methods to prevent charting errors.
- Differentiate between a source record and a problem-oriented record.
- Write a narrative nurses' note.
- Write a SOAP and PIE progress note.
- Describe the purpose of the nursing Kardex.
- Discuss the relationship between documentation and health care financial reimbursement.
- Explain documentation methods used in a home health care setting.

### KEY TERMS

| | |
|---|---|
| *Chart flow sheet* | *Prospective reimbursement* |
| *Incident report* | *Quality assurance* |
| *Invasive* | *Sign* |
| *Objective data* | *SOAP* |
| *PIE* | *Subjective data* |
| *POMR* | *Standardized care plan* |

All health care team members must have the same information about clients to ensure an organized and comprehensive plan of care. Otherwise care becomes fragmented, repetition of tasks occurs, and therapies often become delayed. Records and reports communicate specific information about a client's health care so all interventions are directed toward the same goals.

A report involves an oral or written exchange of information. When nurses complete a shift or tour of duty, they provide an oral report to nurses on the next shift. Support services such as the laboratory or the radiology department issue written reports describing results of diagnostic tests. Information from written reports is incorporated into the client's permanent medical record or chart.

A client's record is a written communication that permanently documents information relevant to that client's health care management. After each clinic visit, information about the reasons a client sought medical care, the medical history, results of diagnostic tests, and the plan of therapy is recorded. With each successive visit the record is available to the physician and nurse. It is a continuing account of the client's health care needs.

Documentation and reporting are two of the most important functions a nurse performs. Unless information about a client's care is communicated with careful thought, serious errors can occur. Legally, if nursing care is not documented it is presumed care was not provided. Good documentation and reporting must accurately reflect the status of the client. All members of the health care team depend on accurate recorded and reported information.

## GUIDELINES

1. *Accuracy*—Information must be correct. Discriminate clearly as to whether objective or subjective data are communicated. (The term objective data pertains to clinical findings that are observed and measurable. The term subjective data pertains to perceptions of the client, nurse, or other health team members and cannot be evaluated by objective standards.) Subjective data can be interpretated differently by different people. Always differentiate between observations of the client's behavior and interpretations of the observations. Chart facts and exact observations. Do not chart opinions. Always chart omissions of nursing procedures that are normally part of the standards of care, for example, if a client refuses a medication, chart the omission. Use precise measurements when document-

***TABLE 2-1*** Examples of Criteria for Reporting and Recording

| Topic | What to Report or Record |
|---|---|
| Symptom (pain, nausea, headache, dizziness). | Description of episode, location of symptom, severity, onset, precipitating factor(s), frequency, duration, aggravating factor(s), relieving factor(s), associated symptom(s). |
| Sign (rash, tenderness on palpation of body part, diminished breath sounds). | Location of sign, description or quality of finding, aggravating or relieving factor(s). |
| Nursing care measures (enema, bath, dressing change). | Time administered, equipment used if appropriate, client's response (positive* or negative†), nurse's observations. |
| Client behavior (anxiety, confusion, hostility). | Time of occurrence, behaviors exhibited, precipitating factor(s), nursing response or action, client response to nursing action. |
| Medication administration (analgesic). | Time administered, any required preliminary observations (pulse, blood pressure), client response (positive‡ or negative) or nursing measures taken if negative response occurs.§ |
| Client teaching. | Information or topic presented, method of instruction (discussion, role-playing, demonstration), resources used (videotape, booklet), and evidence that client understands instruction. |

*For example, client denied pain during dressing change.
†For example, client experienced severe abdominal cramping during enema.
‡For example, client reports pain was reduced by analgesic.
§For example, rash noted on abdomen; Dr Nash notified.

ing. Use correct spelling and the institution's accepted abbreviations and symbols to ensure accurate interpretation of information (see Appendix). Always complete a descriptive entry in the client's record with an accurate signature including first initial, complete surname, and status, such as R.N. or L.P.N. Do not use nicknames. The signature holds a nurse accountable for information recorded.

2. *Conciseness*—Provide precise essential information in a report or written note. A brief, well-written note is more likely to be read than a lengthy, irrelevant one. Avoid unnecessary words and irrelevant detail. For example, do not chart the word "client" or "patient" because it is understood that the chart belongs to the client.
3. *Thoroughness*—Although concise, a record or report must contain complete information about a client. Assumptions about a client cannot be made when data are incomplete. Table 2-1 lists criteria to use when reporting or recording certain topics.
4. *Currentness*—Delays in recording or reporting can result in serious omissions and untimely delays for clients receiving needed care. Decisions about a client's care are based on currently reported information. Activities that must be communicated at the time they occur include administration of medications or other treatments; preparation of clients for diagnostic tests or surgery; change in a client's status; admission, transfer, or discharge of a client; and treatment initiated for sudden changes in a client's condition. Use the institution's accepted time system (Table 2-2) for reporting or recording information.
5. *Organization*—Communicate all information in a chronological and logical format. A health team member will better understand information conveyed in the order in which it occurred. If an institution uses a format such as SOAP or PIE for narrative nurses' notes, follow this format correctly.
6. *Confidentiality*—Information about a client should only be communicated with the understanding that client information will not be disclosed to unauthorized persons. The law protects information about a client that is gathered by examination, observation, conversation, or treatment. The nurse is legally and ethically obligated to keep information pertaining to a client's illness and treatment confidential. Only staff members who are directly involved in a client's care have legitimate access to the client's records.
7. *Legibility*—Use the best penmanship to be sure notes are easy and clear to read. Most institutions require use of black or blue ink. A few agencies may use red ink for the night shift (7:00 PM to 7:00 AM).
8. Always use the client's care plan as a basis for charting.

***TABLE 2-2*** Comparison of Military and Civilian Times

| Military | Civilian | Military | Civilian |
|---|---|---|---|
| 0100 | 1:00 AM | 1420 | 2:20 PM |
| 0200 | 2:00 AM | 1800 | 6:00 PM |
| 0215 | 2:15 AM | 2400 | 12:00 PM |
| 1200 | 12:00 Noon | 0001 | 12:01 AM |
| 1300 | 1:00 PM | | |

## REPORTING

Nurses work professionally to ensure that quality reports are shared so that all team members can make the best decisions about clients and their care. Three types of reports made by nurses are change-of-shift, telephone, and incident reports.

*TABLE 2-3* Intershift Report

| Do | Don't |
|---|---|
| Provide only essential background information about client (i.e., name, sex, age, physician's diagnosis, medical history). | Don't review all routine care procedures or tasks (bathing or I & O). |
| Identify client's nursing diagnosis or health care problems and their related causes. | Don't review all biographical information already available on Kardex. |
| Describe objective measurements or observations about client's condition and response to health problem. Stress any recent changes. | Don't use critical comments about client's behavior. |
| Share significant information about family members as it relates to client's problems. | Don't make assumptions about relationships between family members. |
| Continuously review ongoing discharge plan (e.g., need for resources, client's level of preparation to go home). | Don't engage in idle gossip. |
| Relay to staff any significant changes in the way therapies are given (e.g., different gauze used in dressing change, new medication ordered). | Don't describe basic steps of a procedure. |
| Describe instructions given in teaching plan and client's response. | Don't explain detailed content unless staff asks for clarification. |
| Evaluate results of nursing or medical care measures (e.g., effect of position change, backrub, analgesic administration). | Don't simply describe results as "good" or "poor." Be specific. |
| Be clear on priorities to which the oncoming staff must attend. | Don't force oncoming staff to guess what to do first. |

## Change-of-Shift Report

The change-of-shift report occurs two to three times a day and is a formal exchange of information between the nurse who has completed caring for a client and the nurse ready to assume care for the next shift. The report ensures continuity of care between nurses and provides nurses a chance to share essential information necessary for safe, holistic client care.

A good report includes selection of significant facts about a client (for example, the condition of a wound). Data have little meaning unless a comparison is made with previous information. A nurse cannot make a conclusion about a client unless it is known if a change has occurred (for example, improvement in wound healing). A summary of important data should be objective and concise. Interpretation, the result of selecting, comparing, and summarizing, allows a nurse to report the clinical significance of the shift's events (Table 2-3).

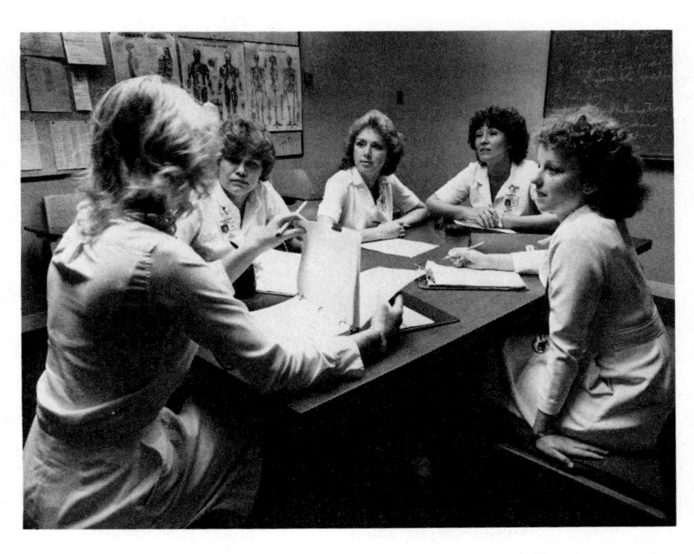

***Fig. 2-1*** Members of nursing team meet at shift change for report on each client's progress and specific health care needs.

A report should be given as quickly as possible. Even though it is the responsibility of a nurse to carefully review a client's Kardex before care begins, it is not necessary to report routine nursing orders or information available in the Kardex. A systematic approach to reporting using the nursing process can provide staff with critical information needed to continue the client's care. The basis for report is the client's health problems. The nursing care plan should be reviewed. At the time of the intershift report the nurse can be in any phase of the nursing process. Thus the actual report should reflect the ongoing, continuous nature of care. It is important that staff assigned to the next shift know exactly what their responsibilities in caring for the client will be.

A report can be given orally in person or by audiotape. An in-person report permits nurses to obtain immediate feedback about unclear or incomplete information. The report may be conducted in a conference room (Fig. 2-1) or during nurses' "walking rounds." During walking rounds the client meets the care giving staff and learns of activities or treatment to expect during the shift, and the nurse meets and observes the client. Information that might alarm a client is reported out of hearing range, usually in the hallway just outside the room. The nurse also takes precautions to ensure that other clients do not hear confidential information.

When giving a report the nurse discusses the client or family in a professional and dignified manner. It is often necessary to describe the interactions between client, nurse, and family members in behavioral terms. The nurse avoids using labels such as "uncooperative," "difficult," or "bad" when describing client behaviors. Any derogatory statements overheard by the client could lead to

**INCIDENT REPORT / Patient-Visitor**

**Barnes Hospital — St. Louis, Missouri**

THIS DATA IS PROVIDED FOR THE LEGAL COUNSEL OF THE DIRECTORS OF BARNES HOSPITAL IN THE EVENT OF POSSIBLE LITIGATION AND IS TO BE CONSIDERED CONFIDENTIAL AND PRIVILEGED INFORMATION.

USE ADDRESSOGRAPH IF PATIENT

REPORT NO.

PERSON INVOLVED: PETERS (Last Name) RON (First Name) L (M.I.)

Age: 68 | Sex: M | Date of Incident: 1/8/-- | Date Reported: 1/8/-- | Time (Military): 0915 | Exact location of incident: ROOM 6201 A | Tele. No.

**PATIENT** ☒

Rm. No. 6201 A | Reason for hospitalization (Diagnosis): ALZHEIMERS WORK UP | Attending Physician: ROGERS

Mental condition of patient before incident: Normal ☐ Senile ☐ Disoriented ☒ Sedated ☐ Other______

Bedrails: Up ☒ Down ☐ Restraints: Yes ☐ No ☒

Activity Orders: Restraints ☐ Bed Rest ☐ Up privileges with assistance ☒ Without assistance ☐

Brief description of incident: PATIENT FOUND ON FLOOR AT SIDE OF BED. SMALL, 2CM ABRASION NOTED OVER Ⓛ FOREHEAD. CONSCIOUS AND RESPONDS TO VOICE.

**VISTOR** ☐ **OTHER** ☐

By whom employed______ Occupation______

Home Address______ Home Phone______

Nature of Incident | Reason in Hospital

**ACCIDENT FACTS**

Name, Address, Tele. No. of Witnesses, if any:

Was patient seen by physician: Yes ☒ No ☐ Not indicated ☐ | Physician's Name.

Time called 1000 a.m. p.m. Time arrived 10:30 a.m. p.m.

Was treatment initiated by physician: Yes ☒ No ☐ X-Rays: Yes ☒ No ☐

I DO NOT WISH TO BE EXAMINED BY A PHYSICIAN: Signed:______

**DESCRIPTION OF INCIDENT**

State what you saw and/or what you were told. Give names and addresses of all individuals who provided information concerning this incident.

ENTERED ROOM. FOUND PT. ON FLOOR AT SIDE OF BED. STATED "WHERE IS MARIE?" NOTED SMALL, 2CM ABRASION OVER Ⓛ FOREHEAD. AREA TENDER TO PALPATION. PT. ABLE TO MOVE ALL EXTREMITIES FULL ROM. ABLE TO RAISE FROM FLOOR INDEPENDENTLY. CALLED DR. ROGERS. SKULL-FILM ORDERED.

Date of Report 1/8/-- Signature of person preparing report Rita Woods RN

**PROPERTY DAMAGE** ☐ **MISSING ARTICLE** ☐

Owner of Property | If theft, what day | and hour | last seen.

Home Address | Tele. No.

Nature and Extent of Damage or Loss

Estimated replacement or repair cost: $

***Fig. 2-2*** Incident report form.
Courtesy Barnes Hospital, St. Louis.

a lawsuit against the nurse. A good report is objective and nonjudgmental. Value-laden terms are not conducive for establishing working relationships between staff members and clients: staff members may unintentionally form a prejudicial opinion about clients before meeting them. The content of reports should be pertinent to clients' health care.

## Telephone Reports

Health care workers frequently communicate orders, or information to one another by telephone. Orders should be documented and include the name of the person giving the order, as well as the name of the person receiving it. Reports may include a nurse informing a physician of changes in a client's condition, a nurse from one unit communicating information to a nurse in another unit about a client transfer, or the laboratory staff or radiologist reporting results of diagnostic tests. Information in a telephone report may not be permanently documented in a written form. Thus the persons involved with a telephone report should be sure the information is clear, accurate, and concise. If any doubt exists about the information conveyed over the telephone, the receiver repeats the message back to the sender.

*Nurse:* This is Ms. Towns from 3200. Do you have the results of Mr. Tom Rush's potassium level?
*Laboratory technician:* Yes. Mr. Tom Rush's potassium is 3.2.
*Nurse:* Let me repeat that, 3.2?
*Laboratory technician:* Yes, that's correct.
*Nurse:* May I have your name, please?
*Laboratory technician:* Yes, it's Mr. Burns.

Clarifying messages is important when nurses accept physician's orders over the telephone. The order is verified by repeating it clearly and precisely. Then the nurse writes the order on the physician's order sheet in the client's permanent record and signs it. The physician later verifies the telephone order by signing it within a set time period (usually 24 hours).

Courtesy is important when making or receiving phone calls. Anyone calling a nursing unit should be treated as a consumer needing a service. Courtesy conveys a sense of professionalism and promotes cooperation of all health team members.

## Incident Reports

An *incident* is any event not consistent with the routine operation of a health care unit or routine care of a client (Blake, 1984). Examples of incidents include client falls or accidental injuries, medication administration errors, accidental deletion of ordered therapies, or carelessness in performance of a procedure that results in actual or potential client injury. When an incident occurs, the nurse involved or the nurse who witnesses the incident completes a report. Most institutions have specific incident report forms (Fig. 2-2). The report documents an unusual situation that may possibly lead to a lawsuit or that indicates a failure to follow an institution's policy and procedures. The nurse describes details of the incident, and the physician examines the client to determine if any effects of the error occurred. The physician documents the examination and findings in the client's medical record. The nurse does not duplicate all information from the incident report in the client's medical record. The fact that an incident report was made is usually not noted. Only an objective description of what happened and any follow-up care is documented (Table 2-4).

The following are guidelines for correctly completing an incident report:

1. The nurse who witnessed the incident or who found the client at the time of the incident should file the report.
2. Describe specifically what happened in concise, objective terms.
3. Do not interpret or attempt to explain the cause of the incident.
4. Describe objectively the client's condition when the incident was discovered.
5. Report any measures taken by you, other nurses, or physicians at the time of the incident.
6. Do not blame any nurse or other health care worker in an incident report.
7. Submit the report as soon as possible to the appropriate administrator.

***TABLE 2-4*** Incident Reports

| Do | Don't |
|---|---|
| Describe exactly what was observed at the time the incident was discovered (e.g., client found on floor, at foot of bed; able to respond to name when called). | Don't interpret what might have caused an incident without supportive data (e.g., client found on floor at foot of bed, probably fell on way to bathroom). |
| Describe objectively any acts involving yourself in the incident (e.g., administered 100 mg Demerol IM at 2 PM; 75 mg Demerol was ordered. Monitored vital signs q 15 min, called Dr. Tiner, vital signs remain stable). | Don't implicate others, make excuses, or lay blame on the individual involved in the incident (e.g., floor short-staffed, administered 100 mg Demerol without checking order before administration, 75 mg Demerol ordered). |
| Describe actions taken at time of incident (e.g., conducted neuro check; client alert and oriented to name, date, and place. Client denies any discomfort. Returned client to bed and called Dr. Wilson). | Don't leave report incomplete, making it difficult for a reader to understand clearly what took place. |

Many nurses are reluctant to file incident reports because they believe such reports are detrimental to their employment record. Actually, incident reports are used by the institution's administration for quality assurance and risk management. By reviewing incident reports, administrators can identify areas of client risk. For example, if incident reports reflect a growing increase in the number of client falls, the risk manager may recommend that nursing service provide inservice training about safety in transferring and ambulating clients. Similarly a quality assurance study may reveal the types of clients most at risk for falls so that a prevention program can be initiated. Incident reports can help identify and eliminate significant problems in nursing practice or delivery of care methods.

## RECORDING

Documentation is very important in health care today. A medical record should be a comprehensive description of the client's health status and needs, as well as the services provided for the client's care. The Joint Commission on Accreditation of Health Care Organizations (JCAHO) sets specific standards for recording information (see box). JCAHO standards ensure the quality and appropriateness of care administered to clients and help clarify what level of nursing personnel is responsible for documenting specific client information. Good documentation reflects not only quality of care but evidence of each health care member's accountability in giving care. Nursing care procedures or treatments, even if considered routine, are assumed not done if they are undocumented. The record is also a document that shows to what extent hospitals should be reimbursed for services and supplies used. The medical record is essentially the client's health care bill.

Several types of records are used to communicate information about clients. Although each agency uses a different record format, all records contain the following basic information:

1. Demographic data
2. Consent forms
3. Admission nursing history
4. Medical history
5. Reports of physical examinations
6. Reports of diagnostic studies
7. Medical diagnosis(es)
8. Therapeutic orders
9. Nursing care plans
10. Nursing progress notes
11. Record of medical care and treatment
12. Discharge plan and summary

The record is a valuable source of data used by all members of the health care team. Its purposes include:

1. *Communication*—The record serves as a means by which health team members communicate their contributions to the client's care. The record should explain measures needed to maintain continuity and consistency of care, as well as the client's response to care.
2. *Education*—A client's history record, clinical course, and response to therapies is an excellent resource for educating nurses, physicians, dietitians, social workers, and members of other health care disciplines about clients with similar problems.
3. *Assessment*—The client's record is an invaluable source of data that nurses use to identify nursing diagnoses and plan proper strategies for care. Information from the record supplements the nurse's own observations and assessment. The record contains data to explain and confirm observations or refute interpretations.
4. *Research*—Statistical data relating to the frequency of

### *EXAMPLES OF JCAHO NURSING SERVICE STANDARDS*

The nursing process (assessment, nursing diagnosis, planning, implementation, and evaluation) is documented for each hospitalized client from admission through discharge.

The plan of care is documented and reflects current standards of nursing practice.

- The plan includes nursing measures that will facilitate medical care prescribed and will restore, maintain, or promote the client's well being.
- As appropriate, such measures include psychological, psychosocial, and environmental factors; client and family education; and client discharge planning.

Documentation of nursing care is pertinent and concise and reflects client status.

- Nursing documentation addresses the client's needs, problems, capabilities, and limitations.
- Nursing intervention and client responses are noted.
- When a client is transfered within or discharged from the hospital, a nurse notes his status in his medical record.
- Evidence of instructions and the client's or family's understanding of these instructions is noted in the medical record.
- The nursing department or service is encouraged to standardize documentation of routine elements of care and repeated monitoring of, for example, personal hygiene and administration of medication.

clinical disorders, complications, use of specific medical and nursing therapies, deaths, and recovery from illness can be gathered from client records. Records are a valuable resource for describing characteristics of the client populations that use a specific health agency.

5. *Auditing*—JCAHO requires hospitals to establish quality assurance programs to conduct objective ongoing and periodic reviews of client care. There are standards for types of information to be found in the client's record, such as indications that discharge planning and client education have occurred. Nurses conduct audits regularly throughout the year to determine the degree to which quality assurance standards are met and to evaluate the level of health care provided in an institution.
6. *Legal documentation*—The client's record is a legal document if it is used as evidence in a court of law. Contents of the record document the level of care. In many agencies, clients have the right to review their records. However, the record is usually the property of the agency. Access to the record is restricted to health care personnel caring for the client. Table 2-5 provides guidelines for a legally sound record.
7. *Financial record*—The chart is a principal source of information about a client's care. Documentation of pertinent observations and nursing actions are crucial to the client's or agency's reimbursement from Medicare and third-party payors (see box). Similarly nurses working in skilled nursing facilities must accurately show that the care provided is skilled and required nursing care. Medicare has set requirements for skilled nursing services that are reimbursable (see box).

**NURSES' NOTES REQUIREMENTS FOR REIMBURSEMENT**

Identification of medical purpose for the visit
Statement of skilled care rendered
Identification of the instruction of skilled activity to client and primary care giver with a return demonstration establishing learner comprehension
Concise and factual information
Elimination of all subjective statements
Avoidance of words that suggest a chronic condition: on-going, repeatedly, continues, monitor, stable

***TABLE 2-5*** Legal Guidelines for Recording

| Guideline | Rationale | Correct Action |
|---|---|---|
| Do not erase, apply correction fluid, or scratch out an error made while recording. | Charting becomes illegible. It may appear as though a nurse was attempting to hide information or deface the record. | Draw a single line through the error, write the word "error" above it and sign your name or initials; then record the note correctly. |
| Do not write retaliatory or critical comments about the client or care of other health care professionals. | Statements can be used as evidence for nonprofessional behavior or poor quality of care. | Enter only objective descriptions of client's behavior and care administered by others. |
| Correct all errors promptly. | Errors in recording can lead to errors in treatment. | Avoid rushing to complete charting; be sure information is accurate. |
| Record only facts. | Record must be accurate and reliable. | Be certain entry is factual; do not speculate or guess. |
| Do not leave blank spaces. | Another person can add incorrect information to the space. | Draw a line horizontally through the space and sign your name at its end. |
| All record entries should be legible and written in ink. | Illegible entries can be misinterpreted, causing errors and lawsuits. Ink cannot be erased. Records are photocopied and stored on microfilm. | Never erase entries or use correction fluid, and never use a pencil. |
| If you question an order, record that a clarification was sought. | If a nurse performs an order known to be incorrect, the nurse is just as liable for prosecution as the physician. | Do not record "physician made an error"; instead chart that "Dr. Smith was called to clarify order for . . . ." |
| Chart only for yourself. | Accountability is that of the nurse entering information into the chart. | Never chart for someone else. |
| Avoid using generalized, empty phrases such as "status unchanged" or "had a good day." | Specific information about a client's condition or case can be accidentally deleted if information is too generalized. | Use complete, concise descriptions of care. |
| Begin each entry with the date and time and end with your signature and title. | Ensures that the correct sequence of events is recorded. Signature documents who is accountable for care delivered. | Do not wait until end of the shift to record important changes that occurred several hours earlier. Be sure to sign. |

## Methods of Recording

The nursing service department of each health care agency selects the method for documentation of client care. The method should consider the philosophy of the nursing service and the way nursing care is given to clients. For example, if a professional model is used to deliver care, a documentation system should be based on the nursing process.

Three common methods of record-keeping are traditional source records, problem-oriented records, and modified problem-oriented records. The primary difference between these types is the manner in which information is organized.

### Source Records

In a source record the client's chart is organized so that each discipline (for example, nursing, medicine, or social work) has a separate section in which to record data. The advantage of a source record is that care givers can easily locate the proper section of the record in which to make entries. Nurses will frequently use sections including flow sheets, medication records, nursing progress notes, and care plans. Physicians will use sections such as physician's order sheets and medical progress records. Table 2-6 lists common sections in a source record.

A disadvantage of the source record is that information is fragmented. Although information may be well organized within each section, it becomes necessary for a care giver to sort out data from several different sections before finding all of the data that relates to one pertinent client problem. The method by which source records are organized does not easily show how information from the various health care disciplines is related or how care is coordinated to meet all of the client's needs.

### Problem-Oriented Medical Records

The problem-oriented medical record (POMR) is a structured method of documentation that places emphasis on the client's problems. The method corresponds to the nursing process and facilitates communication of client needs (Gawlinski and Rasmussen, 1984). Data are organized by problem rather than by source of information. Each member of the health care team contributes to a single list of identified client problems. With the POMR the client's problems are easy to recognize and locate, data are well coordinated, and each discipline records progress notes on the same form. Organizing data by a

**MEDICARE REQUIREMENTS FOR SKILLED NURSING SERVICES**

- Intravenous therapy
- Intramuscular injections required more than once a day (excludes vitamin $B_{12}$)
- Sterile dressing changes
- Care of extensive decubitus ulcers
- Nasogastric or gastrostomy tube feedings (in conjunction with other complications)
- Monitoring an unstabilized condition, such as cardiac or respiratory conditions of an acute nature, for modification of treatment or institution of medical procedures
- Resident teaching for newly diagnosed conditions, such as diabetes, that require insulin administration and blood glucose monitoring
- Pain control for clients with terminal malignancy
- Subcutaneous anticoagulation therapy with weekly lab service

***TABLE 2-6*** Organization of Traditional Source Record

| Section | Contents |
|---|---|
| Admission fact sheet. | Specific demographic data about client: name, identification number, address, date of birth, sex, age, marital status, occupation, employer, health insurance, nearest relative, attending physician, date and hour of admission to health agency, and primary diagnosis. |
| Physician's order sheet. | Record of physician's orders; each order entered with date, time, and physician's signature; orders prescribe specific therapies for client. |
| Graphic/flow sheet. | Record of repeated observations and measurements such as vital signs and weight. |
| Medical data base. | All observations and interpretations of client's condition made by physicians; includes physical examination, history, and progress notes. |
| Nursing notes. | Narrative record of nursing process: assessment, nursing diagnosis, planning, implementation, and evaluation of care provided. |
| Medication records. | Accurate documentation of all medications administered to client; date, time, and signature of nurse are recorded. |
| Health care disciplines: special reports. | Entries made into record by all health-related disciplines: physical therapy, dietary department, radiology, social work, laboratories, surgery, and anesthesia. |
| Discharge summary. | Summary of client's condition, progress, prognosis, rehabilitation, and teaching needs at time of dismissal from hospital or agency. |

POMR format ensures a more coordinated plan of care.

The POMR has four components: data base, problem list, initial plan, and progress notes.

1. *Data base*—Contains all available assessment information pertaining to the client (for example, physician's physical examination and medical history, nurse's admission history and assessment, dietitian's assessment, laboratory reports, and radiological test results). The data base:
   a. Provides a foundation for identifying client problems and planning an effective course of action.
   b. Should remain active and current, with revisions made as new data become available.
   c. Will accompany clients throughout successive hospitalizations or clinic visits.
2. *Problem list*—After data are analyzed, problems are identified and a single list is made (Fig. 2-3). The problems are numbered and listed in chronologic order according to the date each was identified (not in order of priority). The list is an organizing guide by which all health care disciplines plan the client's care. All health care professionals contribute to the list as problems are identified.

   A problem may be well defined, such as a specific medical or nursing diagnosis. Signs, symptoms, or syndromes such as pain or diarrhea may be stated as problems when insufficient data have been recorded to diagnose a problem or when complications of a medical diagnosis arise. Problems include the client's total health care needs and are considered *active* or *inactive.*

   It is important to not list problems that are vague or unsupported by data. However the nurse lists a diagnosis, if one can be established, rather than a less specific term. For example, the nursing diagnosis of ineffective airway clearance is characterized by a cough, dyspnea, and abnormal breath sounds. Coughing or dyspnea would be less acceptable as problems. Characteristics of diagnoses should not be listed separately. This can cause fragmentation of care.

   The list of problems is filed in the front of the client's record to serve as an organizer or table of contents. New problems are added as they are identified. Once a problem has been resolved, the date of resolution is recorded and a line is drawn through the problem and its number on the problem sheet. The number for a resolved or inactive problem is not used again. This system keeps the problem list simple yet meaningful. Once a problem list is developed, succeeding record entries, such as in the progress notes, are coded by the problem number.
3. *Initial plan*—An initial plan is developed for each active problem identified. There are three parts to a plan:

   *Diagnostic workup*—Physician indicates what diagnostic studies should be initiated first. Setting priorities prevents duplication of efforts and delay in dealing with client needs. During a time of cost containment in health care a coordination of diagnostic testing is very important.

   *Proposed therapy*—Physician orders specific therapies by problem. Orders may include medications, activity restrictions, diet, special treatments, precautions, or observations to make. If the original problem is a

| Problem number | Date onset | Problem | Inactive or resolved | Date resolved |
|---|---|---|---|---|
| ~~1~~ | ~~7/8/88~~ | ~~Ⓡ breast mass~~ | ~~Resolved~~ | ~~7/9/88~~ |
| 2 | 7/8/88 | Anxiety over impending surgery | | |
| 3 | 7/9/88 | Ⓡ sub-total mastectomy | | |
| 4 | 7/9/88 | Alteration in comfort related to incisional pain | Controlled | 7/12/88 |

***Fig. 2-3*** POMR problem list.

BARNES HOSPITAL

**Nursing Assessment Flowsheet**

Date 10/14/88 C-10b

Instructions: Circle if Present.
Write in Assessment.
Indicate N/A if not applicable or not assessed.

Code: S - Self, A - Assist, T - Total
I - Instructed, C - Collected

Addressograph

| Section | Item | NIGHT | DAY |
|---|---|---|---|
| NEURO/CEREBRAL | NEURO/CEREBRAL | Alert Confused Memory Loss Agitated; Oriented x 3; ASKS QUESTIONS ABOUT ULCER CARE | Alert Confused Memory Loss Agitated; Oriented x 3; NOTES BURNING @ ULCER SITE DURING DRESSING CHANGE |
| COMFORT/SLEEP | Discomfort / Intervention | N/A | |
| | Sleep Status | Awake Slept at intervals Slept | Awake Slept at intervals Slept |
| ACTIVITY/EXERCISE | MOBILITY | Independent Assist Dependent | Independent Assist Dependent |
| | Limitations/Devices | | |
| | ACTIVITY | UP TO BATHROOM x2 | UP TO CHAIR IN ROOM x3 |
| SKIN/MUCOSA | Appearance | Warm Dry Turgor; SKIN INTACT AROUND BONY PROMINENCES | Warm Dry Turgor REDUCED; SKIN DRY, INTACT EXCEPT FOR ULCER; LOTION APPLIED TO BONY PROMINENCES |
| | Mattress/Equipment | Foam Air Heel Protectors Aqua K pad Teds | Foam Air Heel Protectors Aqua K pad Teds |
| WOUND | LOCATION / Appearance | (L) FOOT ULCER 3CM DIAMETER, DRAINING YELLOW DISCHARGE | (L) FOOT ULCER CONTINUES TO DRAIN YELLOW DISCHARGE, 3CM ULCER INFLAMED ALONG MARGINS |
| | Dressing Change | X1 WET-TO-DRY SALINE, FINE MESH GAUZE | X2 WET-TO-DRY, SALINE AND FINE MESH GAUZE |
| NUTRITION | MEALS | | % Eaten B: 90% S A T L: 80% S A T |
| | Tube Feeding / Infusion Device | Continuous Bolus Flush X | Continuous Bolus Flush X |
| ELIMINATION | URINE | Continent x2 Incontinent Foley; CLEAR, YELLOW URINE | Continent x4 Incontinent Foley; CLEAR, YELLOW URINE |
| | BOWEL | Continent Incontinent Guaiac; Freq X: N/A | Continent Incontinent Guaiac; Freq X: 1 SOFT, FORMED STOOL |
| | Bowel Sounds | Absent Present; Abdomen | Absent Present ALL QUADRANTS; Abdomen SOFT, NON-TENDER |
| RESPIRATORY | Auscultation | N/A | CLEAR TO AUSCULTATION IN ALL LOBES |
| | | O2; Cough/Secretion | O2; Cough/Secretion |
| CIRC | CIRCULATION | FEET COOL, DORSALIS PEDIS PULSES WEAK BILATERALLY | PEDAL PULSES WEAK BILATERALLY |
| OTHER | Specimen | I C Test; GLUCOMETER READING AT 10:00 PM - 110 | I C Test; GLUCOMETER READING AT 8:30 AM - 165; GLUCOMETER READING AT 12:30 PM - 180 |
| | Signature/Status | S. Tucker, RN | |
| | HYGIENE: S A T | Bath Tub Shower; Shave Hair Nails; Oral x1 | Bath Tub Shower; Shave Hair Nails; Oral x2 |
| | SAFETY | ID Band on ✓; Siderails in Use ✓ | ID Band on ✓; Siderails in Use ✓ |

***Fig. 2-4*** Nursing assessment flow sheet.
Courtesy Barnes Hospital, St. Louis.

**Nursing Assessment Flowsheet**

Date 10/14/88 C-10b

Instructions: Circle if Present.
Write in Assessment.
Indicate N/A if not applicable or not assessed.

Code: S - Self, A - Assist, T - Total
I - Instructed, C - Collected

**EVENING**

(Alert) Confused Memory Loss Agitated
Oriented x 3

BURNING AT ULCER SITE MORE INTENSE; PRN ANALGESIC AT 7:00 PM RELIEVED DISCOMFORT

Awake (Slept at intervals) Slept

(Independent) Assist Dependent

UP TO CHAIR x 2

(Warm) (Dry) Turgor

TURNS SELF WELL

Foam Air (Heel Protectors) Aqua K pad Teds

MINIMAL DRAINAGE NOTED AT ULCER SITE. WOUND APPEARS CLEAN. SLIGHT INFLAMMATION ALONG MARGINS
X 1 WET-TO-DRY SALINE, FINE MESH GAUZE

% Eaten D: 90% (S) A T
Continuous Bolus Flush X

(Continent) x 2 Incontinent Foley
CLEAR, YELLOW URINE

Continent Incontinent Guaiac
Freq X: N/A
Absent (Present) ALL QUADRANTS
Abdomen SOFT, NON-TENDER

N/A

$O_2$
Cough/Secretion

PEDAL PULSES WEAK BILATERALLY

I C Test
GLUCOMETER READING AT 5 PM 155

Signature/Status

| HYGIENE: (S) A T | SAFETY |
|---|---|
| Bath Tub Shower | ID Band on ✓ |
| Shave (Hair) Nails | Siderails in Use ✓ |
| (Oral) | |

nursing diagnosis, the nurse outlines the proposed interventions for care. The format of a POMR allows each health care worker to understand the rationale for all orders.

*Client education*—Identifying client educational needs addresses the long-term implications of illness. Health team members identify the types of information or skills required by a client to adapt to any health-related problems.

4. *Progress notes*—Health team members must monitor and record progress of a client's problems. Progress notes follow a special format (for example, SOAP or PIE) so information is communicated clearly to all who read them (Table 2-7). SOAP is an acronym for subjective data, objective data, assessment, and plan. The logic for SOAP notes is similar to that of the nursing process. Data are collected about each of the client's problems, a conclusion is made, and a plan of care is developed. Each SOAP note is numbered and titled according to the problem on the list it addresses. The numbering system makes it easy to find notes about the same problem. The notes help communicate an on-going plan of care.

   S—Subjective data or information gathered from the client. For example, client will describe a symptom such as pain or discuss an interest in learning about a medication. Whether the progress note includes subjective data depends on the acuteness of the client's illness or nature of the problem.

   O—Objective data consists of information that can be observed or measured. Physical findings, laboratory results, observations, or results of x-ray examinations are examples of objective data.

   A—The individual who writes a SOAP note takes subjective and objective data and forms conclusions. The *assessment* is an interpretation of the client's condition or level of progress. It is a statement of the status of the diagnosis or problem. The assessment determines whether the problem has been resolved or if further care is required.

   P—Based on assessment of the situation the health care member develops a *plan of care*. Plans may include specific orders designed to manage the client's problem, collection of additional data about the problem, individual or family education, and goal of care. The plan in each SOAP note is compared with the plan in previous notes. A decision is made to revise, modify, or continue previously proposed interventions.

PIE is an acronym for Problem-Intervention-Evaluation. (Some institutions use the format APIE, in which "A" represents assessment findings.) This format simplifies documentation by unifying the care plan and progress notes into a complete record (Siegrist, 1985). The PIE format differs from SOAP because the narrative note does not include assessment information. Daily assessment data appears instead on special flow sheets (Fig. 2-4) thus pre-

***TABLE 2-7*** **Examples of Progress Notes Written in SOAP and PIE Formats**

| SOAP | PIE |
|---|---|
| **S**—Client states, "My doctor has explained that I will be requiring insulin regularly from now on. I know I need to learn how to give myself shots." | **P**—Knowledge deficit regarding self-administration of insulin related to inexperience. |
| **O**—Client diagnosed as having diabetes, requiring insulin. Asks appropriate questions, is attentive. Has had no experience with administering injections. Has good hand dexterity. | **I**—Instructed client on purpose and action of insulin and parts of syringe. Included wife in teaching session. Will instruct on preparation and administration tomorrow. |
| **A**—Client willing and able to learn insulin administration. | **E**—Client and wife able to describe purpose and action of insulin, ask questions related to client's condition, and able to handle syringe parts correctly. |
| **P**—Instruct client during the following noted days on: 1. Purpose, action of insulin (4/20). 2. Syringe parts (4/20). 3. Principles of asepsis (4/21). 4. Method for drawing up insulin (4/21). 5. Method for administering insulin (4/21). 6. Signs and symptoms of hypoglycemia (4/22). | |

venting duplication of information. PIE notes can be numbered or labeled according to the client's problems. Resolved problems are dropped from daily documentation after the nurse's review. Continuing problems are documented daily.

P—Problem or nursing diagnosis applicable to client.
I—Interventions or actions taken.
E—Evaluation of outcomes of nursing interventions and client's response to nursing therapies.

#### Modified Problem-Oriented Medical Records

In some institutions, the POMR charting method is used only in the nursing notes section of the record. Other disciplines, for example, physicians or dieticians, use narrative notes in their respective sections of the record.

At time of admission, an initial nursing assessment and history (see Chapter 1) identifies the client's problems or nursing diagnoses. Diagnoses may be prioritized in a list or by care plans developed by the nursing staff. The nurse lists the number or name of the problem or diagnosis each time the problem is recorded in the SOAP, PIE, or narrative notes. It is acceptable to underline the number, diagnosis, or problem in the notes so it can be easily spotted. Nurses record notes on each pertinent problem daily or every shift, depending on agency policy. This continues until problems are resolved. When a problem or diagnosis is resolved the nurse enters the date, notes that the problem is resolved, and signs her name. New problems may be added to a problem list or new care plans selected as problems are identified.

#### Alternative Record-Keeping Forms

A client's medical record may use a variety of forms to make documentation easy and quick, yet comprehensive. Many forms eliminate the need to duplicate repeated data in the nursing notes. The forms present special types of information in a format more accessible than reviewing all progress notes.

***Nursing History Forms.*** A nursing history form is a special form completed at the time a client is admitted to a nursing care unit. The form usually contains basic biographic data (i.e., age, method of admission, physician), a brief history (e.g. surgical history, allergies, medication history, previous illnesses), the client's perceptions about illness or hospitalization, and a physical assessment of all body systems. The form allows the admitting nurse to make a thorough client assessment to identify relevant nursing diagnoses or problems. Data on history forms provide baseline data that can be compared with changes that occur later in the client's condition.

***Flow Sheets.*** Flow sheets are forms that allow nurses to record specific measurements or observations that occur on a repeated basis. Examples of flow sheets include nursing assessment sheets (Fig. 2-4), vital signs records (Fig. 2-5), pain flow sheets, postoperative recovery records, and teaching flow sheets (Fig. 2-6). The flow sheet is a rapid, more efficient way to record information. Flow Sheets often remain at the client's bedside, rather than in the chart, because bedside placement offers easy access and prompt recording.

The only time the nurse may wish to duplicate information from a flow sheet into a narrative or progress note is when a significant change that results in specific therapies occurs. For example, if a client's blood pressure becomes dangerously high, the nurse may record the pressure, as well as the medication administered to lower the pressure, in the narrative progress note.

One value of a flow sheet is that it can show important clinical trends graphically without the nurse or physician having to locate the source information in several notes.

***Nursing Kardex.*** Nursing information that is needed for daily care of a client is readily accessible in the nursing Kardex (Fig. 2-7). The Kardex is a flip-over card usually kept in a portable index file or notebook at the central nursing station.) Nurses refer to the Kardex throughout the day. It organizes information in a useful manner as nurses give change-of-shift reports or make walking rounds. An updated Kardex eliminates the need for continual referral to the client's chart for routine information.

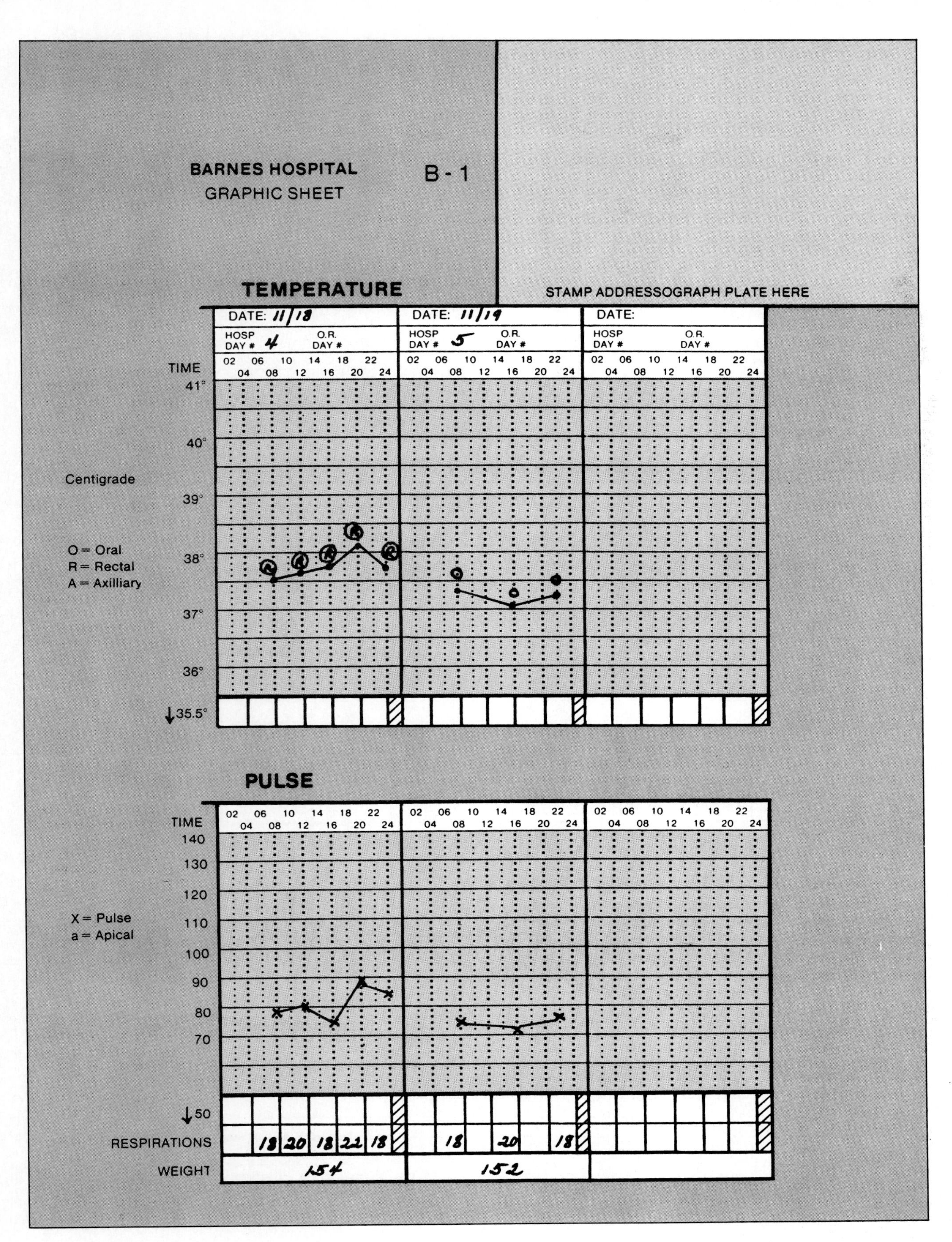


*Fig. 2-5* Vital signs flowsheet.

Courtesy Barnes Hospital, St. Louis.

**BARNES**

C-33

DIABETIC INSTRUCTION RECORD

TI = TEACHING INITIATED
D/V = DEMONSTRATES/VERBALIZES UNDERSTANDING
FI = FAMILY INCLUDED

ADDRESSOGRAPH PLATE

**ASSESSMENT**

1. HIGHEST LEVEL OF FORMALIZED EDUCATION ATTAINED High School
2. VISION Glasses required for reading
3. LITERACY Able to read and explain information in teaching booklet
4. IDENTIFIED BARRIERS TO LEARNING

| | DATE & INITIAL | | | |
|---|---|---|---|---|
| | TI | D/V | FI | COMMENTS |
| **A) DISEASE OVERVIEW** | | | | |
| 1. DEFINITION OF DIABETES | P.L. 3/28 | R.K. 3/29 | P.L. 3/28 | Wife included in teaching session |
| 2. LONGTERM COMPLICATIONS (MICROVASCULAR/MACROVASCULAR/NEUROPATHY) | P.L. 3/28 | R.K. 3/29 | P.L. 3/28 | |
| 3. 3 FACTORS OF CONTROL (DIET, EXERCISE, MEDICATION) | P.L. 3/28 | R.K. 3/29 | P.L. 3/28 | |
| **B) DIET** | | | | |
| 1. TYPE 1800 Cal. ADA | R.K. 3/29 | | | |
| SNACK TIMES 8:00 pm | 3/29 R.K. | | | |
| 2. MEAL TIMING 8am 12N 6pm | 3/29 R.K. | | | |
| 3. FOOD TYPES TO AVOID (FRIED FATTY FOODS, SIMPLE SUGARS) | | | | |
| 4. IMPORTANCE OF WEIGHT CONTROL | | | | |
| **C) EXERCISE** | | | | |
| 1. TYPE | | | | |
| 2. FREQUENCY | | | | |
| 3. DURATION | | | | |
| 4. EFFECTS ON BLOOD SUGAR CONTROL & INSULIN UTILIZATION | | | | |
| **D) MEDICATION** | | | | |
| 1. NAME/DOSAGE | | | | |
| 2. ORAL AGENT | | | | |
| a. WHEN TO TAKE | | | | |
| b. ACTION OF MEDICATION | | | | |
| 3. INSULIN | | | | |
| a. ACTION, KINDS, STORAGE | | | | |
| b. PREPARATION, ADMINISTRATION | | | | |
| c. SITE SELECTION/ROTATION | | | | |

***Fig. 2-6*** Diabetic instruction form.
Courtesy Barnes Hospital, St. Louis.

| | | |
|---|---|---|
| Medical Diagnosis: Diabetes | | |
| Pertinent History: Adult onset, age 41 | | |
| Allergies: (drugs, food & others) Penicillin | | |
| Condition: stable | Isolation: | |
| Code Status: | Service: | |
| Adm. Date: 7/10/90 Age: 45 | Doctor: | |
| **PHYSIOLOGICAL MEASUREMENTS** | **ACTIVITIES** | **NURSING DIAGNOSES** |
| Temp: q̄ shift | Ad Lib ✓ 7/10/90 BRP | Knowledge deficit |
| Pulse & Resp.: q̄ shift | Up, assist of: ☐ ×1 ☐ ×2 ☐ Total lift | related to inexperience |
| BP: q̄ shift | Chair BSC | with insulin therapy |
| Call H.O. T>___, <___ : HR>___, <___; | Bedrest | |
| SPB>___, <___ : DBP>___, <___; | | |
| RR>___, <___ : U/O<___, <___; | ADL: | |
| Neuro/Vascular checks: | (SELF) ASSIST TOTAL | |
| Accuchecks 07-11-17 | BED (SHOWER) TUB | |
| | | |
| **NUTRITION** | **SAFETY PRECAUTIONS** | Primary Nurse: R. Owens |
| Diet: 1800 Calorie ADA T A (S) | ☐ Restraints: | Estimated Discharge Date/Destination: |
| | | 7/15/90 Home |
| Supplements: | ☐ Prosthesis: | Miscellaneous: |
| Calorie Count: | ☐ Blind ☐ HOH ☒ Glasses | Wife included in |
| | ☐ Speech | teaching plan— |
| **FLUID BALANCE** | **ANCILLARY SERVICES** | instructed on insulin |
| I&D q̄ shift | ☐ PT ☐ OT ☐ Speech | administration 7/13/90 |
| Weights Str. | ☒ Dietary ☐ Social Service | (see flow chart) |
| Force/Restraint Total/24 | ☐ Home Health Diabetes Nurse Specialist | |
| Dietary________ Nursing________ | Family/S.O. Phone # 469-2111 | |
| D________ E________ N________ | | |
| IV access: | | |
| ☐ IV ☐ Heplock ☐ Central Line | | |

***Fig. 2-7*** Kardex.

Information commonly found in the Kardex includes:

1. Basic demographic data (e.g., age, religion).
2. Primary medical diagnosis.
3. Current physician's orders to be carried out by the nurse.
4. A written nursing care plan (used when a formal plan is not in the client's record).
5. Nursing orders.
6. Scheduled tests and procedures.
7. Safety precautions to be used in the client's care.
8. Factors related to activities of daily living.

In many institutions, nurses make Kardex entries in pencil because it is usually necessary to make frequent revisions as the client's needs change. However, entries should be made in ink if the Kardex is a permanent part of the client's record.

### Standardized Care Plans

Although it is every professional nurse's responsibility to develop an individualized plan of care for a client, the process of writing the plan is time consuming. Nurses caring for several clients may need to write extensive

**NURSING STANDARD CARE PLAN**

**Nursing Diagnosis:** ALTERATION IN COMFORT

Related to ______
*(inadequate pain relief, fear of drug dependence, vomiting, nausea, other)*

Addressograph

**Expected Outcomes:**

- ☐ Patient will demonstrate increased comfort as evidenced by:
  - ☐ ability to sleep within patient's normal limits.
  - ☐ fewer signs and symptoms of discomfort.
  - ☐ verbalization of comfort level.
  - ☐ participation in self-care activities, i.e., eating, bathing, etc.
- ☐ Patient/support person will demonstrate effective use of medication and/or pain control devices.
- ☐ Patient will verbalize and demonstrate understanding of specific teaching plan.
- ☐ Other: ______
- ☐ Other: ______

| Date Initiated /Initials | Nursing Interventions | Date Inactivated /Initials |
|---|---|---|
| ______ | 1. Evaluate pain/effectiveness of relief measures every ______ | ______ |
| ______ | 2. Establish a trusting relationship with patient, communicate that you know the pain is real by: ______ | ______ |
| ______ | 3. Measure for pain/relief:<br>☐ position ______<br>☐ administer analgesics prior to/during ______<br>☐ minimize negative environmental stimuli by ______<br>☐ administer cutaneous stimulation (TENS, aquakpad, ice bags) of ______ during ______<br>☐ assist patient with relaxation techniques including ______ every ______<br>☐ promote distraction measures including ______<br>☐ possible meditation techniques including ______<br>☐ other ______ | ______ |
| ______ | 4. Assess bowel function and skin integrity every ______ | ______ |
| ______ | 5. Assess potential for injury while receiving therapy by: ______ | ______ |
| ______ | 6. Provide teaching specific to patient/support person needs (e.g. use of medications, other relief measures). Initiate individual plan. ______ | ______ |
| ______ | 7. Initiate consults/referrals. ______ | ______ |
| ______ | 8. Other interventions specific to patient: ______<br>Signature/Initials: ______ | ______ |

***Fig. 2-8*** Standardized nursing care plan.

plans of care. Many institutions have attempted to make documentation easier with standardized care plans. The plans, based on the institution's philosophy of nursing care, are preprinted, established guidelines for the care of clients with similar health problems (Fig. 2-8). After a nursing assessment is completed, the staff nurse identifies the standard care plans appropriate to the client. Care plans are placed in a client's record. Modifications can be made to the standardized plans in ink to individualize nursing therapies. Most standardized plans allow the nurse to write in specific goals or desired outcomes of care, as well as dates when these outcomes should be achieved.

There are several advantages and disadvantages of standardized care plans. One advantage is the establishment of clinically sound standards of care for similar groups of clients. These standards can be useful when quality assurance audits are conducted. Standardized plans are easy to locate in a client's record, and thus all staff can quickly refer to the plan of care. Another advantage is education. Nurses learn to recognize accepted requirements of care for clients. The standardized plans can also improve continuity of care among professional nurses. Finally, even though the plans must be modified for each client, documentation takes less time.

Controversy exists over the use of standardized care

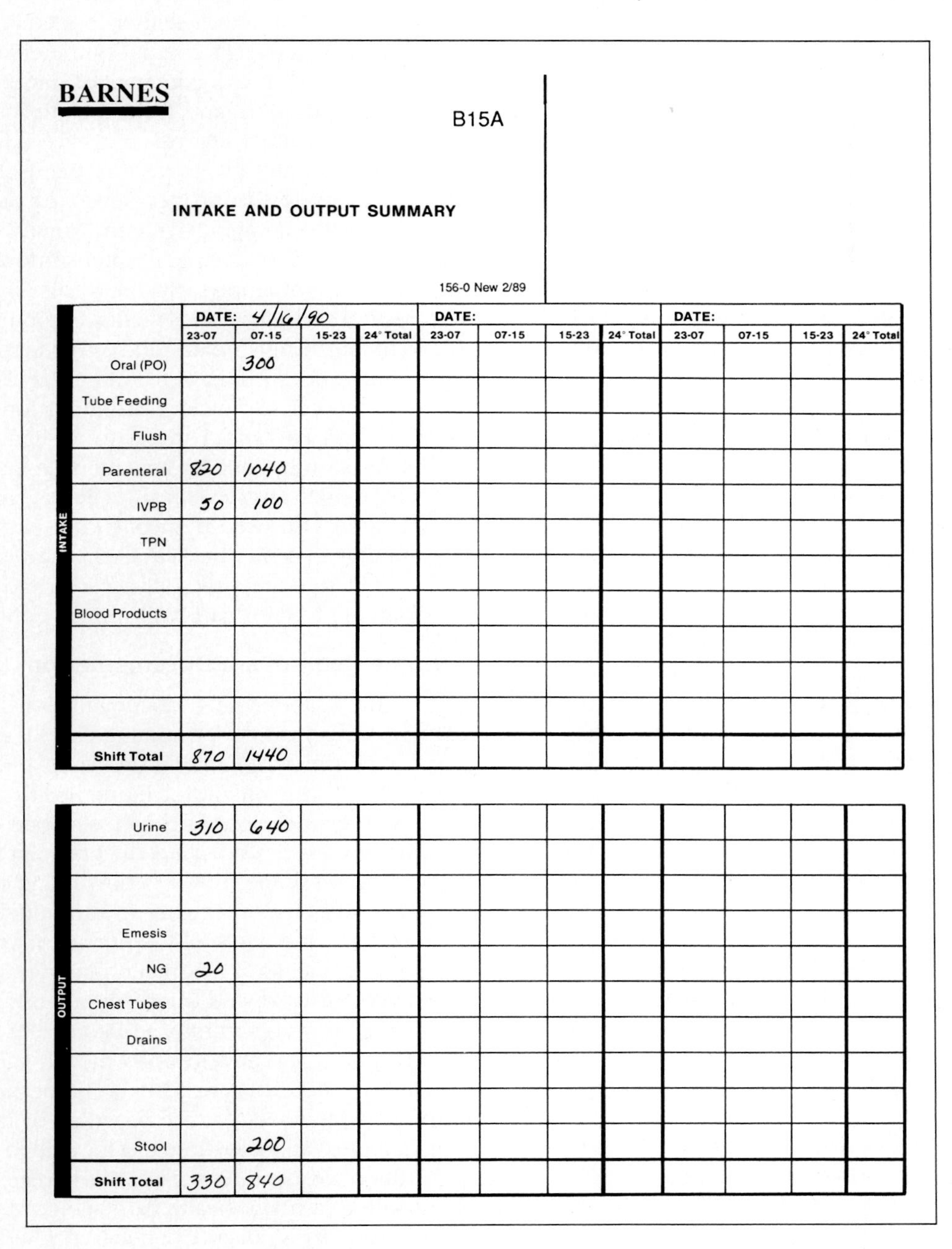

**BARNES**

B15A

INTAKE AND OUTPUT SUMMARY

156-0 New 2/89

| | DATE: 4/16/90 | | | | DATE: | | | | DATE: | | | |
|---|---|---|---|---|---|---|---|---|---|---|---|---|
| | 23-07 | 07-15 | 15-23 | 24° Total | 23-07 | 07-15 | 15-23 | 24° Total | 23-07 | 07-15 | 15-23 | 24° Total |
| **INTAKE** | | | | | | | | | | | | |
| Oral (PO) | | 300 | | | | | | | | | | |
| Tube Feeding | | | | | | | | | | | | |
| Flush | | | | | | | | | | | | |
| Parenteral | 820 | 1040 | | | | | | | | | | |
| IVPB | 50 | 100 | | | | | | | | | | |
| TPN | | | | | | | | | | | | |
| | | | | | | | | | | | | |
| Blood Products | | | | | | | | | | | | |
| | | | | | | | | | | | | |
| | | | | | | | | | | | | |
| | | | | | | | | | | | | |
| Shift Total | 870 | 1440 | | | | | | | | | | |
| **OUTPUT** | | | | | | | | | | | | |
| Urine | 310 | 640 | | | | | | | | | | |
| | | | | | | | | | | | | |
| | | | | | | | | | | | | |
| Emesis | | | | | | | | | | | | |
| NG | 20 | | | | | | | | | | | |
| Chest Tubes | | | | | | | | | | | | |
| Drains | | | | | | | | | | | | |
| | | | | | | | | | | | | |
| | | | | | | | | | | | | |
| Stool | | 200 | | | | | | | | | | |
| Shift Total | 330 | 840 | | | | | | | | | | |

***Fig. 2-9*** Intake and output flowsheet.
Courtesy Barnes Hospital, St. Louis.

plans. The major disadvantage is the risk that standardized plans inhibit nurses' identification of unique, individualized therapies for clients. A second disadvantage is the need to formally update plans on a routine basis to ensure that content is current and appropriate. When standardized care plans are used in a health care facility, the nurse remains responsible for an individualized approach to care.

***24-Hour Intake and Output Records.*** Clients placed on intake and output (I & O) require monitoring of their fluid balance during a 24-hour period. Special forms allow the nurse to document the type and amount of fluid taken in or lost during each 8-hour shift (Fig. 2-9). Forms are divided into sources of intake, such as oral, intravenous, or gastric feeding, and sources of output, such as urine, gastric suction, or emesis. Totals are calculated for each 8-hour shift, as well as for a 24-hour period. Usually I & O records are kept at the client's bedside. At times it is appropriate for clients and family members to be taught how to use I & O records.

***Discharge Summary Forms.*** Ideally, discharge planning begins with a client's admission. The initial nursing history should reflect a client's potential need for referrals, instructions, and special support from health care providers. Nurses revise the plan of care as a client's needs and condition change. Progress toward established goals must be documented to show evidence of discharge planning. There should also be evidence of the client's and family member's involvement in the discharge planning process. Some institutions use discharge summary forms that are signed by the client to demonstrate participation in care and to legally validate the client's having received discharge instructions.

At time of discharge, the nurse reviews the plan of care for the home or extended care facility. The client's status is documented in relation to planned outcomes or discharge criteria. Discharge summary forms (see Chapter 1) make the summary concise and instructive. The nurse may document items, such as diet orders, wound care guidelines, activity restrictions, medication information, the physician's phone number, and signs or symptoms of complications that warrant action. Many forms include a copy that is given to the client or family member at discharge. Other health team members, such as dieticians or social workers, may contribute to the summary.

***Consents and Releases.*** When a client enters a health care institution a consent for examination and treatment must be signed. The consent allows physicians to order necessary diagnostic tests and therapies for clients. Consent forms are usually signed in the admitting office or on a nursing division. In addition to the client's signature, there must also be a signature of a competent witness.

A special consent form must be signed when a client requires surgery or certain invasive procedures. Such a form includes an explanation of the procedure to be performed. It is the physician's responsibility to explain the procedure and its implications. A nurse may witness the consent, thus verifying the client's signature.

A release is a form signed by a client who leaves a hospital without the doctor's consent. When a client leaves a hospital or other health care facility against medical advice, the release frees the physician and agency of neglect.

## Computerized Documentation

Today a variety of computerized forms are available; nurses may document medications, develop and update care plans, and enter data formerly charted on flow sheets. The computer is either located at a central nursing station or in a client's room. Computers can organize data in such a way that documentation time is reduced, there is less duplication, and fewer printed forms are needed for the permanent record.

Most computer programs give the user information that helps to make the proper keyboard or light pen selections on the computer screen. Nurses can enter assessment findings or document interventions that are quickly transmitted for storage. Such systems also improve the accuracy of charging for a client's equipment and supplies. Documentation is timely, and fewer errors occur because the nurse does not have to transcribe data.

A computer can make documentation easier; however, it also can become a threat to a client's confidentiality. The nurse must not let anyone access the computer except for staff involved in the client's care. Special signature codes are used by health care personnel to enter a computer system. The AHA clearly states that clients have the right to expect that all records and communications pertaining to their care will remain confidential.

## Home Health Care Documentation

In the home setting, documentation is the crucial element for continuity of nursing care; it represents the legality of achieving nursing standards and provides the basis for reimbursement for home health care services. The nurse must develop thorough, accurate client care notes. Although this has been a goal, it has not been consistently pursued. In home care it is now being demanded.

Charting of nursing care in the home must reflect the what, why, and when of the nursing process. Documentation must include assessment, nursing diagnoses, medical reasons for care, and interventions used in the home. It must be logical, accurate, and complete.

Terminology used in home health care charting is different from acute care. For the home health care agency to be reimbursed for care provided by the nurse, the language must validate the need for skilled care and the justification for continued care. With greater than 70% of all income to a home health care agency dependent on care delivered to Medicare beneficiaries, and because many health insurance programs are adapting their reimbursement schedules to the Medicare plan, home health care charting focuses on Medicare guidelines.

In 1965, Congress created the Medicare program to offer health care services to a population that had limited access to health care. Expenditures increased dramatically. By the end of the 1960s, the Department of Health, Education and Welfare refined and tightened its definition of health care coverage. By 1970 the level of Medicare health care expenditures began to decline.

In 1983, with the passage of the prospective payment system for hospitals and the establishment of a diagnostic-related-group (DRG) method of paying for hospital care, the future for home health care changed. The purpose of the DRGs was to prompt hospitals to reduce unnecessary tests, avoid overly long hospital stays, and to discharge clients earlier. Many of these clients were older, sicker, and required more intensive care and greater frequency of visits over a longer period of time than was true before 1983. In addition, technologically advanced procedures and equipment, once reserved for hospital rooms, began to appear in the home environment. Changes in payments to hospitals has reduced the cost of care per patient. Recently government cost saving efforts have begun to focus on the home health care industry. In 1985, the government reduced the amount of money paid to home health care, while at the same time increased the amount of documentation required to substantiate the health care services provided.

In home health care, health insurance programs provide reimbursement for care by licensed nurses, physical therapists, speech pathologists, occupational therapists, medical social workers, and home health care aides under very specific and often time-limited circumstances. Not every Medicare beneficiary meets the criteria necessary to qualify for home health care services coverage. Not every health insurance policy provides for home health care. Approval for payment of services is now often obtained by home health care agencies before they will accept a client for care.

Medicare and many health insurance programs do not provide coverage for general health care guidance, maintenance services, preventive illness training, and socioeconomic or emotional needs. Although these aspects of client care are essential and are integral components in providing quality care, they do not constitute skilled services in insurance programs and are not therefore reimbursable unless provided in conjunction with a skilled service visit.

The following criteria distinguish skilled care from unskilled care:

1. The client's condition is such that significant changes may occur that would require the evaluation skills of a professional nurse.
2. The client requires direct service that employs the knowledge, skills, and judgment of a professional.
3. The client and primary care provider require teaching to perform appropriate services and observations.

In addition, most health insurance carriers require that the care of a client be intermittent or part time, that the client be under the care of a physician, and that the client be homebound.

In home care, good documentation is the key to reimbursement (see box). Medicare and health insurance reviewers advise that if care is not written, it is considered not performed, and therefore the service is not reimbursable. Nurses must document observations and interventions for several reasons. There is an increased risk of clients having complications as the result of coming out of the hospital "quicker and sicker." The potential for rehospitalization requires clear and careful documentation of nursing care provided in the home. Furthermore, because of tightening reimbursement, the nurse needs to document the client's or family's ability to provide care; the efforts made to secure additional help to substitute

### SKILLED NURSE'S NOTE

Nursing diagnosis—knowledge deficit in regard to wounds: related to inexperience.

Medical reason for visit—assess wound, wound care, assess s/s wound infection, assess s/s complications PVD, assess pain management.

Nursing services provided—skilled observation, wound care and dressing change, observe and teach medication effects and side effects, teach physiology of disease process.

Plan—visit qd for wound care, assess s/s infection, assess pain control, R/D anatomy and physiology of healing.

Communication with Physician—MD notified of no relief from pain medication, and increased blood drainage from wound site.

Nurse's note: Assessed open wound (L)LE: wound to tibial area 5½" in length ×¼ wide, draining bright red blood, saturating three 4 × 4 gauze pads and topper. Instructed in anatomy and physiology of wound healing: healing occurs in layers and is slow process due to reduced peripheral vascular status. Irrigated wound according to physician's orders: $H_2O_2$ irrigation, followed by betadine solution, three sterile 4 × 4 gauze pads applied, topper taped in place over gauze. Assessed s/s infection: c/o severe pain to (L) leg and foot, not relieved by Demerol. Assessed s/s complications PVD: (L) pedal pulses weak, distal tips of first and second toe necrotic and cool to touch. Assessed pain management: order for Demerol 1 tab q 3½ hours, no relief, obtained good R/D of ASE Demerol. Instructed on acute side effects of Demerol - lethargy, drowsiness, constipation, reduced respirations.

for or supplement care delivered by the agency; and the actions taken to teach clients and families about the disease process, therapies, and technical skills, which demonstrate the ongoing need for skilled care visits by the health professional.

Medicare does not consider the following activities professional nursing skills and therefore will not reimburse for these services:

1. Monitoring medication administration and side effects.
2. Monitoring vital signs when there is no change in client's condition.
3. Assessing client to determine that the client's condition remains stable.
4. Repeating instructions.
5. Reinforcing instructions.
6. Providing emotional support.
7. Checking for fecal impaction.
8. Preventing decubiti or pressure area formations.
9. Observing for circulatory impairment in client with a cast.
10. Providing ROM exercises for the purpose of preventing muscle atrophy.
11. Evaluating client to determine the need to change an indwelling foley catheter.
12. Administering eyedrops or ointments.
13. Administering injectable medications deemed not medically necessary.
14. Administering oral medications.

There are always exceptions to the above list*; however, the provider must prove that the activities require the skills of a nurse.

## GUIDELINES TO ENHANCE REIMBURSEMENT

1. *Medication*—Give instruction on action and side effects of one medication per visit. State name of medication, action, side effects of each medication as it is taught. Document client or primary care giver's comprehension of the instruction. Be sure to write everything out.
2. *Disease process*—Give instruction on signs and symptoms of the primary medical diagnoses. Document each item taught: anatomy and physiology, effect of disease on the normal body, treatment regimen. Document all items presented.
3. *Diet*—Give instruction on the therapeutic diet. Identify menu plan taught. Indicate written material provided to client and primary care giver. Document client's or primary care giver's comprehension of the instruction.
4. *Activity instruction*—Give instruction on all activities permitted the client, e.g., activities of daily living (ADLs), ROM, cane ambulation, walker-assisted ambulation, NWB (nonweight bearing) ambulation with assistance. Document client's or primary care giver's comprehension of the instruction.
5. Points to remember:
   a. Teaching must be in sequence.
   b. Teaching must be logical.
   c. Teaching must be continuous.
   d. Avoid the use of:

| | |
|---|---|
| again instructed | reinstructed |
| re-educated | encouraged |
| reviewed | urged |

Medicare cites examples of teaching and training activities that require skills or knowledge of a nurse or therapist. This is not an inclusive list. Also, any teaching or training activity must be evaluated to determine if it constitutes the skill of a nurse or therapist. Teaching and training activities considered reimbursable by Medicare are:

1. Give injection.
2. Irrigate catheter.
3. Care for colostomy, ileostomy, or gastrostomy (new).
4. Administer medical gases.
5. Prepare and follow a therapeutic diet.
6. Apply dressings to wounds involving prescription medications and aseptic technique.
7. Perform bladder training.
8. Perform bowel training, for incontinence only.
9. Perform self-care activities of daily living through use of special techniques and adaptive devices when client has suffered loss of function.
10. Align and position bed-bound client.
11. Perform transfer activities.
12. Ambulate by means of crutches, walker, cane, etc.
13. Engage in therapeutic exercises after a loss of function.
14. Care for bedridden client.
15. Care for intravenous site.

In home care, the nurse's note should identify the medical reason for each visit. This identification should be consistent with the nursing diagnosis. The nurse's note must be able to stand alone; that is, the reader, usually a reimbursement reviewer, must be able to determine that the care is under the direction of a physician, the client is homebound, and a skilled service is being provided.

## SUMMARY

Recording and reporting are methods of communicating information related to a client's health care management. In any setting the success of a plan of care depends on accurate and complete reporting and precise record documentation. Good reporting and recording create a high level of communication that helps health team members share a common view of the client's problems.

*From Engelbrecht L: Avoiding claims denials documentation service workbook, Jacksonville, Fla, 1987, Health Care Management Consulting, Inc.

Nurses are the primary care providers having the most contact with clients. The use of basic principles for accurate and comprehensive recording and reporting will ensure delivery of safe and effective nursing care.

## BIBLIOGRAPHY


Albrecht CA and Lieske AM: Automating patient care planning, Nurs Manage 16:21, 1985.

Atwood J, et al.: The POR: a system for communication, Nurs Clin North Am 9:229, 1974.

Auerbach M: Changes in home care delivery, Nurs Outlook 33(6):290, 1985.

Balinsky W and Starkman J: The impact of DRG's on the health care industry, Health Care Manage Rev, 12:61, 1987.

Bergerson SR: Charting with a jury in mind, Nursing Life 2:30, 1982.

Bernzweig EP: The nurse's liability for malpractice, ed. 3, New York, 1981, McGraw-Hill Book Co.

Blake P: Incident investigation: a complete guide, Nurs Manage 15:37, 1984.

Bulau JM: Clinical policies and procedures for home health care, Rockville, Md, 1986, Aspen Publishers, Inc.

Casedonte LB: Put something extra in your home care charting, RN 50(9):73, 1987.

Costello S and Summers BY: Documenting patient care: getting it all together, Nurs Manage 16:31, 1985.

Creighton H: Legal implications of home health care, Nurs Manage 18(2):14, 1987.

Crews C, et al.: Computerized central intake: streamlining community health-care admissions, Nurs Econ 4(1):31, 1986.

Curtiss FR: Recent developments in federal reinbursement for home health care, Am J Hosp Pharm 43:132, 1986.

Dobberstein K: Attaching fuzzy documentation, Am J Nurs 86:599, 1986.

Donaghue AM, Reiley PJ: Some do's and dont's for giving report: sometimes knowing what not to say is as important as knowing what to say, Nurs '81 11:171, 1981.

Duespohl T: Nursing diagnosis manual for the well and ill client, Philadelphia, 1986, WB Saunders Co.

Engelbrecht L: Avoiding claims denials documentation service workbook, Jacksonville, Fla, 1987, Health Care Management Consulting, Inc.

Gamberg D, et al.: Outcome charting, Nurs Manage 12:36, 1981.

Gawlinski A and Rasmussen S: Improving documentation through the use of change theory, Focus Crit Care 11:12, 1984.

Georgopoulos BS and Sana JM: Clinical nursing specialization and intershift report behavior, Am J Nurs 71:538, 1971.

Gropper EI: Does your charting reflect your worth? Geriatr Nurs 9:99, 1988.

Harkins B: Keep your eye on the patient's problems, RN 49(12):30, 1986.

Harris MD, et al.: Tracking the cost of home care, Am J Nurs 87(11):1500, 1987.

Hewison NS: Online documentation: keeping up and keeping track, Database 11:67, June, 1988.

Hinson S, et al.: An automated Kardex and care plan, Nurs Manage 15:35, 1984.

Hoke JL: Charting for dollars, Am J Nurs 85:658, 1985.

Iyer P, et al.: Nursing process and nursing diagnosis Philadelphia, 1986, W.B. Saunders Co.

Joint Commission on Accreditation of Healthcare Organizations: accreditation manual for hospitals, Chicago, 1988, JCAHO.

Keating SB and Kelman GB: Home health care; nursing concepts and practice, Philadelphia, 1988, JB Lippincott Co.

Kitto J and Dale B: Designing a brief discharge planning screen, Nurs Manage 16:28, 1985.

Medicare Home Health Agency Manual: HCFA Publication # 11, U.S. Department of Health and Human Services, Health Care Financing Administration.

Morrissey-Ross M: Documentation: If you haven't written it, you haven't done it, Nurs Clin North Am 23:363, June, 1988.

Napiewocki JK: Documentation: a nurse's best defense, Prof Nurs 1:321, 1985.

Omdahl D: Home care charting, do's and dont's, Am J Nurs 88: 203, 1988.

Report Ho 286, National Association for Home Care, Washington, DC, November 4, 1988.

Riegel B: A method of giving intershift report based on a conceptual model, Focus Crit Care 12:12, 1985.

Sanborn CW and Blount M: Standard plans for care and discharge, Am J Nurs 84:1394, 1984.

Siegrist LM, et al.: The PIE system: complete planning and documentation of nursing care, QRB 11:186, 1985.

Stearns L.: Nursing diagnosis: an assessment form, Nurse Manager 19:101, April, 1988.

Vandenbosch TM: How to use a pain flow sheet effectively. Nursing '88 18:50, August, 1988.

Vaughan-Wrobel BD and Henderson BS: The problem-oriented system in nursing, ed 3, St. Louis, 1986, The CV Mosby Co.

# 3
# COMMUNICATION

### OBJECTIVES

*Mastery of content in this chapter will enable the nurse to:*

- Define key terms.
- Identify guidelines to use in therapeutic communication.
- Explain the communication process.
- Identify the purpose of therapeutic communication, communication in the orientation phase, and communication with the anxious and angry client.
- Develop skills for therapeutic communication, communication in the orientation phase, and communication with the anxious and angry client.

### KEY TERMS

*Accurate empathy*
*Attending communication*
*Concreteness*
*Congruent*
*Empathy*
*Genuineness*
*Respect*
*Therapeutic silence*

### SKILLS

**3-1** Establishing Therapeutic Communication
**3-2** Establishing the Orientation Phase of the Nurse-Client Relationship
**3-3** Communicating with the Anxious Client
**3-4** Communicating with the Angry Client

Communication is a basic element of human interactions. The definition of communication relates to its purpose. Webster defines it as "the act or action of imparting or transmitting." Satir (1967) describes communication as nonverbal and verbal behavior in a social context. Since there are many dimensions of communication, an additional definition is the ongoing, dynamic series of events that involves transmission of information or feelings between two or more people.

Nurses must learn good communication skills to convey information and establish and influence the nurse-client relationship. Using specific techniques of communication takes time and commitment. Effective communication is not a skill that becomes rote and repetitious. Communication is always dynamic and an integral part of nurse-client interaction and the nursing process. When a nurse establishes a relationship with a client, communication can provide understanding, assist clients with self-understanding and exploration, and provide feedback in problem solving.

## PATTERNS OF COMMUNICATION

There are three common ways in which people interact with one another: social amenity, informational, and relating. The nurse uses all three patterns during interactions with clients.

1. *Social amenity pattern*—Involves use of social skills. A casual greeting such as "Good morning, Ms. Moore" is a social amenity. Communication takes place, a message is received, but such an exchange is seldom meaningful on a deeper level. Although a nurse's comments or questions to a client center around professional expectations, such as "How are you?" or "Are you having pain?", these statements are ritualistic and without meaning. If social amenity is the main pattern of communication with clients, interaction remains superficial.
2. *Informational pattern*—This pattern is used when a person requests information or gives instruction. Nurses commonly use informational patterns of communication for health teaching or orientation of a client to a health care setting. This pattern can be dehumanizing if it is the only one used. This is especially true if the nurse or client does not perceive the other person as a unique individual with specific needs and means of communicating.
3. *Relating Pattern*—Relating is characterized by meaningful dialogue between two people in which each experience openness, closeness, and understanding of the other. When people relate, both are affected and changed. Nurses who relate effectively establish mutual trust with clients and help clients in problem solv-

ing. Although focus is on the ill person's needs and problems, dialogue is meaningful to the extent that the nurse cares and is genuine. Openness allows clients to experience caring.

### THERAPEUTIC COMMUNICATION

Therapeutic communication helps a nurse form a working relationship with clients and fulfills the purpose of the nursing process. Therapeutic communication is not casual. Instead it is a planned, deliberate, professional act. Several techniques that help develop a therapeutic relationship with a client include attentive listening, conveying acceptance, asking related questions, clarifying, focusing, stating observations, maintaining silence, summarizing, and using assertiveness. Each of these techniques helps focus on the uniqueness of each nurse-client relationship.

Common communication barriers can result in nontherapeutic interpersonal interactions and delay a nurse's ability to build a client relationship. Communication barriers include giving an opinion, offering false reassurance, being defensive, showing approval or disapproval, stereotyping, and asking "why?"

Communication skills in this chapter are designed to help nurses establish effective therapeutic relationships with a variety of clients.

### GUIDELINES

1. Listen to what and how the client communicates, that is, content and verbal and nonverbal messages. Some clients express themselves clearly without difficulty. Often, however, indirect and nonverbal cues communicate a client's needs.
2. Nonverbal communication involves transmission of messages without the use of words. Personal appearance, intonation, facial expression, posture, gait, gestures, and touch are ways to convey nonverbal messages.
3. Know your own attitudes toward the client or situation. Being unaware of personal feelings can lead to negative consequences of communication. To control what and how one communicates, a person must be aware of personal feelings, intrapersonal communication, and the consequences of the interpersonal communication.
4. Control external factors that influence or hinder communication. If the nurse is talking with the client about the client's personal concerns, privacy is important. If teaching, the nurse may want to have a family member present with whom to reinforce the content of the instruction. Controlling noise level and interruptions may also be important.
5. Establish and understand the purpose of the interaction. This is an essential quality of effective communication. Without this quality, the communication is casual and superficial.
6. Guide the interaction dependent on the client's condition and response. Client needs remain the focus of the interaction. For example, a nurse establishes that the purpose of the interaction is client teaching; however, the client just heard of the death of a loved one and expresses a need to talk about the death. The nurse assists the client with grieving and thus remains flexible and creative in the interaction.

### PREREQUISITE KNOWLEDGE

1. Basic principles of behavior.
2. Principles of the therapeutic nurse-client relationship.
3. Basic language, words, and symbols of the client's culture.

## *SKILL 3-1 Establishing Therapeutic Communication*

The primary goal of effective therapeutic communication for the nurse is to promote wellness and growth in clients. Communication assists the client or family to conceptualize problems and to externalize a subjective experience, that is, to share it with another. The health team and other health professionals use communication to share and exchange information about the client and to make joint decisions.

Therapeutic communication is not casual. When learning to communicate a nurse should perceive each client interaction as a positive relationship that results in attainment of nursing care goals.

### Purposes

1. Give and receive information.
2. Understand and be understood.
3. Assist client in problem solving.
4. Facilitate and implement the nursing process and thus accomplish specific and overall objectives of nursing interventions.
5. Provide basis for the nurse-client relationship.

## Procedure 3-1

| Steps | Rationale |
|---|---|
| **Assessment** | |
| 1. Determine client's need to communicate, e.g., client who constantly uses call light; client who is crying; client who does not understand the illness; client who has just been admitted to the hospital. | Clients in need of support, comfort, knowledge, or encouragement can benefit from meaningful communication. |
| 2. Assess reason client requires health care. | Nature of illness can affect client's coping ability and effectiveness in communicating needs or concerns. |
| 3. Assess factors about self and client that normally influence communication: perceptions, values and beliefs, emotions, sociocultural background, knowledge, age level, verbal ability, roles and relationships, environmental setting, physical comfort, physical discomfort. | Communication is a dynamic process influenced by interpersonal and intrapersonal processes. By assessing factors that influence communication the nurse can more accurately assess message and experiences of client. |
| 4. Assess client's language and ability to speak. | Determines need for special communication techniques, e.g., picture boards; aids, such as an interpretor. |
| 5. Observe client patterns of communication and verbal or nonverbal behavior, e.g., gestures, tone of voice, eye contact. | Client's patterns of communication may determine the type and manner of communication used by the nurse. |
| 6. Assess most appropriate type or manner of communication to achieve goal of interaction: | Nurse's task is to guide, direct, and structure interaction. Identifying type and manner of communication assures more effective and therapeutic exchange. |
| a. Active friendliness: nurse initiates consistent interest in other person, does "little things" that are important, acknowledges client's accomplishments. | Increases other person's self-esteem and feeling of being worthwhile. |
| b. Passive friendliness: nurse is available and alert to client's needs but does not push, is always courteous, talks when client demonstrates interest or approaches nurse, avoids exploration or interrogation in areas client finds threatening, avoids whispering or laughing around client because client may believe it is directed at self. | Useful with individuals who are suspicious of nurse's or health team's motive. Nurse may want to use this in beginning of nurse-client relationship with individuals who tend to be distrustful of others, or who isolate themselves. |
| c. Matter-of-factness: nurse responds consistently in casual, calm manner; avoids showing undue concern about complaints; avoids agreeing with unrealistic expectations or complaints but listens to concerns and investigates matter; avoids long explanations or reasons, threats, or overfriendliness. | Aids in dealing with extremely anxious or angry clients. Useful in dealing with clients who have unrealistic expectations of others, themselves, or situation. Also useful in attempting to limit behavior. Avoids judgmental, punitive attitude. |
| d. Kind firmness: nurse uses a kind but firm attitude, instructs client in what has to be done and assists client if it is needed to get client to accomplish task, demonstrates kindness and friendliness but expects client to follow instructions. | Conveys that nurse knows exactly what has to be done and expects request to be carried out. Kind firmness can be helpful in getting cooperation, especially if client is poorly motivated. |
| 7. Assess resources available in selecting communication methods: | Relying totally on information from client can restrict quality of interaction. Additional resources provide insight into best methods to communicate. |
| a. Review information available through chart, care plan, past experience, nursing assessment. | Greater amount of quality information nurse has, greater the ability to understand and communicate with client. |
| b. Consult with physician and other health team members concerning client's condition, symptoms, problems, impression. | Collaboration with other health team members facilitates nurse's response to client based on integration of knowledge. |
| **Nursing Diagnosis** | |
| 1. Cluster data to reveal actual or potential nursing diagnoses: | |
| a. Impaired verbal communication: related to physical barriers. | Client unable to use or understand language and thus requires nurse to use techniques other than verbal. |
| b. Knowledge deficit: related to inexperience with illness. | Nurse will find appropriate way to relate to client to impart information successfully. |
| c. Fear: related to impending surgery. | Effective communication builds sense of trust with nurse so that client can express fear openly. |
| d. Ineffective individual coping: related to unexpected hospitalization. | Client's adaptive behavior and problem-solving abilities are impaired. |

| Steps | Rationale |
|---|---|
| **Planning** | |
| 1. Prepare for communication: | Preparation is part of planned process that facilitates communication and interaction. |
| a. Formulate individualized goals for communicating with client: establish, maintain, terminate nurse-client relationship; teach client; assist in providing physical, psychologic, social, and spiritual care; acknowledge and decrease feelings of anxiety, fear, anger, confusion, helplessness. | Without understanding purpose of interaction there is greater risk of casual nongoal-oriented communication that may fail to assist client in actualizing a greater potential toward physical, psychologic, social, spiritual health. |
| b. Consider time allocation needed to achieve purpose of interaction. | Amount of time required for providing technical skills, giving information, interviewing, problem solving may vary. A greater amount of time may be required initially to meet special needs of client, but this can often save time for nurse later in relationship. Time spent with client depends on needs of client. |
| c. Before interacting with client, formulate initial questions and responses, e.g.: | Assists and directs interaction. |
| ▪ Broad opening (e.g., "Where would you like to begin?"; "Is there something you'd like to talk about?"). | Encourages client to take lead in introducing topic. |
| ▪ Giving information that is needed (e.g., "My name is . . ."; "My purpose in being here is . . ."; "I'm taking you to the . . ."). | Makes facts available to put client at ease. |
| ▪ General leads (e.g., "Go on."; "Tell me more about it."). | Encourages individual to continue and conveys that nurse is interested in hearing more. |
| d. Mentally prepare to keep mind clear of other concerns or distractions during interaction. | Promotes goal achievement of interaction and avoids risk of filtering or misunderstanding message. Also communicates to client that you are listening. |
| 2. Prepare client and environment physically: | |
| a. Determine type and availability of quiet environment conducive to interaction. | Certain environments are more conducive to therapeutic interactions than others. |
| b. Choose private environment for certain tasks and interactions, e.g., discussion of planned therapy, fear of death, concerns over family members. | Privacy is less threatening to client and promotes freer expression of feelings. |
| c. Reduce distractions or interruptions in environment that hinder communication. | Ongoing activity, loud noises, and interruptions may hinder message. |
| d. Take care of client's physical discomfort or needs before beginning discussion, e.g., positioning, liquids or food, pain relief, assistance to bathroom. | Taking care of basic needs will decrease client distractions. |
| **Implementation** | |
| 1. Create initial climate of warmth and acceptance: a. Decrease own anxiety by preparing for interaction, pausing and collecting thoughts before entering room. | Facilitates more open exchange without fear and anxiety; encourages client to express feelings without fear of reprisal or scorn (Egan, 1975). |
| 2. Provide an introduction: | |
| a. Address client by name. | Conveys respect. |
| b. Introduce self and who you are. | Assists client to understand nurse. |
| 3. Use physical attending. | |
| a. Sit in comfortable chair near client, at same eye level, facing each other, and maintaining good eye contact. | Physical attending provides nonverbal message that nurse is interested in what client has to say. |
| b. Maintain "open" position, avoid crossing legs and arms, lean toward client, remain relatively relaxed, avoid distracting movements. | Client is center of attention, attending conveys nurse's interest. |
| 4. Use psychologic attending: a. Listen or observe client's nonverbal behavior, which often carries emotional dimension of messages. Listen to client's verbal behavior, take time to listen, teach yourself to concentrate. Don't interrupt; listen between lines. | Psychologic attending makes nurse more alert to client's true message. It is also congruent with nurse's nonverbal message conveyed in physical attending. |
| 5. Explain purpose of interaction when information is to be shared. Explain how information may be used in care, what client may do to help, plan of interaction. | Information and explanation can decrease anxiety about unknown. |

| Steps | Rationale |
|---|---|
| 6. Encourage client to interrupt at any time to ask questions or clarify something. | Gives client more control and keeps channels of communication open. |
| 7. Use communication techniques to respond to client: | Techniques serve as stepping stones to better understanding that nurtures a trusting relationship. |
| a. Restate or paraphrase main idea, e.g.: Client: Nobody in this place gives a damn about anybody. Nurse: It sounds like you are angry and feel no one here cares about you. | Sends feedback that lets client know if message was understood. Prompts further communication. Ineffective if seeking new information unrelated to topic. |
| b. Reflect by stating last few words of client or feeling expressed, e.g.: Client: I had to go to radiology for my first treatment and I was pretty scared. Nurse: You were scared? | Makes client more aware of feelings and encourages elaboration. |
| Avoid parroting or using reflection repeatedly as primary technique. | Parroting can be annoying. |
| c. When discussion about a client's health becomes vague, focus or refocus on client's statement or central topics or patterns (e.g., "You only mentioned your past hospitalization briefly. Could you tell me more about it?"; "Tell me about the pain in your arm."). | Concentrates on problem areas and avoids wandering or nondirective communication; helps obtain more information in areas that assist the nurse in assessment and care of the client. |
| d. Clarify client's message (e.g., "I'm not sure I understand completely. Could you repeat it?"; "I'm not following you. Can you say it another way?"). | Prevents misunderstanding; sign of interest and attempt to create understanding. |
| Clarify words that have individual meaning, such as "small," "large," "some", "I feel funny". | Information critical to client's care plan can be incomplete unless confusing data are clarified. |
| e. State observations of client's words or nonverbal messages. e.g.: Client: No one comes to see me in the hospital. I live so far away from friends and family. Nurse: It appears that you are feeling lonely. (Avoid observations that may embarrass or anger client.) | Helps client express feelings, which is sometimes difficult to do. |
| f. Use silence to listen to client or to give client time to respond. Silence may be ineffective if nurse and client become uncomfortable or anxious, or if nurse lacks other skills to guide interaction. | Allows client freedom to express wants, think about what was said, organize thoughts, consider alternate actions. Also allows nurse to observe client. |
| To break client's silence: Nurse: Is there anything else you would care to say about . . . ? Can you try to tell me more . . . ? I'm not sure what your silence means. | Shows interest in client's feelings. |
| 8. Use questions carefully: a. Avoid deep probing or forcing information. b. Word questions simply and concisely. c. Begin interview with broad, open question and then, if necessary, close questions. d. Avoid bombarding client with questions. e. Ask one question at a time and allow sufficient time to answer. f. Use terms client understands. | Questions can facilitate or hinder communication. Questioning can put client on defensive. |
| g. Avoid how and why questions. Who, when, where, and what are more desirable, especially when seeking clarification and specific information. | Why and how questions require analytical ability and information the client often does not have. Why questions may be interpreted as a challenge. |
| h. Open-ended questions encourage description and elaboration (e.g., "Tell me about your discomfort or pain"; "What brings you here today?"; "Tell me about ways that have helped you cope with your illness."). | Allows individualistic responses from client's perspective. Ineffective if leads to irrelevant topics. May lead to difficulty in returning to a particular topic. |
| i. Closed or direct questions elicit specific response that usually can be answered with one word (e.g., "Do you take aspirin?"; "Is the pain in your chest?"; "Is your family here?"; "When can you set up an appointment?"). | Provides for limited information and usually focuses on what nurse wants vs what client needs. |

| Steps | Rationale |
|---|---|
| 9. Avoid communication breakdown because of failing to listen; failing to focus on client's problem; giving advice; blaming client; changing topic inappropriately; being defensive ("This hospital has a fine reputation."); giving false reassurance ("Everything will be all right."); disapproving, ("That's bad."; disagreeing "That's wrong."); belittling; interpreting ("What you really mean is . . ."); requesting an explanation ("Why do you think that?"); jumping to conclusions; ignoring or denying client's presence, thoughts, feelings; sending verbal and nonverbal messages that are contradictory. | Communication breakdown occurs when message is not received, is distorted, or not understood by the receiver. Communication and interaction may be hindered by nontherapeutic responses. |
| 10. Summarize with client what was discussed during interaction, e.g.: Nurse: Let me see if I have everything we talked about. We reviewed your treatment plan and what you will need to do. You expressed concern about your length of stay at the hospital and not being able to return to work immediately. Is there anything else? | Summary signals close of interaction, allows nurse and client to depart with same idea, and provides sense of closure at completion of discussion. |

## Evaluation

| Steps | Rationale |
|---|---|
| 1. Observe client's behavioral nonverbal responses toward your communication. | Nonverbal feedback reveals clients' interest and willingness to communicate, as well as emotions. |
| 2. Ask client for feedback regarding message communicated. | Determines if client clearly received message (e.g., teaching instructions). |
| 3. Evaluate content of client's messages in terms of receptivity toward nurse and ability to openly express feelings such as anger, fear, or anxiety. | Spontaneity and ability to clearly verbalize feelings and ideas reflects effective communication pattern. |

### *Expected outcomes*

| Steps | Rationale |
|---|---|
| 1. Client will express fewer verbal and nonverbal messages conveying anxiety, fear, anger, distrust, confusion, or helplessness. | Developing effective communication initiates foundation for sense of trust. |
| 2. Nurse able to understand client's fears, concerns, ideas, and reception of information. | Effective communication enables nurse to collect valuable information about client. |
| 3. Client's nonverbal communication conveys acceptance of nurse. | Nonverbal communication conveying acceptance of nurse may indicate client's readiness to work with nurse regarding health care. |
| 4. Client repeats message or explains information shared in teaching interaction. | Demonstrates message received. |

### *Unexpected outcomes*

| Steps | Rationale |
|---|---|
| 1. Client continues to verbally and nonverbally express feelings of anxiety, fear, anger, confusion, distrust, and helplessness. | Communication between nurse and client has not served to allay these emotions. Client may be responding to internal and external factors and cues. |
| 2. Feedback between nurse and client reveals lack of understanding. | Barriers in communication obviously exist. |
| 3. Nurse is unable to acquire information about client's ideas, fears, and concerns. | Techniques used by nurse fail to promote client's willingness to communicate openly. |

## Recording and Reporting

| Steps | Rationale |
|---|---|
| 1. Record in nurses' notes communication pertinent to client's health, responses to illness or therapies, and responses that demonstrate understanding or lack of understanding. (Include verbal and nonverbal cues.) | Provides information valuable for assessment of client's needs and problems. |

## Follow-up Activities

| Steps | Rationale |
|---|---|
| 1. If there is lack of understanding between client and nurse: | |
| a. Review client and nurse's communication. | Allows nurse to redirect communication efforts. |
| b. Identify factors that hindered communication. | |

### Special Considerations

- For client experiencing sensory impairment or disability, utilization of other senses in communication is important. Interpretors and mechanical aides should be used.
- Communication should be clear and concise with client experiencing altered levels of consciousness; repeat information, orient to surroundings, and offer reassurance.
- Clients experiencing emotionally charged situations may not comprehend message. Focus on understanding the client, provide feedback and assistance in problem-solving, and provide an atmosphere of warmth and acceptance to greatly decrease emotionally charged reactions.
- Confidentiality and respect for client's privacy is always an important consideration in the nurse's communication with others.
- Use less intense attending with client interested in social relationship, manipulative client who uses nurse's interest to obtain personal wants without consideration of others, and suspicious or distrustful client.
- Amount and quality of time for communication depends on needs of the client. Some examples are:
  a. To assist client with problem-solving may require long periods of time that nurse may have available while assisting with bath or after finishing certain tasks, or it may require several interactions over week's period.
  b. Withdrawn, depressed client may require short frequent visits.
  c. As client becomes more independent, less time may be required; or more frequently, focus for the communication may change, i.e., teaching or discharge planning.
  d. Critically ill client often requires greater amount of time for task accomplishment and less time for interpersonal communication.
  e. Client who is acutely ill psychologically requires greater amount of time to meet psychologic and physical needs.
- Nurse must always be flexible and willing to change techniques based on client needs.

### Teaching Considerations

- Present information often and show relationships of portions of information presented to the client.

### Home Care Considerations

- Identify a primary care giver for the client. This individual may be a family member, a friend, or a neighbor.
- Assess level of understanding of the client and primary care giver regarding client's condition.
- Avoid making changes in client's life-style and incorporate client's daily habits into the communication event.
- Speak face-to-face with elderly client and check frequently to determine that the client hears and understands the words.
- Provide only small amount of specific information at a time to the elderly client.
- Plan for identified communication difficulties associated with culture, language, and age. Be alert to literacy status.

## *SKILL 3-2 Establishing the Orientation Phase of the Nurse-Client Relationship*

A nurse can effectively communicate without necessarily seeking actively to establish the orientation phase of the nurse-client relationship. However, once it is apparent that a good working relationship is necessary for structured ongoing interactions with clients, the orientation phase should be established. Skills used in effective communication are similar to those used in the orientation phase. The nurse is purposefully focusing efforts at communication in order to direct the client toward the working phase of a nurse-client relationship.

### Purposes

1. Establish basis for the nurse-client relationship.
2. Promote client understanding of health care goals.
3. Promote a sense of trust between nurse and client.

## *Procedure 3-2*

| Steps | Rationale |
|---|---|
| **Assessment** | |
| 1. Nurse determines that nurse-client relationship is in orientation phase. First interactions with client take place in this phase; interactions may be superficial; nurse may do most of the initiating; communication involves gathering information and observing; testing is done; beginning awareness by nurse of client's problem related to health status begins; understanding and trust begin to develop. | It is difficult to establish working relationship without initial introductions, understanding, testing, and trust. Length and quality of initial phase may take longer with certain clients and nurse cannot push this phase too quickly with them. |

| Steps | Rationale |
|---|---|
| 2. Assess factors that influence communication in orientation phase (Skill 3-1), e.g., past experiences with nurses or health care system, first impressions of nurse, client's expectations of nurse, nurse's impression of client, respect for differences and commonness between them. | Allows nurse to assess relationship and communication process more accurately. Nurse who has negative feelings or internal conflicts toward special clients can hinder orientation phase. |
| 3. Assess most appropriate manner of communicating in orientation phase: | |
| a. Active friendliness (contraindicated with distrustful and angry client). | Demonstrates interest. |
| b. Passive friendliness (contraindicated with depressed clients and warm and caring clients). | Helps with clients reluctant to establish nurse-client relationship. |
| c. Kind firmness (not needed with motivated clients, clients demonstrating health-seeking behavior, clients participating in health care.) | Can assist in establishing confidence in nurse and health team or it can cause upset or anger if client does not wish to cooperate. However, may be necessary in orientation phase if client's cooperation and compliance is necessary for health care. |
| 4. Note patterns of communication (verbal and nonverbal) and any subjective or objective behavioral signs indicating communication problems. | Helps reveal client's existing emotions, openness, and ability to communicate effectively. |

## Nursing Diagnosis

| Steps | Rationale |
|---|---|
| 1. Cluster data to reveal actual or potential nursing diagnoses:<br>a. Impaired verbal communication: related to feelings of mistrust.<br>b. Social isolation: related to feelings of inadequacy.<br>c. Anxiety: related to past and present hospitalization.<br>d. Fear: related to impending surgery or therapy.<br>e. Impaired social interaction: related to communication barriers. | During orientation phase nurse establishes therapeutic relationship that allows client to discuss feelings openly, seek information, and learn about health care problem. Nursing diagnoses will be confirmed or disproved as nurse gathers more information about client. |

## Planning

| Steps | Rationale |
|---|---|
| 1. Prepare for communication during orientation phase. | Initial encounter is very important in "setting stage" for development of relationship. |
| a. Establish individualized goals for purpose of initial interactions with client: | |
| ▪ Establish trust and understanding between nurse and client. | Provides mutual understanding and fosters further communication. |
| ▪ Gather and provide information related to client's condition and needs. This is facilitated by explaining purpose of information (e.g., "I will be asking you some questions to help us understand problems or difficulties you may be having so we can better treat or care for you."). | Assists in identifying actual or potential problems, present health status, and experience. |
| ▪ Perform nursing task related to client's care (giving bath, checking IV, preparing for tests or teaching); e.g., nurse who doesn't say anything or doesn't look at patient and checks IV vs nurse who calls patient by name, explains nursing task, looks at patient, and checks IV. (Each transaction takes same amount of time but communication exchange is significantly different.) | The manner in which a nursing task is performed may influence the relationship. |
| b. Orientation phase may take several minutes and several interactions. Allow ample time for initial interaction and assessment.<br>Warmth and acceptance by nurse often facilitates more rapid achievement of this phase. | Foundation of working relationship. What occurs during first interaction may determine length of time for orientation phase. Initial encounters often set climate for relationship. |
| c. Formulate initial questions and responses. Use broad openings (e.g., "What brings you here?"; "What seems to be the problem?"; "Tell me more about . . . ."). Allow client to ask questions. Provide information. | Assist in directing interaction (Skill 3-1). |
| d. Prepare mentally to keep mind clear of other concerns or distractions during interaction. Attempt to put yourself at ease before interaction. | Promotes goal achievement of interaction and avoids risk of misunderstanding message (Skill 3-1). |

| Steps | Rationale |
|---|---|
| 2. Physically prepare client and environment. | |
| a. Provide relaxed, private environment. Take client to warm, well-ventilated location; e.g., client's room, special interview room, treatment room. | Privacy and avoidance of distractions and interruptions when initially attempting to understand client can help prevent misunderstanding or mixed messages. |
| b. Reduce distractions and interruptions by placing "do not disturb" sign on door, planning interactions before or after scheduled therapies. | |
| c. Attempt to put client at ease by decreasing physical discomforts. | Facilitates more open and free exchange. |

## Implementation

| Steps | Rationale |
|---|---|
| 1. Create initial climate of warmth and acceptance: | Facilitates more open exchange. |
| a. Decrease own anxiety by preparing for interaction, e.g., pausing and collecting thoughts before entering room, relaxing by taking several deep breaths. | Calm, relaxed nurse helps decrease client's anxiety. |
| 2. Assist client to manage anxiety, e.g., provide information regarding what client can expect, encourage client to participate in usual activities as much as possible, assist in expressing concerns and fears. | In orientation phase anxiety may be related to fear of unknown or changes and interruptions in usual activities or life-style. |
| 3. Use physical attending. | Especially important in initial interview or assessment. |
| 4. Use psychologic attending (Skill 3-1). | Client may be testing whether nurse is competent and trustworthy. |
| 5. Introduce self and provide information: | Assists in orientation. |
| a. Information about facilities and environment, e.g., call light, bed adjustments, cabinet space, special equipment. | Increases client's capability of managing the environment. |
| b. Informational pamphlets, e.g., orientation to area of care, services available, treatment and testing information. | Reinforces teaching and allows client to review material. |
| c. Information about beginning plan of care, e.g., procedures that need to be completed, activities, gathering specimens. | Increases client's participation in care because of better understanding. |
| d. Provide general schedule for day. | Helps client and nurse plan their day or alter schedule. |
| 6. Use communication techniques and tools that facilitate orientation phase: | Assists in establishing rapport with client that promotes free exchange of information. |
| a. Accurate empathy (Egan, 1975): listen to message, respond frequently but briefly, respond to both feelings and content, attend carefully to signs that confirm or deny accuracy of your response. | Communicates understanding of client's feelings and experiences. Client senses nurse's interest in communication exchanges. |
| b. Respect (Egan, 1975): be "for" client, be willing and available to work with client, recognize client's uniqueness, use psychologic and physical attending, suspend critical judgments, express warmth, give recognition by greeting client or indicate awareness of change or efforts being made by client. | Communicates positive regard for client. |
| c. Genuineness (Egan, 1975): be nondefensive; be consistent in what you think, feel, and say; be spontaneous but not impulsive; avoid facade. | Allows nurse and client to be basically themselves. |
| d. Concreteness (Egan, 1975): do not let client ramble, ask for more specific information, avoid vagueness ("I noticed that you have been staying in your bed today"), begin to explore ("Tell me more about . . . ."), clarification ("I'm not sure I follow. . . ."), paraphrase or restate client's message. | By speaking about specific experiences, specific behaviors, specific feelings, the client is likely to speak of specific problems with specific solutions. |
| 7. Use questions carefully: | |
| a. Use open-ended and nonthreatening questions as much as possible. | Client is usually more willing to express self. |
| b. Avoid numerous direct questions; avoid using why and how as much as possible. | Numerous direct questions and why and how questions can be intimidating and annoying to client. |
| 8. Avoid communication breakdown in orientation phase, caused by: | Occurs when message is not received, is distorted, or is not understood. |
| a. Rushing into working phase before establishment of initial trust and rapport. | Client may not be ready and resists working with nurse. |
| b. Uncomfortable silence. | Increases client's anxiety. |
| c. Nurse's anxiety increasing with client's anxiety. | May hinder development of trust and confidence in nurse. |
| d. Vagueness in answering client's questions. | Client may begin to lack confidence in nurse's ability. |
| e. Not listening or giving impression of being "too busy." | Blocks communication and client may feel rejected or belittled. |

| Steps | Rationale |
|---|---|
| **Evaluation** | |
| 1. Note client's willingness to discuss information, ask questions, and reveal own feelings. | Reflects client's trust of nurse. |
| 2. Observe nonverbal behaviors. | Nonverbal behaviors may complement or contradict client's verbal communication. |
| 3. Ask client to summarize purpose of interaction. | Ensures client's and nurse's mutual understanding. |
| ***Expected outcomes*** | |
| 1. Client confides in nurse by discussing fears, anxieties, or concerns. | Essential behaviors for nurse to begin working phase of relationship. |
| 2. Verbal and nonverbal cues reflect acceptance of nurse and what is communicated. | |
| ***Unexpected outcomes*** | |
| 1. Client refuses or hesitates to share information, discuss emotions, or respond to nurse's questions. | Reflects mistrust in nurse or difficulty of client to express self. |
| 2. Nonverbal cues, e.g., poor eye contact, facial expressions, and gestures indicate disinterest in conversations. | Client is unwilling to communicate openly. |
| **Recording and Reporting** | |
| 1. Record in nurses' notes communication pertinent to client's health, responses to illness or therapies, and acceptance of health care measures. | Provides data for assessment of client's needs and problems. |
| 2. Record observation of behaviors or nonverbal cues that reflect client's refusal or acceptance of health care measures and response to therapies. | Documents client's response to nursing care. |
| **Follow-up Activities** | |
| 1. If mistrust toward nurse continues: | |
| a. Provide longer period of time for orientation phase. | Clients differ as to when they trust nurse because of previous experiences, fears, and misunderstandings. |
| b. Identify and reinforce areas in which client demonstrates trust toward nurse. | May assist in building trust in other areas. |
| c. Maintain neutral nonthreatening environment, but be available when needed. | Overfriendliness may only increase mistrust. |
| d. Continue to meet client's nursing care needs. | |
| e. Keep promises, such as returning to room at time promised, e.g., "I'll be right back with your pain shot," and be sure to come right back. | |
| f. Clarify factors hindering trust: mistakes in care made by you or other health care providers, lack of information, lack of respect and genuineness by nurse, important others influencing trust, pattern of mistrust by client, anger toward illness directed at nurse, lack of demonstration of care by nurse. | May be able to establish trust only after altering identified factors. |

## Special Considerations

- Orientation phase for some clients may be longer and require special communication skills. Orientation phase may be more difficult with client who is distrustful, angry, shy, or timid; adolescent who may perceive nurse as authority figure; toddler experiencing difficulty with separation and strangers; loner and very private person; person lacking experience in warmth and caring.
- Clients who depend on the nurse, especially when acutely ill, may facilitate orientation phase more quickly. Client rejection of dependency needs may inhibit or prolong orientation phase.
- If client appears preoccupied or adjusting to a new situation, nurse may need to repeat information or limit amount of information.
- Respect for client is facilitated by meeting client's dependency needs, i.e., assistance with physical care and nurturance, respect for independence, and autonomy.

# SKILL 3-3 Communicating with the Anxious Client

Clients in the health care setting may experience anxiety for a variety of reasons. A newly diagnosed illness, separation from loved ones, threat associated with diagnostic tests or surgical procedures, and expectations of life changes are just a few factors that can cause client anxiety. How successfully a client copes with anxiety depends in part on previous experiences, the presence of other stressors, the significance of the event causing anxiety, and the availability of supportive resources. The nurse can be a support to the client. However, unless the nurse knows how to communicate effectively, the client's anxiety may increase. Communication methods reviewed in this skill assist the nurse in helping an anxious client clarify factors causing anxiety and cope more effectively with anxiety-producing situations.

## Purposes

1. Assess client who may be anxious.
2. Reduce level of anxiety experienced by a client.
3. Assist client in understanding nature of one's anxiety.
4. Provide client with coping mechanisms for dealing with anxiety.

## Procedure 3-3

| Steps | Rationale |
|---|---|
| **Assessment** | |
| 1. Assess for signs indicating client is anxious:<br>a. Physical signs, e.g., dry mouth; urinary frequency; diarrhea; oily skin; sweaty palms; increased respiration, heart rate, and blood pressure; headache; nausea or upset stomach.<br>b. Behavioral signs, e.g., tense tone of voice, difficulty concentrating, insomnia, loss of appetite, increased appetite, pacing, inability to sit still, wringing of hands, expanding one aspect of total situation out of proportion, irritability, stuttering. | Anxiety can interfere with usual manner of communication and interaction and thus client's care and treatment. Extreme anxiety can interfere with comprehension, attention, problem-solving. Anxiety can create a sympathetic response resulting in various signs and symptoms that are easily detected. |
| c. Verbal expressions (e.g., "I'm nervous"; "I'm tense"; "I'm scared"; "I can't concentrate"; "I feel like I'm going to suffocate being kept in this room"; "I could feel my heart pounding but they couldn't find anything wrong with me."). | Some clients are able to express anxiety openly or acknowledge its symptoms.<br>Ability to state feelings often depends on previous experiences and acceptance of feelings by others and self. |
| 2. Do not ignore client's anxiety. | Anxiety often continues and increases in intensity if not altered. |
| 3. Assess for possible factors causing client anxiety, e.g., change, loss, or crisis such as death, divorce, loss of job, hospitalization; physical fatigue or weakness; sociocultural factors such as job pressure, economic worries, sexual relationship with partner; the environment (noise, people, new surroundings). | Client's feeling of anxiety may have a source that is nonspecific or unknown to the person. However, understanding source of anxiety can assist nurse in client support and communication. |
| 4. Assess factors influencing communication with the client, e.g., environment, timing, presence of others, values, experiences. | Understanding factors that influence communication helps a nurse identify effective communication strategies. |
| 5. Assess most appropriate manner of communicating with anxious client: | |
| a. Active friendliness: through active listening, staying with client, or making frequent visits. (Contraindicated if anxiety is related to nurse-client relationship, if client is distrustful or shy, or client is overwhelmed by anxious feeling. Try instead matter-of-fact or kind firmness.) | Can increase client's self-esteem and provide feeling of worth. Conveys sense of caring that can decrease anxiety. |
| b. Matter-of-fact manner: be calm; make replies clear, simple, and related to situation; set limits when client feels loss of control. (Contraindicated if client perceives matter-of-factness as distant, cold, and noncaring and is seeking caring atmosphere. Try instead active friendliness.) | Calms client, assists in focusing on immediate situation, and eliminates sense of being overwhelmed. |
| c. Kind firmness: get cooperation of client by using kind but firm attitude and directing client to accomplish task at hand. (Contraindicated if client becomes angry or anxiety is increased significantly. Try instead matter-of-fact or active friendliness.) | Helps when client is having difficulty making decisions or in controlling anxiety. |

| Steps | Rationale |
|---|---|
| 6. Assess resources available to reveal nature of client's anxiety, e.g., input from spouse or family, data in medical record or nursing care plan, physician, and other health team members. | Information will assist nurse in understanding client's problems and selecting best communication methods. |

## Nursing Diagnosis

| Steps | Rationale |
|---|---|
| 1. Cluster data to reveal actual or potential nursing diagnoses: | |
| a. Anxiety: related to alterations in life-style. | Feeling of uneasiness may be unknown or related to recent change such as hospitalization. |
| b. Impaired verbal communication: related to anxiety. | Anxiety inhibits client's ability to communicate clearly. |
| c. Impaired social interaction: related to anxiety. | Individual participates in insufficient, excessive, or ineffective quality of social exchange with others. |

## Planning

| Steps | Rationale |
|---|---|
| 1. Prepare for communication with anxious client: | |
| a. Develop individualized goals. | Anticipating response to client will help convey a rapport that decreases client's anxiety. |
| ▪ Client experiences decreased anxiety. | Effective communication allows client to gain trust in nurse, achieve sense of calm, and begin to analyze source of anxiety. |
| ▪ Identify and alter factors that escalate anxiety. | If uninterrupted, anxiety tends to escalate. |
| ▪ Client gains tolerance for anxiety. | Anxiety can be useful and provide person chance to grow. Individual who learns to tolerate anxiety has energy available for adaptation and pleasure. |
| ▪ Client copes effectively with anxiety. | Effective coping can lead to health promoting behavior. Comprehension and ability to communicate are enhanced. |
| b. Consider time allocation required to achieve purpose of interaction with anxious client. Time required to decrease anxiety depends on: ability to eliminate or alter factors causing anxiety and individual's self-awareness and resources for coping. | Severe anxiety requires more intense period of time for intervention. |
| c. Consider resources to assist in communication with anxious client, i.e., family, mental health professionals, pastoral care. | Client may relate more effectively with significant other or professional counselor, e.g., families can provide support but often may be dealing with their own anxieties. The nurse's guidance with others can be helpful. |
| d. Before interacting with client, formulate initial questions and responses that encourage description of client's experience by: | Beginning with less threatening communication can prevent further escalation of anxiety. |
| ▪ Making observation ("You seem upset by something"). | Encourages expression and sharing of feelings and behavior. |
| ▪ Encouraging description of perception ("What happened?"). | Can help client release anxiety and feelings. |
| ▪ Broad opening ("Where would you like to begin?"). | Encourages client to take lead. |
| ▪ Who, when, where, and what questions that encourage description ("Where were you?"; "Who was there?"; "What did he say?"; "What did you tell him?"). | Encourages clarification and provides information. |
| ▪ Giving information. | Shows nurse's willingness to support client. |
| e. Recognize and control your own anxiety. (Breathe slowly and deeply, spend few minutes alone to collect yourself.) | Anxiety of nurse can increase client's anxiety. |
| 2. Prepare client and environment physically: | |
| a. Provide quiet, calm environment away from groups of people and activity. | Decreased stimuli can have a calming effect. |
| b. Allow ample personal space. Normal personal distance for a conversation is 1½ to 4 ft (Fig. 3-1). If there is increased anxiety with closeness, then provide greater personal space. If there is decreased anxiety with closeness, there may be need for reassurance and less personal space. | There is direct correlation between amount of personal space and level of anxiety. Nature of nurse-client relationship may determine personal space required. |
| c. First acknowledge and take care of anxious client's physical and emotional discomfort but avoid dwelling on physical complaints. | Anxiety can be a very unpleasant emotional experience and sometimes is expressed in physical discomfort or complaints. Relieving physical discomfort is important, but if treated exclusively the underlying cause of anxiety may not be discovered and anxiety continues. |

| Step | Rationale |
|---|---|

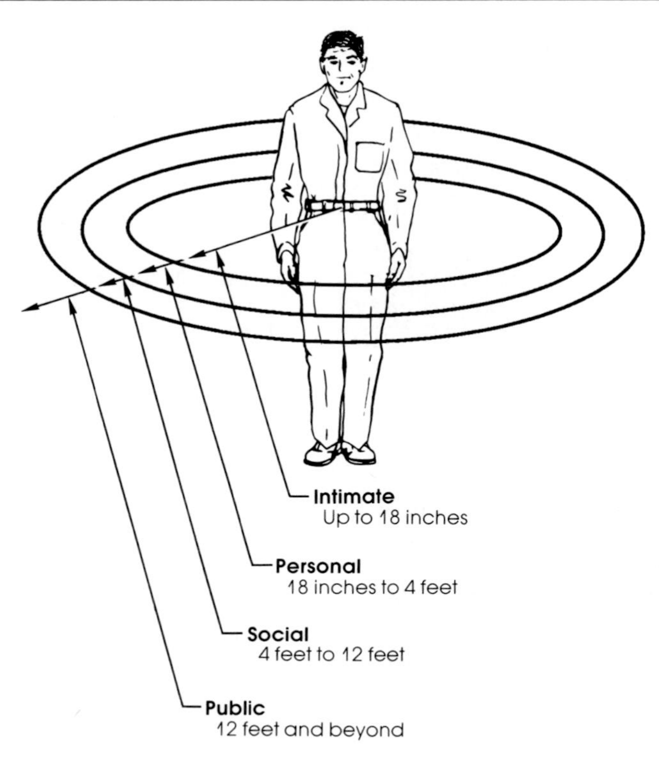


***Fig. 3-1*** Proxemics focuses on four zones of space in human interaction.

(From Beck CK, Rawlins RP, Williams S: Mental health-psychiatric nursing: a holistic life-cycle approach, ed 2, St. Louis, 1988, The CV Mosby Co.)

## Implementation

| Step | Rationale |
|---|---|
| 1. Create climate of warmth and acceptance: | Climate can have a calming effect on the client. |
| a. Maintain composure during interaction. | Nurse's self-control calms client. |
| b. Stay with client or check frequently if client is experiencing extreme anxiety. | Provides reassurance to anxious client. |
| c. Demonstrate genuineness and respect. | Allows client to be self and creates attitude that communicates positive regard between nurse and client. |
| 2. Provide brief, simple introduction: introduce yourself; explain purpose of interaction. Sometimes getting client's attention is all that can be done in introduction. | Anxiety may limit amount of information client can understand. |
| 3. Use physical attending: sit in comfortable chair, maintain eye contact, assume relaxed but attentive posture. | Nonverbal message to client conveys nurse's interest. |
| 4. Use psychologic attending: listen and do not interrupt client. | Enables nurse to be more alert to client's message. |
| 5. Use communication techniques and tools to respond to anxious client: | |
| a. Anticipate needs, e.g., comfort, food or water, hygiene care. | Client may ignore basic needs; meeting needs makes client more comfortable. |
| b. Make replies simple, clear, and related to situation. | Client's perception and attention may be limited. |
| c. Avoid introducing anything new. | Client may become overwhelmed by new situation or experience. |
| d. Limit amount of decision making for client. | Prevents further escalation of anxiety. |
| e. Provide for physical activity, such as walking. | Requires little concentration and can help decrease anxiety. |
| f. Use accurate empathy: state what you understand message to be (e.g., "I understand you to say . . . ."; "I hear you saying . . . ."; "I sense that . . . ."). Move the conversation forward. | Communicating understanding often deescalates anxiety. Empathy involves perceiving the client's feelings and promotes problem-solving. |
| 6. Use questions and responses based on an orderly hierarchy: description of experience, thoughts about experience, feelings experience generates, e.g.,<br>Nurse: I sense that you are upset about something.<br>Client: The doctor was just here. (Describes experience).<br>Nurse: Tell me more about what happened. (Explores experience further). | Aids client in describing event and clarifying thoughts and feelings |

| Steps | Rationale |
|---|---|
| Client: He said I won't be going home tomorrow and that I will have to stay until I am able to eat more.<br>Nurse: What do you think about that? (Requests thoughts about experience).<br>Client: Well, I know he is right. I haven't been eating, but I was counting on going home.<br>Nurse: What are your feelings? (Requests feelings about experience).<br>Client: I'm disappointed and angry, but I need to stay here for now. | |
| 7. Avoid communication breakdown with anxious client: belittling thoughts and feelings associated with anxiety (e.g., "There is no reason why you should feel this way"), ignoring discomfort connected with the anxiety, ignoring client, getting angry with client (e.g., "You have to stop this right now!"), inability to acknowledge and control own anxiety. Nonverbal cues must not communicate conflicting messages. | Communication breakdown can increase anxiety and feelings of isolation. |
| 8. Help client acquire alternate coping mechanisms: | |
| a. Establish trust with client by acting confidently, keeping information confidential, and acting dependably. | Trust provides foundation for effective communication so client can explore causes of anxiety and steps to alleviate problem. |
| b. Assist client in recognizing anxiety by focusing discussion when client's behavior changes or symptoms appear. Convey acceptance. | Client's perception of anxiety is necessary for change to occur. |
| c. Support coping behaviors:<br>▪ Reduce stressful factors in home or work environment.<br>▪ Encourage regular exercise.<br>▪ Maintain diet and regular periods of rest.<br>▪ Encourage relaxation exercises. | Gives client strategies for reducing stressful factors that often initiate or worsen anxiety. |
| d. Have supportive people available for client. | Support system can reduce anxiety and promote physical and mental well-being. |
| 9. Summarize with client what has been discussed in interaction, e.g.:<br>Nurse: Let's review what we have discussed. You seem to have a better idea about what is causing you to feel uneasy. Not knowing how your family will accept you after surgery has been your concern. Is there anything else? | Summary signals close of interaction, allows nurse and client to depart with same idea, and provides sense of closure at completion of discussion. |

## Evaluation

| Steps | Rationale |
|---|---|
| 1. Observe for continuing presence of physical signs and symptoms or behaviors reflecting anxiety. | Determines extent to which planned interaction relieved client's anxiety. |
| 2. Have client discuss ways to cope with anxiety in the future and make decisions about own care. | Measures client's ability to assume more health-promoting behavior. |
| 3. Evaluate client's ability to discuss factors causing anxiety. | Measures client's ability to attend or focus on area of concern. |

### *Expected outcomes*

| Steps | Rationale |
|---|---|
| 1. Client experiences fewer physical signs and symptoms of anxiety. | Signs and symptoms lessen as anxiety is reduced. |
| 2. Client is able to make decisions about care. | Attention to facts can occur when anxiety is relieved. |
| 3. Client is able to describe perceptions and feelings about factor causing anxiety. | Relief of anxiety allows client to analyze situation more objectively. |

### *Unexpected outcomes*

| Steps | Rationale |
|---|---|
| 1. Physical signs and symptoms of anxiety continue. | Nurse's interaction may have increased client's anxiety, or source of anxiety not resolved. |
| 2. Client displays difficulty in decision making, and perception of facts may be altered. | Anxiety continues to prevent client from attending. |
| 3. Client avoids nurse's efforts at focusing discussion or is unable to discuss real concerns. | May result from mistrust; interaction is threatening. |

| Steps | Rationale |
|---|---|
| **Recording and Reporting** | |
| 1. Record in nurses' notes cause of client's anxiety and any exhibited signs and symptoms or behaviors. | Documents nature of client's problem and response. Provides guidelines for other nurses to continue interaction. |
| 2. Record methods used to relieve anxiety and client's response. | Ensures continuity of care between nurses. |
| **Follow-up Activities** | |
| 1. If anxiety continues to escalate: | |
| a. Continue to utilize previous steps. | Time needed for anxiety to lessen varies with clients. |
| b. Refocus or distract client's attention to less anxiety provoking experience. | Removes threat of having to deal with source of anxiety. |
| c. Be very direct and clear when making requests. | Eliminates misunderstanding that can increase anxiety. |
| d. If client needs to deal with stimulus causing anxiety, reintroduce when client is less anxious. | Attempts to minimize extent to which anxiety may increase. |
| e. Antianxiety medication may be necessary. (Requires physician's order; may be last resort when other measures have failed or may be required to prevent further isolation.) | Sometimes client is unable to control anxiety and may need calming effect of antianxiety medication. |

### Special Considerations

- Children often demonstrate anxiety in physical and behavioral signs but are unable to express anxiety verbally. Children may express anxiety by restlessness, agitation, physical complaints, irritability, behavioral regression, e.g., enuresis, school phobia.
- If anxiety results from need to make decision, present facts as simply as possible.
- Sometimes person experiencing anxiety may need to be held or touched, gently but firmly, to control feelings of panic.
- Use client's words to describe feelings, e.g., "scared" "nervous."

## SKILL 3-4 Communicating with the Angry Client

An anxious client can become angry for a variety of reasons. The anger may be directly related to a client's experience with illness or it can be associated with problems that existed before the client entered the health care system. It is common for an angry person to seek a means of expressing the anger. In the health care setting the nurse has frequent contact with a client and thus often becomes the target of the client's anger. It is important for the nurse to understand that in many cases the client's ability to express anger is important to recovery. For example, when a client has experienced a significant loss, anger becomes a means to help cope with grief. A client may express anger toward the nurse, but the anger often hides a specific problem or concern. For example, a client diagnosed as having cancer may voice displeasure with the nurse's care instead of expressing fear of dying.

It can be very stressful for a nurse to deal with an angry client. Anger can represent rejection or disapproval of the nurse's care. A nurse's efforts at satisfying the needs of one angry client can result in a failure to meet the priorities of other clients.

The nurse must allow the client to express anger openly and not feel threatened by the client's words. However, the client's anger should not be allowed to compromise care. Skills for communicating with an angry client will allow a nurse to assist the client in dealing with anger constructively and in refocusing emotional energy toward effective problem solving.

### Purposes

1. Understand client.
2. Establish rapport.
3. Assist in constructive expression of anger.
4. Decrease potentially harmful feelings of anger.

## Procedure 3-4

| Steps | Rationale |
|---|---|
| **Assessment** | |
| 1. Observe for behaviors or expressions that indicate client is angry:<br>a. Behavior (e.g., pacing, clenched fists, tense body, piercing stare, furrowed eyebrows, abrupt and loud movements, loud voice, rigid or fixed jaw, gritting teeth, curt manner, throwing or banging objects).<br>b. Verbal expressions (e.g., anger—"I'm angry"; "I feel like I could explode"; derogatory or blaming remarks—"The nurses are lousy around here"; curse words; "you" rather than "I" statements—"You jerk!"; "You should have been here an hour ago"; threats—"I'll call your instructor [or talk to the head nurse] if you try to change that dressing"; refusal to participate in care—"I'm not going for any more x-rays and you can't make me."). | Anger is a normal expression of frustration or a response to feeling threatened. However, its expression can interfere or block communication and interactions.<br>Anger is often a reaction to:<br>a. Experience of loss (e.g., body appearance, body function, loved one, health, autonomy and independence, material things).<br>b. Frustration (e.g., not achieving goal of getting better; not having needs met, such as getting analgesic, bedpan, meals, water).<br>c. Threat to self-esteem.<br>d. Fear of unknown.<br>e. Previous rejection or disappointment.<br>f. Feelings of inferiority.<br>g. Intrusion of personal space. |
| 2. Assess factors that influence communication of angry client.<br>a. Anger frequently expressed indirectly (e.g., client uses sarcasm; verbally says he is doing fine, but nonverbal behavior indicates anger; client never complains to you and is usually friendly, but you find out from another nurse how upset he is at you).<br>b. Anger may be expressed more frequently in individuals who lack emotional maturity, are impulsive, or have low frustration level (e.g., children, alcohol or drug abusers, clients with organic brain syndrome, clients with emotional or physical illness).<br>c. Individuals who have difficulty expressing anger may be perceived as hostile or aggressive.<br>d. Withdrawn, depressed, timid individuals have difficulty expressing anger directly.<br>e. Reason and logic may be limited during moments of anger.<br>f. Nurse's past relationship with client may increase or decrease feelings of anger.<br>g. Comprehension may be limited during angry state.<br>h. Perception and understanding may be self-centered during angry state.<br>i. Anxious or angry response by nurse can escalate client's feelings of anger. | Allows nurse to accurately assess situation or experiences of client that can hinder or facilitate communication. |
| 3. Assess most appropriate manner of communicating with angry client. | |
| a. Passive friendliness: be available to client to listen to concerns, but do not push. Avoid totally agreeing or disagreeing. Follow through with promises that you make. Acknowledge client's feelings and perceptions. (Contraindicated with client who expresses anger through withdrawal and depression; may require active friendliness.) | Passive friendliness avoids intimidation and allows client to express concerns. |
| b. Matter-of-factness: state what you can and cannot do, remain calm, give direction, but avoid antagonism or defensiveness. (Contraindicated if client's anger is decreasing and client is able to more effectively solve problems by expressing anger.) | Matter-of-factness respects experience of client and nurse and avoids threatening or judgmental approach. |
| 4. Consider resources available to reveal nature of client's anger and assist in communication with client: | |
| a. Use information from health team and family members. | May assist in clarifying cause and intervention required to deal with client's anger. |

| Steps | Rationale |
|---|---|
| b. Use information from chart and care plan. | Assists in identifying larger perspective of client's difficulty. Written information may or may not identify client as angry, but sometimes pattern may be identified, e.g., nurse discovers from chart that client was told on Wednesday that major surgery is needed early next week. Since then, it has been charted that client has lost appetite, become irritable, etc. |

## Nursing Diagnosis

| Steps | Rationale |
|---|---|
| 1. Cluster data to reveal actual or potential nursing diagnoses: | |
| a. Impaired verbal communication: related to feelings of anger. | Client unable to understand communication of others. |
| b. Self-care deficit: related to feelings of anger. | Client unwilling to perform or complete self-care activities. |
| c. Knowledge deficit: related to feelings of anger. | Client unable to attend to information. |
| d. Impaired social interaction: related to anger. | Client ineffective in social exchanges with others. |

## Planning

| Steps | Rationale |
|---|---|
| 1. Prepare for communication with angry client: | Client's anger can be threatening and may interfere with nurse's ability to deal with situation calmly. |
| a. Develop individualized goals including: | |
| ▪ Determine what client is saying. | Effective communication helps nurse understand what has angered client. |
| ▪ Establish rapport. Rapport may be established quickly if client believes nurse is listening, or it may take longer. | Allows honest expression and may assist in decreasing feelings of anger. |
| ▪ Client will constructively express anger by identifying cause of anger, expressing anger directly and honestly, identifying what can and cannot change the situation or feeling, using physical activity to channel energy associated with feelings of anger. | If not expressed through constructive means, anger may be expressed in negative ways, e.g., withdrawal, noncompliance, threats, explosive anger, physical harm, numerous complaints or demands. |
| ▪ Defuse or de-escalate a potentially out-of-control situation. (Client is not able to reason or listen and may become impulsive.) | Prevents harmful behavior and enables client to problem-solve more effectively. |
| b. Consider time required to achieve purpose of interaction with angry client. If suddenly avoiding client or making short infrequent visits, the nurse needs to identify and deal with personal feelings. Greater amount of time required initially until client has worked through anger; dealing with client's anger will often save time later. | Dealing with angry feelings often requires more intensive assistance. Failure to provide adequate time may increase client's anger. |
| c. Before interacting with client, formulate initial questions and responses with angry client. Plan to encourage description of client's experience by: | |
| ▪ Listening. | Allows client to express anger. |
| ▪ Making observation (e.g., "I sense that you are upset about something."). | May assist in providing opportunity to discuss situation. |
| ▪ Encourage description (e.g., "Tell me what happened that you are so angry"; "Tell me what's going through your mind"). Use who, when, where, and what questions. | Beginning exploration of situation. |
| ▪ Focusing (e.g., "Let's look at this situation more closely, since this made you angry."). | Prevents premature change in topic before completing exploration of concern. |
| ▪ Using broad, open-ended statements (e.g., "I would like to hear how you are finding things at present"). | Allows client to explore and share concerns. |
| d. Mentally prepare for interaction with angry client: | Nurse's calm approach may defuse client's anger. |
| ▪ Pause to collect own thoughts, feelings, and reactions. | Awareness and control of nurse's reaction and responses can facilitate more constructive interaction. |
| ▪ Attempt calm, firm, assertive approach. ▪ Attempt to talk in comfortable, reassuring voice. | Uncontrolled responses by nurse may elicit fight or flight response, e.g., unchanneled anger in nurse; power struggle; escalation in client's anger and behavior; increased conflict; blocking of nurse-client relationship; unresolved anger in client; nurse blaming self, avoiding client, taking misplaced anger personally; doubts about ability as nurse; continued anger in client. |

| Steps | Rationale |
|---|---|
| 2. Physically prepare angry client and environment. | |
| a. Encourage other people, particularly those who provoke anger, to leave room or area. | Nurse wants to encourage client's expression of anger rather than provoke it. |
| b. Maintain adequate distance. Normal social distance is 4-12 ft. (see Fig. 3-1). Move nearer as rapport is established. | Avoids pressuring client; also nurse maintains safety distance if anger becomes out of control. |
| c. Maintain open exit. | Prevents feeling of being trapped. |
| d. Make sure gestures are slow and deliberate rather than sudden and abrupt. | Less chance of misinterpretation of message and less threatening. |
| e. When anger begins to disturb others, close door. Particularly important if client is becoming agitated. | Agitation and anxiety can spread to others. |
| f. Reduce disturbing factors in room, e.g., noise, drafts, inadequate lighting. | Reduces irritating factors. |
| g. Take care of client's physical and emotional needs and discomforts, e.g., adjust room temperature and ventilation, offer analgesic for pain. | Physical and emotional needs may be factors in client's anger; sometimes client is not aware of these needs. |

## Implementation

| Steps | Rationale |
|---|---|
| 1. Create climate of acceptance of client. | |
| a. Calm, relaxed atmosphere essential. | Environment of extreme coldness or extreme warmth in approach or surroundings may block communication or escalate anger. |
| b. Demonstrate genuineness and respect. | Communicates positive regard for client's feelings. |
| 2. Introduce self and who you are. Introduction to client should be brief and to the point. | Anger will limit client's receptivitity to a long introduction. |
| 3. Use physical attending. | |
| a. Begin with minimal intensity and gradually increase. | Adequate personal space is very important with angry client. |
| b. Begin with same type of position as client (when possible), e.g., if client is standing, nurse stands; if client is sitting, nurse sits. | Conveys physically being "in tune" with another. |
| c. Gradually move to more relaxed position for both client and nurse, e.g., if standing, eventually sit. | Facilitates less tense or anxious exchange. Sometimes walking can be more relaxing for the angry client than trying to sit quietly. |
| d. Shoulders slightly down or relaxed. | Body language that is less intimidating or threatening. |
| e. Look toward client but avoid glaring or eye contact that is too intense. | Less intimidating. |
| f. Maintain "open" position, avoid crossing legs and arms, keep hands unclenched and relaxed, face slightly toward client. | Provides nonverbal cues of acceptance and listening that is congruent with attitude of acceptance. |
| 4. Practice psychologic attending. | (Skill 3-1) |
| a. Avoid defensive listening with the angry client. | Defensive listening: e.g., instead of listening to client, nurse concentrates on need to defend or thinks of reasons why client should not feel angry. |
| 5. Respond to angry client. | |
| a. Use therapeutic silence, avoid using silence to ignore client. | Often de-escalates anger because anger expands emotional and physical energy; client runs out of momentum and energy to maintain anger at high level. |
| b. Use responses based on hierarchy description of experience, thoughts about experience, feelings experience generated. | Assists client in describing event causing anger and clarifying thoughts and feelings. |
| c. Make vague statements more explicit or specific, e.g.:<br>Client: Nobody cares around here.<br>Nurse: I'm not sure what you mean, Mr. Jones. Could you tell me more?<br>Client: Everybody is just too busy.<br>Nurse: What do you mean, everybody is just too busy?<br>Client: I haven't seen anybody for 3 hours and I need my dressing changed before I go to physical therapy. | Angry client may have difficulty in being specific and needs assistance to do so. In order to change factors contributing to client's anger, nurse often needs specific information. |
| d. Use accurate empathy. | Empathy is ability to accurately comprehend and communicate thoughts, feelings, and experience of client in such a way that client would say, "Yes, that is exactly where I'm coming from." It is a strong anger antidote. |

| Steps | Rationale |
|---|---|
| e. Explore alternatives to situation or feelings of anger.* | May alter factors contributing to anger. |
| f. Present your perspective or point of view calmly and firmly. Use with clients in which nurse needs cooperation and compliance with care. Avoid using until you have listened to angry client. | May assist client to understand whole situation or another point of view; may assist in getting client to comply or follow through with care. |
| g. Use repeated assertion. Firmly repeat original response rather than argue each point. | Can be effective when client ignores, overreacts, or discounts your thoughts or feelings. |
| 6. Use questions carefully. | Questions can either facilitate client's expression of anger or intensify anger. |
| 7. Avoid communication breakdown: | |
| a. Avoid attempts to explain why client should not be angry. | Client reacts more to emotions than reasoning. |
| b. Avoid aggressiveness or oversubmissiveness. | Both tend to escalate client's anger. |
| c. Do not ignore client and anger. | Does not assist client in resolving anger. |
| d. Avoid trying to out-talk or give numerous explanations. | Annoys and irritates client. |

## Evaluation

| Steps | Rationale |
|---|---|
| 1. Observe for continuing behaviors or verbal expressions reflecting anger. | Indicates success of communication efforts. |
| 2. Evaluates client's ability to state feelings clearly. | Determines whether true source of client's anger has been defined. |
| 3. Note client's ability to answer questions. | Determines whether anger has lessened so that client can focus on facts. |

### *Expected outcomes*

| Steps | Rationale |
|---|---|
| 1. Client shows following behaviors: decrease in body tension; more relaxed hands; lower tone of voice; more relaxed facial expression; less pacing, fidgeting, or jerking movement; willingness to work with nurse. | Anger was expressed constructively. |
| 2. Client is able to discuss perceptions of reason(s) for anger. | Client able to attend to reasons for emotional expression(s). |

### *Unexpected outcomes*

| Steps | Rationale |
|---|---|
| 1. Client demonstrates behaviors or verbal expressions of anger. | Nurse unable to assist client in relieving source of anger or in expressing anger openly. |
| 2. Client avoids attempts by nurse to discuss issues related to anger. | |

## Recording and Reporting

| Steps | Rationale |
|---|---|
| 1. Record in nurses' notes observations related to anger; quote client exactly. | Aids in assessment of source of client's anger. |
| 2. Record nursing interventions in response to client's anger. | Documents nurse's actions and promotes continuity of care. |

## Follow-up Activities

| Steps | Rationale |
|---|---|
| 1. If anger continues to escalate: | |
| a. Reassess factors contributing to anger. | Allows nurse to alter behaviors that may cause anger to escalate. |
| b. Remove or alter factors contributing to anger, e.g., if two individuals are arguing and are not able to discuss the situation, ask one individual to leave. | Allows nurse to alter behaviors that may cause anger to escalate. |

*Often the nurse is able to stop at 5e; however, 5f may be required.

## Special Considerations

- Do not touch client indiscriminately. Touch can convey different meaning (warmth, assurance, acceptance), but it can also convey a feeling of intrusion, dependency, or sexual overtones. Taking care of physical needs through touch is necessary and usually gives a message of caring.
- Keep in mind that client may have experiences from the past that perpetuate anger in the present.
- Psychotropic medications may be needed in the agitated client.
- A period of withdrawal or self-isolation may provide a cooling-down period until client is able to talk about the anger.
- Guilt sometimes follows expressions of anger, and the nurse must deal with this reaction as well.
- When people are enraged, they require limits and a here-and-now orientation. Intellectualization and reasoning are usually ineffective during this phase.
- Verbal limits on behavior may be necessary.
- Provide a one-to-one session in a private area.
- Document pattern of acting out, including events that trigger anger.
- Discuss alternate means of releasing tension and physical energy.
- Do not argue, criticize, or threaten punitive action.
- If you are confronted by bitter, angry, accusatory family or client who accuse you of negligence, remember it may be:
  a. Accurate and justified.
  b. Their way of coping with their aggression, helplessness, or guilt at the time.

---

**BIBLIOGRAPHY**

Arnold E, Boggs K: Interpersonal relationships, Philadelphia, 1989, WB Saunders Co.

Beck CK, Rawlins RP, Williams SR: Mental health-psychiatric nursing: a holistic life-cycle approach, ed. 2, St. Louis, 1988, The CV Mosby Co.

Bermosk LS: Interviewing: a key to therapeutic communication in nursing practice, Nurs Clin North Am 1(2):205, 1966.

Bird B: Talking with patients, Philadelphia, 1973, JB Lippincott Co.

Bradley J, Edenberg MA: Communication in the nursing context, New York, 1982, Appleton-Century-Crofts.

Cameron JE: Giant leap forward begins with the nursing interview, Aust Nurses J 12(2):47, 1982.

Coad-Denton A: Therapeutic superficiality and intimacy. In: Longo D, Williams R: Clinical practice in psychosocial nursing, New York, 1978, Appleton-Century-Crofts.

Davis AJ: The skills of communication, Am J Nurs 63(1):60, 1963.

Egan G: The skilled helper, Monterey, Calif, 1975, Brooks/Cole Publishing Co.

Enelow A, Scott S: Interviewing and patient care, ed. 2, New York, 1979, Oxford University Press.

Hein E: Communication in nursing practice, ed. 2, Boston, 1980, Little, Brown & Co.

Hogstel M: Home nursing care for the elderly, Bowie; Englewood Cliffs, NJ, 1985, Prentice-Hall Press.

Iveson-Iveson J: The art of communication, Nurs Mirror, p. 47, Feb, 1983.

Kasch CR: Interpersonal competence and communication in the delivery of nursing care, Adv Nurs Sci 6(2):71, 1984.

Knowles RD: Building rapport through neuro-linguistic programming, Am J Nurs 83(7):1011, July 1983.

McKay M, Davis M, Fanning P: Messages: the communication book, Oakland, Calif, 1983, New Harbinger Publications.

Murray RB: Therapeutic communication for emotional care. In: Murray RB, Huelskoetter MM: Psychiatric mental health nursing giving emotional care, Englewood Cliffs, NJ, 1983, Prentice Hall Inc.

Nelson GB: Assessment and intervention for communication problems in home health care, J Home Health Care Practice 9(1):61, 1988.

Patient Teaching Manual 1, Springhouse, Pa, 1987, Springhouse Corp.

Purtilo R: Health professional/patient interaction, ed. 2, Philadelphia, 1978, WB Saunders Co.

Raudseff E: 7 ways to cure communication breakdowns, Nurs Life, p. 51, Jan/Feb, 1984.

Satir V: Conjoint family therapy, rev ed, Palo Alto, Calif, 1967, Science & Behavior books.

Satir V: Peoplemaking, Palo Alto, Calif, 1972, Science & Behavior Books.

Wilson HS, Kneisel CR: Psychiatric Nursing, ed. 3, Menlo Park, Calif, 1988, Addison-Wesley Publishing Company.

# UNIT II

# SAFETY AND COMFORT

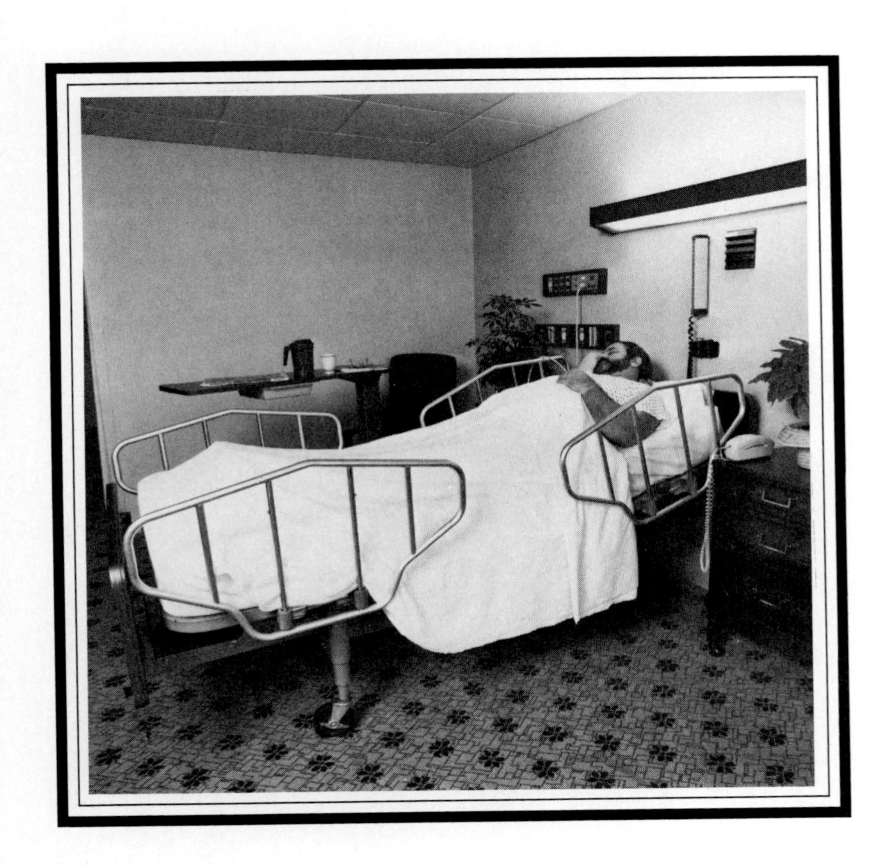

An integral part of caring for any client is taking every possible measure to ensure well-being in sickness and in health. Basic to any client's needs is the provision of a safe and comfortable environment. Chapter 4, "Safety," contains special skills for reducing accidents and other potential threats to safety in the health care setting and the home. Chapter 5, "Comfort," explores various types of noninvasive comfort measures the nurse may independently use for clients with different levels of pain. The various pain relief therapies can easily be used by clients in the home setting to provide them with a sense of control over their pain experience.

# 4

# SAFETY

### OBJECTIVES

*Mastery of content in this chapter will enable the nurse to:*

- Define key terms.
- Discuss methods to reduce physical hazards.
- Discuss specific risks to safety as they pertain to the client's developmental age.
- State nursing diagnoses associated with risk to a client's safety.
- Develop a nursing care plan for clients whose safety is threatened.
- Describe nursing interventions specific to the client's age for reducing risk of falls, fires, poisonings, and electrical hazards.
- Describe methods to evaluate interventions designed to maintain or promote a client's safety.

### KEY TERMS

| | |
|---|---|
| *Aspiration* | *Mummy restraints* |
| *Belt restraints* | *Poison* |
| *Elbow restraints* | *Poison control center* |
| *Extremity restraints* | *Pneumonitis* |
| *Jacket restraints* | *Restraint* |
| *Mitten restraints* | *Syrup of ipecac* |

### SKILLS

**4-1** Reducing Potential Threats to Safety
**4-2** Applying Restraints
**4-3** Preventing Accidental Poisoning
**4-4** Taking Action for Accidental Poisoning

Health promotion and illness prevention involve promotion of the client's safety. Maintenance of a client's safety in the community or within the health care environment is essential.

Promoting client safety reduces the length and cost of treatment, the frequency of treatment-related accidents, the potential for lawsuits, and the number of work-related injuries to personnel. In addition, a safe environment encourages clients to assume a more active role in their health care practices.

Threats to a client's safety are different for each developmental stage. Accidents are the leading cause of death in children at all ages, and the type of injury and the circumstances surrounding the accident are closely related to normal growth and development (Whaley and Wong, 1987). The child's developmental stage can be the basis for accident prevention. For example, an infant should not be placed in a crib with a pillow because of the risk of accidental suffocation. Likewise, a toddler's environment needs to be "child-proofed" to avoid accidental aspiration of foreign bodies, ingestion of household cleaners, or injury from playing with electric outlets. Nurses can assist parents, teachers, and babysitters to prevent accidents and reduce injuries to young children.

As children grow and enter school the potential for accidents is not limited to their home or immediate neighborhood environment. Children become active in contact sports, swimming, and bicycling. Adequate education and supervision can reduce the frequency and severity of accidents occurring with these activities.

Preschool and school-age children must be taught to avoid contact with strangers. Although discussion of these matters is difficult, young children need to learn that there are people in this world who can and do harm children.

As the child continues to develop, threats to his safety expand farther from the home environment. Parents, teachers, and health care professionals need to teach children about potential and actual threats to safety. Adolescents are at risk for exposure to substance abuse, and health education can increase their awareness of the untoward effects of alcohol and drug abuse.

The threats to an adult client's safety are frequently related to life-style habits. The client who abuses alcohol has a greater risk than other persons for motor vehicle accidents. Likewise, the long-term smoker has a greater risk of cardiovascular or pulmonary disease than do nonsmokers. In addition, the adult experiencing a high level of stress is more likely to have an accident because of the impact of stress on decision making. High levels of stress also increase the risk of illnesses such as headaches, gastrointestinal disorders, and infection.

Threats to the safety of older adults focus primarily on accidents. Injuries to older adults can be related to physiologic changes occurring during the aging process, environmental hazards, and relocation stress. Ebersole and Hess (1985) identify the following eight areas for consideration to promote safety in the older adult: housing, relocation stress, institutionalization, migration patterns, transportation and mobility, community and neighborhood supports, adaptational capacity of the aged, and environmental safety and convenience.

A client's safety can also be maintained by preventing a client's self-injury. These accidents are classified as client-inherent accidents. Examples are self-inflicted cuts, injuries, and burns; ingestion or injection of foreign substances; self-mutilation or setting fires; and pinching fingers in drawers or doors. Client-inherent accidents can occur in both oriented and disoriented clients. When a client is at risk of injury from such accidents, or from falling out of bed or a chair, the nurse must ensure that the client is properly restrained and protected from injury.

Measures designed to promote client safety are the result of individualized assessment findings. Frequently, it is the conclusion of the nurse that a client's safety is at risk, and subsequent nursing interventions are implemented. Assessment of a client's safety occurs in a health care environment, as well as a community environment.

***TABLE 4-1*** Expected Motor Development Changes that Increase Risk of Injury in Infants and Toddlers

| Age | Motor Development | Hazard |
|---|---|---|
| 1 mo | Can hold head midline and parallel to body; by age 4 mo infant has good neck control. | If not supported, infant's head flops forward or backward. |
| 2 mo | Grasp reflex present; grasps and holds object for few moments or longer. | Able to grasp electric cords and other dangerous items on floor. |
| 3 mo | May begin to roll from back to abdomen; bears weight on forearms. | Increased risk of falling off bed, changing table, and counter. |
| 4 mo | Increased grasping ability, explores new objects with mouth. | Able to pick up small objects, which usually go immediately into the mouth. |
| | Increased ability to roll from abdomen and from side to side and to move in rocking motion. | Increased risk of falling from surfaces. |
| 5 mo | Ability of locomotion increases by rocking, rolling, twisting. | Able to purposefully move toward objects that may be dangerous. |
| | Able to grasp bottle, but should not be left unattended. | Drinking from bottle in supine position increases risk of choking on contents, increased risk of ear infections and dental caries in baby and permanent teeth. |
| | Increased ability to grasp small objects. | Increased risk of choking on small objects. |
| 6 mo | Scoots by self-propulsion on abdomen, steering with arms and legs. | Able to move to potential dangers, such as electric outlets and household cleaners. |
| 7 mo | May be crawling; able to sit alone for short periods of time. | Able to rapidly move from one spot to another. |
| 8 mo | May be able to pull self to standing position; able to sit unsupported. | Can easily fall unless helped back to sitting or lying position. |
| 9 mo | Begins to crawl up stairs; can stand and move by using furniture for support (walking may occur any time after age 8 mo). | Can lose balance and fall down stairs; can lose balance with wobbly furniture; can bruise self on sharp corners of tables and bookcases. |
| 10 mo | Climbs up and tries to climb down from chairs; able to change from prone to sitting position. | May fall from chair; unable to judge distances or self-limitations. |
| 11 mo | Interested in self-feeding. | Risk of choking, unless foods are cut into small pieces. |
| 12 mo | May climb out of crib (although rare at this age). | Increased risk of falling out of crib or playpen. |
| | Takes covers off plastic and screw-top containers. | Able to open and possibly taste harmful substances. |
| 15 mo | Walks with help; cannot walk around corners or stop suddenly without losing balance. | Loses sense of balance and easily falls. |
| 18 mo | Runs clumsily and falls often. | Falls easily. |
| | Moves furniture and climbs on furniture. | May pull furniture over or fall off furniture. |
| 24 mo | Able to turn door knobs. | Can independently open closed door and may ingest harmful products stored in cabinet, closet, or bathroom. |

Information adapted from Whaley, LF, and Wong, DL: Nursing care of infants and children, ed 3, St. Louis, 1987, The CV Mosby Co.

## GUIDELINES

1. Know the norms for the client's developmental stage (Table 4-1). Threats to safety parallel a client's developmental stage.
2. Know the client's normal activity patterns and activities of daily living.
3. Know the client's medical history and present therapies. Certain illnesses, such as a stroke, and medications, such as tranquilizers, can cause physical or cognitive impairment that increases the risk of injury.
4. Be aware of environmental conditions that can affect the client's safety and increase risk of injury, for example, cluttered hallways.
5. Know proper use of safety devices for a client receiving nursing care in a hospital, extended care facility, or at home.
6. Know what toxic chemicals, such as cleaning solutions, house plants, and medications, may be present in the home.

## PREREQUISITE KNOWLEDGE

1. Normal growth and development.
2. Hazards of immobility.
3. Motor, sensory, and cognitive changes that increase the risk of accidental poisoning.

## PREREQUISITE SKILLS

1. Physical assessment (Chapter 13).
2. Administration of medication (Unit VI).
3. Hygiene measures (Unit III).

# *SKILL 4-1 Reducing Potential Threats to Safety*

Unintentional injuries occur at all ages of the life span. Studies of types and numbers of accidental injuries indicate that specific injuries are more likely to occur at each point of the life span. Knowledge of specific motor and cognitive developmental changes enables the nurse to assess for potential injury for each client. Once the area of potential injury is identified, the nurse designs interventions to eliminate or reduce the threat to the client's safety.

### Purposes

1. Provide the nurse with knowledge of specific motor, sensory, and cognitive developmental changes throughout the life span that influence a person's safety.

## *Procedure 4-1*

| Steps | Rationale |
|---|---|
| **Assessment** | |
| ***Infant and toddler*** | |
| 1. Observe motor activity of infant or toddler. | Provides nurse with knowledge of normal activity patterns, such as crawling and climbing. |
| 2. Compare assessment findings with norms for growth and development for appropriate age in months of infant or toddler (Table 4-1). | Identifies potential threats to safety. |
| 3. Observe home environment to determine presence of potential hazards. | Accidents are major cause of death during infancy, especially for children age 6-12 mo. Accidents can be grouped into following categories: aspiration of foreign objects, suffocation, falls, poisoning, burns, motor vehicle accidents, bodily damage (Whaley and Wong, 1987). |
| 4. Determine family's awareness of potential hazards. | Reflects need for family education. |
| ***School-age child*** | |
| 1. Observe child's home and play environment for threats to safety. | School-age child has greater mobility and frequently explores openings, e.g., caves, closets, cabinets, drawers. Because young child cannot read, "Danger" and "Keep Out" signs are meaningless. Likewise, child may not notice warning labels on household chemicals and poisons. Young child frequently is adventurous without perception of possible injury. Consequently, adult must make environment safe and teach child about potential environmental threats. |
| 2. Determine family's awareness of possible hazards within neighborhood, e.g., potentially unsafe areas en route to school or strangers in neighborhood. | As children grow, potential threats to their safety expand into their neighborhood and community environment. Nurse must determine client's perception of these threats. |

| Steps | Rationale |
|---|---|
| 2. Determine family's awareness of possible hazards within neighborhood, e.g., potentially unsafe areas en route to school or strangers in neighborhood. | As children grow, potential threats to their safety expand into their neighborhood and community environment. Nurse must determine client's perception of these threats. |
| ***Adolescent*** | |
| 1. Observe for signs and symptoms of substance abuse in older school-age child and adolescent: bloodshot eyes, slurred speech, restlessness, sleepiness, erratic appetite, clumsiness, urinary frequency, blackouts, susceptibility to illness, dilated pupils. | Long-term habitual use of drugs or alcohol results in subtle behavioral changes. Parents and nurses must be able to recognize changes especially over time. Parents should also be aware that these signs and symptoms may be associated with medical and emotional disorders. |
| 2. Observe for environmental clues indicating possible substance abuse: drug paraphernalia, drug-oriented magazines, beer and liquor bottles, blood spots on clothing. | During initial experimentation with psychoactive substances, youth is usually consistent about covering any environmental clues. However, carelessness about presence of environmental clues becomes more frequent as substance abuse becomes more chronic. |
| 3. Observe for behavioral clues that correlate with possible substance abuse, such as failing grades, increased absenteeism, changes in interpersonal behavior, avoidance of eye contact, increased time spent in bathroom. | Prolonged substance abuse results in behavioral changes. Subtle changes in behavior may not be noticed by parent until specifically questioned regarding changes. Parents and siblings may be unfamiliar with behavioral changes associated with substance abuse. |
| 4. Determine client's level of knowledge for safe driving practices. | Death rate of adolescents from motor vehicle accidents is increasing at an alarming rate. Assessment of driving practices can lead to driving behaviors aimed at reducing risk of motor vehicle accidents. |
| ***Young and middle adult*** | |
| 1. Observe life-style patterns of young adult to identify risk factors: smoking, stress, drug use, alcohol use, unplanned exercise habits, personal hygiene habits. | Average young adult is usually free of major health concerns. Fast-paced life-style frequently increases risk for developing illnesses or disabilities during middle or older years. |
| 2. Obtain employment history to determine risks within occupational setting. | Occupational inhalants such as asbestos, plastics, dusts, and gases have potential for causing chronic lung diseases or cancers in later life. |
| ***Older adult*** | |
| 1. Observe older adult for physiologic changes common to aging process that increase risk of falling: osteoporosis, decreased hearing, decreased night vision, cataracts or glaucoma, orthostatic hypotension, decreased balance, slowed nervous system response, osteoarthritis. | Physiologic alterations predispose client to falls, e.g., postmenopausal woman is prone to osteoporosis and therefore at risk of breaking hip or ankle as she steps off curb (fall results from stress fracture; fracture is not caused by fall). |
| 2. Assess risk factors in home or community that pose threat to older adult's safety, e.g., improperly lighted stairways or throw rugs. | Provides opportunity to decrease risk of accidents in client's home. |
| 3. Determine actual or potential risk of injury as a result of motor, sensory, or cognitive changes. | Provides opportunity to identify factors that increase older adult's risk of injury. |

## Nursing Diagnosis

| Steps | Rationale |
|---|---|
| 1. Cluster data to reveal actual or potential nursing diagnosis<br>a. Actual or potential risk for injury: related to motor, sensory, or cognitive changes. | Assessment provides subjective and objective data that identify risk factor for potential injury. |

## Planning

| Steps | Rationale |
|---|---|
| 1. Develop individualized goals for client: | |
| a. Maintain environment that is adapted to motor, sensory, and cognitive developmental needs of client. | When client is at either end of life span, changes in environment may be needed every 2-4 weeks. |
| b. Client and family member learn potential threats to safety. | Family must continually review environment to determine level of safety. |

## Implementation

### *Infant, toddler, preschool-age, and school-age child*

| Steps | Rationale |
|---|---|
| Instruct parents or care givers to: | |
| 1. Use cribs, playpens, and portable cribs manufactured after 1976. | Old cribs do not meet current safety codes. It is possible for child to lodge head between mattress or pad and frame, resulting in suffocation. |

| Steps | Rationale |
|---|---|
| 2. Use large soft toys without plastic eyes, nose, or mouth. | Small parts that can be dislodged by baby may be aspirated. |
| 3. Keep all sides of mesh playpen up. | Baby's head can become wedged between playpen pad and lowered mesh side resulting in asphyxiation. |
| 4. Never leave sides of crib down or turn away from infant on changing table. | Child can suddenly roll and fall from crib or changing table. |
| 5. Hold infant at feeding time; do not prop bottle. | Increases bonding and reduces risk of choking. |
| 6. Read instructions before giving formula; most formulas must be diluted with water. | Using undiluted formula can cause fluid and electrolyte imbalances in newborn. |
| 7. Discontinue use of infant seat at age 3 mo or earlier if infant is very mobile. | At 3 mo active infant may be able to propel self out of infant seat and fall. |
| 8. Eliminate small objects, sharp objects, and toxic and poisonous substances from environment. | Infants explore their world with their hands and mouth. Small objects can result in choking. Ingestion of toxic and poisonous substances requires prompt action (Skill 4-4). |
| 9. Cover electric outlets with protective covers. | Electric wall outlets are at infant's eye level and stimulate curiosity. Crawling infant may attempt to play with electric wall plates regardless of number of toys available. |
| 10. Use guardrails at top and bottom of stairs and at doorway of rooms considered off limits to crawling or walking toddler. | Prevents child from falling down stairs. |
| 11. Never leave infant unattended in seat, walker, stroller, or high chair. | Active child can easily slide out of these devices and fall. |
| 12. Never leave infant or child unattended in bathtub or wading pool. | Avoids accidental drowning. |
| 13. Never attach pacifier on string to child. | String may become tangled around child's neck and result in strangulation. |
| 14. Restrain child in back seat of automobile. Children under 4 yr should be in approved car seat (Fig. 4-2). Older children should be restrained with seat belt. | Sudden stop or accident will cause unrestrained child to bounce against hard, sharp surfaces of vehicle's interior, resulting in injuries. |
| 15. Remove from home plastic bags such as those that store fruit or contain dry cleaning. | Bags can cause suffocation. |
| 16. Install strong dead bolt locks on doors well beyond toddler's reach, even if standing on chair. | Prevents child from leaving home without parent's knowledge, which reduces danger of child getting lost, freezing to death, or being abducted. |
| 17. Use "no" and "don't" to convey that object or action increases child's risk to injury. | Improperly using "no" or "don't" renders words meaningless to child; e.g., telling toddler "no" each time environment is explored renders word meaningless when dangerous situation is encountered. |
| 18. Teach child to swim at early age, but always with supervision. | Child will be able to safely enjoy water. |
| 19. Teach child how to cross street and how to walk in parking lots. | Help child learn protection against dangers from automobiles. |
| 20. Teach child not to talk to or accept anything from a stranger and to notify parents if approached by a stranger. | Reduces risk of injury or abduction by stranger; reporting stranger's presence helps law enforcement personnel to investigate and remove threat. |
| 21. Do not allow child to run with sucker or popsicle in the mouth. | Child may fall and stick can cause injury. |
| 22. Teach children not to eat anything found on the street or in the grass. | Substance may be poisonous or may cause severe illness. |
| 23. Use back burners on stove and get into habit of turning pot handles toward back of stove. | Reduces risk of child pulling pot of hot liquid on self. |
| 24. Remove door from unused refrigerators and freezers and instruct child not to hide in these items. | Door may latch; older model doors are not releasable from inside; suffocation can occur. |
| 25. Teach child how to safely use play and work equipment. | Child needs to learn that some equipment is for play and other equipment is for work; improper use can result in injury. |
| 26. Teach child to wear protective helmet and knee and elbow pads when roller or ice skating. | Protective devices reduce risk of serious injury from falls. |
| 27. Teach child how to safely ride bicycle and responsibilities that go with bicycling. | If bicycling is prohibited on sidewalks, child must learn how to obey traffic signals and ride with traffic patterns. |
| 28. Never allow child to operate appliances while alone in house. | If electric or other mishap occurs, no one is available to help child. |
| 29. Keep firearms unloaded and locked out of reach. | Prevents injury from accidental discharge. |

| Steps | Rationale |
|---|---|
| ***Adolescent*** | |
| Encourage parents or guardians to: | |
| 1. Enroll teenager in driver's education course. | Most states require new driver to successfully pass approved driver education program that teaches safe driving and laws that govern driving. |
| 2. Instruct teenager to wear seat belts at all times when in motor vehicle. | Motor vehicle accidents are leading cause of death and severe injury in adolescents. |
| 3. Instruct teenager not to drive when under influence of psychoactive substances. Encourage involvement in Students Against Drunk Driving (SADD). | Most motor accidents involving adolescents result from alcohol or drug use. |
| 4. Learn danger of psychoactive substance abuse and how and where to get help: Alcoholics Anonymous, drug abuse hot lines, substance abuse clinics and hospitals. Provide this information to adolescents. | When substance abuse directly influences one family member, entire family is affected. Family needs to know what type of help is available and how to obtain it. |
| 5. Recognize prolonged changes in adolescent's behavior and mood, as well as changes in academic and social performance. | Behavioral, mood, and performance changes can indicate possible substance abuse, as well as physical or emotional illnesses. |
| ***Young and middle adult*** | |
| 1. Teach health promotional activities in areas of nutrition, exercise, relaxation, smoking cessation. | Health promotional activities in young and middle adult years can reduce risk of certain diseases, e.g., cardiopulmonary diseases, cancer, and obesity, during later years. |
| 2. Teach client how to recognize stress and measures to effectively deal with psychophysiologic effects. | Prolonged stress response can increase client's risk of stress-related illnesses, such as ulcers and migraine headaches. Frequently, person is unable to completely remove self from stressor, but can be taught to change ways to respond to stress. |
| 3. Reinforce illness prevention behaviors and information such as breast self-examination or warning signs for cancer. | Recognition of cancer warning signals can lead to early detection and cure. |
| ***Older adult*** | |
| Teach client or family member to: | |
| 1. Install stair treads with uniform depth of 9 in and 9-in risers (vertical face of steps). | Uniform size of stairs does not require elderly to continually adjust vision. |
| 2. Install uniform-textured or plain-colored surfaces on each tread and mark edge of tread with contrasting color. | Uniform textures or color help decrease vertigo; marking edge of tread provides client with obvious visual clue to end of stair. |
| 3. Ensure proper lighting of each tread. Block sun or lightbulb glare with translucent shades or screen, or use lower wattage bulbs. | Elderly client's vision is unable to quickly accommodate to changes in lighting. |
| 4. Ensure adequate head room so that users need not duck to negotiate stairs. | Sudden changes in client's head position may result in dizziness. |
| 5. Remove protruding objects from walls. | Decreased peripheral vision may prevent client from seeing objects. |
| 6. Maintain outdoor walkways and stairs in firm condition, free of holes, cracks, and splinters, and be sure areas are well lighted at night. | Decreased visual acuity and accommodation can prevent elderly from seeing structural hazard. |
| 7. Install smooth but slip-resistant handrail at least 2 in from wall. Secure handrail firmly so that user's weight is supported especially at bottom and top of stairway. | 2-in distance allows client to firmly grasp handrail for support. Elderly have greatest risk of falling at top and bottom of stairs because center of gravity shifts and balance is unstable. |
| 8. Install grab bars in bathroom near toilet or tub. | Enables elderly to have support while elevating from sitting to standing position. |
| 9. Secure all carpeting, mats, and tile. Place nonskid backing under small rugs. | Sudden slip increases dizziness and decreases ability of elderly to regain balance. |

## Evaluation

| Steps | Rationale |
|---|---|
| 1. Ensure that client's home environment is modified for safety in relation to cognitive and motor developmental needs. | Enables individual modification in care within home or health care agency environment. |
| 2. Ask client to identify safety risks. | Ensures client able to take preventive steps for safety. |
| 3. Reassess motor, sensory, and cognitive developmental status to determine client's response to modification of potential risks. | Determines degree to which nursing interventions have been effective in reducing actual or potential threats to client's safety. |

| Steps | Rationale |
|---|---|
| ***Expected outcomes*** | |
| 1. Client's environment is hazard free. | Reduces environmental hazards that increase risk of injury. |
| 2. Client identifies safety risks. | Demonstrates learning. |
| ***Unexpected outcomes*** | |
| 1. Client is injured. | Not all injuries can be prevented; however, nurse must reassess client in environment to determine if threat could have been reduced. |
| 2. Client unable to identify safety risks. | Requires further instruction. |
| **Recording and Reporting** | |
| 1. Record specific interventions used to promote safety. | Provides written record of specific threats identified and what nurse did to reduce them. |
| 2. Report to all health care personnel specific threat to client's safety and measures taken to reduce threat. | Informs all appropriate personnel that potential risk exists and measures taken to minimize threat. |

## Special Considerations

- Generally, clients whose safety is threatened from environmental factors include infants and toddlers, preschoolers and school-age children, adolescents, older adults, clients with cognitive impairments, clients with sensory impairments, clients with restricted mobility.
- If child spends time in day-care center, with sitters, or with grandparents, these care providers must be aware of actual or potential health hazards.
- As child progresses to adolescence, a developing sense of identity may lead to conflict with parents. Conflict can produce anxiety, and psychoactive substances such as drugs and alcohol may be used to reduce anxiety. Unfortunately, substances used for this purpose leave adolescent at high risk for continued substance abuse (Rice and Kibbee, 1983).
- Presence of drug paraphernalia or drug-oriented magazines can indicate curiosity about rather than actual use of psychoactive substances. Follow-up education and counseling may prevent adolescent from becoming substance abuser.
- Although adolescent client may have passed state-approved driver's education course, practice of safe driving habits may not be consistent.
- Nonfamilial risk factors for young adult include violent death and injury, substance abuse, unwanted pregnancies, sexually transmitted diseases, and environmental or occupational factors (Stanhope and Lancaster, 1988). Familial risk factors include cardiovascular, renal, endocrine, and neoplastic illnesses.
- Clients taking diuretics and hypertensive medication may have increased postural vertigo.
- Older adults, especially postmenopausal women, are at risk for fractured hips. Fractured hip or other weight-bearing bone can cause independent client to become more dependent or immobilized.
- Health promotional and stress-reduction activities are not exclusive to young and middle adults. However, health problems in this age group are frequently related to life-style habits.
- Illness-prevention behavior should be continued into older adult years.
- Any specific intervention is based on child's cognitive and motor development. Parents must be taught that threats to child's safety increase as child grows; however with growth, child can become more active in maintaining safety.
- Encourage parents to allow practice drives in good and bad weather so that teenager can gain confidence. Also permits teenager to demonstrate responsible driving.
- If family has previously set example by wearing seat belts at all times, "buckling up" is habit that adolescent is more likely to keep.
- Encourage parents to make contract stating that if adolescent drinks or uses drugs at party, to call parents for ride home. Parents in return will ask no questions at that time.
- Education of adolescent may bring awareness that parents may be substance abusers and how to seek assistance.

## Home Care Considerations

- Teach parents to childproof their home to reduce risk of accidental poisoning (Skill 4-3).
- If client's visual impairment is severe, additional visual adaptive devices may be required, such as bright color on edge of stair tread.
- Use of grab bars in home bathrooms around toilet and tubs reduces risk of injury.

# SKILL 4-2 Applying Restraints

A restraint is a device used to immobilize a client or an extremity. Restraints serve one or all of the following purposes: (1) Restraints reduce the risk of a client falling out of bed or from wheelchair or chair. (2) Restraints prevent the interruption of therapy such as traction, intravenous infusions, nasogastric tube feedings, or Foley catheterization. (3) Restraints prevent the confused or combative client from removing life support equipment. (4) Restraints reduce the risk of self-inflicted injury and injury to others by the client.

The use of restraints requires physiologic and emotional nursing interventions. The nurse provides emotional support as the client and the family adjust to the restraint. The application of a restraint requires a physician's order. The following information assists the nurse in determining when and what type of restraint device is needed.

When preventing a client from falling out of bed, restraints must be used in conjunction with side rails. A side rail is attached to the side of a bed or stretcher and can be raised or lowered (Fig. 4-1). Side rails should remain up for the unconscious, disoriented, weak, postoperative, postpartum, or immobilized client.

The nurse must know what type of restraint to use and when a restraint is necessary. A client who requires one extremity to be restrained to reduce mobility should not be placed in a jacket restraint. Likewise, a client who is somewhat disoriented immediately postoperatively may need some restraint to prevent accidental removal of postoperative drains. However, once the effects of anesthetics or analgesics decrease and the client's level of orientation improves, the restraint may no longer be necessary.

## Purposes

1. Prevent the client from falling out of bed.
2. Prevent interruption of therapy, such as traction, intravenous (IV) infusions, nasogastric tube feedings, or life support equipment.
3. Reduce the risk of self-inflicted injury and injury to others by the client.

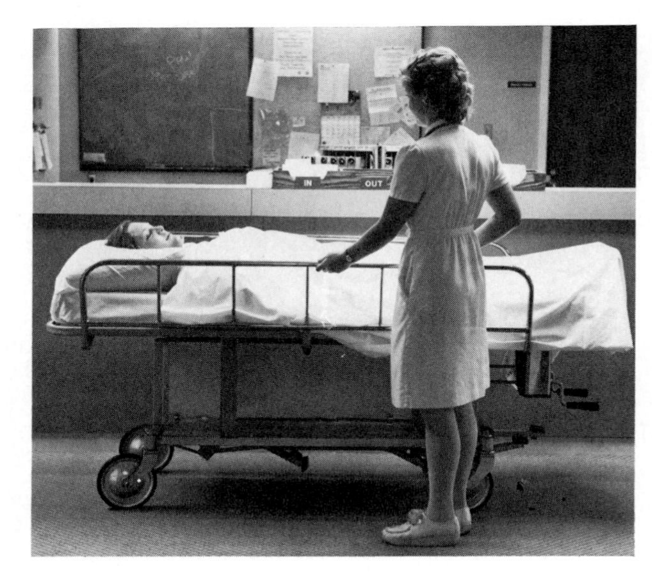


***Fig. 4-1*** Side rails in up position on stretcher.

## Procedure 4-2

| Steps | Rationale |
| --- | --- |
| **Assessment** | |
| 1. Identify clients in need of restraints: confused or disoriented clients, clients requiring immobilization of extremity, children requiring immobilization of elbow joint to prevent dislodgment of therapeutic equipment. | Restraints are used to reduce risk of client falling out of bed, chair, or wheelchair; prevent interruption of therapy such as traction, IV infusions, or nasogastric tube feedings; prevent confused or combative client from injuring himself by removing Foley catheters, surgical drains, or life support equipment; reduce risk of injury to others by client. |
| 2. Check physician's order and assess type of restraint needed. | Nursing assessment aids in determining what type of restraint to use. Physician's order is necessary to apply restraints. |
| **Nursing Diagnosis** | |
| 1. Cluster data to reveal actual or potential nursing diagnoses: | |
| a. Potential for injury: related to absence of restraints. | Restraints are most effective when use is based on client need. |
| b. Potential for impaired skin integrity: related to application of restraint. | Incorrect type of restraint or restraint applied too tightly or too loosely can result in injury. |

| Steps | Rationale |
|---|---|

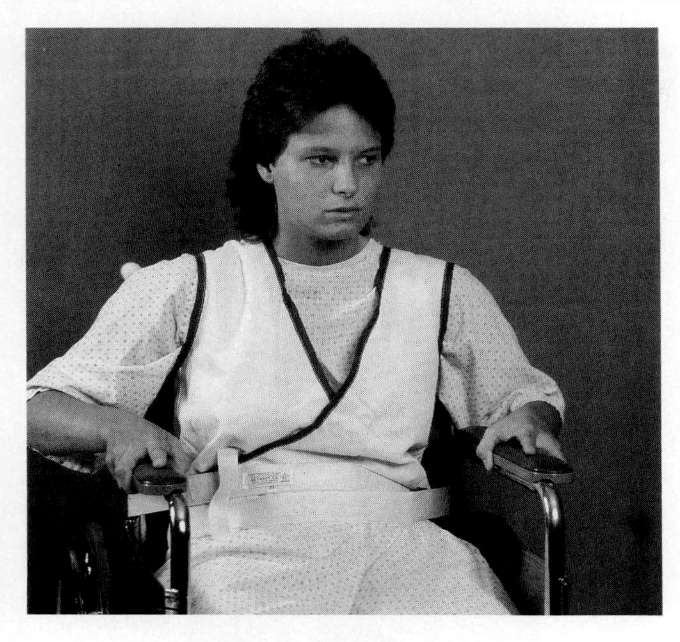

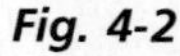

*Fig. 4-2*

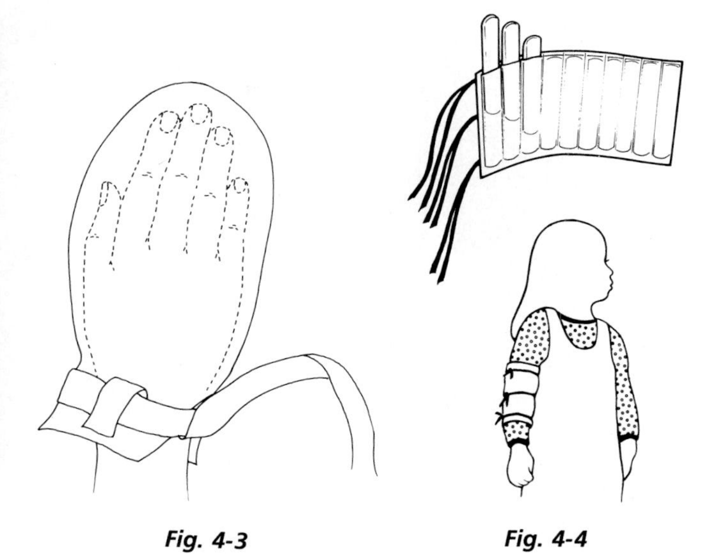

*Fig. 4-3* *Fig. 4-4*

## Planning

1. Develop individualized goals for client:
   a. Prevent injury related to absence of restraints or incorrect use of restraint device. — Lack of appropriate restraint device can result in injury to client.
2. Select restraint that will reduce client's movement only as needed. — Overrestraining client so that activities are unduly restricted can exacerbate hazards of immobility.
3. Explain to client and family why restraint is necessary, type of restraint selected, and anticipated duration of restraint. — Restraints can increase confusion or combativeness in client. Family may express anger about restraint. Explanation and reinforcement can reduce or prevent negative perceptions.
4. Prepare the following equipment for application of selected restraint:
   a. Proper restraint.
   b. Padding to protect bony prominences.

   Nurse is able to complete restraining procedure without leaving client partially restrained. Padding protects circulation to distal portion of extremity when wrist or ankle restraints are used.

## Implementation

1. Wash hands. — Reduces transmission of microorganisms.
2. Apply selected restraint:
   a. Jacket restraint: vestlike garment that usually crosses in back of client but may also cross in front (Fig. 4-2). — Restrains client while lying or reclining in bed and while sitting in chair or wheelchair.
   Jacket restraints are useful in home care settings but should not be used unless other methods to maintain client safety have failed.
   b. Belt restraint: device that secures client on stretcher. Avoid placing belt too tightly across client's chest or abdomen. — Restrains center of gravity and prevents client from rolling off stretcher or sitting up while on stretcher.
   c. Extremity restraints (ankle or wrist restraint): designed to immobilize one or all extremities. Commercially available limb restraints are composed of sheepskin and foam pad that comes in contact with skin. — Maintains immobilization of extremity to protect client from injury from fall or accidental removal of therapeutic device, e.g., an IV tube or Foley catheter.
   d. Mitten restraint: thumbless mitten devices to restrain client's hands (Fig. 4-3). — Prevents client from dislodging invasive equipment, removing dressings, or from scratching.
   e. Elbow restraint: piece of fabric with slots in which tongue blades are placed so that elbow joint remains rigid (Fig. 4-4). — Used with infants and children to prevent elbow flexion.

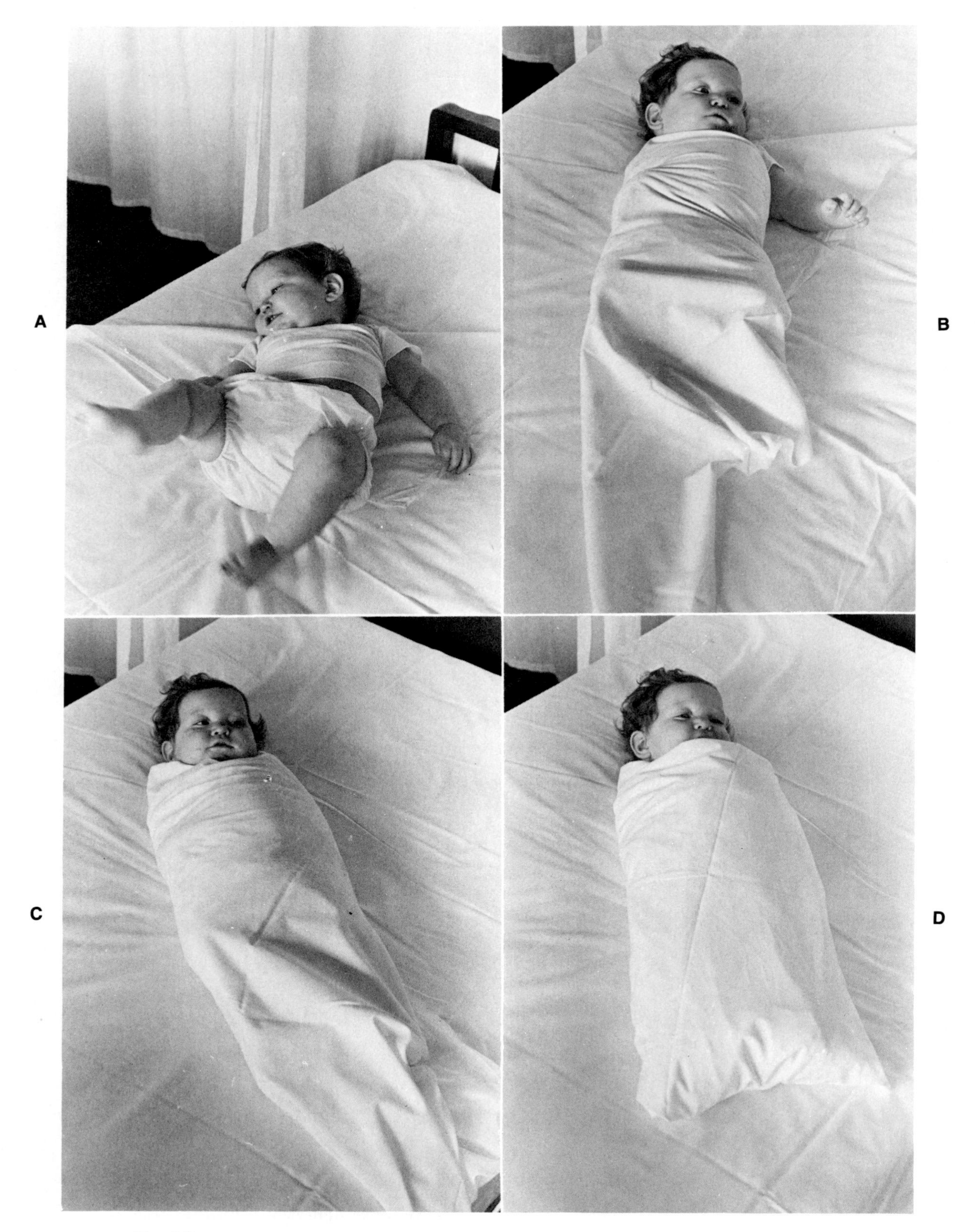


***Fig. 4-5***

From Whaley LF and Wong DL: Nursing care of infants and children, ed 3, St. Louis, 1987, The CV Mosby Co.

| Steps | Rationale |
|---|---|
| f. Mummy restraint (Fig. 4-5): blanket or sheet is opened on bed or crib with one corner folded toward center. Child is placed on blanket with shoulders at fold and feet toward opposite corner. With child's right arm straight down against body, right side of blanket is pulled firmly across right shoulder and chest and secured beneath left side of body. Left arm is placed straight against side, and left side of blanket is brought across shoulder and chest and locked beneath child's body on right side. Lower corner is folded and brought over body and tucked or fastened securely with safety pins (Whaley and Wong, 1987). | Maintains short-term restraint of small child or infant for examination or treatment involving head and neck. Mummy device effectively controls movement of child's torso and extremities. |
| 3. Bony prominences should be padded before applying restraint. | Padding decreases injury to underlying skin. |
| 4. Restraints should be completely removed at least every 4 hrs for 30 min. Client should not be left unattended. | Provides opportunity to assess skin integrity and provide skin care. Areas on which restraints were applied are often massaged. |
| 5. Restraints should be secured so they cannot be undone by client. | When client is able to undo restraints, purpose of restraint is negated. |
| 6. Restraints applied to client in bed or on stretcher should be attached to bed frame, not side rails (Fig. 4-6). | Release of side rails while restraint remains attached can result in injury to client's musculoskeletal system. |
| 7. Wash hands. | Reduces transmission of microorganisms. |

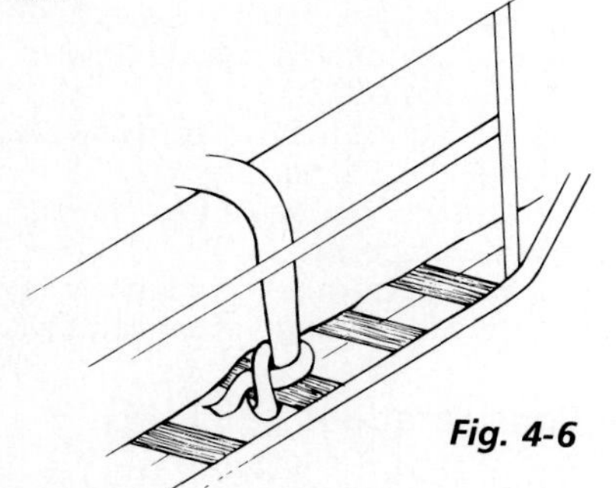

*Fig. 4-6*

## Evaluation

| | |
|---|---|
| 1. Assess adequacy of restraint and presence of any potential injury to musculoskeletal system every 2 hrs. | Timely assessment enables nurse to routinely observe musculoskeletal system and prevent any complications from restraint device. |
| 2. Observe for correct application of restraint every 4 hrs. | Incorrect application of restraints can result in injury to client's musculoskeletal system from falls or muscle strains. |
| 3. Inspect skin for adequate color. Check capillary refill and palpate pulses distal to restraint every 30 min. | Timely identification of impaired circulation related to the restraint device reduces risk of damage to extremities. |

### *Expected outcomes*

| | |
|---|---|
| 1. Client remains in bed or chair without use of restraints. | Continual observation of client's level of orientation and cooperation provides data for determining continued use of restraints. |
| 2. Client remains in bed or chair without use of restraints during daylight hours only. | Evening and nighttime falls are common among older adult clients because of phenomenon known as "sundowning" in which clients become confused or disoriented at end of day. Many of these clients have diminished visual acuity and varying degrees of hearing loss. With less light, they lose visual cues that help them compensate for sensory impairments and they become confused. |

### *Unexpected outcomes*

| | |
|---|---|
| 1. There is impaired skin integrity related to improper or prolonged use of restraint. | Prolonged use of restraints can further increase disorientation and result in musculoskeletal and integumentary changes listed here: pressure sores, contractures, abrasions. |
| 2. There is altered body alignment related to placement of restraint device. | |
| 3. There is increased confusion and disorientation. | |

| Steps | Rationale |
|---|---|
| **Recording and Reporting** | |
| 1. Record in nurses' notes nursing assessment before and after restraints were used, focusing on client's safety, client's level of orientation, type of restraint selected, client's response to restraint. | Documents that client's physical safety was at risk and that specific restraint was warranted. |
| 2. Record in nurses' notes status of client's skin and musculoskeletal system before and after restraints are applied. | Documents presence or absence of any break in skin integrity and status of musculoskeletal system before and after application of restraint. |
| **Follow-up Activities** | |
| 1. Design nursing measures to promote skin integrity and reduce risk of restricted mobility. | Prevents skin breakdown and subsequent decubitus ulcer formation. |
| 2. Develop nursing measures to promote and maintain proper body alignment (Chapter 33). | Prevents development of contractures or dislocations that may result from restricted movement of extremity or region of body. |

## Special Considerations

- Some agencies have very specific guidelines regarding which health professional should order restraints.
- For legal purposes, it is important that nurse be familiar with agency policy and procedures for application of restraints.
- Geriatric specialists believe that nurses skilled in care of confused elderly clients can create safe, comfortable, and structured environment thereby reducing need for restraint (Steffl, 1984; Strumpf and Evans, 1988).
- Restraints are used with elderly to prevent wandering behavior, keep client from sliding out of chair, and to keep client prone or quiet in bed. Indiscriminate use of restraints encourages incontinence (Steffl, 1984; Strumpf and Evans, 1988).
- Clients at risk for injury to underlying musculoskeletal system include immobilized clients, emaciated clients, clients with fever, clients with chronic illnesses, clients with impaired skin integrity.
- Client who is able to undo restraint but remains safely in bed or chair indicates to nursing personnel that restraint is no longer needed. Reassess need for use of restraints daily.
- Frequently some method of restraint is needed for child's safety or comfort, to facilitate examination, or to carry out diagnostic and therapeutic procedures. Restraints are never used as punishment or as substitute for observation (Whaley and Wong, 1987).

## Teaching Considerations

- Teach primary care giver the dangers associated with restraining a client with history of seizures and how to modify environment for client's protection.
- Instruct primary care giver how to correctly restrain a client who is nauseated and vomiting.
- Teach primary care giver to observe for early signs of constriction, pressure, and immobility.
- Instruct primary care giver how to routinely change client's position and utilize passive range of motion (ROM).

## Home Care Considerations

- When jacket restraint is unavailable, create modified restraint by folding bed sheet along bias (Fig. 4-7, *A*). After folding sheet, roll sheet along bias fold until long strip is achieved (Fig. 4-7, *B*). Secure restraint around one thigh and across chest of client. Pass ends of restraint underneath arms of chair and tie in back of chair (Fig. 4-7, *C*). Ties must be secured underneath armrest to prevent client from sliding restraint over back of chair and thus becoming unrestrained.
- Apply limb restraints to prevent removal of supportive equipment (IV lines, indwelling catheters, drainage tubes). Wrap wrist or ankle with soft linen to reduce friction of restraint.
- Form hand mitts out of old socks to prevent removal of supportive equipment and to discourage scratching of skin rashes or sores: wash and dry client's palms, allow client to form loose fist over cloth, and pull sock up over fist.

A
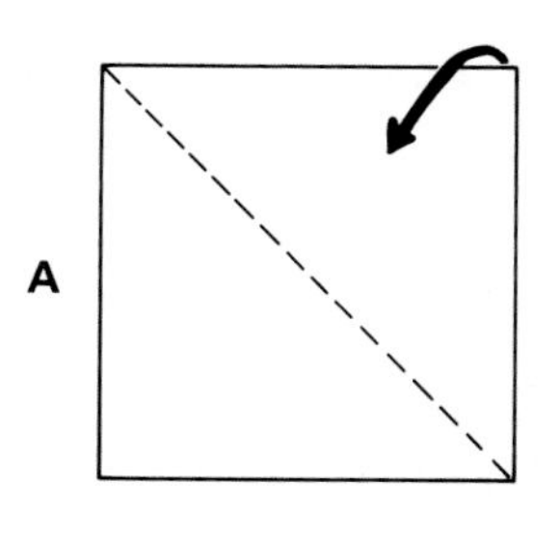
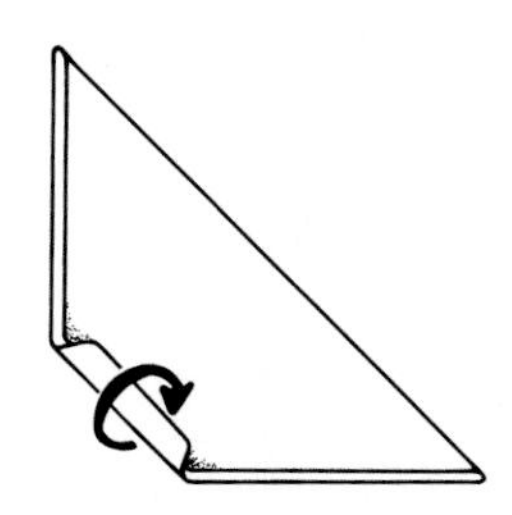
B
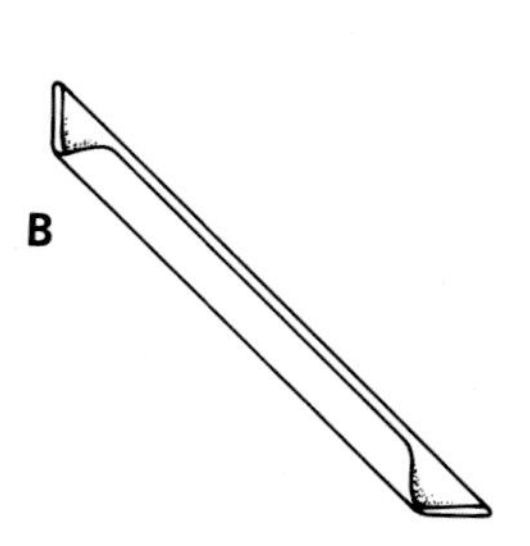
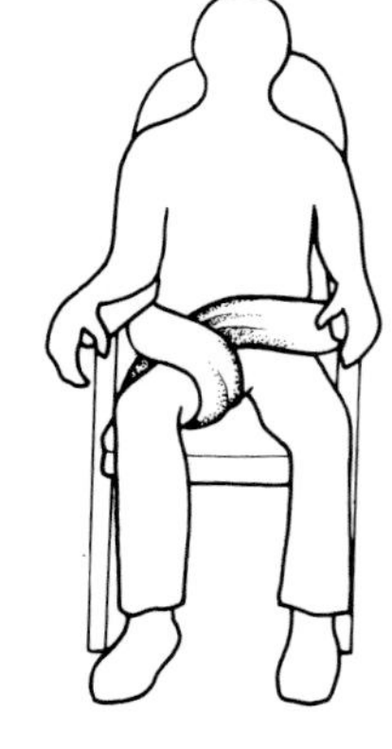
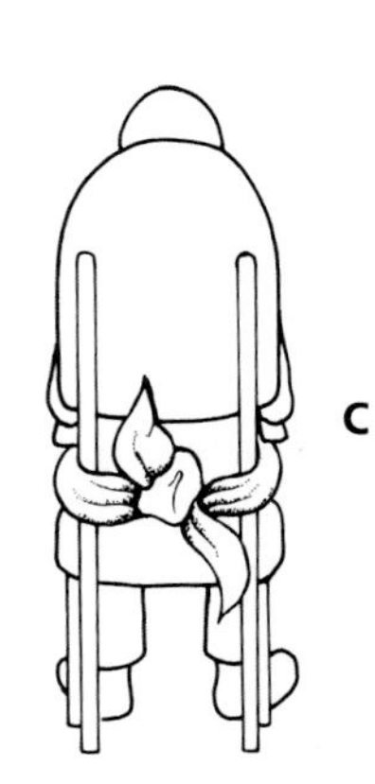
C

*Fig. 4-7*

# SKILL 4-3 Preventing Accidental Poisoning

Accidental poisoning by the ingestion of toxic agents is a common threat to a child's safety. The highest incidence occurs in 2-year-old children (Whaley and Wong, 1987). Although not all childhood poisoning results in death, significant morbidity such as pulmonary complications can follow aspiration of toxic agents.

The child is curious about elements in the environment and frequently puts objects or substances in the mouth. Nonfood substances, such as plants, cleaning solvents, and medication, pose a potential threat to a child's safety. With growth the infant and toddler becomes more mobile and is able to climb and open cabinets that may contain toxic substances. In addition, as fine motor coordination increases the child is able to unscrew bottles, open paint cans, and pry off child-guard tops of medication bottles. No container that holds a potentially toxic substance is safe. Children are capable of opening any jar or bottle and ingesting its contents.

### Purpose

1. Protect the young child and confused client from serious morbidity and death.

## Procedure 4-3

| Steps | Rationale |
|---|---|
| **Assessment** | |
| 1. Observe for presence and storage location of toxic chemicals, cleaning agents, cosmetics, and plants in children's home. | Crawling infant gains mobility as independence and curiosity grow. Infant is also in hand-to-mouth stage and new objects encountered go directly into the mouth. |
| 2. Determine if medications are placed in high, locked cabinet out of reach of toddlers and school-age children. | Child-resistant caps on drugs are required by law, but 4-year-olds and persistent toddlers can open them. |
| 3. Observe dispensing of medicine; toddler or child should be told that it is medication, not candy or juice. | Calling medication candy or juice can confuse young child who may chew pills thinking that they are pieces of candy. |
| 4. Observe for presence of cleaning agents or toxic chemicals in containers that normally hold food (e.g., coffee tins, soda bottles). | Child may associate common food container with safe substance and ingest its contents. |
| 5. Observe for presence of "Mr. Yuk" labels on poisonious substances. | Poison label will be visual cue, even to children who cannot read, that items with such labels should not be swallowed (Woolf, 1987). |
| 6. Determine if there is a poison control center number on or near each phone in home. | Avoids wasting valuable time in event of accidental poisoning. |
| 7. Determine if syrup of ipecac is present in home. | Syrup of ipecac ensures vomiting and emptying of stomach rather than gagging and retching. |
| **Nursing Diagnosis** | |
| 1. Cluster data to reveal actual or potential nursing diagnoses: | |
| a. Potential for poisoning: related to ingestion of a toxic substance. | Hazards for potential injury related to ingestion of poisons are identified from assessment of client's environment. |
| **Planning** | |
| 1. Develop individualized goals for client: | |
| a. Maintain environment with low risk of accidental poisoning. | Removal and locking away of potential poisonous substances in home reduce risk of accidental poisoning. |
| b. Educate family members in making home safe from risk of poisoning. | Reduces risk of future accidents. |
| 2. Keep two 1-oz containers of syrup of ipecac in home at all times. | Frequently poison control personnel instruct parents to administer second dose. Because label directions do not include instruction for second dose, parents mistakenly purchase only one vial. |
| 3. Post poison control phone number and other emergency numbers on or near every phone in house. | Prevents wasting time looking up such numbers if poisoning occurs (Woolf, 1987). |

| Steps | Rationale |
|---|---|
| **Implementation** | |
| 1. Educate parents and babysitters about potential poisonous items in home. | Parents and sitters are often unaware of numerous poisonous plants and substances commonly found in the home. |
| 2. Instruct parents how to securely remove poisons from environment of toddlers and children: | |
| a. Locked cabinets. | It is not sufficient to place potentially toxic substances out of reach of child. Determined toddler or child can climb to top shelf and open cabinet. |
| b. Disposal of out-of-date medications. | Outdated medications can be more harmful if swallowed because of liver and renal toxicity. |
| 3. Instruct children about hazards of poisoning and recognition of "Mr. Yuk" symbol. | "Mr. Yuk" sticker serves as visual cue that substance in container is dangerous. |
| **Evaluation** | |
| 1. Reassess client and family knowledge to determine their response to measures developed to prevent accidental poisoning. | Provides opportunity for nurse to follow up with client and family to determine effectiveness of interventions. |
| ***Expected outcomes*** | |
| 1. Household chemicals are out of reach of children or cognitively impaired clients. | These three expected outcomes objectively document that client and family are attempting to reduce hazard of accidental poisoning. |
| 2. Medications have tamper-resistant packages and are placed out of reach of children. | |
| 3. Children recognize "Mr. Yuk" symbol and relate its importance. | |
| **Recording and Reporting** | |
| 1. Document in nurses' notes specifically what measures were implemented to reduce hazard of accidental poisoning: what was taught, documentation of learning, outcomes of implementation measures. | Provides written record of what was done specifically to reduce risk of poisoning and client's response to intervention. |
| **Follow-up Activities** | |
| 1. Obtain appropriate assistance when accidental poisoning occurs. | Poison control centers are best equipped to inform client or family of specific measures to neutralize or remove poison and if client should be brought to emergency department of hospital. |

## Special Considerations

- Parents and care givers should not try to use home remedies. When ingestion of a dangerous substance is suspected, appropriate medical intervention is immediately sought.
- Removal of poisonous and toxic substances should not take the place of education as a means to prevent accidental poisoning.

## Teaching Considerations

- Parents, relatives, and babysitters should be taught to call poison control or 911 if an actual or suspected ingestion of a toxic substance has occurred.
- Bring container of substance (e.g., cleaning fluid, medication) to the emergency room.
- Syrup of ipecac should be given only on instruction from poison control or a physician.
- Mr Yuk stickers are useful with confused or visually impaired clients.
- Removal of poisonous substances should not replace education as means of preventing poisoning. Child and parent need to learn how to maintain safe environment when visiting relatives and friends (Cooper, 1988).

## Home Care Considerations

- Grandparents, other family members, and friends should remove toxic substances from reach of child.
- Grandparents and friends frequently visited by children should have poison control phone numbers and syrup of ipecac.

# SKILL 4-4 Taking Action for Accidental Poisoning

Accidental poisoning is a risk for the toddler, the preschooler, and the young school-age child. The nurse can help parents take preventive measures to reduce the risk of accidental poisoning. In adolescents and young or middle adults poisoning is usually caused by insect or snake bites. Drug poisoning in these age groups is commonly related to suicide attempts or experimentation with or abuse of drugs. The elderly client is at risk for poisoning because diminished eyesight may cause accidental ingestion of a toxic substance. The impaired memory of some elderly clients may also result in accidental overdosage of prescribed medications.

Specific antidotes or treatments are available for some types of poisons, but for other types there is no treatment. The capacity of body tissue to recover from the poison determines the reversibility of the effect. Poisons can impair the respiratory, circulatory, central nervous, hepatic, gastrointestinal, and renal systems of the body.

Experts recommend that in a case of suspected poisoning, the nurse or parent should call a poison control center, which can provide information regarding all aspects of intoxication, treatment, and referrals. The nurse should teach parents that calling a center for information before attempting home remedies can save their child's life. For example, inducing vomiting after ingestion of corrosive or petroleum-based substances may worsen the victim's condition.

### Purposes

1. Reduce amount of toxic substances in the body.
2. Prevent impairment of major systems of the body.

## Procedure 4-4

| Steps | Rationale |
|---|---|
| **Assessment** | |
| 1. Observe open medication or toxic chemical container in location where child is or was playing. | Indicates that child was at least curious enough to open container and perhaps sample its contents. |
| 2. Determine presence of deep or superficial burns around or within mouth. | Lye and other caustic chemicals result in burns to oral mucosa. |
| 3. Note complaints from child that mouth burns or that something tasted "funny." | After ingestion of poison child frequently will seek out parents or care providers and let them know that pills, liquids, or chemicals were swallowed. |
| **Nursing Diagnosis** | |
| 1. Cluster data to reveal actual or potential nursing diagnoses: a. Potential for injury poisoning: related to ingestion of toxic substance. b. Impaired skin integrity: related to ingestion of caustic poisons. | |
| **Planning** | |
| 1. Note type, amount, and appearance of poisonous substance. | Data needed to determine antidote quickly. |
| 2. Terminate exposure to toxic substance: remove pills, plant parts from mouth; wash eyes and skin with tap water if they were exposed; remove contaminated clothing; in case of inhalation poisoning, bring victim to fresh air (Whaley and Wong, 1987). | Reduction in exposure to toxic substances can decrease overall physiologic effect of poison on victim. |
| 3. Remain close to client and observe for changing symptoms. | Treat client, not poison. |
| **Implementation** | |
| 1. Notify poison control center. | Poison control centers contain information required to treat poisoned client and to offer correct referral to treatment centers. |

| Steps | Rationale |
|---|---|
| 2. If instructed to induce vomiting:<br>a. Infants 0-12 mo—ipecac is administered only under direction of a physician.<br>b. Children (1-12 yr)—1 tbsp (15 ml) of ipecac.<br>c. Adults—2 tbsp (30 ml) of ipecac. | Households should keep syrup of ipecac in an easily accessible place. Ipecac causes vomiting and emptying of the stomach, rather than gagging or retching. Poison control experts recommend these dosages and do not advise inducing vomiting with substances other than ipecac (Aronow, et al. 1985). Vomiting should be induced only under physicians instruction and is not induced with ingestion of gasoline or other caustic poisons. |
| 3. Give oral fluids to assist vomiting:<br>a. Children (1-12 yr)—5 to 15 ml/kg up to 8 oz of water.<br>b. Adults—16 oz of water. | Assists in emptying the stomach and further avoids gagging and retching. |
| 4. If requested to do so, save vomitus and deliver to poison control center. | Laboratory analysis can determine what further treatment is necessary. |
| 5. Place victim with head turned to side. | Reduces risk of aspiration. |
| 6. Vomiting is *never* induced for the following substances: lye, household cleaners, grease or petroleum products, furniture polish. | Vomiting can increase the area of internal burns (in case of lye) and the risk of aspiration. |
| 7. Vomiting is *never* induced in an unconscious victim. | Vomiting increases risk of aspiration. |
| 8. If instructed by the poison control center to bring the person to the emergency room, call an ambulance. | Ambulance personnel can provide emergency measures if needed. In addition, parent or guardian may be too upset to drive safely. |

## Evaluation

| | |
|---|---|
| 1. Measure client's neurologic status and vital signs. | Measures response to nursing interventions aimed at reducing untoward effects of accidental poisoning. |

### *Expected outcomes*

| | |
|---|---|
| 1. Client returns to improved level of consciousness. | Elevated blood levels of toxic substances can result in impaired physiologic, emotional, cognitive, or behavioral functioning. |
| 2. Client's vital signs stabilize. | Return to normal ranges of vital signs provides indicator of response to toxic substance. |

### *Unexpected outcomes*

| | |
|---|---|
| 1. Seizures. | Toxic levels of certain chemicals alter brainwave activity and seizures result. |
| 2. Coma. | Toxic levels of depressants or carbon monoxide can decrease client's level of consciousness. |
| 3. Shock. | |
| 4. Cardiac arrest. | |

## Recording and Reporting

| | |
|---|---|
| 1. Document in nurses' notes or medical record type and quantity of substance, specific interventions taken, and client's response. | Provides written record of type and quantity of poison and how client responds to therapy. |
| 2. Report immediately to physician any unexpected change in client's overall condition. | Indicates presence of untoward event. Early reporting of such observations can lead to intervention that reduces or corrects undesired change. |

## Follow-up Activities

| | |
|---|---|
| 1. Obtain prompt medical assistance when change in client's status occurs. | Provides prompt intervention to correct or reverse undesired change in client's status. |
| 2. Plan education and counseling to prevent recurrence of poisoning. | |

## Special Considerations

- If client is unconscious, immediately call for emergency assistance. Begin CPR (Chapter 18). If foreign body is lodged in client's airway, attempt to remove it (Chapter 18).
- Parents or guardians bringing child to emergency room or poison control center require emotional support during and after crisis.
- Clients at risk for seizure activity include those who have ingested overdose of drugs or insecticides such as malathion.
- Treatment of poisonings is emergent event, and nurse may not have opportunity to completely write nurses' notes until treatment phase is over. However, nurse should keep list of medications and IV fluids administered during emergent phase.

## Teaching Considerations

- Parents and sitters should not assume that by terminating exposure to toxic substance they have treated poisoning and no follow-up is needed.

## Home Care Considerations

- Parents, grandparents, and sitters should never administer anything by mouth to actual or potential poison victim unless instructed to do so by poison control center or physician.

### BIBLIOGRAPHY

Bulau J: Clinical policies and procedures for home health care, Rockville, Md, 1987, Aspen Publishers, Inc.

Bunges ML: Chemical hazards in the household: what every community health nurse should know, J Comm Health Nurs 2(1):31, 1985.

Calfee BE: Are you restraining your patient's rights, Nursing '88, 15(5):148, 1988.

Cooper JM, Widness JA, O'Shea JS: Pilot evaluation of instructing parents of newborns about poison prevention strategies, Am J Dis Child 142(6):627, 1988.

Ebersole P, Hess P: Toward healthy aging: human needs and nursing response, ed. 2, St. Louis, 1985, The CV Mosby Co.

Golden S: Nursing a loved one at home, Philadelphia, 1988, Running Press.

Misnik I: About using restraints with restraint, Nursing '81 11(8)50, 1981.

Nurse's Reference Library: Procedures, Springhouse, Pa, 1985, Intermed Communications, Inc.

Olson M, et al.: Falls: a challenge to home health aides, Home Health Care Nurse 5(5)26, 1987.

Potter PA, Perry AG: Basic nursing, theory and practice, St. Louis, 1987, The C.V. Mosby Co.

Potter PA, Perry AG: Fundamentals of nursing: concepts, principles, and practice, ed 2, St. Louis, 1989, The CV Mosby Co.

Rice MA, Kibbee PE: Review: identifying the adolescent substance abuser, Matern Child Nurs J 8:139, 1983.

Smith S, Duell D: Clinical nursing skills, Los Altos, Calif, 1985, National Nursing Review.

Steffl BM, ed.: Handbook of gerontological nursing, New York, 1984, Van Nostrand Reinhold Co.

Stanhope, Lancaster J: Community health nursing, ed 1, St. Louis, 1984, The CV Mosby Co.

Strumph NE, Evans LK: Physical restraint of the hospitalized elderly: perceptions of patients and nurses, Nurs Res 37(3):132, 1988.

Whaley LF, Wong DL: Nursing care of infants and children, ed 3, St. Louis, 1987, The CV Mosby Co.

Woolf A, Lewander W, Filippome G, et al.: Prevention of childhood poisoning: efficacy of an educational program carried out in an emergency clinic, Pediatrics 80(3):354, 1987.

# 5

# COMFORT

### OBJECTIVES

*Mastery of content in this chapter will enable the nurse to:*

- Define key terms.
- Discuss alternative noninvasive pain relief measures.
- Identify skills appropriate for relieving a client's specific pain complaint.
- Demonstrate ability to assess a client's level of comfort.
- Assist client in positioning and splinting to achieve pain relief.
- Identify common sources of painful stimuli.
- Guide client through a painful procedure using anticipatory guidance.
- Discuss mechanisms by which massage and progressive relaxation relieve pain.
- Correctly assist a client through progressive relaxation.
- Perform a relaxing massage.
- Relieve client's pain through use of guided imagery and distraction.
- Discuss benefits of a patient-controlled analgesia (PCA) device.
- Correctly deliver medication through a PCA device.
- Teach client to use a PCA device.

### KEY TERMS

*Anticipatory guidance*
*Cutaneous*
*Distraction*
*Effleurage*
*Friction*
*Guided imagery*
*Invasive*
*Massage*
*Noninvasive*
*Noxious*
*Pain*
*Pain tolerance*
*Patient-controlled analgesia (PCA)*
*Perception*
*Petrissage*
*Pharmacologic agents*
*Relaxation exercise*
*Sensory discrimination*
*Splinting*

### SKILLS

**5-1** Removing Painful Stimuli
**5-2** Nonpharmacologic Aids to Promote Comfort
**5-3** Patient-Controlled Analgesia

Pain is a complex phenomenon that cannot be defined in a purely physiologic sense. The perception of pain is generally accepted to mean a sensation of unpleasantness having three components. The *sensory-discriminative* component is the recognition of a painful (noxious) sensation. This component involves the individual's perception of pain. The *affective-motivational* component involves the individual's behavioral and emotional responses to the pain experience. The *cognitive* component involves memory of past pain experiences, learned behaviors and responses, and the meaning of the pain to the individual. A helpful working definition is: that pain is whatever the person experiencing the pain says it is, existing whenever he says it does (McCaffery, 1980).

There are several approaches the nurse may use in the management of pain. However, first the nurse must be able to adequately assess the client's pain experience. The pain an individual experiences is personal and therefore requires an individualized approach to management. Through careful assessment, subjective judgments may be avoided. One approach uses pharmacologic agents to diminish the pain an individual experiences. Timely administration is crucial to ensure that the client gains optimal relief. Other approaches use noninvasive techniques that provide a low-risk alternative to the client with pain, an opportunity for the client to assume an active role in achieving a higher level of comfort, and, in some instances, freedom from pain. No single therapy can provide relief for all clients all the time. Therefore, the National Institutes of Health concensus development panel (Emergency Medicine, 1986) recommends an integrated approach that considers both pharmacologic and nonpharmacologic therapies in managing pain.

Providing comfort with noninvasive techniques, as with pharmacologic agents, requires careful attention to assessment and planning. The effectiveness of any therapy will be minimal if clients do not receive what they perceive as helpful. It is important for clients to be active participants in any attempt to alleviate discomfort because they are the best authority about their pain.

The concept or understanding of clients as authoritative participants makes pain control an ethical dilemma. Ethics is a systematic way of making value judgments on human actions; ethical dilemmas occur when there is conflict between values. Pain can dehumanize, destroy autonomy, and create a sense of hopelessness; yet the treatment of pain is regularly and systematically inadequate. The goals of health care—prolonging life and alleviating suffering—often come into conflict when dealing with pain control in the clinical setting. Although pain experience is primarily subjective and qualitative, it is often treated objectively and quantitatively by empirical-minded health care providers who dictate dosage, frequency of administration, and length of treatment. Pain caused or allowed as a result of human values, that is, as a result of nurses' or physicians' attitudes and practices, therefore, becomes a matter of ethics (Lisson, 1987).

Managing a client's pain can be intriguing and exciting if the nurse is knowledgeable about the nature of pain and how it might best be treated. Freedom from pain is not always a realistic goal; pain management, therefore, may have to be directed toward pain control rather than complete pain relief. Although pain management is well researched, research results have not been well implemented in clinical practice. There is still much to learn because of the unique experience pain holds for each client.

The first two skills in this chapter focus on noninvasive comfort measures. Pharmacologic administration of medications through PCA is the focus of the third skill. The skills may be used alone or concomitantly, depending on a client's needs. Many of the measures can be taught to the client and his family for use in the home.

## GUIDELINES

1. Know medical history and type of therapy and medications the client is receiving. Specific types of illnesses or procedures have predictable effects on comfort.
2. Determine client's perception of the pain experience. A thorough assessment of factors contributing to the client's pain will enable the nurse to select appropriate therapies.
3. Control environmental factors that may influence the client's response to discomfort, as well as the effectiveness of comfort measures used.
4. Decide the frequency of making an assessment of a client's comfort. It is the nurse's responsibility to determine the client's response to comfort measures and expression of discomfort. The collection of data leading to establishment of trends and a comparison of changes are useful in making therapeutic decisions.
5. Verify and communicate significant changes in level of comfort. There is no firm guide for the best time to report changes in comfort. However, the nurse who knows the client well can identify when comfort measures are no longer effective, no longer necessary, or when the type and quality of pain have changed.

## PREREQUISITE KNOWLEDGE

1. Principles of body mechanics.
2. Physiology of the nervous system.
3. Pathophysiology of pain.
4. Theories of pain control.
5. Limitations imposed by illness or surgery.
6. Principles of intravenous (IV) fluid therapy.
7. Principles of medication administration.

## PREREQUISITE SKILLS

1. Skills for effective communication (Chapter 3).
2. Proper handwashing techniques (Chapter 37).
3. Dressing changes (Chapter 41).
4. IV therapy (Chapter 23).
5. Administration of IV medications by piggyback (Chapter 21).
6. Care of the surgical client (Chapter 39).

# SKILL 5-1 Removing Painful Stimuli

After assessment of an individual's expression of pain, removal of the painful stimulus may be the approach chosen for management. Although this is a seemingly simple, even obvious, solution, removal of a painful stimulus is often overlooked in the search for a more complicated reason for the pain. Common sources of discomfort are damp or wet dressings, constrictive dressings, wrinkled bed linens, environmental irritants such as the noise of a television, and activity in excess of the individual's tolerance. Maintaining an uncomfortable position for a prolonged period of time is another common source of discomfort, particularly for dependent clients.

If a client is fatigued or anxious even mild irritations can become significant sources of pain. The nurse should always remain observant during any contact with the client for potential sources of painful stimuli.

Removal of painful stimuli combined with careful repositioning can afford clients considerable relief for extended periods of time. The client can often suggest the most comfortable position to assume. The nurse must judge whether any position is contraindicated on the basis of the client's health status.

### Purpose

1. Promote comfort with minimal physical or emotional stress for the client.

## Procedure 5-1

| Steps | Rationale |
|---|---|
| **Assessment** | |
| 1. Assess client's level of comfort (pain relief or tolerable level of pain). | Certain conditions place clients at risk for alterations in comfort, e.g., postoperative clients, those with open wounds or burns, cancer patients, anxious clients, those in labor. |
| 2. Assess physical signs and symptoms of discomfort: | Physiologic response to pain can reveal the existence and nature of pain or need for change in position or environment. |
| a. Acute pain of low to moderate intensity.<br>▪ Increased heart rate.<br>▪ Increased respirations.<br>▪ Increased BP.<br>▪ Pallor.<br>▪ Increased blood glucose.<br>▪ Diaphoresis.<br>▪ Increased muscle tension.<br>▪ Dilated pupils.<br>▪ Decreased GI motility. | Pain of low to moderate intensity or superficial pain stimulates the autonomic nervous system and elicits "flight-or-fight" reaction. |
| b. Severe or deep acute pain:<br>▪ Pallor.<br>▪ Muscle tension.<br>▪ Decreased heart rate.<br>▪ Decreased BP.<br>▪ Rapid irregular respirations.<br>▪ Nausea and vomiting.<br>▪ Weakness.<br>▪ Exhaustion. | Signs and symptoms typically occur with pain originating from involvement of visceral organs and result from stimulation of the parasympathetic nervous system.<br>Sustained physiologic responses could cause serious harm. Most people reach a level of adaptation in which physical signs return to normal. Therefore, a client will not always exhibit physical signs throughout duration of pain. |
| c. Chronic pain:<br>▪ Fatigue.<br>▪ Insomnia.<br>▪ Anorexia.<br>▪ Weight loss.<br>▪ Depression.<br>▪ Hopelessness.<br>▪ Anger. | Client with chronic pain often does not show overt signs and symptoms of acute pain.<br>Signs and symptoms reflect physiologic adaptation and decreased sympathetic response. |
| 3. Assess behavioral responses to discomfort (see box). | Nonverbal behavior is useful in evaluating pain experienced by clients unable or having difficulty communicating verbally.<br>Some nonverbal expressions characterize sources of pain, e.g., assuming fetal position for severe abdominal pain.<br>These responses may not be present in chronic pain. |
| 4. Assess characteristics of pain:<br>a. Onset and duration.<br>b. Location. | Allows nurse to identify possible causative factors from client's description of pain. |
| c. Severity; e.g., ask client to rate pain on a scale of 0 to 10 (*0,* no pain; *10,* worst pain). | Severity or intensity is one of the most subjective characteristics of pain.<br>Numeric or descriptive scales allow client freedom in identifying pain perception. |
| d. Quality; e.g., use open-ended questions such as, "Tell me what your pain feels like."<br>If client cannot describe pain, offer examples such as sharp, dull, pricking, burning, stabbing, gnawing, aching, pounding. | Assessment is more accurate if client can describe sensation in own words.<br>There is consistency in the way people describe certain types of pain, e.g., myocardial infarction: vicelike or crushing, or surgical incision: sharp or stabbing. |
| 5. Assess environment for factors that surround pain experience. | Environmental stimuli can alter client's response to pain.<br>Pain may be aggravated by loud noises, bright lights, strong odors, temperature extremes, high levels of activity. |
| 6. Assess factors that precipitate or aggravate pain and discomfort. | Pain may be precipitated or aggravated by activity, diagnostic or therapeutic procedures, or change in posture. |
| 7. Inspect area of pain. | Clinical observations clarify information received from client. |
| 8. Ask what was used in the past or what client believes will help. | Further assessment may be needed, e.g., palpation, percussion, or auscultation. |
| 9. Check physician's orders for position restrictions. | Client's physical condition may prohibit use of certain positions. |

**Steps** | **Rationale**

### *BEHAVIORAL INDICATORS OF EFFECTS OF PAIN*

**Vocalizations**
Moaning
Crying
Screaming
Gasping
**Facial expressions**
Grimace
Clenched teeth
Open, alert eyes
Biting the lips
Tightened jaw
**Body movement**
Restlessness
Immobilization
Muscle tension
Rhythmic or rubbing motions
Protective movement of body parts
**Social interaction**
Avoidance of conversation
Focus only on activities for pain relief
Avoidance of social contacts
Reduced attention span

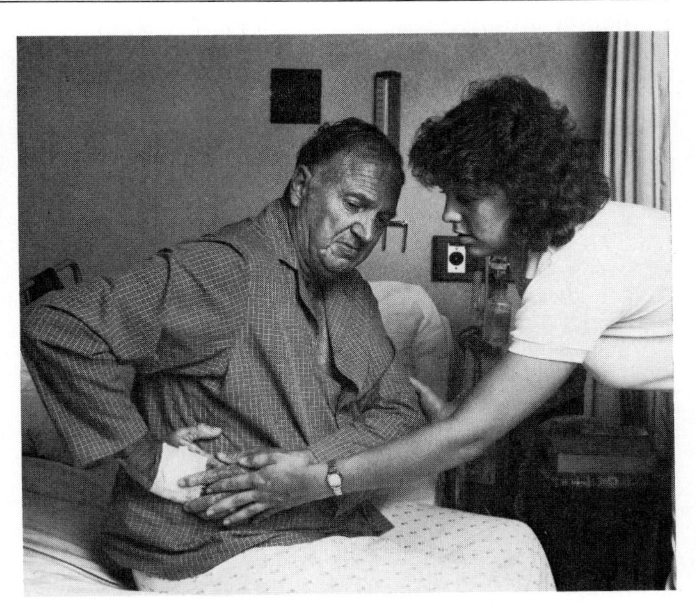

*Fig. 5-1*

## Nursing Diagnosis

1. Cluster data to reveal actual or potential nursing diagnoses:
   a. Pain: related to body position, noxious environmental stimuli, wet or constrictive dressing, postoperative incision, trauma.

   Identification of presence of pain-inducing stimulus or need for position change directs nurse to implement specific measures to remove painful stimulus.

## Planning

1. Develop individualized goals for client based on nursing diagnosis: improve comfort level, help client identify what precipitates pain, and determine what body positions result in comfort.

   Achieving comfort through position change may require several attempts and client will learn over time what is helpful.
   Basic principles of body mechanics apply; what helps one individual may not help another.

2. Prepare environment:
   a. Temperature.

      Temperature extremes can alter client's response to pain.

   b. Lighting.

      Bright or very dim lighting can aggravate pain sensation.
      Whenever possible, allow client to adjust room temperature controls and select amount of available light for maximal comfort.

   c. Activity.

      Prevent unnecessary interruptions; allow for rest periods.

3. Prepare following supplies:
   a. Pillows
   b. Dressings

   To support body parts. May be required if area of discomfort is caused by wet dressings.

4. Close room door or curtain.

   Provides privacy.

| Steps | Rationale |
|---|---|
| **Implementation** | |
| 1. Wash hands. | Reduces spread of microorganisms. |
| 2. Remove painful stimulus: | |
| a. Assist client to position to fully expose area of discomfort. | Improves access to area and minimizes client's need to move. |
| b. Move aside bed linen to expose only area of discomfort. | Maintains client's privacy by preventing unnecessary exposure of body parts. |
| c. Remove wet dressing, if applicable. | Minimizes irritation to wound and surrounding tissues. |
| d. Smooth wrinkles in bed linens. | Reduces pressure and irritation to skin. |
| e. Loosen any constrictive bandage or device, e.g., blood pressure cuff, Ace bandages, upper band of elastic hose, IV dressings, identification (ID) bands, casted extremity. | Bandage that encircles extremity may restrict circulation. |
| f. Remove underlying tubes, wires, or equipment. | Objects apply pressure directly to dependent skin surfaces. |
| 3. Apply splinting (Fig. 5-1): | |
| a. Explain purpose of splinting to client. | |
| b. Assist client to place hands firmly over area of discomfort. | Splinting results in immobilization of painful area. |
| c. Assist client to splint during coughing, deep breathing, and turning. | Splinting decreases movement and subsequent pain during activity. |
| 4. Assist client to comfortable position within normal body alignment. | Turning and repositioning reduces stimulation of pain and pressure receptors. |
| a. Use pillows to support body position. | |
| b. Position to prevent pressure on bony prominences. | |
| 5. Wash hands. | Reduces transmission of microorganisms. |
| **Evaluation** | |
| 1. Evaluate client's comfort level based on original assessment findings. | Determines client's response to stimulus removal and positioning. |
| ***Expected outcomes*** | |
| 1. Client verbalizes full or partial relief from pain. | Removing painful stimulus should result in near immediate relief. Pain may be controlled but not absent, depending on its cause. |
| 2. Nonverbal behaviors reflect comfort is attained. | |
| ***Unexpected outcomes*** | |
| 1. Client verbalizes that discomfort is still present. | Pain may have changed or may have been incompletely evaluated. |
| 2. Client continues to display nonverbal behaviors reflecting pain. | Underlying medical condition may have changed. Positioning over painful site can aggravate discomfort. |
| 3. Client experiences and describes worsening of pain. | Pain complaint must be reassessed. |
| **Recording and Reporting** | |
| 1. Report immediately change in quality or increased intensity of pain, presence of bright red blood saturating dressing, constriction of casted extremity, change in vital signs to nurse in charge or to physician. | If findings indicate worsening of client's condition, physician must be notified so that appropriate medical treatment can be initiated. |
| 2. Record findings of assessment, interventions applied, (including notification of physician, if done), and client's response to interventions. | Documents client's response and provides improved continuity of care for future pain experiences. |
| **Follow-up Activities** | |
| 1. Reassess client's pain complaint. | Pain may have changed or may have been incompletely evaluated. If possible, same nurse should repeat assessment to build on previously obtained information. |
| 2. Review instructions for splinting and positioning with client for understanding and ability to perform. | Splinting and simple position changes can be independent client functions with proper instruction. |
| 3. Implement additional pain-relief measures if pain continues or worsens, e.g., relaxation, massage, imagery, pharmacologic support. | Combined measures reduce pain reception and perception. |

# SKILL 5-2 Nonpharmacologic Aids to Promote Comfort

## USING ANTICIPATORY GUIDANCE

Clients often must undergo a number of painful diagnostic and therapeutic procedures. The degree of discomfort depends in large part on a clients' perceptions of the experience. Perception is largely influenced by higher centers in the brain, and thus the pain experience is a product of a person's past pain experiences, values, cultural expectations, and emotions. The nurse has an excellent opportunity to help clients learn to control their anxieties and fears. Anticipatory guidance is a cognitive strategy that involves use of descriptive sensory words and phrases the client is familiar with to talk through a painful experience or event. The client gains an understanding of what to expect during a procedure. The nurse makes the client as comfortable as possible to eliminate any potential irritants. The client thus is able to direct full attention to the procedure with the end result of improved tolerance to pain.

## USING RELAXATION AND MASSAGE

Modifying the perception of pain, as well as minimizing the reaction to pain, provides a client considerable pain relief. A gentle massage is a form of cutaneous stimulation that activates large-diameter sensory nerve fibers in the skin to prevent painful stimuli from reaching the brain's conscious awareness. The proper use of massage not only blocks perception of pain impulses but also helps a client relax muscle tension that otherwise might increase pain. Massage of a body part is often an instinctual response to pain and thus is a basic but very effective means to control pain. The use of massage often achieves a high state of relaxation that adds to the effects of other pain-relief measures.

Relaxation is a cognitive strategy that provides mental and physical pain relief or reduces pain to an acceptable level. By teaching clients the use of progressive relaxation techniques, the nurse offers the client a sense of self-control when pain occurs. Progressive relaxation may be used independently or with other pain-relief measures. The technique eases pain of muscle tension and reduces anxiety associated with pain. Relaxation techniques often require a physician's order if there is any question as to the stability of a client's condition. A pain therapist often initiates relaxation techniques. The nurse should be available to assist the client in following through with therapy, as well as in timing procedures (such as dressing changes) so that the therapy can be most beneficial. The client's full participation and cooperation are necessary for progressive relaxation to be effective. The techniques are particularly effective for chronic pain, labor pain, and relief of procedure-related pain.

## USING GUIDED IMAGERY AND DISTRACTION

Guided imagery is a creative sensory experience that can effectively reduce pain perception and minimize reaction to pain. It draws on internal experience of memories, dreams, fantasies, and visions; explores the inner world of experience; protects privacy of the client; and fosters the imagination. The goal of imagery is to have the client use one or several of the senses to create an end-result image, that is, an image that consists of the desired result. This creates a positive psychophysiologic response (Droege, 1987; Dossey, et al., 1988). Thus focus of the imagination helps clients change their perceptions about their disease, treatment, and healing ability, which also helps relieve pain, tension, or stress. It is important to choose images that clients find pleasant. The nurse may mistakenly describe images of objects or things that the client fears or dislikes. For example, a scene of rolling waves at the seashore may be restful to one client but desolate or forlorn to another. Imagery may be used with progressive relaxation, massage, or as a distraction.

Distraction is a technique that diverts an individual's attention away from the pain sensation. By introducing meaningful stimuli the nurse helps the client refocus attention. The client's pain tolerance increases as distraction lowers awareness of pain. Typically, distraction is most effective for mild to moderate pain, but with intense concentration even acute pain can be relieved. Characteristically the pain relief lasts only as long as the distraction; therefore, when the distraction is removed, the client may have a heightened awareness of pain. Examples of distraction include music, visitors, television, breathing exercises, or active listening.

### Purposes

1. Provide client a means for controlling pain independently.
2. Reduce pain perception.
3. Stabilize, minimize, or relieve pain.
4. Relieve muscle tension.
5. Reduce anxiety or stress.
6. Promote client sensory awareness.

## *Procedure 5-2*

| Steps | Rationale |
|---|---|
| **Assessment** | |
| 1. Have client identify level of pain or comfort. | Certain conditions place clients at risk for alterations in comfort, e.g., postoperative clients, those with open wounds or burns, cancer patients, those undergoing invasive procedures or dental procedures, anxious clients, those suffering headache or chronic low back pain, clients in labor. |
| 2. Assess physiologic responses to pain or discomfort (see Skill 5-1: Assessment Step 2). | Physiologic responses of individuals vary with severity and duration of pain. Responses serve as means to evaluate effectiveness of pain-relief measures.<br>Overt signs and symptoms may not be present in chronic pain.<br>Physical signs and symptoms may indicate change in level of comfort. |
| 3. Assess intensity and quality of pain: | |
| a. Intensity: ask client to rate pain on scale of 0 to 10 (*0,* no pain; *10,* worst pain). | Numeric scale allows client freedom in identifying pain perception.<br>Allows client opportunity to describe pain from known experience. |
| b. Quality: use open-ended questions, such as, "Tell me what your pain feels like." Seek clarification if description is unclear or uncertain, e.g., sharp vs. dull; aching or burning vs stabbing. | Data serves as baseline to determine change in character of pain. |
| 4. Assess factors related to pain, e.g., environment, previous pain experience, activities, knowledge and experience with scheduled procedures to be done. | Past experiences, noxious environmental stimuli, and activity can affect response to pain. Nurse can control these factors to improve effects of pain-relief therapies. |
| 5. Assess factors that preceded or aggravated pain experience, e.g., diet, exercise, emotional stress. Ask client to describe events leading to pain. Precipitating factors to consider include timing of postoperative analgesics, fatigue, inadequate environmental stimuli, nighttime, immobilization, isolation, end of visiting hours (absence of support persons). | Assisting client to identify what precipitates pain is important for future reference. Allows nurse to control factors adding to client's discomfort.<br>Identification of factors accompanying pain response directs nurse to schedule measures to prevent pain. |
| 6. Examine site of client's pain or discomfort. Include inspection (discoloration, swelling, drainage); palpation (change in temperature, area of altered sensation, painful area, areas that trigger pain, areas that reduce pain); range of motion (ROM) of involved joints (if applicable). | Clinical observations clarify information from client. Site of discomfort may direct nurse to specific types of pain-relief measures. |
| 7. Identify pain management techniques client may be using or has used in past. | Response to current pain management methods must be assessed before planning and implementing pain program. Use of familiar techniques will improve cooperation. Client may be unwilling to try therapy that previously failed. |
| 8. Assess client's willingness to participate in noninvasive, nonpharmacologic pain-relief measures. | Client has right to decide about own care.<br>If client is reluctant about trying activity, accept this uncertainty and provide information regarding suggested therapy so client can make decision. |
| 9. Assess types of activities client participates in at home that may serve as distraction (e.g., jigsaw puzzles, crochet or knitting, board games, music, imagery, relaxation tapes. | Such activities in health care setting will increase likelihood that client will participate. |
| 10. Assess client's language level and identify descriptive terms that will be used when employing relaxation, guided imagery, anticipatory guidance. | Provides clarification of information. |
| **Nursing Diagnosis** | |
| 1. Cluster data to reveal actual or potential nursing diagnoses: | |
| a. Pain: related to invasive procedure (e.g., Foley catheter insertion, blood sample collection, insertion of intravenous catheter). | Anticipatory guidance improves pain tolerance. |
| b. Pain: related to postoperative incision, open wound, chronic joint disease, muscle tension, anxiety, inadequate relief, other. | Potential related factors are numerous. Therapy can be useful for a variety of conditions.<br>If assessment reveals tense, anxious client, it is appropriate to implement relaxation and massage techniques in addition to or independent of pharmacologic support. Client can learn to use progressive relaxation independently. |

| Steps | Rationale |
|---|---|
| c. Knowledge deficit regarding diagnostic or therapeutic procedure and alternative pain relief measures: related to inexperience. | Nurse will explain procedures and sensations client will experience. Client can learn to use most techniques independently. |
| d. Anxiety: related to pain or discomfort. | Anxiety increases pain perception. |
| **Planning** | |
| 1. Develop individualized goals for client based on nursing diagnoses: | Directs nurse and client to identify immediate and long-term needs. |
| a. Pain stabilization or relief. | Provides conscious control of pain. |
| b. Relief of muscle tension and anxiety. | Techniques relieve muscle tension and anxiety that can heighten pain perception. |
| c. Improvement in client's ability to control pain. | |
| d. Promotion of client's understanding of alternative methods of pain control. | Ensures safe measures for pain relief. |
| e. Augmentation of other pain relief therapies. | Combined therapies can be more effective than a single therapy. |
| f. Promotion of effective interpersonal communication. | Important to establish relationship with client to reduce discomfort and anxiety. Client may need to learn to use signals if unable to communicate verbally during procedure. |
| 2. Explain purpose of technique and expectations of client during activity. | Proper explanation of activity results in enhanced client cooperation. |
| 3. If diagnostic or therapeutic procedure is to be performed, plan to explain procedure in advance. | Client will have time to understand nurse's explanations, avoiding anxiety associated with confusion or misunderstanding. |
| 4. Plan to perform technique before client's rest period. | Use 2-hr intervals for rest between pain relief activities whenever possible to maximize effects. |
| 5. Prepare environment by: | |
| a. Controlling lighting in room. | Anticipatory guidance for a procedure: focus bright light on specified area. Relaxation, guided imagery, distraction: use fluorescent lighting if possible. Bright or very dim lighting can aggravate pain perception. |
| b. Controlling distractions by visitors or staff. | Distractions prevent client from attending to pain reduction or pain control techniques. |
| c. Maintaining comfortable room temperature. (Sheet or light blanket prevents chilling.) | Temperature extremes can alter client's response to pain. |
| 6. Close curtains around client's bed or close door. | Maintains client's privacy, helps control lighting. |
| 7. Prepare following supplies: | |
| a. Massage: lotion. | Reduces friction. |
| b. Relaxation: relaxation tape and tape player, if desired. | Encourages client to relax physically and emotionally. |
| c. Distraction: based on type of distraction, i.e., tape player, assorted music tapes, television, books, video games. | Choice will depend on client preference, limitations, or requirements of environment. |
| d. Anticipatory guidance: prepare supplies and equipment for specific diagnostic or therapeutic procedure to be performed. | Choice dictates supplies needed. |
| 8. Assist client to comfortable position for technique chosen. | Client comfort enhances relaxation and participation in skills. Promotes client's ability to relax during procedure. |
| **Implementation** | |
| ***Anticipatory guidance:*** | |
| 1. Use descriptive terms to explain steps of procedure in detail to client. Respect client's limits of listening. | Knowing what to expect helps client cope with painful or uncomfortable procedures. |
| 2. Explain to client approximate length of time procedure will take. Warn client that delays may occur (e.g., in preparing treatment room, transporting client, waiting for physician). | Knowing how long procedure will take helps eliminate anxiety. |
| 3. Prepare by describing sensations client can anticipate during steps of procedure. | Nurse cannot assure client there will be no pain. Ability to anticipate sensation minimizes actual discomfort. |
| 4. Guide client verbally through procedure using terms identified previously (e.g., "Physician is going to clean your skin with a cool liquid."; "Now you will feel a needle stick"; "It will feel like someone is pinching your skin."). | Repetition of explanation of steps during procedure helps orient client to progress. |
| 5. Assist client in returning to comfortable position. | Some procedures require uncomfortable or immobile position; it is desirable to reposition client for comfort. |

| Steps | Rationale |
|---|---|
| ***Relaxation and massage:*** | |
| 1. Wash hands. | Reduces transmission of microorganisms. |
| 2. Instruct client to take several slow, deep breaths. | Increased oxygen can lessen anxiety and prevent feeling short of breath with relaxation. Breaths should be diaphragmatic and deep to avoid hyperventilation. |
| 3. Have client close eyes, if desired. | Client may be less easily distracted. |
| 4. Instruct client to follow verbal cues for relaxation, use calm, soft voice: | Relaxation is guided verbally or by tape until individual is comfortable with sequence and no longer needs verbal guidance. |
| a. Begin series of alternating tightening and relaxing muscle groups: (1) clench right fist, relax; (2) clench left fist, relax; (3) clench both fists, relax; (4) tighten right bicep, relax; (5) tighten left bicep, relax. | Alternating tension and relaxation in muscle groups allows client to feel difference. |
| b. As each muscle group is completed, ask client to enjoy relaxed feeling and allow mind to drift and think how nice it is to be relaxed; ask client to breathe deeply. | Distracts client from perceiving pain. |
| a. Instruct client to repeat each step 2 times: (1) reach with right arm, relax; (2) reach with left arm, relax; (3) reach with both arms, relax; (4) wrinkle forehead, relax; (5) squint eyes, relax; (6) tighten jaw muscles, relax; (7) press head into pillow, relax; (8) bring right shoulder to earlobe, relax; (9) bring left shoulder to earlobe, relax; (10) bring both shoulders to earlobe, relax; (11) inhale deeply and hold breath for 10 counts, exhale; (12) tighten abdominal muscles, relax; (13) tighten hips and buttocks, relax; (14) press right leg into mattress, relax; (15) press left leg into mattress, relax; (16) point right toes and stretch, relax; (17) point left toes and stretch, relax; (18) stretch right leg, relax; (19) stretch left leg, relax; (20) stretch both legs, relax; (21) flex right foot, relax; (22) flex left foot, relax; (23) flex both feet, relax; (24) tense right leg, relax; (25) tense left leg, relax; (26) tense both legs, relax; (27) tense entire body, relax. If muscle group tightens after relaxation has proceeded to other muscles, return to that group and repeat tension-relaxation until relaxation is achieved. | Relaxation response is integrated response associated with diminished sympathetic arousal; decreased muscle tension is desired outcome. Relaxation decreases pulse, respiration rates, and blood pressure and reduces anxiety. |
| b. Calmly instruct during exercise that client may feel sensations of tingling, heaviness, floating, or warmth as relaxation occurs. | Prevents anxiety should sensation occur without warning. |
| c. Continue slow, deep breaths. | |
| 5. Perform massage: | |
| a. Drape client to expose only area to be massaged. | Maintains client's privacy. |
| b. Warm lotion in hands. | Warm lotion is more soothing and less likely than cold to cause muscle tension. |

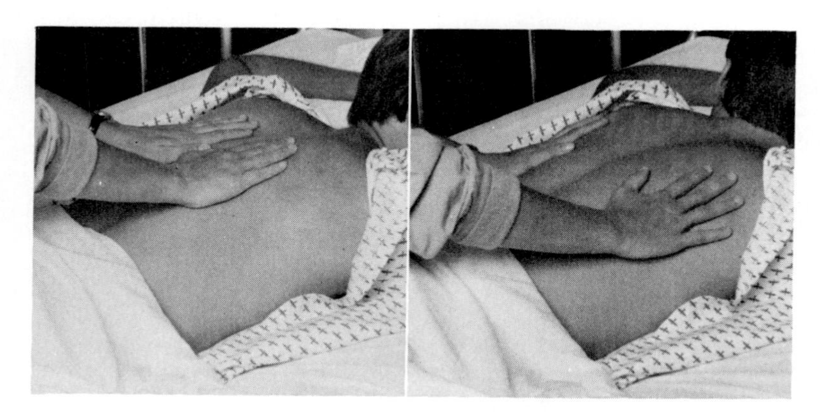

*Fig. 5-2*

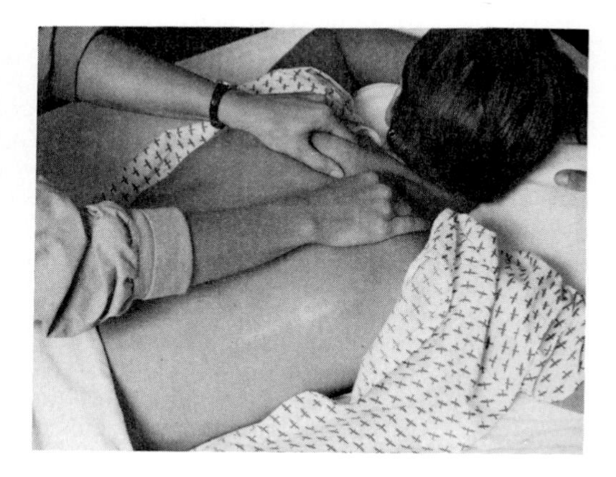

*Fig. 5-3*

| Steps | Rationale |
|---|---|
| c. Choose stroke technique based on desired effect: | |
| ▪ Effleurage (Fig. 5-2). | Gliding stroke used without manipulating deep muscles, smoothes and extends muscles, increases nutrient absorption, improves lymphatic and venous circulation. |
| ▪ Petrissage (Fig. 5-3). | Use on tense muscle groups to "knead" muscles, promote relaxation, and stimulate local circulation. |
| ▪ Friction. | Strong circular strokes that bring blood to surface of skin, thereby increasing local circulation and loosening tight muscle groups. |
| Encourage patient to deep breathe and relax during massage. | |
| d. Massage head and scalp: standing behind client, stimulate scalp and temples; supporting client's head, rub muscles at base of head. | Strong circular strokes (friction) stimulate local circulation and relaxation. |
| e. Massage hands and arms. | Release of tension in hand. |
| ▪ Support hand and apply friction to palm using both thumbs. | |
| ▪ Support base of finger and work each finger in corkscrewlike motion. | |
| ▪ Complete hand massage using effleurage strokes from fingertips to wrist. | |
| ▪ Knead muscles of forearm and upper arm between thumb and forefinger. | Encourages relaxation, enhances circulation and venous return. |
| f. Massage neck. | |
| ▪ Position client in prone position unless contraindicated. | |
| ▪ Knead each neck muscle between thumb and forefinger. | Reduces tension that often localizes in neck muscles. |
| ▪ Gently stretch neck by placing one hand on top and other at base. | Helps relax muscle body. |
| g. Massage back: | |
| ▪ Position client in prone or side-lying position. | Side-lying position is indicated for clients unable to lie prone. |
| ▪ Use long, gliding strokes along muscles of spine in upward and outward motion. | Massage follows distribution of major muscle groups. |
| ▪ Knead muscles of each shoulder toward front of client. | Area often tightens due to tension. |
| ▪ Use palms in upward and outward circular motion from lower buttocks to neck. | |
| ▪ Knead muscles of upper back and shoulder between thumb and forefinger. | These muscles are thick and can be vigorously massaged. |
| ▪ Use both hands to knead muscles up one side of back, then other. | |
| 6. Tell client when massage is over. | Informs and prepares client for inhalation and exhalation (Step 7). |
| 7. When exercise is complete, instruct client to inhale deeply; to exhale; then, to move about slowly initially after resting a few minutes. | Returns client to more awake and alert state. When deeply relaxed, client may experience dizziness on arising too rapidly. |
| 8. Wash hands. | Reduces spread of microorganisms. |
| ***Guided imagery and distraction*** | |
| 1. Direct client's attention away from pain with distraction techniques. | Directing client's attention to something else shields from complete awareness of pain and increases tolerance. Relief continues only as long as client is distracted. |
| 2. Ask client to close eyes or to focus on single object. | Directs attention inward and protects client from external distraction. |
| 3. Instruct client to concentrate on slow, rhythmic breathing. Guide breathing or instruct client to control and concentrate on breathing by thinking: "in, one, two; out, one, two." | Promotes full relaxation. |
| 4. Continue skill using chosen method: | |
| a. Use music client has helped to choose. | |
| ▪ Emphasize rhythm. | Blocks out all other sounds, focusing attention on stimuli other than pain. |
| ▪ Adjust volume as pain increases or decreases. | Provides auditory signal that client controls. |
| b. Direct client to give detailed account of an event or story. | Stress details of event to enhance distraction from pain stimulus. |
| c. Engage client in conversation; encourage participation of family members and visitors. | Visitors can help direct attention away from mild to moderate pain. |

| Steps | Rationale |
|---|---|
| d. Direct client through guided imagery exercise: | |
| ▪ Instruct client to imagine that inhaled air is ball of healing energy. | Development of specific images assists in removal of pain. |
| ▪ Imagine inhaled air travels to area of pain. | Client's ability to concentrate decreases pain perception. |
| e. Alternatively, nurse may direct imagery. | |
| ▪ Suggest client think about going to pleasant place such as beach or mountains. | Direct imagery after selection of restful place by nurse and client. |
| ▪ Direct client to experience all sensory aspects of beach, e.g., warm breeze, warm sand between toes, warmth of sunshine, rhythmic sound of waves, smell of salt air, gulls gliding and swooping in air. | Helps client concentrate and relax. |
| ▪ Continue deep, slow, rhythmic breathing. | |
| ▪ Count to three, inhale, and open eyes. Move about slowly initially. | |
| 5. Provide client time to practice exercise without interruption. | Distraction and guided imagery therapies require level of concentration that may take time to achieve. |

## Evaluation

| Steps | Rationale |
|---|---|
| 1. Evaluate client's physiologic and behavioral response to technique. Observe character of respirations, body position, facial expression, tone of voice, mood, mannerisms, verbalization of discomfort. | Determines effectiveness of anticipatory guidance, level of relaxation, degree of pain relief achieved, and which methods were most effective. |

### *Expected outcomes*

| Steps | Rationale |
|---|---|
| 1. Client is relaxed and comfortable after technique or diagnostic procedure as evidenced by: | Effective guidance before and during procedure assists client to relax and experience less discomfort. |
| a. slow, deep respirations.<br>b. calm facial expressions. | Physiologic response to relaxation procedures and massage is deep relaxation. |
| c. calm tone of voice.<br>d. relaxed muscles.<br>e. relaxed posture. | Distraction promotes comfort by diverting attention from one situation to another. |
| 2. Client verbalizes pain relief. | Although there are objective physiologic indicators to determine pain intensity or relief, they are not as reliable as client's subjective expression (Harrison and Cotanch, 1987). |
| 3. Client demonstrates and describes pain relief measures. | Demonstrates understanding. |

### *Unexpected outcomes*

| Steps | Rationale |
|---|---|
| 1. Client is uncomfortable during diagnostic or therapeutic procedure, requiring procedure to be delayed or stopped. | If sufficiently uncomfortable, client may not be able to cooperate, requiring halt of procedure or technique. |
| 2. Client may be unable to concentrate on technique because of intense pain. | Techniques intended for use with mild to moderate pain. |
| 3. Client indicates continued discomfort: tense posture or muscles, increased or shallow respirations, splinting or holding painful body part, facial grimacing, restlessness or irritability, verbalized discomfort. | Client unable to concentrate on relaxation method, source of distraction, or image. |
| 4. Client unable to describe or use pain relief measures. | Pain may interfere with learning. |

## Recording and Reporting

| Steps | Rationale |
|---|---|
| 1. Record in nurses' notes procedure and technique, preparation given to client, client's response to procedure or technique, and further comfort needs related to event.<br>Record completion date of procedure on Kardex.<br>Incorporate pain-relief technique into nursing care plan. | Documents therapy provided. Data provide continuity of care. Enables nursing staff to continue using effective therapies and provides guidelines to determine client's reaction in future. |
| 2. Report client's response to procedure or technique to charge nurse and to staff at next change of shift. | Directs nurse to continue techniques as needed.<br>Responses to procedure may not be limited to one shift. If further evaluation is necessary, staff members need to be aware of past experiences. |
| 3. Report any unusual responses to techniques, (e.g., uncontrolled or aggravated pain) to charge nurse or physician. | May require monitoring or alternative therapy.<br>Unexpected findings or occurrences during procedure should be reported, since additional assistance or time may be needed. |

| Steps | Rationale |
|---|---|
| **Follow-Up Activities** | |
| 1. Postprocedural client restrictions should be explained to client and family. | Some procedures require client participation or follow-through. |
| 2. Client may desire to talk with nurse about events of procedure or technique. | Talking helps clarify events and reduce anxiety. |
| 3. Client should be instructed to practice relaxation or guided imagery technique two or three times per day. | Practice improves ability to achieve relaxation and increased comfort level more quickly. |
| 4. Client may incorporate guided imagery into relaxation exercise. | Makes relaxation a creative experience. |
| 5. Assess vital signs if dizziness results from relaxation. Encourage bedrest until dizziness subsides. | Dizziness can result from rising too rapidly after deep relaxation when heart rate and blood pressure may be lowered. |
| 6. Continue to provide adequate time for rest between periods of activity. | Fatigue increases pain perception. |
| 7. Do not give up a technique or strategy without adequate trial. Use a combination of techniques for more effective pain control. | |
| 8. Client may need referral to pain or behavioral therapist. Consult with physician regarding referral. | Therapist can individualize pain therapy. |

## Special Considerations

- Individuals may express hearsay about techniques or diagnostic and therapeutic procedures.
- If possible, the nurse who explains procedure or technique should be with client during performance of the procedure or technique.
- Anticipatory guidance:
  a. Do not attempt dialogue during procedure but use brief phrases to provide information and find out how client is tolerating procedures.
  b. Procedure may not be totally pain free but client is able to tolerate brief episodes of discomfort with appropriate explanations.
- Relaxation and massage:
  a. Contraindications to relaxation are not firmly established; research is not conclusive at this time.
  b. Large muscles of the upper arm require more time to massage.
  c. Be certain to massage muscular region, not bones of spine.
  d. If client is unable to tense specific muscle group as a result of illness or injury, omit that muscle group.
  e. Do not use lotion or oils when massaging head and scalp.
  f. If client falls asleep, provide undisturbed time.
- Guided imagery and distraction:
  a. Some clients experience comfort after cessation of distraction; comfort lasts for others only as long as distraction.
  b. Techniques may be difficult with severe pain, are more effective for brief, mild pain.
  c. Pain may have been inadequately assessed, quality or intensity of pain changed since initial assessment, or chosen distraction needs modification.
  d. Client may require variety of distractions depending on level of pain, availability of distraction, and experience.
  e. If client does not like music, substitute ball game or other distraction of client's choice.
  f. Sensation of pain may intensify with removal of distraction, such as when visiting hours are over.
  g. Clients may fall asleep during imagery. If this is not desired, ask client to sit in an upright position, or set timer or alarm.
  h. Image may be vague (i.e., colored light; healthy body image; area of pain is wax, not real body part).
- Techniques may be used in conjunction with other forms of pain management.
- Client may need referral to pain or behavioral therapist. Consult with physician regarding referral.
- If client experiences increased discomfort, stop technique.

## Teaching Considerations

- Clients need information about different pain therapies because participation is essential to successful outcome.
- Some diagnostic and therapeutic procedures conclude with client needing to maintain given position; explain reason and make client as comfortable as possible.
- Sometimes clients experience shortness of breath. If this occurs, ask client to take a deep breath, take shallow breaths, or breathe more slowly.
- Techniques may require more practice before results are achieved. Pharmacologic intervention may be required to lessen pain so that client can achieve relaxation and augment other methods for pain control.
- Techniques may be used as adjunct to other modalities of pain control for clients suffering intense pain.
- Teach client to rest between periods of activity because fatigue increases pain perception.
- Discuss and practice with client possible techniques to use after discharge.

# *SKILL 5-3 Patient-Controlled Analgesia*

Causes of pain are numerous, particularly in the acute care setting. The nurse's awareness of these causes is essential for choosing the best pain control method. Parenteral administration of narcotics is the method of choice when acute or severe pain exists, when high doses of oral drugs are ineffective in providing analgesia, or when patients have obstructive or absorptive gastrointestinal alterations. Advances in modalities for pain control in the past decade include patient-controlled analgesia devices (PCAs), which allow clients to self-administer small continuous doses of intravenous narcotics (usually morphine) as they feel the need.

Although PCAs are used primarily in postoperative clients, they are also effective in controlling pain associated with advanced cancer and sickle cell crises (Panfilli, Brunkhorst, and Dundon, 1988).

There are two variations of PCAs: the electronic computerized pump, which is attached to an IV pole (Fig. 5-4), and the more recent nonelectronic nonbattery-operated pump, which may be attached to an IV pole or placed in a "sleeve" and attached to the client's gown or around the client's wrist (Fig. 5-5). The latter is lightweight, less costly, and more portable.

A PCA consists of three parts: an infusion pump with a chamber that houses a prefilled syringe (infusor), a timing unit linked to a switch or button that is activated by the client to deliver a preset dose of medicine (patient-control module), and tubing that delivers the medication from the infusor through the patient-control module to an indwelling IV. PCAs can be programmed to limit the number of doses within specific predetermined intervals according to the physician's prescription; this prevents overdosing by interposing a "lock-out" or delay time (usually 5 to 10 minutes) between client-initiated doses.

One advantage of a PCA is that it allows more constant serum levels of the narcotic and, therefore, a more constant level of analgesia. Because the blood level is achieved and maintained without peaks and troughs, analgesia is obtained at concentrations below those that produce sedation and respiratory depression (Gaysek, 1987). This results in improved pain control. A second advantage is that fewer postoperative complications occur, probably as a result of diminished sedation. Studies show improved pulmonary function tests and fewer postoperative pulmonary complications (Paice, 1987). Earlier and easier ambulation is another advantage and may also contribute to minimizing postoperative complications. Increased client control and independence is a fourth advantage to a PCA. The device provides medications on demand when the client feels the need and, therefore, reduces narcotic use as a result of immediate response to pain needs. It allows the client to manage pain with minimal nursing intervention and, therefore, also saves nursing time. Clients are not as dependent on the nursing staff for dosing as they are with the more conventional oral or intramuscular and subcutaneous injectable medications. Another advantage is the superiority of PCA-administered medications over IM or SQ injections. One study (Panfilli, Brunkhorst, and Dundon, 1988) shows a significant statistical difference between PCA-dosed and IM-dosed clients: PCA-dosed clients had a smaller mean increase in pain, a smaller increase in sedation, and a smaller drop in incen-

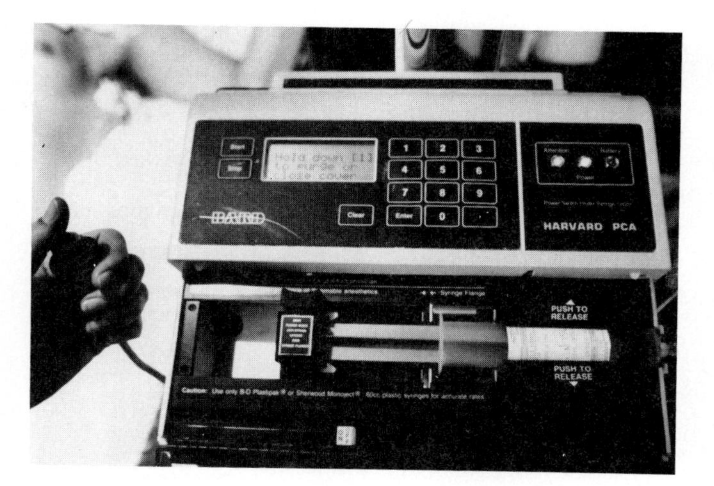


***Fig. 5-4*** Patient-controlled analgesic (PCA) pump.

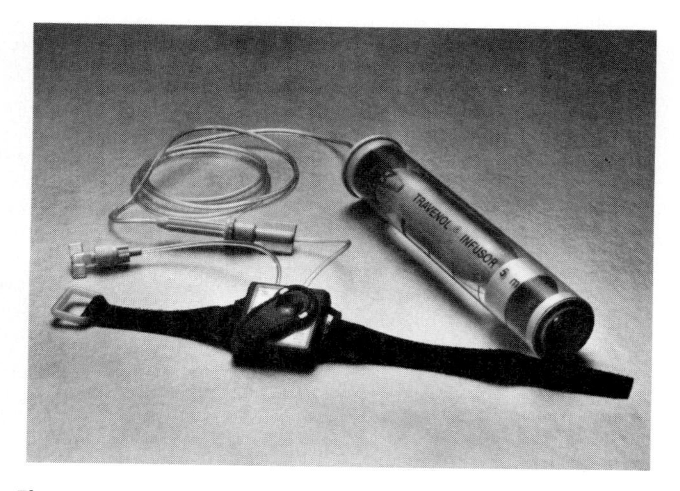


***Fig. 5-5*** Patient-controlled analgesic (PCA) device.

tive spirometry. They were also more able to perform postoperative exercises and had less difficulty with adherence to pulmonary toilet, sleep, self-care, and ambulation. Other studies show that clients discontinue PCA at least as soon as IM injections (Gaysek, 1987). There is also less apprehension and ecchymosis associated with PCA administration. A final advantage is that PCAs offer a more ethical approach to pain control: clients have some autonomy over frequency and timing of the administration of their pain medication and are less dependent on the attitudes and values of health care providers.

### Purposes

1. Relieve or reduce acute or severe pain.
2. Reduce postoperative associated muscle spasms.
3. Provide clients with a mechanism for self-control over pain medication administration.

## *Procedure 5-3*

| Steps | Rationale |
|---|---|
| **Assessment** | |
| 1. Assess comfort level of client. | Certain conditions place clients at risk for alterations in comfort; e.g., trauma, postoperative states, advanced cancer, sickle cell anemia. |
| 2. Assess client's nonverbal responses to pain. | Nonverbal physiologic responses are mediated by autonomic nervous system, vary with severity and duration of pain, and serve as means to evaluate effectiveness of PCA-administered medication. Signs and symptoms include: increased heart rate, blood pressure, respiratory rate and depth; pupil dilation; diaphoresis.<br>Nonverbal behavioral responses are influenced by religion, culture, and beliefs and are useful in evaluating pain experiences. Responses include: immobility; purposeless, inaccurate, or rhythmic movements; grimacing; moaning; restlessness; irritability. |
| 3. Assess characteristics and quality of pain through client's verbal expression. | Allows client to describe pain from experience. Pain is primarily a subjective sensation. Objective indicators are not as reliable as client's subjective expression of pain (Harrison and Cotanch, 1987). |
| 4. Assess environment for factors that surround pain. | Environmental stimuli can aggravate client's response to pain, e.g., loud noises, bright lights, high levels of activity, strong odors, extremes in temperature. |
| 5. If postoperative client, inspect incision. | It is proposed that tissue trauma or damage stimulates peripheral pain receptors to transmit impulses to the cortex to create conscious awareness of pain (Radwin, 1987). |
| 6. Assess patency of existing IV infusion line. | IV line must be patent for medication to reach venous circulation. |
| 7. Assess venipuncture site for infiltration or inflammation (Chapter 23). | Confirmation of placement of IV needle or catheter and integrity of surrounding tissues ensures medication is administered safely. |
| 8. Assess knowledge and effectiveness of previous pain management strategies. | Response to pain control strategies assists in identifying learning needs and affects client's willingness to try therapy. |
| 9. Check physician's order for dose and frequency of PCA-delivered medication. | Narcotic medication administration is a dependent nursing function and requires physician prescription. |
| 10. Check client's history of drug allergies. | Avoids placing client at risk for allergic reaction. |
| **Nursing Diagnosis** | |
| 1. Cluster data to reveal actual or potential nursing diagnoses:<br>a. Pain: related to tissue damage or necrosis, muscle spasm, or tension. | Tissue trauma and reflex muscle spasm result from surgical procedures and body positioning. Cancer pain is due to: infiltration or compression of tissues or nerves by tumor, tissue necrosis, edema or effusions. |
| b. Powerlessness: related to lack of pain control. | Clients who seek control over their situation benefit from PCA: ability to self-administer and manage pain produces sense of control that decreases feelings of powerlessness and vulnerability (Panfilli, Brunkhorst, and Dundon, 1988). |
| c. Knowledge deficit regarding PCA use: related to limited or no exposure to a PCA device. | Proper instruction will allow client to administer medication correctly and according to need. |

| Steps | Rationale |
|---|---|
| **Planning** | |
| 1. Develop individualized goals for client based on nursing diagnoses:<br>a. Improve pain control.<br>b. Increase client control and independence.<br>c. Reduce sedation.<br>d. Reduce narcotic use.<br>e. Reduce postoperative complications. | Nurse and client identify immediate and long-term needs. Provides client control of pain. |
| 2. Explain purpose and demonstrate function of PCA:<br>a. PCA is designed to deliver specific type and dose of pain medication prescribed by physician.<br>b. System has built-in safeguards to help prevent accidental doses or too much medication.<br>c. When medication is needed, client can push medication demand button on timing unit instead of calling the nurse.<br>d. There is no flow of medication between pushes. Explain lock-out time between doses and how client can tell when timing unit is ready to deliver another dose. If pressed before lock-out time is complete, only partial dose will be administered.<br>e. Infusor will be on IV pole, attached to bed clothing or wrist.<br>f. Administers balanced amount of medication to provide comfort and minimize drowsiness.<br>g. If client feels there is not enough medication to control pain or has questions or concerns, check with nurse or doctor. | Effective explanations allow client participation in care and independence in pain-control. |
| 3. Prepare supplies and equipment:<br>a. PCA system: obtain primed infusor and patient-control unit from pharmacy<br>b. Identification label and time tape (may already be attached and completed by pharmacy)<br>c. 18- or 20-gauge needle<br>d. Alcohol swab<br>e. Adhesive tape | Organizing supplies and equipment before implementation of procedure is effective time management; helps assure client that nurse is competent. |
| 4. Check infusor and patient-control module for accurate labeling or evidence of leaking. | To avoid medication error. Damage to system can occur in shipping and handling; inspect to avoid injury or harm to client, self, or others. |
| 5. Draw curtains around client's bed or close door to room. | Maintains client's privacy. |
| 6. Position client comfortably for procedure. | Maintain any postoperative position restrictions.<br>Venipuncture site needs to be accessible.<br>Comfortable position enhances effectiveness of analgesia. |
| **Implementation** | |
| 1. Wash hands. | Reduces nosocomial infections and spread of infections. |
| 2. Follow the "five rights" to be sure of correct medication. Check client's ID band and call client by name. | Minimizes risk of medication error and harm to client. |
| 3. Apply gloves. | Follow universal blood and body fluid precautions: potential contact with blood exists when working with IV. |
| 4. Attach 18- or 19-gauge needle to adapter of exit tubing of patient-control module. | PCA-delivered medication is usually administered by IV piggyback route. |
| 5. Wipe injection port of IV line with alcohol. | Alcohol is a topical antiseptic that minimizes entry of surface microorganisms during needle insertion. |
| 6. Insert needle into injection port nearest IV site. | Establishes route for IV medication to enter main IV line. |
| 7. Secure connection with strip of adhesive tape. Immobilize PCA tubing with adhesive tape. | Prevents dislodging of needle from port. Facilitates ambulation. |
| 8. Discard gloves and supplies in appropriate containers. Wash hands. | Reduces transmission of infection. |
| 9. If client is experiencing pain, demonstrate use of PCA system; if not, have client repeat instructions given earlier (Fig. 5-6). | Repeating instructions reinforces learning. Checking client's understanding through return demonstration helps nurse determine client's level of understanding and ability to manipulate the device. |

| Steps | Rationale |
|---|---|

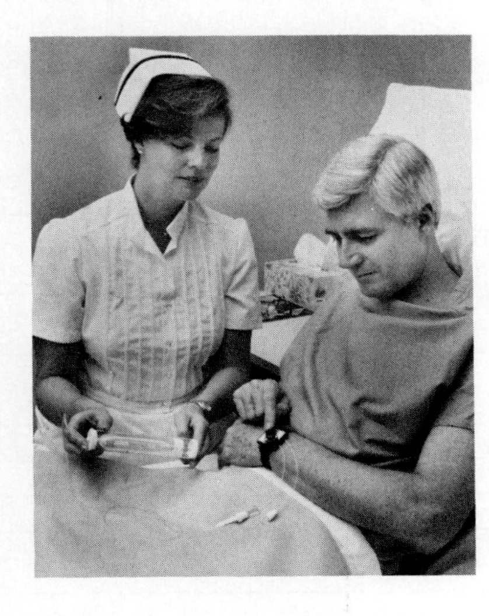

*Fig. 5-6* Client delivers dose of medication.


## Evaluation

| Steps | Rationale |
|---|---|
| 1. Evaluate comfort level based on original assessment data. | Determines response to PCA-administered analgesic. |
| 2. Observe for signs of adverse reactions. | IV medications produce rapid effects. |
| 3. Periodically check infusion rate and condition of site (follow protocol of institution). Infusion rate may be checked by observing movement of the volume indicator on the infusor. | IV must remain patent for proper drug administration. Infiltration necessitates discontinuation of infusion. |

### *Expected outcomes*

| Steps | Rationale |
|---|---|
| 1. Client verbalizes pain relief.<br>2. Client exhibits relaxed facial expression and body position.<br>3. Client alert and oriented.<br>4. Client increasingly participates in activities. | Drug given safely and is effective in providing pain-control. |

### *Unexpected outcomes*

| Steps | Rationale |
|---|---|
| 1. Client verbalizes discomfort is still present or worse. | Underlying medical or postsurgical condition may have changed. |
| 2. Client displays nonverbal behaviors reflective of pain.<br>3. Client is sedated and not readily arousable. | Client may be under- or over-sedated and may need to have dose regulated. |
| 4. Client is unable to manipulate PCA device to maintain pain control. | Alternative medication routes may be needed. |

## Recording and Reporting

| Steps | Rationale |
|---|---|
| 1. Record drug, dose, and time begun on appropriate medication record. Specify concentration and diluent. Note lock-out time (Fig. 5-7). | Timely documentation prevents errors. |
| 2. Record regular periodic assessments of client status on PCA medication record (see Fig. 5-7) or on nurses' notes. Indicate: | Forms may vary from institution to institution, but information recorded is similar. |
| a. Vital signs.<br>b. Sedation status.<br>c. Pain status.<br>d. Status of vascular access site.<br>e. Amount of solution infused.<br>f. Amount of solution remaining.<br>g. Amount of drug received (in mg).<br>h. Number of hr since last status check. | Provides data to evaluate response of client to pain therapy. |

THE UNIVERSITY HOSPITAL
St. Louis University Medical Center

Patient's Dashew

**PCA INFUSOR SYSTEM - DAILY MEDICATION RECORD/PCA REGIMEN**

ALLERGIES: ______ PCA DAY # ______

| DATE/ TIME | DRUG(SPECIFY:Concentration/ Diluent) | LOCKOUT INTERVAL | COMMENTS | NURSE'S SIGNATURE |
|---|---|---|---|---|
| 11/1/88 | 120 mg morphine sul- | 6 min | Dose = 1mg 16 min | K. Thompson, RN |
| 1230 | fate in 60 cc | | | |
| | Normal Saline | | | |

**PATIENT STATUS**

| DATE/ TIME | VITALS RR | HR | BP | SEDATION STATUS (a) | PAIN STATUS (b) | ACCESS STATUS (c) | AMOUNT INFUSED | AMOUNT LEFT | DRUG DOSAGE (in mg) DOSE | # HOURS | NURSES' SIGNATURE |
|---|---|---|---|---|---|---|---|---|---|---|---|
| 11/1/88 1330 | 18 | 84 | 116/72 | 4 | 2 | 1 | 2cc | 58cc | 4 mg | 1 | K. Thompson, RN |
| 11/1/88 1430 | 16 | 80 | 112/70 | 3 | 1 | 1 | 1cc | 57cc | 2 mg | 1 | K. Thompson, RN |
| 11/1/88 1630 | 16 | 82 | 110/70 | 2 | 1 | 1 | 1cc | 56cc | 2mg | 2 | J. Harrigan RN |
| | | | | | | | | | | | |
| | | | | | | | | | | | |
| | | | | | | | | | | | |
| | | | | | | | | | | | |
| | | | | | | | | | | | |
| | | | | | | | | | | | |
| | | | | | | | | | | | |
| | | | | | | | | | | | |
| | | | | | | | | | | | |

(a) SEDATION SCALE 1=AWAKE 2=DROWSY 3=DOZING 4=MOSTLY SLEEPING 5=SLEEPING

(b) PAIN SCALE 1=NO PAIN 2=MILD PAIN 3=MODERATE PAIN 4=SEVERE PAIN 5=UNBEARABLE

(c) ACCESS SITE 1=NORMAL 2=LOCAL TENDERNESS 3=PALPABLE CORD 4=HEAT (associated with site) 5=ERYTHEMA 6=EDEMA 7=PURULENT DRAINAGE

**DRUG WASTAGE RECORD**

| DATE/ TIME | DRUG (SPECIFY: AMOUNT) | COMMENTS (Note: Reason for wastage; if d/c'd chart volume remaining before returning to pharm. | NURSES' SIGNATURE | |
|---|---|---|---|---|
| | | | 1. | 1. |
| | | | 2. | 2. |
| | | | 3. | 3. |

| DATE/ TIME | COMMENTS | NURSE'S SIGNATURE |
|---|---|---|
| | | |
| | | |
| | | |

DISPENSED BY: P. Smith, R.Ph RECEIVED BY: K. Thompson, RN



DATE: ______ RX.NO. ______

***Fig. 5-7*** PCA Infusor system - daily medication record.

3. When PCA syringe is empty, return a copy of PCA Medication Record to pharmacy with used PCA system.
   If discontinued before completely empty, record drug wastage on PCA medication record. Note date, time, amount (in mg) of drug wasted and reason for wastage. Wastage must be witnessed and record signed by two RNs.

   Control and dispensation of narcotics is regulated by the Controlled Substances Act.

4. Report any adverse reactions to nurse in charge or to physician.
   Report client's pain status and response to PCA system during change-of-shift report.

   Reaction may require therapeutic intervention or dosage regulation.

## Follow-Up Activities

1. Reassess comfort level at least every 4 hr or more frequently as condition warrants.

   Client may be under- or over-sedated.

2. When PCA is discontinued or prefilled syringe is empty, remove from infusion port, discard needle in needle box, cap exit tubing and return entire PCA system to pharmacy.

   Control and dispensation of narcotics is regulated by the Controlled Substances Act.

3. Evaluate client's proper use of the PCA. Review instructions if necessary.

   Ability to grasp and follow instructions varies from client to client.

## Special Considerations

- The following are not candidates for using a PCA system: clients with impaired mental status, history of chronic obstructive pulmonary disease (COPD), severe metabolic disorders (i.e., sepsis or severe fluid and electrolyte abnormalities), psychologic disorders, history of narcotic abuse, allergies to morphine (or other prescribed narcotic).
- Because infusor syringe is filled with narcotic analgesia, it must be stored in narcotic box on the clinical division when sent from the pharmacy, if infusion will not be immediately started.
- Some nonelectronic systems must be worn next to the body to maintain correct fluid temperature. Solutions may need to be stored at room temperature before infusion. Follow manufacturer's instructions.
- Determining maximum dose that can be delivered in 1 hour via a PCA is dependent on filling times of medication reservoirs on the patient control module. These times are determined by the model in use; therefore, read the manufacturer's guide to obtain this information. For example, Baxter's most common PCA Infusor System model (Model 2C1073) has a filling time of 6 minutes. When the demand button is pressed, 0.5 ml of drug solution are delivered. Therefore, 5 ml of solution are delivered in 1 hour:

$$60 \text{ min} \div 6 \text{ min} = 10 \text{ doses}$$

thus:

$$0.5 \text{ ml} \times 10 = 5 \text{ ml/hr}$$

Suppose, for example, a prefilled syringe contains 120 mg morphine in 60 ml diluent, or 2 mg/ml. Since 5 ml are delivered in 1 hour (with a filling time of 6 minutes), a maximum of 10 mg morphine could be delivered in 1 hour:

$$2 \text{ mg/ml} \times 5 \text{ ml/hr} = 10 \text{ mg/hr}$$

## Teaching Considerations

- Encourage client to push button on timing unit whenever pain is felt. Tell client not to delay interval if there is pain.
- Instructions are best given during pain-free or pain-reduced states and before initiating therapy. If preoperative client, instruct before surgery.
- Explain regimen to family so they can support and assist client.
- Inform client of pain management strategies that may supplement or enhance pharmacologic intervention.
- Clients need to be alert or readily arousable, oriented, and manually dextrous to use a PCA system.

### BIBLIOGRAPHY


Budiansky S, Carey J, Wellborn SN, et al.: Taking the pain out of pain, US News & World Report, June 29, 1987.

Camp LD: A comparison of nurses' recorded assessment of pain with perceptions of pain as described by cancer patients, Cancer Nursing 1:237, 1988.

Carney R: Clinical application of relaxation training, Hospital Pract 18:83, 1983.

Cook JD: Therapeutic use of music: a literature review, Nurs Forum 20:253, 1981.

Dossey BM, Keegan L, Guzzetta CE, et al.: Holistic nursing: a handbook for practice, Rockville, MD, 1988, Aspen Publishers Inc.

Droege T: Guided grief imagery: a resource for grief ministry and death education, New York, 1987, Paulist Press.

Gaysek J: IV team management of patient-controlled analgesia, NITA 10:142, 1987.

Gedaly-Duff V: Pain theories and their relevance to nursing practices, Nurse Pract 13:66, 1988.

Giuffre M, Keane A, Hatfield SM, et al.: Patient-controlled analgesia in clinical pain research management, Nurs Res 37:254, 1988.

Guyton AC: Textbook of medical physiology, ed 5, Philadelphia, 1976, W.B. Saunders.

Harrison M, Cotanch PH: Pain: advances and issues in critical care, Nurs Clin North Am 22:691, 1987.

Joachim G: Step-by-step massage techniques, Can Nurse 79:32, 1983.

Jones L, Neiswander JA, Perkins M: PCA: patient satisfaction, nursing satisfaction and cost-effectiveness. Nurs Manage 20:16, 1989.

Lederer JR, Marculescu GL, Mocnik B, et al.: Care planning pocket guide: a nursing diagnosis approach, ed 2, Menlo Park, Calif, 1988, Addison-Wesley Publishing Company.

Lisson EL: Ethical issues related to pain control, Nurs Clin North Am 22:649, 1987.

McCaffery M: Relieving pain with noninvasive techniques, Nursing 10:55, 1980.

McCaffery M: Patient-controlled analgesia: more than a machine, Nursing 17:63, 1987.

McCaffery M, Beebe A: Pain: clinical manual for nursing care, St Louis, 1989, The CV Mosby Co.

New gains against pain, Emergency Medicine, p 143 November 30, 1986.

Paice JA: New delivery systems in pain management, Nurs Clin North Am 22:715, 1987.

Panfilli R, Brunkhorst L, Dundon R: Nursing implication of patient-controlled analgesia, J Intrav Nurs 11:75, 1988.

PCA Infusor System: PCA infusor system patient information, Deerfield, IL, 1987, Baxter Healthcare Corporation.

PCA Infusor System: Question and answer reference guide, Deerfield, IL, 1988, Baxter Healthcare Corporation.

Potter P, Perry A: Fundamentals of Nursing: concepts process and practice, ed 2, St. Louis, 1989, The CV Mosby Co.

Radwin LE: Autonomous nursing interventions for treating the patient in acute pain: a standard, Heart and Lung 16:258, 1987.

Watt-Watson JH: What do we need to know about pain? Am J Nurs 11:237, 1988.

Wells N: The effect of relaxation on post-operative muscle tension and pain, Nurs Res 31:236, 1982.

# UNIT III

# HYGIENE

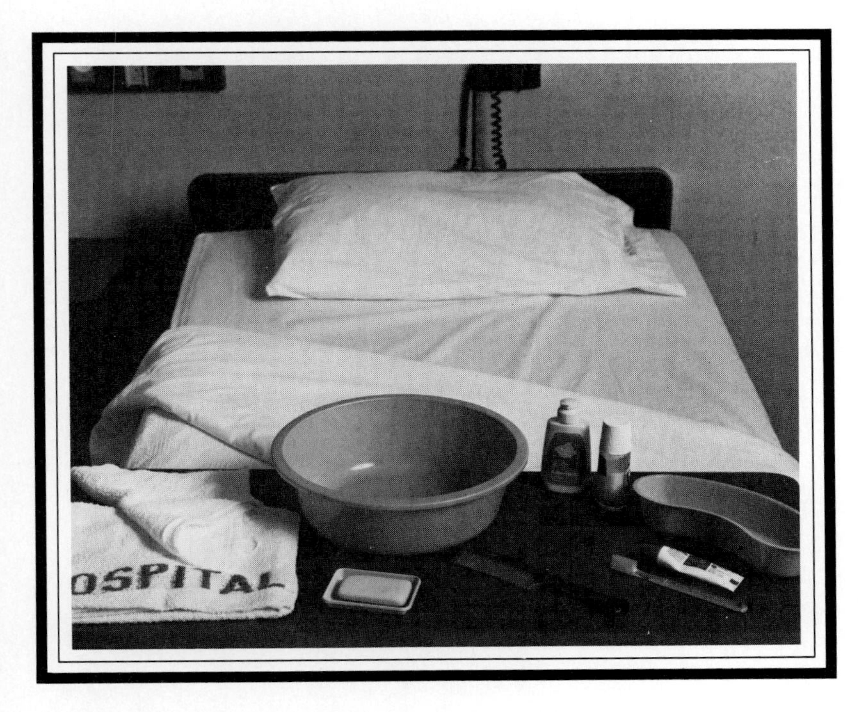


*Health depends in part on the practices a person follows to maintain physical, psychologic, social, spiritual, and cultural well-being. Hygiene is the study or science of health. In nursing, hygiene practices include those measures that maintain an individual's personal cleanliness, good grooming, and the integrity of integumentary structures. Good hygiene is important in promoting a person's self-esteem and in preventing illness.*

*The nurse often works with clients who are unable to meet their own hygiene needs. Infants and young children, the elderly, the seriously ill or disabled, and the mentally ill frequently require the nurse's assistance to carry out routine hygiene practices. The nurse has the responsibilities of assessing the adequacy of a client's hygiene practices and determining the client's ability to perform self-care. As a client's physical condition changes, so too do hygiene needs. The nurse must be sure the client receives thorough hygiene according to needs and preferences.*

*This unit explores a variety of hygiene measures in six separate chapters: Chapter 6, "Bathing and Skin Care"; Chapter 7, "Pressure Ulcer Care"; Chapter 8, "Care of the Mouth"; Chapter 9, "Care of the Hair, Nails, and Feet"; Chapter 10, "Eye Care and Care of Eye and Ear Protheses"; and Chapter 11, "Care of the Client's Environment."*

# 6

# BATHING AND SKIN CARE

## OBJECTIVES

*Mastery of content in this chapter will enable the nurse to:*

- Define key terms.
- Discuss guidelines used to provide proper hygiene care to clients.
- Identify principles of aseptic technique applied while administering a bed bath.
- Administer a complete bed bath.
- Explain precautions to take while assisting clients with a tub bath or shower.
- Record pertinent observations made while bathing clients.
- Administer perineal care to male and female clients.
- Administer a backrub.
- Discuss measures used to prevent heat loss during infant bathing.
- Describe observations parents should learn to make while bathing an infant.
- Bathe an infant.
- Explain the purpose of sponging with tepid water.
- Correctly perform sponging with tepid water.

## KEY TERMS

*Cerumen*
*Debridement*
*Dermatitis*
*Devitalized*
*Episiotomy*
*Exudate*
*Febrile*
*Fontanel*
*Granulation tissue*
*Hygiene*
*Maceration*
*Melanocyte*
*Microvasculature*
*Necrotic*
*Pruritus*
*Tepid*

## SKILLS

**6-1** Bathing a Client
**6-2** Providing Perineal Care
**6-3** Administering a Backrub
**6-4** Bathing an Infant
**6-5** Sponging with Tepid Water

Many clients require assistance with personal hygiene or must learn proper hygiene techniques. Maintenance of personal hygiene is necessary for an individual's comfort, safety, and sense of well-being. The nurse's role is to maintain the integrity of skin surfaces so that cells of the skin receive nutrition and hydration needed to resist injury and disease. To provide proper skin care, the nurse should understand the structure and function of the skin.

The skin is an active organ with the functions of protection, secretion, excretion, temperature regulation, and sensation. Three primary layers make up the skin: the epidermis, dermis, and subcutaneous tissue. The skin covers the entire surface of the body and is continuous with mucous membranes of the mouth, eyes, ears, nose, vagina, and rectum. Thorough hygiene is essential for the integrity and proper function of each skin layer.

The epidermis, or outer skin layer, contains several thin layers of cells undergoing different stages of maturation. The innermost layer continually produces new cells that migrate to the outer layer where dead cells are shed from the epidermal surface.

Bacteria reside on the skin's outer surface. Many of the bacteria are normal flora that inhibit multiplication of disease-causing microorganisms. Transient bacteria that arise from objects coming in contact with the skin are also present. Bathing removes dead cells and bacteria and helps maintain skin integrity.

The dermis contains bundles of collagen and elastic fibers to support the epidermis. Nerve fibers, blood vessels, sweat glands, sebaceous glands, and hair follicles course through the dermis. Sebaceous glands secrete sebum, an oily, odorous fluid, into the hair follicles. Sebum lubricates skin and hair. Two types of sweat glands, the eccrine and the apocrine glands, are distributed over the skin's surface. Eccrine glands secrete a watery fluid that assists in temperature control through evaporation. The apocrine glands secrete sweat in the axillary and genital areas. Bacterial decomposition of sweat from the apocrine glands causes body odor.

The subcutaneous tissue layer contains blood vessels, nerves, lymph, and loose connective tissue filled with fat cells. Fatty tissue serves to insulate the body. Subcutane-

***TABLE 6-1*** Common Skin Problems

| Problem | Characteristics | Implications | Interventions |
|---|---|---|---|
| **Dry skin** | Flaky, rough texture on exposed areas such as hands, arms, legs, or face. | Skin may become infected if epidermal layer is allowed to crack. | Bathe less frequently. Rinse body of all soap well, because residue left on skin can cause irritation and breakdown. Add moisture to air through use of humidifier. Increase fluid intake when skin is dry. Use moisturizing lotion to aid healing process; lotion forms protective barrier and helps maintain fluid within skin. Use creams to clean skin that is dry or allergic to soaps and detergents. |
| **Acne** | Inflammatory, papulopustular skin eruption, usually involving bacterial breakdown of sebum; appears on face, neck, shoulders, and back. | Infected material within pustule can spread if area is squeezed or picked. Permanent scarring can result. | Wash hair and skin each day with hot water and soap to remove oil. Use cosmetics sparingly because oily cosmetics or creams accumulate in pores and tend to make condition worse. Dietary restrictions may need to be implemented. Foods found to aggravate condition should be eliminated from diet. Exposure to ultraviolet rays, either from sunshine or a heat lamp, may help control acne; use caution to prevent burning of skin. Use prescribed topical antibiotics for severe forms of acne. |
| **Hirsutism** | Excessive growth of body and facial hair, especially in women. | Hirsutism may cause negative body image by giving female a male appearance. | The following may be used to remove unwanted hair: depilatories (can cause infection, rashes, or dermatitis), shaving (safest method), electrolysis (permanently removes hair by destroying hair follicles), tweezing (lasts only temporarily), and bleaching of hair (last only temporarily). |
| **Skin rashes** | Skin eruption that may result from overexposure to sun or moisture or from allergic reaction; may be flat or raised, localized or systemic pruritic or nonpruritic. | If skin is continually scratched, inflammation and infection may occur. Rashes can also cause discomfort. | Wash area thoroughly and apply antiseptic spray or lotion to prevent further itching and aid healing process. Warm soaks may relieve inflammation. |
| **Contact dermatitis** | Inflammation of skin characterized by abrupt onset with erythema, pruritus, pain, and appearance of scaly oozing lesions; seen on face, neck, hands, forearms, and genitalia. | Dermatitis is often difficult to eliminate because person is usually in continual contact with substance causing skin reaction. Substance may be hard to identify. | Condition usually disappears when exposure to causative agents (e.g., cleansers and soaps) is avoided. |
| **Abrasion** | Scraping or rubbing away of epidermis; may result in localized bleeding and later weeping of serous fluid. | Infection occurs easily as a result of loss of protective skin layer. | Nurses should be careful not to scratch clients with jewelry or fingernails. Wash abrasions with mild soap and water. Dressing or bandage could increase risk of infection because of retained moisture. |

ous tissue also provides support for upper skin layers.

Because a portion of the skin is usually exposed to environmental irritants and because the skin is an active organ sensitive to physiologic changes within the body, some skin problems commonly occur (Table 6-1). The nurse should assess for the presence of such conditions while providing hygiene and suggest measures to alleviate the symptoms of these conditions. The client is always the best resource to explain the nature and course of skin problems as they develop. Skin problems can cause changes that affect a client's appearance and body image. The nurse should be sensitive to the client's feelings while attempting to care for a skin problem.

## GUIDELINES

1. Bathe any body part as soon as it becomes soiled. Problems such as incontinence, wound drainage, or excess diaphoresis may require bathing several times a day.
2. Attempt to provide baths during the time of day that the client prefers.
3. Protect clients from injury by controlling the bathwater temperature.
4. Wear gloves whenever there is risk of contacting body fluids, such as fecal material, perineal discharge, or wound drainage.
5. Control environmental factors that may alter skin in-

tegrity, such as moisture, heat, and external sources of pressure (wrinkled bed linen, improperly placed drainage tubing).

6. Encourage clients to participate in bathing and skin care to maintain independence with self-care.

## PREREQUISITE KNOWLEDGE

1. Principles of medical asepsis.
2. Principles of safety.
3. Principles of body mechanics and positioning clients.
4. Anatomic structure of body parts.
5. Mechanisms of temperature regulation (Skill 6-5).

## PREREQUISITE SKILLS

1. Proper handwashing techniques (Chapter 37).
2. Physical assessment of the skin and external genitalia (Chapter 13).
3. Assessment of vital signs (Skills 6-3 and 6-5; see Chapter 12).

# *SKILL 6-1 Bathing a Client*

Nurses provide two categories of baths: cleansing and therapeutic. Cleansing baths are usually given early in the morning before scheduled tests or procedures. However, clients may prefer bathing in the evening if this is their routine at home. The type of cleansing bath a nurse provides depends on the client's physical capabilities and the degree of hygiene required. The nurse is responsible for assessing what type of bath is most appropriate for the client's needs.

Types of cleansing baths include:

- *Complete bed bath*—Administered to clients who are totally dependent. The nurse gives the bath with the client in bed.
- *Partial bed bath*—Consists of bathing only body parts that would cause discomfort if left unbathed. Dependent clients in need of partial hygiene or self-sufficient bedridden clients who are unable to reach all body parts receive a partial bed bath.
- *Tub bath*—Client is immersed into a tub of water. The tub bath allows more thorough washing and rinsing than a bed bath. Client may still require the nurse's assistance. There are tubs available to lift dependent clients into the water.
- *Shower*—Client sits or stands under a continuous stream of water. The shower provides more thorough cleansing than a bed bath.

Therapeutic baths are generally ordered by physicians for a specific therapeutic effect. Types of therapeutic baths include:

- *Sitz bath*—Cleanses and reduces inflammation of perineal and anal areas of client who has undergone rectal or perineal surgery or childbirth, or who has local irritation from hemorrhoids or fissures. The client sits in a special tub or basin.
- *Tepid sponge or cooling bath*—Client is immersed in a tub or sponged with tepid water, especially effective in reducing client's body temperature.
- *Medicated baths (oatmeal, cornstarch, sodium bicarbonate, Burow's solution)*—Aid in relief of skin irritation and create an antibacterial and drying effect. Oatmeal has added effect of softening and lubricating the skin.

## Purposes

1. Cleanse the skin.
2. Stimulate circulation.
3. Improve client self-image.
4. Reduce body odors.
5. Promote exercise through joint range of motion (ROM).

## *Procedure 6-1*

| Steps | Rationale |
|---|---|
| **Assessment** | |
| 1. Assess client's tolerance of activity, level of discomfort, cognitive ability, and musculoskeletal function. | Determines client's ability to perform self-care and level of assistance required from nurse. Also determines type of bath to administer, e.g., tub bath or partial bed bath. |
| 2. Assess client's bathing preferences: frequency of and time of day bathing preferred, type of hygiene products used. | Client participates in plan of care. Promotes client's comfort and willingness to cooperate. |
| 3. Ask if client has noticed any problems related to condition of skin. | Allows nurse to direct physical assessment of skin during bathing. |

| Steps | Rationale |
|---|---|
| 4. Identify risks for skin impairment: | Certain conditions increase likelihood of injury to skin or skin breakdown, necessitating more thorough hygiene. |
| a. Immobilized clients (e.g., clients who have paralysis, large casts, or traction, or who are weakened or disabled). | Dependent body parts are exposed to pressure from underlying surfaces. |
| b. Reduced sensation (e.g., circulatory insufficiency, local nerve damage). | Minimizes client's ability to sense injury to skin's surface. |
| c. Nutritional alterations. | Clients with limited caloric and protein intake have impaired tissue synthesis. |
| d. Excessive secretion or excretion on skin, particularly on skin surfaces that rub against each other (under breasts or in perineal area). | Moisture on skin's surface is medium for bacterial growth and causes softening of epidermal cells. |
| e. Vascular insufficiency. | Causes ischemia and breakdown of skin. |
| f. External devices applied to or around skin (e.g., casts, braces, restraints, dressings). | Causes pressure or friction against skin's surface. |
| g. Elderly clients. | Elderly persons may be susceptible to dry skin because of reduced sebaceous gland activity, thinning of epidermis, and poor fluid intake. |
| 5. Assess client's knowledge of skin hygiene in terms of its importance, preventive measures to take, and common problems encountered (Table 6-1). | Determines client's learning needs. |
| 6. Check physician's therapeutic bath order for type of solution, length of time for bath, temperature of solution, body part to be attended. | Therapeutic baths are ordered for specific physical effect. |
| 7. Review orders for specific precautions concerning client's movement or positioning. | Prevent accidental injury to client during bathing activities. Determines level of assistance required by client. |

## Nursing Diagnosis

| Steps | Rationale |
|---|---|
| 1. Cluster data to reveal actual or potential nursing diagnoses: | |
| a. Self-care deficit, bathing or hygiene: related to physical constraints. | Nurse may need to provide total bed bath or offer frequent assistance to client. |
| b. Impaired skin integrity: related to chemical irritant or pressure. | Bathing is a therapy for lubricating and cleansing areas of skin breakdown. |
| c. Potential impaired skin integrity: related to dependent position, body secretions. | Bathing removes secretions or drainage that increase risk of skin breakdown. Turning and positioning during bathing relieves pressure on bony prominences. |
| d. Activity intolerance: related to physical constraints. | Nurse provides total or partial bed bath when client's physical condition prohibits active exercise. |

## Planning

| Steps | Rationale |
|---|---|
| 1. Develop individualized goals for client based on nursing diagnoses: | |
| a. Skin integrity maintained. | Skin surface is cleansed. |
| b. Joint ROM maintained. | Joints are moved through ROM during bathing. |
| c. Client achieves sense of comfort and well-being without fatigue. | Warm bath is relaxing. Nurse assists at a level to minimize client's over-exertion. |
| d. Client participates in and understands methods of skin care. | Bathing is time to discuss hygiene measures and allow client to participate in self-care. |
| 2. Explain procedure and ask client for suggestions or ways to prepare supplies. If partial bath, ask how much of bath client wishes to complete. | Promotes client's cooperation and participation. |
| 3. If shower or tub bath, schedule use of facilities if private bath unavailable. | Prevents unnecessary waiting that can cause client's fatigue. |
| 4. Adjust room temperature and ventilation, and close room doors and windows. | Warm room, free of drafts, prevents rapid loss of body heat during bathing. |
| 5. Draw room divider curtain or close door. | Privacy ensures client's mental and physical comfort. |
| 6. Prepare necessary equipment and supplies: | |
| a. Two bath towels | Separate towel and washcloth are used for face and client's body to enhance feeling of cleanliness. |
| b. Two washcloths | |
| c. Washbasin (for complete or partial bed bath) | |
| d. Soap and soap dish | |
| e. Bath blanket (for complete or partial bed bath) | Bath blanket maintains client's warmth during procedure. |
| f. Clean gown or pajamas | |

| Steps | Rationale |
|---|---|
| g. Hygienic aids, such as skin lotion, deodorant, and powder | |
| h. Bedpan or urinal | For client's use before bath. |
| i. Linen hamper or laundry bag | |
| j. Disposable gloves | Prevents contact with potentially infected body secretions. |

## Implementation

### *Complete or partial bed bath*

| Steps | Rationale |
|---|---|
| 1. Offer client bedpan or urinal. Provide towel and washcloth. | Client will feel more comfortable after voiding. Prevents interruption of bath. |
| 2. Wash hands. | Reduces transmission of microorganisms. |
| 3. Lower side rail and assist client in assuming comfortable position maintaining body alignment. | Aids nurse's access to client. Maintains client's comfort throughout procedure. |
| 4. Bring client toward side closest to you. Place hospital bed in high position. | Nurse does not have to reach across bed; strain on back muscles is minimized. |
| 5. Loosen top covers at foot of bed. Place bath blanket over top sheet. Fold and remove top sheet from under blanket. If possible, have client hold bath blanket while withdrawing sheet. | Removal of top linens prevents their becoming soiled or moist during bath. Blanket provides warmth and privacy. |
| 6. If top sheet is to be reused, fold it for replacement later. If not, dispose in laundry bag, taking care not to allow linen to contact your uniform. | Proper disposal prevents transmission of microorganisms. |
| 7. Remove client's gown or pajamas. If an extremity is injured or has reduced mobility, begin removal from *unaffected* side. If client has intravenous (IV) tube, remove gown from arm *without* IV first, then lower IV container and slide gown covering affected arm over tubing and container. Rehang IV container and check flow rate (Fig. 6-1). | Provides full exposure of body parts during bathing. Undressing unaffected side first allows easier manipulation of gown over body part with reduced ROM. |
| 8. Pull side rail up. Fill washbasin two-thirds full with water between 43°-46° C (110°-115° F). Have client place fingers in water to test temperature tolerance. OPTION: Place plastic container of bath lotion in bath water. | Raising side rail maintains client's safety as nurse leaves bedside. Warm water promotes comfort, relaxes muscles, and prevents unnecessary chilling. Testing temperature prevents accidental burning of client's skin. Bath water warms lotion for application to client's skin. |
| 9. Remove pillow if allowed and raise head of bed 30-45 degrees. Place bath towel under client's head. | Removal of pillow makes it easier to wash client's ears and neck. Placement of towel prevents soiling of bed linen. |
| 10. Place bath towel over client's chest. | Prevents soiling of bath blanket. |
| 11. Fold washcloth around fingers of your hand to form a mitt (Fig. 6-2). Immerse mitt in water and wring thoroughly. | Mitt retains water and heat better than loosely held washcloth, keeps cold edges from brushing against client, and prevents splashing. |
| 12. Wash client's eyes with plain warm water. Use different section of mitt for each eye. Move mitt from inner to outer canthus (Fig. 6-3). Soak any crustations on eyelid for 2-3 min with damp cloth before attempting removal. Dry eye thoroughly but gently. | Soap irritates eyes. Use of separate sections of mitt reduces infection transmission. Bathing eye from inner to outer canthus prevents secretions from entering nasolacrimal duct. Pressure can cause internal injury. |

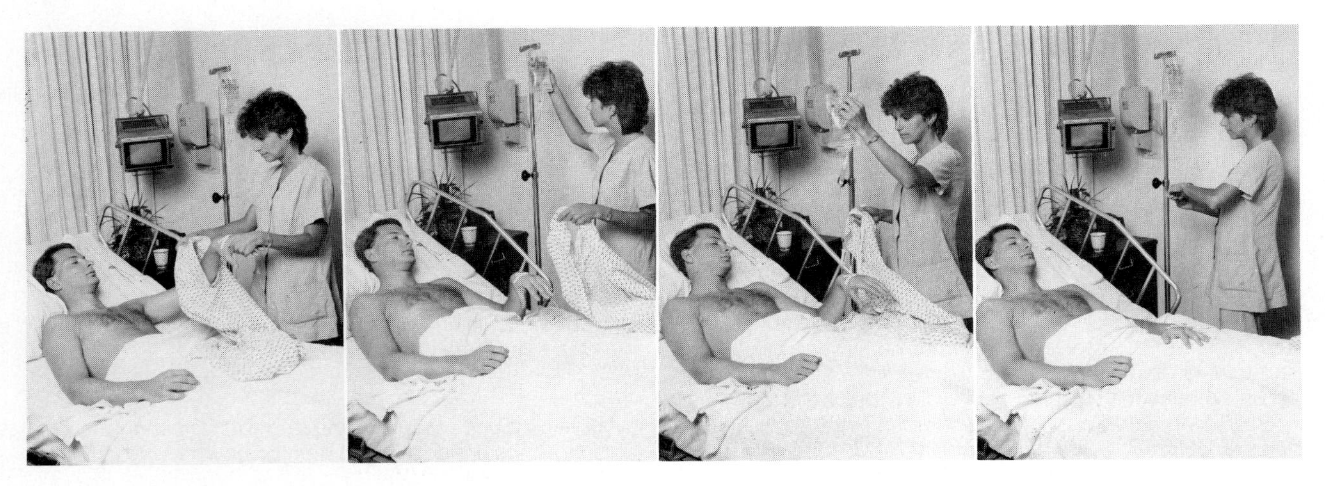

***Fig. 6-1***

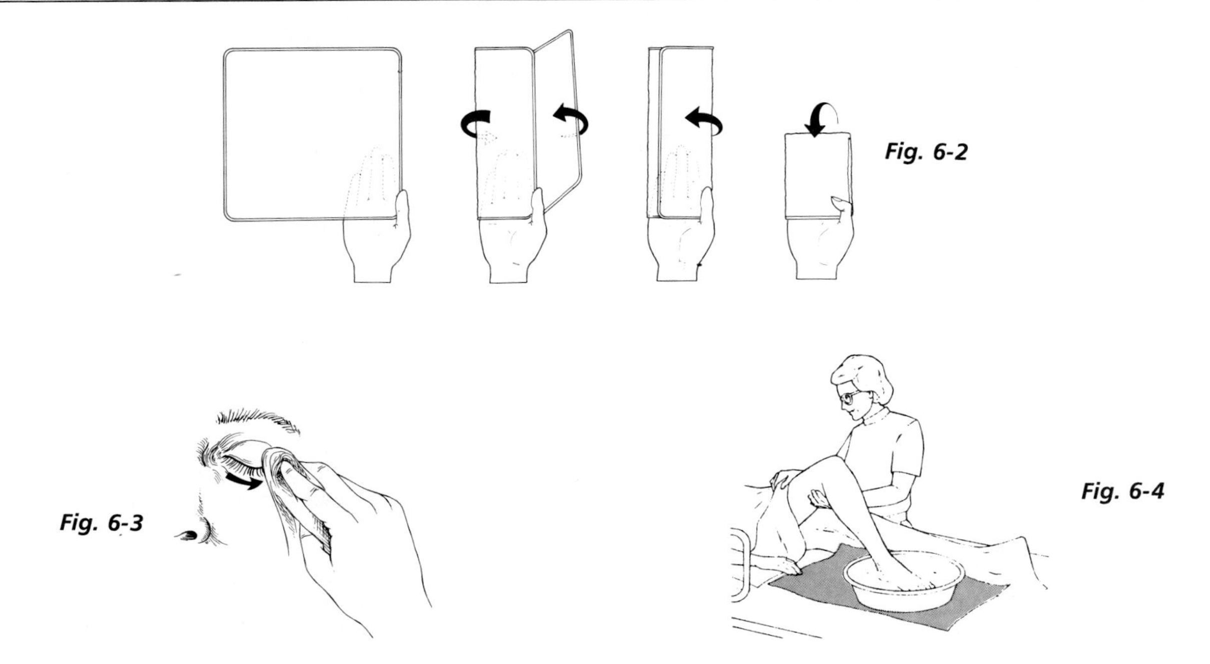

*Fig. 6-2*

*Fig. 6-3*

*Fig. 6-4*

| Steps | Rationale |
|---|---|
| 13. Ask if client prefers to use soap on face. Wash, rinse, and dry well forehead, cheeks, nose, neck, and ears. (Men may wish to shave at this point or after bath). | Soap tends to dry face, which is exposed to air more than other body parts. |
| 14. Remove bath blanket from over client's arm that is farthest from you. Place bath towel lengthwise under arm. OPTION: Raise side rail and move to other side to wash arm. | Bathing far side first prevents reaching over clean area. |
| 15. Lower side rail. Bathe arm with soap and water using long, firm strokes from distal to proximal areas (Fingers to axilla). Raise and support arm above head (if possible) while thoroughly washing axilla. | Soap lowers surface tension and facilitates removal of debris and bacteria when friction is applied during washing. Long, firm strokes stimulate circulation. Movement of arm exposes axilla and exercises joint's normal ROM. |
| 16. Rinse and dry arm and axilla thoroughly. If client uses deodorant or talcum powder, apply it. | Excess moisture causes skin maceration or softening. Deodorant controls body odor. |
| 17. Fold bath towel in half and lay it on bed beside client. Place basin on towel. Immerse client's hand in water. Allow hand to soak for 3-5 min before washing hand and fingernails (see Procedure 9-4). Remove basin and dry hand well. | Soaking softens cuticles and calluses of hand, loosens debris beneath nails, and enhances feeling of cleanliness. Thorough drying removes moisture from between fingers. |
| 18. Repeat Steps 14-17 for other arm. | |
| 19. Check temperature of bath water and change water if necessary. | Warm water maintains client's comfort. |
| 20. Cover client's chest with bath towel and fold bath blanket down to umbilicus. | Prevents unnecessary exposure of body parts. |
| 21. With one hand, lift edge of towel away from chest. With mitted hand, bathe chest using long, firm strokes. Take special care to wash skinfolds under female client's breasts. It may be necessary to lift breast upward while bathing underneath it. Keep client's chest covered between wash and rinse periods. Dry well. | Towel maintains warmth and privacy. Secretions and dirt collect easily in areas of tight skin folds. |
| 22. Place bath towel lengthwise over chest and abdomen. (Two towels may be needed.) Fold blanket down to just above pubic region. | Prevents chilling and exposure of body parts. |
| 23. With one hand, lift bath towel. With mitted hand, bathe abdomen, giving special attention to bathing umbilicus and abdominal folds. Stroke from side to side. Keep abdomen covered between washing and rinsing. Dry well. | Moisture and sediment that collect in skinfolds predispose client to skin maceration and irritation. |
| 24. Apply clean gown or pajama top. If one extremity is injured or immobilized, always dress affected side first. (This step may be omitted until completion of bath; gown should not become soiled during remainder of bath.) | Maintains client's warmth and comfort. Dressing affected side first allows easier manipulation of gown over body part with reduced ROM. |

| Steps | Rationale |
|---|---|
| 25. Cover chest and abdomen with top of bath blanket. Expose far leg by folding blanket over toward midline. Be sure perineum is draped. | Prevents unnecessary exposure. |
| 26. Bend client's leg at knee by positioning your arm under leg. While grasping client's heel, elevate leg from mattress slightly and slide bath towel lengthwise under leg. | Towel prevents soiling of bed linen. Support of joint and extremity during lifting prevents strain on musculoskeletal structures. |
| 27. Ask client to hold foot still. Place bath basin on towel on bed and secure its position next to the foot to be washed. | Sudden movement by client could cause spillage of bathwater. (This step is omitted if client unable to hold leg in basin.) |
| 28. With one hand supporting lower leg, raise it and slide basin under lifted foot. Make sure foot is firmly placed on bottom of basin. Allow foot to soak while you wash leg (Fig. 6-4). | Proper positioning of foot prevents pressure from being applied from edge of basin against calf. Soaking softens calluses and rough skin. (Note if client is unable to hold leg, do not immerse; simply wash with washcloth. |
| 29. Use long, firm strokes in washing from ankle to knee and from knee to thigh. Dry well. | Promotes venous return. |
| 30. Cleanse foot, making sure to bathe between toes. Clean and clip nails as needed (Procedure 9-4). Dry well. If skin is dry, apply lotion. | Secretions and moisture may be present between toes. Lotion helps retain moisture and soften skin. |
| 31. Repeat Steps 25-30 for other leg and foot. | |
| 32. Cover client with bath blanket, raise side rail for client's safety, and change bathwater. | Drop in bathwater temperature can cause chilling. Clean water reduces microorganism transmission. |
| 33. Lower side rail. Assist client in assuming prone or sidelying position (as applicable). Place towel lengthwise along client's side. | Exposes back and buttocks for bathing. |
| 34. Apply disposable gloves. | Prevents contact with microorganisms in body secretions. |
| 35. Keep client draped by sliding bath blanket over shoulders and thighs. | Maintains warmth and prevents unnecessary exposure. |
| 36. Wash, rinse, and dry back from neck to buttocks using long, firm strokes. Pay special attention to folds of buttocks and anus. Give a backrub (Procedure 6-3). | Skinfolds near buttocks and anus may contain fecal secretions that harbor microorganisms. |
| 37. Change bathwater and washcloth. | Prevents transfer of microorganisms from anal area to genitalia. |
| 38. Assist client in assuming side-lying or supine position. Cover chest and upper extremities with towel and lower extremities with bath blanket. Expose only genitalia. (If client can help, covering entire body with bath blanket may be preferable.) Wash, rinse, and dry perineum (Procedure 6-2). Give special attention to skinfolds. | Maintains client's privacy. Clients capable of performing partial bath usually prefer to wash their own genitalia. |
| 39. Dispose gloves in receptacle. | Prevents transmission of infection. |
| 40. Apply any additional body lotion or oil as desired. | Moisturizing lotion prevents dry, chapped skin. |
| 41. Assist client in dressing. | |
| 42. Comb client's hair. Women may want to apply makeup. | Maintains client's body image. |
| 43. Make client's bed (Procedures 11-1 and 11-2). | Provides clean environment. |
| 44. Remove soiled linen and place in dirty-linen bag. Clean and replace bathing equipment. Replace call light and personal possessions. Leave room as clean and comfortable as possible. | Prevents transmission of infection. Clean environment promotes client's comfort. Keeping call light and articles of care within reach promotes client's safety. |
| 45. Wash hands. | Reduces transmission of microorganisms. |
| ***Tub bath or shower*** | |
| 1. Check tub or shower for cleanliness. Use cleaning techniques according to agency policy. Place rubber mat on tub or shower bottom. Place disposable bathmat or towel on floor in front of tub or shower. | Cleaning prevents transmission of infection. Mats prevent slipping and falling. |
| 2. Collect all hygienic aids, toiletry items, and linen requested by client. Place within easy reach of tub or shower. | Placing items close at hand prevents possible falls when client reaches for equipment. |
| 3. Assist client to bathroom if necessary. Have client wear robe and slippers en route to bathroom. | Assistance prevents accidental falls. Wearing robe and slippers prevents chilling. |
| 4. Demonstrate to client how to use call signal for assistance. | Bathrooms are equipped with signaling devices in case client feels faint or weak or needs immediate assistance. Clients prefer privacy during bath if safety is not jeopardized. |
| 5. Place "occupied" sign on bathroom door. | Maintains client's privacy. |
| 6. Fill bathtub halfway with warm water (43° C (109.4° F). Ask client to test water, and adjust water temperature if it is too warm. Explain which faucet controls hot water. If client is taking shower, turn shower on and adjust water temperature before client enters shower stall. | Adjusting water temperature prevents accidental burns. The elderly and clients with neurologic alterations (e.g., spinal cord injury) are high risk for burns as a result of reduced sensation. |

| Steps | Rationale |
|---|---|
| 7. Instruct client to use safety bars when getting in and out of tub or shower. | Prevents slipping and falling. |
| 8. Caution client against use of bath oil in tub water. | Oil causes tub surfaces to become slippery, predisposing client to accidental falls. |
| 9. Instruct client not to remain in tub longer than 20 min. Check on client every 5 min. | Prolonged exposure to warm water may cause vasodilation and pooling of blood, leading to lightheadedness or dizziness. |
| 10. Return to bathroom when client signals, and knock before entering. | Provides client privacy. |
| 11. For client who is unsteady, drain tub of water before client attempts to get out of it. Place bath towel over client's shoulders. | Prevents accidental falls. Client may become chilled as water drains. |
| 12. Assist client in getting out of tub as needed and assist with drying. | Moisture may cause excessive softening of skin and promote spread of infection. |
| 13. Assist client as needed in donning clean gown or pajamas, slippers, and robe. (In home setting client may don regular clothing.) | Maintains warmth to prevent chilling. |
| 14. Assist client to room and comfortable position in bed or chair. | Maintains relaxation gained from bathing. |
| 15. Clean tub or shower according to agency policy. Remove soiled linen and place in dirty-linen bag. Discard disposable equipment in proper receptable. Place "unoccupied" sign on bathroom door. Return supplies to storage area. | Prevents transmission of infection through soiled linen and moisture. |
| 16. Wash hands. | Reduces transfer of microorganisms. |

## Evaluation

| Steps | Rationale |
|---|---|
| 1. Observe behavior and ask if client feels fatigued or uncomfortable. | Determines client's tolerance to bathing activities. |
| 2. If client seems unusually restless or complains of discomfort, assess vital signs. | Factors that may alter pulse, respirations, or blood pressure include anxiety, fatigue from physical exertion, or pain. |
| 3. Note areas on skin that were previously soiled, reddened, or showed early signs of breakdown. | Techniques used during bathing should leave skin clean and clear. |
| 4. Note extent of joint ROM during bath. | Measures joint mobility. |
| 5. Ask client to explain proper hygiene techniques. | Evaluates client's knowledge level. |

### *Expected outcomes*

| Steps | Rationale |
|---|---|
| 1. Client tolerates bath without fatigue, discomfort, or chilling. Client expresses sense of comfort and relaxation. | Bath serves to relax and remove sources of discomfort. |
| 2. Skin is clean, dry, elastic, well hydrated, and without areas of local inflammation. | Indicates intact integument. |
| 3. Previous skin lesions are cleaner, with less drainage. | Size of lesions will not change after one bathing. |
| 4. Joint ROM remains the same or improves from previous measurement. | Important measure for bedrest clients prone to contractures. |
| 5. Client's independence to perform self-care is maintained. | |
| 6. Client describes benefits and techniques of proper hygiene and skin care. | Demonstrates learning. |

### *Unexpected outcomes*

| Steps | Rationale |
|---|---|
| 1. Client becomes excessively fatigued and unable to cooperate or participate in bathing. | Indicates nurse needs to offer more assistance. Client's physical tolerance to any form of exertion is minimal. |
| 2. There are areas of excessive dryness, rashes, or decubitus ulcers on skin. | Previous bathing or skin care measures were ineffective. |
| 3. Joint ROM decreases. | Indicates need for more frequent ROM exercise. |
| 4. Client is unable to identify or discuss methods or advantages of proper hygiene and skin care. | Factors such as anxiety, pain, or fatigue interfere with learning. Client may not be willing or motivated to learn about hygiene care. |

## Recording and Reporting

| Steps | Rationale |
|---|---|
| 1. Record type of bath and client's tolerance of bathing. Also note condition of skin and any significant findings, e.g., reddened skin areas or joint or muscle pain. Record level of assistance required by client. | Timely documentation maintains accuracy of client's record. Condition of skin documents response to therapy, such as turning and positioning. |

| Steps | Rationale |
|---|---|
| 2. Report evidence of alterations in skin integrity to nurse in charge or physician. | May require special medical treatment. |

### Follow-up Activities

| | |
|---|---|
| 1. If decubitus ulcers are present, provide special skin care (Skill 7-1) and position client to avoid further pressure to site of breakdown. | Break in integrity of skin layers provides for entrance of microorganisms. Localized pressure interferes with blood supply to skin and causes further ischemia. |
| 2. If client is predisposed to skin breakdown or shows signs of early decubitus ulcer formation, place on a special mattress or flotation device (Chapter 35). | Mattress and flotation devices are constructed to minimize pressure to skin and dependent body parts. |

### Special Considerations

- Clients with breathing difficulties require a pillow or elevated head of bed during bath.
- Avoid placing soap in washbasin: avoids soapy rinse water.
- Adolescents may require more frequent bathing as a result of active sebaceous glands. Elderly may require less frequent baths, more frequent application of skin lotion, or use of bath oil.
- Diabetic clients require special attention to foot care.
- Conditions placing clients at risk for falls in bath tub include neurologic impairment, arthritis, muscular disease or weakness, amputation, and poor balance or coordination in elderly clients.

### Teaching Considerations

- Family members caring for clients in the home should be included in discussions about hygiene care.
- Instruct elderly or other clients with reduced sensation on how to check temperature of bath water.
- Instruct clients on how to inspect surfaces between skin folds for signs of irritation or breakdown.

### Home Care Considerations

- In home setting, set up equipment according to established routines. Client is best resource for what works in terms of convenience and saving time.
- Clients at risk for falls may wish to have grab bars around the tub installed and the bathroom floor carpeted.
- The three types of bath for the homebound client are the complete bed bath; the abbreviated bed bath during which only parts of the client's body are washed that if neglected might cause illness, odor, or discomfort; and the partial bath, which may take place at the sink, in the tub, or in the shower.
- The kind of bath chosen is dependent on assessment of the home, availability of running water, and condition of the bathing facilities.
- If beds do not have side rails, positioning may be accomplished with pillows or placing bed against the wall.
- Never leave bathing client unattended. Adhesive strips on bottom of tub or shower, handrails, chairs, or stools in tub or shower will further protect the client.
- Follow client's usual bathing and skin care routines.

## *SKILL 6-2 Providing Perineal Care*

Perineal care involves thorough cleansing of the client's external genitalia and the surrounding skin. A client routinely receives perineal care during a bath. The nurse gives special attention to cleansing the skin around the genitalia, since this is a site where secretions can easily accumulate and infection may develop to involve the skin or urinary and reproductive systems. A nurse wears gloves during the procedure because of the risk of contacting infectious microorganisms, such as HIV or herpes, from perineal drainage. Certain clients require perineal care at times other than during a bath, for example, after fecal incontinence or as a part of Foley catheter care.

To minimize embarrassment of both the nurse and the client, it helps for the nurse to be of the same sex as the client. Embarrassment should not cause the nurse to overlook the client's hygiene needs.

### Purposes

1. Prevent and control spread of infection.
2. Prevent skin breakdown.
3. Promote client comfort and cleanliness.
4. Improve client understanding of basic perineal hygiene.
5. Promote healing after surgery or vaginal deliveries.

## Procedure 6-2

| Steps | Rationale |
|---|---|
| **Assessment** | |
| 1. Identify clients at risk for developing infection of genitalia, urinary tract, or reproductive tract, (e.g., presence of indwelling catheter or fecal incontinence). | Secretions that accumulate on surface of skin surrounding female and male genitalia act as reservoir for infection. Tissues traumatized as result of surgery or by presence of foreign object provide route for introduction of infectious organisms. |
| 2. Assess client's cognitive and musculoskeletal function. | Determines client's ability to perform self-care and determines level of assistance required from nurse. |
| 3. Assess genitalia for signs of inflammation, skin breakdown, or infection (Chapter 13). | Determines extent of perineal care required by client. |
| 4. Assess client's knowledge of importance of perineal hygiene. | Clients with risk of infection in perineal area may be unaware of importance of cleanliness. Reflects client's need for education. |
| **Nursing Diagnosis** | |
| 1. Cluster data to reveal actual or potential nursing diagnoses: | |
| a. Potential for infection: related to retained secretions. | Control of secretions through cleansing will minimize risk of infection. |
| b. Impaired skin integrity: related to trauma of surgical incisions. | Hygiene measures become a form of therapy in caring for injured skin (e.g., after an episiotomy). |
| c. Potential impaired skin integrity: related to exposure to fecal, urinary, or wound secretions. | Nurse institutes hygiene measures for preventive care. |
| d. Knowledge deficit regarding basic hygiene care: related to lack of information. | Nurse instructs client regarding proper techniques of care during procedure. |
| **Planning** | |
| 1. Develop individualized goals for client based on nursing diagnoses: | |
| a. Client achieves sense of comfort. | Cleansing removes sources of local irritation. |
| b. Skin integrity maintained. | Cleansing removes secretions that can macerate skin. |
| c. Client remains free of infection. | Any perineal or fecal discharge can be source of urinary tract infection. |
| d. Client participates in and understands methods of perineal hygiene. | Nurse provides instruction during perineal care. |
| 2. Explain procedure and its purpose to client. | Helps minimize anxiety during procedure that is often embarrassing to nurse and client. |
| 3. Prepare necessary equipment and supplies: | Used when administering a bed bath. |
| a. Washbasin | |
| b. Soap dish with soap | |
| c. Two or three washcloths | |
| d. Bath towel | |
| e. Bath blanket | |
| f. Waterproof pad or bedpan | Prevents soiling of bed linen. |
| g. Toilet tissue | |
| h. Disposable gloves | Prevents contact with microorganisms in body secretions |
| Additional supplies when pericare is given other than during a bath: | |
| a. Cotton balls or swabs | Used for cleansing menstruating women or around indwelling catheters. |
| b. A solution bottle or container filled with warm water or prescribed rinsing solution | |
| c. Waterproof bag | For disposal of cotton balls. |
| **Implementation** | |
| 1. Pull curtain around client's bed or close room door. | Maintains client's privacy. |
| 2. Assemble supplies at bedside. | Ensures orderly procedure. |
| 3. Raise bed to comfortable working position. | Facilitates good body mechanics. |
| 4. Lower side rail and assist client in assuming dorsal recumbent (female) or supine (male) position. | Provides easy access to genitalia. |

| Steps | Rationale |
|---|---|

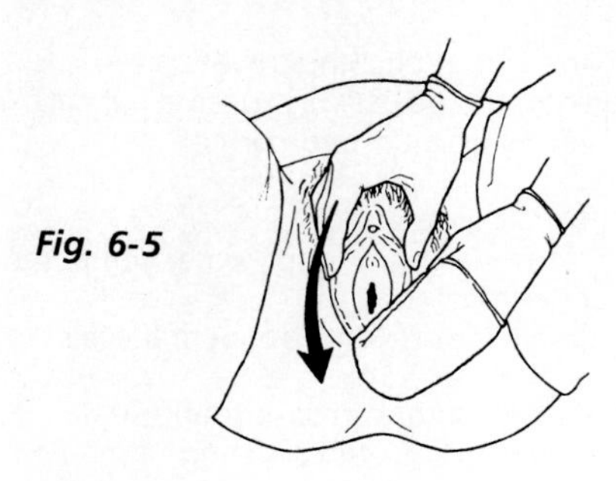

*Fig. 6-5*

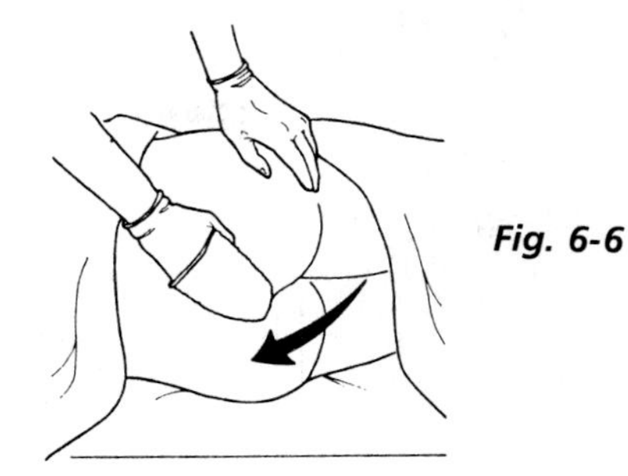

*Fig. 6-6*

***Female perineal care***

| Steps | Rationale |
|---|---|
| 1. Position waterproof pad under client's buttocks or place bedpan under client. | Prevents bed linen from becoming wet. |
| 2. Fold top bed linen down toward foot of bed and raise client's gown up above genital area. | Exposes perineal area for easy accessibility. |
| 3. Drape client by placing bath blanket with one corner between client's legs, one corner pointing toward each side of bed, and one corner over client's chest. Tuck side corners around client's legs and, under hips. | Draping prevents unnecessary exposure of body part and maintains client's warmth and comfort during procedure. |
| 4. Raise side rail. Fill washbasin with water that is approximately 41°-43° C (105°-109.4° F). | Prevents client from falling. Proper water temperature prevents burns to perineum. |
| 5. Place washbasin and toilet tissue on overbed table. Place washcloths in basin. | Equipment placed within nurse's reach prevents accidental spills. |
| 6. Lower side rail and help client flex her knees and spread her legs apart. | Provides full exposure of female genitalia. |
| 7. Don disposable gloves. Fold lower corner of bath blanket up between client's legs onto abdomen. | Minimizes transmission of microorganisms. Keeping client draped until procedure begins minimizes anxiety. |
| 8. Wash and dry client's upper thighs. | Buildup of perineal secretions can soil surrounding skin surfaces. |
| 9. Wash labia majora. Then use your nondominant hand to gently retract labia from thigh; with dominant hand, wash carefully in skinfolds. Wipe in direction from perineum to rectum. Repeat on opposite side using separate section of washcloth. Rinse and dry area thoroughly. | Skinfolds may contain body secretions that harbor microorganisms. Wiping from perineum to rectum reduces chance of transmitting fecal organisms to urinary meatus. |
| 10. Separate labia with your nondominant hand to expose urethral meatus and vaginal orifice. With dominant hand, wash downward from pubic area toward rectum in one smooth stroke (see Fig. 6-5). Use separate section of cloth for each stroke. Cleanse thoroughly around labia minora, clitoris, and vaginal orifice. | Cleansing method reduces transfer of microorganisms to urinary meatus. (For menstruating women or clients with indwelling urinary catheters, cleanse with cotton balls.) |
| 11. If client is on bedpan, pour warm water over perineal area. | Rinsing removes soap and microorganisms more effectively than wiping. |
| 12. Dry perineal area throughly. | Retained moisture harbors microorganisms. |
| 13. Fold lower corner of bath blanket back between client's legs and over perineum. Ask client to lower legs and assume side-lying position. | Side-lying position provides access to anal area for cleansing. |
| 14. Clean anal area by first wiping off fecal material with toilet tissue. Wash by wiping from vagina toward anus with one stroke (Fig. 6-6). Discard washcloth. Repeat with clean cloth until skin is clear of fecal material. | Fecal material contains large numbers of microorganisms that can cause vaginal or urinary tract infection. |
| 15. Rinse area well and dry with bath towel. | Rinsing removes soap and microorganisms. |
| 16. Remove disposable gloves and dispose in proper receptacle. | Moisture and body secretions on gloves can harbor microorganisms. |
| 17. Assist client in assuming comfortable position and cover with sheet. | Client's comfort minimizes emotional stress of procedure. |
| 18. Remove bath blanket and dispose of all soiled bed linen. Return unused equipment to storage area. | Reduces transmission of infection. |
| 19. Raise side rail and lower bed to proper height. Return client's room to its condition before procedure. | Prevents client from accidentally falling. Clean environment enhances client's comfort. |
| 20. Wash hands. | Reduces transmission of infection. |

| Steps | Rationale |
|---|---|
| ***Male perineal care*** | |
| 1. Position waterproof pad under client's buttocks. | Prevents bed linen from becoming wet. |
| 2. Drape client by placing bath blanket with one corner between client's legs, one corner pointing toward each side of bed, and one corner over client's chest. Tuck side corners around client's legs and under hips. | Draping prevents unnecessary exposure of body parts and maintains client's warmth and comfort. |
| 3. Raise side rail. Fill washbasin with water that is approximately 41°-43° C (105°-109.4° F). | Prevents client from falling. Proper water temperature prevents burns to perineum. |
| 4. Place washbasin and toilet tissue on overbed table. Place washcloths in washbasin. | Easy access to supplies prevents accidental spills. |
| 5. Lower side rail and don disposable gloves. | Prevents nurse's exposure to microorganisms. |
| 6. Lower top corner of bath blanket below client's perineum. Gently raise penis and place bath towel underneath. | Towel prevents moisture from collecting in inguinal area. |
| 7. Gently grasp shaft of penis. If client is uncircumcised, retract foreskin. If client has an erection, defer procedure until later. | Gentle handling reduces chance of client having an erection. Secretions capable of harboring microorganisms collect underneath foreskin. |
| 8. Wash tip of penis at urethral meatus first. Using circular motion, cleanse from meatus outward (Fig. 6-7). Discard washcloth and repeat with clean cloth until penis is clean. Rinse and dry gently. | Direction of cleansing moves from area of least contamination to area of most contamination, preventing microorganisms from entering urethra. |
| 9. Return foreskin to its natural position. | Tightening of foreskin around shaft of penis can cause local edema and discomfort. |
| 10. Wash shaft of penis with gentle but firm downward strokes. Pay special attention to underlying surface of penis. | Vigorous massage of penis can lead to erection, which can cause embarassment for client and nurse. Underlying surface of penis may have greater accumulation of secretions. |
| 11. Rinse and dry penis thoroughly. Instruct client to spread legs apart slightly. | Abduction of legs provides easier access to scrotal tissues. |
| 12. Gently cleanse scrotum. Lift it carefully and wash underlying skinfolds. Rinse and dry. | Pressure on scrotal tissues can be very painful to client. Secretions collect between skinfolds. |
| 13. Fold bath blanket back over client's perineum and assist client in turning to side-lying position. | Draping promotes comfort and minimizes client's anxiety. Side-lying position provides access to anal area. |
| 14. Clean anal area by first wiping off fecal material with toilet tissue. Wash by wiping carefully around anal area. Discard washcloth. Repeat with clean cloth until all skinfolds are clear of fecal material. | Fecal material contains large numbers of microorganisms that can cause urinary tract infection. |
| 15. Rinse area well and dry with bath towel. | Rinsing removes soap and microorganisms. |
| 16. Follow Steps 16-20 of female perineal care. | |

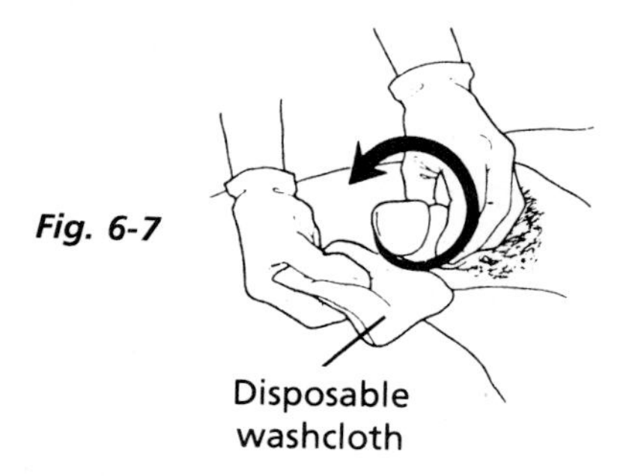

***Fig. 6-7***

## Evaluation

| | |
|---|---|
| 1. Inspect surface of external genitalia and surrounding skin after cleansing. | Thick secretions may cover underlying skin lesions or areas of breakdown. Evaluation determines need for additional therapy. |
| 2. Ask if client feels a sense of cleanliness. | Evaluates clients level of comfort. |
| 3. Note presence of any abnormal drainage or discharge from genitalia. | Evaluates presence of infection. |
| 4. Observe client's ability to perform hygiene and ask questions about its importance. | Evaluates client's self-care ability and knowledge level. |

***Expected outcomes***

| | |
|---|---|
| 1. Skin and surrounding genitalia are clean, pink, intact, and without discharge. | Absence of skin irritation. |

| Steps | Rationale |
|---|---|
| 2. Client expresses sense of cleanliness and is able to describe or perform steps of perineal hygiene. | Perineum is clean. Self-care measures are understood. |
| ***Unexpected outcomes*** | |
| 1. Skin and genitalia may be inflamed with localized tenderness, swelling, and presence of foul-smelling discharge. | Signs of infection or maceration of skin layers. |
| 2. Client expresses discomfort. | Perineal area not thoroughly cleansed, or irritation present as a result of infection. |
| 3. Client unable to describe or perform perineal hygiene. | Further instruction required at a later time. |
| **Recording and Reporting** | |
| 1. Record procedure and presence of any abnormal findings, e.g., character and amount of discharge or condition of genitalia. | Ensures accurate and timely documentation of care (flow sheet may be used). |
| 2. Record appearance of suture line, if present. | Documents nurse's observations of client's postoperative recovery. |
| 3. Report any break in suture line or presence of abnormalities to nurse in charge or physician. | Additional therapy may be required as result of altered wound healing or altered skin integrity. |
| **Follow-up Activities** | |
| 1. Client with localized inflammation of genitalia or suture line may have sitz baths ordered. | Warm water bath cleanses and reduces inflammation of perineal and anal areas (Chapter 43). |
| 2. Suture line care may involve application of antibiotic ointments. | Prevents onset of tissue infection. |
| 3. Continued skin irritation from repeated incontinence may necessitate application of protective ointment and a more aggressive bowel or urinary control program. | Voluntary control of micturition and defecation will prevent incontinence. |

### Special Considerations

- Clients with urinary or fecal incontinence, rectal or perineal surgery, or surgery involving the lower urinary tract, and women who are recovering from normal childbirth require special attention with perineal care. It may be necessary to offer care frequently.
- Young adolescent girls should learn basic perineal hygiene measures and know why they are predisposed to urinary tract infections.

### Teaching Considerations

- Clients most at-risk for infection of the perineum are taught signs and symptoms of early infection, as well as principles and techniques for cleansing the perineum correctly. Clients who are physically unable to perform hygiene and who rely on family members for care must have family instructed on hygiene techniques.

### Home Care Considerations

- For clients who require bathing assess perineum at every visit because clients are at risk for infection and skin breakdown.

## SKILL 6-3 Administering a Backrub

A massage of the back, shoulders, and lower neck is a backrub. A nurse usually offers a backrub after a bath or before a client prepares for sleep. The backrub promotes relaxation, relieves muscular tension, and stimulates skin circulation. Gentle massage prevents trauma to the skin. The nurse can assess condition of the client's skin during a backrub.

An effective backrub takes 3 to 5 minutes. The nurse should inquire if the client would like a backrub, since some clients dislike physical contact.

### Purposes

1. Promote client relaxation and comfort.
2. Relieve muscular tension.
3. Stimulate circulation to the skin.

## Procedure 6-3

| Steps | Rationale |
|---|---|
| **Assessment** | |
| 1. Identify any restrictions or limitations in client's positioning. | Determine type of position client can best assume during backrub. |
| 2. Determine client's potential for benefit from a backrub: signs of fatigue, movement reflecting muscle stiffness. | Backrub relieves muscular tension and improves relaxation. |
| 3. Identify factors or conditions, such as rib or vertebral fractures, burns, or open wounds, that contraindicate a backrub. | Massage of sensitive tissues might lead to further tissue injury. |
| 4. Assess pulse and blood pressure of clients with history of hypertension or arrhythmias. | Massage may cause autonomic nervous system stimulation that induces changes in heart rate and blood pressure. Research has not shown consistent relationships between human touch and the cardiac response of those being touched. |
| 5. Ask if client would like a backrub. | Some clients dislike close physical contact of a backrub. |
| **Nursing Diagnosis** | |
| 1. Cluster data to reveal actual or potential nursing diagnoses: | |
| a. Pain: related to muscle or joint stiffness. | Backrub can effectively reduce discomfort. |
| b. Impaired skin integrity: related to pressure or altered circulation. | Disruption in skin layers contraindicates massage over affected area. |
| c. Potential impaired skin integrity: related to immobility and pressure. | Immobilized clients benefit from frequent massage to areas of skin at risk for developing decubitis. |
| d. Anxiety: related to threat of physical touch. | Contraindicates use of backrub. |
| **Planning** | |
| 1. Develop individualized goals for client based on nursing diagnoses: | |
| a. Achieve relaxation. | Attained by reducing muscle tension. |
| b. Minimize anxiety. | Backrub distracts client and enhances relaxation. |
| c. Increase local circulation. | Massage improves circulation to muscles. |
| 2. Prepare needed equipment and supplies: | |
| a. Bath blanket | |
| b. Bath towel | Removes excess moisture. |
| c. Skin application (lotion, alcohol, or powder) | Lotion lubricates skin and prevents friction during massage. Alcohol cools skin but has drying effect. Powder reduces friction during massage. |
| 3. Explain procedure and desired position to the client. | Helps promote relaxation. |
| **Implementation** | |
| 1. Adjust bed to high, comfortable position. | Ensures proper body mechanics and prevents strain on nurse's back muscles. |
| 2. Adjust light sources, temperature, and sound within room. | Environmental distractions can prevent client from relaxing. |
| 3. Lower side rail and help client assume either prone or side-lying (Sims') position with back toward nurse. Close curtain around bed. | Facilitates application of pressure to back muscles. Privacy promotes client's relaxation. |
| 4. Expose client's back, shoulders, upper arms, and buttocks. Cover remainder of body with bath blanket. Lay towel alongside client's back. | Prevents unnecessary exposure of body parts. |
| 5. Wash and warm hands in warm water. | |
| 6. Warm lotion in hands or by placing container in warm water. | Cold causes muscle tension. |
| 7. Place lotion in hands. Explain to client that lotion will feel cool and wet. | Warning client reduces startle response. |
| 8. Apply hands first to sacral area, massaging in circular motion (Fig. 6-8, *A*). Stroke upward from buttocks to shoulders. Massage over scapulas with smooth, firm stroke. Continue in one smooth stroke to upper arms and laterally along sides of back down to iliac crests. Do not allow hands to leave client's skin. Continue massage pattern for 3 min. | Gentle, firm pressure applied to all muscle groups promotes relaxation. Continuous contact with skin's surface is soothing and stimulates circulation to tissues. |

| Steps | Rationale |
|---|---|

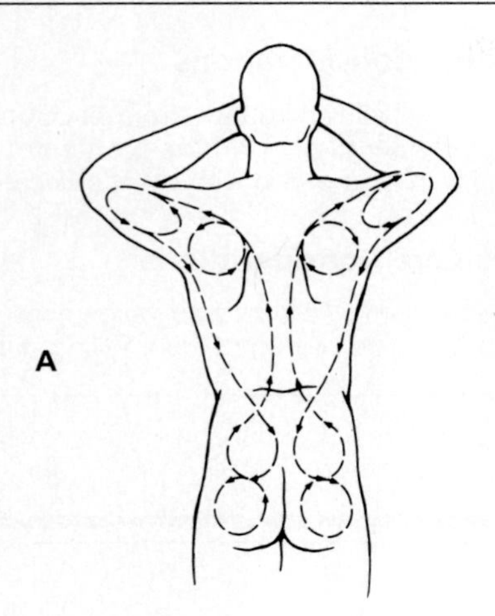


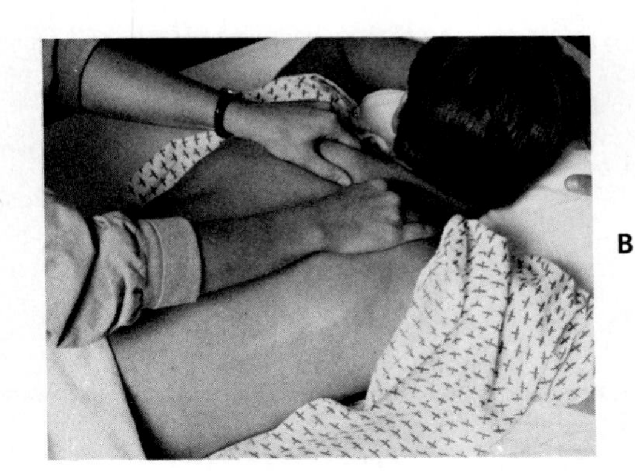


*Fig. 6-8*

| Steps | Rationale |
|---|---|
| 9. Knead skin by grasping tissue between thumb and fingers. Knead upward along one side of spine from buttocks to shoulders and around nape of neck. Knead or stroke downward toward sacrum. Repeat along other side of back (Fig. 6-8, *B*). | Kneading increases circulation to muscles. Continuous motion is soothing and relieves muscle tension. |
| 10. End massage with long stroking movements and tell client you are ending massage. | Long stroking is most soothing of massage movements. |
| 11. If lying on side, ask client to turn to opposite side, and massage other hip. | |
| 12. Wipe excess lotion from client's back with bath towel. Retie gown or assist with pajamas. Help client to comfortable position. Open curtain and raise side rails as needed. | Excess lotion can be an irritant. Comfortable position enhances backrub's effects. |
| 13. Dispose of soiled towel and wash hands. | These measures promote infection control. |

## Evaluation

| | |
|---|---|
| 1. Ask if client feels comfortable or has any areas of muscle pain or tension. | Degree of relief will depend on length of massage, client's ability to relax, and degree of discomfort before massage. |
| 2. Reassess pulse. Check blood pressure if change in pulse is noted. | Gentle back massage may increase heart rate and systolic blood pressure. |

### *Expected outcomes*

| | |
|---|---|
| 1. Client reports feeling relaxed, with less muscle tension. | Backrub effectively promoted relaxation. |
| 2. Heart rate and blood pressure remain stable. | No cardiovascular changes. |

### *Unexpected outcomes*

| | |
|---|---|
| 1. Client may continue to express discomfort or muscular tension. | Pain or source of anxiety unrelieved. |
| 2. There may be slight elevations in heart rate and systolic blood pressure (Longworth, 1982). | Result of increased sympathetic stimulation. |

## Recording and Reporting

| | |
|---|---|
| 1. Record client's condition of skin and response to massage. | Accurate documentation describes client's response to therapy. |
| 2. Record massage on flow sheet. | Quicker method for documenting procedure. |

## Follow-up Activities

| | |
|---|---|
| 1. Initiate necessary care measures for areas of redness, abrasion, or breakdown. | Extent of tissue injury determines type of care nurse administers (Chapters 7 and 35). |
| 2. Position client off pressure sites. | Prevents pressure ulcer formation. |

### Special Considerations

- Clients with respiratory disease, back alterations, or abdominal wounds or incisions should avoid lying prone. Clients who have had surgery involving an arm, leg, or lobes of the lung may be restricted from turning on operative side.
- If client notes tender muscular area, apply additional gentle massage. Avoid direct massage over areas of abrasions.

### Teaching Considerations

- If client achieves relaxation from backrub teach a family member how to perform the procedure. A backrub can become a routine part of the client's sleep hygiene.

### Home Care Considerations

- Position client in proper body alignment, using pillows.
- Client must be protected from falling during backrub.

# *SKILL 6-4 Bathing an Infant*

An infant can be bathed by sponge bath or in a small tub. Because the infant's skin is immature, the epidermis and dermis are loosely bound together. Precautions must be taken to avoid applying friction against skin layers. The skin remains prone to bruising until the child reaches toddler age.

Because an infant's temperature control mechanisms are immature, prolonged exposure of body parts may cause rapid cooling. The nurse keeps the infant well covered when giving a sponge bath. When giving a tub bath, the nurse works quickly to be sure the water stays warm enough to prevent chilling.

In hospitals where the infant stays in the same room with the mother, the infant's bath is an excellent opportunity to involve parents in the child's care. Parents can examine the infant's body parts and learn about normal variations in skin characteristics and infant behavior.

### Purposes

1. Promote cleanliness and integrity of the skin and umbilical cord stump.
2. Minimize changes in body temperature.
3. Assess infant's skin and general behavior.
4. Provide pleasant tactile stimulation.

## *Procedure 6-4*

| Steps | Rationale |
|---|---|
| **Assessment** | |
| 1. Inspect integrity of neonate's umbilical cord. Look for redness or foul smelling discharge. | Tub bath is contraindicated if umbilical cord has not healed. Immersion of umbilicus in water before skin heals can cause serious infection. |
| 2. Assess general condition and cleanliness of skin. | Except for face, genitalia, and anal areas, infant may not require complete daily bath. Peeling of skin usually occurs 2-4 weeks after birth. |
| 3. Assess parents' knowledge of how to give bath, as well as their knowledge of common features and characteristics of infant's integument. | Determines extent of client education nurse must provide. |
| 4. Check agency policy for need to weigh infant, measure body temperature, or administer cord care. | Agency policies will differ. |
| **Nursing Diagnosis** | |
| 1. Cluster data to reveal actual or potential nursing diagnoses: | |
| a. Impaired skin integrity: related to rashes or dryness. | Dryness, rashes, or vernix caseosa are normal alterations that influence extent of bathing. |
| b. Knowledge deficit regarding infant hygiene needs: related to inexperience. | Bathing procedure provides excellent opportunity for nurse to instruct parents on bathing techniques. |
| c. Self-care deficit, bathing and hygiene: related to immaturity. | Infant requires total assistance with bathing. |

| Steps | Rationale |
|---|---|
| **Planning** | |
| 1. Develop individualized goals for client based on nursing diagnoses: | |
| a. Protecting infant from injury. | Nurse protects infant from accidental burns and falls during procedure. |
| b. Maintaining skin integrity. | Bath cleans skin of irritants. |
| c. Providing meaningful tactile stimulation. | Gentle touch stimulates infant. |
| d. Increasing parents' understanding of bathing techniques. | Instructions given throughout bath procedure. |
| 2. Prepare needed equipment and supplies: | |
| a. Washbasin or small tub | Selection depends on whether infant is to receive sponge or tub bath. |
| b. Rubber bath pad | Bath pad placed in tub prevents accidental falls. |
| c. Mild soap, e.g., Dove or Ivory | Soap is used to cleanse only soiled areas such as joint creases or anal area. Harsh soaps will irritate skin. |
| d. Shirt | |
| e. Diaper (disposable or plain cloth) | |
| f. Additional clothing or sleeper | |
| g. Safety pins | |
| h. Soft washcloth | |
| i. Soft-bristled brush or fine-toothed comb | |
| j. Cotton balls | |
| k. Towel (adult sized) | Covers infant more completely to prevent chilling. |
| l. Facial tissue | |
| m. Optional supplies: | |
| ▪ Lotion | Provides pleasurable tactile stimulation. |
| ▪ Alcohol, 70% (cord care only) | Promotes drying and cleansing of umbilical cord. |
| ▪ Petrolatum jelly | Reduces incidence of diaper rash. |
| 3. Control room temperature and ventilation. | Infant's temperature control mechanisms are immature. Room should be warm and without drafts. |
| 4. Move safety pins away from infant's reach. | Infant might suddenly reach for pointed object and injure self. |
| **Implementation** | |
| ***Sponge bath*** | |
| 1. Wash hands. | Reduces transmission of microorganisms. |
| 2. Prepare washbasin with warm water at 38°-40.5° C (100°-105° F). Test water temperature by placing drops on inside surface of your forearm. Water should feel comfortably warm. | Prevents accidental burns. |
| 3. Keep infant clothed in shirt and diaper with bath towel wrapped around shoulders. | Keeping infant clothed and draped prevents chilling. |
| 4. Begin by cleansing eyes with plain water, with infant lying supine. Wash each eye gently using separate cotton ball or clean portion of washcloth. Wipe from inner to outer canthus. | Prevents spread of microorganisms. Cleansing movement prevents microorganisms from entering tear duct. |
| 5. If crustations are present on eyelid margins, apply moistened cotton ball for 1-2 min before cleansing. | Softening of crustations promotes easy removal and thus prevents trauma to eye. |
| 6. Roll dampened cotton ball or use twisted end of washcloth to clean nares and ears. Note presence of crusts in nares. | Avoids trauma to mucous membranes and internal ear structures. |
| 7. Use moistened portion of washcloth to cleanse infant's face thoroughly. Give special attention to areas behind ears and around neck. Small amount of soap may be used for soiled creases. | Face becomes easily soiled during feeding. Neck may collect regurgitated food. Body creases are sites for secretions to accumulate and harbor microorganisms. |
| 8. Dry face and neck thoroughly. | Excess moisture causes skin softening. |
| 9. Cleanse infant's scalp by gently wiping off secretions with mild soap and water. | Usually an infant's scalp does not become excessively soiled. Excess pressure over fontanels should be avoided. |
| 10. Shampoo infant's hair in cases of excess soiling: | Shampooing scalp is best prevention against cradle cap—a seborrheic dermatitis characterized by thick, adherent, yellowish, scaly, oily patches of scalp. |
| a. Drape infant's trunk with large bath towel. | |
| b. Hold infant's head securely in one hand while positioning it over washbasin. | Infants are not able to hold their necks erect until approximately 5 mo of age. |
| c. Lather scalp gently with small amount of mild soap. | Excess soap may accidentally enter infant's eyes. |

| Steps | Rationale |
|---|---|
| d. Rinse by pouring water from small cup or container over infant's scalp, into basin. | Thoroughly removes soap that becomes irritating to scalp on drying. |
| e. Dry thoroughly and cover infant's head with towel. | Prevents evaporative heat loss. |
| 11. Comb or brush infant's hair gently. | Helps remove any loosened crusts in hair. |
| 12. Undress infant and remove diaper. Use lower portion of towel or additional towel to drape areas not being washed. | Prevents chilling. |
| 13. Wipe off any fecal material from anal area or around genitalia with facial tissue. | Prevents spread of microorganisms during bathing. |
| 14. With washcloth and small amount of soap, gently cleanse arms, hands, and axilla. Proceed to chest, abdomen, and back. Rinse and dry thoroughly. | Infant's skin is sensitive. Minimal friction should be used for cleansing. |
| 15. Cleanse umbilicus thoroughly with soap and water. Rinse and dry thoroughly. Apply alcohol with cotton ball to cord or stump if it remains unhealed. | Until cord closes, it is excellent site for growth and entrance of microorganisms. Alcohol promotes drying and prevents infection. |
| 16. Apply clean shirt. | Prevents chilling and promotes infant's comfort. |
| 17. Use plain water to cleanse infant's lower legs and feet. Dry thoroughly. | Area is usually not excessively soiled. |
| 18. For female infant: | |
| a. Wash folds of groin. | Area where secretions easily collect. |
| b. Gently retract labia fully and wash from front to back toward anus. Use separate portion of washcloth or moistened cotton ball for each wipe. | Provides full exposure. Direction of cleansing reduces chance of transmitting fecal organisms to urinary meatus. |
| c. Pay particular attention to removal of vernix caseosa (in newborns) but do not apply excess friction to skin. | Vernix caseosa is grayish white, cheeselike substance on skin at time of infant's birth. Often it becomes thick and adherent. |
| 19. For male infant: | |
| a. Use plain water to wash gently around penis and scrotum. | Soap can be irritating. |
| b. In uncircumcised newborns do not retract foreskin until it has been initially retracted by physician, usually when infant is 6 weeks old. | Foreskin of infants is initially too tight. |
| c. In older infants retract foreskin and cleanse around glans penis in circular motion with moist cotton ball, moving from tip of urethra outward. | Once foreskin is loose, it should be retracted to remove underlying secretions that serve as source of irritation and infection. |
| d. Dry and return foreskin to its normal position. | Foreskin can constrict blood flow to penis if it remains retracted. |
| 20. With facial tissue remove fecal material around buttocks or anus. Gently place infant on back on top of towel, keeping upper body draped. Grasp both ankles with your nondominant hand and lift buttocks. Wash, rinse, and dry anal area thoroughly. Apply thin layer of petrolatum jelly as desired. | Fecal contents, especially in liquid form, can be irritating to skin. Retained moisture on buttocks can cause rash and irritation. Petrolatum jelly retains skin moisture and prevents diaper rash. |
| 21. Apply body lotion to dry, cracked skin areas. | Provides lubrication and tactile stimulation. |
| 22. Apply a clean diaper: | |
| a. Be sure it fits snugly around thighs and abdomen. | Snug fit prevents urine leakage. |
| b. If umbilicus is not healed, keep top edge of diaper below site. | Prevents friction from being applied to sensitive tissues. |
| c. If infant is circumcised, secure diaper loosely. | Prevents friction against penis. |
| d. Fasten diaper with back overlapping front. | Permits full hip flexion. |
| 23. Dress infant in sleeper or regular clothing. | Maintains warmth and comfort. |
| 24. Place infant in crib, playpen, or basinette. | Protects infant from injury while cleaning work site. |
| 25. Store reusable supplies. Empty, rinse, and dry washbasin. Dispose of soiled linen and diaper in proper receptacle. Wash hands. | Reduces transmission of microorganisms. |
| ***Tub bath*** | |
| 1. Place rubber mat in bottom of tub. | Mat can be placed securely before tub is filled with water. |
| 2. Follow Steps 1-11 of sponge bath procedure before immersing infant into tub. | Eases ability of nurse to securely hold younger infant during bath. |
| 3. Undress infant and slowly immerse into tub of water. | Minimizes startling of infant. Bathing by immersion causes less heat loss. |
| 4. Hold infant securely with one hand positioned behind neck and upper back (Fig. 6-9). | Prevents slipping and sinking of infant's head beneath water. |
| 5. Move from shoulders and arms to lower extremities. Use soap only in areas of soiling or in body creases. Rinse areas thoroughly. | Body creases are easier to clean from soaking effects of tub bath. |

| Steps | Rationale |
|---|---|

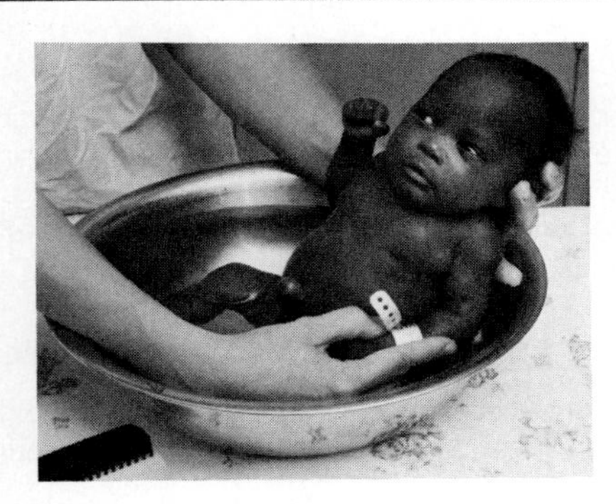

*Fig. 6-9*

| Steps | Rationale |
|---|---|
| 6. Allow older infants to briefly play in water; do not leave unattended. | Infant derives pleasurable sensation from water. |
| 7. Remove infant from tub and wrap completely in large bath towel. Gently pat body parts dry, paying special attention to body creases. | Maintains warmth and prevents chilling. Retained moisture causes softening and maceration of skin. |
| 8. Apply body lotion to any dry, cracked areas of skin. | Lotion soothes, lubricates, and provides important tactile stimulation. |
| 9. Apply clean diaper and clothing as described in Steps 22 and 23 of sponge bath procedure. | |
| 10. Place infant in crib or playpen. | Prevents falls when infant is unattended. |
| 11. Store reusable supplies. Empty, rinse, and dry washbasin. Dispose of soiled linen and diaper in proper receptacle. Wash hands. | Reduces transmission of microorganisms. |

## Evaluation

| Steps | Rationale |
|---|---|
| 1. Inspect areas of infant's skin after cleansing. | Soiling or body secretions may cover underlying skin lesions or signs of irritation. |
| 2. Question parents about bathing techniques and have them return demonstrate a bath. | Evaluates parents' learning and ability to manage infant's hygiene. |

### *Expected outcomes*

| Steps | Rationale |
|---|---|
| 1. Infant's skin is soft, clean, and well lubricated. Perineal area is pink and clear. Umbilicus is intact without drainage or inflammation. | Absence of skin irritation. Umbilical stump usually dries and falls off in 7-10 days. Base of cord may take a few weeks to heal. |
| 2. Infant demonstrates pleasurable behaviors, e.g., cooing, smiling, or simple vocalization. | Bath provided pleasurable stimulation. |
| 3. Parents are able to explain and demonstrate proper bath procedure. | Bathing technique is learned. |

### *Unexpected outcomes*

| Steps | Rationale |
|---|---|
| 1. Presence of inflammation in perineal area with small vesicopustules. | Signs of diaper rash or dermatitis. |
| 2. Presence of cradle cap. | Normally it takes several days for cradle cap to disappear. |
| 3. Open umbilical stump with drainage or localized redness. | Signs of infection. |
| 4. Parents unable to explain and demonstrate proper bath procedure. | Further instruction is necessary. |

## Recording and Reporting

| Steps | Rationale |
|---|---|
| 1. Record procedure and note any unusual findings, e.g., condition of umbilicus, presence of cradle cap, skin lesions. | Accurate documentation includes recording of procedures. |
| 2. Include description of infant's behavior during bath. | Bath time provides opportunity to observe and document infant's behaviors and reflexes. |
| 3. Report any unusual findings, e.g., drainage from umbilical stump, to nurse in charge or physician. | Alterations in infant's skin integrity can easily lead to infection. |

## Follow-up Activities

| Steps | Rationale |
|---|---|
| 1. Apply any topical preparation ordered by physician to affected perineal area. | Topical steroids reduce inflammation. |

### Special Considerations

- Avoid use of oils that clog pores and act as media for infection. Powder can cake with moisture and irritate skin. Never use cotton-tipped swabs to clean infant's nose or ears because infant's sudden movement may injure eardrum or mucosa.

### Teaching Considerations

- Demonstrate bathing procedure and allow parents to practice techniques. Emphasize the following: fontanels on head will not puncture or tear with mild pressure; avoid running water too deep in tub if infant cannot sit upright; do not leave infant unattended during bath. Parents should practice diaper changing and cleansing techniques for the perineum. Inform parents about signs of infection of umbilical cord, for example, presence of drainage, foul odor, localized redness or swelling.

### Home Care Considerations

- Supervise family member during infant's bath.
- Assess bathing techniques for safety precautions of the infant.

# *SKILL 6-5 Sponging With Tepid Water*

Bathing can provide specific therapeutic benefits because of the nature of the skin's structure and function. Tepid sponging is used when a client's temperature is very high. It can be soothing, but also uncomfortable, depending on the client's skin temperature. Using tepid water avoids the chilling effect of cold water and promotes slow cooling, which reduces temperature fluctuations in the client. Tepid water promotes heat loss through evaporation. Parents must be taught the skill of providing a tepid bath because infants can develop high fevers suddenly, and the tepid bath can reduce temperatures quickly.

### Purpose

1. Lower body temperature during times of febrile episode.

## *Procedure 6-5*

| Steps | Rationale |
|---|---|
| **Assessment** | |
| 1. Assess client's body temperature and pulse. | Provides baseline for evaluating response to therapy. Sudden circulatory changes may alter pulse. |
| 2. Assess parents' understanding of sponging with tepid water procedure and dangers of high fever. | Identifies parents' learning needs and motivation to learn. |
| **Nursing Diagnosis** | |
| 1. Cluster data to reveal actual or potential nursing diagnoses: | |
| a. Hyperthermia: related to illness or increased metabolism. | High fever can result from a variety of infectious diseases or metabolic changes. |
| b. Knowledge deficit regarding fever and tepid sponging: related to misinformation. | Instruction will enable parents to perform skill at home. |
| **Planning** | |
| 1. Develop individualized goals for client based on nursing diagnoses: | |
| a. Minimize heat loss during sponging. | Chilling can cause increase in body temperature. |
| b. Control sources of anxiety. | Fever can cause confusion, irritability. |
| c. Reduce body temperature gradually. | Rapid drop in temperature can be dangerous. |
| d. Improve parents' understanding of nature of fever and technique to use in sponging. | Promotes home health maintenance. |
| 2. Prepare needed equipment and supplies: | |
| a. Bath basin | Infants or small children can be immersed in tubs more easily. |
| b. Tepid water (37° C [98.6° F]) | Use of tepid water prevents sudden heat loss and chilling. |

| Steps | Rationale |
|---|---|
| c. Bath thermometer | Use to check water temperature. |
| d. Washcloths | |
| e. Waterproof pads | |
| f. Bath blanket | |
| g. Ethyl alcohol (optional) | Increases evaporative heat loss. |
| h. Thermometer | |
| 3. Explain to client that purpose of sponging with tepid water is to cool body slowly. Briefly describe steps of procedure. | Procedure can be uncomfortable because of cool applications. Anxiety over procedure can increase body temperature. |
| 4. Obtain physician's order if client has history of heart disease or cardiac arrhythmias. | Changes in blood flow that occur during heat loss may induce arrhythmias. |

## Implementation

| Steps | Rationale |
|---|---|
| 1. Wash hands. | Reduces transfer of microorganisms. |
| 2. Place waterproof pads under client and remove gown. | Pads prevent soiling of bed linen. Removing gown provides access to all skin surfaces. |
| 3. Keep bath blanket over body parts not being sponged. Close windows and door to prevent drafts in the room. | Bath blanket prevents chilling. |
| 4. Check water temperature. | Tepid water prevents chilling. |
| 5. Immerse washcloths in water and apply wet cloths under each axilla and over groin. If using tub, immerse client for 20-30 min. | Axilla and groin contain large superficial blood vessels. Application of sponges promotes cooler temperature of body's core by conduction. Immersion provides more effective heat loss. |
| 6. Gently sponge an extremity for 5 min. Note client's response. The opposite extremity may be covered by a cool washcloth. In tub, gently squeeze water over client's back and chest. | Prevents sudden temperature fall and minimizes risk of developing chills. |
| 7. Dry extremity and reassess client's pulse and body temperature. Observe client's response to therapy. | Client's response to therapy is monitored to prevent a sudden temperature change. |
| 8. Continue sponging other extremities, back, and buttocks for 3-5 min each. Reassess temperature and pulse every 15 min. | |
| 9. Change water and reapply sponges to axilla and groin as needed. | Water temperature rises as a result of exposure to client's warm body surface. |
| 10. When body temperature falls to slightly above normal, discontinue procedure. | Prevents a temperature drift to a subnormal level. Follow institutional guidelines. |
| 11. Dry extremities and body parts thoroughly. Cover client with light bath blanket or sheet. | Drying and covering the client prevent chilling. Excessively heavy covering may increase body temperature. |
| 12. Dispose of equipment and change bed linen if soiled. Wash hands. | Reduces transmission of infection. |

## Evaluation

| Steps | Rationale |
|---|---|
| 1. Measure client's body temperature and pulse. | Temperature indicates response to therapy. Arrythmias may be a complication of therapy. |

### *Expected outcomes*

| Steps | Rationale |
|---|---|
| 1. Client's body temperature drops to normal range. | Sponging effectively lowers body temperature. |
| 2. Pulse rate is regular and within normal range for client's age. | No cardiac complications develop. |

### *Unexpected outcomes*

| Steps | Rationale |
|---|---|
| 1. Client's temperature remains elevated. | Shivering may occur or febrile state continues unrelieved. |
| 2. Chilling may develop during procedure, requiring discontinuation of therapy. | Risk of fever increases. |
| 3. Pulse rate may become irregular. | Circulatory changes result in pulse alteration. |

## Recording and Reporting

| Steps | Rationale |
|---|---|
| 1. Record temperature change on graphic flow sheet. | Documents temperature variations and provides visual record of response to therapy. |
| 2. Record in nurses' notes length of procedure and client's response to sponging, e.g., onset of chills or arrhythmias. | Accurate documentation includes timely description of client's response to therapy. |
| 3. Report any complications (e.g., arrhythmias or failure of body temperature to fall) to nurse in charge or physician. | May require additional therapy such as administration of antipyretics or use of hypothermia blanket. |

| Steps | Rationale |
|---|---|
| **Follow-up Activities** | |
| 1. Provide opportunity for parents to discuss procedure and ask questions. | Feedback measures parents' level of understanding. |
| 2. Administer antipyretics or initiate other fever control measures as ordered Unit VI. | Antipyretics lower body temperature by reducing hypothalamic "set point." |
| 3. Monitor client's vital signs within 30 min and thereafter according to physician's orders. | Temperature may rise again after therapy, particularly if infectious process continues to raise hypothalamic set point. |

## Special Considerations

- Physicians will disagree as to what body temperature warrants sponging. Fever is believed to be a beneficial physiologic response. Generally body temperature should be above 39°-40° C (102°-104° F) before sponging is necessary. Stop procedure immediately if chilling starts. Avoid rubbing skin too briskly when sponging, since this may cause increased heat production.

## Teaching Considerations

- Instruct parents on importance of keeping water tepid and not cold. Warn parents not to add alcohol to water as there is a risk of poisoning an infant by inhalation. Also explain necessity of supporting infant's head and shoulders if infant is immersed in tub. (Immersion increases rate of heat loss).

### BIBLIOGRAPHY


Donahue AM: Tepid sponging, J Emerg Nurs 9:78, 1983.

Ebersole P, Hess P: Toward healthy aging: human needs and nursing response, ed 3, St. Louis, 1990, The CV Mosby Co.

Golden S: Nursing a loved one at home, Philadelphia, 1988, Running Press Book Publishers.

Henningson A, Nystrom B, Tunnell R: Bathing or washing babies after birth? Lancet 2:1401, 1981.

Longworth JCD: Psychophysiological effects of slow stroke back massage in normotensive females, Annals Nurs Sci. 4:44, 1982.

Michelson D: How to give a good back rub, Am J Nurs 78:1197, 1978.

Potter PA, Perry AG: Fundamentals of nursing, ed 2, St. Louis, 1989, The CV Mosby Co.

Potter, PA, Perry AG: Basic nursing, theory and practice, St. Louis, 1987, The CV Mosby Co.

Rose J: Back to basics: skin care in the elderly, J Practical Nurs 30:20, 1980.

Thomas DO: Fever in children, RN 48:18, 1985.

Walsh J, Persons C, Wieck L: Manual of home health care nursing, Philadelphia, 1987, JB Lippincott Co.

Whaley LF, Wong DL: Nursing care of infants and children, ed 3, St. Louis, 1987, The CV Mosby Co.

Wilson CB, et al.: When is umbilical cord separation delayed? J Pediatr 107:292, 1985.

Winslow EH: Oxygen uptake and cardiovascular response in control adults and acute myocardial infarction patients during bathing, Nurs Res 34:164, 1985.

# 7

# PRESSURE ULCER CARE

### OBJECTIVES

*Mastery of content in this chapter will enable the nurse to:*

- Define key terms.
- Describe guidelines to follow in preventing pressure ulcer formation.
- Identify risks for development of pressure ulcers.
- Discuss implications for the use of topical agents in the treatment of pressure ulcers.
- Apply topical agents correctly to a pressure ulcer.

### KEY TERMS

*Astringent*
*Debride*
*Excoriation*
*Exudate*
*Hyperemia*
*Hypoxemia*
*Maceration*
*Pressure ulcer*
*Tissue ischemia*
*Topical agents*

### SKILL

**7-1** Risk Assessment and Prevention Strategies
**7-2** Treatment of Pressure Ulcers

A pressure sore, or decubitus ulcer, is an inflammation or ulcer that develops in the skin as a result of a prolonged period of ischemia in the tissues. It results when the client remains in one position for an extended period of time. Usually the ulcer forms over a bony prominence. Ischemia develops when pressure on the skin is greater than the pressure inside the small peripheral blood vessels supplying blood to the skin. Any shearing force, the force that stretches the skin during turning or moving up in bed, increases the reduction in blood flow. Damage to the skin in the form of minor abrasions leaves thromboses in peripheral vessels, further compromising blood flow. Circulatory impairment often is compounded by altered body metabolism and negative nitrogen balance that commonly occurs in immobilized clients.

Pressure ulcers pose serious risks to a client's health status. A break in the skin, seen in advancing stages of pressure ulcers, eliminates the body's first line of defense against infection. When an ulcer invades subcutaneous tissues there is loss of protein- and electrolyte-rich body fluids from the wound; with large ulcers serious electrolyte imbalances can occur. A pressure ulcer can prolong morbidity and interfere with the rehabilitative and supportive care the client receives.

Nursing care requires aggressive prevention including meticulous hygienic care. Care is complex because of the many variables involved in each client's risk for developing pressure sores. Even high-risk clients who receive thorough nursing care may develop ulcers in spite of the nurse's efforts. When a pressure sore develops the nurse must use diligent aseptic techniques and apply wound care principles in management of the ulcer based on the ulcer stage (Chapters 38 and 41).

### GUIDELINES

1. A diet high in calories, vitamins, and protein maintains normal tissue status and promotes healing. A daily protein intake of 0.35 g/kg of body weight in young persons and 0.6 g/kg for older adults will maintain a proper nitrogen balance (Munro, 1972).
2. Frequently turn and position client to relieve pressure around superficial capillaries and allow tissues to compensate for temporary ischemia. Classic research (Kosiak, 1961) found that tissue ischemia begins within 1 to 2 hours after onset of pressure in paraplegic animals. Turning clients every 1 to 2 hours will minimize formation of pressure sores.
3. Specialized beds and mattresses (Chapter 35) distribute pressure on dependent body parts more evenly. Clients at high risk for pressure ulcer formation should be placed on these devices as soon as possible.
4. Do not expose client's skin to moisture and increased temperature. Incontinence, diaphoresis, and wound drainage are factors that promote maceration of superficial skin layers. Thorough washing and drying will help maintain skin integrity.
5. Frequently inspect linen and bed clothes to be sure they are clean, dry, and wrinkle free. Uneven underlying bed linen or bed clothing can create pressure against skin layers.

6. Carefully monitor any form of treatment with regard to the process of healing. Changes in therapy often become indicated. Prescribed treatment for a client's bedsore will vary depending on the extent of the ulcer and the client's underlying condition.

Most clients will require a variety of therapies depending on whether nursing care is preventive or directed toward treatment of an existing ulcer. Because a client with one sore can develop another, preventive care is always important. Chapter 41 describes the use of dry, wet-to-dry, and occlusive transparent dressings and their applicability to pressure ulcer care. Chapters 33 and 35 review specific positioning techniques and how to use special mattresses and beds. This chapter reviews risk assessment of pressure ulcer formation and the use of topical agents for treatment of pressure ulcers.

**PREREQUISITE KNOWLEDGE**

1. Effects of immobilization on the skin and musculoskeletal system.
2. Principles of medical asepsis.
3. Principles of wound healing.

**PREREQUISITE SKILLS**

1. Bathing techniques (Chapter 6).
2. Handwashing techniques (Chapter 37).
3. Physical assessment of the skin (Chapter 13).
4. Nutritional assessment (Chapter 26).
5. Techniques for changing dressings (Chapter 41).
6. Application of sterile gloves (Chapter 38).
7. Opening sterile packages (Chapter 38).
8. Techniques for positioning (Chapter 33).
9. Use of pressure relief mattresses or beds (Chapter 35).

## *SKILL 7-1 Risk Assessment and Prevention Strategies*

The best treatments for pressure ulcers are the early identification of the high-risk client and the implementation of prevention strategies. The three populations of clients who are known to be at high risk are: (1) the client with a neurologic impairment that decreases sensation, (2) the chronically-ill long-term-care client, and (3) orthopedic patients. These groups can be readily identified, but *any* client exposed to the right conditions for pressure sore development may be at risk. Conditions for pressure sore development include, but are not limited to, pressure, friction, shear, and moisture.

Techniques for identification of the individual at risk and basic prevention strategies are described in the skill.

**Purposes**

1. Identify clients at risk for breakdown.
2. Identify clients with existing breakdown.
3. Develop plan for prevention of breakdown in the at-risk population.

### *Procedure 7-1*

| Steps | Rationale |
|---|---|
| **Assessment** | |
| 1. Identify client's risk for pressure ulcer formation: | Determines need to administer preventive care in addition to use of topical agents for existing ulcers. |
| a. Paralysis or immobilization caused by restrictive devices. | Client unable to turn or reposition independently. |
| b. Sensory loss. | Client feels no discomfort from pressure. |
| c. Circulatory disorders. | Disorders reduce perfusion of skin's tissue layers. |
| d. Fever. | Causes increase in metabolic demands of tissues. Accompanying diaphoresis leaves skin moist. |
| e. Anemia. | Decreased hemoglobin reduces oxygen-carrying capacity of blood and amount of oxygen available to tissues. |
| f. Malnutrition. | Inadequate nutrition can lead to weight loss, muscle atrophy, and reduced tissue mass. Less tissue is available to pad between skin and underlying bone. Poor protein, vitamin, and caloric intake limit person's wound-healing capabilities. |
| g. Incontinence. | Skin becomes exposed to moist environment containing bacteria. Moisture causes skin maceration. |
| h. Heavy sedation and anesthesia. | Client is not mentally alert; does not turn or change position independently. Sedation can also alter sensory perception. |
| i. Elderly. | Skin is less elastic and drier; tissue mass is reduced. |
| j. Dehydration. | Results in decreased skin elasticity and turgor. |

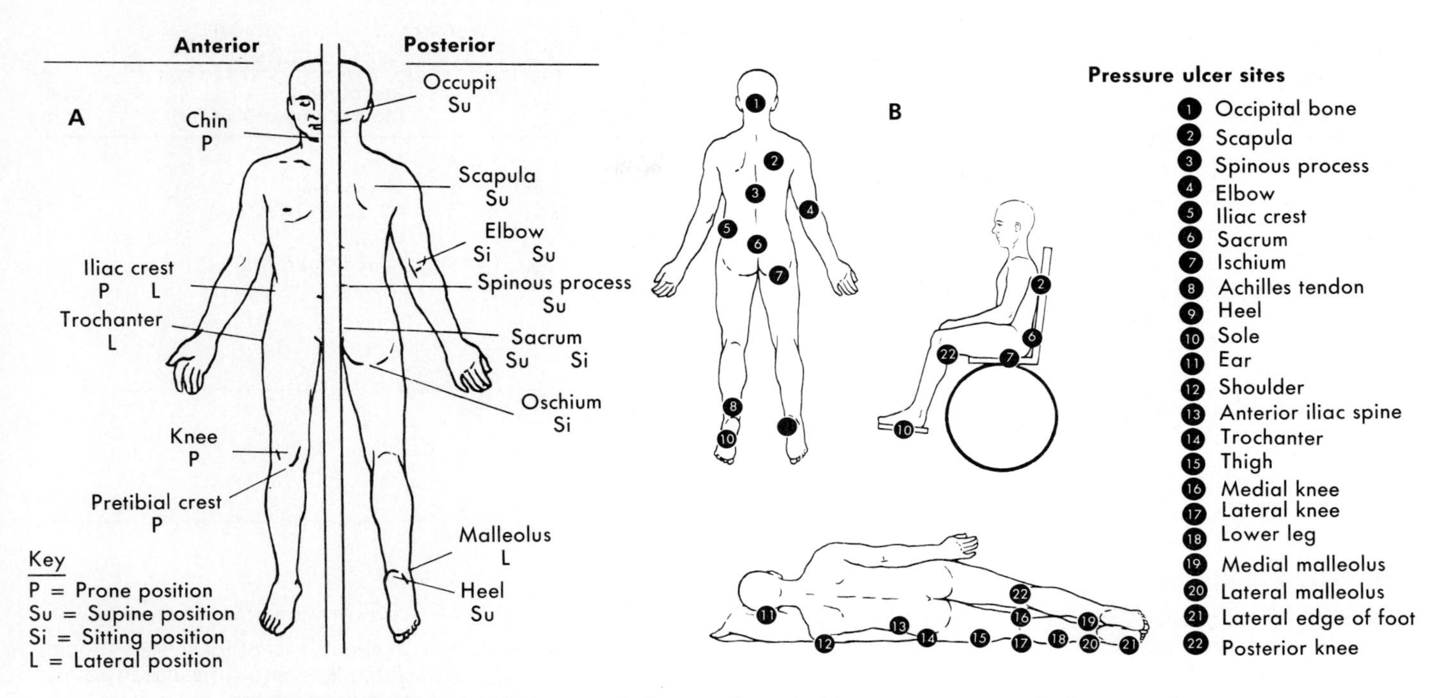


***Fig. 7-1*** **A,** Bony prominences most frequently underlying pressure sores. **B,** Pressure ulcer sites.

From Trelease CC: Developing standards for wound care, Ostomy/ Wound Management 20:46, 1988.

| Steps | Rationale |
|---|---|
| k. Edema. | Edematous tissues are less tolerant of pressure, friction, and shear. |
| l. Existing pressure ulcers. | Limits surfaces available for position changes, placing available tissues at increased risk. |
| 2. Assess condition of client's skin over regions of pressure (Fig. 7-1). Look for areas of: | Body weight against bony prominences places underlying skin at risk for breakdown. |
| a. Redness, warmth. | May indicate tissue was under pressure, hyperemia is normal physiologic response to hypoxemia in tissues. |
| b. Pallor and mottling. | Persistent hypoxia in tissues that were under pressure; an abnormal physiologic response. |
| c. Absence of superficial skin layers. | Represents early pressure ulcer formation. |
| 3. Assess client for additional areas of potential pressure: | Clients at high risk have multiple sites in addition to bony prominences for pressure necrosis: |
| a. Nares. | NG tube. |
| b. Tongue, lips. | Oral airway, endotracheal (ET) tube. |
| c. Intravenous (IV) sites (especially long-term access sites). | Stress on catheter at exit site. |
| d. Drainage tubes. | Stress against tissue at exit site. |
| e. Foley catheter. | Pressure against labia, especially with edema. |
| 4. Observe client for preferred positions when in bed or chair. | Weight of body will be placed on certain bony prominences. Presence of contractures may result in pressure exerted in unexpected places. This phenomenon is best assessed through observation. |
| 5. Observe ability of client to initiate and assist with position changes. | Potential for friction and shear increases when client is completely dependent for position changes. |
| 6. Obtain "Risk Score" (Table 7-1). | Risk score will depend on instrument used, and predicts client's need for preventive care. |
| 7. Assess client's and support persons' understanding of risks for pressure ulcers. | Provides opportunity to begin prevention education. |

***TABLE 7-1*** Norton Scale

| **Physical Condition** | | **Mental Condition** | | **Activity** | | **Mobility** | | **Incontinent (Bowel and/or Bladder)** | | **Total Score** |
|---|---|---|---|---|---|---|---|---|---|---|
| Good | 4 | Alert | 4 | Ambulant | 4 | Full | 4 | Not | 4 | |
| Fair | 3 | Apathetic | 3 | Walk/Help | 3 | Slightly limited | 3 | Occasional (< 2 per 24 hours) | 3 | |
| Poor | 2 | Confused | 2 | Chairbound | 2 | Very limited | 2 | Usually (> 2 per 24 hrs) | 2 | |
| Very Bad | 1 | Stupor | 1 | Bed | 1 | Immobile | 1 | Always | 1 | |

Maximum score = 20 (good physical condition)
Minimum score = 5
High risk for pressure ulcers = 12 or below

From Trelease CC: Developing standards for wound care. Ostomy/Wound Management, 20:46, 1988.

| **Steps** | **Rationale** |
|---|---|

## Nursing Diagnosis

| Steps | Rationale |
|---|---|
| 1. Cluster data to reveal actual or potential nursing diagnoses: | |
| a. Potential impaired skin integrity: related to malnutrition, immobilization. | Client will not require topical agents except for more thorough cleansing. Nurse must institute preventive measures against ulcer formation. |
| b. Sensory alteration, tactile: related to neurologic injury. | Client will require preventive care as a result of inability to feel discomfort. |
| c. Impaired physical mobility: related to bedrest. | Client will require preventive care as a result of inability to change position independently. |
| d. Altered tissue perfusion, peripheral: related to poor arterial perfusion. | Reduced perfusion to tissues enhances ischemia. |
| e. Knowledge deficit regarding decubitus prevention: related to inexperience. | Nurse incorporates instruction during assessment and positioning techniques. |

## Planning

| Steps | Rationale |
|---|---|
| 1. Develop individualized goals for client based on nursing diagnoses: | |
| a. Skin remains intact without breakdown. | Prevention strategies reduce pressure, friction, shear, and moisture on skin. |
| b. Client attains rest and increased mobility. | A regular schedule for position changes coupled with rest relieves pressure on bony prominences and restores client's energy stores. |
| c. Maintain adequate blood flow in affected vessels. | Pressure relief maneuvers facilitate adequate blood flow. |
| 2. Explain procedure(s) and purpose to client and family. | Relieves anxiety and provides opportunity for education. |
| 3. Prepare necessary equipment and supplies: | |
| a. Pressure relief mattress, bed or chair cushion. | Provides pressure relief to bony prominences (see Chapter 35). |
| b. Positioning aids, such as pillows, foam wedges, orthotic splints. | A variety of devices assist with position changes without adding pressure to dependent parts. |
| c. Documentation record. | Documenting areas of risk and a schedule for position changes may be helpful for consistent care. |

## Implementation

| Steps | Rationale |
|---|---|
| 1. Wash hands. | Reduces transmission of infection. |
| 2. Close room door or bedside curtain. | Maintains client privacy. |
| 3. Assist client to change of position: | See Chapter 33 for specifics. Avoid positions that place client directly on an area of existing ulceration. |
| a. Supine. | |
| b. Prone. | |
| c. Side-lying. | |
| d. 30° oblique. Achieved with one pillow under shoulder and one pillow under leg on the same side. | Protects sacrum and trochanters. |
| 4. Observe for redness in area that was under pressure. Initial flushing is expected. | Early detection of pressure indicates need for more frequent position change. |

| Steps | Rationale |
|---|---|
| 5. Monitor length of time any area of redness persists. | Redness usually persists for 50% of the time hypoxia actually occurred. |
| a. Determine appropriate turning interval. | E.g.: turning interval is 2 hr, redness lasts 15 min, hypoxia was therefore approximately 30 min. |
| b. A turning interval of <1.5-2 hr may not be realistic, therefore use of a pressure relief device would be recommended (Chapter 35). | Recommended turning interval should be: turning interval − hypoxia time = suggested interval, e.g.: 2 hr − 30 min = 1.5 hr |
| 6. Wash hands. | Reduces spread of microorganisms. |

## Evaluation

| | |
|---|---|
| 1. Observe client's skin for areas at risk for change in color, texture. | Monitors for success of prevention techniques. |
| 2. Observe tolerance of client for position change. | Position changes may interfere with client's sleep and rest pattern. |
| 3. Compare subsequent risk assessment scores. | Provides ongoing comparison of client's risk level to facilitate appropriateness of plan of care. |

### *Expected outcomes*

| | |
|---|---|
| 1. Skin is intact without erythema or breakdown. | Prevention strategies are successful. |
| 2. Client reports sense of well-being and minimal sleep disruption. | Turning schedule has not disrupted sleep pattern. |
| 3. Peripheral circulation is maintained as evidenced by absence of pallor, mottling, or persistent redness. | Adequate blood flow maintained. |

### *Unexpected outcomes*

| | |
|---|---|
| 1. Skin becomes mottled, reddened. | Early signs of pressure ulcer. |
| 2. Client reports sense of fatigue and inability to sleep. | Turning schedule needs to be modified to promote sleep. |
| 3. Areas under pressure develop persistent redness and induration. | Impaired blood flow to an area of the skin. |

## Recording and Reporting

| | |
|---|---|
| 1. Record appearance of skin under pressure. | Baseline observations and subsequent inspections reveal success of prevention program. |
| 2. Describe positions, turning intervals, and other prevention measures. | Documents care. |
| 3. Report need for additional consultations for the high-risk client. | Preventing and treating pressure ulcers requires a multidisciplinary approach. Resources include: physical therapist, occupational therapist, social worker, dietician, home health nurse, clinical nurse specialist. |

## Special Considerations

- Body regions that receive greatest pressure in specific positions:
  1. *Sitting*—ischial tuberosities, sacrum.
  2. *Supine*—back of skull, elbow, sacrum, ischial tuberosities, heels.
  3. *Prone*—elbows, knees, toes.
  4. *Side-lying*—knees, greater trochanters.
- Clients may tolerate 30° oblique for longer intervals, which would allow minimal disturbance at night.

## Teaching Considerations

- Explain risks of pressure ulcer formation.
- Assist client (and family) to understand multiple factors involved in preventing and treating pressure ulcers.
- Explain and demonstrate positioning options to achieve pressure relief.
- Explain purpose(s) and maintenance of pressure relief device(s).
- When teaching clients to change position for pressure relief, suggest using television programming and commercial intervals or a watch with an alarm as reminders.

## Home Care Considerations

- Have family learn and demonstrate positioning techniques, using pillows and rolled towels.

# SKILL 7-2 Treatment of Pressure Ulcers

There is no conclusive research on a single topical agent as the most effective agent in the treatment of pressure sores. Topical agents, however, are popular because of their ease of application and the fact that therapy takes little time. Some agents are harmful when applied over superficial pressure ulcers. For example, massaging reddened skin with soap produces swelling, drying, and loss of natural oils leading to epidermal damage (Bettley, 1960). Astringents such as alcohol and witch hazel can also harm skin layers through excessive drying and vasoconstriction, which can reduce local blood flow to tissues.

Topical agents that are beneficial in pressure ulcer care include enzymes, antiseptics, oxidizing agents, and dry dextranomer beads. The choice of agents depends on the depth of the ulcer. A deeper ulcer containing necrotic tissue may benefit from enzyme application. The nurse frequently uses antiseptic solutions for more superficial ulcers. There are basic techniques the nurse uses to apply each type of topical agent.

Local treatment of pressure ulcers includes use of a variety of dressings. Occlusive dressings are used with increasing frequency to treat pressure ulcers. The occlusive dressings (transparent dressings, hydrocolloid dressings, the hydrogels) may be used in combination with topical agents or by themselves.

### Purposes

1. Promote cleansing and debriding of skin layers.
2. Prevent infection of tissue.
3. Stimulate granulation of healthy tissue.

## Procedure 7-2

| Steps | Rationale |
|---|---|
| **Assessment** | |
| 1. Assess pressure ulcer and surrounding skin: | |
| a. Note color and appearance of skin around ulcer. | Retained moisture causes maceration. Skin condition may indicate progressive tissue damage. |
| b. Measure diameter of pressure ulcer. | Provides an objective measure of wound size. May influence the size and type of dressing chosen. |
| c. Measure depth of pressure ulcer using sterile cotton-tipped applicator or other device that will allow measurement of wound depth. | Depth measure is important for staging the ulcer. Also assists in making volume measurement. |
| d. Measure depth of undermining of skin by lateral tissue necrosis. Use a cotton-tipped applicator and gently probe under skin edges. | Undermining may indicate progressive tissue necrosis. |
| 2. Determine stage of pressure ulcer (Table 7-2). | Determine form of therapy to be used. |
| 3. Assess client's level of comfort and need for pain medication. | Dressing change procedure is better tolerated if pain is controlled. |
| 4. Determine if client has allergies to topical agents. | Topical agents contain elements that may cause localized skin reactions. |
| 5. Assess client's and support persons' understanding of purpose of treatment. | Explanations relieve anxiety and promote cooperation during procedure. |
| 6. Review physician's order for topical agent or dressing. (In many cases physician follows nurse's recommendations for pressure ulcer care.) | Ensures that proper medication and treatment are administered. |
| **Nursing Diagnosis** | |
| 1. Cluster data to reveal actual or potential nursing diagnoses: | |
| a. Impaired skin integrity: related to immobility, exposure to wound drainage. | Stage and etiology of ulcer influence choice of treatment options. |
| **Planning** | |
| 1. Develop individualized goals for client based on nursing diagnoses: | |
| a. Promote wound healing and tissue repair. | Cleansing, proper use of topical agents and appropriate dressings promote healing. |
| b. Prevent trauma to tissue around ulcer. | Some agents may be irritating to intact skin. |

***TABLE 7-2*** Pressure Ulcer Stages

| Stage | Appearance |
|---|---|
| **Stage 1**  | Region of pallor, mottling, followed by erythema.<br>Early lesion: erythema blanches, lesion may be painful.<br>Late lesion: erythema does not blanch, may be soft or indurated; edge is usually irregular. |
| **Stage 2** 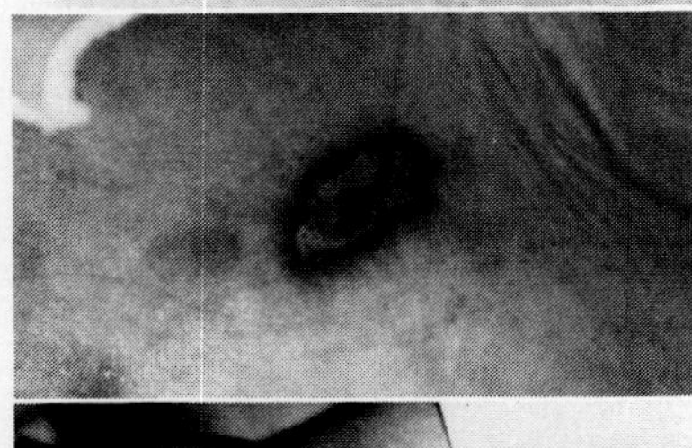 | Superficial epithelial damage, may range from a heel blister to as much as a 4 mm tissue loss over the buttocks. Surrounding area is red and scaley with irregular borders. |
| **Stage 3** 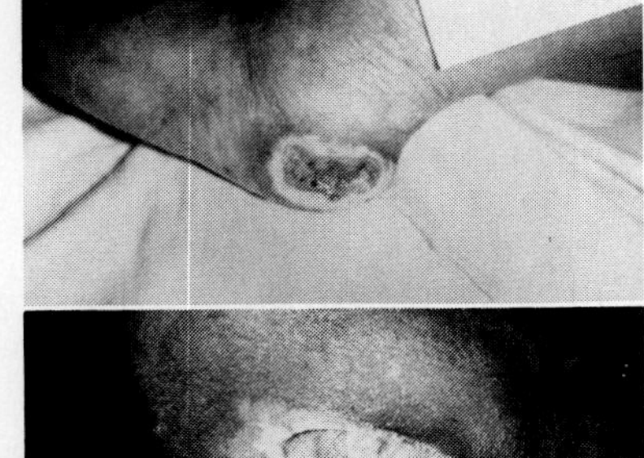 | Destruction of tissue has involved the subcutaneous layers. Surface of ulcer will likely be smaller than internal diameters. |
| **Stage 4** 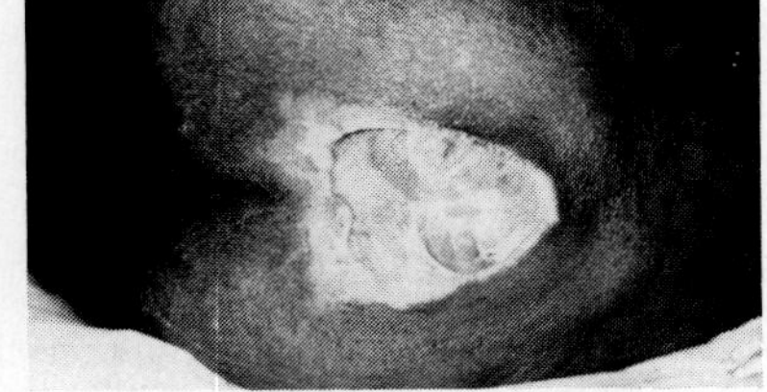 | Tissue destruction extends through subcutaneous layers into muscle and bone. Ulcer edge appears to "roll over" into the defect and is a tough fibrinous ring. |
| **Eschar** | Lesion is covered by a tough membranous layer that may be rigidly adherent to the ulcer base. Stage is difficult to determine until eschar has sloughed or has been surgically removed. |

| Steps | Rationale |
|---|---|
| 2. Explain procedure and its purpose to client and family. | Preparatory explanations relieve anxiety and offer opportunity for client and family education. |
| 3. Prepare necessary equipment and supplies: | |
| a. Wash basin, warm water, soap, wash cloth, bath towel. | Used to bathe surrounding skin. |
| b. Normal saline or other cleansing agent (Table 7-3) in sterile cup. | Ulcer surface must be cleansed before application of topical agents and new dressing. |
| c. Prescribed topical agent: | |
| ▪ Enzymes: collagenase, fibrinolysin desoxyribonuclease, or sutilains. | Proteolytic enzymes debride dead tissue to clean ulcer surface. |
| ▪ Antiseptics: povidone-iodine, ointment or solution; merbromin, 5% or 10% solution; sodium hypochlorite, 1:12 or 1:20 solution. | Antiseptic reduces bacterial growth in presence of necrotic tissue, pus, serum, or blood. Reduces infection in weeping ulcers. |
| ▪ Oxydizing agents: benzoyl peroxide, 20%; hydrogen peroxide, half strength. | Cleans wounds, especially in presence of anaerobic bacteria. Increases oxygen supply to devitalized tissues. |
| ▪ Dextranomer beads: Debrisan. | Cleans wounds with heavy exudate. Absorbs fluid, protein, fibrin, fibrinogen, and all products of tissue breakdown and bacterial infection. |

***TABLE 7-3*** Topical Cleansing Solutions

| Name | Type | Comments |
|---|---|---|
| **Acetic acid** | Antimicrobial. | Effective against *Pseudomonas aeruginosa.* Discontinue use when infected organisms are gone. |
| **Biolex** | Detergent. | Non-ionic surfactant for wound cleansing. |
| **Cara-Klenz** | Detergent. | Wound cleanser. |
| **Hydrogen peroxide** | Oxidizing agent. | Facilitates removal of necrotic debris, crusting. Will oxidize healthy tissue. *Do not use* in clean, healing ulcers. Do not use in deep ulcers as gas emboli may result. |
| **Povidone-iodine** | Antimicrobial. | Potentially irritating to intact skin. If used undiluted may cause toxicity to granulating tissues. |
| **Sodium hypochlorite (Dakins)** | Antimicrobial. | Effective for odor control. Protect intact skin with zinc oxide. Discontinue use when necrotic tissue is gone. |

***TABLE 7-4*** Dressings by Ulcer Stage

| Ulcer Stage | Dressing | Comments* |
|---|---|---|
| **Stage 1** | Film dressing. | Tegaderm, Bioclusive, Op-site, Uniflex, etc.<br>Protect from shear. May be left in place up to 7 days if occlusive seal remains. Will facilitate softening of eschars on deeper ulcers. |
| | Hydrocolloid dressing. | DuoDerm, Comfeel, IntraSite, etc.<br>Absorbent, may be left in place up to 7 days if occlusive seal remains. Unable to assess wound with dressing in place. |
| **Stage 2** | Hydrocolloid dressing. | See Stage 1. |
| | Composite dressing. | Viasorb, film dressing over Telfa, etc.<br>Provides absorbent, nonadherent layer over wound with occlusive cover. |
| | Hydrogel dressing. | Vigilon, Geliperm, J&J Gel Dressing, etc.<br>Absorbent for draining ulcers, usually requires gauze dressing cover. |
| | Burn dressing. | Exu-dry.<br>Absorbent, nonadherent; protects from shear; may be used with topical agents; not an occlusive dressing. |
| **Stage 3** | Hydrocolloid dressing. | See Stage 1.<br>Use of hydrocolloid granules or paste will increase absorbency and wear time. Frequent removal (every day or more often) may cause tissue damage. Recommend other dressing. |
| | Hydrogel dressing. | See Stage 2.<br>May be used as "carrier" for topical agents including topically applied growth factors. |
| | Burn dressing. | See Stage 2. |
| **Stage 4** | Hydrocolloid dressing. | See Stages 1 to 3.<br>May be contraindicated due to location of ulcer, exposed bone, amount of drainage. |
| | Hydrogel dressing. | See Stages 2 to 3. |
| | Gauze dressing. | Kerlix type, absorbent, not occlusive. Generally require dressing changes every 8-12 hr. |

*Note: As with *all* occlusive dressings, wounds should *not* be clinically infected.

| Steps | Rationale |
|---|---|
| d. Sterile dressing (Table 7-4): | |
| ▪ Gauze type: 4 × 4 pads fluffs. | Applied over ulcers treated with enzymes, oxidizing agents, and dextranomer beads. |
| ▪ Transparent dressings. | Applied over superficial ulcers and skin subjected to shear. |
| ▪ Hydrocolloid type. | Maintains moist environment to facilitate wound healing. |
| ▪ Hydrogel type. | Maintains moist environment to facilitate wound healing. May be used to apply topical agents. |
| e. Hypoallergenic tape or adhesive dressing sheet (Hypofix). | Used to apply gauze dressing. Prevents skin irritation and tearing. |
| f. Disposable or sterile gloves. | Used to apply topical agents. Prevents contact with infectious material. |
| g. Protective paste such as zinc oxide (optional). | Used over nonaffected skin areas to protect from irritating solutions. |
| h. Tools to measure wound size: | Wound measurement provides objective methods to evaluate progress toward wound healing. |
| ▪ transparency film and marker. | |
| ▪ metric ruler. | |

## Implementation

| Steps | Rationale |
|---|---|
| 1. Wash hands. | Reduces transmission of infection. |
| 2. Close room door or bedside curtains. | Maintains client privacy. |
| 3. Position client comfortably with area of pressure ulcer and surrounding skin easily accessible. | Area should be accessible for cleansing of ulcer and surrounding skin. |
| 4. Assemble needed supplies at bedside. Open sterile packages and topical solution containers. | Sterile supplies should be ready for easy application so that nurse can use sterile gloves without contaminating them. |
| 5. Remove bed linen and client's gown to expose ulcer and surrounding skin. Keep remaining body parts draped. | Prevents unnecessary exposure of body parts. |
| 6. Gently wash skin surrounding ulcer with warm water and soap. | Cleansing of skin surface reduces bacteria. |
| 7. Rinse area thoroughly with water. | Soap can be irritating to skin. |
| 8. Gently dry skin thoroughly by patting lightly with towel. | Retained moisture causes maceration of skin layers. |
| 9. Apply sterile gloves. | Aseptic technique must be maintained during cleansing, measuring, and application of dressings. |
| 10. Cleanse ulcer thoroughly with normal saline or cleansing agent: | Removes wound debris. Previously applied enzymes may require soaking for removal. |
| a. Use irrigating syringe for deep ulcers. | |
| b. Cleansing in the shower may be done with a hand-held shower head. | |
| c. Whirlpool treatments may be used to assist with wound cleansing and debridement. | |
| 11. Measure wound diameters and depth: | Provides objective record of wound size against which subsequent measurements can be compared. |
| a. Tracing wound diameters may be done using transparency film. | |
| b. Ruler measures wound diameter. | |
| 12. Apply topical agents, if prescribed (see Table 7-3): | |
| a. Enzymes: | |
| ▪ Keeping gloves sterile, place small amount of enzyme ointment in palm of hand. | Thick layer of ointment is not necessary. Thin layer absorbs and acts more effectively. Excess medication can irritate surrounding skin. |
| ▪ Soften medication by rubbing briskly in palm of hand. | Makes ointment easier to apply. |
| ▪ Apply thin, even layer of ointment over necrotic areas of ulcer. Do not apply enzyme to surrounding skin. | Proper distribution of ointment ensures effective action. Enzyme can cause burning, paresthesia, and dermatitis to surrounding skin. |
| ▪ Moisten gauze dressing in saline and apply directly over ulcer. | Protects wound. Moist ulcer surface reduces time needed for healing. Skin cells normally live in moist environment. |
| ▪ Cover moistened gauze with single dry gauze and tape securely in place. | Prevents bacteria from entering moist dressing. |
| b. Antiseptics: | |
| ▪ Superficial ulcers: | |
| Moisten sterile gauze with antiseptic solution and paint surface of ulcer. | Distributes antiseptic over entire area to effectively reduce bacterial growth. |
| Leave ulcer open to air. | If superficial epidermal skin layer is only layer affected, keeping wound dry promotes better healing. |

| Steps | Rationale |
|---|---|
| ▪ Deep ulcers: Apply antiseptic ointment to dominant gloved hand and spread ointment in and around ulcer. | Antiseptic ointment causes minimal tissue irritation. All surfaces of wound must be covered to effectively control bacterial growth. |
| Apply sterile gauze pad over ulcer and tape securely in place. | Protects ulcer and prevents removal of ointment during turning or repositioning. |
| c. Oxidizing agents: ▪ Spread zinc oxide paste over skin surface surrounding ulcer. | Oxidizing agents can be caustic to normal tissues. |
| ▪ Apply single layer of gauze dressing moistened in oxidizing solution over ulcer (do not apply full-strength peroxide). | Coats wound surface and retains exposure to tissue surface. |
| ▪ Apply dry gauze dressing over ulcer. | Protects ulcer and prevents loosening or pulling away of moist dressing. |
| d. Dextranomer beads: ▪ Hold container of beads approximately 1 in (2.5 cm) above ulcer site and lightly sprinkle 5 mm-diameter layer over wound. | Layer of insoluble powder is needed to absorb wound exudate. |
| ▪ Apply gauze dressing over ulcer. | Holds beads in place and protects wound. |
| e. Hydrocolloid beads or paste: ▪ Fill ulcer defect to approximately half of the total depth with hydrocolloid beads or paste. | Hydrocolloid beads or paste assist in absorbing wound drainage. Highly draining wounds are best treated with hydrocolloid beads or granules. |
| ▪ Cover with hydrocolloid dressing, extend dressing 1-1.5 inches beyond edges of wound. | Maintains wound humidity. May be left in place up to 7 days. |
| f. Hydrogel agents: ▪ Cover surface of ulcer with hydrogel using sterile applicator or gloved hand. | Provides maintenance of wound humidity while absorbing excess drainage. May be used as carrier for topical agents. |
| ▪ Apply dry fluffy gauze over gel to completely cover ulcer. | Holds hydrogel against wound surface; absorbant. |
| 13. Reposition client comfortably off pressure ulcer. | Avoids accidental removal of dressings. |
| 14. Remove gloves and dispose of soiled supplies. Wash hands. | Reduces transmission of microorganisms. |

## Evaluation

| | |
|---|---|
| 1. Observe skin surrounding ulcer for inflammation, edema, and tenderness. | Contact dermatitis may result from exposure to certain topical agents. Without proper preventive care, ulcer can spread to involve neighboring tissue. |
| 2. Inspect dressings and exposed ulcers, observing for drainage, foul odor, and tissue necrosis. | Ulcers can easily become infected. |
| 3. Compare subsequent ulcer measurements. | Allows comparison of serial measurements to assess wound healing. |

### *Expected outcomes*

| | |
|---|---|
| 1. Skin surrounding ulcer remains healthy, intact. | No irritation of surrounding tissues. |
| 2. Ulcer drainage decreases. | Ulcer shows signs of healing. |
| 3. Ulcer measurements and tracings are progressively smaller. | Signs of healing. |

### *Unexpected outcomes*

| | |
|---|---|
| 1. Skin surrounding ulcer becomes macerated. | Neighboring tissues involved from exposure to topical agents, moisture. |
| 2. Ulcer becomes deeper with increased drainage and development of necrotic tissue. | With further ischemia, chances of infection increase. |
| 3. Pressure ulcer extends beyond original margins. | Continued ischemia to tissue layers. |

## Recording and Reporting

| | |
|---|---|
| 1. Record appearance of ulcer in nurses' notes. | Baseline observations and subsequent inspections reveal progress of healing. |
| 2. Describe type of topical agent used, dressing applied, and client's response. | Documents care. |
| 3. Report any worsening in ulcer's appearance to nurse in charge or physician. | Worsening of condition may indicate need for additional therapy. |

## Special Considerations

- Preventing and treating pressure ulcers requires a multidisciplinary approach. Resources for prevention and management include physical therapist, occupational therapist, social worker, dietician, clinical specialist.
- Agents containing iodine commonly cause contact dermatitis.
- If wound is large, irrigating with plain water from irrigating syringe may be helpful. A useful irrigating device is a 35 cc syringe with a 19-gauge needle attached.
- If necrotic tissue is present in ulcer, physician should debride area thoroughly before cleansing.
- The Kundin scale is a tool for wound volume calculations.
- Early ulcers tend to have irregular borders; with time, borders become smooth and rounded.

## Teaching Considerations

- Discuss treatment and identify individual(s) who will assist in care at home.
- Discuss process of wound healing and expected wound appearance.
- Identify signs, symptoms, and four stages of ulcers to report to health care team.
- Review prevention guidelines to halt further breakdown.
- Discuss options for maintaining good nutrition.

## Home Care Considerations

- Identify clean storage area for dressing supplies.
- Identify ability and availability of required supplies.
- Discuss need for home health nurse.

---

### BIBLIOGRAPHY

Bettley FR: Some effects of soap on the skin, Br Med J 1:1675, 1960.

David JA: Pressure sore treatment: a literature review, Int J Nurs Stud 19:183, 1982.

Ebersole P, Hess P: Toward healthy aging: human needs and nursing response, ed 3, St. Louis, 1990, The C.V. Mosby Co.

Ek A, Boman G: A descriptive study of pressure sores: the prevalence of pressure sores and the characteristics of patients, J Adv Nurs 7:51, 1982.

Fowler E, Goupil DL: Comparison of the wet-to-dry dressing and copolymer starch in the management of debrided pressure sores, J Enterostomal Ther 11:22, 1984.

Fowler EM: Equipment and products used in management and treatment of pressure ulcers, Nurs Clin North Am 22(7):449, 1987.

Kerr JC, et al.: Pressure sores: distinguishing fact from fiction, Can Nurse 77:23, 1981.

Kosiak M: Etiology of decubitus ulcers, Arch Phys Med Rehab 42:19, 1961.

Lineaweaver W, et al.: Topical antimicrobial toxicity, Arch Surg 120:267, 1985.

Meyers D: Client teaching guides for home health care, Rockville, Md, 1989, Aspen Publishers, Inc.

Morley M: 16 steps to better decubitus ulcer care, Can Nurse 77:29, 1981.

Munro HN: Protein requirements and metabolism in aging. In Carlson LA, ed: Symposium on nutrition in old age, Uppsala, Sweden, 1972, Almqvist & Wiksell.

Norton D: Nursing care of the immobile patient. In Walker W, ed: Intensive Care, New York, 1975, Churchill Livingstone, Inc.

Potter PA, Perry AG: Fundamentals of nursing, ed 2, St. Louis, 1989, The CV Mosby Co.

Thomason SS: Pressure ulcers: considerations of intervention strategies. Ostomy/Wound management 19:48, 1988.

Tooman T, Patterson J: Decubitus ulcer warfare: product versus process, Geriat Nurs 5:166, 1984.

Trelease CC: Developing standards for wound care. Ostomy/Wound Management 20:46, 1988.

Tudhope M: Management of pressure ulcers with a hydrocolloid occlusive dressing: results in twenty-three patients, J Enterostomal Ther 11:102, 1984.

Young ME: Malnutrition and wound healing, Heart and Lung, 17(1):60, 1988.

# 8

# CARE OF THE MOUTH

### *OBJECTIVES*

*Mastery of content in this chapter will enable the nurse to:*

- Define key terms.
- Identify guidelines to follow when administering mouth care.
- Explain differences in providing oral care to dependent versus unconscious clients.
- Administer oral hygiene correctly to a client.
- Explain the purposes of dental flossing.
- Floss a client's teeth correctly.
- Discuss precautions used to prevent breakage of dentures.
- Administer denture care correctly.

### *KEY TERMS*

*Aspiration*
*Buccal*
*Caries*
*Cheilosis*
*Dentifrice*
*Flossing*
*Gag reflex*
*Gingiva*
*Gingivitis*
*Halitosis*
*Mastication*
*Periodontal*
*Periodontitis*
*Plaque*
*Tarter*

### *SKILLS*

***8-1*** Brushing and Flossing Teeth
***8-2*** Performing Mouth Care for the Unconscious or Debilitated Client
***8-3*** Cleaning Dentures

The oral cavity, which is lined with a normally moist, intact mucous membrane, contains the teeth and gums. The membrane is an epithelial tissue that lines and protects organs, secretes mucous to keep the cavity moist and lubricated, and absorbs nutrients. Normally the mucosa is light pink and moist. The teeth are organs of chewing, or mastication. Dentin, a hard, ivory-like substance that surrounds the pulp cavity (Fig. 8-1), forms the major part of a tooth. A layer of enamel, visible in the oral cavity, covers the upper portion of the tooth or crown. The periodontal membrane, just below the gum margins, surrounds the tooth root and holds it firmly in place. A tooth receives its blood, lymph, and nerve supply from the base of the tooth socket within the jaw. Healthy teeth are white, smooth, shiny, and properly aligned.

The gums, or gingivae, are mucous membranes with underlying supportive fibrous tissue. They encircle the neck of erupted teeth to hold them firmly in place. The gums are normally pink, moist, firm, and relatively inelastic.

Structures of the oral cavity must remain healthy for a person's comfort, maintenance of nutrition, protection from infection, and sense of well-being. Even a minor alteration of the oral cavity, such as inflammation of the gums, can create a significant health problem. A person's appetite is diminished, and the discomfort from inflammation can become an annoying irritant. Complete oral hygiene including regular brushing and flossing maintains the integrity of oral cavity structures.

The nurse's responsibilities in oral hygiene are maintenance and prevention. The nurse assists clients in maintaining good oral hygiene by teaching them correct techniques or by actually performing hygiene for weakened or disabled clients. It may be necessary for the nurse to refer clients to a dentist for problems requiring special care. Educating clients about common gum and tooth disorders and methods of prevention can motivate them to follow good oral hygiene practices.

## GUIDELINES

1. Establish a regular routine that the client can easily follow at home. Good dental hygiene requires brushing at least four times daily and flossing at least once a day. Even a client who works can brush regularly during meal breaks.
2. Encourage clients to continue visits to their dentist every six months. Even though a client may establish an effective preventive program, a dentist should screen for serious dental or periodontal problems.

3. Use dental hygiene products of the client's choice whenever possible.
4. Remember that dental hygiene can be a means for improving the client's level of comfort. Persons who are unable to eat or drink, who have nasogastric tubes inserted, or who have had trauma or surgery of the mouth will benefit from frequent oral care.
5. Use the time spent providing mouth care to teach clients about factors that increase the incidence of dental or gum disease and the proper techniques that ensure good oral hygiene practices.
6. Wearing gloves while administering oral hygiene is recommended, especially if there is active bleeding within the oral cavity or there is a risk of injury to the hands from biting.

### PREREQUISITE KNOWLEDGE

1. Principles of medical asepsis.
2. Anatomy and physiology of the mouth.

### PREREQUISITE SKILLS

1. Proper handwashing techniques (Chapter 37).
2. Physical assessment of the mouth (Chapter 13).
3. Proper positioning techniques (Skill 8-2; see Chapter 33).

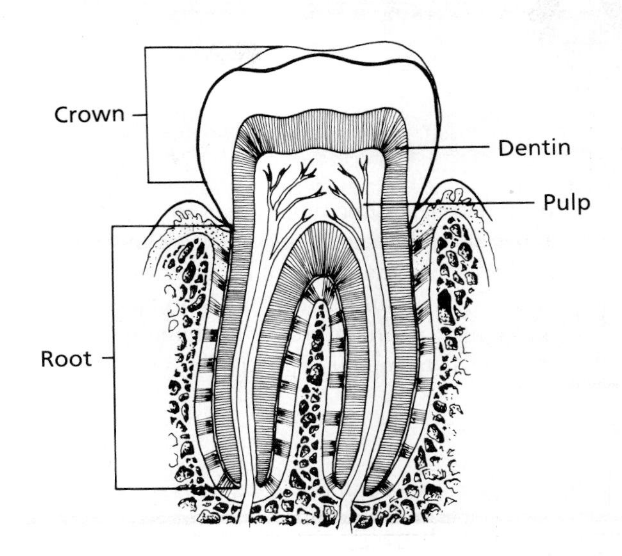


***Fig. 8-1*** A normal tooth.

## *SKILL 8-1 Brushing and Flossing Teeth*

Brushing, flossing, and irrigation are necessary for proper cleansing of teeth. Brushing removes food particles, loosens plaque, and stimulates gums. Flossing removes tartar that collects at the gum line. Irrigation removes dislodged food particles and excess toothpaste. When a client becomes ill a regular dental hygiene routine is difficult if not impossible to follow. The nurse offers whatever assistance is required, from preparing needed supplies to actually brushing the client's teeth. Techniques for brushing ensure the complete removal of food particles and stimulation of the gums.

The nurse's responsibility includes judging the frequency with which clients require brushing. Certain conditions resulting from illness or therapy cause the oral cavity to become excessively dry or irritated. For example, clients restricted from eating or drinking often develop thick, foul-tasting secretions in their mouths because of reduced hydration. Frequent oral hygiene provides clients considerable relief. Frequency of care should be based on condition of the oral cavity and the client's level of comfort. This may require oral care as often as every 1 to 2 hours.

### Purposes

1. Cleanse and irrigate tooth surfaces and stimulate gums and mucosa.
2. Prevent infection and dental caries.
3. Promote self-esteem and comfort.
4. Maintain client's appetite.
5. Develop client understanding of importance of oral hygiene.
6. Develop client skills in performing toothbrushing.

## *Procedure 8-1*

| Steps | Rationale |
|---|---|
| **Assessment** | |
| 1. Inspect integrity of lips, teeth, buccal mucosa, gums, palate, and tongue. (Wear gloves during inspection.) | Determines status of client's oral cavity and extent of need for hygiene. Gloves prevent contact with blood or saliva that may harbor infectious microorganisms. |
| 2. Assess client's risk for oral hygiene problems: | Certain conditions increase likelihood of impaired oral cavity integrity and need for preventive care. |
| a. Dehydration, inability to take fluids or food by mouth (NPO).* | Causes excess drying and fragility of mucous membranes; increases accumulation of secretions on tongue and secretions on tongue and gums. |
| b. Presence of nasogastric tubes; mouth-breathers. | Causes drying of mucosa. |
| c. Chemotherapeutic drugs. | Drugs cause death of rapidly multiplying cells, including cancerous tumors, as well as cells lining oral cavity and gastrointestinal tract. |
| d. Presence of artificial airway. | Increases irritation to gums and mucosa. Excess secretions accumulate on teeth and tongue. |
| e. Blood clotting disorders, (e.g., leukemia, aplastic anemia). | Clients are predisposed to inflammation and bleeding of gums. |
| f. Oral surgery, trauma to mouth. | Break in mucosa resulting from incision or trauma increases risk of infection. Vigorous brushing can disrupt suture lines. |
| g. Aging. | Physiologic changes of aging (e.g., reduced gum vascularity; loss of periodontal tissue elasticity; atrophy of jaw bone; teeth becoming dry, brittle, and thinner) require frequent preventive oral hygiene. |
| h. Diabetic clients. | Prone to dryness of mouth, gingivitis, periodontal disease, and loss of teeth. |
| 3. Identify presence of common oral problems:<br>a. *Dental caries*—chalky white discoloration of tooth or presence of brown or black discoloration.<br>b. *Gingivitis*—inflammation of gums.<br>c. *Periodontitis*—receding gum lines, inflammation, gaps between teeth.<br>d. *Halitosis*—bad breath.<br>e. *Cheilosis*—cracking of lips. | Helps determine type of hygiene client requires and information client requires for self-care. |
| 4. Determine client's oral hygiene practices:<br>a. Frequency of tooth brushing and flossing.<br>b. Type of toothpaste or dentifrice used.<br>c. Client's last dental visit.<br>d. Frequency of dental visits. | Allows nurse to identify errors in technique, deficiencies in preventive oral hygiene, and client's knowledge regarding dental care. |
| e. Use of mouthwash or lemon-glycerine preparation. | Lemon-glycerine preparations can be detrimental. Glycerine is an astringent that dries and shrinks mucous membranes and gums. Lemon exhausts salivary reflex and can erode tooth enamel. Mouthwash provides only pleasant aftertaste and can dry mucosa after extended use. |
| 5. Assess client's ability to grasp and manipulate toothbrush. | Elderly clients or persons with musculoskeletal or nervous system alterations may be unable to hold toothbrush with firm grip or manipulate brush. Assessment determines level of assistance required from nurse. |
| **Nursing Diagnosis** | |
| 1. Cluster data to reveal actual or potential nursing diagnoses: | |
| a. Altered oral mucous membrane: related to dehydration. | Thorough brushing can help maintain mucous membrane integrity and restore changes resulting from dehydration or inflammation. |
| b. Pain: related to inflammed oral cavity. | Requires gentle brushing to avoid injuring fragile gums. |
| c. Altered nutrition—less than body requirements: related to oral pain or absence of teeth. | Frequent mouth care can improve appetite. |
| d. Knowledge deficit regarding oral hygiene care: related to request for information. | Client requires instructions given during care. |

*No food/fluids by mouth.

| Steps | Rationale |
|---|---|
| e. Self-care hygiene deficit: related to reduced dexterity. | Nurse encourages involvement by allowing client to make choices of hygiene products. |

## Planning

| Steps | Rationale |
|---|---|
| 1. Develop individualized goals for client based on nursing diagnoses: | |
| a. Client achieves sense of comfort. | Moist mucosa is less irritating. |
| b. Oral mucosa is intact and well hydrated. | Removal of coating and crustations moistens mucosa. |
| c. Teeth are without new dental caries. | Brushing aids removal of plaque. |
| d. Client understands oral hygiene techniques. | Oral care instruction may include client and family. |
| e. Client retains sense of independence. | Client participates in care by selecting hygiene aids. |
| 2. Prepare needed equipment and supplies: | |
| a. Toothbrush with straight handle and small, soft rounded bristles | Brush should reach all areas of mouth. Rounded soft bristles stimulate gums without causing bleeding. |
| b. Toothpaste or dentifrice | Fluoride is preferred. |
| c. Dental floss | |
| d. Water glass with cool water | |
| e. Mouthwash (optional) | Some clients dislike taste of mouthwash. |
| f. Straw | |
| g. Emesis basin | |
| h. Face towel and paper towels | |
| i. Disposable gloves | Prevents contact with oral secretions and blood. |
| 3. Explain procedure to client and discuss preferences regarding use of hygienic aids. | Some clients feel uncomfortable about having the nurse care for their basic needs. Client involvement with procedure minimizes anxiety. |

## Implementation

| Steps | Rationale |
|---|---|
| 1. Wash hands. | Reduces transmission of microorganisms. |
| 2. Place paper towels on overbed table and arrange other equipment within easy reach. | Towels collect moisture and spills from emesis basin. |
| 3. Pull curtain or close room door (optional if client only brushing teeth). | Provides client privacy. When brushing is part of bathing and total hygiene, privacy is essential. |
| 4. Raise bed to comfortable working position. Raise head of bed (if allowed) and lower side rail. Move client or help client move toward you. Side-lying position can be used. | Raising bed and positioning client prevent nurse from acquiring muscle strain. Semi-Fowler's position helps prevent client from choking or aspirating. |
| 5. Place towel over client's chest. | Prevents soiling of gown and bed linen. |
| 6. Position overbed table within easy reach and adjust height as needed. | Easy accessibility of supplies ensures smooth, safe procedure. |
| 7. Apply gloves. | Prevents contact with microorganisms in saliva. |
| 8. Apply toothpaste to brush, holding brush over emesis basin. Pour small amount of water over toothpaste. | Moisture aids in distribution of toothpaste over tooth surfaces. |
| 9. Hold toothbrush bristles at 45° angle to gum line (Fig. 8-2). Be sure tips of bristles rest against and penetrate under gum line. Brush inner and outer surfaces of upper and lower teeth by brushing from gum to crown of each tooth. Use short vibrating strokes and brush each tooth separately. Clean biting surfaces of teeth by holding top of bristles parallel with teeth and brushing gently back and forth (Fig. 8-3). Brush sides of teeth by moving bristles back and forth (Fig. 8-4). | Angle allows brush to reach all tooth surfaces and to clean under gum line where plaque and tartar accumulate. Back-and-forth motion dislodges food particles caught between teeth and along chewing surfaces. |

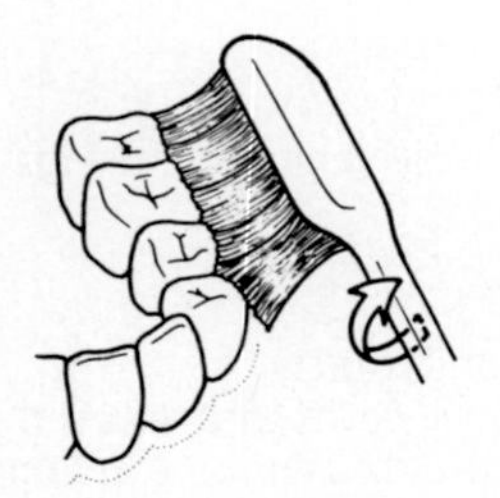

*Fig. 8-2*

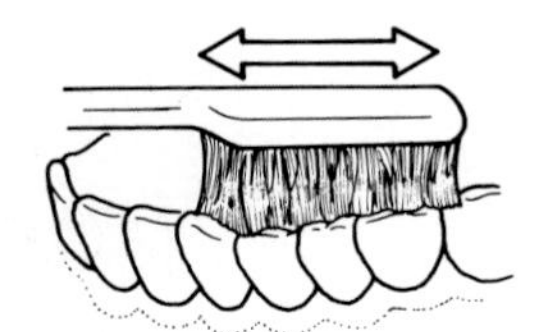

*Fig. 8-3*

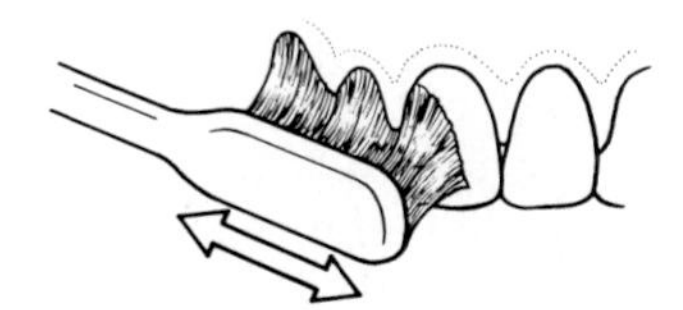

*Fig. 8-4*

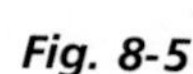
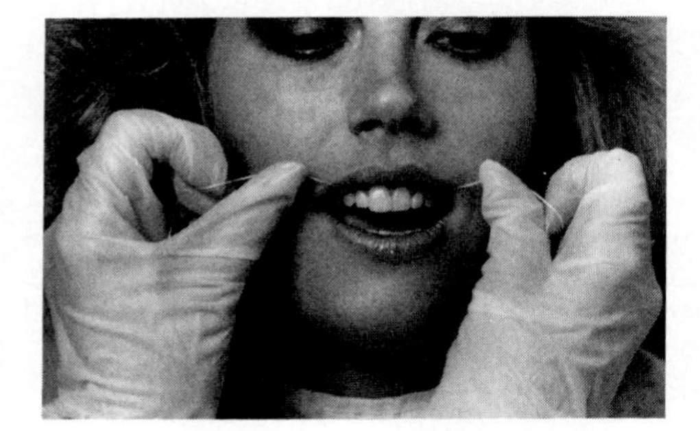
*Fig. 8-5*

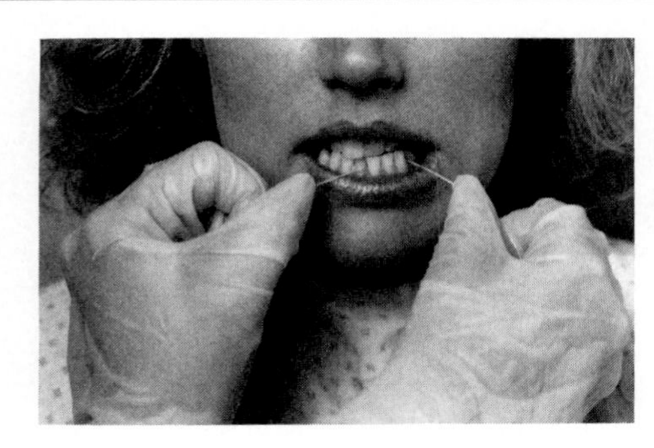
*Fig. 8-6*

| Steps | Rationale |
|---|---|
| 10. Hold brush at 45° angle and lightly brush over surface and sides of tongue. Avoid initiating gag reflex. | Microorganisms collect and grow on tongue's surface. Gagging is uncomfortable and may cause aspiration of toothpaste. |
| 11. Allow client to rinse mouth thoroughly by taking several sips of water, swishing across all tooth surfaces, and spitting into emesis basin. | Irrigation removes food particles. |
| 12. Allow client to gargle or rinse mouth with mouthwash. | Mouthwash leaves pleasant taste in mouth. |
| 13. Remove emesis basin and assist in wiping client's mouth. | Promotes sense of comfort. |
| 14. Prepare for flossing by having client wash hands, if client is to floss independently. | Reduces transmission of microorganisms. |
| 15. Prepare two pieces of dental floss approximately 25 cm (10 in) in length. Opinion differs over use of waxed vs unwaxed floss. Waxed floss frays less easily. Food particles adhere to unwaxed floss. | Need adequate length to grasp floss firmly and insert over surfaces of teeth. |
| 16. Wrap ends of floss around the third finger of each hand. Using thumb and index finger, stretch floss and insert between two upper teeth (Fig. 8-5). Move floss up and down in seesaw motion between teeth from under gum lines up to top of each tooth's crown. Be sure to clean outer surface of back molar. Make a figure **C** around the edge of the tooth being flossed. Work systematically along each set of teeth. | Proper insertion and movement of floss along tooth surfaces mechanically removes plaque and tartar. |
| 17. Take a clean piece of floss and wrap around third finger of each hand. Using index fingers stretch floss and insert between two lower teeth (Fig. 8-6). | Frayed floss becomes caught between teeth and can be torn off. This can lead to gum inflammation and infection. Position of hands helps reach lower tooth surfaces. |
| 18. Move floss up and down, between gum lines and crown of lower teeth one at a time. | Upward motion of floss removes plaque and tartar. |
| 19. Allow client to rinse mouth thoroughly with tepid water and spit into emesis basin. Assist in wiping client's mouth. | Irrigation removes plaque and tartar from oral cavity. |
| 20. Assist client to comfortable position, remove bedside table, raise side rail, and lower bed to original position. | Provides client comfort and safety. |
| 21. Wipe off overbed table, discard soiled linen and paper towels in appropriate containers, remove soiled gloves, and return equipment to proper place. | Proper disposal of soiled equipment prevents spread of infection. |
| 22. Wash hands. | Reduces transmission of microorganisms. |

## Evaluation

| | |
|---|---|
| 1. Ask client if any area of oral cavity feels uncomfortable or irritated. | Pain is indication of more chronic problem. |
| 2. Inspect condition of oral cavity. | Determines effectiveness of hygiene and rinsing. |
| 3. Ask client to describe proper hygiene techniques. | Evaluates client's learning. |

### *Expected outcomes*

| | |
|---|---|
| 1. Client expresses feeling of comfort. | Mucosa and gums moist and intact. |
| 2. Oral mucosa is moist, intact, and normal color. | Normal characteristics of oral cavity structures. If client had degree of alteration before brushing, condition should not worsen after brushing. |
| 3. Gums are pink, firm, and adherent to neck of teeth. | |
| 4. Teeth are clean, white, smooth, and shiny. | |
| 5. Tongue is pink and without secretions or coating. | |

| Steps | Rationale |
|---|---|
| 6. Client describes correct oral hygiene techniques and necessary frequency. | Demonstrates understanding of nurse's instructions. |
| ***Unexpected outcomes*** | |
| 1. Mucosa is dry and inflamed. | Signs of dehydration and changes resulting from local trauma, infection, or chemotherapy. |
| 2. Gum margins are retracted from teeth with localized areas of inflammation. Bleeding occurs around gum margins. | Bleeding of gums or mucous membranes may result from too-vigorous brushing or client's underlying bleeding tendency. |
| 3. Teeth show signs of dental caries. | Client's personal dental hygiene is poor. |
| 4. Tongue continues to have thick coating. | Several brushings required to remove thick coating. |
| 5. Client unable to describe correct oral hygiene techniques. | Further instruction required. |
| **Recording and Reporting** | |
| 1. Record procedure on flow sheet. Note condition of oral cavity in nurses' notes. | Documents client's response to hygiene measures and status of oral cavity. |
| 2. Report bleeding or presence of lesions to nurse in charge or physician. | Bleeding may indicate serious systemic problems. Certain oral lesions may be cancerous. |

### Special Considerations

- All postoperative clients who receive general anesthesia are initially NPO after surgery and thus require frequent mouth care. Brushing is often contraindicated for these clients.
- Clients with sensitive gums or bleeding tendencies benefit from use of unflavored oral care sponges. A swab stick containing an aqueous solution of sorbital, sodium, carboxymethylcellulose, and electrolytes may be used.
- Clients unable to grasp a toothbrush can have an enlarged handle placed on toothbrush, e.g., push handle through center of small plastic ball.

### Teaching Considerations

- Educate clients about methods to prevent tooth decay, e.g., reduce intake of carbohydrates, especially sweet snacks between meals; brush within 30 minutes of eating sweets; rinse mouth thoroughly with water or eat acid-containing fruit (e.g., an apple); use fluoridated water.
- Cheilosis can be prevented by applying lip ointment or lubricant and avoiding licking of lips.

### Home Care Considerations

- During the initial admission visit document the condition of the client's mouth, teeth, and gums, thus providing a reference point for assessment of the client's ability to comply with special diets and fluid intake.
- Assess oral cavity during each visit to determine effects of medication regimen.
- Assess the state of dental health of family members and attitudes toward oral hygiene.

## *SKILL 8-2 Performing Mouth Care for the Unconscious or Debilitated Client*

Unconscious or debilitated clients pose challenges for the nurse because of their risk for having alterations of the oral cavity and because of their total dependence on the nurse for care. The nurse should recognize that these clients cannot eat or drink orally; frequently they are mouth-breathers, and they often have nasogastric or oxygen tubing exiting from the nose or mouth. All of these factors contribute to drying of the mucosa and the formation of secretions and crusts on the tongue and mucous membranes. Sometimes clients require mouth care as often as every 1 to 2 hours until the mucosa returns to normal. Many unconscious clients have no gag reflex as a result of neurologic injury. The accumulation of salivary secretions in the mouth can easily lead to aspiration. Because oral secretions usually contain gram-negative bacteria, aspiration may result in development of pneumonia. Proper oral hygienic care requires keeping the oral mucosa moist and removing secretions that can lead to infection.

### Purposes

1. Maintain an intact, well-hydrated oral mucosa.
2. Prevent injury from aspiration.
3. Maintain cleanliness of tooth surfaces, mouth, and lips.
4. Prevent infection and dental caries.

## Procedure 8-2

| Steps | Rationale |
|---|---|
| **Assessment** | |
| 1. Test for presence of gag reflex by placing blade on back half of client's tongue. | Reveals whether client is at risk for aspiration. |
| 2. Inspect condition of client's oral cavity. | Determines condition of oral cavity and client's need for hygiene. |
| 3. Assess client's risk for oral hygiene problems (Skill 8-1, Assessment): | Certain conditions increase likelihood of client having alterations in integrity of oral cavity structures. These clients may require more frequent care. |
| a. Dehydration, inability to take food or fluids by mouth. | |
| b. Presence of nasogastric tubes or artificial airways. | |
| c. Chemotherapeutic drugs. | |
| d. Blood clotting disorders. | |
| e. Oral surgery or trauma. | |
| f. Aging. | |
| **Nursing Diagnosis** | |
| 1. Cluster data to reveal actual or potential nursing diagnoses: | |
| a. Altered oral mucous membrane: related to mouthbreathing, retained secretions, etc. | Oral hygiene measures help maintain oral mucosa integrity and restore changes caused by dehydration or inflammation. |
| b. Potential altered oral mucous membrane: related to presence of airway, etc. | Exposure to drying and irritation can injure mucosa. |
| c. Potential for injury: related to absent gag reflex. | Client at risk for aspiration. |
| **Planning** | |
| 1. Develop individualized goals for client based on nursing diagnoses: | |
| a. Protect client from aspiration. | Positioning and use of suction will prevent aspiration. |
| b. Prevent injury to sensitive mucous membranes. | Debilitated clients are more likely to suffer from conditions causing injury to mucosa. |
| c. Increase hydration of mucosa. | Frequent care moistens mucous membranes. |
| d. Promote client's sense of comfort. | Clean oral cavity eliminates painful stimuli. |
| 2. Prepare needed equipment and supplies: | |
| a. Anti-infective solution, (e.g., hydrogen peroxide diluted in equal parts of mouthwash and water) | Loosens crustations and acts as anti-infective agent; mouthwash makes taste palatable. |
| b. Sponge toothette or tongue blade wrapped in single layer of gauze; small toothbrush | Brush cleans teeth most effectively. Toothette or swab stimulates and cleans gums and mucosa. |
| c. Padded tongue blade | Used to keep mouth open and teeth separated during procedure without traumatizing oral structures. |
| d. Face towel | |
| e. Curved emesis basin | |
| f. Paper towels | |
| g. Water glass with cool water | |
| h. Petrolatum jelly | |
| i. Portable suction machine; with rubber suction catheter (optional) | Removes retained oral secretions while oral cavity is cleansed. |
| j. Small bulb syringe (optional) | Can be used for rinsing oral cavity. |
| k. Disposable gloves | Infections of mouth may involve organisms such as *Neisseria gonorrhea,* herpesvirus, and *Mycobacterium tuberculosis* (MacMillan, 1981). |
| 3. Position client on side (Sim's position) with head turned well toward dependent side and head of bed lowered. Raise side rail. | Allows secretions to drain from mouth instead of collecting in back of pharynx. Prevents aspiration. |
| 4. Explain procedure to client. | Unconscious client may retain ability to hear. |
| **Implementation** | |
| 1. Wash hands and apply disposable gloves. | Reduces transfer of microorganisms. |
| 2. Place paper towels on overbed table and arrange equipment. Turn on suction machine and connect tubing to suction catheter. | Prevents soiling of table top. Equipment prepared in advance ensures smooth, safe procedure. |

| Steps | Rationale |
|---|---|

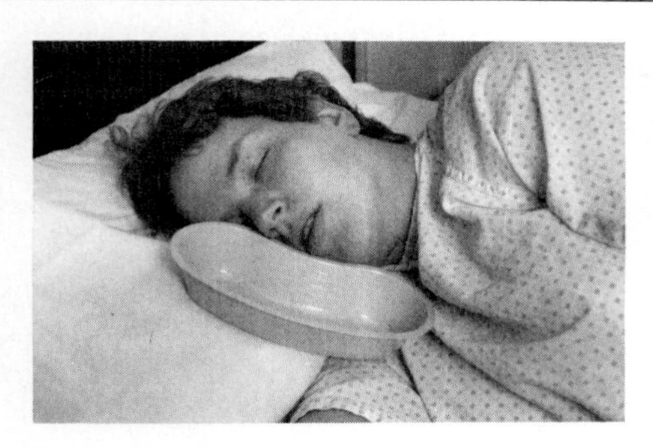

*Fig. 8-7*

| Steps | Rationale |
|---|---|
| 3. Pull curtain around bed or close room door. | Provides privacy. |
| 4. Raise bed to its highest horizontal level; lower side rail. | Use of good body mechanics with bed in high position prevents injury to nurse and client. |
| 5. Position client close to side of bed and near you; turn client's head toward mattress. | Proper positioning of head prevents aspiration. |
| 6. Place towel under client's face and emesis basin under client's chin (Fig. 8-7). | Prevents soiling of bed linen. |
| 7. Carefully retract client's upper and lower teeth with padded tongue blade by inserting blade, quickly but gently, between the back molars. Insert when client is relaxed, if possible. | Prevents client from biting down on nurse's fingers and provides access to oral cavity. |
| 8. Clean mouth using brush or tongue blade moistened with peroxide and water. Have second nurse suction as secretions accumulate during cleansing. Clean chewing and inner tooth surfaces first. Clean outer tooth surfaces. Swab roof of mouth and inside cheeks. Gently swab or brush tongue but avoid stimulating gag reflex (if present). Moisten clean swab or toothette with water to rinse. (Bulb syringe may also be used to rinse.) Repeat rinse several times. Suction any remaining secretions. | Brushing action removes food particles between teeth and along chewing surfaces. Swabbing helps remove secretions and crustations from mucosa and moistens mucosa. Suction removes secretions and fluid that can collect in posterior pharynx. Repeated rinsing removes peroxide that can be irritating to mucosa. |
| 9. Apply thin layer of petroleum jelly to lips. | Lubricates lips to prevent drying and cracking. |
| 10. Explain to debilitated client that procedure is completed. | Provides meaningful stimulation to unconscious or less-responsive client. |
| 11. Remove gloves and dispose in proper receptacle. | Prevents transmission of microorganisms. |
| 12. Reposition client comfortably, raise side rail, and return bed to original position. | Maintains client's comfort and safety. |
| 13. Clean equipment and return to its proper place. Place soiled linen in proper receptacle. | Proper disposal of soiled equipment prevents spread of infection. |
| 14. Wash hands. | Reduces transmission of microorganisms. |

## Evaluation

| Steps | Rationale |
|---|---|
| 1. Inspect oral cavity. | Determines efficacy of cleansing. Once thick secretions are removed, underlying inflammation or lesions may be revealed. |
| 2. Ask debilitated client if mouth feels clean. | Evaluate client's level of comfort. |
| 3. Observe patency of oral pharynx on an ongoing basis. | Ensures early recognition of aspiration. |

### *Expected outcomes*

| Steps | Rationale |
|---|---|
| 1. Buccal mucosa and tongue are pink, more moist, and intact. Gums are moist and intact. Teeth are cleaner, smooth, and shiny. Tongue is pink and without coating. Lips are moist, smooth, and without cracks. | Degree of improvement in condition of oral cavity structures will depend on extent of secretions or changes that existed before care. |
| 2. Client expresses feeling of cleanliness. | Comfort achieved. |
| 3. Oral pharynx remains clear. | Secretions removed, thus avoiding aspiration. |

### *Unexpected outcomes*

| Steps | Rationale |
|---|---|
| 1. Coating of secretions or crusts remains on mucosa, tongue, or gums. | Frequent cleansing needed. |
| 2. Localized inflammation of gums or mucosa is present. | May indicate a chronic problem. |
| 3. Teeth appear dull. | |
| 4. Lips are cracked or inflamed. | Repeated lubrication needed. |

| Steps | Rationale |
|---|---|
| 5. Client reports source of discomfort in mouth. | Continued care is needed. |
| 6. Client aspirates secretions. | Secretions accumulate in pharynx and enter airway. |

### Recording and Reporting

| | |
|---|---|
| 1. Record procedure, including pertinent observations, (e.g., presence of bleeding gums, dry mucosa, ulcerations, or crusts on tongue). | Documents response of client to nursing therapy. |
| 2. Report any unusual findings to nurse in charge or physician. | Bleeding may indicate more serious systemic problems. Lesions of oral cavity can be cancerous. |

### Follow-up Activities

| | |
|---|---|
| 1. Change oral airways as secretions accumulate every 8 hr (see Chapter 16). | Maintains patency of airway. |

### Special Considerations

- Clients who are unconscious often cannot be tested for gag reflex because they may have reflex response to bite on any object placed in mouth. Consult physician's note or history to determine presence of reflex.
- Side-lying position is routinely used for unconscious clients. If head cannot be lowered, turn to side.
- If unconscious client becomes agitated from insertion of tongue blade, repeated attempts to insert blade toward back of mouth will be useless. Smooth quick insertion of tongue blade while client is relaxed with mouth open works best.
- Chemotherapy, radiation, and nasogastric tube intubation can cause stomatitis. Clients should rinse their mouths before and after each meal using a solution containing .5 to 1 teaspoon of salt to 1 pint of water (Wilson, 1986). To remove thick mucous, use sodium bicarbonate solution, 1 teaspoon to 1 pint of water.
- Clients with diabetes require visits to the dentist every 3 or 4 months. All tissues should be handled gently with a minimum of trauma. Clients should be taught to follow rigid cleansing schedules.

### Teaching Considerations

- Family members may care for debilitated client in the home. Instruction in mouth care is needed so that the family understands how to protect client from aspirating, yet still ensure thorough cleansing of the oral cavity.

### Home Care Considerations

- Irrigate oral cavity with a bulb syringe; if unavailable, a gravy baster may be substituted. A large syringe may also be used.
- Encourage primary care giver to cleanse client's mouth at least twice a day. If client breathes through mouth, gauze or soft linen may be wrapped around a tongue blade, moistened, and used every 1 to 2 hours to keep mouth moist and fresh.

## *SKILL 8-3 Cleaning Dentures*

Clients should be encouraged to clean their dentures as frequently as natural teeth to prevent gingival infection and irritation. Dentures can cause some special problems. Loose, ill-fitting dentures can cause discomfort and embarrassment to the client. Poorly fitting dentures also make it difficult for clients to chew food thoroughly and to speak clearly. Clients who have poorly fitting dentures that cause gum or mucosal irritation should be referred to a dentist. The nurse can explore reasons why the client does not seek help.

Dentures are the client's personal property and should be handled with care because they can be easily broken. Dentures should be stored in an enclosed, labeled cup for soaking or when dentures are not worn (e.g., during surgery or a diagnostic procedure). Clients who return from surgery or a test usually prefer to have their dentures reinserted as quickly as possible. The change in appearance that results when dentures are removed can be embarrassing.

Most clients prefer to clean their dentures themselves. However, when it becomes necessary for the nurse to assist, the client's preferences for denture care should always be considered.

### Purposes

1. Maintain an intact, well-hydrated oral mucosa and gums.
2. Promote client comfort.
3. Control onset of halitosis.
4. Maintain client self-esteem.

## *Procedure 8-3*

| Steps | Rationale |
|---|---|
| **Assessment** | |
| 1. Ask if client has noticed loose fitting dentures and if there is any gum or mucous membrane tenderness or irritation. (After dentures are removed, nurse should inspect oral cavity and surfaces of dentures.) | Ill-fitting dentures rub against gums and mucous membranes. |
| 2. As client speaks, observe how well dentures fit. | Indicates potential problem with chewing food. |
| 3. Assess type of hygiene aids client uses to clean dentures. | Use of client's preferences individualizes care. |
| 4. Assess client's home routines for denture care. | Determines need for client teaching. |
| **Nursing Diagnosis** | |
| 1. Cluster data to reveal actual or potential nursing diagnoses: | |
| a. Pain: related to gum irritation. | Will often require referral to dentist. |
| b. Potential altered nutrition: related to loose dentures. | Loose-fitting dentures make chewing difficult; however, nurse may be able to offer foods that are easy to chew. |
| c. Potential altered oral mucous membrane: related to ill-fitting dentures. | Ill-fitting dentures can cause mucosal irritation. |
| d. Knowledge deficit regarding denture care: related to unfamiliarity with proper techniques. | Client will require instruction on care. |
| **Planning** | |
| 1. Develop individualized goals for client based on nursing diagnoses: | |
| a. Gums and mucosa are well hydrated. | Client cleans dentures and brushes and rinses oral cavity. |
| b. Client has access to necessary resources for properly fitting dentures. | Client may not visit dentist regularly. |
| c. Minimal irritation occurs to sensitive gums and mucosa. | Dentist may need to adjust denture fit. |
| d. Client understands denture care. | Nurse offers instruction during procedure. |
| 2. Prepare needed equipment and supplies: | |
| a. Soft-bristled toothbrush | For client to brush gums and tongue. |
| b. Denture toothbrush | |
| c. Emesis basin or sink | |
| d. Denture dentifrice or toothpaste | |
| e. Water glasses (for warm and cool water) | |
| f. Single 4 × 4 gauze pad (optional) | Used to remove tight-fitting dentures. |
| g. Washcloth | |
| h. Plastic denture cup | For storage of dentures. |
| i. Disposable gloves | Avoids contact with infectious microorganisms. |
| 3. Explain procedure to client and assure that individual hygiene aids will be used (as appropriate). | Promotes client's understanding and cooperation. |
| **Implementation** | |
| 1. Wash hands. | Reduces transmission of microorganisms. |
| 2. Arrange supplies on bedside table or near sink. | Accessibility of supplies ensures smooth, organized procedure. |
| 3. Pour emesis basin half full with tepid water or place washcloth in sink and run water until it is approximately 1 in deep. | Water aids in distribution of dentifrice over denture surfaces. Cloth in bottom of sink protects dentures against breakage. Hot water can cause warping or softening of dentures. |
| 4. Apply disposable gloves. | Reduces transmission of infection. |
| 5. Ask client to remove dentures and place them in emesis basin. If client is unable to remove dentures, grasp upper plate at front with thumb and index finger wrapped in gauze. Use steady downward pull. Gently lift lower denture from jaw and rotate one side downward to remove from client's mouth. Place dentures in emesis basin. | Gauze prevents accidental slipping while handling dentures. Rotating denture at angle reduces pulling of lips during removal. |
| 6. Apply dentifrice to denture and brush surfaces of dentures (Fig. 8-8). Hold dentures close to water. Hold brush horizontally and use back-and-forth motion to cleanse biting surfaces. Hold brush horizontally and use short strokes from top of denture to biting surfaces of teeth to clean outer tooth surface. Hold brush vertically and use short | Cleansing prevents food and bacteria from collecting on denture surfaces and prevents odor and stain buildup. Holding dentures close to water reduces chance of breakage, because water will break fall if dentures slip. |

| Steps | Rationale |
|---|---|

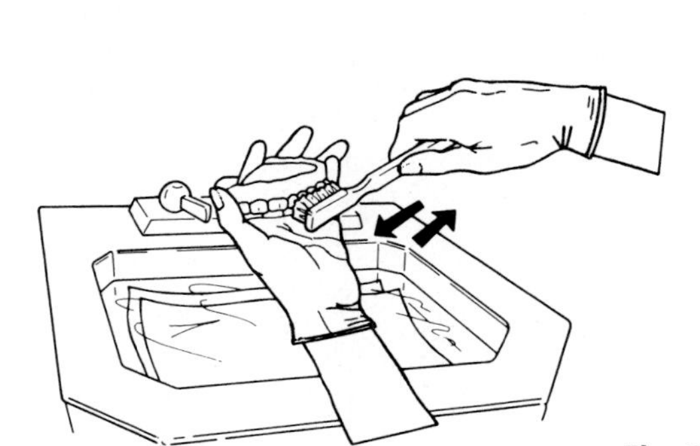
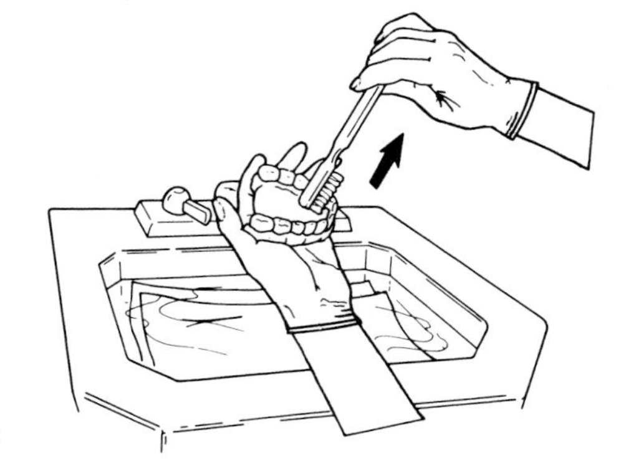

*Fig. 8-8*

| Steps | Rationale |
|---|---|
| strokes to clean inner tooth surfaces. Hold brush horizontally and use back-and-forth motion to clean undersurface of dentures. | |
| 7. Rinse dentures thoroughly in tepid water. | Warm water dilutes and rinses dentrifice more effectively than cool water. |
| 8. Return dentures to client or store in tepid water in denture cup. | Storage protects dentures from breakage. Tepid water keeps dentures well-moistened to make eventual insertion easier. Plastic dentures become brittle and warp if not kept moist. |
| 9. Empty emesis basin and add fresh cool water. Apply toothpaste to soft toothbrush and gently brush client's gums, palate, and tongue. | Brushing helps stimulate circulation to gums and removes residual film of debris on gums and mucosa. |
| 10. Have client rinse mouth thoroughly. | Rinsing removes food particles and secretions. |
| 11. Reinsert dentures if client desires or allow client to do so. Begin by gently inserting moistened upper denture. Have client use finger to press denture firmly in place, then insert moistened lower denture. | Bulkier upper denture easier to insert first when client has both upper and lower plates. Moistening lubricates denture for easier insertion. Applying gentle pressure to upper denture seals it against palate. |
| 12. Dispose of gloves in proper receptacle. Clean and store supplies. Wash hands. | Reduces spread of infection. |

## Evaluation

| | |
|---|---|
| 1. Ask client if dentures feel comfortable. | Cleansing of food particles from dentures removes source of irritation. |
| 2. Inspect condition of oral cavity. | Determines presence of chronic inflammation and adequacy of hygiene. |
| 3. Ask client to explain steps of denture care. | Measures understanding of procedure. |

### *Expected outcomes*

| | |
|---|---|
| 1. Client expresses feeling that mouth is refreshed and clean. | Irritating food particles removed. |
| 2. Gums and mucosa are pink, moist, and intact. | Hygiene adequate. |
| 3. Client explains steps in denture care. | Demonstrates cognitive learning. |

### *Unexpected outcomes*

| | |
|---|---|
| 1. Client continues to complain of poorly fitting dentures and tenderness in mouth. | Continued irritation from dentures requires that dentist evaluate fit and presence of any cracks or irregularities. |
| 2. Inflammation or ulceration of gums and mucosa are present. | Temporary removal of dentures may be necessary. Additional explanation or practice required. |
| 3. Client unable to explain steps in denture care. | Additional explanation or practice required. |

## Recording and Reporting

| | |
|---|---|
| 1. Record procedure on flow sheet or nurses' notes. Include any problems client may be having with dentures. | Accurate documentation is timely. |

## Follow-up Activities

| | |
|---|---|
| 1. Refer client who has local irritation from ill-fitting denture to dentist. | Dentist can smooth out roughened edges of dentures. |

## Special Considerations

- While cleansing give special attention to underlying denture plate where food particles often accumulate, especially if dentures are loose. If clients prefer to use an adhesive to seal dentures in place, apply a thin layer to undersurface of each denture before reinserting.

## Teaching Considerations

- Inform client about proper storage methods. Stress techniques of cleansing that avoid damage to dentures.
- Instruct primary care giver in safety factors associated with denture care, e.g., use brush with soft bristles, avoid unnecessary pressure on gums, carry dentures in container, hold dentures with cloth to avoid dropping.
- Instruct primary care giver on signs and symptoms of infection or irritation including reddened or whitened areas, bleeding, and lesions.
- Instruct primary care giver to include foods in client's diet that will not interfere with dentures and chewing.

## Home Care Considerations

- On regular visits, assess for signs and symptoms of infection or irritation including reddened, bleeding lesions.
- Provide special care to clients undergoing head and neck radiation as the gums may be dry, swollen, and interfere with proper denture fit.

**BIBLIOGRAPHY**

Bersani G, et al: Oral care for cancer patients, Am J Nurs 83:533, 1983.
Bulau J: Clinical policies and procedures for home health care, Rockville Md, 1986, Aspen Publishers, Inc.
Deliefde B: The dental care of pregnant women, NZ Dent J 80:41, 1984.
Ebersole P, Hess P: Toward healthy aging: human needs and nursing response, ed 3, St. Louis, 1985, The CV Mosby Co.
Gannon EP, Kadezabek E: Giving your patients meticulous mouth care, Nursing '80 10:14, 1980.
Golden S: Nursing a loved one at home. Philadelphia, 1988, Running Press Book Publishers.
MacMillan K: New goals for oral hygiene, Canad Nurse 77:40, 1981.
Maurer J: Providing optimal oral health, Nurs Clin North Am 12:4, 1977.
Napierski GE, et al.: Oral hygiene for the dentulous total care patient, Spec Care Dent 2:257, 1982.
Ostchega Y: Preventing and treating cancer chemotherapy's oral complications, Nursing '80, 10:47, 1980.
Poland JM: Comparing Moi-Stir to lemon glycerine swabs, Am J Nurs 87:422, 1987.
Potter PA, Perry AG: Fundamentals of nursing, ed 2, St. Louis, 1988, The CV Mosby Co.
Ramos LY: Oral hygiene for the elderly, Am J Nurs 81:1468, 1981.
Schweiger JL, et al.: Oral assessment: how to do it, Am J Nurs 80:654, 1980.
Suomi JD: Methods for the prevention of periodontal diseases, Fam Comm Health 3:41, 1980.
Walsh J, Persons C, Wiech L: Manual of home health care nursing, Philadelphia, 1987, JB Lippincott Co.
Wilson D: Make mouth care a must for your patients, RN 49:39, 1986.

# 9

# CARE OF THE HAIR, NAILS, AND FEET

### OBJECTIVES

*Mastery of content in this chapter will enable the nurse to:*

- Define key terms.
- Identify guidelines used in administering hair, nail, and foot care.
- Explain the importance of identifying a client's hygiene practices before caring for the client's hair.
- Comb and brush a client's hair.
- Shampoo the hair of a bedridden client.
- Shave a male client.
- Identify risk factors for foot and nail problems.
- Safely administer nail care.

### KEY TERMS

*Alopecia*
*Conjunctivitis*
*Cuticle*
*Dandruff*
*Orthopedic*
*Pediculosis*
*Podiatrist*
*Sebaceous gland*
*Sebum*
*Seborrheic dermatitis*
*Vellus*

### SKILLS

**9-1** Brushing and Combing Hair
**9-2** Shampooing the Hair of a Bedridden Client
**9-3** Shaving a Client
**9-4** Performing Nail and Foot Care

Bathing of skin surfaces affords a client considerable comfort. However, depending on the condition of the client's hair and nails a client may not sense a total feeling of cleanliness. When illness and disability cause a person to ignore care of the hair and nails, it becomes the nurse's responsibility to assist with cleaning and grooming hair, shaving, and soaking and trimming nails. Many of the procedures can be done during or immediately after a bath. Clients may appreciate having their hair combed or feet soaked anytime during the day to maintain an attractive appearance or to promote comfort. The client should be encouraged to make decisions regarding need and frequency for hygienic care.

## GUIDELINES

1. Consider clients' cultural preferences in regard to grooming techniques. Hair styles differ, for example. Women of some cultures shave the hair on their legs whereas others prefer to keep their legs unshaved.
2. Respect client's preferences for the use of grooming products. However, there may be opportunities for the nurse to caution against use of products that can damage or injure hair and nails.
3. Consider client's normal grooming routines. Incorporate client's schedule into the plan of care.

## HAIR CARE

Hair grows from follicles located within the dermis of the skin (Fig. 9-1). Tiny blood vessels supply each follicle with nourishment necessary for normal hair growth. Each hair has a shaft extending from the follicle. Sebaceous glands secrete sebum, an oil substance, into each follicle, which serves to lubricate the hair and scalp. The hair shaft is normally shiny and pliant and is not excessively oily, dry, or brittle.

Two types of hair cover the body. Terminal hair is the long, coarse, thick hair that is easily visible on the scalp, axilla, and pubic area. Special hair care practices focus primarily on care of terminal hair. Vellus hair is the soft tiny hair that covers the entire body except for the palms of the hands, fingertips, soles of the feet, tips of the toes, and part of the genitalia. Hair growth, distribution, and pattern can be indicators of a person's health status. Hormonal changes, emotional and physical stress, aging, infection, and certain diseases can affect hair characteristics. The hair shaft is an inert structure; any change in its color

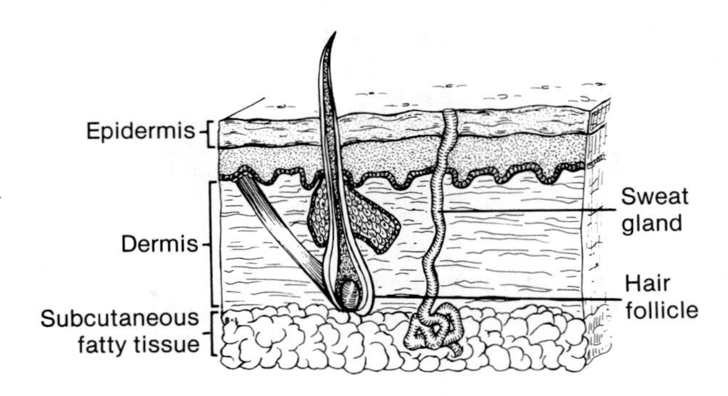


***Fig. 9-1*** Cross section of hair follicle and supporting structures.

or condition occurs as a result of hormonal activity and nutrient supply to the hair follicle. For example, a reduction in serum protein will result in hair becoming dry and brittle.

A person's appearance and feeling of well-being often depend on the way the hair looks and feels. Illness or disability often prevent clients from maintaining daily hair care. An immobilized client's hair soon becomes tangled if not brushed or combed regularly. Dressings of the face or neck may leave sticky adhesive, blood, or antiseptic solutions on the hair. Diaphoresis leaves hair oily and unmanageable. Proper hair care is very important to a person's body image. Brushing, combing, shampooing, and shaving are basic hygiene measures.

### PREREQUISITE KNOWLEDGE

1. Principles of medical asepsis.
2. Cultural factors influencing hair grooming.

### PREREQUISITE SKILLS

1. Proper handwashing techniques (Chapter 37).
2. Physical assessment of hair, scalp, nails, and feet (Chapter 13).

## *SKILL 9-1 Brushing and Combing Hair*

Brushing and combing hair can promote integrity of the scalp and enhance a client's self-esteem. Frequent brushing helps keep hair clean and distributes oil along hair shafts. Combing prevents hair from tangling. Combing and brushing may also improve a client's range of motion (ROM) in the upper extremities.

Clients requiring the nurse's assistance appreciate having their hair groomed before they are seen by others. For example, the nurse should offer to brush the client's hair before a physician's visit, a diagnostic test, or the arrival of family members or visitors.

### Purposes

1. Maintain cleanliness and integrity of the hair.
2. Stimulate circulation to the scalp.
3. Promote or maintain client self-esteem.

## *Procedure 9-1*

| Steps | Rationale |
|---|---|
| **Assessment** | |
| 1. Assess condition of client's hair and scalp. Note distribution of hair, degree of oiliness, and hair texture. Inspect scalp for lesions, areas of inflammation, and presence of infection or infestation (Table 9-1). | Determines need for additional interventions (e.g., medicated shampoo for dandruff, Kwell shampoo for lice). |
| 2. Assess client's routine hair care practices: preferred hairstyle, type of hair care products used, type of comb or brush used, time of day hair care is usually performed. | Cultural factors may influence methods for grooming and hair styling. Use of client's preferences individualizes nursing care. |
| 3. Assess adequacy of hygiene practices: ask client about frequency of shampooing, combing, and other practices. | Determines type of hair care required and client's need for health teaching. |
| 4. Assess client's physical ability to care for hair. Ask client to grasp comb and brush, raise arm above head, and brush hair. | Determines level of assistance needed from nurse. |

***TABLE 9-1*** Hair and Scalp Problems

| Problem | Characteristics | Implications | Interventions |
|---|---|---|---|
| **Dandruff** | Scaling of the scalp accompanied by itching; in severe cases, dandruff on eyebrows. | Dandruff causes embarrassment; if dandruff enters the eyes, conjunctivitis may develop. | Shampoo regularly with a medicated shampoo; in severe cases a physician's advice may be needed. |
| **Ticks** | Small gray-brown parasites that burrow into skin and suck blood. | Ticks transmit several diseases to people; most common are Rocky Mountain spotted fever and tularemia. | Do not pull ticks from skin because the sucking apparatus remains and may become infected; placing a drop of oil or ether on the tick or covering it with petrolatum jelly eases removal; oil suffocates the tick. |
| **Pediculosis capitis (head lice)** | Tiny grayish white parasite insects that infest mammals. Found on the scalp attached to hair strands; eggs look like oval particles, similar to dandruff; bites or pustules may be observed behind ears and at hairline. | Head lice are difficult to remove and if not treated may spread to furniture and other people. | Shampoo with a shampoo for eliminating lice and repeat 12-24 hr later; change bed linens. |
| **Pediculosis corporis (body lice)** | Tend to cling to clothing so may not be easily seen; body lice suck blood and lay eggs on clothing and furniture. | Client itches constantly; scratches on skin may become infected; hemorrhagic spots may appear on skin where lice are sucking blood. | Client should bathe or shower thoroughly; after skin is dried, apply a lotion for eliminating lice; after 12-24 hr another bath or shower should be taken; bag any infested clothing or linen until laundered |
| **Pediculosis pubis (crab lice)** | Found in pubic hair; crab lice are grayish white with red legs. | Lice may spread through bed linen, clothing, or furniture or between persons via sexual contact. | Shave hair off affected area; cleanse as for body lice; if lice were sexually transmitted, partner must be notified. |
| **Alopecia** | Occurs in all races, mostly women. Balding patches in periphery of hair line, hair becomes brittle and broken, caused from use of hair curlers, Afro picks, tight braiding, and use of hot comb. | Patches of uneven hair growth and loss alter client's appearance. | Stop hair care practices that damage hair. |

| Steps | Rationale |
|---|---|
| **Nursing Diagnosis** | |
| 1. Cluster data to reveal actual or potential nursing diagnoses: | |
| a. Self-care hygiene deficit: related to impaired mobility. | Motor or sensory deficit interferes with client's ability to handle equipment. |
| b. Knowledge deficit regarding hair care practices: related to lack of recall. | Nurse includes instructions on proper care. |
| **Planning** | |
| 1. Develop individualized goals for client based on nursing diagnoses: | |
| a. Client attains independence within physical limitations. | Client may assist in actual grooming or by suggesting ways to style hair. |
| b. Client understands proper hair care techniques. | Will allow client to maintain own hygiene. |
| c. Integrity of hair and scalp is maintained. | Regular grooming maintains integrity of hair. |
| d. Client attains self-esteem. | Hair should be styled attractively. |

| Steps | Rationale |
|---|---|

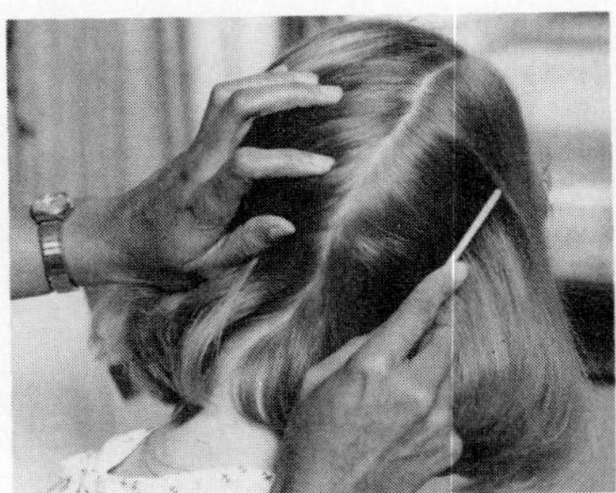

*Fig. 9-2*

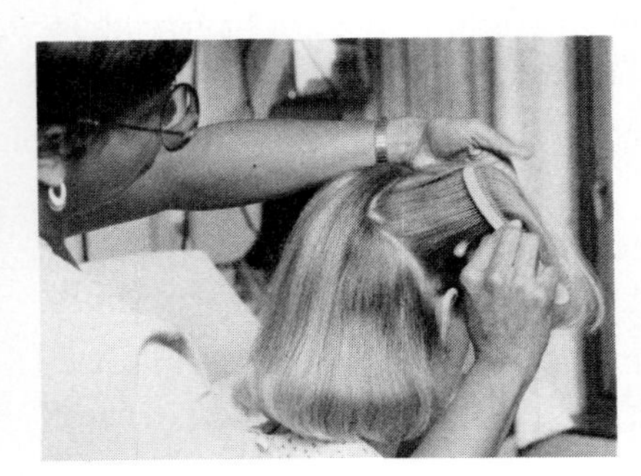

*Fig. 9-3*

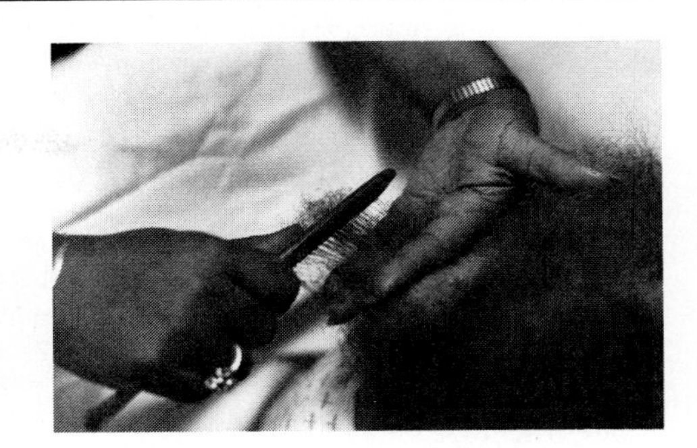

*Fig. 9-4*

| Steps | Rationale |
|---|---|
| 2. Prepare needed equipment and supplies: | |
| a. Comb (short-toothed for short hair; large-toothed for curly or long hair) | Combing eliminates tangles. |
| b. Brush (stiff bristles) | Brushing stimulates scalp circulation and distributes sebum evenly along hair shafts. |
| c. Bath towel | |
| d. Hair clips or ribbons (optional, as requested by client) | |
| e. Mirror | Allows client to view styling and make suggestions during procedure. |
| f. Baby oil, vaseline hair oil, or water (optional) | Preparations used by black clients to prevent pulling during combing. |
| 3. Ask client for final suggestion on how to style or arrange hair (e.g., location of part, braiding, or creating bun). | Offers client opportunity to decide about own care and participate in care plan. |

## Implementation

| Steps | Rationale |
|---|---|
| 1. Wash hands. | Reduces transmission of microorganisms. |
| 2. Arrange equipment on bedside table. | Ensures smooth, orderly procedure. |
| 3. Pull curtain around bedside or close room door (if client desires). | Provides client privacy. |
| 4. Assist client to sitting position in bed or on chair. (If activity is restricted, assist client to alternate side-lying position and raise bed to comfortable working height). | Sitting provides easiest access to client's hair. (Side-lying position allows nurse to comb and brush out half of hair at a time.) |
| 5. Place towel over client's shoulders or over pillow if client is lying down. | Towel collects loosened hair, debris, or material from scalp. |
| 6. Remove hair clips, pins, or ribbons. | Ensures all hair is thoroughly combed. |
| 7. Comb and brush hair one side at a time. | |
| 8. Part hair into two sections, taking edge of comb and parting from top of scalp down toward back of neck (Fig. 9-2). | It is easier to comb and brush small sections of hair. |
| 9. Separate each side into two more sections, front and back, by parting down along the side of the client's head (Fig. 9-3). | Ensures thorough combing of all hair. |
| 10. Gently grasp section of parted hair. Comb carefully from scalp toward hair ends. | Prevents tangle formation. |
| 11. Brush same section of parted hair. | Rotation of brush distributes sebum evenly along hair shaft. Brushing stimulates circulation to scalp. |
| 12. If tangles are present, separate with fingers lock of hair that is matted. Grasp hair near scalp and gently brush and comb tangled end loose (Fig. 9-4). | Anchoring tangled hair prevents painful pulling of scalp during combing. |
| 13. For black clients, apply a lubricant as needed. Lift open fingers through hair. | Gentle lifting of fingers eases tangles free. |
| 14. Repeat brushing and combing for each major section of parted hair. | |
| 15. Style hair as client desires. If client has long hair and is confined to bed, ask permission to braid hair. (Client may request nurse to use setting gel, spray, or oil). Steps for braiding: | Braiding reduces need for repeated grooming when client is bedridden for extended periods. |

| Steps | Rationale |
|---|---|
| a. For one braid, divide hair into three equal strands. For two braids, part hair down the middle and then divide each section into three strands. | Equal strands ensure even braiding. |
| b. Hold left strand in left hand, center strand by the second finger and thumb of the left hand, and right strand in the right hand. Do not pull strands but hold firmly. | Prevents client discomfort and hair damage. |
| c. Place right strand (a) over the middle strand (b). Then while holding hair taut, cross the left strand (c) over the middle strand (a). | |
| d. The left hand now holds strand a, the right fingers hold strand c, and the right hand holds strand b. Cross the right strand (b) over the center strand (c). Then cross the left strand (a) over the middle strand (b). | |
| e. Continue braiding by crossing side strands over the center strand. Alternate right and left strands until all hair is braided. | |
| f. Secure end of braid with ribbon or elastic band. | Keeps braid intact. |
| 16. Have client view hair after styling. | A means to positively reinforce client's self-esteem. |
| 17. Discard towel in proper receptacle. Store brush and comb in client's bedside stand. | Reduces spread of infection. Neat, clean environment promotes sense of well-being. |
| 18. Wash hands. | Reduces transmission of microorganisms. |

## Evaluation

| | |
|---|---|
| 1. Inspect appearance of hair after combing. | Determines need for additional hygiene measures (e.g., shampooing). |
| 2. Ask client to describe hair care techniques. | Evaluates client's understanding of hygiene practices. |
| 3. Observe client's verbal or nonverbal response to appearance. | Evaluates level of self-esteem. |

### *Expected outcomes*

| | |
|---|---|
| 1. Hair is straight, neatly styled, without tangles or matting. | Clean hair grooms easily. |
| 2. Client describes hair care techniques correctly. | Learning achieved. |
| 3. Client states satisfaction with appearance, views self spontaneously in mirror. | Client perceives body image positively. |

### *Unexpected outcomes*

| | |
|---|---|
| 1. During combing or brushing nurse observes problems (e.g., dandruff or infestation of lice). | Indicates need for additional intervention. |
| 2. Client unable to describe or explain hair care techniques. | Further instruction needed or client unwilling to learn. |
| 3. Client avoids looking at hair, becomes preoccupied with appearance, states dissatisfaction of appearance. | Client perceives disruption in body image. |

## Recording and Reporting

| | |
|---|---|
| 1. Record presence of any alterations in condition of hair or scalp. | Documents presence of alterations requiring further intervention. |

## Follow-up Activities

| | |
|---|---|
| 1. For specific hair or scalp problems, obtain physician's order to initiate appropriate interventions. | Specific types of conditions require special therapies (Table 9-1). |

## Special Considerations

- Female clients who have had mastectomies may have reduced ROM in arm on affected side for several days. Presence of intravenous (IV) tubes, bulky dressings, casts, or other encumbrances will impair client's ability to handle comb or brush.
- Avoid combs with sharp irregular teeth that may scratch scalp.
- Never cut client's hair without written consent (agency policies may differ).
- Thick, coarse, curly hair of black clients often becomes dry and brittle. To comb natural or "afro" styles, use an open-toothed comb. Start at the client's neckline and slowly lift and fluff hair outward until the forehead is reached (Fig. 9-5).

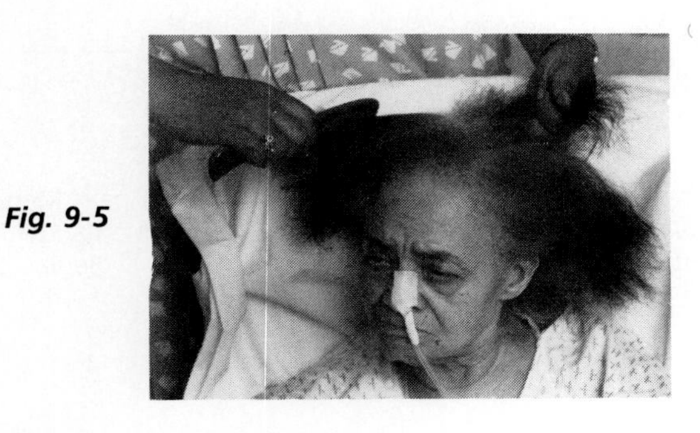
*Fig. 9-5*

### Teaching Considerations

- Caution black clients against using petroleum jelly and hot combs for straightening hair. Inflammation and scarring of the scalp may occur.
- If client has lice, instruct on proper measures to prevent spread of infection (Table 9-1).
- Instruct primary care giver on methods to cut or braid hair to prevent discomfort.

## *SKILL 9-2 Shampooing the Hair of a Bedridden Client*

Frequency of shampooing depends on condition of the hair and the person's daily routines. Dry hair, which commonly results from aging and protein deficiency, requires less frequent shampooing than oily hair or hair of people who exercise actively. The nurse should remind hospitalized clients that staying in bed, excess perspiration, or treatments that leave blood or solutions in the hair may require more frequent shampoos. For clients in the home setting the nurse's greatest challenge is to find ways the client can shampoo the hair without causing injury. For example, a client with a long leg cast may need to wash hair at a sink until it is safe to shower or until the cast is removed and tub baths can be resumed. In a hospital setting it may be necessary to transport a client by stretcher to a special facility where a spray nozzle and sink are available for shampooing.

Clients who are allowed to sit in a chair can usually be shampooed in front of a sink. The individual should be positioned facing away from the sink with the head and neck hyperextended over the sink's edge. A folded towel placed under the neck on the edge of the sink provides added comfort. If the client is forced to sit at bedside, it is possible to shampoo the hair as the client leans forward over a wash basin. Caution is needed with clients who have suffered neck injuries, since hyperextension of the neck could cause further injury.

If the client is unable to sit in a chair or to be transferred to a stretcher, shampooing must be done with the client in bed. The nurse may choose to do this after the bath, common in the care of infants, or later as a separate procedure.

### Purposes

1. Maintain integrity of hair and scalp.
2. Promote client comfort.
3. Maintain client self-esteem.
4. Apply medicated solutions to hair or scalp.

## *Procedure 9-2*

| Steps | Rationale |
|---|---|
| **Assessment** | |
| 1. Determine if risks exist that might contraindicate shampooing. Physician's order may be needed to shampoo (consult agency policy). | Certain medical conditions could place client at risk for injury during shampooing because of positioning, exposure to moisture, or manipulation of head and scalp. |
| 2. Determine if there are restrictions for positioning client. | Influences manner in which nurse prepares and positions client for procedure. |
| 3. Review physician's orders to determine whether to use medicated shampoo. | Special shampoos may be ordered for conditions such as lice or dandruff. |
| 4. Assess client's preference for hair care products. | Maintains client's independence through decision making. |
| 5. Assess condition of hair and scalp. Note presence of lacerations, abrasions, masses, painful areas, sites of inflammation, or preexisting skin conditions. | Determines need for further interventions and assesses effectiveness of previous hygiene measures. |

| Steps | Rationale |
|---|---|
| **Nursing Diagnosis** | |
| 1. Cluster assessment data to reveal actual or potential nursing diagnoses: | |
| a. Impaired skin integrity: related to local inflammation. | Shampooing improves cleanliness of scalp and hair. Medicated shampoos may be used to treat specific problems. |
| b. Self-care hygiene deficit: related to physical immobility. | Client dependent on nurse for assistance with hygiene. |
| **Planning** | |
| 1. Develop individualized goals for client based on nursing diagnoses: | |
| a. Hair and scalp are clean. | |
| b. Client experiences minimal discomfort during shampooing. | Tangled hair is combed before shampooing. |
| 2. Prepare needed equipment and supplies: | |
| a. Two bath towels | |
| b. Face towel or washcloth | |
| c. Shampoo (hair conditioner and cream rinse, optional) | Shampoo removes oil and sediment. Conditioner reduces tangles. |
| d. Water pitcher | |
| e. Plastic shampoo trough or board (Fig. 9-6) | Diverts water to basin to prevent soiling of bed linen. |
| f. Washbasin | |
| g. Bath blanket | |
| h. Waterproof pad | |
| i. Clean comb and brush | |
| j. Hair dryer | |

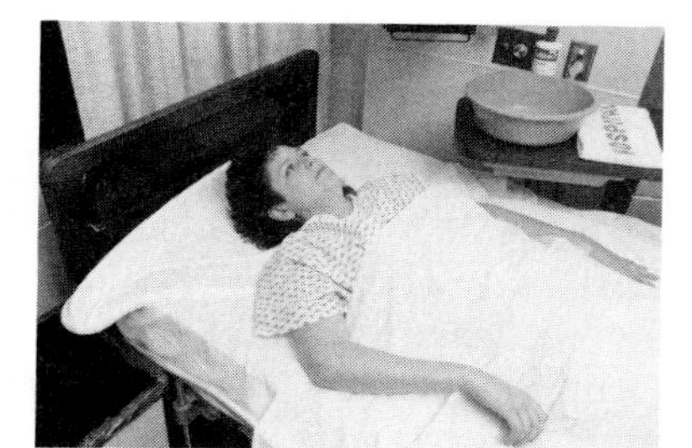

*Fig. 9-6*

| Steps | Rationale |
|---|---|
| k. Bottle of hydrogen peroxide and saline (optional) | To clean hair matted with blood. |
| 3. Explain procedure to client. | Client may be apprehensive about positioning or water entering eyes. |
| **Implementation** | |
| 1. Wash hands. | Reduces transmission of microorganisms. |
| 2. Arrange equipment in convenient place and lower side rail. | Easy access to equipment and client prevents interruptions during procedure. |
| 3. Place waterproof pad under client's shoulders, neck, and head. Position client supine with head and shoulders at top edge of bed. Place plastic trough under client's head and washbasin at end of trough. Be sure trough spout extends beyond edge of mattress. | Prevents soiling of bed linen. |
| 4. Place rolled towel under client's neck and bath towel across client's shoulders. | Hyperextension of neck minimizes problem of water draining down back of neck. |
| 5. Brush and comb client's hair. | Removing tangles results in more thorough cleansing. |
| 6. Obtain water at about 110° F (43°-44° C). | Proper water temperature prevents burns to face and scalp. |
| 7. Ask client to hold face towel or washcloth over eyes. | Prevents shampoo or water from entering eyes. |
| 8. Slowly pour water from water pitcher over hair until it is completely wet. If hair contains matted blood, apply peroxide to dissolve clots, then rinse hair with saline. Apply small amount of shampoo. | Water aids in distribution of shampoo suds over hair. |
| 9. Work up lather with both hands. Start at hairline and work toward back of neck. Lift head slightly with one hand to wash back of head. Shampoo sides of head. Massage scalp by applying pressure with fingertips. | Systematic progression over hair and scalp ensures thorough cleansing. Massage increases scalp circulation. Use of fingernails during massage can cause scratching of scalp. |
| 10. Rinse hair with water. Make sure water drains into basin. Repeat rinsing until hair is free of soap. To speed drainage from trough, press down on its spout. | Retained soap leaves dull finish on hair. Dried soap may cause scalp irritation. |

| Steps | Rationale |
|---|---|
| 11. Repeat Steps 8-10. | Ensures thorough cleansing. |
| 12. Apply conditioner or rinse if requested and rinse hair thoroughly. | Conditioner prevents excess drying. Cream rinse makes combing and brushing easier. |
| 13. Wrap client's head in bath towel. Dry client's face with cloth used to protect eyes. Dry off any moisture along neck or shoulders. | If client is ill, retained moisture may cause cooling and chills. |
| 14. Dry client's hair and scalp. Use second towel if first becomes saturated. | |
| 15. Comb hair to remove tangles and dry with dryer or remaining towel as quickly as possible. | Drying prevents chilling. |
| 16. Assist client to comfortable position and complete styling of hair. | Promotes client's sense of well-being. |
| 17. Return equipment to its proper place. Discard soiled linen in linen hamper. Wash hands. | Maintains cleanliness of environment and reduces transmission of infection. |

## Evaluation

| | |
|---|---|
| 1. Ask client how hair feels. | Client will experience sense of cleanliness after shampooing. |
| 2. Inspect condition of hair. | Shampooing should leave hair in clean condition. |

### *Expected outcomes*

| | |
|---|---|
| 1. Client states that hair feels clean. | All soap, oil, and sediment removed. |
| 2. Hair is shiny and pliant. | |
| 3. Scalp is clean. | |

### *Unexpected outcomes*

| | |
|---|---|
| 1. Nurse may note presence of scalp lesions, dry flaky scalp, or localized areas of inflammation. | Chronic scalp conditions will not be alleviated by single shampooing. |

## Recording and Reporting

| | |
|---|---|
| 1. Record any pertinent findings related to condition of hair or scalp. | Documents client's response to therapy and condition of hair or scalp if further treatment is necessary. |

## Special Considerations

- Shampooing may be contraindicated for clients with open incisions of face, head, or neck; cervical neck injuries; presence of tracheostomy; severe facial edema; respiratory distress.
- Trendelenburg position (head is positioned lower than trunk and legs) is ideal for promoting drainage of water away from client's face. However, many clients cannot tolerate this position.
- Hyperextension must be avoided if client has any form of neck injury.
- Black clients may choose to apply oil preparations to hair before or after shampooing. Oil prevents drying and breaking of hair at ends of follicles.
- Black clients normally need to shampoo their hair only once or twice a week.

## Teaching Considerations

- Clients who are permanently disabled, e.g., from spinal cord injury, may require family member or friend to learn shampooing techniques.
- Teach client lice preventive measures to avoid further exposure to lice.

## Home Care Considerations

- Assess temperature of the room, availability of water, and the most satisfactory position of the client for the procedure.
- Provide extra protection from wetness for clients with casts.
- Obtain dry shampoo preparations when a wet shampoo is contraindicated.
- Construct a trough by arranging a plastic shower curtain or tablecloth under the client's head and then tapering the cloth to form a narrow end that can drain into a bucket or basin next to the client's bed.

# SKILL 9-3 Shaving a Client

Shaving of facial hair can be done after a bath or shampoo. It is a task most men prefer to do for themselves. However when a client is physically unable, the nurse should be able to perform the procedure as quickly and comfortably as possible. Men without beards usually shave daily. The facial hair of older clients does not grow as quickly and thus a shave might not be necessary each day. Clients with mustaches and beards require daily grooming. Keeping these areas clean is important because food particles easily collect in the hair. The beard or mustache should be trimmed, combed, or washed as needed or at client request. The nurse never shaves off a mustache or beard without client consent.

Some women may wish to shave the hair under their arms or on their legs. Generally, it is not necessary for women to shave each day but some may prefer it. The technique used to shave the male client's facial hair is the same as that for the woman who shaves axillary or leg hair.

### Purposes

1. Maintain client's neat, well-groomed appearance.
2. Promote client's comfort.

## Procedure 9-3

| Steps | Rationale |
|---|---|
| **Assessment** | |
| 1. Assess if client has a bleeding tendency. Review medical history or laboratory values (e.g., platelet counts, prothrombin time). | Determines need to use electric razor for client's safety. |
| 2. Assess client's ability to manipulate razor. | Determines level of assistance required from nurse. |
| 3. Assess client's preferences for shaving products (e.g., after-shave lotion, skin conditioner, shaving cream). | Promotes client's independence through decision making. |
| **Nursing Diagnosis** | |
| 1. Cluster data to reveal actual or potential nursing diagnoses: | |
| a. Potential for injury: related to bleeding tendency. | Indicates need to use electric razor. |
| b. Self-care grooming deficit: related to impaired mobility. | Client dependent on nurse for assistance. |
| **Planning** | |
| 1. Develop individualized goals for client based on nursing diagnoses: | |
| a. Minimize trauma to areas being shaved. | Precaution used to avoid cuts. |
| b. Client attains sense of independence. | Client may assist with shave or offer suggestions on shaving techniques. |
| 2. Prepare needed equipment and supplies: | |
| a. Straight razor | |
| ▪ Razor with new blade | New blade has sharper cutting surface, which minimizes pulling of hair and face. |
| ▪ Bath towel(s) | |
| ▪ Washcloth | |
| ▪ Wash basin | |
| ▪ Shaving cream or soap | Soap is more drying than cream. |
| ▪ After-shave (optional) | |
| ▪ Mirror (optional) | Have mirror available if client able to perform any portion of shave. |
| b. Electric razor | |
| ▪ Razor (with clean cutting heads) | Used as a client's preference or if client has bleeding tendency. |
| ▪ Bath towel | |
| ▪ Skin or beard conditioner | |
| ▪ After-shave lotion (optional) | |
| c. Mustache care | |
| ▪ Pair of sharp scissors | Trims edges of mustache. |
| ▪ Brush or comb | |

| Steps | Rationale |
|---|---|
| ▪ Bath towel | |
| ▪ Mirror | |
| ▪ Gooseneck lamp or overhead light | Ensures proper illumination of face. |
| 3. While performing actual procedure, ask client to explain steps he uses to shave. Ask client to indicate if shave becomes uncomfortable. | Client can become very apprehensive about being accidentally cut. |
| **Implementation** | |
| ***Straight razor*** | |
| 1. Arrange supplies at bedside table and adjust lighting. | Easy access to supplies prevents interruption of procedure. Lighting provides clear view of client's face. |
| 2. Assist client to sitting or supine position with head of bed elevated. | Provides easy access to all sides of client's face. |
| 3. Place bath towel over client's chest and shoulders. | Prevents shaving cream or water from soiling gown. |
| 4. Run water in wash basin at approximately 110° F (43°-44° C). If client is reliable ask him to test water for desired temperature. | Warm water will soften beard. Proper temperature prevents accidental burns. |
| 5. Place washcloth in basin and wring out thoroughly. Apply cloth over client's entire face for several seconds. | Warm cloth helps soften skin and beard. Sensation of warmth can be relaxing. |
| 6. Apply shaving cream or soap to client's face. Smooth cream evenly over sides of face, chin, and under nose. | Cream creates additional softening effect to skin and lubricates skin for application of razor. |
| 7. Take razor in dominant hand and hold at 45° angle to the client's skin. Begin by shaving across one side of the client's face. Use nondominant hand to gently pull skin taut while shaving. Use short firm strokes in direction hair grows (Fig. 9-7). Short downward strokes work best over upper lip. | Holding skin taut prevents razor cuts and discomfort during shaving. |

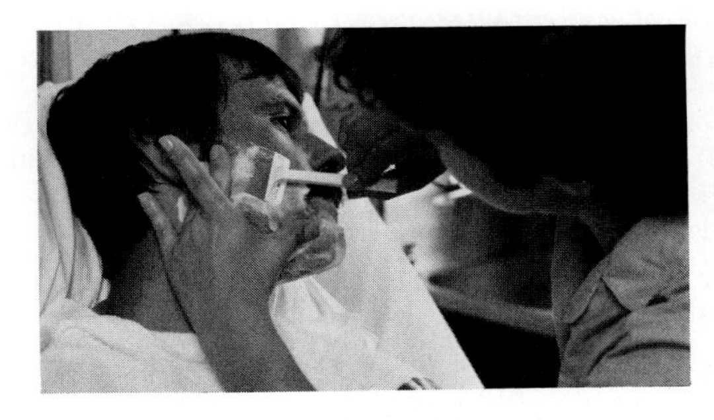

***Fig. 9-7***

| Steps | Rationale |
|---|---|
| 8. Dip razor blade in water as cream accumulates on blade's edge. | Keeps cutting surface of razor blade clean. |
| 9. After all facial hair is shaved, rinse face thoroughly with moistened washcloth. | Prevents accumulation of cream that can cause drying of skin. |
| 10. Dry face thoroughly and apply after-shave lotion if desired. | Retained moisture may cause chapping of skin. |
| 11. Assist client to comfortable position. | |
| 12. Return equipment to proper place. Discard soiled linen in hamper. Wash hands. | Maintains cleanliness of client's environment and reduces transmission of infection. |
| ***Electric razor*** | |
| 1. Perform Steps 1-3 for straight razor. | |
| 2. Apply skin conditioner or pre-shave preparation. | Softens skin and beard to reduce friction from razor head. |
| 3. Turn razor on and begin by shaving across side of face. Gently hold skin taut while shaving over skin's surface. Use gentle downward stroke of razor in direction of hair growth. | Prevents pulling of beard and skin. |
| 4. After completing shave, apply after-shave as desired. | Stimulates and lubricates skin. |
| 5. Perform Steps 11-12 for straight razor. | |
| ***Mustache and beard care*** | |
| 1. Perform Steps 1-3 for straight razor. | |
| 2. If necessary, gently comb mustache or beard. | Straightens hair that requires trimming. |
| 3. Allow client to use mirror and direct areas to trim with scissors. | Allows client to make decisions in care; maintains sense of independence. |
| **Evaluation** | |
| 1. Inspect condition of shaved area and skin underneath beard or moustache. | Nurse looks for areas of localized bleeding from cutting skin's surface, and areas of dryness. |
| 2. Ask client if face feels clean and comfortable. | Evaluates level of client's comfort. |

| Steps | Rationale |
|---|---|
| ***Expected outcomes*** | |
| 1. Client expresses sensation of face feeling clean and refreshed. | Hair and soap lather removed. |
| 2. Skin's surface is smooth, well hydrated, free of cuts. | Client free from injury. |
| ***Unexpected outcomes*** | |
| 1. There may be small isolated nicks or cuts of skin. | Result of dull blade or improper shaving technique. |
| 2. Skin's surface may appear dry. | Result of soap residue. |
| 3. Client reports burning or stinging sensation. | Result of cuts or rubbing of skin surface. |

## Recording and Reporting

1. It is not necessary to record shaving procedure.

## Follow-up Activities

| | |
|---|---|
| 1. If client's face remains dry, apply lotion as desired. | Lubricates skin to maintain its integrity. |

### Special Considerations

- Conditions that place clients at risk to bleed excessively if cut include use of anticoagulants, use of high doses of aspirin, bleeding disorders (e.g., leukemia, hemophilia, disseminated intravascular coagulation).
- Some institutions have special policies restricting use of client's own electrical equipment. Check electrical cord for any safety hazards.

### Teaching Considerations

- Shaving is a simple procedure that can be taught to a family member. Instruct primary care giver in safety precautions for shaving, especially if client is on anticoagulant therapy.
- Instruct technique to follow in the event the client is accidently nicked.

### Home Care Considerations

- Provide adequate toweling around client's neck to avoid spilling shaving cream or water on chest or bed.
- Provide adequate lighting for the procedure.
- Perform procedure in comfortable setting, such as bathroom or bedroom.

# *SKILL 9-4 Performing Nail and Foot Care*

Feet and nails often require special care to prevent infection, odors, and injury to soft tissues. Often people are unaware of foot or nail problems until discomfort or pain occurs. Common foot and nail problems are listed in Table 9-2. Problems often result from abuse or poor care of the feet and hands, such as biting nails or trimming them improperly, exposure to harsh chemicals, or wearing ill-fitting shoes. There are also changes in the shape, color, and texture of nails that may result from various nutritional, infectious, and circulatory disorders. The normal process of aging causes changes in the nails and feet. The elderly often have dry feet because of a decrease in sebaceous gland secretion and dehydration of skin cells. The nails become opaque, tougher, scaly, brittle, and hypertrophied.

The feet are important to a person's physical and emotional health. Foot pain may cause a person to change gait, resulting in strain on different muscle groups. If job performance requires a person to walk or stand comfortably, a foot disorder can become a serious problem.

Nails are epithelial tissues that grow from the root of the nail bed located in the skin at the nail groove. A normal healthy nail is transparent, smooth, and convex with pink nail beds and translucent white tips. In black clients a brown or black pigmentation is normally present between the nail and nail base. The nail is surrounded by a cuticle, which slowly grows over the nail and must be regularly pushed back. The skin around the nail beds and cuticles should be smooth and without inflammation.

Nail and foot care should be included in a client's daily hygiene; the best time is during the client's bath.

### Purposes

1. Maintain integrity of skin surfaces surrounding nails.
2. Promote client comfort and sense of cleanliness.
3. Maintain proper function of the feet.

***TABLE 9-2*** Common Foot and Nail Problems

| Condition | Characteristics | Implications | Interventions |
|---|---|---|---|
| **Callus** | Thickened portion of epidermis, consisting of a mass of horny, keratotic cells; usually flat, painless, and found on undersurface of foot or on palm of hand; caused by local friction or pressure. | Condition may cause discomfort when wearing tight-fitting shoes. | Advise client to wear gloves when using tools or objects that may create friction on palmar surfaces. Encourage client to wear comfortable shoes. Soak callus in warm water and Epsom salts to soften cell layers. Use pumice stone to remove callus after it softens. Applications of creams or lotions can reduce reformation. |
| **Corns** | Keratosis caused by friction and pressure from shoes; mainly on toes, over bony prominence; usually cone shaped, round, and raised. | Conical shape compresses underlying dermis, making it thin and tender. Pain is aggravated when tight-fitting shoes are worn. Tissue can become attached to bone if allowed to grow. Client may suffer alteration in gait owing to pain. | Surgical removal may be necessary depending on severity of pain and size of corn. Avoid use of oval corn pads, which increases pressure on toes and reduces circulation. |
| **Plantar warts** | Fungating lesion that appears on sole of foot; caused by *Papillomavirus.* | Warts may be contagious, are painful, and make walking difficult. | Treatment ordered by physician may include applications of salicylic acid, electrodesiccation (burning with an electric spark), or freezing with solid carbon dioxide. |
| **Athlete's foot (tinea pedis)** | Fungal infection of foot; scaliness and cracking of skin between toes and on soles of feet; small blisters containing fluid may appear, apparently induced by constricting footwear, e.g., sneakers. | Athlete's foot can spread to other body parts, especially hands. It is contagious and frequently recurs. | Feet should be well ventilated. Drying feet well after bathing and applying powder help prevent infection. Wearing of clean socks or stockings reduces incidence. Physician may order application of griseofulvin, miconazole nitrate, or tolnaftate. |
| **Ingrown nails** | Toe or fingernail growing inward into soft tissue around nail; often results from improper nail trimming. | Ingrown nails can cause localized pain when pressure is applied. | Treatment is frequent hot soaks in antiseptic solution and removal of portion of nail that has grown into skin. Instruct client on proper nail trimming techniques |
| **Ram's horn nails** | Unusually long curved nails. | Attempt by nurse to cut nails may result in damage to nail bed with risk of infection. | Refer client to podiatrist. |
| **Paronychia** | Inflammation of tissue surrounding nail after hangnail or other injury; occurs in people who frequently have their hands in water; common in diabetic clients. | Area can become infected. | Treatment is hot compresses or soaks and local application of antibiotic ointments. Paroynchia can be prevented by careful manicuring. |
| **Foot odors** | Result of excess perspiration promoting microorganism growth. | | Frequent washing, use of foot deodorants and powders, and clean footwear will prevent or reduce this problem. |

## Procedure 9-4

| Steps | Rationale |
|---|---|
| **Assessment** | |
| 1. Inspect all surfaces of fingers, toes, feet, and nails. Pay particular attention to areas of dryness, inflammation, or cracking. Also inspect areas between toes, heels, and soles of feet. | Assesses integrity of feet and nails to determine frequency and level of hygiene required. Heels, soles, and sides of feet are prone to irritation from ill-fitting shoes. |
| 2. Assess color and temperature of toes, feet, and fingers. Assess capillary refill of nails. Palpate radial and ulnar pulse of each hand and the dorsalis pedis pulse of the foot; note character of pulses. | Assesses adequacy of blood flow to extremities. Circulatory alterations may change integrity of nails and increase client's chance of localized infection when a break in skin integrity occurs. |
| 3. Observe client's walking gait. Have client walk down hall or walk straight line (if able). | Painful disorders of feet can cause limping or unnatural gait. |
| 4. Ask female clients about whether they use nail polish and polish remover frequently. | Chemicals in these products can cause excessive dryness. |
| 5. Assess type of footwear worn by clients: are socks worn? are shoes tight or ill-fitting? are garters or knee-high nylons worn? is footwear clean? | Types of shoes and footwear may predispose client to foot and nail problems (e.g., infection, areas of friction, ulcerations). |
| 6. Identify client's risk for foot or nail problems: | Certain conditions increase likelihood of foot or nail problems. |
| a. Elderly. | Poor vision, uncoordination, obesity, or inability to bend over contribute to difficulty elderly have in performing foot and nail care. Normal physiologic changes of aging also result in nail and foot problems. |
| b. Diabetes. | Vascular changes associated with diabetes reduce blood flow to peripheral tissues. Break in skin integrity places diabetic at high risk for skin infection. |
| c. Heart failure; renal disease. | Both conditions can have symptoms of increased tissue edema, particularly in dependent areas (e.g., feet). Edema reduces blood flow to neighboring tissues. |
| d. Cerebrovascular accident, or stroke. | Presence of residual foot or leg weakness or paralysis results in altered walking patterns. Altered pattern causes increased friction and pressure on feet. |
| 7. Assess type of home remedies clients use for existing foot problems: | Certain preparations or applications may cause more injury to soft tissue than initial foot problem. |
| a. Over-the-counter liquid preparations to remove corns. | Liquid preparations can cause burns and ulcerations. |
| b. Cutting of corns or calluses with razor blade or scissors. | Cutting of corns or calluses may result in infection caused by break in skin integrity. |
| c. Use of oval corn pads. | Oval pads exert pressure on toes and can decrease circulation to surrounding tissues. |
| d. Application of adhesive tape. | Skin of older adult is thin and delicate and prone to tear when adhesive tape is removed. |
| 8. Assess client's ability to care for nails or feet: visual alterations, fatigue, musculoskeletal weakness. | Determines client's ability to perform self-care and degree of assistance required from nurse. |
| 9. Assess client's knowledge of foot and nail care practices: how to cut nails, use of over-the-counter-products, value of soaking before foot care. | Determines client's need for health teaching. |
| **Nursing Diagnosis** | |
| 1. Cluster assessment data to reveal actual or potential nursing diagnoses: | |
| a. Impaired skin integrity: related to thickening and keratosis of toe surfaces. | Soaking during foot care helps to eliminate dead skin layers. |
| b. Pain: related to inflammation of nail bed. | Proper nail care eliminates sources of irritation. |
| c. Altered tissue perfusion: related to arterial insufficiency. | Client's risk requires nurse to use extra caution in avoiding cutting skin surrounding nails. |
| d. Impaired physical mobility: related to foot discomfort. | Nail care may remove source of discomfort. |
| e. Self-care hygiene deficit: related to reduced mobility. | Family member may require instruction on hygiene techniques. |
| f. Knowledge deficit regarding foot and nail care: related to inexperience. | Procedure for foot and nail care takes several minutes and is an excellent time for client teaching. |

| Steps | Rationale |
|---|---|
| **Planning** | |
| 1. Develop individualized goals for client based on nursing diagnoses: | |
| a. Skin and nail surfaces remain intact and smooth. | Caution is used when trimming nails to avoid cuts in skin. |
| b. Client's comfort and ambulation improve through use of appropriate footwear. | Nurse instructs client about proper footwear. |
| c. Client understands proper nail care practices. | Client predisposed to foot or nail problems should know risks. |
| 2. Prepare needed equipment and supplies: | |
| a. Wash basin<br>b. Emesis basin<br>c. Washcloth<br>d. Bath towel or face towel<br>e. Nail clippers<br>f. Orange stick<br>g. Emery board or nail file<br>h. Body lotion<br>i. Disposable bath mat<br>j. Paper towels<br>k. Disposable gloves | Used to soak and soften tissues around fingernails, toes, and feet. |
| 3. Explain procedure to client, including fact that proper soaking requires several minutes. | Client must be willing to place fingers and feet in basins for 10-20 min. Client may become anxious or fatigued. |
| 4. Obtain physician's order for cutting nails if agency policy requires it. | Client's skin may be accidentally cut. Certain clients are more at risk for infection depending on their medical condition. |
| **Implementation** | |
| 1. Wash hands. Arrange equipment on overbed table. | Easy access to equipment prevents delays. Reduces transmission of infection. |
| 2. Pull curtain around bed or close room door (if desired). | Maintaining client's privacy reduces anxiety. |
| 3. Assist ambulatory client to sit in a bedside chair. Help bedrest client to a supine position with head of bed elevated. Place disposable bath mat on floor under client's feet or place towel on mattress. | Sitting in chair facilitates immersing feet in basin. Bath mat protects feet from exposure to soil or debris. |
| 4. Fill wash basin with water at 100°-110° F (43°-44° C). Test temperature of water. | Warm water softens nails and thickened epidermal cells, reduces inflammation of skin, and promotes local circulation. Proper water temperature prevents burns of skin. |
| 5. Place basin on bath mat or towel and help client place feet in basin. Place call light within client's reach. | Clients with muscular weakness or tremors may have difficulty positioning feet. Client's safety is maintained. |
| 6. Adjust overbed table to low position and place it over client's lap. (Client may sit in chair or lie in bed.) | Easy access prevents accidental spills. |
| 7. Fill emesis basin with water at 100°-110° F (43°-44° C) and place basin on paper towels on overbed table. | Warm water softens nails and thickened epidermal cells. |
| 8. Instruct client to place fingers in emesis basin and place arms in a comfortable position. | Prolonged positioning can cause discomfort unless normal anatomic alignment is maintained. |
| 9. Allow client's feet and fingernails to soak for 10-20 min. Rewarm water in 10 min. | Softening of corns, calluses, and cuticles ensures easy removal of dead cells and easy manipulation of cuticle. |
| 10. Clean gently under fingernails with orange stick while fingers are immersed (Fig. 9-8). Then remove emesis basin and dry fingers thoroughly. | Orange stick removes debris under nails that harbors microorganisms. Thorough drying impedes fungal growth and prevents maceration of tissues. |
| 11. With nail clippers, clip fingernails straight across and even with tops of fingers (Fig. 9-9). Shape nails with emery board or file. If client has circulatory problems file the nail only. | Cutting straight across prevents splitting of nail margins and formation of sharp nail spikes that can irritate lateral nail margins. Filing prevents cutting nail too close to nail bed. |

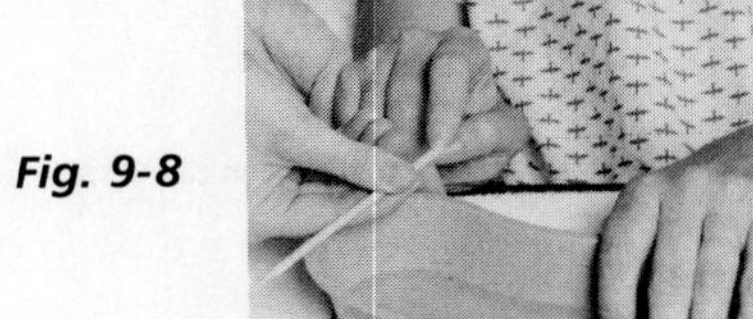

*Fig. 9-8*

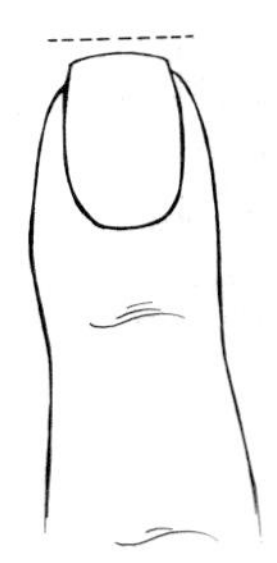

*Fig. 9-9*

| Steps | Rationale |
|---|---|
| 12. Push cuticle back gently with orange stick. | Reduces incidence of inflamed cuticles. |
| 13. Move overbed table away from client. | Provides easier access to feet. |
| 14. Put on disposable gloves and scrub callused areas of feet with washcloth. | Gloves prevent transmission of fungal infection. Friction removes dead skin layers. |
| 15. Clean gently under nails with orange stick. Remove feet from basin and dry thoroughly. | Removal of debris and excess moisture reduces chances of infection. |
| 16. Clean and trim toenails using procedures in Steps 11 and 12. Do not file corners of toenails. | Shaping corners of toenails may damage tissues. |
| 17. Apply lotion to feet and hands and assist client back to bed and into comfortable position. | Lotion lubricates dry skin by helping to retain moisture. |
| 18. Remove disposable gloves and dispose in receptacle. Clean and return equipment and supplies to proper place. Dispose of soiled linen in hamper. Wash hands. | Reduces transmission of infection. |

## Evaluation

| | |
|---|---|
| 1. Inspect nails and surrounding skin surfaces after soaking and nail trimming. | Evaluates condition of skin and nails. Allows nurse to note any remaining rough nail edges. |
| 2. Ask client to explain or demonstrate nail care. | Evaluates client's level of learning techniques. |
| 3. Observe client's walk after toe nail care. | Evaluates level of comfort and mobility achieved. |

### *Expected outcomes*

| | |
|---|---|
| 1. Nails are transparent, smooth, and convex with pink nail bed and translucent white tip. | Nail integrity and cleanliness maintained. |
| 2. Cuticles and tissues surrounding nail are clear and of normal color. Surfaces of feet are smooth. | Excess skin layers removed. |
| 3. Client explains or demonstrates nail care correctly. | Client learns skill. |
| 4. Client walks freely, without pain or unusual gait. | Sources of pressure or irritation are removed. |

### *Unexpected outcomes*

| | |
|---|---|
| 1. Nails discolored, rough, and concave or irregular in shape. | A single hygiene measure will not improve nail condition. |
| 2. Cuticles and surrounding tissues may be inflamed and tender to touch. Localized areas of tenderness on feet with calluses or corns at point of friction. | Repeated soakings are necessary to help relieve inflammation and remove layers of cells from calluses or corns. Change in footwear or corrective foot surgery may be needed for permanent improvement in corns or calluses. |
| 3. Ulcerations involving toes or feet may remain. | Foot care will not eliminate ulcers caused by vascular disease but will aid in keeping areas clean. |
| 4. Client unable to explain or perform foot care. | Further instruction required. |
| 5. Client complains of pain while walking and has unsteady gait. | Pressure or irritation on foot remains. |

## Recording and Reporting

| | |
|---|---|
| 1. Record procedure and observations (e.g., breaks in skin, inflammation, or ulcerations). | Documents procedure, client's response, and presence of abnormalities requiring additional therapy. |
| 2. Report any breaks in skin or ulcerations to nurse in charge or physician. | These abnormalities can seriously increase client's risk of infection and must be carefully observed. |

## Follow-up Activities

| | |
|---|---|
| 1. Clients with severe hypertrophy of nails should be referred to podiatrist for care. | During nurse's attempt to remove or cut hardened nails there is risk of additional tissue injury. |
| 2. Clients with chronic foot pain should be seen by physician. | Underlying problem could be of musculoskeletal nature, requiring care by orthopedic surgeon. |

## Special Considerations

- Clients with diabetes and peripheral vascular disease may have peripheral neuropathies that reduce sensation. Test water temperature carefully.
- Never cut nails of clients with diabetes and other circulatory problems. File only.

## Teaching Considerations

- Wash and soak feet daily using lukewarm water. Thoroughly pat feet dry and dry well between the toes.
- Do not cut corns or calluses or use commercial removers. Consult a physician or podiatrist.
- If feet tend to perspire, apply a bland foot powder.

- If dryness is noted along the feet or between the toes, apply lanolin, baby oil, or even corn oil and rub gently into skin.
- Teach client to avoid wearing elastic stockings or constricting garters and do not cross legs. Both impair circulation to the lower extremities.
- Inspect feet daily: tops and soles, heels, and area between toes.
- Wear clean socks or stockings daily. Socks should be free of holes or darns that might cause pressure.
- Do not walk barefoot.
- Wear proper-fitting shoes. Soles of shoes should be flexible and nonslipping. Shoes should be sturdy, closed in, and not restrictive to the feet.
- Any minor cuts should be washed immediately and dried thoroughly. Only mild antiseptics, e.g., neosporin ointment, should be applied to the skin. Avoid iodine or merbromin. Notify a physician.

## Home Care Considerations

- Alternative therapies: moleskin applied to areas of feet that are under friction does not cause local pressure as do corn pads; spot adhesive bandages can guard corns against friction but do not have padding to protect against pressure; wrapping small pieces of lamb's wool around toes reduces irritation of soft corns between toes.
- Assess use of client's bathroom sink for soaking client's hands and the tub for soaking client's feet.

---

**BIBLIOGRAPHY**

Bulau J: Clinical policies and procedures for home health care, Rockville, Md, 1986, Aspen Publishers, Inc.

Care of the ingrowing toenail: guidelines in technique, Hosp Med 19:204, 1983.

Davis M: Getting to the root of the problem: hair grooming techniques for black patients, Nursing '77 7:60, 1977.

Ebersole P, Hess P: Toward healthy aging: human needs and nursing response, ed 3, St. Louis, 1989, The CV Mosby Co.

Forbes K, Stokes SA: Saving the diabetic foot, Am J Nurs 84:884, 1984.

Graham S, Morley M: What "foot care" really means, Am J Nurs 84:889, 1984.

Grier ME: Hair care for the black patient, Am J Nurs 76:1781, 1976.

Nurse's Reference Library: Procedures. Springhouse, Pa, 1985, Intermed Communications, Inc.

Potter PA, Perry AG: Fundamentals of nursing, ed 2, 1989, St. Louis, The CV Mosby Co.

Rosen T, et al.: What nails can tell, RN 45:32, 1982.

Walsh J, Persons C, Wiech L: Manual of home health care nursing, Philadelphia, 1987, JB Lippincott Co.

Wells R, Trostle K: Creative hair washing techniques for immobilized patients, Nursing '84 14:47, 1984.

Whaley LF, Wong DL: Nursing care of infants and children, ed 3, St. Louis, 1987, The CV Mosby Co.

# 10

# EYE CARE AND CARE OF EYE AND EAR PROSTHESES

## *OBJECTIVES*

*Mastery of content in this chapter will enable the nurse to:*

- Define key terms.
- Explain why proper care of prostheses is important to a client's self-esteem.
- Identify guidelines used in caring for lenses and prostheses.
- Explain differences in the care of soft and rigid contact lenses.
- Correctly remove, store, cleanse, and insert a contact lens.
- Explain the rationale for maintaining aseptic technique during care of an artificial eye.
- Describe techniques that determine whether a hearing aid functions properly.
- Correctly remove, cleanse, and reinsert a hearing aid.

## *KEY TERMS*

*Astigmatism*
*Contact lens*
*Enucleation*
*Hyperopia*
*Myopia*
*Ophthalmologist*
*Optometrist*
*Prosthesis*
*Refractive error*

## *SKILLS*

**10-1** Taking Care of Contact Lenses
**10-2** Taking Care of an Artificial Eye
**10-3** Taking Care of a Behind-the-Ear Hearing Aid

Many clients rely on artificially constructed devices to replace or restore lost or impaired body functions. Eyeglasses and contact lenses help restore visual loss, and hearing aids can improve sound reception. Clients often depend on these devices to maintain attractive appearances, as well as to improve sensory function. Artificial eyes, in particular, help clients maintain appearances when an eye has been lost because of injury or disease.

Prostheses and contact lenses must fit and function properly so that clients can function normally within their environments. Clients can be extremely sensitive about lens or prosthesis care. Accidental breakage or malfunction can seriously impair sensory function and threaten self-esteem when a client becomes dependent on others for assistance.

Lenses and prostheses must be cleaned regularly to ensure proper function. Most clients have an established routine for cleaning their contact lenses or prostheses. When clients are unable to care for themselves, the nurse must understand the correct way to clean, handle, and store contact lenses and prostheses. Clients usually show great interest in the manner in which the nurse performs cleaning and maintenance procedures. Careful handling of lenses, an artificial eye, or a hearing aid is vital to avoid damage to these devices or to the client's eye or ear.

## GUIDELINES

1. Let the client be a resource in the care of each device. Unless receiving lenses or a prosthesis for the first time, a client is likely to have an established routine for care and maintenance, and have adapted special care techniques as well. It is the nurse's responsibility to be sure clients are not damaging the devices or injuring themselves.
2. Always protect the device from breakage. Replacement can be costly.
3. Use techniques that facilitate interaction with the client when a sensory loss exists. For example, if a client wears a hearing aid, the nurse should use communication techniques that ensure the client's ability to hear and understand. If visual function is reduced, the nurse should provide visual aids to improve the client's interaction within the environment.

4. Encourage clients to express feelings about changes in body image, such as feeling unusual or different, because of reliance on an artificial device for function or appearance. For example, clients with hearing impairments are often treated as though they are mentally impaired because they do not understand what is said to them. Families become frustrated when they cannot communicate with the client whose hearing aid malfunctions. The nurse must be supportive and demonstrate understanding when communicating with these clients. Likewise, nurses can teach families methods for interacting more effectively.

### PREREQUISITE KNOWLEDGE

1. Principles of medical asepsis.
2. Normal structures of the eye and ear.
3. Effects of visual and auditory impairment.
4. Existence of variations in contact lens care systems.
5. Principles of communicating with persons who have hearing loss.

### PREREQUISITE SKILLS

1. Proper handwashing techniques (Chapter 37).
2. Physical assessment of the eye and ear (Chapter 13).

## *SKILL 10-1 Taking Care of Contact Lenses*

A contact lens is a thin, transparent, oval disc that fits directly over the cornea of the eye. Contact lenses are designed specifically to correct refractive errors of the eye or abnormalities in the cornea's shape. They are relatively easy to apply and remove.

There are two major types of contact lenses: rigid and soft. Rigid lenses are thick and approximately 6 to 11 mm in diameter. Soft lenses are approximately 12.5 to 16.5 mm in diameter, large enough to cover the cornea completely. Soft lenses are flimsy because they consist primarily of water, 30% to 79% by weight (Carden, 1985). Both types are available as clear (untinted) or tinted lenses.

The normal eye needs oxygen and receives most of it through air and tears. (OxyFlow EW, 1987). Although soft lenses and newer rigid lenses are gas permeable and therefore allow oxygen to pass directly through the lens, all contact lenses still restrict the flow of oxygen to the eye's surface. Consequently, all lenses must be removed periodically to prevent ocular infection and corneal abrasions or ulcers (Stehr-Green, et al., 1987). A major difference between rigid and soft lenses is the length of time each can be safely worn. Rigid and daily wear soft lenses should be removed overnight and should not be worn more than 12 to 14 hours daily. It is not recommended that extended-wear soft lenses be left in place longer than one week (Egan, Soft Lens Care 1988). Pain, tearing, discomfort, and redness of the conjunctiva may be symptoms of lens overwear. Persistence of symptoms even after lens removal is abnormal, however, and may indicate serious ocular damage.

As contact lenses are worn by clients they accumulate secretions and foreign matter. This material deteriorates and then irritates the eye, causing distorted vision and risk for infection. Once removed, contact lenses should be cleaned and thoroughly disinfected.

Care of contact lenses includes cleaning, proper application and removal, and storage. Many clients wear contact lenses today. It is extremely important that nurses determine whether clients wear contact lenses, particularly when clients are admitted to hospitals or agencies in unresponsive or confused states. If a seriously ill client is wearing contact lenses and this goes undetected, serious corneal injury can result.

Clients usually have a preferred method for caring for their lenses. When it is necessary for the nurse to assist with lens care, the client's preferences should be considered.

### Purposes

1. Promote client's optimal visual acuity with use of lenses.
2. Prevent corneal injury or ocular infection.
3. Prevent breakage or loss of lenses.

## *Procedure 10-1*

| Steps | Rationale |
|---|---|
| **Assessment** | |
| 1. Place towel just below client's face. | Catches lens if one should accidently fall from eye. |
| 2. Inspect eye or ask client if contact lens is in place. | Lenses are generally comfortable to wear, and client may forget they are in place. Prolonged wear may cause injury to eye. |

| Steps | Rationale |
|---|---|
| 3. Ask if client feels any eye discomfort. | Contact lens fits over cornea of eye. Scratched lens can cause corneal irritation and abrasion. Accumulation of dust or debris between lens and cornea causes irritation. |
| 4. Assess length of time client normally wears lenses. | Continuous wearing of certain types of lenses can irritate cornea. |
| 5. Assess client's ability to manipulate and hold contact lens. | Determines level of assistance required in care. |
| 6. Assess client for any unusual visual symptoms. | May indicate underlying visual alteration or need to change lens prescription. |
| 7. Assess type of medications prescribed for client: sedatives, hypnotics, muscle relaxants, antihistamines, anticholinergics, and antidepressants. | Sedatives, hypnotics, and muscle relaxants reduce blink reflex and thus reduce lubrication of cornea. Antihistamines, anticholinergics, and antidepressants can reduce tear production. |
| 8. After lenses are removed, inspect eye for signs of corneal irritation, e.g., redness, pain, swelling around conjunctiva, and excess tearing. | Signs and symptoms indicate corneal irritation or abrasion. |

## Nursing Diagnosis

| Steps | Rationale |
|---|---|
| 1. Cluster data to reveal actual or potential nursing diagnoses: | |
| a. Pain: related to corneal irritation. | May require removal of lenses. |
| b. Changes in sensory perception: related to visual alterations. | Proper cleansing and placement of lens should improve visual acuity. |
| c. Self-care hygiene deficit: related to impaired hand movement. | Client may require assistance in removal, care, and insertion of lenses. |
| d. Knowledge deficit regarding contact lens care: related to inexperience. | Nurse offers instructions during care. |

## Planning

| Steps | Rationale |
|---|---|
| 1. Develop individualized goals for client based on nursing diagnoses: | |
| a. Promote comfort. | Cleansing removes debris on lens. |
| b. Improve client's knowledge of lens care. | During procedure nurse explains tips regarding care. |
| c. Promote improved visual perception. | Properly cleaned lenses improve visual acuity. |
| d. Prevent injury to the eye. | Lenses are inserted carefully and removed gently to prevent damage to eye structures. |
| 2. Prepare equipment and supplies for removal of lenses: | |
| a. Contact lens storage container | Separate cups labeled *R* for right lens and *L* for left lens hold lenses and protect from breakage. |
| b. Suction cup (optional) | Used to remove hard lenses from unconscious, debilitated, or confused clients. |
| c. Sterile saline solution | Used to moisten cornea before lens removal. |
| d. Bath towel | |
| 3. Prepare equipment and supplies for cleansing and insertion: | |
| a. Lenses in storage container | |
| b. Thermal disinfecting kit (optional) | Heats up to 80° C to sterilize soft lenses. |
| c. Surfactant cleaner | |
| d. Rinsing solution | |
| e. Sterile lens disinfectant and/or enzyme solution | Cleans lens surfaces and reduces number of microorganisms present. |
| f. Sterile wetting solution for rigid lenses | Wetting solution allows lens to glide easily over cornea during insertion. |
| g. Cotton ball or cotton-tipped applicator | Use to spread lens cleaner over surface of rigid contact lens. |
| h. Bath towel | |
| i. Emesis basin | |
| j. Glass of warm tap water | |
| 4. Discuss procedure with client. | Client can assist in planning by explaining technique that may aid removal and insertion. Client may be anxious as nurse retracts eye-lids and manipulates lenses. |
| 5. Have client assume supine or sitting position in bed or chair. | Provides easy access for nurse while retracting eyelids and manipulating lens. |

## Implementation

### *Removing soft lenses*

| Steps | Rationale |
|---|---|
| 1. Wash hands. | Reduces transmission of microorganisms. |
| 2. Place towel just below client's face. | Catches lens if one should accidentally fall from eye. |

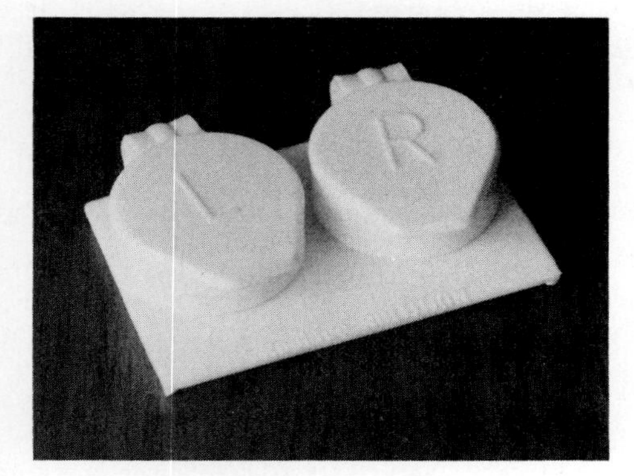

Fig. 10-1

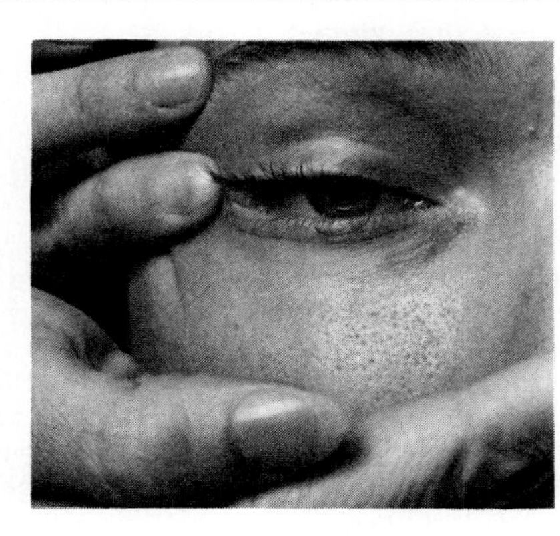
Fig. 10-2

| Steps | Rationale |
| --- | --- |
| 3. Add a few drops of sterile saline to client's eye. | Lubricates eye to facilitate lens removal. |
| 4. Tell client to look straight ahead. | Eases tipping of lens during removal. |
| 5. Using middle finger, retract lower eyelid. | Exposes lower edge of lens. |
| 6. With pad of index finger of same hand, slide lens off cornea onto white of eye. | Positions lens for easy grasping. Use of finger pad prevents injury to cornea and damage to lens. |
| 7. Pull upper eyelid down gently with thumb of other hand and compress lens slightly between thumb and index finger. | Causes soft lens to double up. Air enters underneath lens to release suction. |
| 8. Gently pinch lens and lift out. | Protects lens from damage. Avoid lens edges from sticking together. |
| 9. If lens edges stick together, place lens in palm and soak thoroughly with sterile saline. Gently roll lens with index finger in back and forth motion. If gentle rubbing doesn't separate edges, soak lens in sterile solution. | Assists in returning lens to normal shape. |
| 10. Clean and rinse lens (see "Cleansing and disinfecting contact lenses"). Place lens in proper storage case compartment: *R* for right lens and *L* for left lens (Fig. 10-1). Be sure lens is centered. | Ensures proper lens will be reinserted into correct eye. Proper storage prevents cracking or tearing. |
| 11. Repeat Steps 3-10 for other lens. Secure cover over storage case. | Proper storage prevents damage to lens. |
| 12. Dispose of towel and wash hands. | Reduces transmission of infection. |
| ***Removing rigid lenses*** | |
| 1. Wash hands. | Reduces transmission of microorganisms. |
| 2. Place towel just below client's face. | Catches lens if one should accidentally fall from eye. |
| 3. Be sure lens is positioned directly over cornea. If it is not, close the eyelids, place index and middle fingers of one hand behind the lens, gently but firmly massage lens back into place. | Correct position of lens allows easy removal from eye. |
| 4. Place index finger on outer corner of client's eye and draw skin gently back toward ear (Fig. 10-2). | Maneuver tightens lids against eyeball. |
| 5. Tell client to blink. Do not release pressure on lids until blink is completed. | Maneuver should cause lens to dislodge and pop out. Lid margins must clear top and bottom of lens until the blink. |
| 6. If lens fails to pop out, gently retract eyelid beyond edges of lens. Press lower eyelid gently against lower edge of lens. | Pressure causes upper edge of lens to tip forward. |
| 7. Allow both eyelids to close slightly and grasp lens as it rises from eye. | Maneuver causes lens to slide off easily. |
| 8. Cup lens in your hand. | Protects lens from breakage. |
| 9. Cleanse and rinse lens (see Cleansing and disinfecting contact lenses). Place lens in proper storage case compartment: *R* for right lens and *L* for left lens. Center lens in storage case, convex side down. | Both lenses may not have the same prescription. Proper storage prevents cracking, tearing, or chipping. |
| 10. Repeat Steps 3-9 for other lens. Secure cover over storage case. | Proper storage prevents damage to lens. |
| 11. Dispose of towel and wash hands. | Reduces spread of infection and keeps client's environment neat. |

| Steps | Rationale |
|---|---|
| ***Cleansing and disinfecting contact lenses*** | |
| 1. Wash hands. | Reduces transmission of microorganisms. |
| 2. Assemble supplies at bedside. | Provides easy access to supplies. |
| 3. Place towel over work area. | Towel helps prevent lens breakage. |
| 4. Open lens container carefully, taking care not to flip lens caps open suddenly. | Prevents lenses from being accidentally spilled or flipped out of case. |
| 5. After removal of lens from eye, apply 1-2 drops of daily surfactant cleaner on the lens in palm of your hand (use cleanser recommended by lens manufacturer or eye care practitioner). | Removes tear components, including mucous, lipids, and proteins that collect on lens. |
| 6. Rub lens gently but thoroughly on both sides for 20-30 sec. Use index finger (soft lenses) or little finger or cotton tip applicator soaked with cleaner (rigid lenses) to clean inside lens. Be careful not to contact or scratch lens with fingernail. | It is easier to manipulate and clean lenses using fingertips. Cleans all surfaces for microorganisms. |
| 7. Holding lens over emesis basin, rinse thoroughly with manufacturer-recommended rinsing solution (soft lenses) or cold tap water (rigid lenses). | Removes debris and cleaning agent from lens surface. |
| 8. Place lenses in storage case and fill with storage solution recommended by manufacturer or eye care practitioner. | Disinfects lenses, removes residue, enhances wettability of lenses, and prevents scratches from a dry case. |
| ***Inserting rigid lenses*** | |
| 1. Wash hands thoroughly with mild noncosmetic soap. Rinse well. Dry with clean lint-free towel or paper towel. | Lint or film on hands from soaps containing perfumes, deodorants, or complexion creams can be transferred to lenses and cause eye irritation. |
| 2. Place towel over client's chest. | Towel will catch dropped lens and avoid breakage, scratching, or tearing. |
| 3. Remove right lens from storage case, attempt to lift lens straight up (Fig. 10-3). | Sliding lens out of case can cause scratches on the surface. |
| 4. Rinse with cold tap water. | Hot water causes lens to warp. |
| 5. Wet lens on both sides using prescribed wetting solution. | Lubricates lens so that it slides easily over and adheres to cornea. |
| 6. Place right lens concave side up on tip of index finger of dominant hand (Fig. 10-4). | Proper manipulation of lens ensures easy insertion. Inner surface of lens should face up so that it is applied against cornea. |
| 7. Instruct client to look straight ahead, while retracting both upper and lower eyelids; place lens gently over center of cornea. | Hard lens is rigid and can be placed as client looks straight ahead. Retraction of lids promotes easy insertion between lid margins. |
| 8. Ask client to close eyes briefly and avoid blinking. | Helps to secure position of lens. |
| 9. Be sure lens is centered properly by asking client if vision is blurred. | If lens slips to side of cornea or into conjunctival sac, vision will blur. |
| 10. Repeat Steps 3-9 for left eye. | |
| 11. Assist client to comfortable position. | Promotes client's comfort. |
| 12. Discard soiled supplies; discard solution in storage case; rinse case thoroughly and allow to air dry; wash hands. | Use of fresh solution daily prevents infection. |
| ***Inserting soft lenses*** | |
| 1. Wash hands with mild noncosmetic soap, rinse well, dry with clean lint-free or paper towel. | Lint or film left on hands from cosmetic or deodorant soaps can be transferred to lenses and irritate eye. |
| 2. Place towel over client's chest. | Towel will catch dropped lens and avoid breakage, scratching, or tearing. |

***Fig. 10-3***

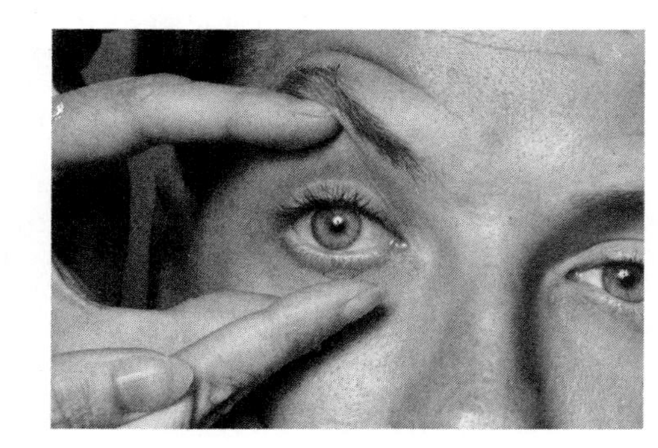

***Fig. 10-4***

| **Steps** | **Rationale** |
|---|---|
| 3. Remove right lens from storage case and rinse with recommended rinsing solution; inspect lens for foreign materials, tears, or other damage. | Removes disinfectant solution. Prevents irritation or damage to eye. |
| 4. Check that lens is not inverted (inside out). | Soft lens is inverted if bowl has a lip; it is in proper position if curve is even from base to rim. |
| 5. Using middle or index finger of opposite hand, retract upper lid until iris is exposed. | Soft lenses do not adhere as easily as hard lenses. Separating lids as much as possible allows room for lens to contact cornea without touching lids or lashes. |
| 6. Use middle finger or the hand holding the lens to pull down lower lid. | |
| 7. Tell client to look straight ahead and "through" the lens and finger, gently place lens directly on cornea, and release lens slowly, starting with lower lid. | Assures secure fit and comfort. |
| 8. If lens is on sclera rather than cornea, tell client to slowly close eye and roll it towards the lens. | Maneuver centers soft lens over cornea. |
| 9. Tell client to blink a few times. | Ensures lens is centered, free of trapped air, and comfortable. |
| 10. Be sure lens is centered properly by asking client if vision is blurred. | If lens slips to side of cornea or into conjunctival sac vision will blur. |
| 11. If client's vision is blurred: | |
| a. Retract eyelids.<br>b. Locate position of lens.<br>c. Ask client to look in direction opposite of lens and with your index finger, apply pressure to lower eyelid margin and position lens over cornea.<br>d. Have client look slowly toward lens. | Technique repositions lens over center of cornea as client looks toward lens. |
| 12. Repeat Steps 3-10 for other eye. | |
| 13. Assist client to comfortable position. | Promotes client's comfort. |
| 14. Discard soiled supplies; discard solution in storage case; rinse case thoroughly and allow to air dry; wash hands. | Prevents infection. |

## Evaluation

| | |
|---|---|
| 1. Ask client if lens feels comfortable after reinsertion. | Determines if any debris is caught between lens and cornea. Lens should be removed if client experiences severe discomfort. |
| 2. Assess client's visual acuity. | Determines improvement in visual perception. |
| 3. Have client discuss or demonstrate lens care. | Evaluates client's understanding of techniques. |

### *Expected outcomes*

| | |
|---|---|
| 1. Client will verbalize lens feels comfortable.<br>2. Client will be able to see clearly. | Lens cleaned and positioned correctly. |
| 3. Client will describe and demonstrate lens care. | Learning acheived. |

### *Unexpected outcomes*

| | |
|---|---|
| 1. Client's vision may be blurred. | Improper lens placement is likely cause of blurred vision. |
| 2. Client may complain of burning, pain, or sensation of having foreign body in eye. | Lens must be removed. |
| 3. Client unable to explain or perform lens care. | Further instruction required. |

## Recording and Reporting

| | |
|---|---|
| 1. Record or report any signs or symptoms of visual alterations noted during procedure. | May indicate presence of eye injury or disease. |
| 2. Record on nursing care plan or Kardex times of lens insertion and removal if client is going to surgery or special procedure. | In most institutions it is not necessary to record procedure unless it was ordered or client is going to surgery. |

## Follow-up Activities

| | |
|---|---|
| 1. If client continues to feel foreign body sensation, remove, clean, rinse, and reinsert lenses. | It is often difficult to remove all debris from lens surface on first cleaning. |

### Special Considerations

- Never apply direct downward pressure to eyeball because this may cause serious injury.
- Unconscious or confused client entering health care setting should be carefully assessed.
- Malpositioning of lens is common in clients who are comatose, confused, or in less responsive state.
- When removing or inserting lens, client may assume side-lying position if movement and position are restricted.
- Lenses are often difficult to locate if clear (untinted).
- For unconscious or confused client, a suction cup may be used for removing lenses. Gently apply suction cup to lens surface and lift lens out.
- Special heat-resistant cases can be placed in electric heating units for soft lens sterilization; however, units usually are not available in hospital.
- Soft lenses are more pliable than rigid lenses and thus less irritating. Chronic irritation should be reported to physician.
- Wearers of contact lenses, especially soft lenses, are at risk for developing ocular infections and corneal ulcers. Common infectious agents are *pseudomonas aeruginosa* and staphylococci. Acanthamoeba is a rarer, but more serious, agent that can cause protozoal infections (Kirn, 1987; Stehr-Green, et al., 1987). Adherence to recommended methods of lens care should be emphasized.
- Some women experience discomfort with contact lens wear during menstrual periods, pregnancy, menopause, or while taking oral contraceptives. Hormonal-related fluid retention may cause corneal swelling and result in ill-fitting lenses.

### Teaching Considerations

- Nurse should encourage client to see ophthalmologist regularly.
- Teach clients with weak pincer grasp to place lens in palm of hand.
- Plastic lenses scratch easily. Special cleansing solutions and drying tissues are recommended.
- Never use fingernail to remove dirt or debris that does not loosen during washing.
- Follow recommendations of lens manufacturer or eye practitioner when cleaning and disinfecting lenses.
- Caution client against using saliva, homemade saline solution, or tap water as wetting solutions because they can cause infection.
- Lenses become very slippery once cleaner is applied.
- If lens is dropped on a hard surface, moisten finger with cleaning or wetting solution and gently touch lens to pick it up. Then clean, rinse, and disinfect lens.
- Lens should be kept in a moist, wet state when not worn.

### Home Care Considerations

- Rigid lenses and daily wear soft lenses should be removed for sleeping, sunbathing, swimming, and showering.
- Clients in the home setting should be cautioned against working over sink unless towel is placed in sink or sink stopper is in place.
- Lenses must be both cleaned and disinfected. One procedure does not replace the other.
- Use fresh solution daily when storing and disinfecting lenses.
- Soft lenses need to be cleaned weekly with an enzymatic cleaner to remove protein.
- Check expiration dates of solutions. Discard outdated solutions to avoid adverse effects or infections.
- Do not use nonsterile water (distilled, mineral, well, or tap) on soft lenses. Such use increases chances of infection and can discolor a soft lens.
- Do not wipe lens with tissue or towel.
- Thoroughly wash and rinse lens storage case on a daily basis. Clean periodically with soap or liquid detergent; rinse thoroughly with warm water and air dry.
- To avoid mix-up, always start with the same lens when removing or inserting lenses.
- Do not wear lenses in presence of noxious or irritating vapors or fumes.
- Use hair spray before lenses are inserted.
- Apply makeup after lenses are inserted and use water-based or water-soluble eyeliners only; cosmetics trapped under a lens can cause irritation.
- Do not use eye drops or medications without consulting an eye care practitioner.
- Assess level of understanding of the client and primary care giver regarding application of contact lenses.
- Assess willingness and ability of client and primary care givers to apply contact lenses.

## *SKILL 10-2 Taking Care of an Artificial Eye*

As a result of tumor, infection, congenital blindness, or severe trauma to the eye, clients often must undergo an enucleation, a procedure involving the complete removal of the eyeball. Surgery is indicated when there is danger of an infectious or malignant process spreading to the neighboring eye or brain tissue, or when trauma has caused disruption of the entire globe of the eye. All that remains after an enucleation is the socket and eyelids. For obvious cosmetic purposes, clients who have had an enucleation are often fitted with an artificial eye, or prosthesis.

Artificial eyes are made of glass and plastic. The common plastic prosthesis is smooth and assumes the shape of the normal eyeball's anterior curvature. The prosthesis fits just behind the client's eyelids. Each prosthesis is designed to take on the appearance of the client's natural iris, pupil, and sclera. Prostheses are relatively easy to remove and insert, and cleansing with soap and water is all that is necessary. Artificial eyes can be worn day and night. Some clients may wear their prosthesis several months between cleansings. Others may prefer daily cleansing. Some nurses may find caring for an artificial eye distasteful. However, it is a necessary element of good basic hygiene.

## Purposes

1. Maintain integrity of the eye socket and eyelids.
2. Prevent infection of neighboring tissues.
3. Maintain client self-image.

# *Procedure 10-2*

| Steps | Rationale |
|---|---|
| **Assessment** | |
| 1. Determine from client, family, or medical record which eye is artificial. | Artificial eye is made to look like normal eye. |
| 2. Inspect surrounding tissues of eyelid and eye socket for inflammation, tenderness, swelling, or drainage. (Inspect socket after removal of prosthesis.) | Infection can spread easily to neighboring eye, underlying sinuses, or brain tissue. |
| 3. Assess client's routines for prosthetic care: frequency of cleaning and cleaning methods. | Provides client with sense of independence in influencing own care. Prosthesis is important to client's appearance. Allows nurse to assess adequacy of hygiene practices. |
| 4. Assess client's ability to remove prosthesis. | Determines level of assistance required during care. |
| **Nursing Diagnosis** | |
| 1. Cluster data to reveal actual or potential nursing diagnoses: | |
| a. Potential for infection: related to impaired tissue integrity. | If infection is serious, it may be necessary to remove prosthesis for extended period of time. |
| b. Self-care hygiene deficit: related to decreased motor function, decreased strength, or visual disturbance. | Client dependent on nurse for assistance. |
| c. Knowledge deficit regarding hygiene practices: related to inexperience. | Nurse will provide instructions on care. |
| **Planning** | |
| 1. Develop individualized goals for client based on nursing diagnoses: | |
| a. Promote client's self-concept. | Avoids showing any revulsion toward procedure. |
| b. Clean external lid margins and eye socket. | Complete eye care provided. |
| c. Improve client's knowledge of prosthesis care. | Nurse discusses importance of regular cleansing during procedure. |
| 2. Prepare following equipment and supplies: | |
| a. Soft washcloth or cotton gauze square | |
| b. Wash basin with warm water or saline | |
| c. 4×4" gauze pads | |
| d. Mild soap | |
| e. Facial tissues | |
| f. Bath towel | |
| g. Suction device, such as rubber bulb syringe or medicine dropper bulb (optional) | Syringe removes prosthesis by suction if manual removal is not successful. |
| h. Covered plastic storage case | Case used to store prosthesis if eye not reinserted. |
| 3. Discuss procedure with client. | Allows client opportunity to suggest further ideas about procedure. |
| 4. Assist client to supine position with head slightly elevated. | Position facilitates removal of prosthesis with less chance of breakage. |
| **Implementation** | |
| 1. Wash hands. | Reduces transmission of microorganisms. |

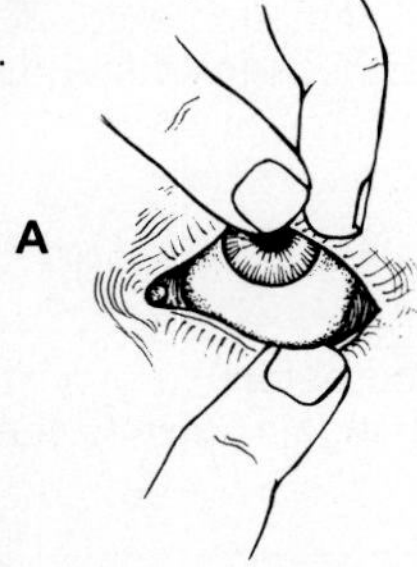

A B *Fig. 10-5*

| Steps | Rationale |
|---|---|
| 2. With thumb, gently retract lower eyelid against lower orbital ridge (Fig. 10-5, *A*). | Exposes lower edge of eye prosthesis. |
| 3. Exert slight pressure below eyelid (Fig. 10-5, *B*). | Maneuver causes break in suction and prosthesis to rise and slide out of socket. |
| 4. If prosthesis does not slide out, use bulb syringe or medicine dropper bulb to apply direct suction to prosthesis. | |
| 5. Place prosthesis in palm of hand. | Protects prosthesis from breakage. |
| 6. Clean prosthesis. | Tears and secretions containing microorganisms may have collected on surface of prosthesis. |
| a. Wash with mild soap and water or plain saline by rubbing it well between thumb and index finger. | |
| b. Rinse well with tap water. | Removes soap and residue. |
| c. Dry and polish prosthesis with soft washcloth or facial tissue. | Maintains shiny appearance of prosthesis to resemble normal eye. |
| 7. If client is not to have prosthesis reinserted, store it in water in plastic storage case. Label container and place in bedside stand. | Maintains condition of plastic. Label prevents accidental loss of container. |
| 8. Clean eyelid margins and socket. | |
| a. Retract upper and lower eyelid margins with thumb and index finger. | Exposes eye socket. |
| b. Wash socket with washcloth or gauze square moistened in warm water or saline. | Removes secretions that contain microorganisms. |
| c. Dry socket well with gauze pads. | Removes moisture that can harbor microorganisms. |
| d. Wash eyelid margins with mild soap and water. Wipe from inner to outer canthus, using a clean section of cloth with each wipe. | Prevents secretions from entering tear duct in inner canthus. |
| e. Dry eyelids by wiping from inner to outer canthus. | |
| 9. Dampen prosthesis in water. | Makes insertion easier, i.e., dry plastic rubs against tissue surfaces. |
| 10. Retract client's upper eyelid with index finger or thumb of nondominant hand. | Retraction of lid will ease prosthesis insertion. |
| 11. With dominant hand hold prosthesis so that notched edge is positioned toward nose. | Correct positioning of prosthesis ensures proper fit. |
| 12. Slide prosthesis up under upper eyelid as far as possible. Then depress lower lid to allow prosthesis to slip into place. | Prosthesis will fit evenly into socket. |
| 13. Wipe prosthesis toward nose if wiping is necessary. | Prevents prosthesis from dislodging. |
| 14. Help client assume comfortable position. | Maintains client's comfort. |
| 15. Dispose of soiled supplies, store all equipment and supplies, and wash hands. | Controls infection and maintains neat environment. |

## Evaluation

| | |
|---|---|
| 1. Observe position of prosthesis. | Determines whether prosthesis fits properly. |
| 2. Inspect condition of eyelids. | Evaluates cleanliness and position of eyelids. |
| 3. Ask client to explain or demonstrate prosthetic care. | Evaluates clients ability to perform techniques. |

### *Expected outcomes*

| | |
|---|---|
| 1. Client states prosthetic eye fits comfortably. | Prosthesis inserted correctly. |
| 2. Eyelid margins clean and of normal color with lashes turned away from prosthesis. | Eyelids clean and positioned correctly. |
| 3. Absence of redness, tenderness, or swelling of socket or eyelid margins. | Eyelid margins and socket free of infection. |
| 4. Client able to perform prosthetic care. | Learning achieved. |

### *Unexpected outcomes*

| | |
|---|---|
| 1. Client states prosthesis feels uncomfortable. | Prosthesis may require repositioning. |
| 2. Tissues of socket or lid margins are red, tender, or swollen. | If area of tenderness or inflammation exists in socket, it may be necessary to remove prosthesis for a few days. |
| 3. Excessive, purulent, or foul drainage. | Indicates infection. |
| 4. Client unable to explain or perform prosthetic care. | Further instruction required. |

## Recording and Reporting

| | |
|---|---|
| 1. Record removal of prosthesis for client going to surgery. | Prostheses must be removed before surgery to prevent loss. |
| 2. Record or report any alterations in integrity of tissues surrounding eye. | Documents condition of change in client's status. |

| Steps | Rationale |
| --- | --- |
| **Follow-up Activities** | |
| 1. If eyelid or socket is infected, prosthesis should remain out. Provide client with comfortable eye patch. | Maintains client's sense of positive body image. |

### Special Considerations

- Artificial eye will not move in socket nor will pupil respond to light reflex or accommodation.
- Most clients prefer to remove, clean, and insert prosthesis themselves.
- Soap is not used when cleansing socket because it is difficult to rinse off thoroughly and may cause irritation to tissues.
- If crustations are difficult to remove, during cleansing place moistened cloth over eyelids for several minutes. This will loosen all crustations.

### Teaching Considerations

- Never use alcohol or chemicals for cleansing; these agents can damage plastic prosthesis.
- Look for rough edges of prosthesis after removal. These may abrade tissue surfaces.
- Instruct primary care giver not to force artificial eye into socket.

### Home Care Considerations

- Client in home setting should use available equipment, e.g., clean washcloth. Procedure need not be sterile.
- Some clients may wear a prosthesis for several months before removing or cleaning. Excess tearing or crusting indicates need to clean eye and socket.
- Assess level of understanding of client and primary care giver regarding client's condition and need for a prosthesis.
- Assess ability and willingness of client and primary care giver to administer eye care.
- Assess physical condition for which client is being treated and determine special precautions necessary.
- Assess ability of client to cooperate with eye procedures.

## *SKILL 10-3 Taking Care of a Behind-the-Ear Hearing Aid*

Hearing loss is a common problem. In the United States, 16.4 million persons suffer from hearing loss. Although 14.4 million admit to a hearing problem, only 3.9 million own a hearing aid (Wilson and Wilson, 1988). This is in spite of technologic advances that have made hearing aids more acceptable to clients. Hearing is vital for normal communication and for people to orient themselves to the sounds of their environment.

Market sales (Wilson and Wilson, 1988) indicate that there are three popular types of hearing aids:

1. An in-the-canal (ITC) aid is the newest, smallest, and least visible and fits entirely in the ear canal. It has cosmetic appeal, is easy to manipulate and place in the ear, does not interfere with the wearing of eyeglasses or telephone use, and can be worn during most physical exercise. However, disadvantages are that it requires adequate ear diameter and depth for proper fit; does not accommodate to progressive hearing loss; and requires manual dexterity to operate, insert and remove, and change batteries. Also, cerumen tends to plug this model more than the others.
2. An in-the-ear (ITE or intra-aural) aid fits into the external auditory ear and allows more fine-tuning. It is more powerful and stronger and therefore is useful for a wider range of hearing loss than the ITC aid. It is also easy to position and adjust, and does not interfere with eyeglass wearing. It is, however, slightly more noticeable than the ITC aid and is not recommended for persons with moisture or skin problems in the ear canal.
3. A behind-the ear (BTE or postaural) aid hooks around and behind the ear and is connected by a short, clear, hollow plastic tube to an ear mold inserted into the external auditory canal (Fig. 10-6). It also allows for

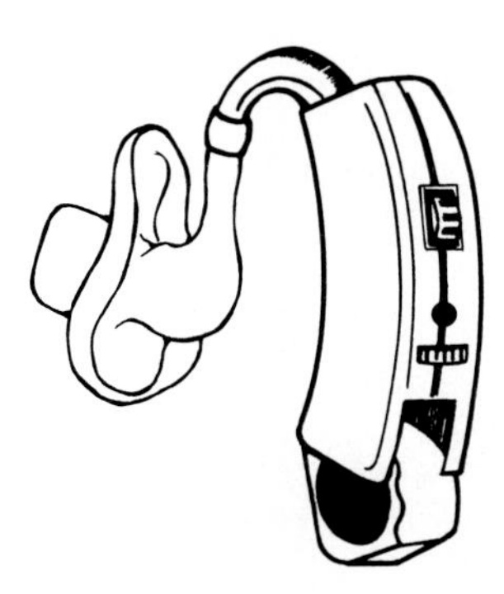

***Fig. 10-6*** Behind-the-ear hearing aid.

fine-tuning adjustment. It is the largest of the three and is useful for clients with rapidly progressive hearing loss, manual dexterity difficulties, or those who find partial ear occlusion intolerable. Disadvantages are that it is more visible (depending on hairstyle), may interfere with eyeglasses and telephone use, and is more difficult to keep in place during physical exercise.

Two other styles are less popular:

1. The eyeglass aid is a hearing aid that fits in the ear canal and attaches to a battery located on the arm of the eyeglass frame. The frame must be bulky to accommodate the equipment; therefore style selection is limited.
2. The body aid is a bulky instrument used for severe hearing loss. A fitted ear mold attaches to a round receiver that connects to a transmitter the size of a cigarette case. The case may be hidden in the clothing but the receiver and wire cannot. This type of aid is rarely used today.

Hearing aids amplify so that sound is heard at a more effective level. All aids have four basic components:

1. A microphone that receives and converts sound into electrical signals.
2. An amplifier that increases strength of the electrical signal.
3. A receiver that converts strengthened signal back into sound.
4. A power source (batteries) that energizes the components.

The devices can be tailored to a client's specific amplification need. Anyone caring for a hearing aid should know the device is delicate and must be protected from moisture, heat, and breakage. The skill in this section describes the care of a behind-the-ear hearing aid.

### Purposes

1. Improve client hearing reception.
2. Improve client communication capabilities.
3. Maintain function of the hearing aid.
4. Educate client about proper care of the hearing aid device.

## *Procedure 10-3*

| Steps | Rationale |
|---|---|
| **Assessment** | |
| 1. Assess client's knowledge of and routines for cleansing and caring for hearing aid. | Determines client's understanding and need for health education. Nurse will adapt method of care to client's procedure. |
| 2. Determine whether client can hear clearly with use of aid by talking slowly and clearly in normal voice tone. | Inability to hear may indicate faulty function of hearing aid. |
| 3. Assess whether hearing aid is working by removing from client's ear. Close battery case and turn volume slowly to high. Cup hand over earmold. If squealing or a whistling sound (feedback) is heard, it is working. If no sound is heard, replace batteries and test again. | Determines need for new battery. Feedback squeal will cause harsh whistling sound. |
| 4. Check that plastic connecting tube is not twisted or cracked. | Cracked or twisted tube prevents transmission of sound. |
| 5. Check earmold for cracked or rough edges. | Can cause irritation to external ear canal. |
| 6. Check for accumulation of cerumen around earmold and plugging of opening in mold. | Prevents clear sound reception and transmission. |
| **Nursing Diagnosis** | |
| 1. Cluster data to reveal actual or potential nursing diagnoses: | |
| a. Sensory and perceptual alterations: related to hearing loss. | |
| b. Knowledge deficit regarding hearing aid care: related to unfamiliarity with care of hearing aid. | Nurse has client explain techniques of care; reinforces proper techniques. |
| c. Impaired verbal communication: related to hearing deficit. | Nurse uses effective communication techniques during care. |
| d. Potential for injury: related to hearing loss or damaged earmold. | Client at risk in environment if hearing is poor. Damaged earmold may injure sensitive ear tissues. |
| **Planning** | |
| 1. Develop individualized goals for client based on nursing diagnoses: | |
| a. Improve client's hearing reception. | Obstruction of ear canal or malfunction of parts of hearing aid device will reduce sound amplification and transmission. |
| b. Improve client's ability to care for hearing aid independently. | Client's routines and knowledge of hearing aid care may reveal poor understanding of care techniques. |

| Steps | Rationale |
|---|---|
| 2. Prepare equipment and supplies: | |
| a. Emesis basin | Use to soak earmold. |
| b. Mild soap and warm water | |
| c. Pipe cleaner (optional) | Use to clean plastic connecting tube. |
| d. Syringe needle (optional) | Use to clean opening in earmold. |
| e. Soft towel | |
| f. Washcloth | |
| g. Storage case | |
| 3. Have client suggest any additional tips for care; explain that you are going to clean and replace hearing aid. | Client becomes uncomfortable when unable to hear clearly. Explain all steps before removing aid to minimize confusion and anxiety. |

## Implementation

### *Cleaning hearing aid*

| Steps | Rationale |
|---|---|
| 1. Wash hands. | Reduces transmission of microorganisms. |
| 2. Assemble supplies at bedside table or sink area. | Procedure can be performed without delays. |
| 3. Detach earmold from battery device. | Moisture entering battery and transmitter will cause permanent damage to aid. |
| 4. Add warm water and soap to emesis basin. Soak ear mold for several min. | Soaking removes cerumen that can accumulate on mold. |
| 5. Wash ear canal with washcloth moistened in soap and water. Rinse and dry. | Removes cerumen and debris. |
| 6. If cerumen has built up in hole of earmold, carefully clean hole with tip of syringe needle. | Wax will prevent normal sound transmission. |
| 7. Rinse earmold thoroughly with clear water. | Soap may form residue that blocks opening in mold. |
| 8. Allow mold to dry thoroughly after wiping with soft towel. | Water droplets left in connecting tube could enter hearing aid and damage parts. |
| 9. Clean connecting tube with pipe cleaner (optional). | Removes moisture and debris that can interfere with sound transmission and hearing aid function. |
| 10. Reconnect earmold to hearing aid device before inserting or storing hearing aid. | Reassembly allows nurse to check functioning. |
| 11. Store hearing aid in storage case if client is about to do any of following: bathe, use a hair dryer, go to surgery or major procedure, sleep, or if client is diaphoretic. | Protects hearing aid against damage and breakage. |

### *Inserting hearing aid*

| Steps | Rationale |
|---|---|
| 1. To reinsert hearing aid, first check batteries (Assessment, Step 3); replace batteries (if necessary) over soft surface, e.g., towel or bed. | Necessary for proper sound amplification. Protects hearing aid against damage and breakage. |
| 2. Turn aid off and turn volume control down. | Will protect client from sudden exposure to sound. |
| 3. Place ear mold in external ear canal. Be sure ear bore (hole) in mold is placed into canal first. Shape of mold indicates correct ear. Gently press and twist until mold feels snug. | Proper fit ensures optimum sound transmission. |
| 4. Gently bring connecting tube up and over toward back of ear, avoid kinking. Battery device fits around upper ear. | Ensures correct function of hearing aid device and maintains client's comfort. |
| 5. Adjust volume gradually to comfortable level for talking to client in regular voice at a 1-1.25 m (3-4 ft) distance. | Gradual adjustment prevents exposing client to harsh squeal or feedback. Client should hear nurse comfortably. |
| 6. Remove soiled equipment from bedside. Dispose of used supplies. Wash hands. | Maintains clean environment and reduces risk of infection. |

## Evaluation

| Steps | Rationale |
|---|---|
| 1. Return to client to assess whether hearing is clear and hearing aid is producing inappropriate feedback sound. | If ear mold is not securely in place, it will squeal or not function. |
| 2. Have client explain or perform insertion and cleansing. | Reveals client's understanding of techniques. |

### *Expected outcomes*

| Steps | Rationale |
|---|---|
| 1. Client is able to hear conversation spoken in normal tone of voice and responds appropriately. | Batteries are operational. Earmold is secure and unobstructed. Connecting tube is intact. |
| 2. Client states aid fits comfortably. | Earmold positioned correctly. |
| 3. Client able to clean and insert hearing aid. | Demonstrates learning. |

### *Unexpected outcomes*

| Steps | Rationale |
|---|---|
| 1. Feedback squeal or harsh whistling is heard from hearing aid. | Result of loose earmold, cracked tubing, or weak batteries. |

| Steps | Rationale |
|---|---|
| 2. Client is unable to hear conversations clearly. | Ear canal may be obstructed. Hearing aid device malfunctioning. |
| 3. Client's verbal responses are inappropriate. | Hearing is impaired. |
| 4. Client unable to clean or insert hearing aid. | Further instruction is required. |

## Recording and Reporting

| | |
|---|---|
| 1. Document that aid is removed and stored if client is going to surgery or special procedure. | Protects nurse from liability of loss of hearing aid. |
| 2. Report to nursing staff difficulties client has in communicating. | Improves continuity of care in communication techniques for client. |

## Follow-up Activities

| | |
|---|---|
| 1. Nurse should discuss with client guidelines for hearing aid use and tips for care. | Improves client's ability for self-care. |

## Special Considerations

- Hearing aids offer the greatest benefit in conductive hearing loss. Common causes of conductive loss include chronic otitis media, otosclerosis, or congenital anomalies.
- Contrary to some perceptions, amplification of sound through a hearing aid may substantially help clients with sensorineural hearing loss that may be caused by presbycusis, lesions of the cochlea or auditory nerve, or that may be noise-induced.
- The earlier a diagnosis of hearing impairment is made and accepted, the better the prognosis for acceptance of a hearing aid.
- Development of digital aids is being given high priority in the research laboratory (Wilson and Wilson, 1988).
- Hearing aid users may find that background noises are bothersome and when amplified tend to mask speech. A tone control to reduce low-frequency amplification may help.
- Two aids (binaural) may be better than one: listening with both ears increases discrimination in noisy surroundings and improves sound localizations.
- As degree of hearing loss increases, need for a good seal to the ear also increases in order to prevent feedback (Knight, 1987).
- When cleaning the earmold, do not force the syringe needle into the mold or insert it further than 0.6 cm (.25 in).

## Teaching Considerations

- Never use alcohol or other chemicals as cleaning agents because they can cause cracking and drying of the mold.
- If hearing is less than "normal" after cleaning, check for the following:
  a. Earmold blocked with cerumen or fitted to wrong ear.
  b. Batteries worn or dead.
- Suggest assistive listening devices for specific situations, e.g., telephone or television amplifiers.
- Teach clients methods for managing their environment through improved listening techniques, e.g., speech reading, listening in a quiet environment, close proximity to the speaker.
- Refer clients to an audiologist or hearing specialist for consultation if appropriate.
- A dealer or specialist must clean actual hearing aid device.

## Home Care Considerations

- In home setting client may use clean plastic container for soaking and cleaning hearing aid.
- Toothpick may be used to clean earmold opening; pipe cleaner may be used to clean connecting tube.
- Client may use blow dryer on cool setting to dry tubing.
- Avoid exposure of aid to extreme heat or cold. Do not leave aid in case near stove, heater, or sunny window. Do not use with hair dryer on hot settings or with a sun lamp. In humid climate, storage case with silica gel is ideal for absorbing moisture.
- Remove aid for bathing or when at hair stylist.
- Hair spray tends to clog the aid; therefore, apply hair spray *before* fitting the aid.
- Store batteries in cool, dry place. Keep spares on hand (especially on holidays). Batteries can last a few days to a few weeks depending on the type of battery, frequency of use, volume setting, and power of the aid.
- Volume controls are numbered 1 to 4, with 4 the loudest. Various brands of aids use different sizes of batteries, and thus batteries are not interchangeable. Insert batteries only when aid is turned off.
- Assess level of understanding of client and primary care giver regarding care required for the hearing aid.
- Assess willingness and ability of client or primary care giver to perform necessary care of the hearing aid.
- Assess physcial conditions for which the client is being treated and determine necessary special precautions.
- Assess ability of client to cooperate with procedures to care for the hearing aid.

## BIBLIOGRAPHY


Carden RG: The ins and outs of contact lenses, RN 48:48, 1985.

Corrado OJ: Hearing aids, Br Med J 296:33, 1988.

Egan D, Bennett E, Davis: Rigid lens care and handling, Bethesda Eye Institute and St. Louis University School of Medicine, Department of Ophthalmology, St. Louis, 1988, Unpublished.

Egan D, Bennett E, Davis L: Soft lens care and handling, Bethesda Eye Institute and St. Louis University School of Medicine, Department of Ophthalmology, St. Louis, 1988, Unpublished.

Hitzeman SA, Meyers CO: Comparison of the acceptance of progressive addition multifocal vs a standard multifocal lens design, J Am Optom Assoc 56:706, 1985.

Kirn TF: Contact lens need tender, loving care, opthalmologists warn, or infection may result, JAMA 258:18, 1987.

Kirn, T.F.: As number of contact lens users increases, research seeks to determine risk factors, how best to prevent potential eye infections, JAMA 258:17, 1987.

Knight JJ: Hearing aids, Practitioner 231:1121, 1987.

Nursing Reference Library: Procedures, Springhouse, Pa, 1985, Springhouse Corp.

OxyFlow EW, Rigid permeable contact lens: instructions for wearers, Product Development Corporation. The PDC Contact Lens Network, Little Rock, Ark, 1987.

Potter PA, Perry AG: Fundamentals of nursing, ed 2, St. Louis, 1989, The CV Mosby Co.

Stehr-Green JK, Bailey TM, Brandt FH, et al.: Acanthamoeba keratitis in soft contact lens wearers: a case-control study, JAMA 258:57, 1987.

Walsh J, Persons C, Wieck L: Manual of home health care nursing, Philadelphia, Pa, 1987, JB Lippincott Co.

Wilson LA, Wilson KS: Hearing aids: who can benefit? what's new? one or two? Postgrad Med 83:249, 1988.

Zucnick M: Care of an artificial eye, Am J Nurs 75:835, 1975.

# 11

# CARE OF THE CLIENT'S ENVIRONMENT

*OBJECTIVES*

*Mastery of content in this chapter will enable the nurse to:*

- Define key terms.
- Describe typical types of room equipment found in a hospitalized client's room.
- Explain bed safety features.
- Describe common bed positions.
- Make an occupied bed.
- Make an unoccupied bed.

*KEY TERMS*

| | |
|---|---|
| *Drawsheet* | *Reverse Trendelenburg position* |
| *Fowler's position* | *Semi-Fowler's position* |
| *Mitered corner* | *Trendelenburg position* |

*SKILLS*

***11-1*** Making an Unoccupied bed
***11-2*** Making an Occupied bed

A typical hospital room contains certain basic pieces of furniture: overbed table, bedside stand, storage space, chairs, lights, and bed with call light. Behind each bed is a wall unit that contains various power outlets, as well as receptacles for connecting oxygen and suction equipment. In most hospitals a mercury sphygmomanometer with cuff is attached to the wall. Special intensive care units often have poles extending from the ceiling on which to hang intravenous (IV) fluids. The room is generally designed so that all necessary supplies and equipment can be easily accessible for the nurse and physician's use.

## ROOM EQUIPMENT

### Chairs

Most hospital rooms contain two types of chairs: an armless straight-backed chair and an upholstered lounge chair with arms. When clients are recovering from surgery or illnesses resulting in abdominal pain, they often prefer the straight-backed chair because less effort is needed to get in or out of it. The lounge chair often has a deeper seat and may require more effort on the part of the client to sit comfortably. Straight-backed chairs are convenient when temporarily transferring the client from the bed, as during bed making. The straight-backed chair is also easier to maneuver than the heavy lounge chair.

### Lights

Each room has an overbed light that focuses on the client's bed. The light controls are usually in the call light apparatus. Each room also has a floor or table lamp. Special examination lights may extend over the bed from the wall or ceiling. These lights are useful during procedures such as a dressing change. They are often movable and should be positioned for easy reach but moved aside when not in use. Portable gooseneck lamps provide extra illumination for bedside procedures. These are especially useful to focus light on hard-to-reach areas, for example, during urinary catheter insertion.

A call light (Fig. 11-1) is at each client's bedside. When a client presses a button located on the side rail of the bed or at the end of an extension cord a light goes on at the nurses' station or just outside the client's room. The call light signal indicates a client needs assistance. It is important for the nurse to respond to a call light as soon as possible. In addition to call lights, most hospitals have intercoms that allow clients to talk to a staff person at the nurses' station. Many hospital units also have emergency signal lights that nurses use to call for assistance when clients are in trouble.

### Overbed Tables

The overbed table is a long narrow table with wheels that can be adjusted to various heights over the client's

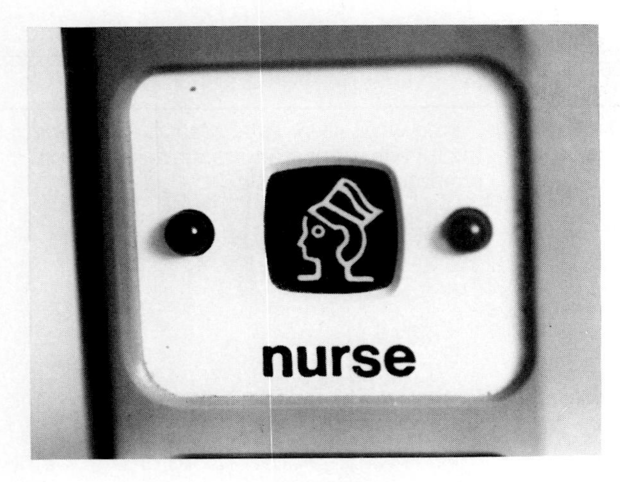


*Fig. 11-1*

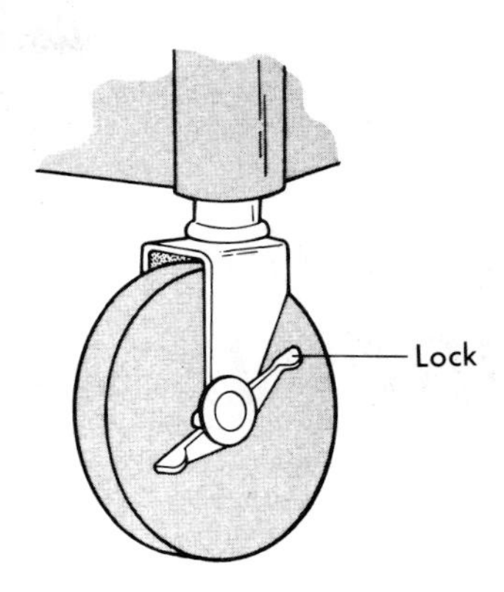


*Fig. 11-2*

bed or chair. It usually contains two storage drawers. The table provides ideal working space for the nurse and serves as a surface to place meal trays, toiletry items, and objects frequently used by the client.

### Bedside Stand

The bedside stand or table is a small table or cabinet located next to the bed. It is used to store the client's personal articles and hygiene equipment such as the bath basin, towels, or an emesis basin. Each table usually contains a drawer above and a cupboard below. The telephone, water pitcher, and drinking cup are commonly placed on the bedside table.

### Beds

Because a bed is the piece of equipment used most by a client, it should be designed for comfort, safety, and adaptability for changing positions.

The typical hospital bed consists of a firm mattress on a metal frame that can be raised and lowered horizontally. The frame is divided into three sections so the operator can raise and lower the head and foot of the bed, in addition to inclining the entire bed with the headboard up or down. Table 11-1 lists common bed positions. Most beds are powered by electric motors, but some beds are run manually or by hydraulic power.

Hospital beds come in two different lengths. Standard length is approximately 6 feet; a longer bed is available for taller patients. Each bed sits on four rollers or coasters that allow the nurse to move the bed easily. Often clients who are critically ill or who are immobilized in traction are transported to different locations, such as the x-ray department, in bed.

The position of a bed is usually changed by electric controls on the side of the bed, at the foot of the bed, or in a bedside cable. Clients can thus raise or lower sections of the bed without expending much energy. It is important for nurses to instruct clients on the proper use of controls and to caution them against raising the bed to a position that might cause harm. A hospital bed is usually 65 to 70 cm (26 to 28 inches) above the floor at its lowest level. In the home most beds are 50 to 55 cm (20 to 22 inches) high. The greater height of a hospital bed prevents undue musculoskeletal strain on the nurse and the client. It is unnecessary for the nurse to reach across or bend down while caring for clients, and clients can move from bed to a chair with minimal stress on hips and knees.

Beds contain a number of safety features. Locks located on the wheels or casters should be used whenever the bed is stationary to prevent accidental movement during performance of a procedure (e.g., transferring client from bed to a stretcher). Side rails, located on both sides of a bed protect clients from accidental falls, help clients position themselves, and provide upper extremity support as a client gets out of bed. Side rails are adjustable metal frames that raise and lower by pushing or pulling a knob. The nurse never leaves the bedside when a siderail is lowered with the client still in bed. Each bed also has a special headboard that is removable. This feature is important in emergency situations when the medical team must have easy access to the client's head during cardiopulmonary resuscitation (see Chapter 18).

#### Mattresses

Most beds have firm, water-repellent mattresses. A mattress should have an even surface for the client's comfort. Most mattresses have handles on the sides, to be used when the mattresses are removed or turned over. A rubber or plastic surface permits easy cleaning.

Special mattresses provide extra comfort and support for clients and relieve pressure on bony prominences. Chapter 35 reviews a variety of special mattresses and their indications for use.

***TABLE 11-1*** Common Bed Positions

| Position | Description | Uses |
|---|---|---|
| **Fowler's** | Head of bed raised to angle of 45°-90° or more; semisitting position (Knees raise on most beds approximately 15°). | Preferred while client eats; used during nasogastric tube insertion and nasotracheal suction; promotes lung expansion. |
| **Semi-Fowler's** | Head of bed raised approximately 30°-45°; incline is less than Fowler's position. (Knees raise on most beds approximately 15°). | Promotes lung expansion; relieves strain on abdominal muscles. |
| **Trendelenburg** | Entire bed frame tilted downward with head of bed down. | For postural drainage; facilitates venous return in clients with poor peripheral perfusion. |
| **Reverse Trendelenburg** | Entire bed frame tilted downward with foot of bed down. | Used infrequently; promotes gastric emptying and prevents esophageal reflux. |
| **Flat** | Entire bed frame horizontally parallel with floor. | For clients with vertebral injuries and in cervical traction. Position used for clients who are hypotensive, and generally preferred by clients for sleeping. |

## Special Equipment

There is special equipment that may be added to a bed or room. Examples of equipment available are listed in the box.

## GUIDELINES

1. Keep the environment as comfortable as possible by controlling ventilation and temperature. Depending on client's age and physical condition, room temperature should be maintained between 20° and 23° C (68° and 74° F). Infants, the elderly, and the acutely ill may need a warmer temperature. However, certain critically ill clients require cooler room temperatures to lower the body's metabolic demands. Controlling drafts and eliminating lingering odors from draining wounds, vomitus, bedpans, or urinals will also improve a client's comfort. Many hospitals are now prohibiting smoking in client's rooms.
2. Control extraneous noises in a client's room. Ill clients are sensitive to noises in a hospital environment. A nurse should try to control noise levels by handling equipment properly, making sure equipment is in

## SPECIAL ROOM EQUIPMENT

**Footboard** A flat plastic or wood panal placed at the foot of the bed above mattress level (Fig. 11-3). It keeps feet in the dorsiflexion position to prevent foot drop. A footboard also keeps bed covers up and off client's feet.

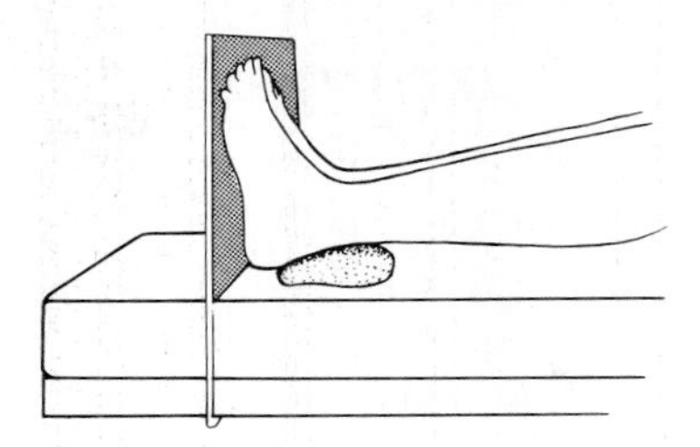

*Fig. 11-3*

**Foot boots** Sheepskin-lined boots made of smooth plastic that support each foot in dorsiflexion (Fig. 11-4); preferred over the footboard because they allow clients a variety of positions. The boot stays tied with velcro strips.

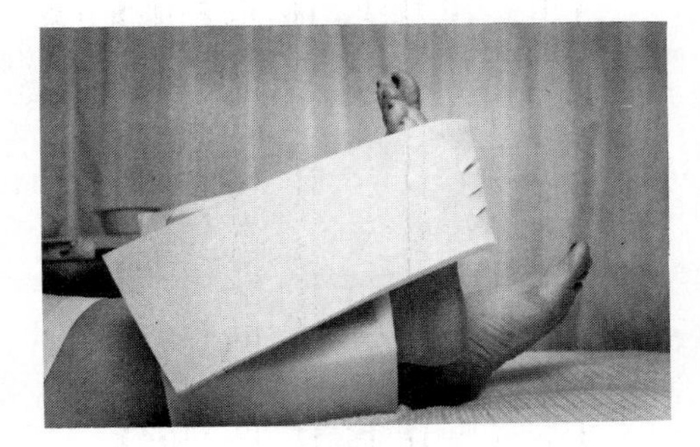

*Fig. 11-4*

**Bed boards** A long wooden or plexiglass board, the length of a regular bed mattress, that is placed under a mattress to provide added support. Clients with back pain frequently use bed boards. The boards are either rigid or hinged so that the foot or end of the bed can be elevated.

**Bed cradle** A curved, semicircular device, made of metal, that can be placed over a portion of the client's body. The cradle keeps top bed linens off of the client's feet, legs, or abdomen. Bed cradles come in a variety of sizes.

**Intravenous rods** A metal pole or stand that supports an IV fluid container while fluid is administered to a client. The rod may fit into the metal frame of a client's bed, stand on the floor, or attach to an overhead tract (Fig. 11-5).

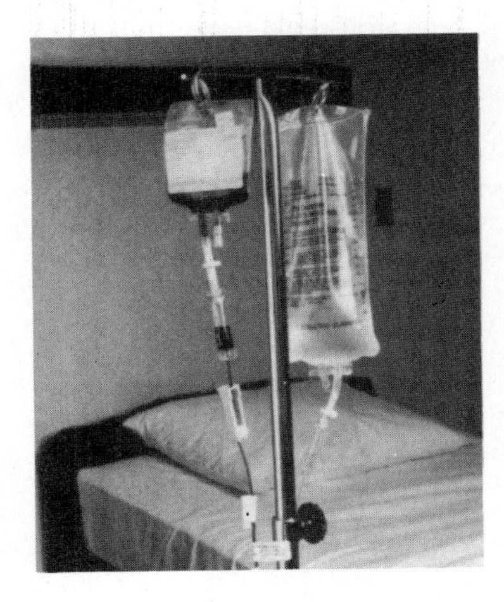

*Fig. 11-5*

proper working order, and controlling voice volume.

3. Make the environment as safe as possible. Keep all personal care items within client's reach. If client must leave bed to go to the bathroom, be sure there are no objects obstructing the way.
4. Make the environment personal for the client. Do not clutter client's environment with so many articles that make it impossible to arrange nursing care equipment and supplies. However, a picture of family members, a few get well cards, or even a small table radio helps the client feel more at home.
5. Be sure client is easily accessible. Often a client will have numerous IV lines and drainage tubes connected to portable poles and suction machines. At times of emergency the health care team must reach the client easily and quickly. Keep intravenous poles and portable equipment in positions that do not obstruct access to the client.

### PREREQUISITE KNOWLEDGE

1. Principles of medical asepsis.
2. Principles of body mechanics.

### PREREQUISITE SKILLS

1. Proper handwashing techniques (Chapter 37).

# SKILL 11-1 Making an Unoccupied Bed

Clients spend much of their time in bed, eating, bathing, using bedpans or urinals, and undergoing numerous therapeutic procedures. It is essential for the nurse to keep the bed as clean and comfortable as possible. Frequent inspections are necessary during the day to be sure linen is clean, dry, and wrinkle free. Bed linen that becomes wet or soiled should always be changed immediately.

Whenever possible the nurse should make the bed while it is unoccupied. Having the client get out of bed is an ideal way to promote ambulation. The nurse usually makes a bed in the morning after the client's bed bath or as the client is up bathing and showering. Another convenient time for bed making is when the client is out of the room for tests or procedures.

By making an unoccupied bed the nurse can be assured that linen is smooth and free of wrinkles. It is also easier to insert any extra waterproof pads or special foam rubber mattresses (Chapter 36) when a bed is unoccupied.

### Purposes

1. Provide a neat, clean environment for the client.
2. Eliminate sources of irritation to the client's skin.
3. Promote client comfort and relaxation.

## Procedure 11-1

| Steps | Rationale |
|---|---|
| **Assessment** | |
| 1. Assess potential for client being incontinent or having excess drainage on bed linen, e.g., postoperative clients with wounds or drainage tubes, clients receiving soak applications, diaphoretic clients. | Determines need for protective waterproof pads or bath blankets on bed. |
| 2. Check client's activity orders. | Physician's assessment of client's medical condition determines level of activity allowed, including whether client should be out of bed. |
| 3. Assess client's ability to get out of bed, e.g., level of fatigue or discomfort, status of vital signs, coordination, strength, nausea, or dizziness. | Nurse is responsible for judging whether it is safe for client to get out of bed and if additional assistance is needed. |
| 4. Determine need for any special position precautions once client is out of bed, e.g., elevation of leg or arm. | Position must be maintained as client is sitting to prevent any physical complications. |
| **Planning** | |
| 1. Prepare needed equipment and supplies: | |
| a. Linen bag | Collecting linen (top to bottom) in order of use makes it easier to make bed without delays. |
| b. Mattress pad (need only be changed when soiled) | |
| c. Bottom sheet (flat or fitted) | |
| d. Drawsheet | Used to help lift or move client and to protect bottom sheet from soiling. |
| e. Top sheet (flat) | |
| f. Blanket | |
| g. Bedspread | |
| h. Waterproof pads or bath blankets (optional) | To lay under client at points where drainage is expected. Reduces soiling of bed linen. |
| i. Pillow cases | |
| j. Bedside chair or table | To place linen on in order of use. |
| 2. If client is in bed, explain that you wish to change bed while client is sitting up. Ask if client feels able to sit in chair and assist as necessary. | Client should not feel inconvenienced by procedure, may feel anxious if uncomfortable or fatigued. |
| **Implementation** | |
| 1. Wash hands. | Reduces transmission of microorganisms. |
| 2. Assemble and arrange equipment on bedside chair or table. Remove all unnecessary equipment, such as overbed table. | Assembling all equipment provides smooth flow of procedure and ensures client's comfort. Placing linen on clean surface minimizes spread of infection. |

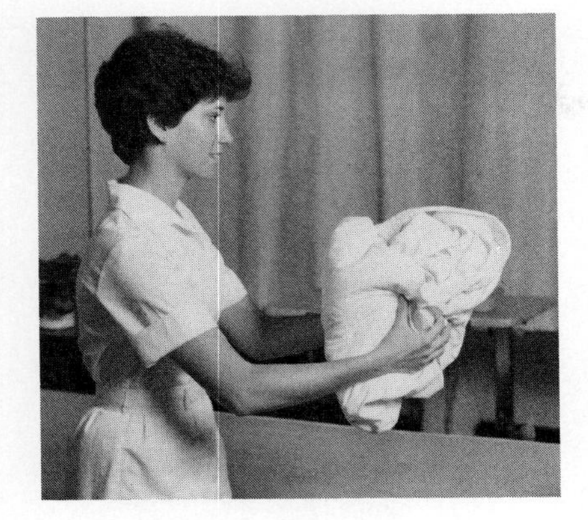

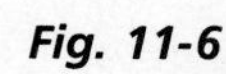

*Fig. 11-6*

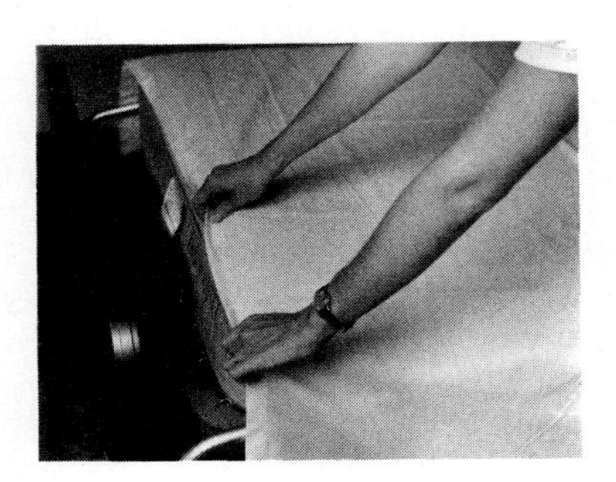

*Fig. 11-7*

| Steps | Rationale |
|---|---|
| 3. Lower side rail on your side of bed and remove call light. | Provides easy access to bed. |
| 4. Adjust bed height to comfortable working position. | Raising bed minimizes strain on nurse's back and muscles. |
| 5. On your side, loosen linen, starting at top of bed. Move along sides and then down toward foot. Move to other side of bed; loosen all linen. | Loosening linen makes it easier to remove. |
| 6. Remove bedspread and blanket separately by folding each into ball or folded square and discarding into linen bag if they are not to be reused. Do not allow uniform to come in contact with soiled linen (Fig. 11-6). Avoid fanning or shaking linen. | Reduces transmission of microorganisms. |
| 7. If spread or blanket is to be reused, fold as follows: grasp top edge with both hands: one hand at center, other hand at end. Fold top edge down and even with the bottom edge. Pick up spread at center and fold so that farthest side comes even with nearest side. Bring top and bottom edges together again. Place folded spread or blanket over back of chair. | Folding method facilitates replacement and prevents wrinkling. |
| 8. Remove soiled pillow cases by grasping closed end with one hand and slipping pillow out with other. Discard pillow cases in linen bag and place pillows on table. | Pillows slide out easily, minimizing chance of contact with soiled linen. |
| 9. Fold each piece of remaining bed linen separately into ball or folded square and discard into linen bag. | Attempting to fold all soiled linen at once creates bulky bundle that is difficult to discard and may easily come in contact with the nurse's uniform. |
| 10. Slide mattress toward head of bed. | If mattress slides toward foot of bed when head of bed is raised, it is difficult to tuck in linen. |
| 11. Wipe off any moisture on mattress with washcloth moistened in antiseptic solution; dry thoroughly. | Reduces transmission of microorganisms. |
| 12. Stand at side of bed where linen is placed. Spread mattress pad over mattress. | Time is saved by making half of bed first and then moving to opposite side. |
| 13. Smooth out all wrinkles in pad. | Wrinkles or folds of linen are source of chronic irritation against client's skin. |
| 14. Unfold bottom sheet lengthwise and place vertical center crease of the sheet lengthwise along center of the bed. Fold sheet's top layer over toward opposite side of bed. Smooth bottom layer of sheet across mattress on your side; bring edge over side of mattress. Allow it to hang 25 cm (10 in) over mattress edge. Hem of bottom edge of sheet should lie seam down, even with bottom edge of mattress (Fig. 11-7). Pull remaining top portion of sheet over top edge of mattress. | Method of unfolding linen saves nurse time and energy. Making one side of bed at a time avoids excess movement. Proper placement of linen ensures adequate length will be available to cover opposite side of bed. Keeping seam edge down eliminates source of irritation to client's skin. If bottom edge of sheet is not tucked in, it can later be changed without removing top linen. |
| 15. While standing at head of the bed, miter top corner of bottom sheet.<br>a. Face head of bed diagonally. Place hand that is away from head of bed under top corner of mattress near mattress edge and lift.<br>b. With other hand, tuck top edge of bottom sheet smoothly under mattress so side edges of sheet above and below mattress would meet if brought together. | Mitered corner is not loosened easily. |

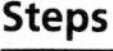

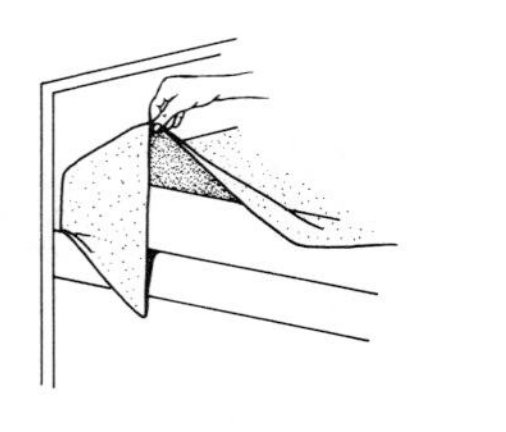

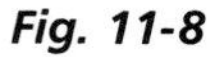

*Fig. 11-8*

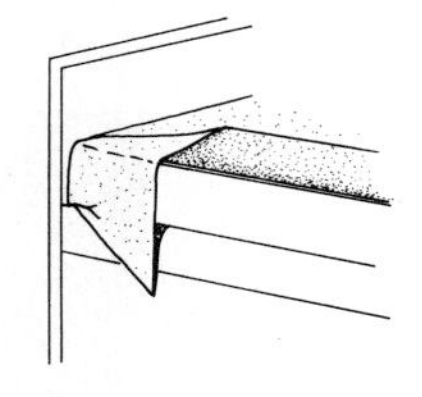

*Fig. 11-9*

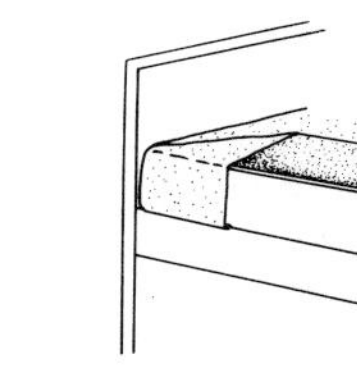

*Fig. 11-10*

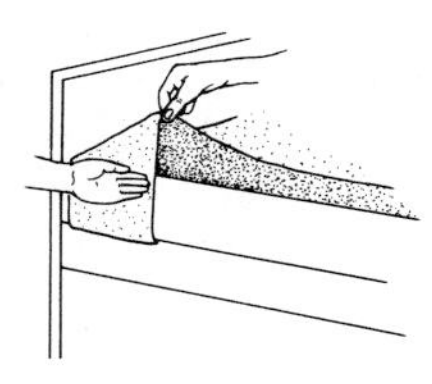

*Fig. 11-11*

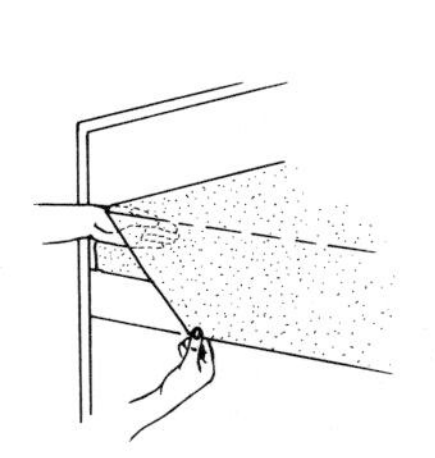

*Fig. 11-12*

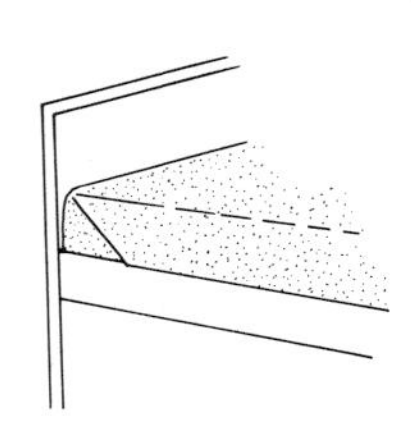

*Fig. 11-13*

| Steps | Rationale |
|---|---|
| c. Face side of bed and pick up top edge of sheet approximately 45 cm (18 in) down from top of mattress (Fig. 11-8). | |
| d. Lift sheet and lay it on top of mattress to form neat, triangular fold, with lower base of triangle even with mattress side edge (Fig. 11-9). | |
| e. Tuck lower edge of sheet, hanging free below mattress, under mattress. Tuck with your palms down. Do this without pulling triangular fold (Fig. 11-10). | |
| f. Hold portion of sheet covering side edge of mattress in place with one hand. With other hand, pick up top of triangular linen fold and bring it down over side of mattress. Tuck this portion of sheet under mattress (Figs. 11-11 and 11-12). | |
| 16. Tuck remaining portion of sheet under mattress. Keep linen smooth (Fig. 11-13). | Folds of linen can irritate client's skin. |
| 17. Open drawsheet so it unfolds in half. Lay center fold along middle of bed lengthwise. Fanfold top layer at center of bed. Smooth bottom layer of drawsheet over mattress. | Drawsheet is used to lift and reposition client. Placement under client's torso distributes most of body weight over sheet. |
| 18. Tuck excess edge under mattress, keeping palms down. | Anchors sheet in place to prevent sliding and wrinkling. |
| 19. Move to opposite side of bed. | One side of bed is completed before nurse moves to other side. |
| 20. Spread fanfolded bottom sheet smoothly over edge of mattress from head to foot of bed. | Wrinkles can cause irritation. |
| 21. Miter top corner of bottom sheet (Step 15). When tucking corner be sure sheet is taut. | Taut sheet eliminates wrinkles and folds that can rub client's skin. |
| 22. Facing side of bed, grasp remaining edge of bottom sheet, lean back, keeping back straight, and pull as you tuck excess linen tightly under mattress. Proceed from head to foot of bed. (Avoid lifting mattress during tucking to ensure tight fit.) | Proper use of body mechanics while tucking linen prevents injury to nurse. |
| 23. Smooth folded drawsheet over bottom sheet. Grasp edge of drawsheet with palms down, lean back, and tuck sheet tightly under mattress. Tuck first at middle, then at top, and then at bottom (Fig. 11-14). | Tucking first at top or bottom may pull sheet sideways, causing poor fit. |
| 24. If needed, apply waterproof pad or bath blanket over drawsheet. | Pad collects body secretions and drainage, protecting linen from becoming soiled. |
| 25. Move to side of bed where linen is located. Place top sheet over bed with vertical center fold lengthwise down middle of bed. Open sheet out from head to foot, being sure top edge of sheet is seam up and even with top edge of mattress. Spread excess sheet over bottom edge of mattress. (Do not fan top sheet over the bed.) | Placement ensures equal distribution of sheet over bed. Positioning sheet with seam up prevents irritation of client's skin. Avoid fanning because it creates air currents, which can spread microorganisms throughout room. |
| 26. Make horizontal toe pleat: stand at foot of bed and form fold in sheet 5-10 cm (2-4 in) across bed. Pull sheet up from bottom to make fold. Fold should be approximately 15 cm (6 in) from bottom edge of mattress (Fig. 11-15). | Allows free movement of client's feet and prevents friction against surface of toes. |
| 27. Tuck in remaining portion of sheet on one side of foot of mattress (optional). | Anchors top sheet so that client can move freely. |
| 28. Place blanket on bed, unfolding it so that crease runs lengthwise along middle of bed. Top edge should be parallel with edge of top sheet and 15-20 cm (6-8 in) down from top mattress edge. Bottom edge should hang over mattress edge. Spread blanket evenly over bed. | Blanket provides adequate warmth. Cuff will be formed with sheet folded over top edge of blanket and spread. |

| Steps | Rationale |
|---|---|

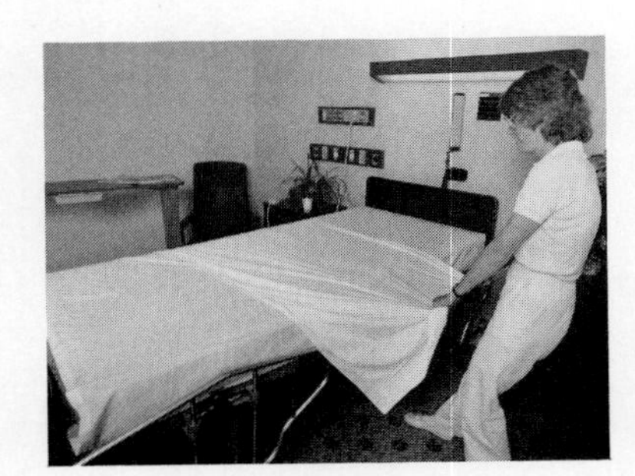

*Fig. 11-14*

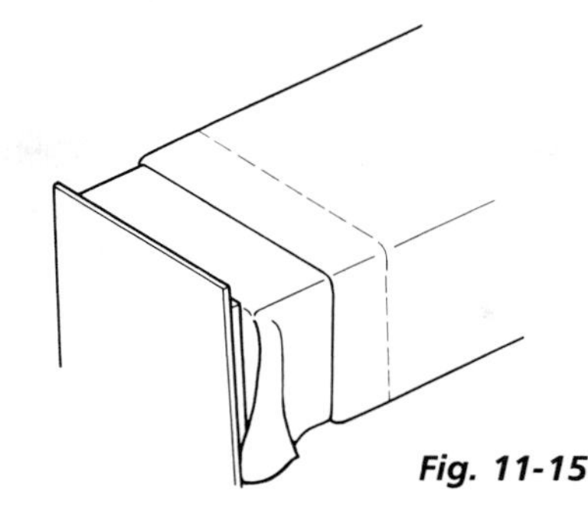

*Fig. 11-15*

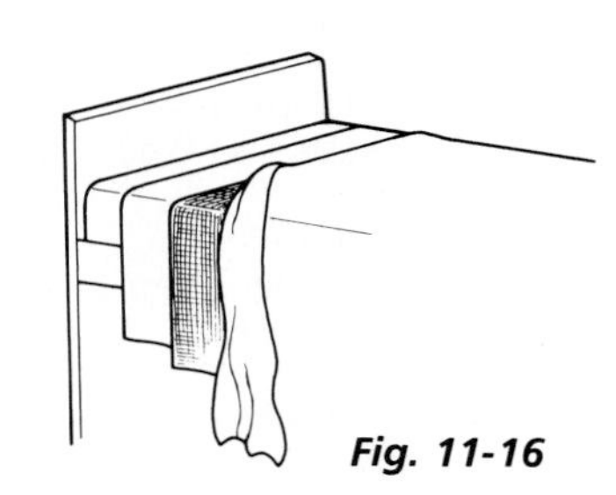

*Fig. 11-16*

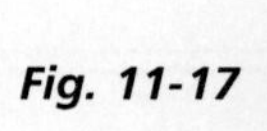

*Fig. 11-17*

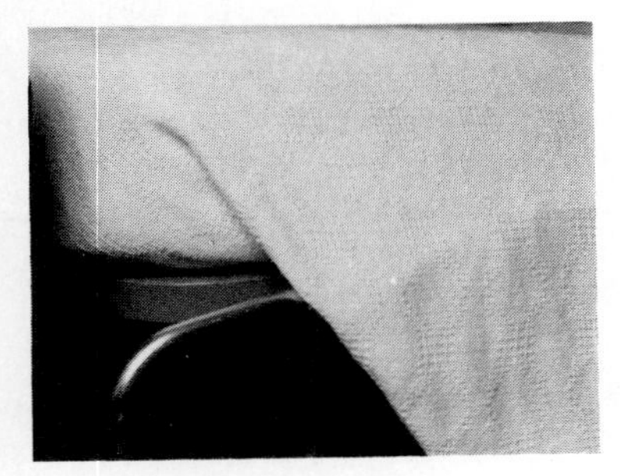

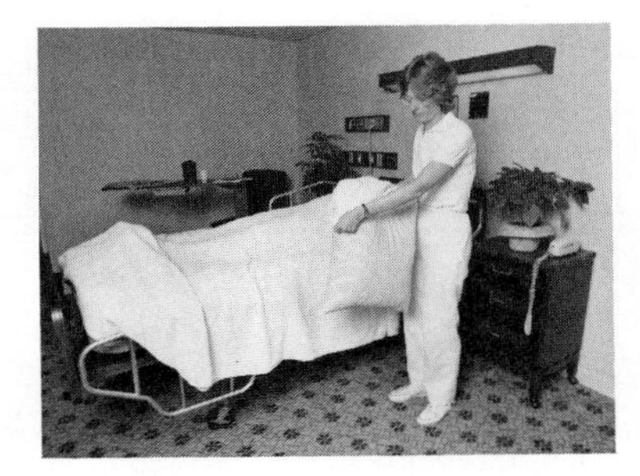

*Fig. 11-18*

| Steps | Rationale |
|---|---|
| 29. Place spread over bed according to Step 28. Be sure top edge of spread extends about 2.5 cm (1 in) above blanket's edge. Then tuck top edge of spread over and under top edge of blanket (Fig. 11-16). | Spread gives bed a neat appearance and provides extra warmth. |
| 30. Make a cuff by running edge of top sheet down over top edge of blanket and spread. | Smooth cuff protects client's face from irritation. |
| 31. Standing on one side at foot of bed, lift mattress corner slightly with one hand and with other hand tuck top sheet, blanket, and spread together under mattress. Be sure you have not pulled out toe pleat of sheet so linens are loose enough for client to move. | Pressure sores can develop on client's toes and heels if feet rub between tight-fitting bed sheets. Lifting mattress too high can loosen bottom linen. |
| 32. Make modified mitered corner with top sheet, blanket, and spread: pick up side edge of top sheet, blanket, and spread approximately 45 cm (18 in) up from foot of mattress. Lift linens to form triangular fold and lay it on bed. Tuck loose edge hanging down under side of mattress. Pick up triangular fold and bring it down over mattress, holding linen in place along side of mattress. Do not tuck tip of triangle (Fig. 11-17). | Modified mitered corner secures top linen but keeps even edge of top sheet, blanket, and spread draped over mattress. |
| 33. Go to other side of bed: spread sheet, blanket, and spread out evenly. Fold top edge of spread over blanket and make cuff with top sheet (Step 29). Make modified mitered corner at foot of bed (Step 32). | Nurse saves time and energy by completing one side of bed at a time. |
| 34. Apply clean pillowcase. With one hand, grasp pillowcase at center of closed end. Gather case, turning it inside out over hand holding it. With same hand, pick up middle of one end of pillow. Pull pillowcase down over pillow with other hand. Be sure corners of case fit evenly over pillow (Fig. 11-18). | This method makes it easy to slide case smoothly over pillow. |
| 35. Position pillow(s) at center of head of bed. | Maintains neat appearance. |
| 36. Place call light within client's reach and return bed to comfortable height. | Provides client safety. |
| 37. If client is to return to bed, fold back top covers to one side or fanfold them down to bottom third of bed. | Folding back covers makes it easy for client to return to bed. |
| 38. Rearrange furniture and place personal items within easy reach. | Neat environment promotes sense of well-being. |
| 39. Discard dirty linen in linen hamper or chute. Wash hands. | Reduces transmission of microorganisms. |

| Steps | Rationale |
|---|---|
| **Evaluation** | |
| 1. Evaluate client's tolerance to sitting up in chair: compare heart rate to previous resting rate; ask if client feels weak, dizzy, or fatigued; assess blood pressure if client complains of dizziness or weakness. | Client's inability to tolerate exertion or low level exercise may be reflected in changes in vital signs or subjective report of symptoms. |
| ***Expected Outcomes*** | |
| 1. Client's vital signs remain stabilized and client denies fatigue or dizziness. | Client tolerates sitting in chair. |
| ***Unexpected Outcomes*** | |
| 1. Client's blood pressure falls below baseline and heart rate is elevated. | Sitting in upright position may cause orthostatic hypotension; exertion may raise heart rate. |
| 2. Client complains of weakness or dizziness. | Symptoms of poor activity tolerance and orthostatic changes. |
| **Recording and Reporting** | |
| 1. Bedmaking need not be documented. Record client's vital signs and symptoms only if there are changes. | Documents client's response to activity and position change. |

## Special Considerations

- If client has a circulatory impairment, elevate affected extremity while client is out of bed. This promotes venous return.
- Agency policy determines types of solutions to use in cleaning mattress surface.
- Bedpads are ideal for collecting secretions, e.g., urine under a small area. If client is diaphoretic, bath blankets spread across bottom sheets can collect moisture.
- Use waterproof pads with caution. Accumulation of moisture creates a risk for skin maceration and breakdown.
- When client is in surgery the nurse may choose to prepare an unoccupied surgical bed. Top linen is arranged in a manner that faciliates easy transfer of client from stretcher to bed. Bottom sheet is placed on the bed in same manner as making an unoccupied bed. Because client often returns from surgery with a dressing, the nurse places a plastic or cloth drawsheet and absorbent pad on the bed. After top sheet, blanket, and spread are applied over the bed, the nurse prepares the linen by performing the following steps:
  a. Fan fold all top linen back from head of bed toward foot of mattress. Linen fold should be just above bottom edge of mattress.
  b. Leave bed in high position for easy transfer of client from stretcher. (Fig. 11-19).
  c. Optional
     - Fold all top linen back from foot of bed toward center of mattress. Linen fold should be flush with bottom edge of mattress.
     - Fold all top linen that is down over sides of bed toward center of mattress. Linen folds should be flush with side edges of mattress.
     - Face one side of bed, pick up bottom corner of linen nearest you and fold back and over toward opposite side of bed, forming a triangle.
     - Repeat Step c with top corner of linen to form other side of triangle.
     - Grasp apex of triangle and fanfold top linen over to side of bed.

## Home Care Considerations

- Assess primary care giver's ability and willingness to maintain a clean environment for the client.
- Assess home laundry facilities to plan with the primary care giver the frequency with which linens could reasonably be laundered.
- Assess amount of linen in the home to establish with the primary care giver the number of changes of sheets that could be reserved for the client's use.

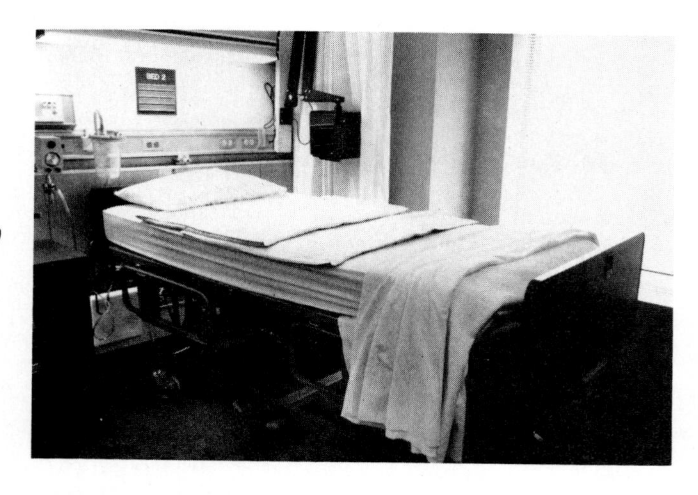

*Fig. 11-19*

# SKILL 11-2 Making an Occupied Bed

At times it is necessary to make a bed when it is occupied by a client. The client may be too weak to get out of bed; the illness may prohibit sitting up; or the client may be restricted to bed by traction or heavy body or leg casts. If a client is confined to bed, bed making should be done in a way that conserves time and the client's energy.

Even though the client remains in bed the nurse encourages self-help as much as possible. For example, the client can turn, assist in moving up in bed, or hold top sheets while linen is applied. These activities keep the client active and a participant in hygiene care.

Making an occupied bed poses some difficulties; it is harder to keep newly applied linen smooth and wrinkle free. The procedure can be done quickly, however, if the nurse organizes actions effectively.

### Purposes

1. Minimize client's physical exertion.
2. Protect client from potential injury.
3. Provide a neat, clean environment for the client.
4. Eliminate sources of irritation to the client's skin.
5. Promote client comfort and relaxation.

## Procedure 11-2

| Steps | Rationale |
|---|---|
| **Assessment** | |
| 1. Assess potential for client being incontinent or having excess drainage on bed linen, e.g., postoperative clients with wounds or drainage tubes, clients receiving soak applications, diaphoretic clients. | Determines need for protective waterproof pads or extra bath blankets on bed. |
| 2. Check client's chart for orders or specific precautions for movement and positioning, e.g., unstable cervical neck injury, fracture of pelvis, placement of lower extremities in weighted traction, severe hypotension, severely painful conditions. | Ensures client's safety, as well as use of proper body mechanics for nurse and client. |
| **Planning** | |
| 1. Prepare needed equipment and supplies: | |
| a. Linen bag | Collecting linen (top to bottom) in order of use makes it easier to make bed without delays. |
| b. Bath blanket | |
| c. Mattress pad (need only be changed when soiled) | |
| d. Bottom sheet (flat or fitted) | |
| e. Drawsheet | Used to help lift or move client and to protect bottom sheet from soiling. |
| f. Top sheet (flat) | |
| g. Blanket | |
| h. Bedspread | |
| i. Waterproof pads (optional) | Lay under client at points where drainage is expected. Reduces soiling of bed linen. |
| j. Pillow case(s) | |
| k. Bedside chair or table | |
| 2. Explain procedure to client, noting that client will be asked to turn on side to roll over linen. | Minimizes anxiety and promotes client's cooperation. |
| **Implementation** | |
| 1. Wash hands. | Reduces transmission of microorganisms. |
| 2. Assemble equipment and arrange it on bedside chair or table. Remove all unnecessary equipment. | Assembling all equipment provides for smooth procedure and ensures client's comfort. Placing linen on clean surface minimizes spread of infection. |
| 3. Draw room curtain around bed or close door. | Maintains client's privacy, thus promoting emotional and physical comfort. |
| 4. Lower side rail on your side of bed. Remove call light. | Provides easy access to bed and linen. |
| 5. Adjust bed height to comfortable working position. | Raising bed horizontally minimizes strain on nurse's back. It is easier to remove and apply linen evenly when bed is in flat position. |

| Steps | Rationale |
|---|---|
| 6. Loosen top linen sheet at foot of bed. | Loosening linen makes it easier to remove. |
| 7. Remove bedspread and blanket separately by folding them into squares and placing them in linen bag (if not to be reused). Do not allow linen to contact uniform. Do not fan or shake linen. | Reduces transmission of microorganisms. |
| 8. If blanket and spread are to be reused, fold by bringing top and bottom edges together. Fold side farthest from your working side over onto nearer bottom edges together again. Place folded linen over back of chair. | Folding method facilitates replacement and prevents wrinkling. |
| 9. Cover client with bath blanket in following manner: unfold bath blanket over top sheet. Ask client to hold top edge of bath blanket. If client is unable to help, tuck top of bath blanket under client's shoulders. Grasp top sheet under bath blanket at client's shoulders and bring sheet down to foot of bed. Remove sheet and discard it in linen bag. | Bath blanket provides warmth and keeps body parts covered during linen removal. |
| 10. With assistance from another nurse slide mattress toward head of bed. | If mattress slides toward foot of bed when head of bed is raised, it is difficult to tuck linen and is uncomfortable for client. |
| 11. Assist client to side-lying position on far side of bed, facing away from you. Adjust pillow under client's head. Be sure side rail is up. | Moving client to side provides space for placement of clean linen. Side rail ensures client's safety. |
| 12. Loosen bottom linens, moving from head to foot of bed. | Prepares for removal of all bottom linen simultaneously. |
| 13. Fanfold bottom sheet and drawsheet toward client; first drawsheet, then bottom sheet. Tuck edges of linen just under client's buttocks, back, and shoulders (Fig. 11-20). Do not fanfold mattress pad if it is to be reused. | Provides maximum work space for placing clean linen. Later, when client turns to other side, soiled linen can be easily removed. |
| 14. Wipe off any moisture on mattress with towel and appropriate disinfectant. | Reduces transmission of microorganisms. |
| 15. Apply clean linen to exposed half of bed. | |
| a. Place clean mattress pad on bed by folding it lengthwise with center crease in middle of bed. Fanfold top layer over mattress. (If pad is reused, simply smooth out wrinkles.) | Applying linen over bed in successive layers minimizes energy and time nurse uses in bed making. |
| b. Unfold bottom sheet lengthwise so center crease is lengthwise along center of bed. Fanfold sheet's edge toward center of bed alongside client. Smooth bottom half of sheet over mattress and bring edge over your side of mattress. Allow sheet's edge to hang about 25 cm (10 in) over mattress edge. Hem of bottom sheet should lie seam down and even with bottom edge of mattress (Fig. 11-21). | Proper positioning of linen on one side ensures that adequate linen will be available to cover opposite side of bed. Keeping seam edges down eliminates irritation to client's skin. |
| 16. Miter bottom sheet at head of bed: | Mitered corner cannot be loosened easily even if client moves about frequently in bed. |
| a. Face head of bed diagonally. Place hand that is away from head of bed under top corner of mattress, near mattress edge, and lift. | |
| b. With other hand, tuck top edge of bottom sheet smoothly under mattress so side edges of sheet above and below mattress would meet if brought together. | |
| c. Face side of bed and pick up top edge of sheet at approximately 45 cm (18 in) down from top of mattress. | |
| d. Lift sheet and lay it on top of mattress to form neat triangular fold, with lower base of triangle even with mattress side edge. | |

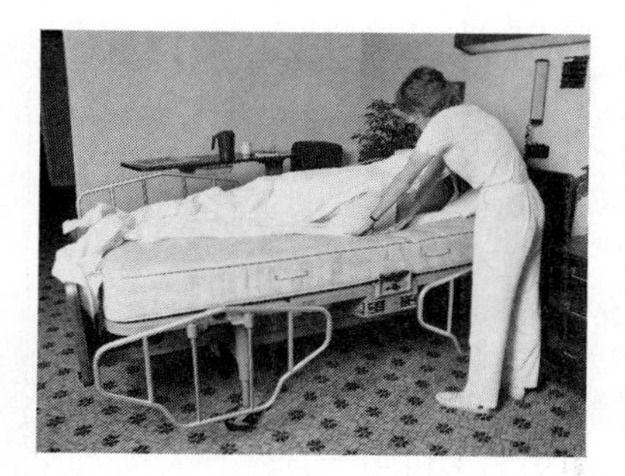

*Fig. 11-20*

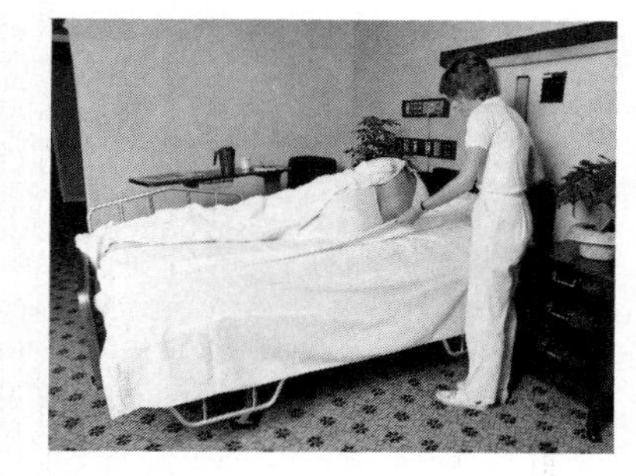

*Fig. 11-21*

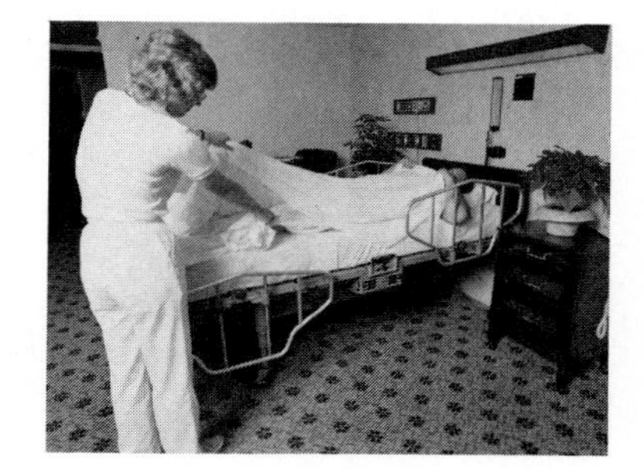

*Fig. 11-22*

| Steps | Rationale |
|---|---|
| e. Tuck lower edge of sheet, which is hanging free below mattress, under mattress. Tuck with palms down. Do this without pulling triangular fold. | |
| f. Hold portion of sheet covering side edge of mattress in place with one hand. With other hand, pick up top of triangular linen fold and bring it down over side of mattress. Tuck this portion of sheet under mattress. | |
| 17. Tuck remaining portion of sheet under mattress, moving toward foot of bed. Keep linen smooth. | Folds of linen are source of irritation. |
| 18. Open drawsheet so it unfolds in half. Lay center fold along middle of bed lengthwise and position sheet so it will be under client's buttocks and torso. Fanfold top layer toward client with edge alongside client's back. Smooth bottom layer over mattress and tuck excess edge under mattress (keep palms down). | Drawsheet is used to lift and reposition client. Placement under client's torso distributes most of client's body weight over sheet. |
| 19. Place waterproof pad over drawsheet with center fold against client's side. Fanfold far half toward client. | Protects bed linen from soiling. |
| 20. Raise side rail on working side and go to other side. | Maintains client's safety during turning. |
| 21. Lower side rail. Assist client to slowly roll over to other side, over folds of linen. | Exposes opposite side of bed for removal of soiled linen and placement of clean linen. |
| 22. Loosen edges of soiled linen from underneath mattress. | Loosening linen makes it easier to remove. |
| 23. Remove soiled linen by folding it into a bundle or square, with soiled side turned in. Discard in linen bag. | Reduces transmission of microorganisms. |
| 24. Spread clean fanfolded linen smoothly over edge of mattress from head to foot of bed. | Smooth linen will not irritate client's skin. |
| 25. Assist client in rolling back into supine position. Reposition pillow. | Client's comfort is maintained. |
| 26. Miter top corner of bottom sheet (Step 16). When tucking corner be sure sheet is taut. | Taut sheet eliminates irritating wrinkles and folds. |
| 27. Facing side of bed, grasp remaining edge of bottom sheet. Lean back, keeping back straight, and pull as you tuck excess linen tightly under mattress. Proceed from head to foot of bed. (Avoid lifting mattress during tucking to ensure tight fit.) | Proper use of body mechanics while tucking linen prevents injury to nurse. |
| 28. Smooth fanfolded drawsheet over bottom sheet. Grasp edge of sheet with palms down, lean back, and tuck sheet tightly under mattress. Tuck from middle to top and then to bottom. | Tucking first at top or bottom may pull sheet sideways, causing poor fit. |
| 29. Place top sheet over client with center fold lengthwise down middle of bed. Open sheet from head to foot and unfold it over client. | Sheet should be equally distributed over bed by correctly positioning center fold. |
| 30. Ask client to hold clean top sheet, or tuck sheet around client's shoulders (Fig. 11-22). Remove bath blanket and discard it in linen bag. | Sheet prevents exposure of body parts. Having client hold sheet encourages client participation in care. |
| 31. Place blanket on bed, unfolding it so that crease runs lengthwise along middle of bed. Unfold blanket to cover client. Top edge should be parallel with edge of top sheet and 15-20 cm (6-8 in) down from top sheet's edge. | Blanket should be placed to cover client completely and provide adequate warmth. |
| 32. Place spread over bed according to Step 31. Be sure top edge of spread extends about 2.5 cm (1 in) above blanket's edge. Tuck top edge of spread over and under top edge of blanket. | Spread gives bed neat appearance and provides extra warmth. |
| 33. Make cuff by turning edge of top sheet down over top edge of blanket and spread. | Smooth cuff protects client's face from rubbing against blanket or spread. |
| 34. Standing on one side at foot of bed, lift mattress corner slightly with one hand and tuck top linens under mattress. Top sheet and blanket are tucked under together. Be sure linens are loose enough to allow movement of client's feet. (You may make horizontal toe pleat [Procedure 11-1, Step 26]). | Tucking all top linens together makes neat-appearing bed. Pressure sores can develop on client's toes and heels from feet rubbing between tight fitting bed sheets. |
| 35. Make modified mitered corner with top sheet, blanket, and spread: | |
| a. Pick up side edge of top sheet, blanket, and spread approximately 45 cm (18 in) up from foot of mattress. Lift linens to form triangular fold and lay it on bed. | Modified mitered corner secures top linen but keeps an even edge of blanket and top sheet draped over mattress. |

| Steps | Rationale |
|---|---|
| b. Tuck lower edge of sheet, which is hanging free below mattress, under mattress. Do not pull triangular fold. | |
| c. Pick up triangular fold and bring it down over mattress while holding linen in place along side of mattress. Do not tuck tip of triangle. | |
| 36. Raise side rail. Make other side of bed; spread sheet, blanket, and bedspread evenly; fold top edge of spread over blanket and make cuff with top sheet (Step 33); make modified corner at foot of bed (Step 35). | Side rail protects client from accidental fall. |
| 37. Change pillowcase. | |
| a. Have client raise head. While supporting neck with one hand, remove pillow. | Support of neck muscles prevents injury during flexion and extension of neck. |
| b. Remove soiled case by grasping pillow at open end with one hand and pulling case over pillow with other hand. Discard case in linen bag. | |
| c. Grasp clean pillowcase at center of closed end. Gather case, turning it inside out over hand holding it. With same hand pick up middle of one end of pillow. Pull pillowcase down over pillow with other hand. | Method makes it easy to slide pillowcase over pillow. |
| d. Be sure pillow corners fit evenly in corners of pillowcase. | Poorly fitting case constricts fluffing and expansion of pillow. |
| 38. Support client's head under neck and place pillow under head. | Support prevents hyperextension of neck muscles. |
| 39. Place call light within client's reach and return bed to comfortable position. | Ensures client's safety and comfort. |
| 40. Open room curtains. Rearrange furniture. Place personal items within easy reach on overbed table or bedside stand. Return bed to comfortable height. | Neat environment promotes sense of well-being. |
| 41. Discard dirty linen in linen hamper or chute and wash hands. | Reduces transmission of microorganisms. |

## Evaluation

| | |
|---|---|
| 1. Ask if client feels comfortable. | Evaluates sense of comfort. |

***Expected outcomes***

| | |
|---|---|
| 1. Client expresses feeling of relaxation and comfort. | Bed linen is smooth and without wrinkles. |

***Unexpected outcome***

| | |
|---|---|
| 1. Client feels source of discomfort from linen fold. | Linen not properly smoothed. |

## Recording and Reporting

1. Making an occupied bed need not be recorded.

## Special Considerations

- Assure client that client will not fall off bed during turning procedure.
- Client with respiratory distress may be unable to tolerate lying flat during bedmaking.

## Teaching Considerations

- Explain steps of procedure involving client's participation.

### BIBLIOGRAPHY

Ebersole P, Hess P: Toward healthy aging: human needs and nursing response, ed. 3, St. Louis, 1989, The CV Mosby Co.

Golden S: Nursing a loved one at home, Philadelphia, 1988, Running Press Book Publishers.

Potter PA, Perry AG: Basic nursing, theory and practice, St. Louis, 1987, The CV Mosby Company.

Potter PA, Perry AG: Fundamentals of nursing, ed 2, St. Louis, 1989, The CV Mosby Co.

Smith S, Duell D: Clinical nursing skills, Los Altos, Calif, 1985, National Nursing Review.

# *UNIT* IV

# *VITAL SIGNS AND PHYSICAL ASSESSMENT*

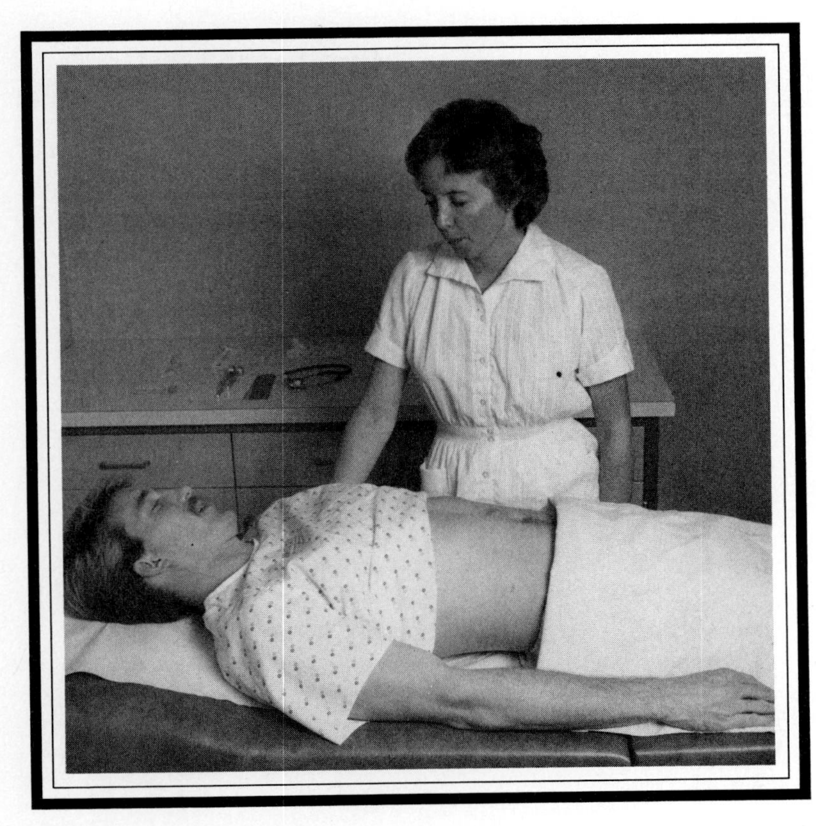

*To be an effective practitioner the nurse must be competent in a variety of skills. The ability of a nurse to accurately measure vital signs and perform a physical assessment is very important. Skills in these areas are used more often and on more clients than any other skills the nurse might need. Vital sign assessment and physical assessment provide data to determine a client's state of health and to formulate nursing diagnoses, plan for the client's care, implement nursing actions properly, and evaluate a client's response to medical and nursing therapy. Chapter 12, "Vital Signs," includes procedures for measuring the four basic vital signs: temperature, pulse, respirations, and blood pressure, with special considerations for infants and the elderly. Chapter 13, "Physical Assessment," presents a head-to-toe approach to physical assessment of the client. Teaching sections for clients and family are important features of both chapters.*

# 12

# VITAL SIGNS

## OBJECTIVES

*Mastery of content in this chapter will enable the nurse to:*

- Define key terms.
- Correctly record vital sign values.
- Identify when it is appropriate to assess each vital sign.
- Correctly assess a client's oral, rectal, and axillary temperature.
- Identify factors to assess in determining potential alterations in body temperature.
- Discuss factors in selecting temperature measurement sites.
- Explain nursing measures to initiate when a client's temperature is above or below normal.
- Instruct a client on techniques for self-measurement of temperature.
- Assess a client's radial and apical pulses correctly.
- Identify factors to assess in determining potential alterations in pulse character.
- Explain indications of a pulse deficit.
- Instruct a client on techniques for self-assessment of pulse.
- Assess a client's respirations correctly.
- Identify factors to assess in determining potential alterations in respirations.
- Correctly measure a client's blood pressure (BP) using techniques of auscultation and palpation.
- Identify factors to assess in determining potential alterations in BP.

## KEY TERMS

*Anoxia*
*Antiarrhythmic*
*Antipyretic*
*Apical*
*Apnea*
*Axillary*
*Bradycardia*
*Cardiotonic*
*Coronary bypass surgery*
*Diastolic pressure*
*Dyspnea*
*Dysrhythmia*
*Fever*
*Hypothermia*
*Hypoxia*
*Immunosuppressive*
*Myocardial infarction*
*Orthopnea*
*Premature ventricular contraction (PVC)*
$S_1$
$S_2$
*Stroke volume*
*Sympathomimetic*
*Systolic pressure*
*Tachycardia*
*Thermoregulation*

## SKILLS

**12-1** Measuring Body Temperature
**12-2** Teaching Clients to Measure Body Temperature
**12-3** Assessing a Client's Pulse
**12-4** Teaching Clients to Assess Their Own Pulse
**12-5** Assessing a Client's Respirations
**12-6** Assessing Arterial Blood Pressure

Temperature, pulse, respirations, and blood pressure (BP) are known as vital signs or life signs. Vital signs are indicators of the body's physiologic status and response to physical, environmental, and psychologic stressors. Temperature, pulse, respiratory rates, and BP reveal the client's current ability to maintain body temperature regulation, to maintain local and systemic blood flow, and to provide oxygenation of body tissues. Any difference between a client's normal baseline measurement and actual present vital signs poses implications for the nurse to pursue necessary medical care and initiate appropriate nursing therapies. Vital signs may reveal sudden changes in a client's condition, as well as changes that occur progressively over a lengthy period of time.

The nurse may measure all four vital signs as part of a routine physical assessment (Chapter 13). The nurse's findings aid in determining whether it is necessary to assess specific body systems more thoroughly. For example, after assessing an abnormal respiratory rate, the nurse will also auscultate lung sounds. Vital sign assessment may be limited to measurement of a single vital sign for the purpose of reviewing a specific aspect of a client's

### *TAKE VITAL SIGNS*

1. On client's admission to a health care facility.
2. In hospital, on routine schedule according to physician's order or hospital policy.
3. During client's visit to clinic or physician's office.
4. Before and after any surgical procedure.
5. Before and after any invasive diagnostic procedure.
6. Before and after administration of medications that affect cardiovascular, respiratory, and temperature control function.
7. When the client's general physical condition changes, for example, loss of consciousness or increased intensity of pain.
8. Before and after nursing interventions influencing any one of the vital signs, for example, before ambulating client previously on bed rest or before client performs range of motion (ROM) exercises.
9. Whenever client reports to nurse any nonspecific symptoms of physical distress, for example, "feeling funny or different."

condition. For example, after administering an antihypertensive medication, the nurse measures the client's BP to evaluate the drug's effects. Part of the nurse's clinical judgment involves deciding which vital signs to measure, when measurements should be made, and the frequency of assessment (see box). The nurse should always obtain a baseline measurement of vital signs at initial contact with a client to provide a means for comparison with subsequent vital sign values.

Taking vital signs is an individualized (rather than routine) approach to assessment. The nurse's judgment is essential in determining the need for assessment.

## GUIDELINES

1. The primary nurse caring for the client is the best one to take vital signs, interpret their significance, and make decisions about care.
2. Equipment used to measure vital signs must be appropriate and work properly to ensure accurate findings.
3. Knowing the normal range for all vital signs helps the nurse detect abnormalities.
4. A client's normal range may differ from the standard range for that age or physical state. Normal values for a client serve as a baseline for comparison with findings taken later. Thus a nurse can detect a change in condition over time.
5. Know client's medical history and therapies or medications prescribed. Some illnesses or treatments cause predictable vital sign changes.
6. Control or minimize environmental factors that may affect vital signs. Measuring a pulse after a client exercises or experiences an emotional upset may yield values that are not clear indicators of the client's current status.
7. An organized, systematic (step-by-step) approach when taking vital signs ensures accuracy of findings.
8. Decide the frequency of vital sign assessment on the basis of the client's condition. The physician orders a minimum frequency of vital sign measurements for each client, but the nurse judges if more frequent assessments are needed. If a client's physical condition begins to worsen the nurse takes vital signs more often, perhaps as often as every 5 to 10 minutes. After a client returns from surgery or major diagnostic examination, such as a cardiac catheterization, frequent measurements are taken until the vital signs stabilize to the before-procedure range. Changes or trends in vital signs are useful in making therapeutic decisions for client care.
9. Analyze results of vital sign measurements. The nurse is often in the best position to assess all clinical findings about a client. Vital signs are not assessed in isolation. The nurse assesses physical signs or symptoms, as well as vital signs to be aware of the client's ongoing health status.
10. Verify and communicate significant changes in vital signs. Baseline measurements allow a nurse to identify changes in vital signs. When vital signs reach an abnormal range, it may help to have another nurse or a physician repeat a measurement to verify it. The nurse tells a physician when vital signs become abnormal. It is also important for the nurse to record and report any changes to the nurses working the next shift.

## PREREQUISITE KNOWLEDGE

1. Principles of medical asepsis.
2. Physiologic mechanisms of temperature control, ventilation, and circulation.
3. Anatomic pulse sites and sites for auscultating BP.
4. Principles of communication.
5. Principles of teaching and learning.

## PREREQUISITE SKILLS

1. Proper handwashing techniques (Chapter 37).
2. Techniques for using a stethoscope (Chapter 13).

# SKILL 12-1 Measuring Body Temperature

In health the body's tissues and cells function best within a relatively narrow temperature range. Under the control of the hypothalamus the body's core temperature is maintained within ± 0.6° C (1° F) of the average normal body temperature of 37° C (98.6° F). In contrast, the body's surface temperature rises and falls as the temperature of the surrounding environment changes. Skin temperatures may fluctuate between 20° C (68° F) and 40° C (104° F) without causing tissue damage.

No single temperature is normal for all people. The temperature range for a normal active adult is larger than might be expected (Fig. 12-1), depending in part on a person's range of activity.

The balance of body temperature is precisely regulated by physiologic and behavioral mechanisms, for example, vasodilation, vasoconstriction, sweating, and avoidance of heat or cold. For body temperature to stay constant, heat produced in the body must equal heat lost to the environment. When temperature control mechanisms fail the nurse may initiate measures such as controlling environmental temperatures, removing or adding external coverings, and administering ordered antipyretics to achieve better temperature control.

Three types of thermometers measure body temperature: mercury-in-glass, electronic, and disposable. The common inexpensive mercury-in-glass consists of a glass tube sealed at one end and a mercury filled bulb at the other. Exposure of the bulb to heat causes the mercury to expand and rise in the enclosed tube. The length of the thermometer is marked with either Fahrenheit or centigrade calibrations (Fig. 12-2). Three types of glass thermometers are available: oral or slim tipped, stubby, and pear-shaped rectal (Fig. 12-3). All are available in centigrade or Fahrenheit.

The electronic thermometer consists of a battery-powered display unit, a thin wire cord, and a temperature sensitive probe covered by a disposable plastic sheath (Fig. 12-4). Separate probes are available for oral and rectal use. The oral probe has a blue tip, and the rectal probe has a red tip. An electronic thermometer is not

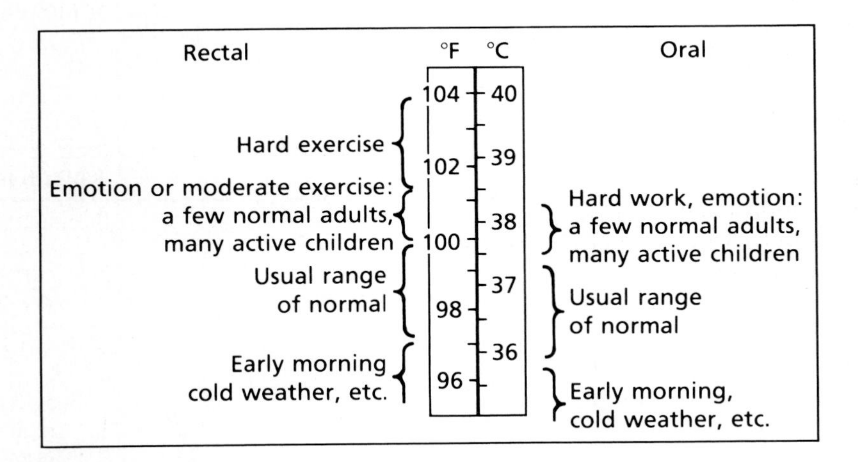


*Fig. 12-1* Ranges of rectal and oral temperatures found in normal persons.
Redrawn from Mountcastle VB: Medical physiology, vol 2, ed 14, St. Louis, 1980, The CV Mosby Co; based on Dubois EF: Fever and the regulation of body temperature, Springfield, Ill, 1948, Charles C Thomas, Publisher.

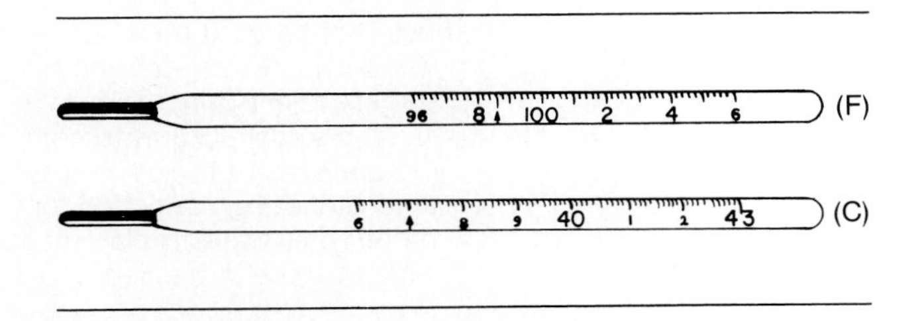


*Fig. 12-2* Comparison of Fahrenheit and centigrade calibrations.

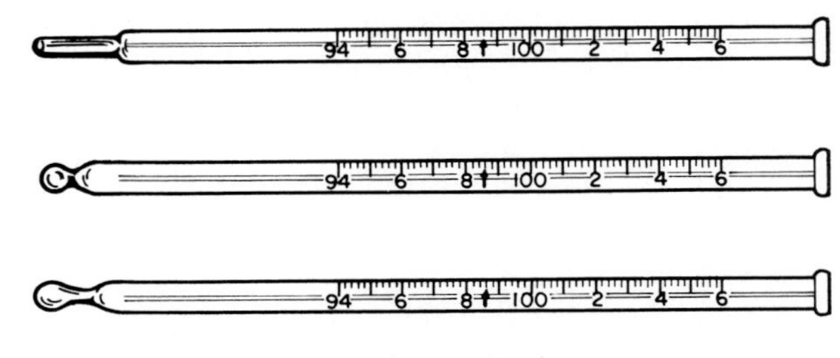


*Fig. 12-3*

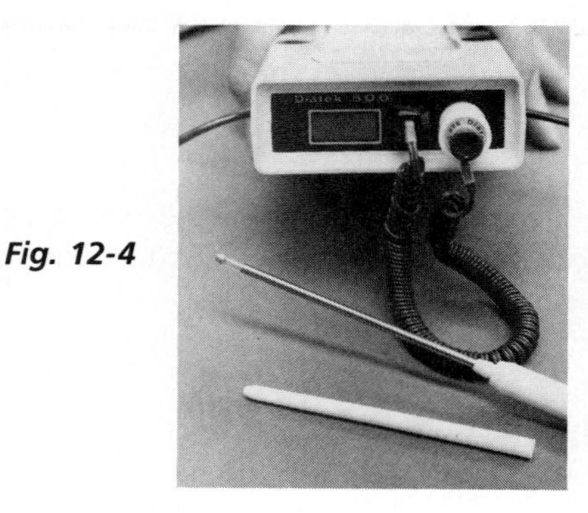

*Fig. 12-4*

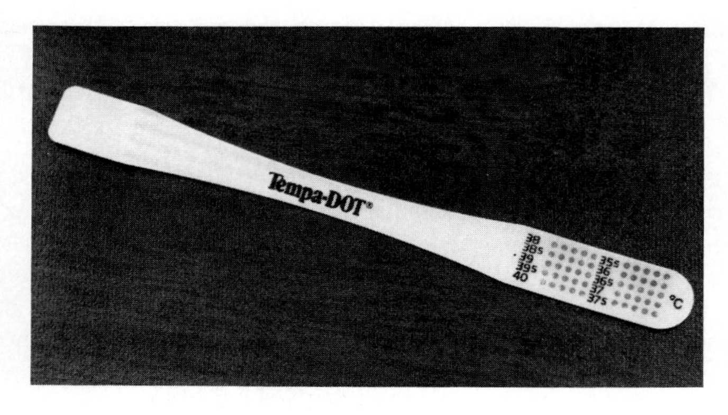


*Fig. 12-5*

necessarily more accurate than a glass thermometer (Baker, et al, 1984). However, the electronic thermometer can be inserted immediately, readings appear within seconds, they are easy to read, and client discomfort is minimized.

Disposable, single use thermometers are thin strips of plastic with chemically impregnated paper (Fig. 12-5). They are used for oral or axillary temperatures, particularly with children. Chemical dots on the thermometer change color to reflect temperature reading, usually within 45 seconds. The dot that changes color represents the highest reading and indicates the client's body temperature. There is also temperature sensitive tape that can be applied to the skin of the abdomen or forehead. Color change of the tape indicates normal temperature by one color and elevated temperature by another color.

A relatively new form of thermometer is the tympanic membrane thermometer, which consists of a temperature sensitive probe inserted into the opening of the external ear canal. Within seconds the probe registers the temperature of the blood flowing near the tympanic membrane, which shares blood supply with the hypothalamus.

## Purposes

1. Determine status of thermoregulation.
2. Screen for temperature alterations.
3. Assess clients at risk for elevated temperature.

***TABLE 12-1*** Sites for Temperature Measurement

| Common Sites | Advantages | Disadvantages |
|---|---|---|
| **Mouth** | Most accessible site; more comfortable for client. | Should not be used for clients who could be injured by thermometer, who are unable to hold thermometer properly, or who might bite down on thermometer: infants or small children; confused or unconscious clients; clients who have had nasal or oral surgery, trauma to face or mouth; clients with oral pain, a shaking chill, a nasogastric tube in place, history of convulsions, who breathe only with mouth open or who have a nasal oxygen catheter in place. |
| **Rectum** | Thought to provide most reliable measurement. | Should not be used for newborns, clients after rectal surgery, clients who have a rectal disorder such as tumor or severe hemorrhoids, clients who cannot be positioned for proper thermometer placement such as those in traction. |
| **Axilla** | Safest method because noninvasive. | Requires nurse to hold thermometer in position. |

## *Procedure 12-1*

| Steps | Rationale |
|---|---|
| **Assessment** | |
| 1. Determine need to measure client's body temperature, e.g., clients with expected or diagnosed infections, open wounds or burns, white blood cell count below 5,000 or above 12,000, immunosuppressive drug therapy, injury to hypothalamus, exposure to temperature extremes, blood product infusion, hypothermia or hyperthermia therapy, or postoperative clients. | Certain conditions place clients at risk for temperature alterations. |
| 2. Assess for other signs and symptoms of temperature alteration:<br>a. Fever: (depending on stage) pale or flushed skin; skin warm or hot to touch; skin dry or diaphoretic; visible shivering with chills; piloerection or "gooseflesh" of skin; tachycardia; malaise with muscle or joint pain; nausea, vomiting, or diarrhea; feeling hot or cold; restlessness.<br>b. Hypothermia: pale skin; skin cool or cold to touch, bradycardia or arrhythmias, visible shivering, reduced level of consciousness, shallow respirations. | Physical signs and symptoms may indicate elevation or decline in body temperature. |
| 3. Assess for factors that normally influence temperature:<br>a. Age: newborns and infants are subject to wide fluctuations; elderly persons experience deterioration in temperature regulation.<br>b. Exercise: muscle activity raises heat production.<br>c. Hormones: women have wider temperature fluctuations than men because of menstrual cycle hormonal changes.<br>d. Stress: stress elevates temperature.<br>e. Environmental temperature.<br>f. Medications: some drugs impair sweating.<br>g. Daily fluctuations: body temperature is lowest during early morning; peaks in late afternoon; falls gradually during night. | Allows nurse to accurately assess temperature variations. |
| 4. Assess site most appropriate for temperature measurement (Table 12-1): | |
| a. Oral site. | Oral site is most accessible and more comfortable for client. Provides accurate core temperature reading. |
| b. Rectal site. | Rectal site provides reliable measure of body core temperature. Used as preferable site when oral site is contraindicated. |
| c. Axillary site. | Axillary site is safest method for temperature measurement. |
| 5. Determine baseline temperature (if available) from client's record. | Allows nurse to identify if change has occurred in client's status. |
| **Nursing Diagnosis** | |
| 1. Analyze client's physical signs and symptoms with temperature values to identify actual or potential nursing diagnoses: | |
| a. Hyperthermia: related to exposure to hot environment. | Heat production increased or body is unable to lose heat. |
| b. Hypothermia: related to trauma or exposure to cold. | Result of excess loss of body heat or client's inability to take measures to conserve heat. |
| c. Ineffective thermoregulation: related to aging. | Temperature fluctuates between hypothermia and hyperthermia. |
| d. Potential for infection: related to altered immunity. | Client is at increased risk for invasion of fever causing pathogenic organisms. |
| **Planning** | |
| 1. Develop individualized goals for assessing client's body temperature: | |
| a. Establish baseline temperature level. | Provides comparison with future temperature measurements. |
| b. Identify abnormalities in temperature regulation. | Directs nurse to pursue supportive therapies. |
| c. Detect changes in body temperature in response to selected therapies. | Directs nurse to initiate preventive therapies. |

| Steps | Rationale |
|---|---|
| 2. Prepare needed equipment and supplies: | |
| a. Appropriate thermometer | Thermometer is chosen on basis of nurse's assessment of preferred site. |
| b. Soft tissue | Reduces transmission of organisms from body secretions. |
| c. Lubricant (rectal only) | Prevents trauma to mucosa with rectal insertions. |
| d. Pen, pencil, and flowsheet or record form | Provides for timely documentation of assessment findings. |
| e. Disposable gloves | Prevents contact with body fluids. |
| 3. Identify client and explain how temperature is to be taken and importance of maintaining proper position until reading is complete. | Clients are often curious about their temperatures and should be cautioned against prematurely removing thermometer to read results. |
| 4. Wait 20 to 30 min before measuring oral temperature if client has smoked or ingested hot or cold liquids or foods. | Smoking and hot or cold substances can cause false temperature readings in oral cavity (Erickson, 1980). |

## Implementation

| Steps | Rationale |
|---|---|
| 1. **Oral temperature—glass thermometer.** | |
| a. Wash hands. | Reduces transmission of microorganisms. |
| b. Assist client to comfortable position that provides easy access to mouth. | Ensures client's comfort and accuracy of temperature reading. |
| c. Apply disposable gloves. | Gloves can be worn for handling items soiled with body fluids, e.g., saliva (Centers for Disease Control [CDC], 1987). |
| d. Hold color-coded end of glass thermometer with fingertips. | Reduces contamination of thermometer bulb. |
| e. If thermometer is stored in disinfectant solution, rinse in cold water before using. | Removes solution irritating to oral mucosa. Hot water can cause mercury to expand and break bulb. |
| f. Take soft tissue and wipe thermometer bulb end toward fingers in rotating fashion. Dispose of tissue. | Reduces contamination of bulb end. |
| g. Read mercury level while gently rotating thermometer at eye level (Fig. 12-6). | Mercury should be below 35.5° C (96° F). Thermometer reading must be below client's actual temperature before use. |
| h. If mercury is above desired level, shake down thermometer. Grasp tip of thermometer securely and stand away from any solid objects. Sharply flick wrist downward as though cracking a whip. Continue shaking until reading is below 35.5° C (96° F). | Brisk shaking lowers mercury level in glass tube. Standing in open spot avoids breakage of thermometer. |
| i. Ask client to open mouth and gently place thermometer under tongue in posterior sublingual pocket lateral to center of lower jaw (Fig. 12-7). | Heat from superficial blood vessels in sublingual pocket produces temperature reading. |
| j. Ask client to hold thermometer with lips closed. Caution against biting down on thermometer. | Maintains proper position of thermometer during recording. Breakage of thermometer may injure mucosa and cause mercury poisoning. |
| k. Leave thermometer in place for 2 min according to agency policy. | Studies vary as to proper length of time for recording. Graves and Markarian (1980) found that glass thermometers kept in place for 8 min recorded values averaging only 0.7° F higher than those kept in place for 3 min. Baker, et al. (1984) found that 2-min insertions did not cause clinically significant variations. |
| l. Carefully remove thermometer and read at eye level. Gently rotate until scale appears. | Ensures accurate reading. |

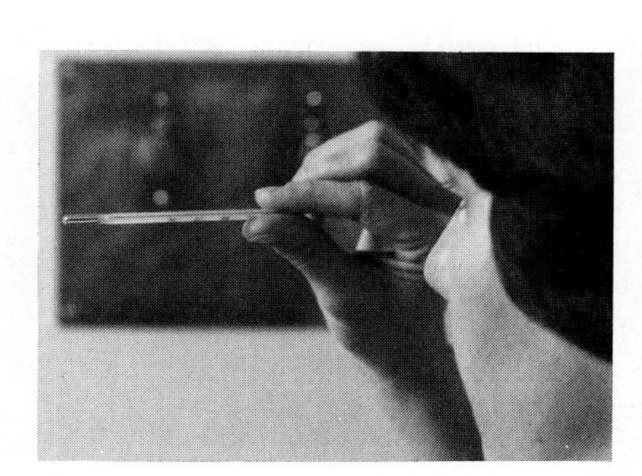

*Fig. 12-6*

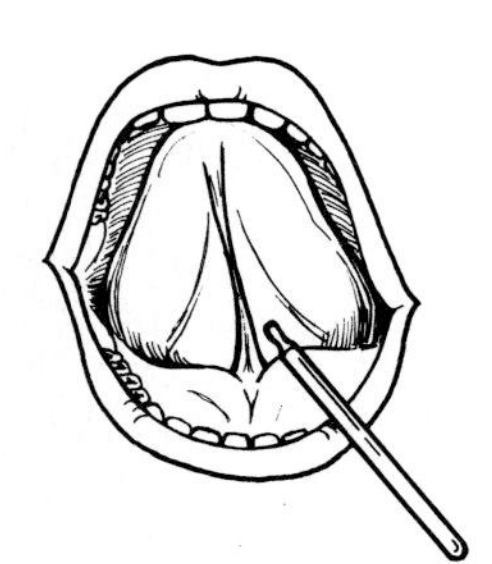

*Fig. 12-7*

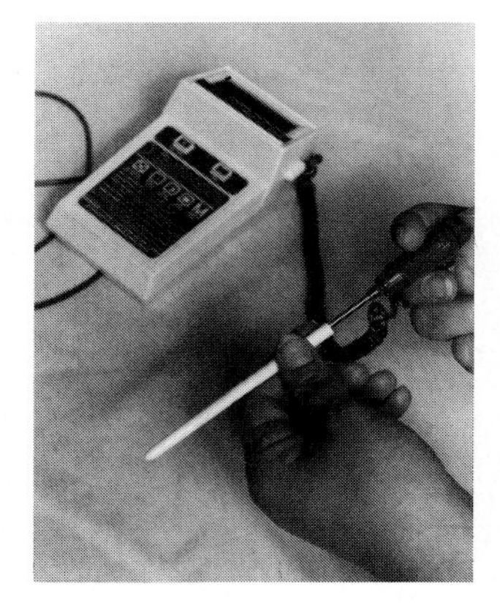

*Fig. 12-8*

| Steps | Rationale |
|---|---|
| m. Inform client of temperature reading. | Promotes participation in care and understanding of health status. |
| n. Wipe secretions from thermometer with soft tissue. Wipe in rotating fashion from fingers toward bulb. Dispose of tissue. | Avoids contact of microorganisms with nurse's hands. Wipe from area of least contamination to area of most contamination. |
| o. Wash thermometer in lukewarm soapy water, rinse in cool water, dry, and replace in storage container. | Mechanically removes organic material that can harbor microorganisms and hinder action of disinfectant. Storage container prevents breakage. |
| p. Remove and dispose of gloves. Wash hands. | Reduces transmission of microorganisms. |
| 2. **Oral temperature—electronic thermometer.** | |
| a. Wash hands. | Reduces transmission of microorganisms. |
| b. Assist client to position of comfort that provides easy access to mouth. | Ensures client's comfort and accuracy of temperature reading. |
| c. Apply disposable gloves. | Gloves can be worn for handling items soiled with body fluids (CDC, 1987). |
| d. Attach oral probe (blue tip) to thermometer unit. Grasp top of stem, being careful not to apply pressure to ejection button. | Ejection button releases plastic cover from probe. |
| e. Slide disposable plastic probe cover over thermometer probe until it locks in place (Fig. 12-8). | Soft plastic cover will not break in client's mouth, and prevents transmission of microorganisms between clients. |
| f. Ask client to open mouth and gently place probe under tongue in posterior sublingual pocket lateral to center of lower jaw. | Heat from superficial blood vessels in sublingual pocket produces temperature reading. With electronic thermometer, temperatures in right and left posterior sublingual pocket are significantly higher than in area under front of tongue (Erickson, 1980). |
| g. Ask client to hold thermometer with lips closed. | Maintains proper position of thermometer during recording. |
| h. Leave probe in place until audible signal occurs. Client's temperature appears on digital display. | Probe must stay in place until signal occurs to ensure accurate reading. |
| i. Remove probe from under client's tongue and inform client of temperature reading. | Promotes participation in care and understanding of health status. |
| j. Push ejection button on thermometer probe to discard plastic probe cover into proper receptacle. | Reduces transmission of microorganisms. |
| k. Return probe to storage well. | Protects probe from damage. Automatically causes digital reading to disappear. |
| l. Remove and dispose of gloves. Wash hands. | Reduces transmission of microorganisms. |
| m. Return thermometer to charger after temperature reading. | Maintains battery charge. |
| 3. **Rectal temperature—glass thermometer.** | |
| a. Wash hands. | Reduces transmission of microorganisms. |
| b. Draw curtain around client's bed or close room door. Keep client's upper body and lower extremities covered with sheet or blanket. | Maintains client's privacy, minimizes embarrassment, and promotes comfort. |
| c. Assist client to Sim's position with upper leg flexed. Move aside bed linen to expose only anal area. | Exposes anal area for correct thermometer placement. |
| d. Prepare thermometer following Steps 1d-h for oral temperature measurement with glass thermometer. | Mercury must be below client's temperature level before insertion. |
| e. Squeeze liberal portion of lubricant on tissue. Dip thermometer's blunt end into lubricant, covering 2.5 to 3.5 cm (1 to 1.5 in) for adult or 1.2 to 2.5 cm (0.5 to 1 in) for infant. Apply disposable gloves. | Lubrication minimizes trauma to rectal mucosa during insertion. Use of tissue avoids contamination of all lubricant in container. Gloves can be worn for handling items soiled by body fluids (CDC, 1987). |
| f. With nondominant hand, separate client's buttocks to expose anus. | Fully expose anus for thermometer insertion. |
| g. Ask client to breathe slowly and relax. | Relaxes anal sphincter for easier thermometer insertion. |
| h. Gently insert thermometer into anus in direction of umbilicus. Insert 1.2 cm (0.5 in) for infant and 3.5 cm (1.5 in) for adult. Do not force thermometer. | Ensures adequate exposure against blood vessels in rectal wall. |
| i. If resistance is felt during insertion, withdraw thermometer immediately. Never force thermometer. | Prevents trauma to mucosa. Glass thermometers can break. |
| j. Hold thermometer in place for 2 min according to agency policy. | Hold thermometer to prevent injury to client. Recommended times vary among institutions. Nichols and Kucha (1972) identified optimal placement time as 2 min. |
| k. Carefully remove thermometer and wipe off secretions with tissue. Wipe in rotating fashion from fingers toward bulb. Dispose of tissue. | Avoids nurse's contact with microorganisms. Wipe from area of least contamination to area of most contamination. |
| l. Read thermometer at eye level. Rotate until scale appears. | Ensures accurate reading. |

| Steps | Rationale |
|---|---|
| m. Inform client of temperature reading. | Promotes participation in care and understanding of health status. |
| n. Wipe client's anal area to remove lubricant or feces. Dispose of gloves. Wash hands. | Provides for client's comfort. Reduces transmission of microorganisms. |
| o. Help client return to comfortable position. | Restores client's comfort. |
| p. Wash thermometer in lukewarm soapy water, rinse in cool water, dry, and replace in storage container. | Mechanically removes organic material that can harbor microorganisms and hinder action of disinfectant. Storage container prevents breakage. |
| q. Wash hands. | Reduces transmission of microorganisms. |
| 4. **Rectal temperature—electronic thermometer.** | |
| a. Wash hands. | Reduces transmission of microorganisms. |
| b. Draw curtain around client's bed or close room door. Keep client's upper body and lower extremities covered with sheet or blanket. | Maintains client's privacy, minimizes embarrassment, and promotes comfort. |
| c. Assist client to Sim's position with upper leg flexed. Move aside bed linen to expose only anal area. | Exposes anal area for correct thermometer placement. |
| d. Attach rectal probe (red tip) to thermometer unit. Grasp top of stem, being careful not to apply pressure to ejection button. | Ejection button releases plastic cover from probe. |
| e. Slide disposable plastic cover over thermometer probe until it locks in place. | Probe cover prevents transmission of microorganisms between clients. |
| f. Squeeze liberal portion of lubricant onto tissue. Dip probe cover into lubricant, covering 2.5 to 3.5 cm (1 to 1.5 in) for adult or 1.2 to 2.5 cm (0.5 to 1 in) for infant. (Optional to apply disposable gloves.) | Lubrication minimizes trauma to rectal mucosa during insertion. |
| g. With nondominant hand, separate client's buttocks to expose anus. | Fully exposes anus for thermometer insertion. |
| h. Ask client to breathe slowly and relax. | Relaxes anal sphincter for easier thermometer insertion. |
| i. Gently insert probe into anus in direction of umbilicus. Insert 1.2 cm (0.5 in) for infant and 3.5 cm (1.5 in) for adult. | Ensures adequate exposure against blood vessels in rectal wall. |
| j. If resistance is felt during insertion, withdraw thermometer immediately. Never force thermometer. | Prevents trauma to mucosa. |
| k. Hold electronic probe until audible signal occurs. Read temperature on digital display. | Reading occurs within seconds after insertion. |
| l. Carefully remove probe from rectum and inform client of temperature reading. | Promotes participation in care and understanding of health status. |
| m. Push ejection button to discard plastic probe cover into receptacle. | Reduces transmission of microorganisms. |
| n. Return probe to storage well. | Protects probe from damage. Automatically causes digital reading to disappear. |
| o. Wipe client's anal area to remove lubricant or feces. Remove and dispose of gloves. | Provides for client's comfort. Reduces transmission of microorganisms. |
| p. Help client return to comfortable position. | Restores client's comfort. |
| q. Wash hands. | Reduces transmission of microorganisms. |
| 5. **Axillary temperature—glass thermometer.** | |
| a. Wash hands. | Reduces transmission of microorganisms. |
| b. Draw curtain around client's bed or close room door. | Provides privacy and minimizes client's embarrassment. |
| c. Position client lying supine or sitting. | Provides easy access to axilla. |
| d. Move clothing or gown away from client's shoulder and arm. | Provides optimal exposure of axilla. |
| e. Prepare glass thermometer following Steps d-h of oral measurement, glass thermometer. | Mercury must be below client's temperature level before insertion. |
| f. Insert thermometer into center of axilla with bulb directed toward client's head, lower client's arm over thermometer, and place arm across client's chest. | Maintains proper position of thermometer against blood vessels in axilla. |
| g. Hold thermometer in place for 5-10 min. | Recommended time varies among institutions. Eoff and Joyce (1981) recommend 5 min for children. |
| h. Remove thermometer and wipe off any secretions with tissue. Wipe in rotating fashion from fingers toward bulb. Dispose of tissue. | Avoids nurse's contact with microorganisms. Wipe from area of least contamination to area of most contamination. |
| i. Read thermometer at eye level. Rotate until scale appears. | Ensures accurate reading. |
| j. Inform client of temperature reading. | Promotes participation in care and understanding of health status. |

| Steps | Rationale |
|---|---|
| k. Wash thermometer in lukewarm soapy water, rinse in cool water, dry, and replace in storage container. | Mechanically removes organic material that can harbor microorganisms and hinder action of disinfectant. Storage container prevents breakage. |
| l. Assist client in replacing clothing or gown. | Restores client's sense of well-being. |
| m. Wash hands. | Reduces transmission of infection. |
| 6. **Axillary temperature—electronic thermometer.** | |
| a. Wash hands. | Reduces transmission of microorganisms. |
| b. Draw curtain around client's bed or close room door. | Provides privacy and minimizes client's embarrassment. |
| c. Position client lying supine or sitting. | Provides easy access to axilla. |
| d. Move clothing or gown away from client's shoulder and arm. | Provides optimal exposure of axilla. |
| e. Attach rectal probe (red) to thermometer unit. Prepare electronic thermometer following Steps 6d and 6e for electronic oral temperature measurement. | Probe cover prevents transmission of microorganisms between clients. |
| f. Insert probe into center of axilla, lower client's arm over thermometer, and place arm across client's chest. | Maintains proper position of thermometer against blood vessels in axilla. |
| g. Hold electronic probe in place until audible signal occurs. Read temperature on digital display. | Reading occurs within seconds after insertion. |
| h. Remove probe from axilla and inform client of temperature reading. | Promotes participation in care and understanding of health status. |
| i. Push ejection button to discard plastic probe into proper receptacle. | Reduces transmission of microorganisms. |
| j. Return electronic probe to storage well. | Protects probe from damage. Automatically causes digital reading to disappear. |
| k. Assist client in replacing clothing or gown. | Restores client's comfort. |
| l. Wash hands. | Reduces transmission of infection. |

## Evaluation

| | |
|---|---|
| 1. If temperature is within normal range establish it as baseline. | To use for comparison with future temperature readings. |
| 2. Compare temperature reading with client's baseline and normal temperature range for client's age group. | Normal body temperature fluctuates within narrow range; comparison reveals presence of abnormality. |

### *Expected outcomes*

| | |
|---|---|
| 1. Body temperature is within normal range for client's age-group. | Nurse controlled for environmental factors that could normally alter temperature. Thermoregulation is stable. |

### *Unexpected outcomes*

| | |
|---|---|
| 1. Body temperature is above normal upper expected range. | Client has fever. |
| 2. Body temperature is below normal lower expected range. | Client is hypothermic. |

## Recording and Reporting

| | |
|---|---|
| 1. Record temperature on vital sign flowsheet (Fig. 12-9) or nurses' notes. Also record any signs or symptoms of temperature alterations. | Vital sign measurements should be recorded promptly on flowsheets to avoid omissions from client's record. Abnormalities may require therapy. |
| 2. Report abnormal findings to nurse in charge or physician. | Abnormalities may require immediate implementation of therapy. Measurement of body temperature after administration of specific therapy should be documented in narrative form in nurses' notes. |

## Follow-up Activities

| | |
|---|---|
| 1. For temperature above normal upper expected range initiate following nursing measures: | |
| a. Increase fluid intake to at least 3 L daily, (unless contraindicated by client's condition). | Restores fluids lost from insensible loss, sweating, or increased metabolism. |
| b. Control environmental temperature at 21°-27° C (70°-80° F). | Higher room temperatures may increase body temperature. Room temperature lower than body temperature promotes loss by radiation. |
| c. Remove excess blankets or bed coverings. | Promotes heat loss through radiation and conduction. |
| d. Reduce frequency of exhaustive care activities. | Minimizes body's oxygen demands. |
| e. Keep clothing and bed linen dry. | Potentiates heat loss through conduction and convection. |

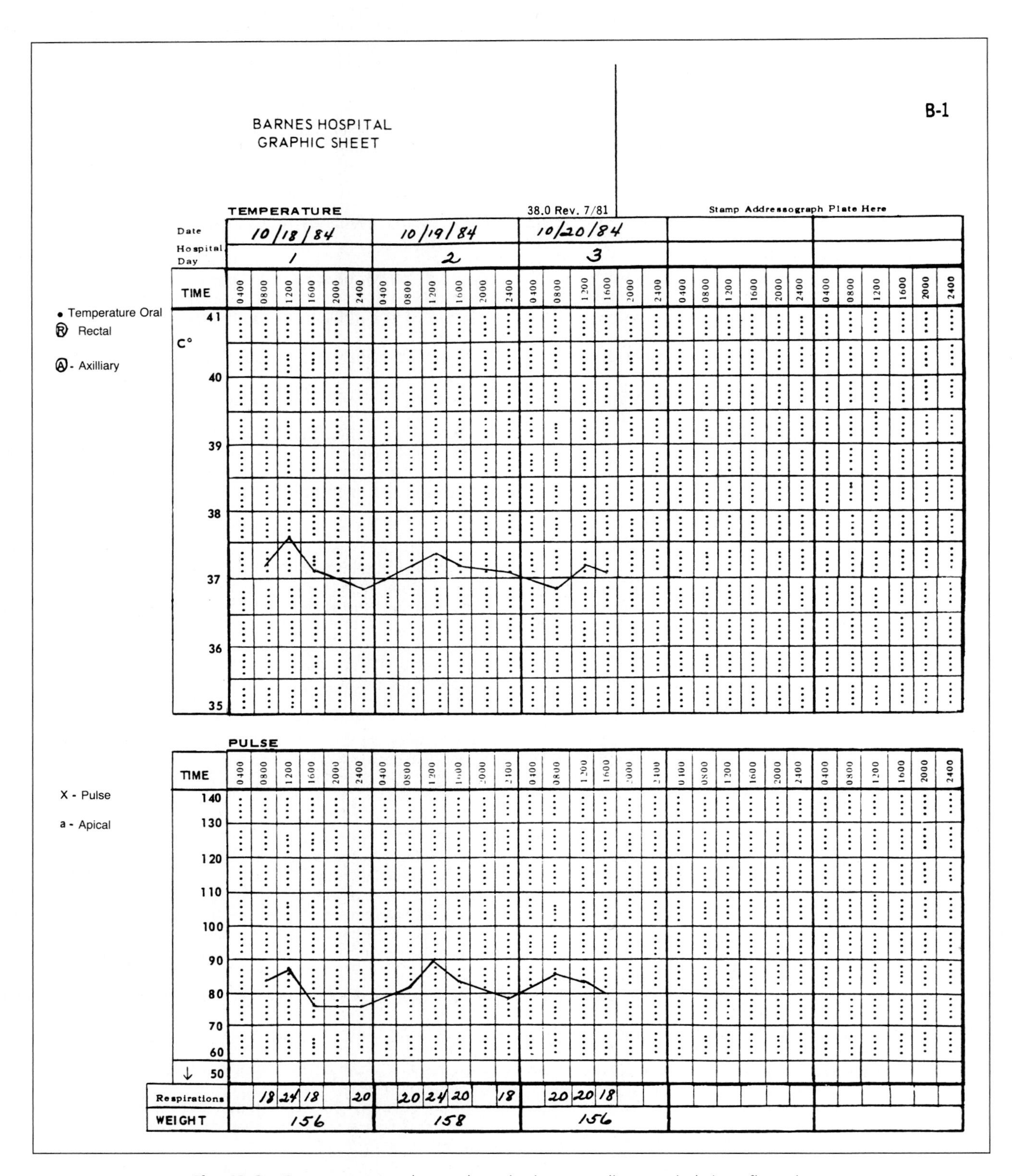


*Fig. 12-9* Temperature, pulse, and respiration recording on vital signs flow sheet.
Courtesy Barnes Hospital, St. Louis.

| Steps | Rationale |
|---|---|
| f. Implement measures to prevent or control spread of infection, e.g., pulmonary hygiene and postural drainage (Chapter 15), wound care (Chapter 42), and adequate urinary elimination (Chapter 30). | Pulmonary hygiene promotes removal of secretions that can harbor microorganisms. Cleansing and drainage of wounds prevent accumulation of drainage that harbors microorganisms. Promotion of normal bladder emptying prevents urine retention. |
| 2. If fever persists or reaches unacceptable level defined by physician, implement sponging with tepid water (Chapter 6), administer antipyretics as ordered, apply hypothermia blanket, administer antibiotics as ordered. | No set temperature is accepted by all clinicians as level for initiating more aggressive therapy. Fever is adaptive response of body and seems to form host defense. Recent studies show fever has beneficial effects, including inhibition of bacterial growth, enhanced motility of white blood cells, and improved phagocytosis (Shaver, 1982). |
| 3. For temperature below normal lower expected range initiate following nursing measures: | |
| a. Cover client with warm blankets. | Provides gradual rewarming, thus preventing wide fluctuations in body temperature. |
| b. Close room doors or windows to eliminate cool drafts. | Room temperature below that of body temperature promotes heat loss by radiation. |
| 4. For temperature below 35° C (95° F) initiate the following measures: | |
| a. Turn client every 1-2 h and place extremities through passive ROM. | Prevents venous stasis and potential skin breakdown. |
| b. Monitor apical pulse rate and rhythm (Skill 12-3). | Hypothermia causes bradycardia and cardiac arrhythmias. |

## Special Considerations

- It is best to compare temperatures taken during same time of day.
- Temperature should be taken within 30 min after administering antipyretics.
- Do not remove bed coverings if client has chills. Chills increase heat production.
- Clients with musculoskeletal alterations may be able to suggest to nurse ways for positioning to avoid discomfort during rectal insertion. Children may assume prone position. Infants may lie supine with knees flexed toward abdomen as nurse holds infant's ankles during entire insertion. Elderly clients unable to flex their legs may lie on their sides with legs straight.
- Caution clients using oral thermometer against moving mouth or repositioning thermometer.
- Do not allow client to insert rectal thermometer. Tissue trauma may easily occur if thermometer is forced.
- If client complains of rectal pain after insertion, notify physician and observe for rectal bleeding. Localized discomfort may result from irritation of hemorrhoids.
- With children who cry or become restless, it is helpful to reverse order for taking vital signs, i.e., measure respirations and pulse before temperature (BP may be optional).
- Axillary temperature is safest for newborn. In infant or young child it may be necessary to hold arm against child's side.
- Normal temperature ranges are:
  a. Newborns and infants: 35.5°-37.5° C (96°-99.5° F).

## Teaching Considerations

- Clients with febrile illnesses or conditions that increase risk of infection or who have young children or family members unable to measure temperature must learn techniques for body temperature measurement (Skill 12-2).

## Home Care Considerations

- Assess temperature and ventilation of client's room to determine existence of any environmental condition that may influence outcome of the client's temperature.

# *SKILL 12-2 Teaching Clients to Measure Body Temperature*

To practice health maintenance for themselves and their family members, clients need to know how to measure body temperature. An elevation in body temperature can be an early warning sign of serious health problems. Clients susceptible to temperature alterations should know how to measure their temperatures correctly so that they can seek medical attention early when alterations occur. Parents must know how to measure their children's temperature, since children can develop seriously high fevers very quickly. Because the elderly have impaired temperature control mechanisms, the care giver should know the techniques for temperature measurement. Nurses can teach clients the skills of measuring body temperature and lowering temperature when a febrile episode occurs at home and medical care is not immediately accessible.

### Purposes

1. Assist clients in early detection of fever.
2. Increase client knowledge of nature, signs, and symptoms of fever.
3. Improve family members' ability or client's ability to care for self when temperature alterations develop.

## *Procedure 12-2*

| Steps | Rationale |
|---|---|
| **Assessment** | |
| 1. Assess client's ability to manipulate and read thermometer by having client read temperature values and shake thermometer down. Client who wears eyeglasses should wear them while reading thermometer. | Physical restrictions in handling or reading thermometer may necessitate nurse instructing family member or significant other instead of client. Visual acuity impairment may prevent client from being able to read thermometer. |
| 2. Assess client's knowledge of normal temperature range and symptoms and common causes of fever and hypothermia. | Identifies client's ability to initiate preventive health measures and recognize alterations in body temperature. |
| 3. If client has had experience in measuring temperature ask for demonstration of technique. | Allows nurse to assess client's knowledge and use of safety precautions, aseptic technique, and time period for insertion. |
| **Nursing Diagnosis** | |
| 1. Cluster data to reveal client's learning capabilities and needs and identify appropriate nursing diagnoses: | |
| a. Altered health maintenance: related to inability to manipulate thermometer. | Family member must learn skill. |
| b. Knowledge deficit regarding temperature measurement; related to limited experience or practice. | Client should have opportunity to practice skill. |
| c. Knowledge deficit regarding cause and nature of temperature alterations: related to lack of information. | Nurse will discuss cause and implications of fever and hypothermia. |
| **Planning** | |
| 1. Identify learning objectives for teaching plan. Client will be able to: | Ensures that information for performing procedure safely and correctly is presented. |
| a. Read temperature levels on thermometer accurately and know normal temperature value. | |
| b. Correctly shake down thermometer. | |
| c. Insert thermometer correctly in chosen measurement site without causing injury. | |
| d. Follow safety precautions during insertion. | |
| e. Use clean technique during handling of thermometer. | |
| f. Clean and store thermometer correctly. | |
| g. Identify effects of cold or hot liquids and foods on oral temperature readings. | |
| h. Identify three common symptoms of fever and hypothermia. | Hypothermia needs to be discussed only when elderly client is involved. |
| i. Identify two ways to control or reduce fever. | |
| 2. Prepare needed equipment and supplies: | |
| a. Instruct client on purchase and selection of glass thermometer. | Glass thermometer is inexpensive and available in any drug store. Newborn infants require oral or stubby thermometer for axillary use. Infants and young children require rectal thermometer or oral thermometer for axillary use. Older children and adults use oral thermometers. |
| b. Assemble soft tissue and lubricant (if rectal measurement). | |
| c. Instruct client on use of lubricating jelly for rectal thermometer. | Prevents trauma to mucosa with rectal thermometer insertion. |
| 3. Select setting in home that client is most likely to use when measuring temperature. | Practice in same environment where skill is routinely performed facilitates comprehension and learning. |

| Steps | Rationale |
|---|---|
| 4. Discuss and demonstrate with client proper way to position self or family member before thermometer insertion. | Promotes client's understanding of comfort and safety principles, as well as technique to ensure accurate measurement. |

## Implementation

| Steps | Rationale |
|---|---|
| 1. Demonstrate steps and state rationale for preparation and insertion of thermometer: handwashing, reading thermometer, shaking thermometer down, reading thermometer, inserting thermometer, holding thermometer in place (rectal and axillary), timing placement, removing thermometer, reading thermometer, cleansing and storing. | Demonstration is best technique for teaching psychomotor skill. |
| 2. Have client perform each step with guidance from nurse. Do not rush client. | Nurse is able to correct errors in technique as they occur and discuss implications. |
| 3. Discuss what normal temperature is for adult or child. | Client must be able to identify temperature alterations. |
| 4. Discuss effects of smoking and hot and cold liquids or foods on oral temperature readings. | Client must understand factors that falsely alter temperature readings. |
| 5. Discuss common symptoms of fever: warm, dry, flushed skin; feeling warm; chills; pilo-erection; malaise, restlessness. | Client must be able to recognize onset of fever in self or family member. |
| 6. When elderly clients are involved discuss common signs and symptoms of hypothermia: cool skin, uncontrolled shivering, loss of memory, signs of poor judgment. | Persons with inadequate home heating or those unaware of potential dangers of cold conditions are at risk. |
| 7. Discuss importance of notifying physician when temperature elevations occur and review common therapies for temperature reduction that are safe to perform at home. | Clients must understand danger of high temperature elevations. Use of antipyretics, sponging with tepid water (Chapter 6), and drinking fluids are unlikely to cause complications. |

## Evaluation

| Steps | Rationale |
|---|---|
| 1. Have client independently demonstrate technique for temperature measurement. | Feedback through independent demonstration of psychomotor skill is best means of evaluating mastery of skill. |
| 2. Ask client to identify normal temperature range and influence of smoking and hot and cold liquids or foods on oral readings; discuss safety implications for temperature measurement. | Measures cognitive learning. |
| 3. Have client describe common signs and symptoms of fever and hypothermia and methods for control. | Measures cognitive learning. |

### *Expected outcomes*

| Steps | Rationale |
|---|---|
| 1. Client is able to correctly measure own or family members' temperature and clean thermometer. | Indicates skill effectively learned. |
| 2. Client knows factors affecting temperature, signs and symptoms of fever and hypothermia, and measures to lower fever. | Cognitive learning achieved. |

### *Unexpected outcomes*

| Steps | Rationale |
|---|---|
| 1. Client is unable to measure temperature or clean thermometer correctly. | May be result of physical weakness, visual alterations, poor motor coordination, poor memory or concentration, anxiety, or lack of interest. |
| 2. Client is not able to explain factors affecting temperature, common signs and symptoms of fever and hypothermia, or measures to lower fever. | Anxiety, lack of interest, language barrier, or method of instruction may interfere with learning. |

## Recording and Reporting

| Steps | Rationale |
|---|---|
| 1. Record information taught and client's response in nurses' notes. | Joint Commission on Accreditation of Health Care Organizations (JCAHO) requirement for health agencies is to document client education. Provides for continuity of care when other nurses teach client. |

## Follow-up Activities

| Steps | Rationale |
|---|---|
| 1. If home health nurse is visiting client, plan for a repeat demonstration during a scheduled visit. | Provides excellent measure of client's ability to retain information. |

### Special Considerations

- Arthritis or other joint conditions, weakness in finger grasping, or conditions causing pain in upper extremities may prohibit client from being able to shake down thermometer properly.
- Clients unable to shake down thermometer may use chemical single-use thermometer strips.

### Teaching Considerations

- Nurse may demonstrate on self or family member. Using client for demonstration prevents client from being able to observe entire procedure.
- Caution parents of infants and young children about child's predisposition to sudden temperature elevations and danger of convulsions.
- Use caution in recommending aspirin or acetaminophen (Tylenol) in clients whose conditions contraindicate their use (e.g., gastric ulcer, bleeding tendencies).
- Pay extra attention to method parent uses to insert rectal thermometer in child. Do not allow parent to insert thermometer too far or to force it. Note if parent holds thermometer after it is inserted in child's oral or rectal cavity. Instruct parent to use axillary route until child can safely hold thermometer in mouth.
- Explain to parent that temperature should be taken anytime a child's skin feels warm.
- Instruct client or family to never leave child or client unattended when rectal thermometer is in place.
- Teach elderly when they are alert and rested. Keep teaching session short but involve client actively in discussion or activity.
- Instruct client and family in proper cleaning and storage of the thermometer in the home.
- Instruct client not to take temperature after smoking or eating hot or cold foods.
- Hold a rectal thermometer in place, never leaving the client unattended.

### Home Care Considerations

- Assess the priority client and family give to taking the client's body temperature on a regular basis.
- Bedroom provides comfort and privacy for temperature measurement.

## *SKILL 12-3 Assessing a Client's Pulse*

A peripheral pulse is a wave that travels through the arterial system following the ejection of the ventricle's stroke volume against the aorta's walls. With each stroke volume the walls of the aorta distend, creating a pulse wave that travels rapidly to the most distal arteries. The nurse palpates a pulse wave by lightly compressing the artery against underlying bone or muscle. Occasionally a nurse has difficulty palpating a pulse. A Doppler or ultrasound stethoscope is designed to amplify sounds so that low-velocity blood flow can be heard (Chapter 13). The stethoscope has a special probe applied over the pulse site. A thin layer of transmission gel covers the skin. The stethoscope transmits a "whooshing" sound that indicates arterial blood flow.

The apical pulse is not a wave at all. Instead, it is the sound auscultated during contraction of the heart (Chapter 13). Each heartbeat is the combination of heart sounds $S_1$ and $S_2$, which correspond with heart valve closure before and after each ventricular contraction. The apical pulse is the most accurate measure of the frequency and rhythm of heart contraction.

Assessing a client's pulse offers valuable data for determining the integrity of the cardiovascular system. Pulse rate, for example, indirectly measures the heart's cardiac output. The volume of blood pumped by the heart during 1 minute is equal to the cardiac output. The cardiac output (CO) equals the product of the ventricle's stroke volume (SV) and the heart rate (HR) for 1 minute:

$$CO = HR \times SV$$

An abnormally slow, rapid, or irregular pulse may indicate the heart's inability to deliver an adequate cardiac output. Another example of how pulse assessment measures cardiac function is in the assessment of pulse strength. The strength or amplitude of a pulse reflects the volume of blood ejected against the arterial wall with each heart contraction. If the heart's stroke volume falls, the pulse often becomes weak and difficult to palpate. In contrast, a full bounding pulse is an indication of increased stroke volume.

The integrity of peripheral pulses indicates the status of blood perfusion to the area distributed by the pulse (Table 12-2). For example, assessment of the right femoral pulse determines whether blood flow to the right leg is adequate. If a peripheral artery feels weak on palpation, the volume of blood reaching tissues distal to the pulse site may be inadequate. Chapter 13 describes techniques for assessing the peripheral pulses. This chapter describes techniques for assessing radial and apical pulses.

### Purposes

1. Radial pulse:
   a. Obtain a baseline measure of heart rate and rhythm.
   b. Assess a client's cardiovascular status.

***TABLE 12-2*** Pulse Sites

| Site | Location | Assessment Criteria |
|---|---|---|
| **Temporal** | Over temporal bone of the head, above and lateral to the eye. | Easily accessible site to assess pulse in children. |
| **Carotid** | Along medial edge of sternocleido-mastoid muscle in the neck. | Easily accessible site to assess character of pulse peripherally. Used during physiologic shock or cardiac arrest when other sites are not palpable. |
| **Apical** | Fourth to fifth intercostal space at midclavicular line. | Site for auscultation of heart sounds. |
| **Brachial** | Groove between biceps and triceps muscles at the antecubital fossa. | Assess status of circulation to lower arm.<br>Site used to auscultate blood pressure. |
| **Radial** | Radial or thumb side of forearm at the wrist. | Common site to assess character of pulse peripherally. Assess status of circulation to hand. |
| **Ulnar** | Ulnar side of forearm at the wrist. | Assess status of circulation to ulnar side of hand. Used to assess an Allen test. |
| **Femoral** | Below the inguinal ligament, mid-way between symphysis pubis and anterior superior iliac spine. | Assess character of pulse during physiologic shock or cardiac arrest when other pulses are not palpable. Assess status of circulation to the leg. |
| **Popliteal** | Behind the knee in popliteal fossa. | Assess status of circulation to the lower leg. |
| **Posterior tibial** | Inner side of each ankle, below medial malleolus. | Assess status of circulation to the foot. |
| **Dorsalis pedis** | Along top of foot between extension tendons of great and first toe. | Assess status of circulation to the foot. |

c. Monitor heart response to various pathologic conditions and therapies.
d. Assess local blood flow to the hand.

2. Apical pulse:
   a. Assess a client's cardiovascular status.
   b. Monitor heart response to various pathologic conditions and therapies.
   c. Assess the nature of irregularities in the radial pulse.

## *Procedure 12-3*

| Steps | Rationale |
|---|---|
| **Assessment** | |
| 1. Determine need to assess client's pulse. | |
| a. Note risk factors for alterations in pulse: history of heart disease; history of cardiac arrhythmias, e.g., bradycardia, tachycardia, or heart block; onset of sudden chest pain, after invasive cardiovascular diagnostic tests, e.g., cardiac catheterization or arteriograms; postoperative; sudden infusion of large volume of IV fluid; internal or external hemorrhage; acute pain (from any site). | Certain conditions place clients at risk for pulse alterations. |

| Steps | Rationale |
|---|---|
| b. Assess for signs and symptoms of cardiovascular alterations: dyspnea (on exertion), fatigue, chest pain, orthopnea, syncope, palpitations (person's unpleasant awareness of heartbeat), jugular venous distention, edema of dependent body parts, cyanosis or pallor of skin. | Physical signs and symptoms may indicate alteration in cardiac or vascular status. |
| 2. Assess for factors that normally influence character of pulse: | Allows nurse to accurately assess presence and significance of pulse alterations. |
| a. Age: infant's heart rate at birth ranges from 100-180 beats/min at rest; by age 2, pulse rate slows to 70-110 beats/min; with adolescence rate varies between 55 and 90 beats/min and remains so throughout adulthood; no changes occur in elderly persons at rest and in absence of disease. | |
| b. Medications: antiarrhythmics, sympathomimetics, and cardiotonics affect rate and rhythm of pulse; large doses of narcotic analgesics can slow heart rate; general anesthetics slow heart rate; central nervous system stimulants may increase heart rate. | |
| c. Exercise: physical activity normally increases heart rate; person who is physically well conditioned has slower than normal resting heart rate and quicker return to resting rate after exercise. | |
| d. Postural changes: heart rate increases from lying to sitting or standing position. | |
| e. Fever or exposure to warm environment: heat increases heart rate. | |
| 3. Assess site most appropriate for pulse assessment (Table 12-2) (see Chapter 13). | Ensures accurate measurement of pulse characteristics. |
| 4. Determine previous baseline heart rate (if available) from client's record. | Will allow nurse to identify if change has occurred in client's status. |

## Nursing Diagnosis

| | |
|---|---|
| 1. Analyze client's physical signs and symptoms along with pulse findings to identify potential nursing diagnoses: | |
| a. Decreased cardiac output: related to conduction defect or reduced contractility. | Additional data must be gathered to confirm nursing diagnoses. However, nurse's initial findings can direct a more thorough assessment. |
| b. Altered tissue perfusion: related to arterial obstruction. | Risk identified by weak or absent peripheral pulse. |

## Planning

| | |
|---|---|
| 1. Develop individualized goals for assessing client's pulse: | |
| a. Establish baseline heart rate. | Provides comparison with future pulse assessments. |
| b. Identify abnormalities in pulse character. | Directs nurse to pursue supportive therapies. |

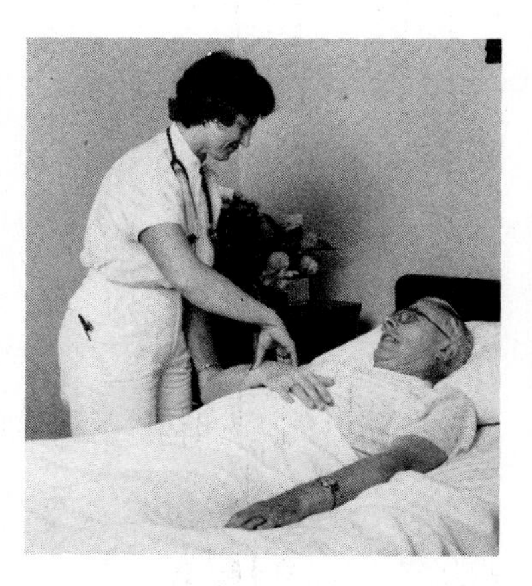

*Fig. 12-10*

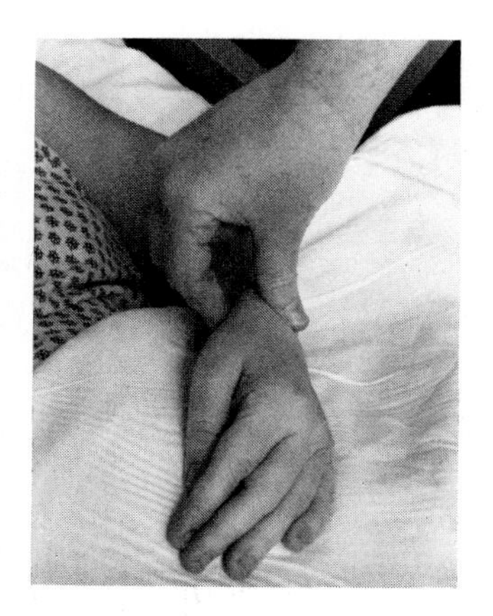

*Fig. 12-11*

| Steps | Rationale |
|---|---|
| c. Detect changes in pulse in response to selected therapies. | Directs nurse to initiate preventive therapies. |
| 2. Prepare needed equipment and supplies: | |
| a. Stethoscope | Used to auscultate apical pulse. |
| b. Pen, pencil, and vital sign flow sheet or record form | Provides for timely documentation of assessment findings. |
| c. Wristwatch with second hand or digital display | Necessary for accurate calculation of rate. |
| d. Alcohol swab | To cleanse stethoscope. |
| 3. Explain to client that pulse or heart rate is to be assessed. Encourage client to relax as much as possible. Ask client to not speak while assessing pulse. Wait 5-10 min before assessing pulse if client has been active. | Anxiety can cause elevation in heart rate. Client's speech interferes with nurse's ability to hear sounds when apical pulse is measured. |
| 4. Have client assume sitting or supine position. Child may sit in parent's lap. | Provides easy access to pulse sites. |

## Implementation

| Steps | Rationale |
|---|---|
| 1. Radial pulse. | |
| a. Wash hands. | Reduces transmission of microorganisms. |
| b. If supine, place client's forearm across lower chest with wrist extended and palm down (Fig. 12-10). If sitting, bend client's elbow 90° and support lower arm on chair or on your arm. Slightly extend wrist with palm down. | Relaxed position of lower arm and extension of wrist permits full exposure of artery to palpation. |
| c. Place tips of first 2 or middle 3 fingers of your hand over groove along radial or thumb side of client's inner wrist (Fig. 12-11). | Fingertips are most sensitive parts of hand to palpate arterial pulsation. Nurse's thumb has pulsation that may interfere with accuracy. |
| d. Lightly compress against radius, obliterate pulse initially, and then relax pressure so pulse becomes easily palpable. | Pulse is more accurately assessed with moderate pressure. Too much pressure occludes pulse and impairs blood flow. |
| e. When pulse is felt regularly, look at watch's second hand and begin to count rate: when sweep hand hits number on dial, start counting with zero, then one, etc. | Rate is determined accurately only after assessor is assured pulse can be palpated. Timing begins with zero. Count of one is first beat palpated after timing begins. |
| f. If pulse is regular, count rate for 15 sec and multiply total by 4. | Regular heart rate can be accurately assessed in 15 sec. |
| g. If pulse is irregular, count for full min. | Longer time period ensures accurate count. |
| h. Assess regularity and frequency of any dysrhythmia. | Inefficient contraction of heart fails to transmit pulse wave and can interfere with cardiac output. Determines need to assess for pulse deficit. |
| i. Determine strength of pulse. Note thrust of vessel against fingertips. | Strength reflects volume of blood ejected against arterial wall with each heart contraction. |
| j. Palpate with 2 fingers along course of artery toward wrist to determine elasticity of arterial wall. | Degree of elasticity reflects quality of arterial wall and reveals general condition of peripheral vascular system. Normal artery is straight, smooth, round, and elastic. |
| k. Assist client in returning to comfortable position. | Promotes sense of well-being. |
| l. Discuss findings with client. | Promotes client's participation in care and understanding of health status. |
| 2. Apical pulse | |
| a. Clean earpieces and diaphragm of stethoscope with alcohol swab as needed (optional). | Controls transmission of microorganisms when nurses share stethoscope. |
| b. With client in supine or sitting position, turn down bed linen and raise gown to expose sternum and left side of chest. | Exposes portion of chest wall for selection of auscultatory site. |
| c. Palpate Louis' angle, located just below suprasternal notch at point where horizontal ridge is felt along body of sternum. Place index finger just to right (client's left) of sternum and palpate second intercostal space. Place next finger in intercostal space below and proceed downward until fifth intercostal space is located. Move index finger horizontally along fifth intercostal space to left midclavicular line (Fig. 12-12). Palpate point of maximal impulse (PMI), also called Erb's point. | Use of anatomic landmarks allows nurse to place stethoscope over apex of heart, which lies just under fifth intercostal space along left midclavicular line. This position enhances ability to hear heart sounds clearly. PMI is over apex of heart. |
| d. Place diaphragm of stethoscope in palm of your hand for 5-10 sec. | Warming of metal or plastic diaphragm prevents client from being startled and promotes comfort. |
| e. Place diaphragm over PMI and auscultate for normal $S_1$ and $S_2$ heart sounds (heard as "lub dub") (Fig. 12-13). | Heart sounds are caused by movement of blood through heart valves. |
| f. When occurrence of $S_1$ and $S_2$ is heard with regularity, use watch's second hand and begin to count rate: when sweep hand hits number on dial, start counting with zero, then one, etc. | Rate is determined accurately only after nurse is able to auscultate sounds clearly. |

| Steps | Rationale |
|---|---|

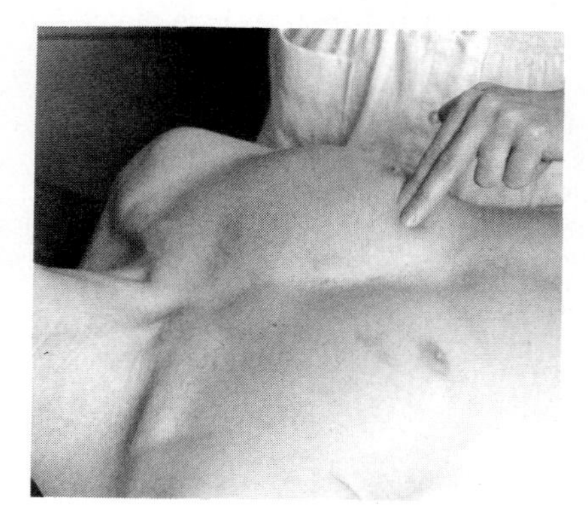

*Fig. 12-12*

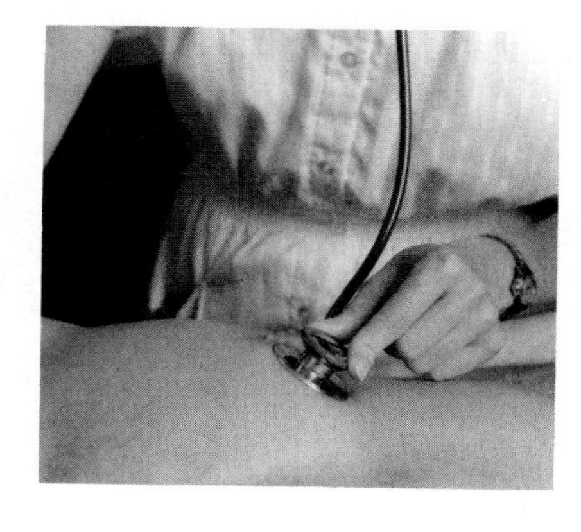

*Fig. 12-13*

| Steps | Rationale |
|---|---|
| g. If heart rate is regular, count for 30 sec and multiply by 2. | Regular apical rate can be assessed within 30 sec. |
| h. If heart rate is irregular, count for 1 min. | Rate determined is more accurate when measured over longer interval. |
| i. Note regularity of any dysrhythmia ($S_1$ and $S_2$ occurs early or later after previous sequence of sounds; $S_1$ or $S_2$ is absent for a beat). | Regular occurrence of dysrhythmia within 1 min may indicate inadequate cardiac function. |
| j. Replace client's gown and bed linen. Assist client in returning to comfortable position. | Maintains client's comfort. |
| k. Discuss findings with client. | Promotes client's participation in care and understanding of health status. |

## Evaluation

| Steps | Rationale |
|---|---|
| 1. If pulse is assessed for first time, establish as baseline. | Used to compare future pulse assessments. |
| 2. Compare client's pulse rate and character with previous baseline and normal pulse range for age group. | Allows nurse to assess for change in client's condition and for presence of cardiac alteration. |
| 3. Assess pulse again by having another nurse conduct measurement, if pulse character is abnormal. | Original measurement may result from error by assessor. Second measurement confirms finding of pulse alteration. |

### *Expected outcomes*

| Steps | Rationale |
|---|---|
| 1. Pulse and heart rate are within normal range for client's age. | Cardiovascular status is stable. |
| 2. Rhythm is regular. | |
| 3. Radial pulse is strong, firm, and elastic. | Condition of radial artery is normal. |

### *Unexpected outcomes*

| Steps | Rationale |
|---|---|
| 1. Pulse and heart rate are above or below normal range for client's age. | Indicates potential for poor cardiac output, resulting from variety of causes: e.g., heart disease, medication side effect, blood loss. |
| 2. Rhythm is irregular. | Indicates need to assess for pulse deficit. |
| 3. Radial pulse may be weak and difficult to palpate. | Reduced cardiac output will cause weak pulse. Local obstruction to blood flow, e.g., clot or edema of hand and wrist, may cause pulse to be difficult to palpate. |

## Recording and Reporting

| Steps | Rationale |
|---|---|
| 1. Record characteristics of pulse in medical record or vital sign flow sheet (see Fig. 12-9). Also, record any accompanying signs and symptoms of pulse alterations. | Vital signs should be recorded immediately for accuracy and inclusion in medical record. |
| 2. Report abnormal findings to nurse in charge or physician. | Abnormalities may necessitate immediate medical therapy. |

## Follow-up Activities

| Steps | Rationale |
|---|---|
| 1. Nurse may perform or assist technician in performing electrocardiogram (ECG) (Chapter 46). | Diagnostic test measures electrical activity of heart to detect conduction alterations. |

| Steps | Rationale |
|---|---|
| 2. Assess client for pulse deficit: | |
| a. One nurse measures client's radial pulse. | Indicated when irregularity in rhythm is assessed. |
| b. At same time, another nurse measures client's apical pulse. | Deficit usually involves radial pulse being slower than apical pulse. Results from failure of heart contraction to generate pulse wave to periphery or from interference in blood flow to peripheral artery. |
| c. The two rates are compared. | Reveals degree of deficit. |

## Special Considerations

- If radial pulses are inaccessible because of dressings, bandages, casts, or IV placement, use apical pulse. Also use apical pulse when radial pulse reveals irregularities. Apical pulse is best site for assessing infant's or young child's heart rate. Client with history of heart disease should have apical assessment.
- Normal pulse range for given age is best basis for comparison if client's baseline rate has been abnormal.
- Do not palpate radial pulse with thumb because own pulse may be felt.
- PMI in an infant is usually located at third to fourth intercostal space to left of midclavicular line.
- Premature ventricular contraction (PVC) is common in most persons. However, its frequency increases with heart disease. Nurse will hear premature sequence of $S_1$ and $S_2$ and then short pause before normal $S_1$ and $S_2$ return. Multiple PVCs or repeated coupling of normal heartbeats followed by PVCs should be reported to physician.
- It is often difficult to palpate the pulse of an elderly or obese client. A Doppler device will provide a more accurate reading.

## Teaching Considerations

- Identify client's need to learn how to assess own pulse in home setting (Skill 12-4).
- Clients taking certain prescribed cardiotonic or antiarrhythmic medications should learn to assess their own pulse rates to detect side effects of medications. Clients undergoing cardiac rehabilitation should learn to assess their own pulse rates to determine their response to exercise.

## Home Care Considerations

- Assess home environment to determine the room that will afford the fewest disruptions for taking of vital signs.
- Palpate client's radial, femoral, pedal, and carotid pulse rates each visit, reporting discrepancies between rates.

# SKILL 12-4 Teaching Clients to Assess Their Own Pulse

Certain clients can benefit from knowing how to assess their own pulse. Persons taking medications that specifically affect heart function are already symptomatic of heart disease and are susceptible to side effects of the medications. By being able to assess their own pulse rate and rhythm correctly, these clients can detect complications of their disease, as well as any undesirable effects of their medications. Clients can thus seek medical attention before serious problems occur.

Another group of clients who should learn how to assess their own pulse are those undergoing cardiovascular rehabilitation. For example, clients who have had myocardial infarction undergo exercise training to improve the strength of their heart muscle. Pulse rate and rhythm are the criteria used to determine how well these clients tolerate exercise.

There are also many healthy persons who actively exercise and who can learn about their health from measuring their own pulse. Exercise tolerance can vary depending on environmental conditions, intake of certain foods, and the overall physical condition of a person. By measuring pulse rate and rhythm, a person can learn how the body responds to strenuous exercise and when to cease further physical activity.

## Purposes

1. Assist clients in early detection of cardiovascular alterations.
2. Improve client understanding of the effects of medications on heart function.
3. Improve client understanding of the effects of exercise on heart function.

## *Procedure 12-4*

| Steps | Rationale |
|---|---|
| **Assessment** | |
| 1. Assess client's ability to feel arterial pulsation by having client palpate own or nurse's artery. (Nurse palpates pulse of client or self simultaneously to see if client can successfully feel pulse wave.) | Physical impairment in sensation may necessitate nurse instructing family member or significant other instead of client. |
| 2. Identify client's knowledge of purpose for assessing pulse and level of interest in performing skill. | Aids in identifying client's motivation to regularly assess pulse after learning skill. Also allows nurse to assess client's understanding of physical condition and knowledge of medications prescribed. |
| 3. If reportedly measured own pulse before, ask client to demonstrate technique for assessing pulse. | Reveals client's level of skill in assessing pulse. |
| **Nursing Diagnosis** | |
| 1. Identify nursing diagnoses appropriate to client's learning capabilities and needs. Nursing diagnoses might include: | |
| a. Knowledge deficit regarding pulse assessment skill: related to limited experience. | Client lacks information to perform skill correctly. |
| b. Sensory and perceptual alteration (tactile): related to altered sensory reception. | Client's inability to perform skill requires family member to be involved in teaching plan. |
| **Planning** | |
| 1. Identify learning objectives for teaching plan. Client or family member will be able to: | Ensures that information required for performing procedure safely and correctly is presented. |
| a. Correctly palpate arterial pulsation. | |
| b. Accurately calculate pulse rate and determine rhythm. | |
| c. Identify normal range for pulse rate. | Physician may designate normal pulse range for client. Desired range depends on client's cardiac status and medication. |
| d. Discuss steps to take when pulse is above or below desired range. | Client will recognize complications. |
| 2. Select setting in home that client is most likely to use when assessing pulse. | Practice in same environment in which skill is routinely performed facilitates comprehension and learning. |
| 3. Prepare needed equipment and supplies: | |
| a. Wristwatch or clock with second hand. | |
| b. Paper, note card, or notebook and pencil. | Client can keep daily record of pulse rate. |
| **Implementation** | |
| 1. Discuss with client best sites for assessing pulse: radial and carotid. | Most accessible sites are easiest to palpate for accuracy of assessment. |
| 2. If carotid site is chosen, caution client against vigorously massaging the neck while attempting to locate pulse. | Stimulation of carotid sinus could lead to reflex slowing of heart rate. |

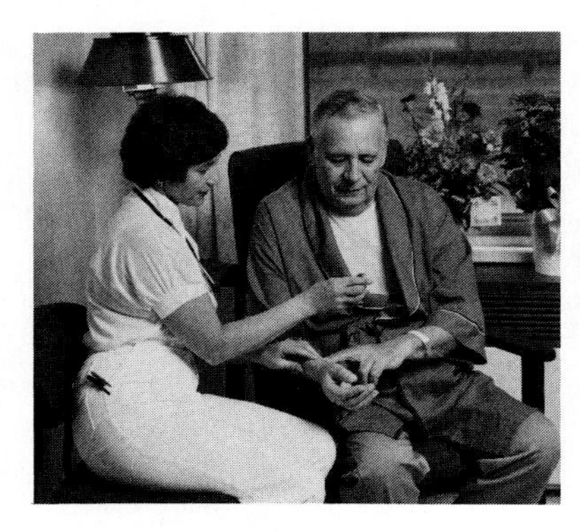

***Fig. 12-14***

| Steps | Rationale |
|---|---|
| 3. Demonstrate steps for palpating pulse: position body part, locate artery, use fingertips for palpation, compress artery, identify regular rate before counting, count pulse (method), calculate pulse (method). | Demonstration is best technique for teaching psychomotor skill. |
| 4. Have client perform each step with nurse's guidance (Fig. 12-14). | Nurse can correct any errors in technique as they occur. |
| 5. Discuss normal desired pulse range, purpose for monitoring pulse, and best time to assess pulse. | Client must be able to identify pulse alterations. |
| 6. Discuss importance of notifying physician and withholding medication dosage when pulse alterations occur. | Client must understand preventive measures to take if alterations in pulse develop. |

## Evaluation

| Steps | Rationale |
|---|---|
| 1. Have client independently demonstrate technique for pulse assessment and calculate pulse rate and rhythm. (Family member may assess client's pulse.) | Feedback through independent demonstration of psychomotor skill is best means of evaluating learning of skill. |
| 2. Ask client to identify reasons for assessing pulse, normal pulse rate range, and steps to take when abnormalities are found. | Measures client's cognitive learning. |

### *Expected outcomes*

| Steps | Rationale |
|---|---|
| 1. Client is able to measure own pulse rate and rhythm correctly. | Indicates skill effectively learned. |
| 2. Client identifies normal range of pulse rate. | Cognitive learning achieved. |
| 3. Client discusses importance of assessing pulse and best time for measurement. | |

### *Unexpected outcomes*

| Steps | Rationale |
|---|---|
| 1. Client is able to palpate pulse or count rate correctly. | May result from sensory alteration or inability to locate artery or palpate it correctly. Clients with preexisting arrhythmias often have difficulty learning to count pulse correctly. |
| 2. Client is unable to discuss information related to pulse assessment. | Anxiety, lack of interest, language barrier, or method of instruction may interfere with learning. |

## Recording and Reporting

| Steps | Rationale |
|---|---|
| 1. Record information taught and client's response in nurses' notes. | JCAHO requirement of health agencies is to document all client education: provides continuity between teaching sessions. |

## Follow-up Activities

| Steps | Rationale |
|---|---|
| 1. If home health nurse is visiting client, plan a repeat demonstration during a scheduled visit. | Provides excellent measure of client's ability to retain information. |

## Special Considerations

- Most difficult step is usually that of palpating artery. Client tends to obliterate pulse at first. Taking client's pulse can be effective way of showing how light palpation works best.
- Pulse rate is usually assessed before medications are taken and before and during exercise.
- Physician will recommend whether drug dosage should be withheld in event of pulse alteration.

## Teaching Considerations

- Nurse may demonstrate on self or family member. Using client for demonstration prevents client from being able to observe entire procedure. Nurse explains rationale for each step during demonstration.
- Instruct client or primary care giver to use finger tips, never to use thumb.
- Instruct use of gentle pressure, not to press hard over pulses.
- Instruct use of watch with a second hand to assess pulses.

## Home Care Considerations

- Bedroom or bath are two areas that provide privacy and are likely locations for client to store medications that require pulse measurement before administration.

# SKILL 12-5 Assessing a Client's Respirations

The movement of air between the environment and the lungs involves four complex but interrelated processes: *ventilation,* mechanical movement of air to and from the lungs; *conduction,* movement of air through the lungs' airways; *diffusion,* movement of $O_2$ and $CO_2$ between the alveoli and red blood cells; and *perfusion,* distribution of blood through the pulmonary capillaries. The nurse can directly assess ventilation only by observing the rate, depth, and rhythm of ventilatory movements.

Normal breathing is active and passive. The respiratory center in the brainstem regulates involuntary control of respirations. During quiet breathing the chest wall gently rises and falls. More energy is required during inspiration than during expiration. On inspiration impulses along the phrenic nerve cause the thin-walled diaphragm to contract, causing abdominal organs to move downward and forward thereby increasing the vertical dimension of the chest cavity. At the same time, the ribs lift upward and outward and the sternum lifts outward to aid the transverse expansion of the lungs. On expiration the diaphragm relaxes, the ribs and sternum return to their relaxed position, and the abdominal organs return to their original position (Fig. 12-15). Little energy is needed to expire air out of the lungs. Expiration is an active process only during exercise, voluntary hyperventilation, and certain disease states.

The nurse's assessment of respirations depends on recognition of normal thoracic and abdominal movements. Passive breathing is more diaphragmatic as the abdominal cavity slowly rises and falls. Contraction of the intercostal muscles between the ribs or of the accessory muscles in the neck and shoulders is not normally visible. During more active breathing the intercostal and accessory muscles work actively to move air in and out. The shoulders may rise and fall, and accessory muscles in the neck visibly contract.

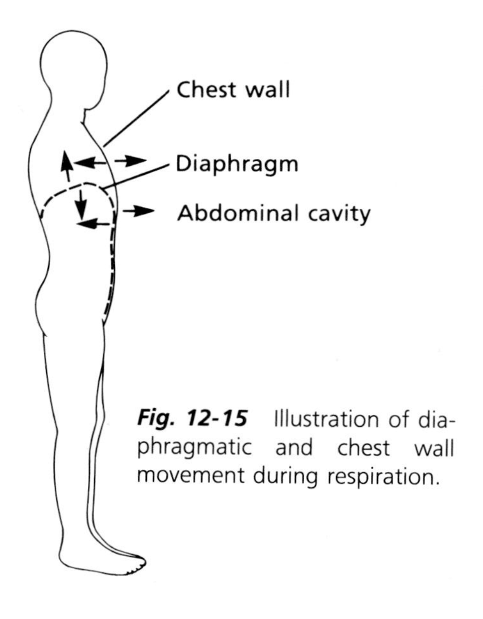


***Fig. 12-15*** Illustration of diaphragmatic and chest wall movement during respiration.

### Purposes

1. Obtain a baseline measure of respiration.
2. Assess respiratory status in relationship to respiratory and cardiovascular function.
3. Determine the influence of various pathologic conditions and therapies on respirations.

## Procedure 12-5

| Steps | Rationale |
| --- | --- |
| **Assessment** | |
| 1. Determine need to assess client's respirations: | |
| a. Note risk factors for alterations: fever, pain and anxiety, diseases of chest wall or muscles, constrictive chest or abdominal dressings, gastric distention, chronic obstructive pulmonary disease (emphysema, chronic bronchitis, asthma), traumatic injury to chest wall with or without collapse of underlying lung tissue, respiratory infection (pneumonia, acute bronchitis), pulmonary edema and emboli, head injury with damage to brainstem. | Certain conditions place client at risk for respiratory alterations and thus aid in early detection of alterations. |
| b. Assess for signs and symptoms of respiratory alterations: bluish or cyanotic appearance of nail beds, lips, mucous membranes, and skin; restlessness, irritability, confusion, reduced level of consciousness; pain during inspiration; dyspnea (labored or difficult breathing); adventitious breath sounds (Chapter 13); client feeling "short of breath"; thick or copious sputum produced on coughing. | Physical signs and symptoms may indicate alterations in respiratory status. |

| Steps | Rationale |
|---|---|
| 2. Assess for factors that normally influence character of respirations. | Allows nurse to accurately assess for presence and significance of respiratory alterations. |
| a. Age: newborn infant breathes at rate of 30-60 respirations min; child 2 yr old breathes 20-30 respirations min; child 6 yr old has rate of 18-26 respirations min; adults average 12-20 respirations min; with advancing age average respiratory rate increases. | |
| b. Exercise: respirations increase in rate and depth to improve oxygen delivery. | |
| c. Anxiety: respirations increase in rate, depth, with change in rhythm. | |
| d. Pain: alters rate, depth, and rhythm. | |
| e. Smoking: long-term smoking can cause permanent increase in average respiratory rate. | |
| f. Medications: narcotic analgesics, general anesthetics, and sedative-hypnotics depress respirations; bronchodilators cause dilation of airways that ultimately can slow respiratory rate. | |
| g. Postural changes: standing or sitting erect promotes full ventilatory movement and lung expansion; stooped or slumped posture impairs ventilatory movement; lying flat prevents full chest expansion. | |
| 3. Assess pertinent laboratory values: | |
| a. Arterial blood gases (ABGs): Normal ABGs (values may vary within institutions): pH 7.35-7.45; $Paco_2$ 35-45; $Pao_2$ 80-100; $Sao_2$ 94%-98%. | ABGs measure arterial blood pH, partial pressure of $O_2$ and $CO_2$, and arterial $O_2$ saturation, which reflects client's oxygenation status. |
| b. Complete blood count (CBC). Normal CBC for adults (values may vary within institutions): <br>▪ Hemoglobin: 14-18 g/100 ml males; 12-16 g/100 ml females. <br>▪ Hematocrit: 40%-54% males; 38%-47% females. <br>▪ Red blood cell count: 4.6-6.2 × $10^6$ microliter males; 4.2-5.4 × $10^6$ microliter female. | CBC measures red blood cell count, volume of red blood cells, and concentration of hemoglobin, which reflects client's capacity to carry $O_2$. |
| 4. Determine previous baseline respiratory rate (if available) from client's record. | Will allow nurse to identify if change has occurred in client's status. |

## Nursing Diagnosis

| Steps | Rationale |
|---|---|
| 1. Analyze client's physical signs and symptoms with respiration assessment findings to identify potential nursing diagnoses: | Additional data must be gathered to confirm nursing diagnoses. However, nurse's initial findings can direct more thorough assessment. |
| a. Ineffective airway clearance: related to fatigue. | Client unable to clear secretions. |
| b. Ineffective breathing pattern: related to pain, tracheobronchial obstruction. | Pattern of inhalation or exhalation is abnormal. |
| c. Impaired gas exchange: related to reduced hemoglobin levels. | An imbalance occurs between $O_2$ uptake and $CO_2$ elimination. |

## Planning

| Steps | Rationale |
|---|---|
| 1. Develop individualized goals for assessing client's respirations: | Provides for comparison with future assessments. |
| a. Establish baseline respiratory rate. | |
| b. Identify abnormalities in respiratory rate and rhythm. | Directs nurse to initiate supportive therapies. |
| c. Detect changes in respirations in response to selected therapies. | Directs nurse to initiate preventive therapies. |
| 2. Prepare needed equipment and supplies: | Necessary for accurate calculation of rate. |
| a. Wristwatch with second hand or digital display. | |
| b. Pen, pencil, and flow sheet or record form. | For timely recording. |
| 3. If client has been active, wait 5-10 min before assessing respirations. | Exercise increases respiratory rate and depth. Respirations should be assessed at rest to allow for objective comparison of values. |
| 4. Assess respirations as first vital sign in infant or child. | Avoids startling or arousing infant or child, which can falsely increase respiratory rates. |
| 5. Assess respirations after pulse measurement in adult. | Inconspicuous assessment of respirations immediately after pulse assessment prevents client from conscious attempt to control breathing. |

| Steps | Rationale |
|---|---|
| 6. Be sure client is in comfortable position, preferably sitting. | Position of discomfort may cause client to breathe more rapidly. Sitting erect promotes full ventilatory movement. |

## Implementation

| Steps | Rationale |
|---|---|
| 1. Be sure client's chest is visible. If necessary, move bed linen or gown. | Ensures clear view of chest wall and abdominal movements. |
| 2. Place client's arm in relaxed position across the abdomen or lower chest, or place your hand directly over client's upper abdomen (Fig. 12-16). | This position used during assessment of pulse allows nurse to be inconspicuous. Client's or nurse's hand rises and falls during respiratory cycle. |
| 3. Observe complete respiratory cycle (one inspiration and one expiration). | Rate is accurately determined only after nurse has viewed respiratory cycle. |
| 4. After cycle is observed, look at watch's second hand and begin to count rate: when sweep hand hits number on dial, begin time frame, counting *one* with first full respiratory cycle. | Timing begins with count of one. Respirations occur more slowly than pulse; thus timing does not begin with zero. |
| 5. If rhythm is regular in adult, count number of respirations in 30 sec and multiply by 2. In infant or young child count respirations for full min. | Respiratory rate is equivalent to number of respirations per min. Young infants and children normally breathe irregularly. |
| 6. If adult's respirations have irregular rhythm or are abnormally slow or fast, count for full min (Table 12-3). | Accurate interpretation with irregularities requires assessment for at least 1 min. |
| 7. Note depth of respirations. This can be assessed subjectively by observing degree of chest wall movement while counting rate. Nurse can also objectively assess depth by palpating chest wall excursion (Chapter 13) after rate has been counted. Depth is shallow, normal, or deep. | Depth of respirations helps reveal volume of air moving to and from lungs. Character of ventilatory movements may reveal specific alterations or disease status. |
| 8. Note rhythm of ventilatory cycle (Table 12-3). Normal breathing is regular and uninterrupted. Infants breathe less regularly. Young child may breathe slowly for a few sec and then suddenly breathe faster. Sighing should not be confused with abnormal rhythm. Periodically people unconsciously take single deep breaths or sighs to expand small airways prone to collapse. | Character of ventilations can reveal specific types of alterations. |

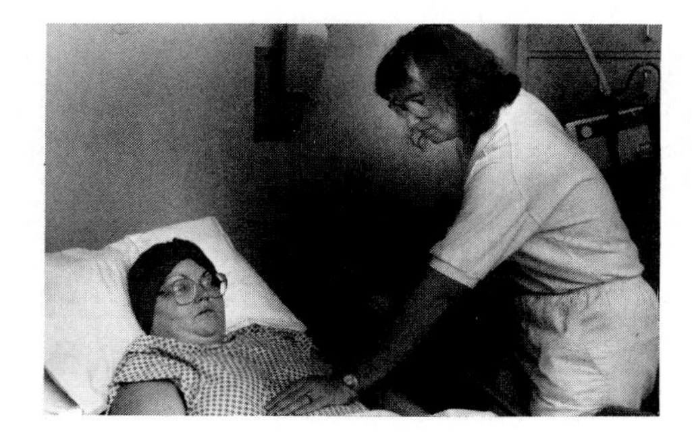

***Fig. 12-16***

| Steps | Rationale |
|---|---|
| 9. Replace client's gown and cover with bed linen. | Restores client's comfort. |
| 10. Wash hands. | Reduces transmission of microorganisms. |
| 11. Discuss findings with client as needed. | Promotes client's participation in care and understanding of health status. |

## Evaluation

| Steps | Rationale |
|---|---|
| 1. If respirations are assessed for first time establish as baseline. | Used to compare future respiratory assessments. |
| 2. Compare client's respirations with previous baseline and normal respiratory rate for age group. | Allows nurse to assess for change in client's condition and for presence of respiratory alterations. |

### *Expected outcomes*

| Steps | Rationale |
|---|---|
| 1. Respiratory rate is within normal range for client's age. Respirations are deep and regular. | Respiratory status is stable. |

### *Unexpected outcomes*

| Steps | Rationale |
|---|---|
| 1. Respiratory rate is above or below normal range for client's age.<br>2. Rhythm may be irregular.<br>3. Depth of respirations may be increased or decreased. | May indicate ventilatory or respiratory problems caused by pain, chest trauma, pulmonary or heart disease, medication side effects, neurologic disease. May result from pathologies or client's position. |

## Recording and Reporting

| Steps | Rationale |
|---|---|
| 1. Record respiratory rate on vital sign flow sheet (see Fig. 12-9) or medical record. | Vital signs should be recorded immediately for accuracy and inclusion in medical record. |

**TABLE 12-3** Alterations in Respiration

| Term | Description |
|---|---|
| **Bradypnea** | Rate of breathing is abnormally slow but regular. |
| **Tachypnea** | Rate of breathing is abnormally rapid but regular. |
| **Hyperpnea** | Respirations are increased in depth and rate. This occurs normally with exercise. |
| **Apnea** | Respirations cease for several seconds. Persistent cessation is called respiratory arrest. |
| **Hyperventilation** | Rate of ventilation exceeds normal metabolic requirements for exchange of respiratory gases. Rate and depth of respirations increase. There is an excessive intake of $O_2$ and blowing off of $CO_2$. |
| **Hypoventilation** | Volume of air entering the lungs is insufficient for the body's metabolic needs. Respiratory rate is below normal and depth of ventilation is depressed. There is decreased $O_2$ intake and $CO_2$ exhalation. |
| **Cheyne-Stokes respiration** | Respiratory rhythm is irregular, characterized by alternating periods of apnea and hyperventilation. The respiratory cycle begins with slow, shallow breaths that gradually increase to abnormal depth and rapidity. Gradually breathing slows and becomes shallower, climaxing in a 10-20 second period of apnea before respiration resumes. |
| **Kussmaul respiration** | Respirations are abnormally deep but regular, similar to hyperventilation. This is characteristic of clients with diabetic ketoacidosis. |
| **Dyspnea** | Breathing is difficult and characterized by increased effort to inhale and exhale. Active use of intercostal and accessory muscles. |
| **Sighing** | Not to be confused with abnormal ventilatory rhythm, a sigh is a protective physiologic mechanism for expanding small airways and alveoli not used during a normal tidal breath. |
| **Orthopnea** | Respiratory condition in which a person must sit or stand in order to breathe deeply or comfortably. |

| Steps | Rationale |
|---|---|
| 2. Record any accompanying signs and symptoms of respiratory alterations in nurses notes on flow sheet. | |
| 3. Report abnormal findings to nurse in charge or physician. | Abnormalities may indicate need for immediate medical therapy. |

## Follow-up Activities

| Steps | Rationale |
|---|---|
| 1. If abnormalities are present, physician may order diagnostic tests, e.g., chest x-ray examination (Chapter 46) or arterial blood gas determinations (Chapter 45). | Diagnostic tests provide additional evidence for determining cause or nature of abnormalities. |
| 2. Assist client to semi-Fowler's or Fowler's position (unless contraindicated by client's condition). | Position maximizes ventilatory movement. |
| 3. If client has artificial airway, maintain its patency (Chapter 16). | Maintains delivery of $O_2$ to airways. |
| 4. If client exhibits signs or symptoms of respiratory distress, provide $O_2$ as ordered by physician. | With increased concentration of $O_2$ to alveoli, gas diffusion is improved. |

## Special Considerations

- Client's physical condition may restrict positioning for assessment.
- Nurse can simply observe infant or young child while chest and abdomen are exposed.
- Infant's respirations are primarily diaphragmatic and thus observed by abdominal movement.
- Clients with chest or abdominal pain frequently splint chest wall movement to minimize discomfort, thus decreasing depth of breathing. Aging causes ossification of costal carti-

lage and downward slant of ribs, resulting in more rigid rib cage, which reduces chest wall expansion. Normal kyphosis and scoliosis that occur with aging may also restrict chest expansion.
- Normal respiratory rate for given age is best basis for comparison if client's baseline rate has been abnormal.
- *Do not* administer high concentrations of $O_2$ to client with chronic lung disease. This may depress respirations.
- Normal average respiratory rates by age:

| AGE | RATE/MIN |
|---|---|
| Newborn | 35 |
| 1-11 mo | 30 |
| 2 years | 25 |
| 4 years | 23 |
| 6 years | 21 |
| 10 years | 19 |
| 14 years | 18 |
| 18 years | 16-18 |
| Adult | 19-20 |

### Teaching Considerations

- Clients who demonstrate decreased ventilation may benefit from being taught deep breathing and coughing exercises (Chapter 39)
- Advise family member to count client's respiratory rate when client is unaware of being observed. If client is aware of the assessment, respiratory rate may be altered.
- Instruct family member to contact home care nurse if unusual fluctuations in respiratory rate occur.

### Home Care Considerations

- Assess for environmental factors in the home that may influence client's respiratory rate.

## *SKILL 12-6 Assessing Arterial Blood Pressure*

Blood pressure (BP) is the force exerted by the blood against the vessel wall. The standard unit for measuring BP is millimeters of mercury (mm Hg). The measurement indicates the height to which the BP can raise a column of mercury. During a normal cardiac cycle BP reaches a peak that is followed by a trough or low point in the cycle. The peak or maximum pressure occurs during systole as the left ventricle pumps blood into the aorta. The trough occurs during diastole as the ventricles relax. Diastolic pressure is the minimal pressure exerted against the arterial walls at all times. The nurse records BP with the systolic reading before the diastolic (for example, 120/80). The difference between systolic and diastolic pressure is the pulse pressure. If the BP is 120/80 the pulse pressure is 40 mm HG.

BP reflects various hemodynamic factors within the circulatory system. It is a product of cardiac output (CO) and peripheral vascular resistance (R):

$$BP = CO \times R.$$

When volume increases in an enclosed space, pressure in that space rises. As cardiac output increases, more blood is pumped against the arterial walls, causing BP to rise.

When vascular resistance increases, BP rises. The size of arteries and arterioles changes to adjust blood flow to the needs of local tissues. The smaller the lumen of a vessel, the greater its peripheral vascular resistance to blood flow. When blood flow to a major organ falls sharply, peripheral arteries constrict to shunt blood to the major vessels supplying the organ. Arterial pressure rises to push blood through narrowed vessels. In contrast, as vessels dilate and vascular resistance falls, BP drops.

The volume of blood circulating within the vascular system affects BP. Normally blood volume remains constant; 5000 ml in an adult. However, if volume increases, such as after a rapid IV infusion, pressure exerted against arterial walls rises. When circulating blood volume falls, as in the case of hemorrhage or dehydration, BP falls. Other hemodynamic variables that can affect BP include blood viscosity and arterial distensibility.

### HYPERTENSION

In certain diseases such as arteriosclerosis the arterial walls lose their elasticity and are replaced by fibrous tissue that cannot stretch well. With reduced elasticity there is greater resistance to blood flow. As blood is forced through rigid arterial walls, BP rises. Systolic pressure is more significantly elevated than diastolic because of reduced arterial elasticity.

Hypertension is a major factor underlying death, heart attack, and strokes in the United States and Canada. The American Medical Association's Joint National Committee on Detection, Evaluation, and Treatment of High Blood Pressure (1984) has set criteria for determining categories of hypertension (Table 12-4). The diagnosis of hypertension in adults is made when an average of two or

***TABLE 12-4*** Classification of Blood Pressure

| Range (mm Hg) | Category |
|---|---|
| **Diastolic** | |
| <85 | Normal blood pressure |
| 85-89 | High normal blood pressure |
| 90-104 | Mild hypertension |
| 105-114 | Moderate hypertension |
| ≥115 | Severe hypertension |
| **Systolic, when diastolic BP is <90** | |
| <140 | Normal blood pressure |
| 140-159 | Borderline isolated systolic hypertension |
| ≥160 | Isolated systolic hypertension |

From The Joint National Committee on Detection, Evaluation, and Treatment of High Blood Pressure: The 1984 report of the Joint National Committee on Detection, Evaluation, and Treatment of High Blood Pressure, Arch Intern Med 144:1045, May 1984. Copyright 1984, American Medical Association.

***TABLE 12-5*** Follow-Up Criteria for First-Occasion Measurement

| Range (mm Hg) | Recommended Follow-Up |
|---|---|
| **Diastolic** | |
| <85 | Recheck within 2 years |
| 85-89 | Recheck within 1 year |
| 90-104 | Confirm promptly (not to exceed 2 months) |
| 105-114 | Evaluate or refer to source of care (not to exceed 2 weeks) |
| ≥115 | Evaluate or refer immediately to a source of care |
| **Systolic, when diastolic pressure is 90** | |
| <140 | Recheck within 2 years |
| 140-199 | Confirm promptly (not to exceed 2 months) |
| ≥200 | Evaluate or refer promptly to source of care (not to exceed 2 weeks) |

From The Joint National Committee on Detection, Evaluation, and Treatment of High Blood Pressure: The 1984 report of the Joint National Committee on Detection, Evaluation and Treatment of High Blood Pressure, Arch Intern Med 144:1045, May 1984. Copyright 1984, American Medical Association.

more diastolic readings on at least two subsequent visits is 90 mm Hg or higher or when the average of multiple systolic BP on two or more subsequent visits is consistently higher than 140 mm Hg. One BP recording does not qualify as a diagnosis of hypertension. However, if the nurse assesses a high reading (for example, 150/90 mm HG), the client should be encouraged to return for another checkup within 2 months (Table 12-5).

## BLOOD PRESSURE EQUIPMENT

Special mention is needed for describing the equipment used in measuring arterial BP. A sphygmomanometer is a pressure manometer with an occlusive cloth cuff that encloses an inflatable rubber bladder (Fig. 12-17). A pressure bulb with a release valve inflates the bladder. There are two types of manometers: aneroid and mercury.

The aneroid manometer has a glass-enclosed circular gauge containing a needle that registers millimeter calibrations. A metal bellows within the gauge expands and collapses in response to pressure variations in the inflated bladder. Metal parts in the aneroid manometer are subject to temperature expansion and contraction; thus the instrument is not as reliable as a mercury manometer. Before a nurse can use an aneroid manometer, the needle should point to zero and the instrument should be correctly calibrated.

The mercury manometer is an upright tube containing mercury. Pressure created by inflation of the bladder moves the column of mercury upward against the force of gravity. Millimeter calibrations mark the height of the mercury column. The instrument is the most accurate of the sphygmomanometers. To ensure accurate readings,

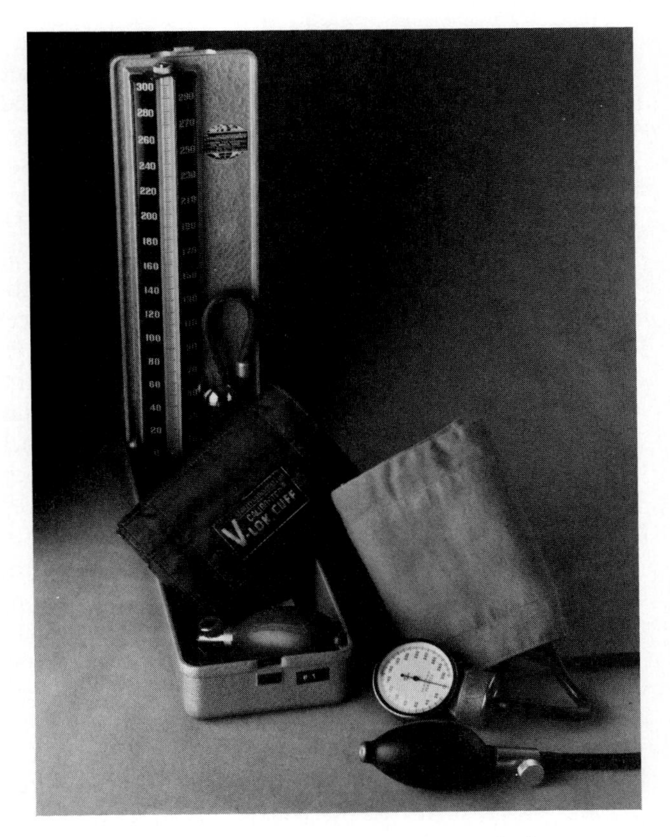


***Fig. 12-17*** Sphygmomanometer is composed of pressure manometer, cloth cuff with rubber bladder, and pressure bulb. Mercury manometer is at left, aneroid manometer at right.

**TABLE 12-6** Common Mistakes in Blood Pressure Assessment

| Error | Effect |
|---|---|
| Bladder or cuff too wide | False low reading |
| Bladder or cuff too narrow | False high reading |
| Cuff wrapped too loosely | False high reading |
| Deflating cuff too slowly | False high diastolic reading |
| Deflating cuff too quickly | False low systolic and false high diastolic reading |
| Stethoscope that fits poorly or impairment of the examiner's hearing, causing sounds to be muffled | False low systolic and false high diastolic reading |
| Inaccurate inflation level | False low systolic reading |
| Multiple examiners using different Korotkoff sounds for diastolic readings | Inaccurate interpretation of systolic and diastolic readings |

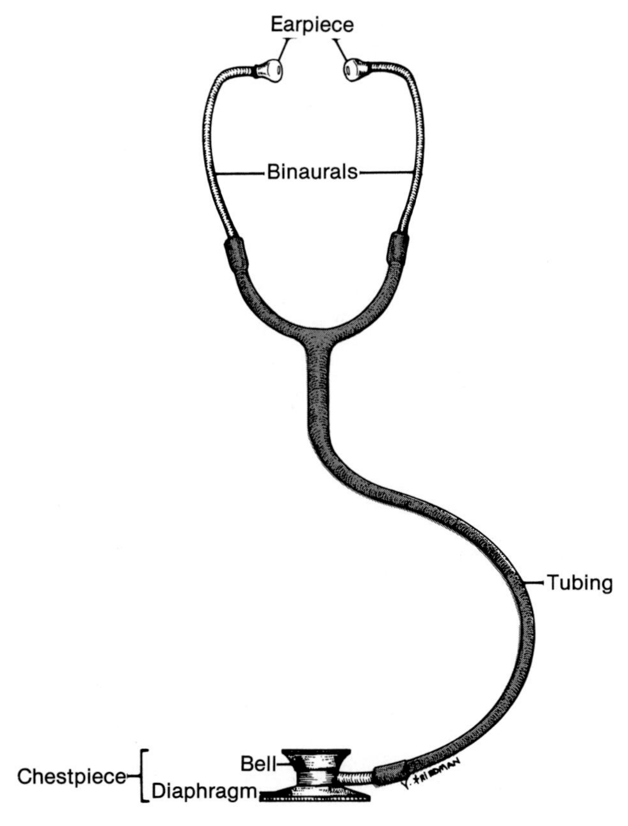


*Fig. 12-18* Acoustical stethoscope.

the mercury column should always be at zero when the cuff is deflated, and it should fall freely when pressure is released.

Cuffs come in several different sizes (newborn to extra large). Ideally width of the cuff should be 40% of the circumference (or 20% wider than the diameter) of the midpoint of the limb on which the cuff is to be used (American Heart Association, 1980). Length of the enclosed bladder should be approximately twice the recommended width. A bladder of this length nearly encircles the arm and minimizes the risk of misapplication. In an adult the average bladder width is 12 to 13 cm and the length is 22 to 23 cm. An improperly fitting cuff produces inaccurate BP readings (Table 12-6).

The stethoscope is used to auscultate sound waves created by the arterial pulse (Fig. 12-18). It is a closed cylinder that prevents dissipation of sound waves as they reach the body's surface and amplifies them for the examiner. The four major parts of the stethoscope are the earpieces, binaurals, plastic or rubber tubing, and chestpiece.

Earpieces should fit snugly and comfortably in the nurse's ears. Binaurals should be angled and strong enough to keep the earpieces in place without causing discomfort. The earpieces follow the contour of the ear canal for best sound reception. For most persons the earpieces should point toward the face when put on.

The tubing should be flexible and 30 to 40 cm (12 to 18 in) in length. Longer tubing decreases sound transmission through the stethoscope. The tubing should be thick walled to help eliminate transmission of noises caused by rubbing of the tubing against other surfaces.

The chestpiece consists of a bell and diaphragm. The diaphragm is a circular flat-surfaced portion of the chestpiece and has a thin plastic disk on its end. It transmits high-pitched sounds best, such as bowel and lung sounds. The examiner holds the diaphragm firmly against the skin for full sound amplification. The bell is the cone-shaped portion of the chestpiece. It transmits low-pitched sounds, such as heart and vascular sounds. The bell must be held lightly against the skin for sound amplification. The bell and diaphragm are rotated into position on the chestpiece depending on which part the nurse chooses to use.

## Purposes

1. Maintain a baseline measure of arterial pressure.
2. Assess the hemodynamic status of a client.
3. Monitor response of the circulatory system to various pathologic conditions and therapies.

## Procedure 12-6

| Steps | Rationale |
|---|---|
| **Assessment** | |
| 1. Determine need to assess client's BP. | |
| a. Note risk factors: history of cardiovascular disease, history of renal disease, history of diabetes mellitus, circulatory shock (hypovolemic, septic, cardiogenic, or neurogenic), acute or chronic pain, rapid IV infusion of fluids or blood products, increased intracranial pressure, postoperatively. | Certain conditions place clients at risk for BP alterations. |
| b. Observe for signs and symptoms of BP alterations. ▪ High BP (hypertension): often asymptomatic until pressure is very high, headache (usually occipital), flushing of face, nosebleed, elderly client notices fatigue. ▪ Low BP (hypotension): dizziness; mental confusion, restlessness; pale, dusky, or cyanotic skin and mucous membranes; cool, mottled skin over extremities. | Physical signs and symptoms may indicate alterations in arterial BP. |
| c. Determine client's age. | BP is not a routine part of assessment in children under 3 yr. |
| 2. Assess for factors that normally influence BP. a. Age: normal average BP varies throughout life. b. Stimulation: sympathetic nerve stimulation resulting from pain, anxiety, or fear causes arterial pressure to rise. c. Sex: no difference in BP exists between preadolescent boys and girls. Postpubescent males have higher readings because of hormonal influences; during and after menopause women have higher pressures than men of same age. d. Medications: antihypertensives and antiarrhythmics lower BP, narcotic analgesics and general anesthetics can also cause hypotension, diuretics reduce body's fluid volume and thus lower pressure. e. Daily (diurnal) variation: BP varies throughout day; pressure is lowest in early morning, rises during morning and afternoon, and peaks in late afternoon or evening. f. Exercise: increase in cardiac output raises BP. g. Postural change: BP can fall as person moves from lying to sitting or standing position; normally, variations are minimal. h. Smoking: resultant vasoconstriction causes BP to rise. | Allows nurse to accurately assess presence and significance of BP changes. |
| 3. Determine best site for BP assessment. Avoid applying cuff to arm when IV catheter is in antecubital fossa and IV fluids are infusing, in the presence of arteriovenous shunt, when breast or axillary surgery has been performed on that side, if arm or hand has been traumatized or diseased, in presence of lower arm cast or bulky bandage. | Inappropriate site selection may result in poor amplification of sounds, causing inaccurate readings. Application of pressure from inflated bladder can temporarily impair blood flow and compromise circulation in extremity that already has impaired circulation. |
| 4. Determine previous baseline BP (if available) from client's record. | Will allow nurse to identify if change has occurred in client's status. |
| **Nursing Diagnosis** | |
| 1. Assess client's history and physical signs and symptoms. If client is taking antihypertensives, review medication schedule. Potential nursing diagnoses may include: | Additional data must be gathered to confirm diagnoses. |
| a. Altered health maintenance: related to poor compliance with therapies. | Medications to control BP not taken regularly. |
| b. Knowledge deficit regarding BP control: related to inexperience. | Client will require education. |
| c. Altered tissue perfusion: related to reduced BP. | Results when BP is critically low. |
| **Planning** | |
| 1. Develop individualized goals for assessing client's BP: | |
| a. Establish baseline systolic and diastolic readings. | Provides comparison with future BP assessment. |

| Steps | Rationale |
|---|---|
| b. Identify abnormalities in BP. | Directs nurse to provide supportive care. |
| c. Detect changes in BP in response to selected therapies. | Directs nurse to pursue preventive therapies. |
| 2. Prepare needed equipment and supplies and make sure they are in working order: | |
| a. Mercury sphygmomanometer: control valve should be clear and freely adjustable; when closed, valve should hold mercury constant; when released, valve allows controlled fall in mercury level; air vent at top of mercury manometer should be patent; rubber tubing connecting bladder to manometer should be at least 80 cm (32 in) long and with airtight connections. | Used to measure arterial BP indirectly. Accurate measurements depend on functional equipment. |
| b. Bladder and cuff: bladder should completely encircle arm without overlapping; tapering cuff should be long enough to encircle arm several times. | Secure-fitting cuff and proper-sized bladder are required to exert equal pressure around artery being auscultated. Too narrow bladder causes false high reading. |
| c. Stethoscope. | Auscultates arterial pressure waves. |
| d. Pen, pencil, and flow sheet or record form. | Provide for timely documentation of findings. |
| 3. Encourage client to avoid exercise and smoking for 30 min before assessment. | These factors can cause false elevations in BP. |
| 4. Have client assume sitting or lying position. Be sure room is warm and quiet. | Maintains client's comfort during measurement. |
| 5. Explain procedure to client and have client rest at least 5 min before measurement. | Reduces anxiety that can falsely elevate readings. BP readings taken at different times can be objectively compared when all are assessed with client at rest. |
| **Implementation** | |
| ***Auscultation*** | |
| 1. Wash hands. | Reduces transmission of microorganisms. |
| 2. Support client's forearm (while client is sitting or lying) at heart level with palm turned up (Fig. 12-19). | If arm is unsupported, client may perform isometric exercise that can increase diastolic pressure 10%. Placement of arm above heart level causes false low reading. |
| 3. Expose upper arm fully by removing constricting clothing. | Ensures proper cuff application. |
| 4. Palpate brachial artery (Fig. 12-20). Position cuff 2.5 cm (1 in) above site of brachial pulsation (antecubital space). Center bladder of cuff above artery (Fig. 12-21). | Inflating bladder directly over brachial artery ensures proper pressure is applied during inflation. |
| 5. With cuff fully deflated, wrap cuff evenly and snugly around upper arm (Fig. 12-22). | Loose-fitting cuff causes false high readings. |
| 6. Be sure manometer is positioned vertically at eye level. Observer should be no further than 1 m (approximately 1 yd) away. | Eye level placement ensures accurate reading of mercury level. |
| 7. Palpate brachial or radial artery with fingertips of one hand while inflating cuff rapidly to pressure 30 mm Hg above point at which pulse disappears. Slowly deflate cuff and note point when pulse reappears. | Identifies approximate systolic pressure and determines maximal inflation point for accurate reading. Prevents auscultatory gap. |
| 8. Deflate cuff fully and wait 30 sec. | Prevents venous congestion and false high readings. |
| 9. Place stethoscope earpieces in ears and be sure sounds are clear, not muffled. | Each earpiece should follow angle of ear canal to facilitate hearing. |
| 10. Relocate brachial artery and place bell or diaphragm chestpiece over it. Do not allow chestpiece to touch cuff or clothing (Fig. 12-23). | Proper stethoscope placement ensures optimal sound reception. Stethoscope improperly positioned causes muffled sounds that often result in false low systolic and false high diastolic readings. |
| 11. Close valve of pressure bulb clockwise until tight. | Tightening of valve prevents air leak during inflation. |
| 12. Inflate cuff to 30 mm Hg above palpated systolic pressure. | Ensures accurate measurement of systolic pressure. |
| 13. Slowly release valve and allow mercury to fall at rate of 2 to 3 mm Hg/sec. | Too rapid or slow a decline in mercury level can cause inaccurate readings. |
| 14. Note point on manometer when first clear sound is heard. | First Korotkoff sound indicates systolic pressure. |
| 15. Continue to deflate cuff gradually, noting point at which muffled or dampened sound appears. | Fourth Korotkoff sound involves distinct muffling of sounds and is recommended by American Heart Association as indication of diastolic pressure in children. |
| 16. Continue cuff deflation, noting point on manometer at which sound disappears. (Note pressure to nearest 2 mm Hg.) | American Heart Association recommends recording fifth Korotkoff sound as diastolic pressure in adults. |
| 17. Deflate cuff rapidly and completely. Remove from client's arm unless you plan to repeat measurement. | Continuous cuff inflation causes arterial occlusion, resulting in numbness and tingling of client's arm. |

**Steps** | **Rationale**

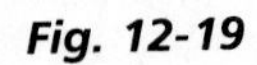
*Fig. 12-19*

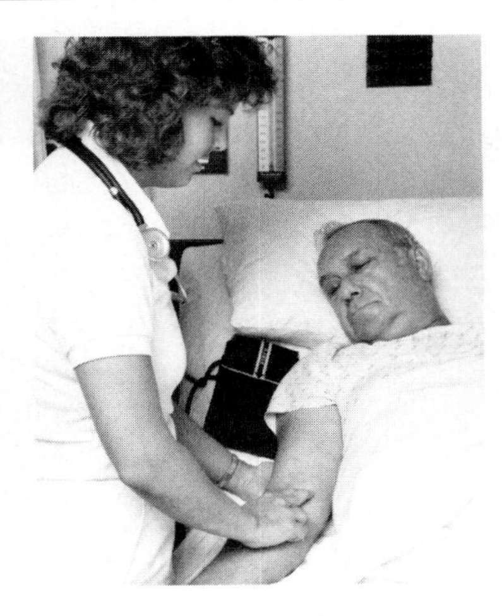
*Fig. 12-20*

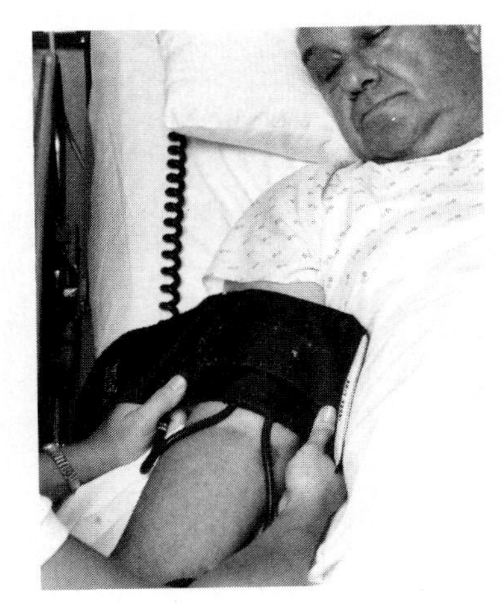
*Fig. 12-21*

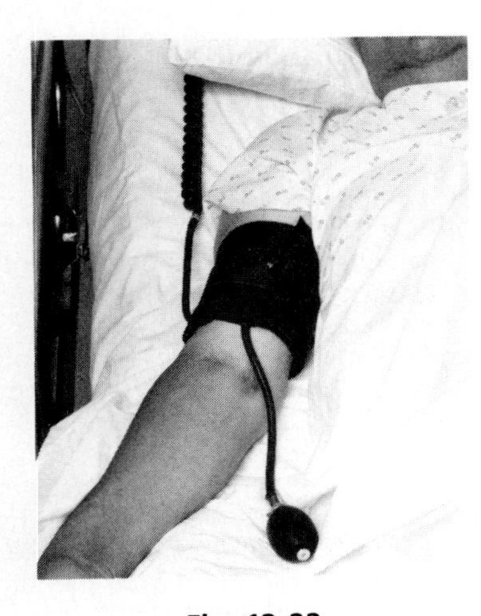
*Fig. 12-22*

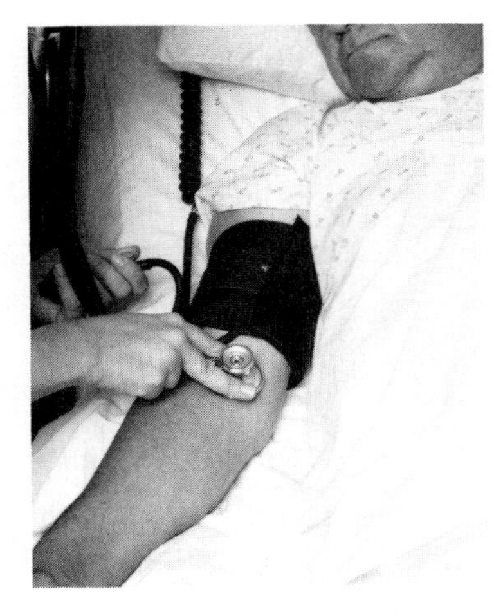
*Fig. 12-23*

18. If this is first assessment of client, repeat procedure on other arm.
    Comparison of pressure in both arms serves to detect any circulatory problems. (Normal difference of 5-10 mm Hg exists between arms.) First measurement should be an average of 2 or more measurements with the client positioned comfortably.
19. Assist client in returning to comfortable position and cover upper arm if previously clothed.
    Restores client's comfort.
20. Inform client of BP reading.
    Promotes participation in care and understanding of health status.
21. Wash hands.
    Reduces transmission of microorganisms.

### *Palpation*

1. Follow Steps 1-6 of auscultation method.
2. Palpate brachial or radial artery with fingertips of one hand. Inflate cuff to a pressure 30 mm Hg above point at which pulse disappears.
   Ensures accurate detection of true systolic pressure once pressure valve is released.
3. Slowly deflate cuff, allowing mercury to fall 2 mm Hg per sec.
   Too rapid or slow a decline can result in inaccurate readings.
4. As soon as pulse is again palpable, note manometer reading.
   Reading is the systolic pressure by palpation.
5. Deflate cuff rapidly and completely. Remove from client's arm unless reassessment is necessary.
   Continuous cuff inflation causes arterial occlusion, resulting in numbness and tingling of client's arm.
6. Assist client in returning to comfortable position and cover upper arm if previously clothed.
   Restores client's comfort.
7. Wash hands.
   Reduces transmission of microorganisms.

| Steps | Rationale |
|---|---|

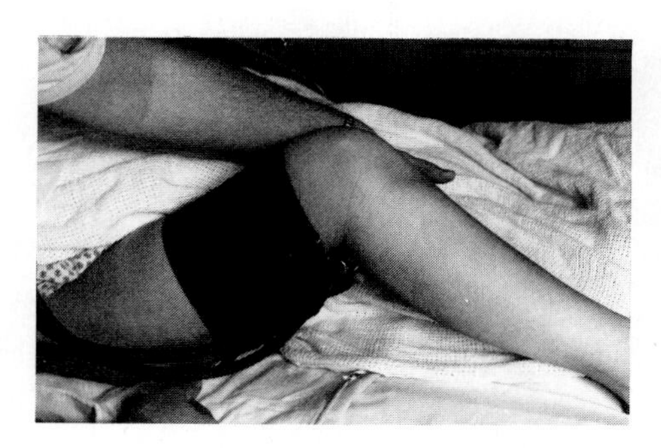

*Fig. 12-24*

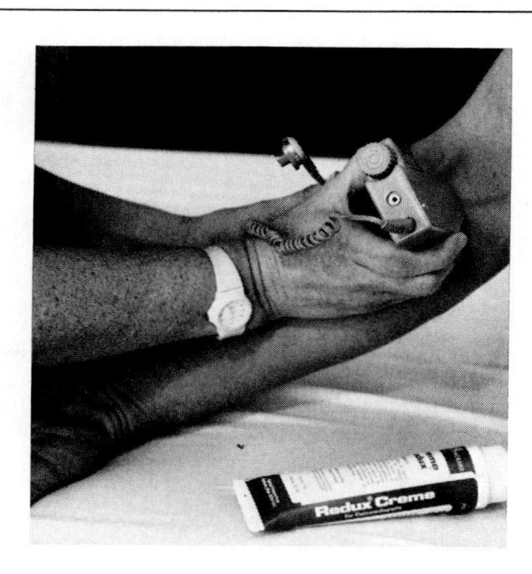


*Fig. 12-25*

***Auscultation in lower extremities***

| Steps | Rationale |
|---|---|
| 1. Wash hands. | Reduces transmission of microorganisms. |
| 2. Assist client to prone position. If unable to assume position, assist client to supine position with knee slightly flexed. | Prone position provides best access to popliteal artery. |
| 3. Remove any constricting clothing from leg. | Ensures proper cuff application. |
| 4. Locate popliteal artery behind knee (Fig. 12-24). | Artery palpation site lies just below client's thigh, making it suitable site for application rather than more distal artery such as dorsalis pedis. |
| 5. Apply large leg cuff 2.5 cm (1 in) snugly above artery around posterior aspect of middle thigh. Center arrows marked on cuff over artery. | Proper cuff size is necessary for accurate reading. Cuff that is too narrow causes false high readings. |
| 6. Follow Steps 6-18 of auscultation method, using popliteal artery. | |
| 7. Note systolic and diastolic pressures. | Systolic BP in legs may be 10-40 mm Hg higher than in upper extremities because of pressure needed for blood to reach periphery. Diastolic BP may be the same or lower. |
| 8. Assist client in returning to comfortable position. | Restores client's comfort. |
| 9. Inform client of BP reading. | Promotes client's participation in care and understanding of health status. |
| 10. Wash hands. | Reduces transmission of microorganisms. |

## Evaluation

| Steps | Rationale |
|---|---|
| 1. If BP is inaudible or difficult to obtain, wait 1-2 min and repeat assessment. | Prevents venous congestion and false high readings. |
| 2. If pressure is still inaudible or difficult to obtain, try alternative methods: use other arm, attempt palpation, measure pressure in legs, use Doppler or ultrasound stethoscope (Fig. 12-25). | Alternative methods can provide accurate measurements of arterial pressure. |
| 3. Identify reading as baseline or compare BP reading with previous baseline and normal average pressure for client's age. | Initial reading establishes baseline. Comparison reveals change in client's condition and presence of BP alterations. |

## Expected Outcomes

| Steps | Rationale |
|---|---|
| 1. BP is within normal average range for client's age. | Cardiovascular status is normal. |

## Unexpected Outcomes

| Steps | Rationale |
|---|---|
| 1. BP is above or below expected normal range for client's age. | Indicates potential for alterations in peripheral vascular resistance, blood volume, and cardiac function, e.g., circulatory shock. |

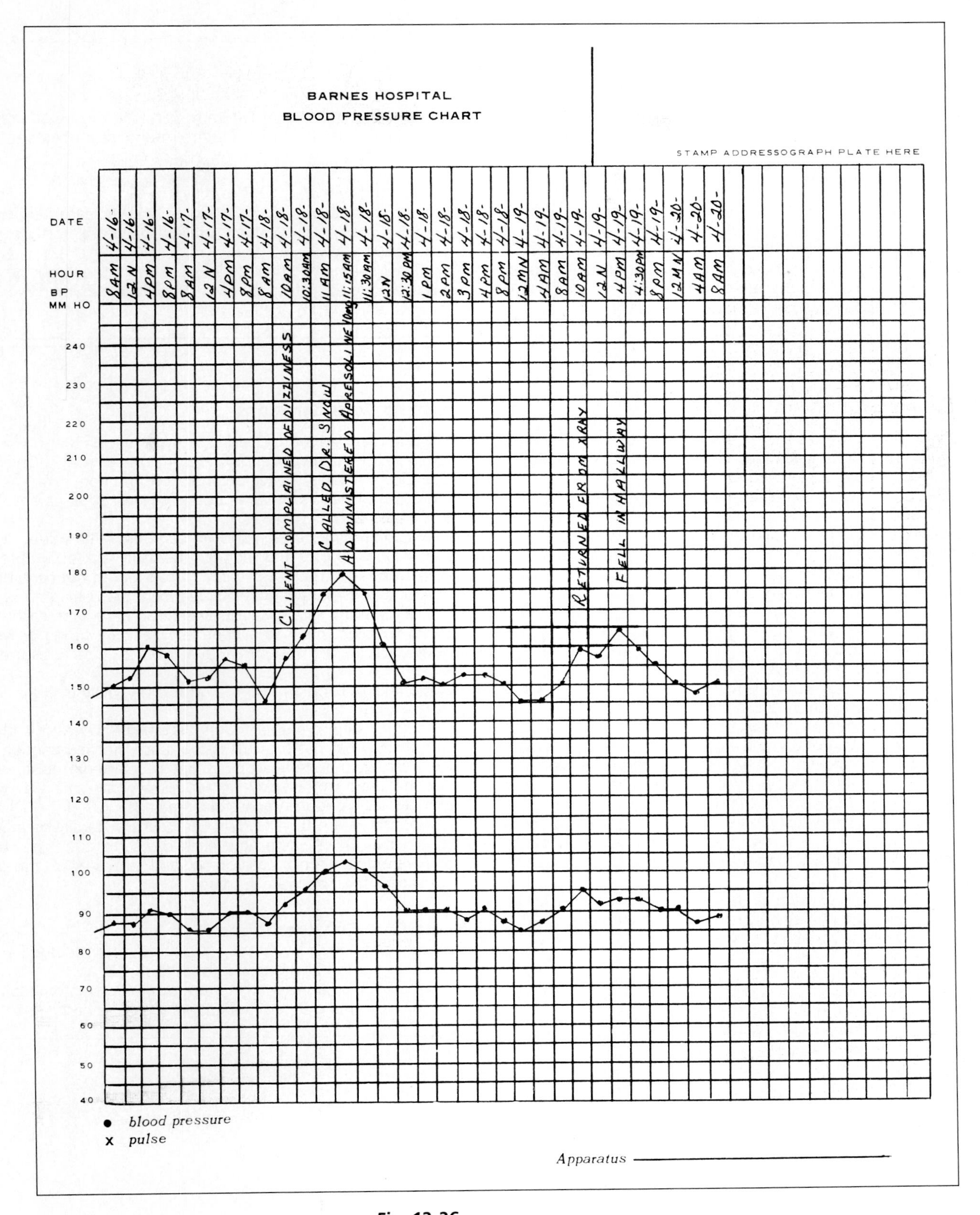


**Fig. 12-26**
Courtesy Barnes Hospital, St. Louis.

| Steps | Rationale |
|---|---|
| **Recording and Reporting** | |
| 1. Record BP in medical record or flow sheet (Fig. 12-26). | Vital signs should be recorded immediately to ensure accuracy. |
| 2. Report abnormal findings to nurse in charge or physician. | Abnormalities may necessitate immediate medical therapy. |
| **Follow-up Activities** | |
| 1. Client who is hypotensive may have various therapies ordered by physician, e.g., increased infusion of IV fluids or vasopressor medications. Client is placed in supine position. | Fluids increase blood volume. Vasopressors increase peripheral vascular resistance. Position prevents postural (orthostatic) hypotension. |
| 2. Client with hypertension may have various therapies ordered by physician, e.g., antihypertensives, control or reduction in IV fluid infusion, or administration of diuretics. | Individual or combined therapy lowers BP by either reducing peripheral vascular resistance or circulating blood volume. |

## Special Considerations

- Take BP in child before anxiety-producing tests or procedures are performed. At times it may be unrealistic to wait 5 min to assess BP. In emergency situations, do not wait.
- As long as cuff is inflated client will feel numbness or tingling in arm due to reduced blood flow.
- Pressures should be recorded to near 2 mm Hg.
- Average measurements:
  1. Width of bladder:
     a. Adult: 12-13 cm (4.8-5.2 in)
     b. Obese arm: 15-16 cm (6-6.4 in)
     c. Infant: 6.8 cm (2.4-3.2 in)
  2. Length of bladder:
     a. Adult: 22-24 cm (8.8-9.6 in)
     b. Obese arm: 30 cm (12 in)
     c. Infant: 12-13 cm (4.8-5.4 in)
- When a child reaches adolescence, BP varies by body size. Normal range for 13-18 yr olds at the 90th percentile is 124-136/77-84 for boys and 124-127/63-74 for girls. The standard norm for a healthy middle aged-adult is 120/80. An older adult's BP range is normally 140-160/80-90.
- Auscultation in lower extremities is also used when brachial artery is inaccessible, e.g., with casts or IV lines. Also used in clients with certain BP abnormalities so that nurse can compare BP in arms and legs.
- Average leg cuff for adult is 18 cm (7.2 in) wide and 36 cm (14.4 in) long. Child may only require adult's arm cuff.

## Teaching Considerations

- Educate client about their risks for hypertension. Persons with family history of hypertension are at significant risk. Obesity, cigarette smoking, heavy alcohol consumption, high blood cholesterol levels, and continued exposure to stress are factors linked to hypertension.
- Clients with hypertension should learn about BP values, long term follow-up care and therapy, the usual lack of symptoms (it can't be felt), therapy's ability to control but not cure, benefits of a consistently followed treatment plan.
- Instruct primary care giver to take BP at same time each day and after client has had a brief rest. Take BP sitting or lying down, use same position and arm each time pressure is taken.
- Avoid taking BP on arm with IV, arm injury, dialysis shunt, and mastectomy.
- Instruct primary care giver that if it is difficult to hear the pressure, it may be that the cuff is too loose, not big enough or too narrow, the stethoscope is not over arterial pulse, cuff was deflated too quickly or too slowly, or cuff was not pumped high enough for systolic readings.
- Clients may learn to take own BP. Client or family members should take BP at same time each day, after client has had brief rest. Instruction, positioning, and selection of arm site are causes for inaccurate readings.

## Home Care Considerations

- Assess home noise level to determine the room that will provide the quietest environment for assessing BP.
- Assess family's financial ability to afford a sphygmomanometer for performing BP evaluations on a regular basis.

## BIBLIOGRAPHY

American Heart Association: Recommendations for human blood pressure determination by sphygmomanometers, Dallas, 1980, The Association.

American Medical Association: The 1984 report of the Joint National Committee on detection, evaluation, and treatment of high blood pressure, Arch Intern Med 144:1045, May 1986.

Baker NC, et al: The effect of type of thermometer and length of time inserted on oral temperature measurements of afebrile subjects, Nurs Res 33:109, March-April, 1984.

Blainey CG: Site selection in taking body temperatures, Am J Nurs 74:1859, 1974.

Bulau J: Clinical policies and procedures for home health care, Rockville, 1986, Aspen Publishers, Inc.

Centers for Disease Control: Recommendations for prevention of HIV transmission in health care settings, Morbidity and Mortality Weekly Report (Suppl) 36:55, Aug 1987.

Ebersole P, Hess P: Toward healthy aging: human needs and nursing response, ed 3, St. Louis, 1989, The CV Mosby Co.

Electronic thermometers, the better alternative? Health Dev. 12:18, 1982.

Eoff MJ, Joyce B: Temperature measurements in children, Am J Nurs 81:1010, 1981.

Erickson R: Oral temperature differences in relation to thermometer and technique, Nurs Res 29:157, 1980.

Felton CL: Hypoxemia and oral temperatures, Am J Nurs 78:57, 1978.

Golden S: Nursing a loved one at home, Philadelphia, 1988, Running Press Book Publishers.

Graves RD, Markarian MF: Three-minute time interval when using an oral mercury-in-glass thermometer with or without J-temp sheaths, Nurs Res 29:323, 1980.

Guerevich I: Fever; when to worry about it, RN 48:14, Dec. 1985.

Guyton AC: Textbook of medical physiology, ed 6, Philadelphia, 1986, WB Saunders Co.

Higgins P: Can 98.6° be a fever in disguise? Geriatr Nurs 4:101, 1983.

Nichols GA, Kucha DH: Taking adult temperatures: oral measurement, Am J Nurs 72:1090, 1972.

Petersdorf RC: Disturbances of heat regulation. In Isselbacher KJ, et al, editors: Harrison's principles of internal medicine, ed 9, New York, 1980, McGraw Hill Book Co.

Potter PA, Perry AG: Fundamentals of nursing, ed 2, St. Louis, 1989, The CV Mosby Co.

Shaver JF: The basic mechanisms of fever: considerations for therapy, Nurse Pract 7:15, 1982.

Smith S, Duell D: Clinical nursing skills, Los Altos, Calif, 1985, National Nursing Review.

Task force on Blood Pressure Control in Children: Report of second task force on blood pressure control in children, 1987, Pediatrics 79:1, Jan. 1987.

Thibodeau GA: Textbook of Anatomy and Physiology, ed 12, St. Louis, 1987, The CV Mosby Co.

Thompson DR: Recording patients' blood pressure: a review, J Adv Nurs 6:283, 1981.

Walsh J, Persons C, Wieck L: Manual of home health care nursing, Philadelphia, Pa, 1987, JB Lippincott Company.

Westra B: When your patient says, "I can't breathe," Nursing '82 84:34, 1984.

Whaley LF, Wong DL: Nursing care of infants and children, ed 3, St. Louis, 1987, The CV Mosby Co.

Working group on hypertension in the elderly: statement on hypertension in the elderly, JAMA 256:70, 1986.

Zinn WJ: Hypothermia in the critical care unit, Heart Lung 2:58, 1973.

# 13 PHYSICAL ASSESSMENT

## OBJECTIVES

*Mastery of content in this chapter will enable the nurse to:*

- Define key terms.
- Discuss purposes of the physical assessment.
- Discuss common guidelines to follow while performing physical assessments on clients.
- Explain how physical assessment can be incorporated into routine nursing care.
- Identify differences in assessing children, young adults, and older adults.
- Explain importance of maintaining client comfort while performing a physical examination.
- Describe examples in which patient education can be conducted during physical assessment.
- Discuss types of historical information to be reviewed before each portion of a physical assessment.
- Successfully complete a physical assessment of each major body system.

## KEY TERMS

*Accommodation reflex*
*Alopecia*
*Anthropometry*
*Atrophy*
*Borborygmus*
*Bruit*
*Buccal*
*Carcinoma*
*Cerumen*
*Conjunctiva*
*Consensual light reflex*
*Crackle*
*Dorsal*
*Edema*
*Exophthalmos*
*Friction rub*
*Gait*
*Gurgle*
*Hirsutism*
*Hyperpigmentation*
*Integument*
*Melanin*
*Nares*
*Pallor*
*Palpebra*
*PERRLA*
*Pleura*
*Point of maximal impulse (PMI)*
*Sebaceous gland*
*Sign*
*Speculum*
*Systemic*
*Tinnitus*
*Tracheostomy*
*Ventral*

## SKILLS

**13-1** Performing a General Survey
**13-2** Assessing the Skin
**13-3** Assessing the Hair and Scalp
**13-4** Assessing the Nails
**13-5** Assessing the Eyes
**13-6** Assessing the Ears
**13-7** Assessing the Nose and Sinuses
**13-8** Assessing the Mouth and Pharynx
**13-9** Assessing the Structures of the Neck
**13-10** Assessing the Thorax and Lungs
**13-11** Assessing the Heart and Vascular System
**13-12** Assessing the Breasts
**13-13** Assessing the Abdomen
**13-14** Assessing the Female Genitalia and Rectum
**13-15** Assessing the Male Genitalia and Rectum
**13-16** Assessing the Musculoskeletal System
**13-17** Assessing the Neurologic System

Physical assessment skills are tools that enable the nurse to make intelligent and precise clinical judgments relating to a client's physical condition. Through inspection, palpation, auscultation, and percussion the nurse carefully examines the client's body parts to review their integrity and to determine if abnormalities exist. No one assessment finding conclusively reveals an abnormality. The nurse relies on data from a variety of sources to reveal patterns of abnormalities, which, when validated with physical assessment findings, can indicate significant clinical problems.

The initial physical assessment performed on a client provides a baseline measurement of the client's existing functional abilities. Successive examinations serve to reveal information used to plan the client's care. Physical assessment findings help the nurse to diagnose client problems and determine the best nursing measures for their management.

Inspection, palpation, percussion, and auscultation are skills or techniques that enable the nurse to collect a broad range of physical data about clients. Inspection involves visual examination of body parts to detect significant physical signs. An examiner methodically takes the time necessary to carefully inspect body parts. Inspection is the easiest assessment skill to perform but if an examiner becomes hurried, significant signs may be overlooked, and incorrect conclusions may be made about a client's condition. Good lighting and full exposure of body parts are essential for inspection. Each area is inspected for size, shape, color, symmetry, position, and the presence of abnormalities. If possible, each area inspected is compared with the same area on the opposite side of the body. When necessary use additional light (a penlight for example) to inspect body cavities such as the mouth and throat.

Palpation involves use of the sense of touch to detect characteristics such as texture, temperature, perception of vibration or movement, and consistency. Different parts of the hand are best suited for detecting specific characteristics. For example, the dorsum of the hand is sensitive to temperature variations. Pads of the fingertips detect subtle changes in texture, shape, size, consistency, and pulsatility of body parts. To measure vibration the nurse uses the palm of the hand. Often it becomes necessary to assess the condition of underlying body organs, as in the case of the abdominal assessment. First the nurse uses light palpation, depressing an area of the skin approximately 1 cm (0.5 in) to assess an organ's condition. The client should be relaxed and positioned comfortably so that muscle tension does not interfere with assessment findings. Any tender areas are palpated last. If an abnormality is detected through light palpation it may become necessary to use deep palpation for a more thorough examination. In this case the nurse may use one or both hands to depress the skin 2 cm (1 in). With bimanual palpation one hand is placed over the other. The upper hand exerts downward pressure as the other hand feels the subtle characteristics of deep organs and masses. A student should not attempt deep palpation without a qualified instructor's assistance to ensure that the client does not suffer internal injury.

The nurse further assesses body parts through percussion. Percussion denotes location, size, and density of underlying structures. Percussion requires dexterity. The nurse strikes the body's surface with a finger to create a vibration that travels through body tissues. The character of sound from the vibration depends on the density of underlying tissues. There are two methods of percussion: direct and indirect. The direct method involves striking the body surface directly with one or two fingers. The indirect technique is performed by placing the middle finger of the examiner's nondominant hand (pleximeter hand) firmly against the body surface. With palm and fingers remaining off the skin, the tip of the middle finger of the dominant hand (plexor hand) strikes the base of the distal joint of the pleximeter (Fig. 13-1). The examiner uses a quick, sharp stroke with the plexor finger, keeping the forearm stationary. The wrist must remain relaxed to deliver the proper blow. If the blow is not sharp or if the pleximeter hand is held loosely, a dampened sound results and the nurse cannot detect the presence of underlying structures. A light, quick blow produces the clearest sounds. Table 13-1 describes the five different percussion sounds.

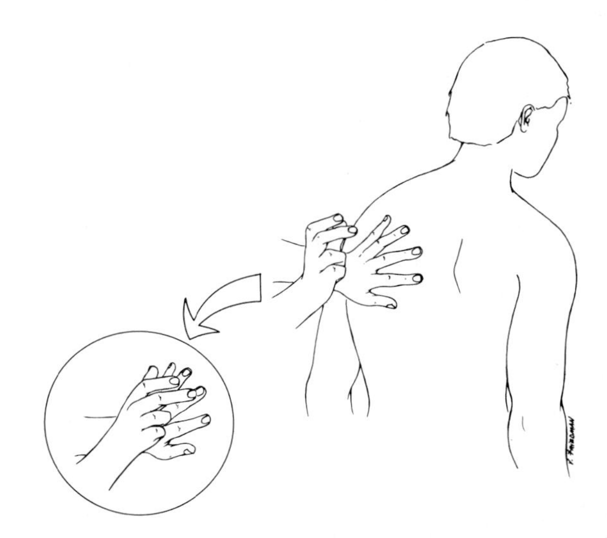

***Fig. 13-1*** To perform indirect percussion nurse places middle finger of nondominant hand against body's surface. Tip of middle finger of dominant hand strikes tip of middle finger of nondominant hand.

***TABLE 13-1*** Sounds Produced by Percussion

| Percussion Sound | Intensity | Pitch | Duration | Quality | Anatomic Location Where Examiner Hears Sounds |
|---|---|---|---|---|---|
| Tympany | Loud | High | Moderate | Drumlike | Enclosed air-containing space: gastric air bubble, puffed-out cheek |
| Resonance | Moderate to loud | Low | Long | Hollow | Normal lung |
| Hyperresonance | Very loud | Very low | Longer than resonance | Booming | Emphysematous lung |
| Dullness | Soft to moderate | High | Moderate | Thudlike | Liver |
| Flatness | Soft | High | Short | Flat | Muscle |

Auscultation is listening to sounds created in various body organs to detect variations from normal. Although some sounds can be heard with the unaided ear, most sounds are heard only with a stethoscope. It is important for a student to recognize normal sounds, such as the passage of blood through an artery, heart sounds, and movement of air through the lungs, in order to detect abnormal sounds. The nurse is more successful in auscultation after knowing what type of sounds arise from each body structure and the location in which they can most easily be heard.

Through auscultation the nurse notes the following characteristics of sound:

*Frequency*—Number of sound wave cycles generated per second by a vibrating object. The higher the frequency, the higher the pitch of a sound and vice versa.

*Loudness*—Amplitude of a sound wave. Auscultated sounds are described as *loud* or *soft*.

*Quality*—Sounds of similar frequency and loudness from different sources. Terms such as *blowing* or *gurgling* describe quality of sound.

*Duration*—Length of time that sound vibrations last. Duration of sound is short, medium, or long. Layers of soft tissue dampen the duration of sounds from deep internal organs.

A nurse cannot be successful at auscultation without knowing how to properly use a stethoscope. Chapter 12 describes the parts of the acoustic stethoscope and use of the bell and diaphragm. Useful exercises for the nurse to practice in order to become more familiar with a stethoscope are described in the box.

The final skill a nurse may use during assessment is olfaction. Certain alterations in body function create characteristic body odors (Table 13-2). The sense of smell can detect abnormalities that go unrecognized by any other means.

### *EXERCISES TO INCREASE FAMILIARITY WITH THE STETHOSCOPE*

1. Place earpieces in your ears with tips of earpieces turned toward the face. *Lightly* blow into the stethoscope's diaphragm. Again place earpieces in your ears, this time with ends turned toward the back of the head. *Lightly* blow into the stethoscope's diaphragm. The earpiece should follow contour of the ear canal. Comparing amplification of sounds with earpieces in both directions helps you learn what fit is best for you. After you learn the right fit for loudest amplification, wear stethoscope the same way each time.
2. Put stethoscope on and *lightly* blow into the diaphragm. If sound is barely audible, *lightly* blow into the bell. Sound is carried through only one part of the chestpiece at a time. If sound is greatly amplified through the diaphragm, the diaphragm is in position for use. If sound is barely audible through the diaphragm, the bell is in position for use.
3. Put stethoscope on and place diaphragm over a friend's arm. Move diaphragm lightly over hair on the arm. The bristling sound created by rubbing of hair against the diaphragm mimics a sound heard in the lungs. The diaphragm should be held firmly and stationary to eliminate extraneous sounds.
4. Place diaphragm over anterior part of your chest. Ask a friend to speak in a conversational tone. Environmental noise seriously detracts from hearing noise created by body organs. Whenever a stethoscope is used, both client and examiner should remain quiet.
5. Place stethoscope on and gently tap tubing. It is often difficult to avoid stretching or movement of the stethoscope's tubing. The examiner should be in a position so that tubing hangs free. Moving or touching tubing creates extraneous sounds.

***TABLE 13-2*** Assessment of Characteristic Odors

| Odor | Site or Source | Potential Causes |
|---|---|---|
| Alcohol | Oral cavity | Ingestion of alcohol |
| Ammonia | Urine | Urinary tract infection |
| Body | Skin, particularly in areas where body parts rub together (under arms, beneath breasts) | Poor hygiene, excess perspiration (hyperhidrosis), foul-smelling perspiration (bromhidrosis) |
| Fecal | Wound site | Wound abscess |
| | Vomitus | Bowel obstruction |
| | Rectal area | Fecal incontinence |
| Foul-smelling stools in infant | Stool | Malabsorption syndrome |
| Halitosis | Oral cavity | Poor dental and oral hygiene, gum disease |
| Sweet fruity, ketones | Oral cavity | Diabetic acidosis |
| Stale urine | Skin | Uremic acidosis |
| Sweet, heavy, thick | Draining wound | *Pseudomonas* (bacterial) infection |
| Musty | Casted body part | Infection inside cast |
| Fetid sweet | Tracheostomy or mucous secretions | Infection of bronchial tree (*Pseudomonas* bacteria) |

Performing the skills of physical assessment is a relatively simple task. The difficult challenge is to relate actual findings to anatomic, physiologic, and pathologic knowledge. The nurse is accountable for evaluating the results of nursing care. Physical assessment skills enable the nurse to monitor the physiologic outcomes of care.

Continuity in health care management improves when the nurse is able to make ongoing, objective, and comprehensive assessments of clients. Knowledge gained from a complete physical examination enables all health team members to deliver care as the client's needs change.

The process of physical assessment involves actual measurement of a specific body part's integrity and function. The nurse will perform a complete examination:

1. For routine screening to promote preventive health care.
2. As a requisite for a client's eligibility for health insurance, military service, or a new job.
3. During a client's admission to a health care agency.

The nurse will perform only portions of an examination to:

1. Gather baseline data about the client's health.
2. Refute, confirm, or supplement data obtained in the nursing history.
3. Confirm and identify nursing diagnoses.
4. Make clinical judgments about a client's changing health status and management.
5. Evaluate the physiologic outcomes of care.

## GUIDELINES

1. Set priorities for assessment procedures based on a client's presenting signs and symptoms or health care needs. For example, a client who develops sudden shortness of breath should first undergo an assessment of the lungs and thorax.
2. Use physical assessment findings to establish a baseline of the client's existing health status or as a means to evaluate changes in a client's condition.
3. Always use a systematic process when performing a physical assessment. When performing a complete examination, most nurses use a head-to-toe approach, beginning with assessment of head and neck structures and ending with assessment of musculoskeletal or neurologic function. Follow the sequence of inspection, palpation, percussion, and auscultation (except for abdominal assessment). This sequence ensures a comprehensive assessment and improves accuracy of findings.
4. Correlate knowledge of anatomy and physiology while performing the assessment. This improves the nurse's ability to recognize normal findings and to identify abnormalities. It also improves the nurse's understanding of various maneuvers to use during assessment.
5. Allow client to be a participant in assessment as much as possible. The client is usually most knowledgeable about his physical condition. Often the client can let the nurse know when certain findings are normal or when actual changes have occurred.
6. Consider client's race, sex, and age. These are three very important variables that influence assessment findings as well as the techniques used to perform an assessment.
7. Integrate physical assessment into routine nursing care measures. The nurse learns to use all physical assessment skills during activities such as bathing, administration of medications, or while conversing with a client.
8. Describe assessment findings in specific anatomical terms.

This chapter discusses physical assessment techniques for each body system. A head-to-toe organizational format is presented to provide guidelines for the nurse wishing to perform a total physical examination. Skills for assessing each body system describe normal findings, potential signs and symptoms of system alterations, equipment necessary for examination, methods for preparing clients, step-by-step assessment procedures, and potential nursing diagnoses resulting from the nurse's findings. Because the skills of physical assessment involve collecting assessment data, nursing diagnoses for each skill will follow the evaluation.

## PREREQUISITE KNOWLEDGE

1. Normal anatomy and physiology.
2. Principles of nonverbal and verbal communication.
3. Purposes for vital sign assessment and expected normal vital sign values.
4. Principles of medical asepsis.
5. Principles of body mechanics and range of joint motion.
6. How to conduct a nursing history.
7. Behavioral effects of sensory loss, e.g., impaired vision, hearing, touch.
8. Teaching and learning principles.
9. Principles of hygiene.
10. Principles of human sexuality.

## PREREQUISITE SKILLS

1. Proper handwashing techniques (Chapter 37).
2. Techniques for assessing vital signs (Chapter 12).
3. Correct transfer techniques (Chapter 33).
4. Inspection, palpation, percussion, and auscultation.

## PREEXAMINATION PREPARATIONS

Before beginning a physical assessment, the nurse should make necessary arrangements to properly prepare the examination room, the equipment, and the client. Poor preparation may result in a haphazard examination that yields incomplete or inaccurate assessment findings.

### Preparing the Environment

To promote client comfort and ensure an efficient examination, the examination room should have the following features: privacy for the client (a separate examination room; curtains or dividers to enclose the client's bed); adequate lighting; control of outside noises; precautions to prevent interruptions by visitors or other health care personnel; a bed or table set at examiner's waist level.

### Preparing Equipment

The nurse will use a variety of equipment throughout the assessment process (see box). To facilitate the examination the equipment should be readily accessible, in proper working order (check batteries and light of ophthalmoscope), and warmed, (if possible run warm water over speculum blades, rub diaphragm of stethoscope briskly between hands before applying to client's skin).

### Preparing the Client

An examination will not occur smoothly if the client is ill prepared. The client's physical and psychologic comfort is essential to ensure accurate assessment findings. A tense, anxious client will not be able to go through many of the physical maneuvers required during an assessment or to cooperate with the nurse's instructions. To prepare a client properly the nurse:

1. Provides for client's physical comfort by allowing the opportunity to empty the bowel or bladder (a good time to collect needed specimens).
2. Provides privacy while client changes into a gown (allows for greater accessibility to body parts).
3. Drapes body parts that need not be exposed.
4. Provides thorough explanation of each portion of the examination including what will be done, what client should expect to feel, and how client can cooperate.
5. Uses simple terminology while describing procedures.
6. Has a third person present in examination room when client and nurse are of opposite sex.
7. Paces or times examination process according to client's physical and emotional tolerance.
8. Assists in proper positioning to minimize discomfort and embarrassment (Table 13-3).

## PHYSICAL ASSESSMENT OF VARIED AGE GROUPS

The nurse uses different interview styles when talking with clients of different ages and with parents of clients. The following tips will assist in data collection during physical examination:

1. When obtaining histories on infants and children, gather all or part of information from the parent or guardian.
2. Parents may think they are being tested by the examiner. Offer support during examination and do not pass judgment.
3. Call children by their first name, and address parents as "Mr. and Mrs. Brown" rather than by first names.
4. Open-ended questions often allow parents to share more information and to describe more of the child's problems.
5. Interviewing older children allows the nurse to observe parent-child interactions.
6. Older children often can provide details about their health history and severity of symptoms.
7. Adolescents tend to respond best when treated as adults and individuals.
8. The adolescent has a right to confidentiality. After talking with parents about historical information the nurse speaks alone with the adolescent.
9. Do not stereotype aging clients. Most are able to adapt to change and learn about their health.
10. Sensory or physical limitations can affect how quickly the nurse is able to interview older clients and conduct examinations. Plan for more than one examination session.

**_EQUIPMENT AND SUPPLIES FOR PHYSICAL ASSESSMENT_**

Cotton applicators
Disposable pad
Drapes
Eye chart (e.g., Snellen chart)
Flashlight and spotlight
Forms (e.g., physical, laboratory)
Gloves (sterile or clean)
Gown for client
Lubricant
Ophthalmoscope
Otoscope
Papanicolaou (Pap) smear slides
Paper towels
Percussion hammer
Safety pin
Scale with height measurement rod
Specimen containers and microscope slides
Sphygmomanometer and cuff
Stethoscope
Swabs or sponge forceps
Tape measure
Thermometer
Tissues
Tongue depressor
Tuning fork
Vaginal speculum
Wristwatch with second hand

***TABLE 13-3*** Positions for Examination

| Position | Areas Assessed | Rationale | Limitations |
|---|---|---|---|
| **Sitting** | Head and neck, back, posterior thorax and lungs, anterior thorax and lungs, breasts, axilla, heart, vital signs, and upper extremities. | Sitting upright provides full expansion of lungs and better visualization of symmetry of upper body parts. | A physically weakened client may be unable to sit. Use supine position with head of bed elevated instead. |
| **Supine** | Head and neck, anterior thorax and lungs, breasts, axilla, heart, abdomen, extremities, pulses. | Most normally relaxed position. Prevents contraction of abdominal muscles and provides easy access to pulse sites. | If client becomes short of breath easily, examiner may need to raise head of bed. |
| **Dorsal recumbent** | Head and neck, anterior thorax and lungs, breasts, axilla, heart. | Certain clients with painful disorders are more comfortable with knees flexed. | Position is not used for abdominal assessment because it promotes contraction of abdominal muscles. |
| **Lithotomy** | Female genitalia and genital tract. | Position provides maximal exposure of genitalia and facilitates insertion of vaginal speculum. | Embarrassing and uncomfortable position, so minimize time client spends in this position. Keep client well draped. Client with severe arthritis or other joint deformity may be unable to assume this position. |
| **Sim's** | Rectum. | Flexion of hip and knee improves exposure of rectal area. | Joint deformities may hinder client's ability to bend hip and knee. |
| **Prone** | Musculoskeletal. | Position is used only to assess extension of hip joint. | Position is intolerable for client with respiratory difficulties. |

## *SKILL 13-1 Performing a General Survey*

The general survey is the preliminary portion of the examination during which the client's vital signs, height and weight, skinfold thickness, and general appearance are recorded. Data for the survey can also be acquired as the nurse collects the nursing history. If abnormalities or signs of problems are revealed during the survey the nurse can direct attention to specific body systems later in the examination. The survey can reveal important information about the client's behavior that can influence how the nurse communicates instructions to the client and conducts portions of the examination.

### Purposes

1. Screen clients for obvious abnormalities that may require more detailed assessment.
2. Measure vital signs before positioning or movement of the client interferes with accuracy of findings.
3. Determine client's physical development by height and weight.
4. Determine client's nutritional status by height, weight, and skinfold thickness.
5. Assess for obvious behavioral alterations.

## *Procedure 13-1*

| Steps | Rationale |
|---|---|
| **Assessment** | |
| 1. Ask if client knows personal normal pulse rate and blood pressure at rest. | Provides means to compare nurse's assessment findings to detect change. |
| 2. Assess factors or conditions that may normally alter vital sign reading. | See Chapter 12. |
| 3. Ask what client's normal height and weight are. | Client's response may reveal degree of satisfaction with weight and size. |
| 4. Determine if sudden gain or loss in weight has occurred, amount, and period of time in which weight change occurred. | Sudden loss in weight can indicate presence of serious disease or significant change in dietary habits and exercise. |
| 5. Review client's past fluid intake and output (I & O) records. | Fluid and electrolyte balance within the body is necessary to maintain health and function in all body systems. Intake includes all liquids taken orally, by feeding tube, and parenterally. Liquid output includes urine, diarrhea, vomitus, gastric suction, and drainage from postsurgical tubes, such as chest tubes or Penrose drains. |
| 6. Assess if client has recently been dieting or following exercise program. | Regular strenuous exercise and changes in dietary habits promote weight loss. |
| 7. Determine type of client's diet. | Certain diets can result in serious nutrient losses. |
| 8. Assess client's general perceptions about personal health. | Nurse's assessment of client's general appearance coupled with client's own perceptions may reveal specific problem areas. |
| **Planning** | |
| 1. Develop individualized goals for assessment, including: | |
| a. Establish baseline vital sign values. | General survey may be first time vital signs are measured, or it may provide findings for comparison with previous measurements. |
| b. Detect presence of abnormalities in vital signs. | |
| c. Correctly determine client's height and weight and compare with normal for client's size. | |
| d. Assess client's nutritional status. | Revealed by height, weight, and skinfold thickness. |
| e. Identify client's emotional status before examination. | Client's behaviors will reveal acceptance of examination procedure. |
| f. Direct physical assessment toward specific problem areas. | Client's general appearance often reveals signs of potential problems involving specific body systems. |
| 2. Prepare needed equipment and supplies: | |
| a. Stethoscope | Equipment used to assess vital signs. |
| b. Sphygmomanometer and cuff | |
| c. Thermometer | |
| d. Standing platform scale | Used for adults or children who can bear weight. |
| e. Stretcher scale | Used for clients who are unable to bear weight. |
| f. Table model or basket scale | Used to weigh infants and toddlers. |
| g. Calibrated calipers | Used to measure skinfold thickness. |
| 3. Prepare client: | |
| a. Explain procedure to client, noting that vital sign and height and weight measurements require individual to assume certain positions. | Understanding promotes client's cooperation. |
| b. Be sure client removes shoes and any heavy clothing. | Ensures accurate weight measurement. |
| **Implementation** | |
| 1. Assess temperature, pulse, respiration, and blood pressure (BP). | See Chapter 12. |

| Steps | Rationale |
|---|---|
| 2. Calibrate scale by setting weight at zero and noting if balance beam registers in middle of mark. | Calibrated scales ensure accurate measurements. |
| 3. Weigh client (client is able to bear weight): | |
| a. Place paper towel on scale platform. | Reduces transmission of microorganisms. |
| b. Ask client to stand on platform facing scale and to remain still (Fig. 13-2). | Client's movement causes balance beam to oscillate and may result in inaccurate reading. |
| c. Slowly adjust scale weight until balance beam registers in middle of mark. | Scale weight used to balance beam is equal to client's weight. |
| 4. Measure height (client is able to bear weight): | |
| a. Have client remain standing on scale platform, facing toward or away from scale.<br>▪ Raise metal rod on back of scale and swing rod over top of client's head.<br>▪ Instruct client to stand erect, exercising good posture (Fig. 13-3). Read height in in/cm as recorded on height scale. | Height is measured by placing smooth, flat surface against crown or vertex of head. Client's position encourages keeping head erect. Erect posture ensures accurate reading. |
| b. Alternative for measuring height of child in home: attach metal or paper measuring tape perpendicular against wall; have child stand against wall, adjacent to tape; place thick book on child's head so that end of book forms right angle with wall; note point of juncture of tape measure and underside of book. | |
| 5. Weigh client (client is unable to bear weight): | |
| a. Prepare stretcher scale by placing light cloth or paper covering over stretcher platform. | Reduces transmission of microorganisms. |
| b. Calibrate scale to zero with covering in place. | Covering adds to weight measured on scale. |
| c. Raise height of client's bed to level of stretcher scale. With one or two nurses assisting, transfer client to scale using proper body mechanics and transfer techniques (Chapters 32 and 33). | Prevents muscular strain on nurse and client during transfer. Prevents client from accidentally falling. |
| d. Instruct client to be still while weight is measured. | Movement can cause inaccurate reading. |
| 6. Measure height (client is unable to bear weight): | Height is measurement from vertex of head to soles of feet. |
| a. Position client supine in bed with legs extended and soles of feet supported upright. | |
| b. With tape measure determine height from soles of feet to vertex of head. | |

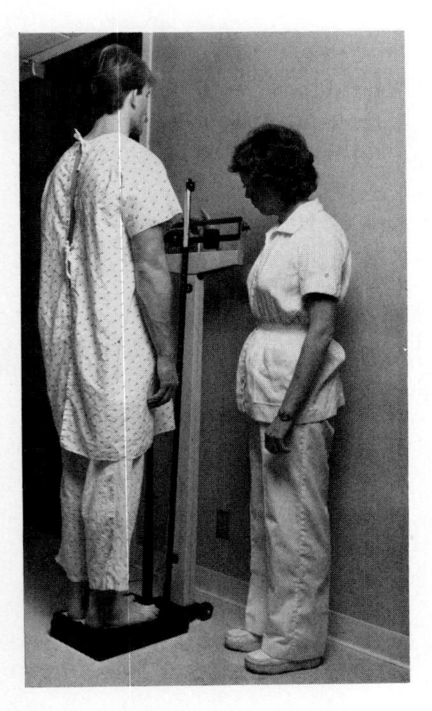

*Fig. 13-2*

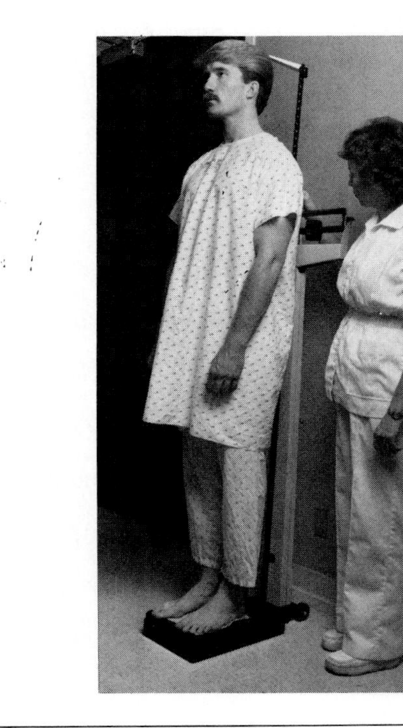

*Fig. 13-3*

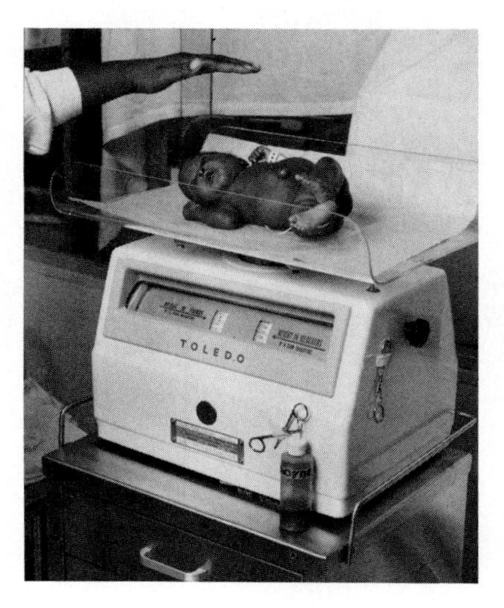


*Fig. 13-4*

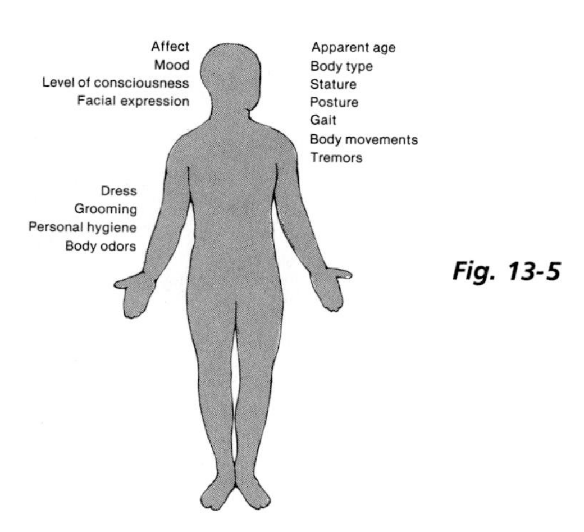


*Fig. 13-5*

| Steps | Rationale |
|---|---|
| 7. Weigh and measure height of infant or toddler: | |
| a. Be sure room temperature is warm. | Infants are weighed nude and are susceptible to temperature fluctuations because of immature thermoregulation. |
| b. Place light cloth or paper covering on basket or platform. | Reduces transmission of microorganisms. |
| c. Place unclothed infant in basket or on platform. Hold hand lightly above infant during measurement (Fig. 13-4). | Nurse's hand prevents accidental fall off scale. |
| d. Note weight in grams (pounds) and ounces. | Standard for measurement. |
| e. Measure infant's length. Place infant supine on table. Hold head in midline. Gently grasp knees and extend fully against table. Keep feet in normal flexed position with toes pointed to ceiling. Measure from vertex of head to heel of foot with tape measure. | Accurate measurement requires full extension of infant's legs and upright position of head and feet. |
| 8. Measure skinfold thickness (Chapter 26): | |
| a. Select area of skinfold over upper abdomen, subscapular region, or deltoid triceps of upper arm. | Subcutaneous areas of fat are most commonly found in these regions. |
| b. Grasp fold of skin so that both sides run parallel; do not pinch bone or muscle. | Ensures accurate measurement of actual thickness of adipose tissue. |
| c. Apply calipers over skinfold, using constant but not extreme pressure. Note thickness in millimeters. | Excessive pressure applied with calipers causes inaccurate readings. Millimeters are standard for measurement. |
| 9. Throughout assessment note client's verbal and nonverbal behaviors. | Behaviors may reflect specific physical abnormalities. |
| 10. Observe client's appearance (Fig. 13-5). | Preliminary survey of client's general appearance can provide clues to significant health problems. |

## Evaluation

| Steps | Rationale |
|---|---|
| 1. Compare client's vital signs with baseline or normal range for client's age (Chapter 12). | Determines baseline physiologic status and presence of alterations. |
| 2. Compare client's height and weight with normal standards on height and weight chart (Table 13-4). | Determines client's size with desirable height and weight for client's age and size. |
| 3. Compare client's skinfold thickness with 50th percentile for men and women. | Reveals general nutritional status by presence or absence of body fat. |

### *Expected outcomes*

| Steps | Rationale |
|---|---|
| 1. Client's vital signs will be within average normal range for clients of same age (Chapter 12). | Vital signs stable. |
| 2. Client's height and weight will be within desired range for height and weight of client of same age. | Normal body size. |
| 3. Client's skinfold thickness will be within normal desired value (50th percentile) for client of same age and size. | Normal nutritional status. |
| 4. Client's behaviors or appearance will not demonstrate signs of physical or emotional stress (e.g., unkept appearance, inappropriate affect, poor posture). | |

***TABLE 13-4*** 1983 Metropolitan Height and Weight Tables*

| Men | | | | | Women | | | | |
|---|---|---|---|---|---|---|---|---|---|
| Height | | Small Frame | Medium Frame | Large Frame | Height | | Small Frame | Medium Frame | Large Frame |
| Feet | Inches | | | | Feet | Inches | | | |
| 5 | 2 | 128-134 | 131-141 | 138-150 | 4 | 10 | 102-111 | 109-121 | 118-131 |
| 5 | 3 | 130-136 | 133-143 | 140-153 | 4 | 11 | 103-113 | 111-123 | 120-134 |
| 5 | 4 | 132-138 | 135-145 | 142-156 | 5 | 0 | 104-115 | 113-126 | 122-137 |
| 5 | 5 | 134-140 | 137-148 | 144-160 | 5 | 1 | 106-118 | 115-129 | 125-140 |
| 5 | 6 | 136-142 | 139-151 | 146-164 | 5 | 2 | 108-121 | 118-132 | 128-143 |
| 5 | 7 | 138-145 | 142-154 | 149-168 | 5 | 3 | 111-124 | 121-135 | 131-147 |
| 5 | 8 | 140-148 | 145-157 | 152-172 | 5 | 4 | 114-127 | 124-138 | 134-151 |
| 5 | 9 | 142-151 | 148-160 | 155-176 | 5 | 5 | 117-130 | 127-141 | 137-155 |
| 5 | 10 | 144-154 | 151-163 | 158-180 | 5 | 6 | 120-133 | 130-144 | 140-159 |
| 5 | 11 | 146-157 | 154-166 | 161-184 | 5 | 7 | 123-136 | 133-147 | 143-163 |
| 6 | 0 | 149-160 | 157-170 | 164-188 | 5 | 8 | 126-139 | 136-150 | 146-167 |
| 6 | 1 | 152-164 | 160-174 | 168-192 | 5 | 9 | 129-142 | 139-153 | 149-170 |
| 6 | 2 | 155-168 | 164-178 | 172-197 | 5 | 10 | 132-145 | 142-156 | 152-173 |
| 6 | 3 | 158-172 | 167-182 | 176-202 | 5 | 11 | 135-148 | 145-159 | 155-176 |
| 6 | 4 | 162-176 | 171-187 | 181-207 | 6 | 0 | 138-151 | 148-162 | 158-179 |


Source of basic data: 1979 Build Study, Society of Actuaries and Association of Life Insurance Medical Directors of America, 1980.
*Weights at ages 25-59 based on lowest mortality. Weight in pounds according to frame (in indoor clothing weighing 5 lb for men and 3 lb for women; shoes with 1-in heels).

| Steps | Rationale |
|---|---|
| ***Unexpected outcomes*** | |
| 1. Client's vital signs are above or below normal expected range for client of same age. | Vital sign alterations can be result of a number of pathologic conditions. |
| ***Potential nursing diagnoses*** | |
| ▪ Actual or potential fluid volume deficit: related to fever. | Higher metabolism poses risk for fluid loss through dehydration. |
| ▪ Decreased cardiac output: related to dysrhythmias and hypotension. | Dysrhythmias impair heart's pumping action. |
| ▪ Ineffective breathing pattern: related to altered respiratory rate. | Respirations do not enable adequate ventilation. |
| ***Unexpected outcomes*** | |
| 1. Client's height is above or below normal desired range for person of same age. | Characteristic of growth disorder (e.g., dwarfism or gigantism). |
| 2. Client's weight is above or below normal desired range for person of same age and height. | Nutritional problems may be attributed to changes in eating habits, sources of nutrients, or pathologic conditions. |
| 3. Client's skinfold thickness is above or below desired normal range for person of same size and age. | |
| ***Potential nursing diagnoses*** | |
| ▪ Altered nutrition—more than body requirements: related to high carbohydrate, high fat diet. | |
| ▪ Altered nutrition—less than body requirements: related to restricted diet intake, loss of appetite. | |

## Recording and Reporting

| Steps | Rationale |
|---|---|
| 1. Record client's vital signs on vital sign flow sheet. | Provides graphic representation of changes in vital sign values. |
| 2. Record height and weight in nurses' notes or flow sheet. | Repeated weight measurements entered in flow sheet for comparison. |
| 3. Record description of client's general appearance and skinfold thickness in nurses' notes. | Provides means for determining changes in client's condition. |
| 4. Describe client's behavior using objective terminology. | Used to compare subsequent behavioral responses. |
| 5. Report abnormalities in vital signs to nurse in charge or physician. | May require immediate therapy. |

### Special Considerations

- Normally, person's weight can fluctuate daily because of fluid loss or retention (1 L of water weighs 1 kg or 2.2 lb).
- Fasting induces rapid weight loss but causes serious protein and electrolyte imbalance.
- Client should be weighed on same scale, at same time, with same clothing each day.
- If client is standing the movable measuring rod must be parallel to floor when resting on client's head in order to obtain a correct height.
- When client is unresponsive, nurse may need assistance to maintain plantar flexion of feet to correctly determine client's height. In critically ill, height becomes important measure to determine body surface area; measurement used to compute hemodynamic factors.
- Body fat can be estimated from results. Generally, weight of 15%-20% above standard indicates excess body fat.

### Teaching Considerations

- Best form of weight reduction is to achieve gradual weight loss by increasing energy expenditures and decreasing caloric intake.
- It is preferable to weigh person in morning after voiding and before food or drink is taken.
- Parents may wish to find spot inside closet or in inconspicuous area to mark child's height on wall. Successive measurements graphically show child's growth over period of time.

### Home Care Considerations

- Perform a complete nursing assessment during the initial home visit to the client, utilizing findings to develop client's plan of care.
- Consult referring physician as to the assessment findings and proposed plan of care based on the assessment findings.

## *SKILL 13-2 Assessing the Skin*

The skin provides the body's external protection, regulates body temperature, and acts as a sensory organ for pain, temperature, and touch. It is the largest organ of the body and thus requires careful and thorough assessment. The nurse may initially examine the skin in parts as other body systems are assessed. The skin is a mirror that reflects an individual's general health and well-being. Valuable information can be obtained by assessing skin surfaces to reveal potential problems affecting other body systems.

### Purposes

1. Determine integrity of the skin.
2. Determine client's hygiene status.
3. Identify physical signs reflecting client's nutritional and hydrational status.
4. Identify physical signs and alterations in other body systems.

## *Procedure 13-2*

| Step | Rationale |
|---|---|
| **Assessment** | |
| 1. Ask if client has noted any changes in skin color. | Client is best judge to determine skin color change. |
| 2. Determine if client works or spends excess time outside. | Exposed areas such as face and arms will be more pigmented than rest of body. |
| 3. Determine if client has noted any lesions or changes in skin. | Most skin changes do not develop suddenly. Change in character of skin lesion might indicate cancerous lesion. |
| 4. Question client regarding frequency of bathing and type of soap used. | Excessive bathing and use of certain harsh soaps contribute to dry skin. |
| 5. Ask if client has experienced recent trauma to skin. | Traumatic injury can cause changes in skin texture and result in certain types of lesions. |
| 6. Ask if client has history of allergies. | Skin rashes commonly occur from allergies. |
| **Planning** | |
| 1. Develop individualized goals for assessment, including: | |
| a. Maintain client's comfort. | Various position changes are necessary to inspect all skin surfaces. |
| b. Provide client's privacy. | When assessing all skin surfaces it will be necessary to systematically expose different body parts. |
| c. Improve client's knowledge of hygiene practices. | Nurse discusses hygiene practices during assessment. |
| d. Determine presence of abnormalities in skin. | Nurse will initiate preventive or therapeutic nursing measures. |

| Step | Rationale |
|---|---|
| 2. Prepare needed equipment and supplies: | |
| a. Gooseneck or high-intensity lamp. | Assessment of skin requires good illumination. |
| b. Disposable gloves | Prevents contact with microorganisms when palpating moist or draining skin lesions. |
| 3. Prepare client: | |
| a. Client may sit initially. | Position allows nurse to inspect upper trunk anteriorly and posteriorly and upper and lower extremities. |
| b. Ask client to lie supine and turn to side. | Position allows visualization of buttocks and genital area. |
| c. Explain to client that it is necessary to inspect all skin surfaces to ensure normal skin integrity. If lesions are found, explain need to palpate lesions gently. | Client may become embarrassed because skin condition is often associated with hygiene. |
| d. Expose only single body part to be inspected at one time. | Minimizing exposure of body parts reduces client anxiety. |
| e. Nurse may request client to clean skin with soap and water or remove cosmetics. | Makeup, body secretions, or soil may cover areas of skin requiring inspection and mask true determination of characteristics such as skin color or presence of lesions. |
| **Implementation** | |
| 1. Inspect color of skin surfaces, comparing color of symmetric body parts. | Skin color varies from body part to body part. Changes in color can be indicative of pathologic alterations (Table 13-5). |
| 2. Carefully inspect color of oral mucosa, nail beds, lips, palms of hands, sclerae, and conjunctivae. | Nurse can more readily identify abnormalities in areas of body where melanin production is least. |
| 3. Using fingertips, palpate skin surfaces to feel moisture of skin. Note character of any secretions by describing color, odor, amount, and consistency (e.g., thin and watery or thick and oily). | Skin hydration helps to indicate body fluid imbalances, changes in skin environment, and body temperature regulation. Character of secretions from skin lesions helps to indicate type of lesion. |
| 4. Using dorsum (back) of hand, palpate temperature of skin surfaces. Compare symmetric body parts. Compare upper and lower body parts. Note distinct temperature differences. | Increased or decreased skin temperature reflects increase or decrease in blood flow. Skin on dorsum of hand is thin, which allows detection of subtle temperature changes. |
| 5. Stroke skin surfaces lightly with fingertips to detect texture of skin's surface. Note whether skin is smooth or rough and if there are localized areas of hardness or lesions. | Skin texture changes result from alterations in hydration, as well as from localized trauma or skin lesions. |
| 6. Palpate deeply any areas that appear irregular on light palpation. | Deep palpation allows nurse to detect localized areas of hardness within subcutaneous skin layers. |

***TABLE 13-5*** Skin Color Variations

| Color | Condition | Cause | Assessment Location |
|---|---|---|---|
| **Blue** (cyanosis) | Increased amount of deoxygenated hemoglobin, associated with hypoxia. | Heart or lung disease, cold environment. | Nail beds, lips, mouth, skin (severe cases). |
| **Pallor** (decrease in color) | Reduced amount of oxyhemoglobin. Reduced blood flow. | Anemia. | Face, skin, nail beds, conjunctivae, lips. |
| | | Shock. | Skin, nail beds, conjunctivae, lips. |
| | Congenital or autoimmune condition causing lack of pigment. | Vitiligo. | Patchy areas on skin. |
| **Yellow-orange** (jaundice) | Increased deposition of bilirubin in tissues. | Liver disease, destruction of red blood cells. | Sclera, mucous membranes, skin. |
| **Red** (erythema) | Dilation of blood vessels or increased blood flow. | Fever, direct trauma, blushing, alcohol intake. | Face, area of trauma. |
| **Tan-brown** | Increased amount of melanin. | Suntan, pregnancy. | Areas exposed to sun, face, areola, nipples. |

***TABLE 13-6*** Types of Skin Lesions

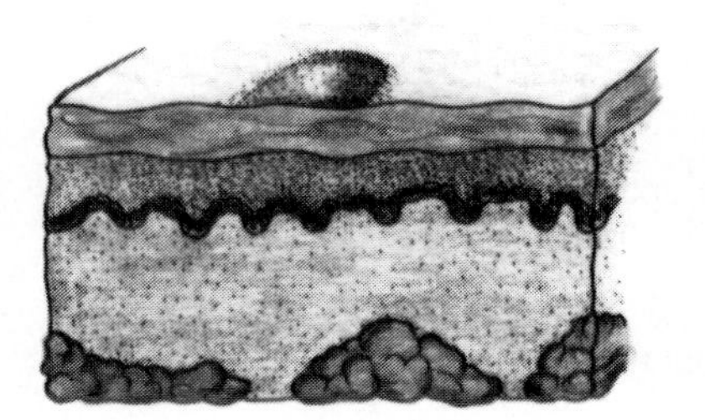

**Macule:** flat, nonpalpable, change in skin color, smaller than 1 cm (e.g., freckle, petechia).

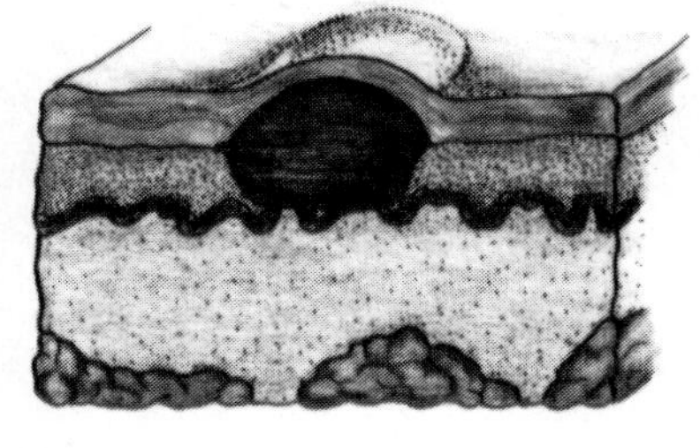

**Papule:** palpable, circumscribed, solid elevation in skin, smaller than 0.5 cm (e.g., elevated nevus).

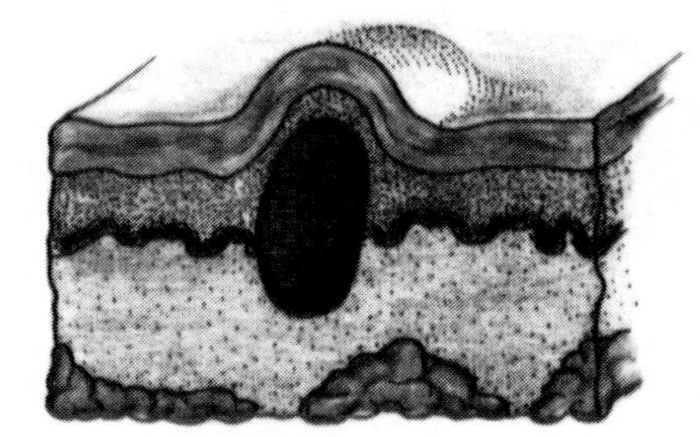

**Nodule:** elevated solid mass, deeper and firmer than papule, 0.5-0.2 cm (e.g., wart).

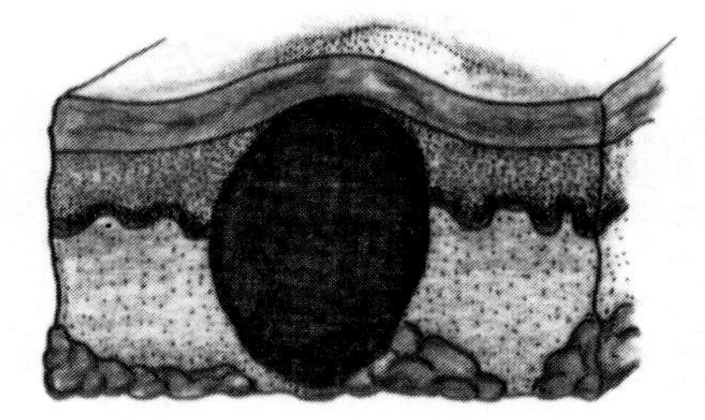

**Tumor:** solid mass that may extend deep through subcutaneous tissue, larger than 1-2 cm (e.g., epithelioma).

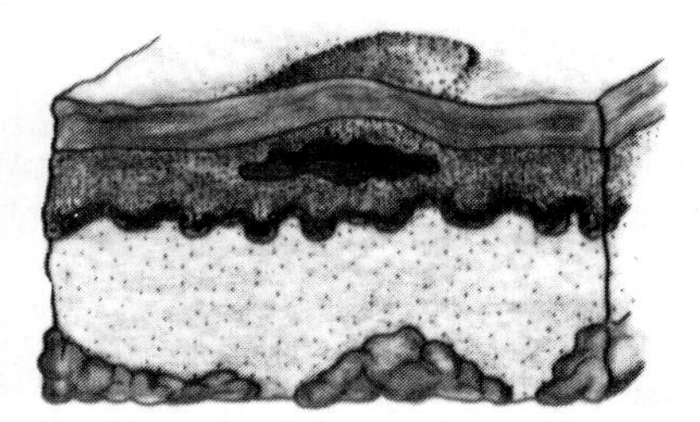

**Wheal:** irregularly shaped, elevated area or superficial localized edema; varies in size (e.g., hives, mosquito bite).

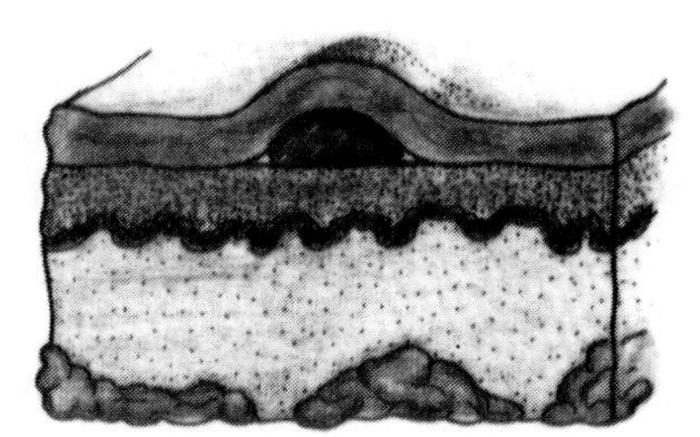

**Vesicle:** circumscribed elevation of skin filled with serous fluid, smaller than 0.5 cm (e.g., herpes simplex, chickenpox).

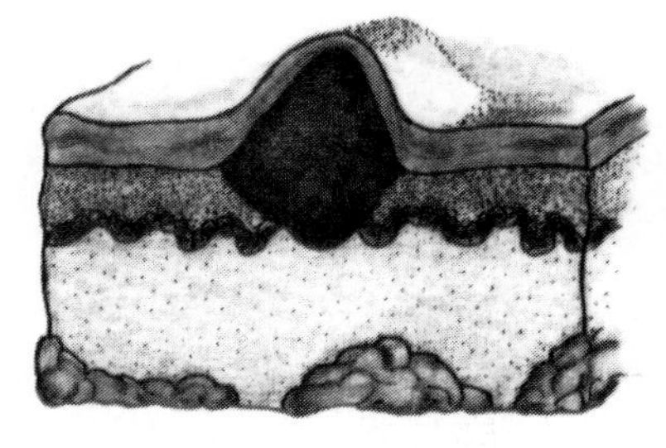

**Pustule:** circumscribed elevation of skin similar to vesicle but filled with pus, varies in size (e.g., acne, staphylococcal infection).

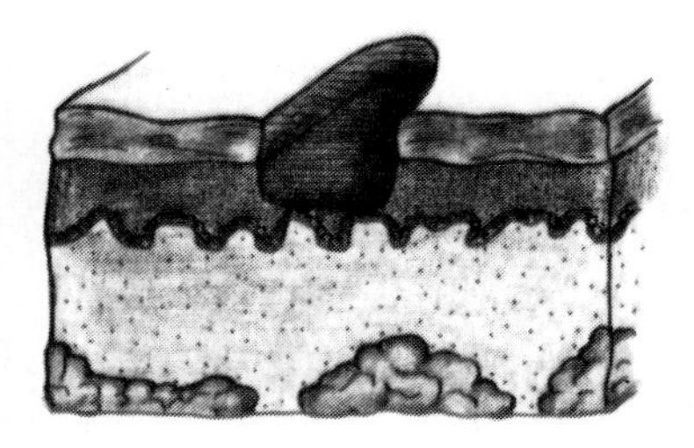

**Ulcer:** deep loss of skin surface that may extend to dermis and frequently bleeds and scars, varies in size (e.g., venous stasis ulcer).

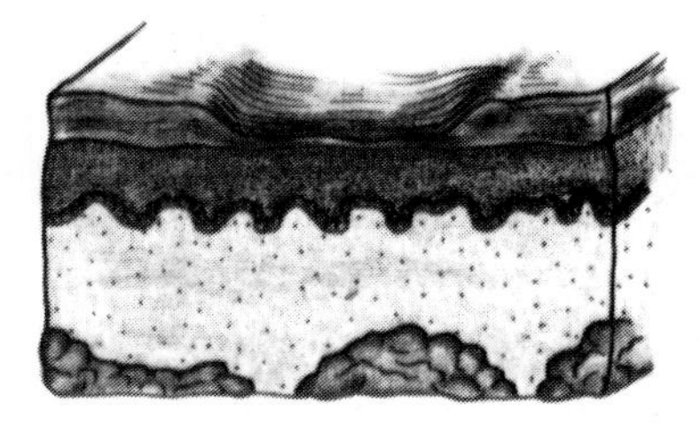

**Atrophy:** thinning of skin with loss of normal skin furrow and skin appearing shiny and translucent, varies in size (e.g., arterial insufficiency).

| Step | Rationale |
|---|---|
| 7. Assess skin turgor by first grasping fold of skin on back of client's hand, on sternum, forearm, or abdomen. Release skinfold and note ease and speed at which skin returns to place (Fig. 13-6). | Turgor is measure of skin's elasticity. |
| 8. When lesion is detected, don gloves, inspect color, location, size, type (Table 13-6), grouping (e.g., clustered or linear), and distribution (localized or generalized). | Certain skin lesions can be identified by a characteristic pattern of features. Gloves reduce transmission of microorganisms. |
| 9. Gently palpate any lesion to determine mobility, contour (flat, raised, or depressed), and consistency (soft or hard). If lesion is moist or draining, don disposable gloves before palpation. | Gentle palpation prevents accidental rupture of underlying cysts. Gloves reduce transmission of microorganisms. |
| 10. Note if client complains of tenderness during palpation. | Tenderness may be indicative of inflammation or pressure to body part. |

| Step | Rationale |
|---|---|
| 11. Inspect areas of skin for edema, paying particular attention to dependent body parts such as feet and ankles, sacrum, and scapular areas. Note color, location, and shape of area. | Edema is result of accumulation of fluid in tissues. Poor venous return causes edema in dependent body parts. Direct trauma causes localized edema. |
| 12. Palpate edematous areas noting mobility, consistency, and tenderness. | Assists in determining extent of edema. |
| 13. Assess for pitting edema by pressing edematous area firmly with thumb for 5 seconds.<br>1 cm indentation = 1+ edema<br>2 cm indentation = 2+ edema<br>3 cm indentation = 3+ edema<br>4 cm indentation = 4+ edema | Depth of pitting determines degree of edema. |

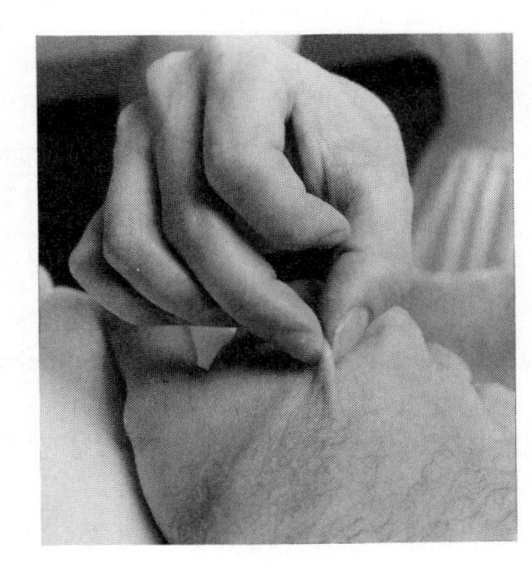

***Fig. 13-6***

## Evaluation

1. Compare assessment findings with previous observations of skin and normal skin characteristics. — Detects change in client's condition and determines skin integrity.

### *Expected outcomes*

1. Skin has normal color, is warm and smooth on palpation, with no excess dryness or areas of edema. Turgor is normal. — Normal findings.
2. There may be primary lesions such as freckles. — Normal findings.

### *Unexpected outcomes*

1. Client's skin demonstrates abnormal coloring, dry texture, reduced turgor, and temperature variations. — Abnormalities may result from factors such as dehydration, improper hygiene measures, fever, or circulatory alterations.
2. Skin lesions will be present. — Lesions may result from trauma or underlying pathology.

### *Potential nursing diagnoses*

- Impaired skin integrity: related to dehydration, poor hygiene, etc. — Indications for hygiene measures, nutritional therapy, proper positioning, and possibly pressure ulcer or wound care.
- Potential impaired skin integrity: related to nutritional alterations, positioning, etc. — Indicates need for preventive care.
- Altered peripheral tissue perfusion: related to impaired arterial flow.

## Recording and Reporting

1. Describe condition of client's skin in nurses' notes. — Provides means to assess changes in client's condition and provides data to evaluate effect of nursing therapies.
2. Report abnormalities in skin (e.g., pressure ulcer, draining lesion, or wound) to nurse in charge or physician. — May require initiation of medical therapy.

## Special Considerations

- Skin changes commonly occur in different age groups. Infants develop rashes from food allergies. Adolescents develop acne. Adults notice reduced firmness of skin. Elderly develop wrinkling of skin, reduced elasticity, spotty pigmentation ("liver spots") in areas exposed to sun, and excessively dry skin.
- Well-lit room may be satisfactory but examination light allows nurse to see less accessible areas more clearly.
- Elderly clients are sensitive to glaring lights.
- Infants should be kept covered as much as possible to prevent temperature changes.
- Normal skin in light-skinned persons varies from milky white and rosy color to deep pink. Dark-skinned persons have various brown, red, olive green, yellow, and blue skin tones.
- Dry skin may indicate dehydration, use of harsh soaps, too frequent bathing, or lack of humidity in room.

- Repeated intramuscular and subcutaneous injections often cause localized areas of hardness.
- With reduced turgor, skin remains suspended or "tented" for few sec before slowly returning to place. Poor hydration and nutrition, plus process of aging cause reduced turgor.
- Cancerous tumor is usually hard, localized, and immobile.
- Child's skin is normally smooth and soft. Skin texture of adult is normally not uniform throughout. Irregularities in texture may be result of scarring from recent trauma.

### Teaching Considerations

- Instruct client how to prevent skin cancer by avoiding overexposure to the sun: wear wide-brimmed hats and long sleeves, use sunscreens before going into the sun and after swimming or perspiring, avoid tanning under direct sun at midday (11 AM to 2 PM).
- Teach client to conduct a monthly self-examination of the skin, noting any moles, blemishes, or birth marks.
- Tell client to report any changes in size, shape, or color of lesions. If a sore does not heal, report it to a physician.
- The elderly tend to have delayed wound healing. Instruct client to report any lesion that bleeds or fails to heal to a physician.
- Teach client to avoid applying drying agents such as rubbing alcohol or soap to the skin.
- Tell client to apply lotion and moisturizers to the skin regularly to reduce itching and drying.

# *SKILL 13-3 Assessing the Hair and Scalp*

The nurse assesses condition and distribution of the two types of body hair—terminal and vellus. Terminal hair is long, coarse, thick hair that is easily visible on the scalp, axilla, and pubic areas. Vellus hairs are soft, tiny hairs covering the whole body except for palms and soles. As in skin assessment, the nurse may inspect body hair all at one time or at different points during the examination. For example, the nurse can inspect hair on the scalp while assessing all head and neck structures and inspect pubic hair during the genitalia examination. This approach minimizes any embarrassment the client might experience.

### Purposes

1. Determine condition of the hair and supportive structures.
2. Determine client's hair care practices.
3. Identify changes in hair growth or conditions that may reveal underlying local or systemic diseases.

## *Procedure 13-3*

| Steps | Rationale |
|---|---|
| **Assessment** | |
| 1. Ask if client is wearing a wig or a hairpiece and request that it be removed. | Interferes with complete inspection of hair and scalp. |
| 2. Determine if client has noted recent change in growth or loss of hair or lesions of scalp. | Changes may occur subtly over time. |
| 3. Identify type of shampoo or hair care products used. | Excessive use of shampoo or other chemical agents may cause drying or brittleness. |
| 4. Determine if client has experienced recent trauma to scalp. | Trauma may be cause of bruising or localized lesions. |
| **Planning** | |
| 1. Develop individualized goals for assessment, including: | |
| a. Respect client's body image. | During assessment, maintain neat appearance of hair when possible. |
| b. Determine cleanliness of hair and condition of scalp. | May indicate need for improved hygiene practices. |
| c. Assess integrity of hair shaft. | Condition of hair may reveal nutritional status, existence of systemic or local disease, or exposure to environmental irritants. |
| d. Improve client's knowledge of proper hair care. | Nurse may discuss proper ways for combing or shampooing hair during assessment. |
| 2. Prepare needed equipment and supplies: | |
| a. Examination light | Illuminates hair shafts. |
| b. Disposable gloves | Prevents nurse's contact with microorganisms, lice, or other vermin. |

| Steps | Rationale |
|---|---|
| 3. Prepare client: | |
| a. Client may sit initially. | Position allows nurse to inspect scalp thoroughly. |
| b. Client may be asked to lie supine. | Allows for inspection of distribution of body hair. |
| 4. Explain to client that inspection of hair and scalp requires separation of hair shafts. If lesions or lice are found, explain need to wear gloves. | Client may be sensitive about personal appearance. Embarrassment may occur because condition of hair reflects client's overall hygiene. |
| **Implementation** | |
| 1. Inspect distribution, thickness, color, elasticity, texture, and lubrication of hair. | Changes in hair distribution may reflect hormonal changes. Excessive dryness, coarseness, or brittleness may result from aging, poor nutrition, or use of certain hair care products. Disturbances in body function such as febrile illness or exposure to general anesthesia can cause hair loss. |
| 2. Wash hands and don gloves. | Reduces transmission of microorganisms. |
| 3. Focus inspection to areas of baldness or thinning of hair. | Alopecia (baldness) may be related to genetic tendency or be caused by skin disorders such as tinea capitis (ringworm). |
| 4. Inspect scalp for cleanliness and presence of lesions by carefully separating shafts of hair. Inspect each lesion using same guidelines described in Skill 13-2. | Pulling of hair can cause client discomfort. Lesions can easily go unnoticed with thick hair growth. |
| 5. Inspect scalp contour and palpate for unusual masses or prominences. In newborns, fontanels should feel flat, firm, and well-demarcated against skull's bony edges. | Lumps may result from localized trauma. In newborns, change in contour results from overlapping of cranial bones that have not yet fused. |
| 6. If hair is in poor condition inspect hair follicles to determine presence of lice. Stand away from client during inspection. | Head and crab lice attach their eggs to hair shafts and follicles, are difficult to see, and can easily attach to clothing and be transmitted to other persons. |
| 7. Inspect for bites or pustular eruptions in areas where skin surfaces meet (i.e., behind ears). | Lice gather in areas of body where exposure is limited. |
| 8. Inspect hair over perineal area for crab lice (pediculosis pubis). | Site where lice develop after contact with infested clothing or people. |
| 9. Remove gloves and dispose in appropriate container. Wash hands. | Reduces transmission of microorganisms and vermin. |
| 10. Inspect hair distribution over lower extremities. | Reduction in hair covering extremities may be caused by arterial insufficiency. |
| **Evaluation** | |
| 1. Compare findings with previous observations and normal characteristics of hair. | Detects change in condition or presence of abnormalities. |
| ***Expected outcomes*** | |
| 1. Hair will be evenly distributed over scalp and pubic areas. | Normal findings. |
| 2. Terminal scalp hair will be soft, strong, lustrous, and without areas of local discoloration. | Evidence of good hygienic practices. |
| 3. Scalp will be smooth, without lesions or presence of vermin. | Skin integrity maintained. |
| 4. Vellus hair evenly distributed over symmetric body parts. | Normal findings. |
| ***Unexpected outcomes*** | |
| 1. Terminal scalp hair will be dry, brittle, discolored, coarse, or stringy. There may be localized areas of baldness (alopecia). | May result from poor hygiene, nutritional deficiencies, hormonal changes, or alterations from chemotherapy. |
| 2. Scalp will be scaly or have lesions or vermin present. | May result from poor hygiene or trauma. |
| 3. Vellus hair will be absent or unevenly distributed over symmetric body parts. | May result from aging or local circulatory alterations. |
| ***Potential nursing diagnoses*** | |
| ▪ Self-care hygiene deficit: related to physical immobility.<br>▪ Body image disturbance: related to hair loss.<br>▪ Impaired skin integrity: related to scalp lesions. | Indications for hygiene measures, nutritional therapy, promotion of self-concept, and client education. |
| ▪ Altered peripheral tissue perfusion: related to arterial insufficiency. | Change in hair growth is one of several signs indicative of this diagnosis. |
| **Reporting and Recording** | |
| 1. Describe condition of hair and scalp in nurses' notes. | Documents changes in condition of hair and scalp. Means of evaluating results of hygiene care and other therapies. |

### Special Considerations

- Some hairpieces require considerable effort to remove. Client may request nurse to defer this portion of assessment.
- If hair is in obviously good condition, it is not necessary to inspect entire scalp. Client is often best guide in locating lesions.
- With onset of puberty, change in amount and distribution of hair growth occurs. Women with hirsutism, a hormone disorder, have hair growth on upper lip, chin, and cheeks, with coarse body hair.
- Scaling or dryness of scalp may be caused by dandruff or psoriasis.
- Newborns have anterior and posterior fontanels (spaces of unossified tissue where cranial bones have not closed).
- Tiny eggs look like oval particles of dandruff. Head lice (pediculosis capitis) and body lice (pediculosis corporis) are small with grayish white bodies.
- Chemotherapeutic drugs (Chapter 21) cause alopecia as a side effect.

### Teaching Considerations

- Some hair products contain oils or lubricants that can clog sebaceous glands and promote scalp infections.
- If moles are found, warn client that combing or brushing can cause bleeding.
- Instruct clients who have lice about the importance of using Kwell shampoo or soap.
- Instruct clients who have lice about the risks of transmitting the infestation.

***TABLE 13-7*** Abnormalities of the Nail Bed

| Type | Description | Associated Causes |
|---|---|---|
| **Normal nail** | | |
| **Clubbing** (180°; >180°) | Change occurs in angle between nail and nail base; nail bed softens, with nail flattening. Eventually angle is greater than 180 degrees; fingertips often become enlarged. | Chronic lack of oxygen; heart disease; pulmonary disease. |
| **Beau's lines** | Transverse depressions in the nails, indicates that nail growth was temporarily disturbed; grows out over several months | Systemic illness, such as severe infection; injury to nail. |
| **Koilonychia (spoon nail)** | Concave curves. | Iron deficiency anemia; syphilis; use of strong detergents. |
| **Splinter hemorrhages** | Red or brown linear streaks in nail bed. | Minor trauma; subacute bacterial endocarditis; trichinosis. |
| **Paronychia** | Inflammation of skin at base of nail. | Local infection; trauma. |

# SKILL 13-4 Assessing the Nails

The condition of the nails can reflect a person's general state of health. Poor nutritional habits, presence of systemic disease, recent trauma to hands, and infection of nails are examples of conditions that can cause abnormalities of the nail and nail bed (Table 13-7). Normally, nails are transparent, smooth, and convex with pink nail beds and translucent white tips. The angle between the nail bed is normally about 160 degrees. Nails normally grow at a constant rate. The client is the best resource for reporting changes in nail appearance and growth.

### Purposes

1. Determine condition of the nail and nail bed.
2. Determine presence of underlying systemic or local disease.
3. Determine quality of nail care the client practices.

## Procedure 13-4

| Steps | Rationale |
|---|---|
| **Assessment** | |
| 1. Ask if client has experienced any recent trauma to the nails. | Trauma results in change in nail growth and potential loss of all or portion of nail. |
| 2. Question client's nail care practices and use of nail polish remover. | Chemical agents can cause excessive drying of nails. Improper nail care can damage nails and cuticles. |
| 3. Determine if client has noted recent changes in nail appearance or growth. | Many alterations in nail growth and appearance occur slowly over time. |
| **Planning** | |
| 1. Develop individualized goals for assessment, including: | |
| a. Improve client's knowledge of nail care practices. | Nurse can discuss hygiene practices while inspecting nails. |
| b. Determine presence of abnormalities in nails. | Changes may reveal systemic disease. May pose implications for education. |
| 2. Prepare client: | |
| a. Client may assume sitting or lying position. | Promotes client comfort. |
| b. Explain need to inspect nails and cuticles. | Promotes client relaxation. |
| 3. If necessary to view color of nails, ask client to remove polish. | Allows full visualization of nail features. |
| **Implementation** | |
| 1. Inspect nails for quality, color, thickness, shape, and curvature. Inspect entire nail surface and sides of nails and fingers. | Color of nails indicates status of blood oxygenation. Thin nails are indicative of nutrition (vitamin) deficiency. Changes in shape and curvature of nails indicate systemic disease. Contour can best be inspected by viewing side of nail and finger. |
| 2. Grasp client's finger and observe color of nail bed. Apply gentle firm pressure with thumb to client's nail bed. Release pressure quickly. (With pressure applied nail bed appears white or blanched; pink color should return immediately.) | Assesses capillary refill. Failure of color to return promptly indicates circulatory insufficiency. |
| **Evaluation** | |
| 1. Compare condition of nails with normal nail characteristics. | Determines presence of abnormalities. |
| ***Expected outcomes*** | |
| 1. Nails will be transparent, smooth and convex, with pink nail beds and translucent white tips; tips should extend over fingers; capillary return is brisk. | Normal findings. |
| 2. In black clients brown or black pigmentation between fingernail and nail base is present. | Normal findings. |

| Steps | Rationale |
|---|---|
| ***Unexpected outcomes*** | |
| 1. Nails will appear thin, brittle, rough, or pale. | Capillary return is poor. |
| ***Potential nursing diagnoses*** | |
| ▪ Self-care hygiene deficit: related to poor knowledge.<br>▪ Altered peripheral tissue perfusion: related to reduced arterial flow. | Indications for hygiene measures, nutritional therapy, and client education. |
| **Recording and Reporting** | |
| 1. Describe condition of nails in nurses' notes. | Data used for future comparison and to document response to hygienic measures. |

## Special Considerations

- Cyanosis is best observed in the nail beds.
- Exposure to cold temperatures causes vasoconstriction and may impair refill. Local circulatory alterations (i.e., pressure from cast or bandage) will impair refill. Vascular disease also may impair refill.
- Ragged, short nails may indicate nail biting.

## Teaching Considerations

- Discuss dietary sources of protein.
- Instruct clients to cut nails only after soaking them about 10 min in warm water.
- Caution clients against use of over-the-counter preparations to treat corns, calluses, or ingrown toe nails.

# *SKILL 13-5 Assessing the Eyes*

The ability to see clearly is often taken for granted. Vision is vital to performing activities of daily living, communicating effectively with others, and analyzing and learning about events that occur within our world daily. The nurse often cares for clients with preexisting visual alterations, as well as clients undergoing diagnostic or therapeutic procedures that may impair vision. The nurse must be familiar with typical symptoms of eye disease. Assessment of visual symptoms may lead to identification of specific eye disorders.

Examination of the eye includes skills for assessing visual acuity, visual fields, extraocular movements, and external and internal eye structures (Fig. 13-7).

## Purpose

1. Screen for preexisting eye disease.
2. Assess extent to which visual impairment affects activities of daily living and need for nursing care.
3. Determine condition of eye structures.

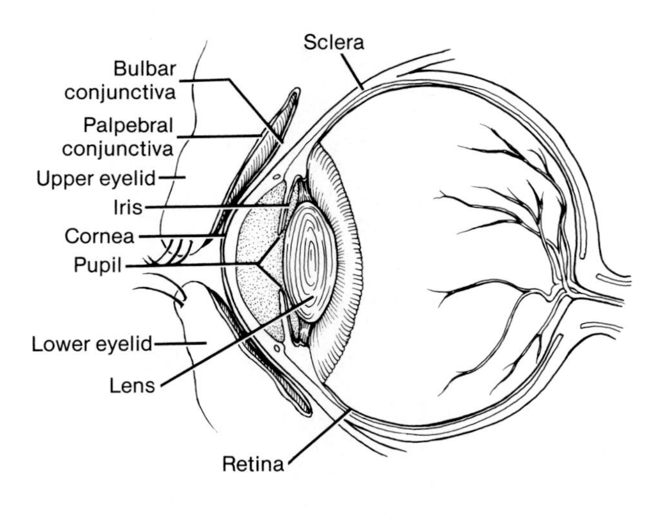


***Fig. 13-7*** Cross section of eye.

## *Procedure 13-5*

| Steps | Rationale |
| --- | --- |
| **Assessment** | |
| 1. Question if client has history of eye disease, diabetes, or hypertension. | Diseases that create significant risk for partial or complete loss of vision. |
| 2. Ask if client has experienced eye pain, photophobia (sensitivity to light), burning, itching, excess tearing or crusting, diplopia (double vision), blurred vision, spots or floaters, flashing lights, halos around lights. | Identification of common symptoms of eye disease may lead client to pursue medical care or follow preventive health care practices. |
| 3. Determine client's occupational history. | Clients who perform close, intricate work often experience eye fatigue. Clients working outdoors are at greater risk for foreign bodies in eye. |
| 4. Ask if client has visited an eye doctor recently. | Date of last examination reveals level of preventive care taken by client. |
| **Planning** | |
| 1. Develop individualized goals for assessment, including: | |
| a. Maintain client's comfort. | Clients often become anxious when eye structures are examined and manipulated. |
| b. Prevent injury to eye. | Gentle technique is needed when inspecting or palpating eye structures to avoid injury. |
| c. Identify presence of abnormalities. | Reveals localized or systemic alterations. |
| d. Improve client's knowledge of signs and symptoms of eye disease. | Nurse may discuss this topic while assessing client. |
| 2. Prepare needed equipment and supplies: | |
| a. Newspaper or magazine | For testing visual acuity. |
| b. Snellen chart | |
| c. Opaque index card | |
| d. Cotton-tipped applicator | To retract upper eyelid for visualization. (Usually only done by nurses with advanced training in eye examinations.) |
| e. Penlight or flashlight | To assess pupillary response. |
| f. Ophthalmoscope | To visualize internal eye structures. |
| 3. Prepare client: | |
| a. Ask client to stand during assessment of visual acuity. | Client stands prescribed distance from Snellen chart to test visual acuity. |
| b. During remainder of examination client may sit. | Promotes client's comfort and improves nurse's access to eye structures being examined. |
| c. Explain to client each portion of examination. When examining external eye structures, explain how nurse's hands and equipment will be positioned. | Client may be apprehensive during eye examination, particularly if there are symptoms of alterations. Fear of loss of sight causes anxiety. |
| d. Use confident but gentle approach. Ask client to inform you if there is discomfort. | Minimizes client anxiety. |
| **Implementation** | |
| 1. Test visual acuity: | |
| a. If client wears glasses or contact lenses, ask client to read print from newspaper or magazine while wearing lenses or glasses. | Cursory assessment of visual acuity. |
| b. If client is unable to see print clearly, test each eye separately by placing index card over one eye at time. | Determines extent of involvement of each eye. |
| c. For clients with severe visual impairment ask them to count nurse's upraised fingers. | Client with severe impairment has difficulty seeing large objects. |
| d. If client unable to see objects, shine light into eye, then turn light off. Determine if client can tell when light is on and off. | Tests light perception. |
| e. For more accurate assessment test visual acuity by using Snellen chart: | |
| ▪ Client wears glasses (but not if glasses are intended only for reading). | Reading glasses are prescribed only for distances of 1.2 to 14 in. |
| ▪ Position client 20 ft away from chart. | Allows for standardization of findings. |

**Steps** | **Rationale**

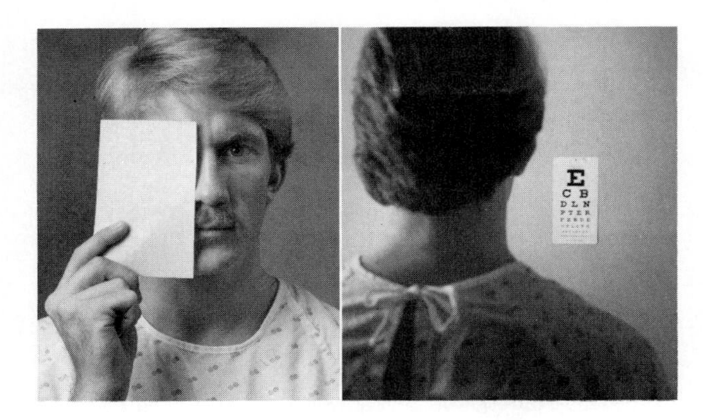


*Fig. 13-8*

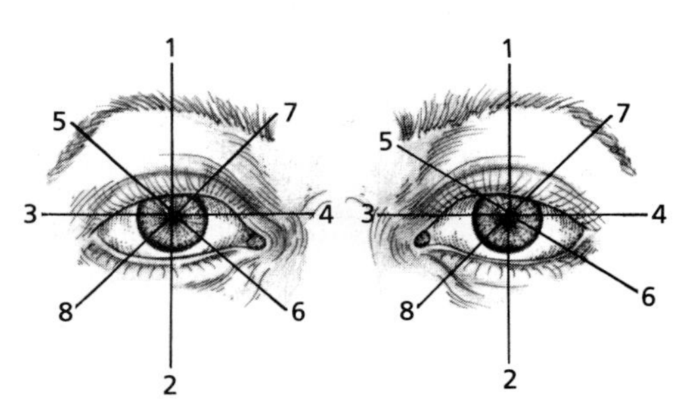


*Fig. 13-9*

- Instruct client to read smallest line of print possible three times; once with both eyes and then with each eye separately, alternating by covering each eye with opaque card (Fig. 13-8).
- With **E** chart ask client to point in direction each **E** is pointing. Ask children to identify images on chart. **E** chart is used for clients unable to read.

Client is successful if able to read more than half of letters or figures in line. Normal visual acuity indicates central vision (macular function) is intact.

2. Test visual fields:
   a. Ask client to stand or sit 2 ft away, facing nurse.
   b. Have your eyes at eye level of client.

   Superimposes nurse's field of vision (assuming it is normal) on that of client.

   c. Ask client to gently close or cover one eye and to look at nurse's eye directly opposite.

   Allows for measurement of visual field of each eye.

   d. Nurse closes other eye, opposite client's closed eye.
   e. Nurse moves finger outside of own field of vision. Slowly brings finger back into field, asking client to state when finger is first seen. Procedure repeated for all directional fields.

   Point at which finger can first be viewed indicates farthest limit of visual field for that direction.

3. Test extraocular movements:
   a. Instruct client to look straight ahead toward you, keeping head motionless throughout examination.

   Assessment tests for parallel eye movement. Movement of head interferes with accurate assessment.

   b. Nurse holds finger 6-12 in (15-30 cm) from client.

   Keeping finger comfortable distance from client prevents blurring and eye strain.

   c. Nurse asks client to follow movement of finger with eyes, keeping head still. Nurse moves finger slowly through each of eight cardinal gazes (Fig. 13-9).

   Assesses movement of each of six pairs of extraocular muscles.

   d. Nurse keeps finger within normal field of vision.

   Forcing client to look beyond visual field may cause nystagmus (rhythmic oscillation of eyes).

   e. Nurse observes parallel eye movement, position of upper eyelid in relation to iris, and presence of nystagmus (Fig. 13-10).

   Eyes move together in parallel. Upper eyelid should cover iris only slightly. Eyelid does not cover pupil.

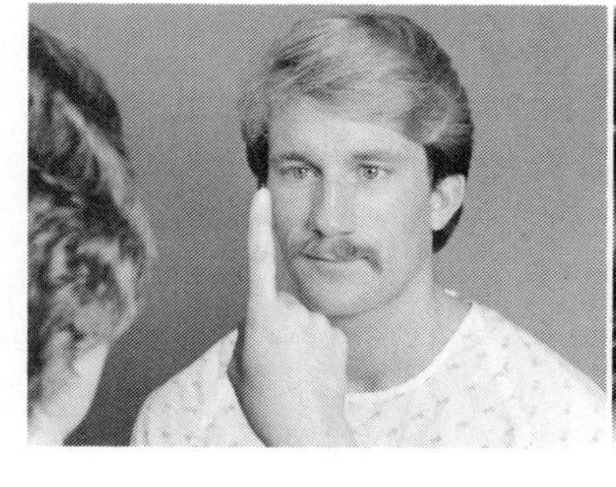

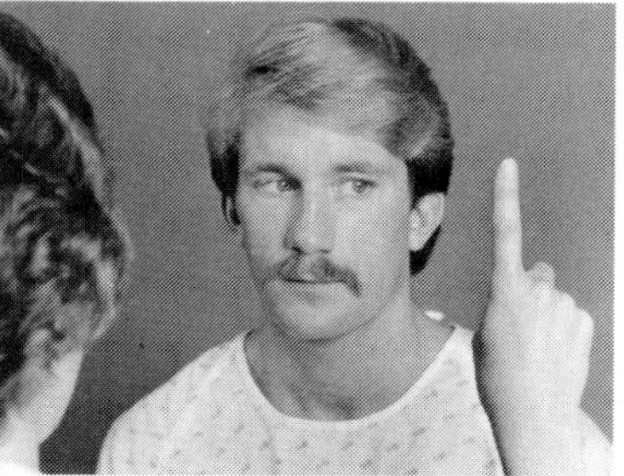

4. Assess external eye structures:
   a. If client wears contact lenses request their removal.

   Palpation of eye structures during examination could cause breakage of lens and injury to eye.

   b. Stand or sit in front of client at eye level. Instruct client to look at nurse's face.

   Allows nurse to clearly inspect position and alignment of eyes in addition to characteristics of all external eye structures.

**Steps** | **Rationale**

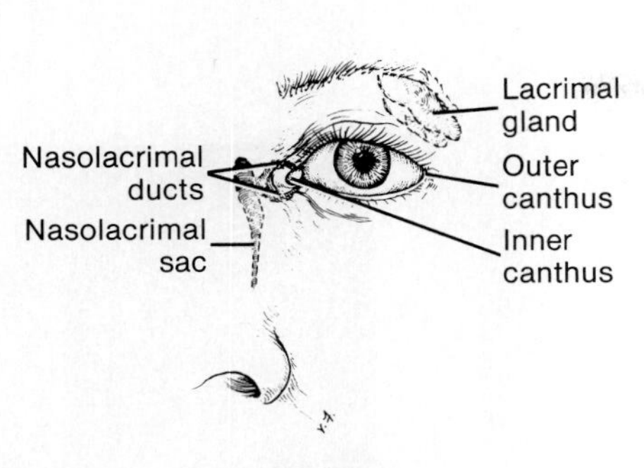


*Fig. 13-11*

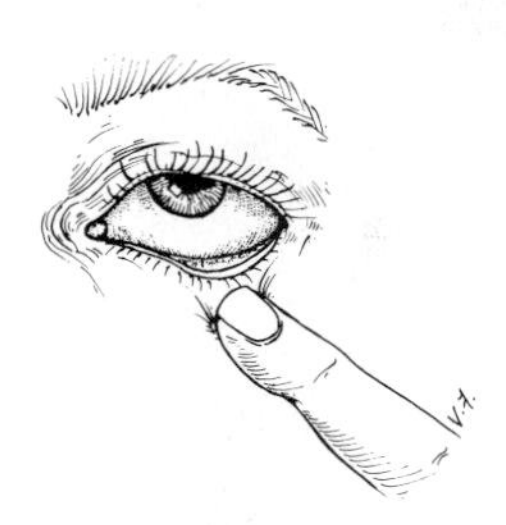

*Fig. 13-12*

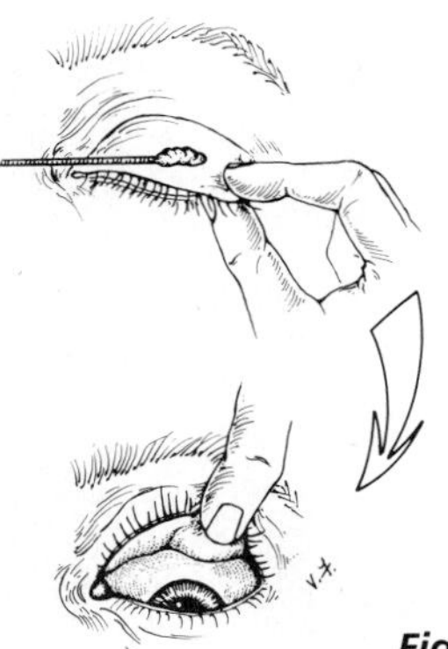

*Fig. 13-13*

c. Inspect position and alignment of eyes.
May indicate genetic, neurologic, or metabolic alterations.

d. If abnormal placement is suspected, measure distance between two pupils by placing small ruler at bridge of nose and asking client to gaze straight ahead.
Large spacing between eyes (hypertelorism) may indicate mental retardation. Normal distance between pupils is 4.5-5.5 cm (1.75-2.25 in).

e. Observe eyebrows for symmetry, quantity of hair, and movement.
Eyebrows are normally symmetric with equal distribution of hair growth. Client should be able to move eyebrows easily. Inability to move eyebrows indicates paralysis of facial nerve.

f. If flaking of skin is seen around eyebrows, ask if client has experienced eye irritation.
Form of dandruff may affect eyebrows with particles of skin entering eyes and irritating eyelids or conjunctivae.

g. Inspect eyelid position with eyes open.
Normally eyelids do not cover pupil, and sclera cannot be seen above iris. Abnormal drooping of lid over pupil (ptosis) is caused by localized edema, impairment of third cranial nerve, or myasthenia.

h. Note if any portion of lower conjunctiva is visible.
With eyelids open or closed no palpebral conjunctiva should be visible. Malposition of lid margins may lead to conjunctival irritation.

i. Ask client to close eyes and inspect eyelid positions.
Eyelids should close completely. Failure to close exposes cornea to dryness and irritation.

j. Inspect eyelids for color, edema, and presence of lesions. If inflammation or lesion is present, ask if client is experiencing any discomfort.
Normally lids are same color as client's skin. There should be no inflammation, drainage, edema, or lesions.
Common forms of inflammation of eyelid:

- *Hordeolum or stye:* small sebaceous glands near eyelashes become inflamed; localized painful, reddened area usually on lower lid.
- *Chalazion:* cyst of internal sebaceous glands; usually localized, nontender, and firm with freely movable skin.
- *Marginal blepharitis:* Inflammation of eyelid margin, lids become inflamed, scaly, and crusted.

k. Inspect distribution and direction of growth of eyelashes.
Determines risk of irritation to conjunctivae. Normally upper lashes curl upward and lower lashes curve downward.

l. Inspect lacrimal apparatus (Fig. 13-11). Note presence of edema or inflammation at upper outer wall of anterior part of each orbit. Palpate gently to detect tenderness.
Normally lacrimal gland cannot be seen or palpated.

m. Inspect for excess tearing of eyes and edema of inner canthus.
Obstruction of nasolacrimal duct causes blockage to flow of tears.

n. Gently palpate lower eyelid just inside orbital rim if tearing is noted.
Palpation will cause regurgitation of tears if duct is blocked.

o. Inspect conjunctiva. Gently depress lower lid with thumb pressed against bony orbit. Ask client to look up (Fig. 13-12). Inspect color of conjunctivae and note any edema or lesions. To retract upper eyelid ask client to look down, relax eyes, and avoid any sudden movement. Gently grasp upper lid, pulling it down and forward. Place end of cotton-tipped applicator 1 cm (0.5 in) above lid margin. Push down on eyelid with applicator, turning lash inside out (Fig. 13-13). Light grasp of lashes keeps lid inverted. After inspection pull eyelashes gently forward and instruct client to look up. Eyelid returns to normal position.
Gentle retraction prevents pressure from being applied directly to eyeball. Retraction provides full exposure. Normal palpebral conjunctiva lining the lids is light pink in color. Sclera is seen under bulbar conjunctiva and normally is white color of porcelain. Exposure of upper palpebral conjunctiva allows inspection for foreign bodies. Client's ability to relax prevents accidental trauma during use of applicator.

| Steps | Rationale |
|---|---|

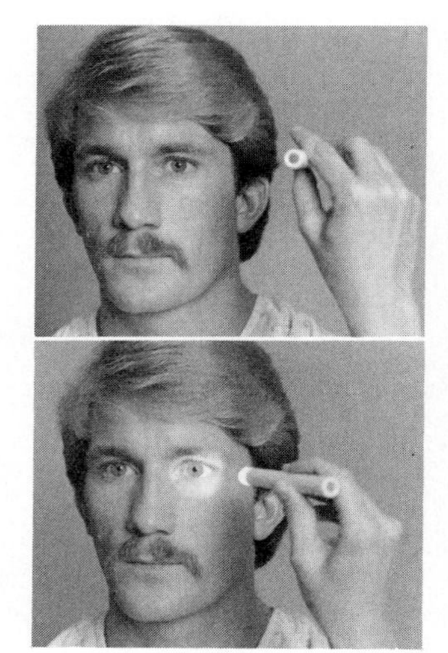

*Fig. 13-14*

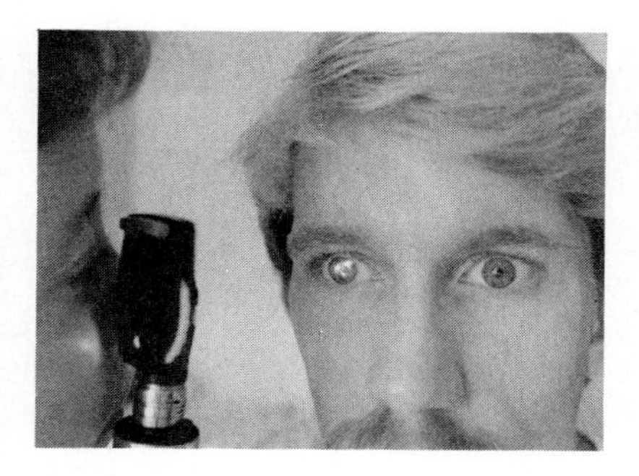

*Fig. 13-15*

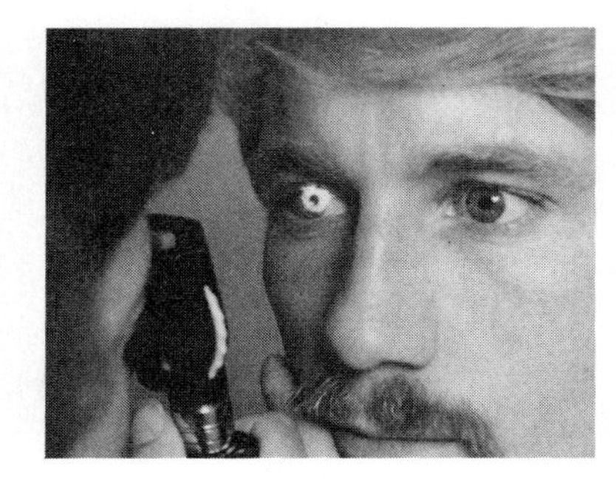

*Fig. 13-16*

| Steps | Rationale |
|---|---|
| p. Inspect pupils for size, shape, and equality. | Normal pupils are round, clear, and equal in size and shape. |
| q. Inspect surrounding iris for symmetry of shape. | Defects along inner margins of iris may be result of surgical correction for glaucoma. |
| r. Test pupillary reflexes. To test reaction to light dim room lights. Nurse should still be able to see client's pupils. As client looks straight ahead, move penlight from side of client's face and direct light on pupil. Observe pupillary response of both eyes (Fig. 13-14). | In normal client ensures brisk response of pupils to light. Pupil that is illuminated constricts (direct light reaction). Pupil in other eye should constrict equally (consensual light reaction). Pupils should constrict briskly. |
| s. Test accommodation by first asking client to look at wall in distance. Then quickly bring finger within 10-15 cm (4-6 in) of client's nose and ask client to look at finger. | When focusing on near object, pupils of both eyes should constrict. |
| 5. Perform ophthalmoscopic examination: | |
| a. Have client sit in front of nurse with eyes at same height as nurse's. | Provides nurse easy access to illuminate eye structures. |
| b. Darken room. | Promotes pupil dilation, allowing more light from ophthalmoscope to enter eye. |
| c. Turn ophthalmoscope on by rotating dial at top of battery tube. Adjust lens to setting of 0. Shine light on palm of hand. By reading newsprint through ophthalmoscope nurse can determine if objects can be seen clearly. Lens setting can be adjusted at that time. | Lens settings depend on whether examiner or client has errors in refraction (nearsightedness or farsightedness). Setting of 0 is good starting point but may require adjustment for examiner to see eye structures clearly. |
| d. Ask client to keep both eyes open during examination and to focus on distant object behind nurse. | Nurse's ability to visualize eye structures requires that client keep eyelids open and head still. |
| e. Nurse examines client's right eye by holding ophthalmoscope in right hand against right eye. | Permits easiest access to illuminate pupil and view structures. |
| f. Nurse rests ophthalmoscope against face over right eye and keeps both eyes open. Index finger remains on lens disc. At distance of 25 cm (10 in) from client and lateral to line of vision, focus light on pupil. Bright orange glow ("red reflex") can be seen in pupil (Fig. 13-15). | Red reflex indicates light is directed onto pupil and internal structures are illuminated. Orange color is same as that of retina. Focusing light from distance allows nurse to accurately aim ophthalmoscope. |
| g. Nurse keeps light focused on red reflex and slowly brings head and ophthalmoscope toward client's face from side at 15° angle and not directly toward eye. As light approaches pupil, nurse begins to see structures of fundus. Rotation of lens disc brings structures into focus. Nurse systematically scans fundus in detail, beginning with optic disc, and moving outward toward blood vessels and nerve fibers (Fig. 13-16). | Visualization of internal structures requires clear focusing and proper illumination. Accurate inspection requires nurse to view each part of fundus separately. Optic disc is most prominent structure and serves as point from which inspection begins. Normal fundus: clear, creamy pink, or yellow optic nerve disc, 1.5 mm in size, flat and round; reddish orange retina; light red arteries and dark red veins; 3:2 vein-to-artery ratio in size proportion; avascular macula. Presence of any abnormalities requires referral to ophthalmologist. |
| h. Repeat procedures for left eye. | |

## Evaluation

| | |
|---|---|
| 1. Compare findings with normal assessment characteristics of eye. | Determines presence of abnormalities. |

| Steps | Rationale |
|---|---|
| ***Expected outcomes*** | |
| 1. Client has normal visual acuity with or without correction. | Normal findings. |
| 2. Client has full visual fields and parallel eye movement in each cardinal gaze. | |
| 3. Position of eyes, eyelids, and eyebrows is normal. | |
| 4. Clarity noted in sclera with conjunctiva clear and pink. | |
| 5. Pupils equal and round, react briskly to light and accommodation. Abbreviation for this response is PERRLA. | |
| 6. Internal eye structures normal in color, size, and shape. | |
| ***Unexpected outcomes*** | |
| 1. Visual acuity reduced, client unable to see objects or perceive light. | May be caused by an acute or long-term problem. |
| 2. Visual fields are narrowed. | Indicative of optic nerve problem. |
| 3. Eye movements unequal in all or in specific gazes. | May be due to alteration in neurologic or muscular function. |
| 4. Ptosis noted of eyelids. | Drooping of lid due to edema or possibly nerve paralysis. |
| 5. Conjunctivae may be inflamed or pale. | Infection results in inflammation. Anemia causes pale conjunctivae. |
| 6. Pupils may be unequal in size or shape. | Usually indicates intracranial alteration. |
| 7. Abnormalities noted in fundus and vessels of retina. | Requires follow-up by ophthalmologist. |
| ***Potential nursing diagnoses*** | |
| ▪ Self-care deficit: related to reduced visual acuity. | Client may require assistance with activities of daily living (ADL). |
| ▪ Potential for injury: related to visual impairment. | Nurse maintains safe environment. |
| ▪ Disturbance in self-concept: related to impaired vision. | Client's independence should be maintained. |
| ▪ Fear: related to threat of loss of vision. | Client must understand implications of findings. |

## Recording and Reporting

| | |
|---|---|
| 1. Record score of Snellen test, note sc (without correction) or cc (with correction). | Documents status of acuity with or without corrective lenses. |
| 2. Record observations made of eye structures and results of functional assessments. | Provides data for comparison with subsequent assessments. Abbreviations: right eye, OD; left eye, OS; both eyes, OU. |
| 3. Report serious abnormalities to nurse in charge or physician. | Immediate medical attention may be required. |

## Follow-up Activities

| | |
|---|---|
| 1. Refer client to ophthalmologist or optometrist for further testing of visual acuity. | Provides for timely correction of visual acuity or other visual impairments. |
| 2. If client's vision is severely impaired obtain information about community resources for visually impaired clients. | Enables client with visual impairments an opportunity to use community resources to learn braille, or obtain talking tapes and large-print books and magazines. |

## Special Considerations

- Presence of foreign object or corneal abrasion is very painful. Client may have difficulty relaxing.
- The three varieties of Snellen charts are:
  1. Chart with alphabet, used by client able to read English.
  2. **E** Chart, used by illiterate clients.
  3. Chart with series of familiar objects, used for children.
- Normally, only portion of the eye examination that may cause some discomfort is ophthalmoscopic examination (bright light focused on the fovea centralis can be uncomfortable).
- Visual acuity score is recorded in 2 numbers. Standardized numbers (fraction) are located at end of each line of chart. Numerator is 20, standard distance client stands from chart. Denominator is distance from which normal eye can read chart. Normal vision is 20/20. High denominator indicates poor vision. 20/200 means client can read letter 20 ft away that normal person could read standing 200 ft away.
- Optic nerve injury, retinal disorders, and intracranial tumors cause loss of portions of visual fields.
- Disturbances in eye movement reflect local injury to eye muscles and supporting structure or pathologic condition of cranial nerves that innervate muscles.
- Clients with decreased levels of consciousness, who are comatose, or who have neurologic alterations (e.g., stroke, facial nerve injury) are at risk for corneal exposure and will require frequent lubrication of cornea and perhaps application of protective eye patch.
- Elderly clients commonly have reduced tearing and are prone to corneal irritation.
- If you observe a foreign body that appears embedded in the eye, *do not attempt to remove it.* Notify physician immediately.
- Dilated or constricted pupils can result from neurologic disorders (e.g., increased intracranial pressure, glaucoma, effects of eye medications).

- Arcus senilis, a halo around the cornea, is common in older adults.
- *Xanthoma palpebrarum,* deposits of fat (lipid) on eyelids, is associated with clients who have hyperlipidemia.

### Teaching Considerations

- Clients under age 40 should have complete eye examinations every 3-5 yr (or more often if family histories reveal risks, such as diabetes or hypertension).
- Clients over age 40 should have eye examinations every 2 yr to screen for glaucoma.
- Clients over age 65 should have yearly eye examinations.
- Describe typical symptoms of eye disease.
- Instruct elderly client to take the following precautions because of normal visual changes: avoid driving at night, increase lighting in home to reduce risk of falls, paint the first and last steps of a staircase and the edge of each step in between a bright color to aid depth perception.
- Any client with eyelid inflammation should be cautioned against rubbing eyes because of risk of spreading inflammation or infection to uninvolved eye.
- To reduce anxiety show child ophthalmoscope and how light shines. Explain that procedure is painless.
- Do not let client focus on light of ophthalmoscope because bright light can become irritating.

### Home Care Considerations

- Measure of visual acuity helps nurse determine level of assistance client requires with daily living activities and ability of client to safely ambulate independently.
- Examination assesses client's ability to read educational materials.
- Clients with visual field loss may require safety precautions, instruction to look down or to side for obstacles, or placing articles of care in field of vision.

# *SKILL 13-6* Assessing the Ears

The nurse assesses condition of ear structures (Fig. 13-17) and performs measurements of hearing acuity when examining the ears. Ears are easily accessible, and the otoscope provides a means to visualize internal middle ear structures. Generally the client experiences only minor discomfort during the assessment unless there is preexisting inflammatory conditions of outer ear structures.

A hearing disorder is caused by one of four types of problems: (1) mechanical dysfunction (blockage of external ear by cerumen or a foreign body), (2) trauma (foreign bodies or excess noise exposure), (3) neurologic disorders (auditory nerve damage), and (4) acute illnesses affecting inner ear function (viral infection). Conduction deafness results from sound waves failing to pass through external or middle ear structures. This type of deafness often is curable. Nerve deafness is more serious, because it involves sensitive internal ear or auditory nerve structures.

### Purposes

1. Determine client risk for developing hearing loss.
2. Determine condition and function of ear structures.
3. Assess client hearing acuity.

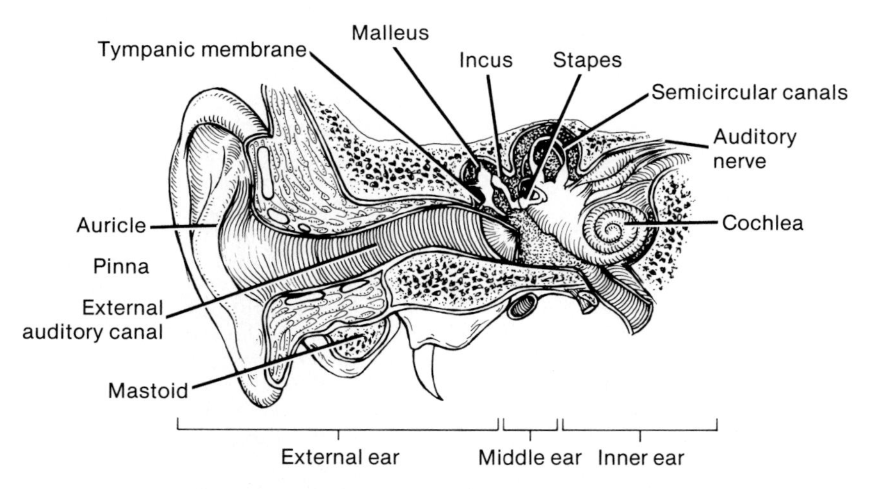


***Fig. 13-17*** Ear structures. External ear consists of auricle and external auditory canal. Middle ear structures include tympanic membrane and bony ossicles (malleus, incus, and stapes). Semi-circular canal, cochlea, and auditory nerve are inner ear structures.

## Procedure 13-6

| Steps | Rationale |
|---|---|
| **Assessment** | |
| 1. Ask if client has experienced ear pain, itching, discharge, tinnitus (ringing in ears), or change in hearing ability. | Signs and symptoms indicative of infection or hearing loss. |
| 2. Determine risks for hearing problems: hypoxia at birth, meningitis, birth weight less than 1500 g, family history of hearing loss, nonbacterial intrauterine fetal infections (rubella, herpes, syphilis), frequent ear infections, congenital anomalies of skull or face, hyperbilirubinemia. | These factors can increase risk of permanent hearing loss caused by associated hypoxia or congenital predisposition. |
| 3. Assess client's occupation in terms of exposure to loud noises and availability of protective devices. | Prolonged exposure to loud noises can cause temporary and permanent hearing loss. |
| 4. Note behavior during earlier assessments that may indicate hearing problem: failure to respond when spoken to; repetition of statement, "What did you say?"; complaint of people mumbling; leaning forward to hear; hearing better when watching speaker's face. Children also may be inattentive, interrupt nurse without being aware of it, have monotonous voice tone, or use gestures to communicate. | Clients with hearing loss cope with sensory deficit through a variety of behavioral cues. |
| 5. Determine if client takes antibiotics or large doses of aspirin. | These medications can cause hearing disorders, e.g., aminoglycosides (gentamicin, vancomycin). |
| 6. Determine whether client uses a hearing aid. | Determination allows nurse to assess client's ability to care for device and allows nurse to adjust voice tone to communicate with client. |
| 7. If client has had a recent hearing problem, note onset, contributing factors, and effect on activities of daily living. | Determines nature and severity of hearing problem. |
| **Planning** | |
| 1. Develop individualized goals for assessment, including: | |
| a. Maintain client's comfort. | Client can become anxious when nurse inserts otoscope. External ear structures are sensitive when inflamed. |
| b. Promote effective communication. | Clients have various degrees of hearing loss. |
| c. Improve client's knowledge of risks for hearing loss. | Topic discussed during assessment. |
| d. Identify presence of abnormalities. | Findings may initiate therapeutic measures of care. |
| 2. Prepare needed equipment and supplies: | |
| a. Otoscope. Speculums for otoscope come in various sizes to conform to ear canal. Choose largest one that fits comfortably. | Used to visualize outer and middle ear structures. |
| b. Tuning fork. | Used to assess hearing acuity. |
| 3. Prepare client: | |
| a. Explain steps of procedure, particularly when otoscope is inserted, and assure client that procedure normally is painless. | Introduction of otoscope is painless unless ear canal is inflamed. |
| b. Have adult client sit through examination. | Sitting offers easy access to ear structures. |
| c. Allow infant or young child to sit on parent's lap, or if necessary, restrain child in side-lying position for otoscopic examination. | Restraining child prevents accidental injury to internal ear structures during procedure. |
| **Implementation** | |
| ***External ear*** | |
| 1. Inspect auricle for placement, size, and symmetry. Auricles are normally level with each other, and upper point of attachment to head is in straight line with lateral outer canthus of eye to occipital bone of skull. | Abnormal placement of ears may result from mental retardation or other congenital anomalies. |
| 2. Inspect skin around and behind auricle for scratches, inflammation, lesions, or swelling. In children, note small openings or sinuses. | Scratches or lesions may predispose to infection. Sinus or opening may reveal fistula that drains into area of ear or neck. |
| 3. If client complains of pain or ear appears inflamed, pull gently on auricle or press inward on tragus (soft, tongue-like projection just below entrance to external ear canal). | If palpation of external ear increases client's pain, external ear infection is present. If pain does not increase, discomfort may originate in middle ear. |

| Steps | Rationale |
|---|---|
| 4. Observe opening of ear canal for lesions, discharge, swelling, foreign bodies, or inflammation. Palpate any lesions gently. Nurse should wear gloves when palpating draining lesion. | Narrowing of ear canal by obstruction reduces client's hearing acuity. Skin of ear canal rests closely against underlying cartilage and thus is extremely tender when inflamed. |
| 5. Inspect canal for buildup of cerumen. If canal is clear, ask how client usually cleans ears. | Allows nurse to assess client's hygiene practices. Small amount of cerumen normally should be in ears. Absence of cerumen indicates client uses special method for cleaning canal. |
| ***Otoscopic examination*** | |
| 1. Be sure canal is clear of foreign objects. Instruct client about importance of holding head still during insertion of otoscope. Turn on light by rotating disk at top of battery tube. Young child or infant can be restrained by having child sit sideways in parent's lap with one arm hugging parent and other at child's side. Parent holds child by restraining arm with one hand and holding child's head against parent's shoulder with other (Fig. 13-18, *A*). Child also can be restrained in side-lying position, with arms at sides and head turned with ear pointed toward ceiling (Fig. 13-18, *B*). | If foreign object is present, inserting otoscope can embed object deeper into canal. Sudden movement by client can damage canal or eardrum. |
| 2. Ask client to tip head slightly toward shoulder opposite ear being examined. Pull auricle gently upward and backward in adult, backward and downward in infant. | Tilting head better exposes ear. Pulling auricle straightens ear canal for proper insertion of otoscope. |
| 3. Insert speculum, taking care not to abrade lining of canal (Fig. 13-19). | Skin of canal is sensitive to minor trauma. Inflamed ear canal can be very sensitive. |
| 4. Brace hand against client's head during insertion of otoscope. | Prevents accidental, sudden movement of otoscope. |
| 5. Inspect inner canal for proper color, lesions, foreign bodies, or discharge. | Disorder of inner canal interferes with sound conduction. |
| 6. Inspect eardrum by observing one quadrant at a time. Observe for light reflex, umbo of malleus, and any tears (Fig. 13-20). Normal eardrum is translucent or pearly gray. Eardrum angles away from ear canal, and thus light of otoscope creates cone of light. Absence of light reflex indicates bulging of membrane. Umbo of malleus (knoblike structure at top of ear) attaches to center of eardrum. | Allows visualization of entire eardrum and its periphery to detect middle ear abnormalities. |
| ***Hearing acuity*** | |
| 1. Ask client to close eyes and occlude one ear with finger. Standing approximately 30 cm (1 ft) away, exhale fully and | Provides cursory screening of hearing acuity. Closing eyes prevents client from lipreading. |

A

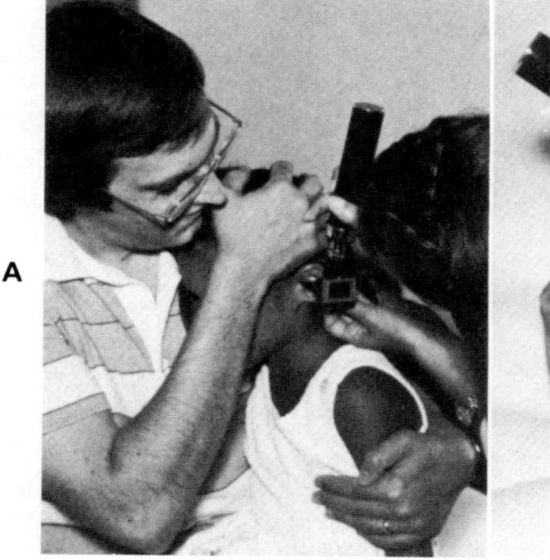

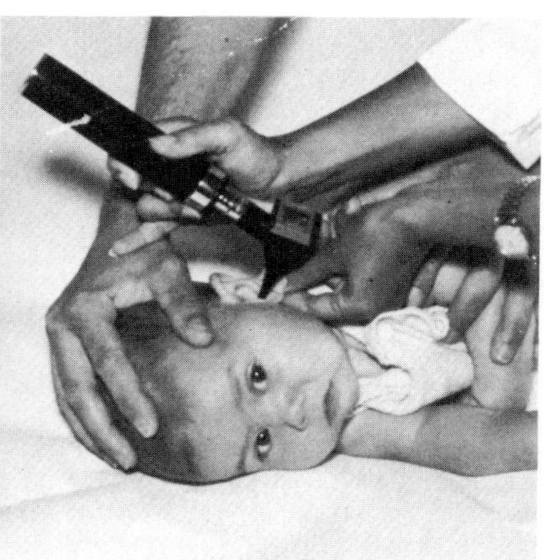

B

***Fig. 13-18***

From Whaley L and Wong D: Nursing care of infants and children, ed 3, 1987, St Louis, The CV Mosby Co.

**Steps** | **Rationale**

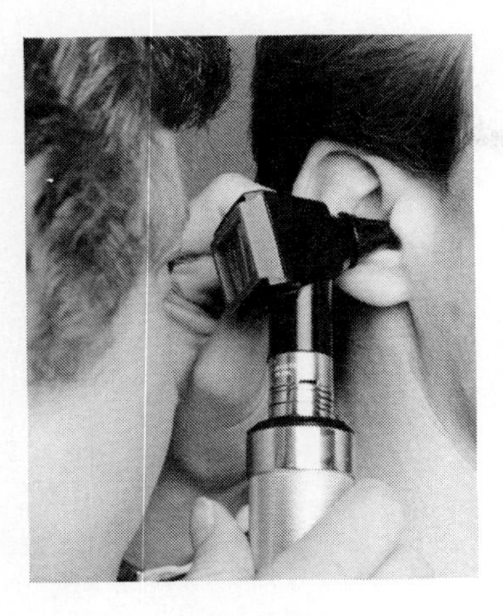

***Fig. 13-19***

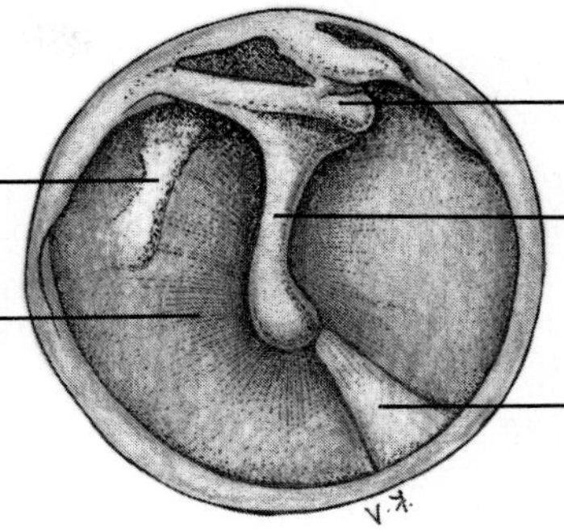

Short process of malleus
Incus
Handle of malleus
Pars tensa
Cone of light

***Fig. 13-20*** Normal tympanic membrane.

softly whisper sequence of numbers toward unoccluded ear for client to identify. Do not use consecutive numbers, so there is no doubt client can hear. Repeat for opposite ear.

2. Perform tuning fork test:

Checks for lateralization of sound. Vibrating fork transmits sound through bone directly to inner ear structures, bypassing external and middle ear structures. Client with normal hearing hears sound equally in both ears or in midline of head.

   a. Weber's test: hold fork at base and strike ends against palm of hand. Place base of vibrating fork on top of client's head and ask client where sound is heard (Fig. 13-21).

Normally client can hear sound equally in both ears. Provides measure to lateralize any hearing loss:
Conductive loss: vibration noted in deaf ear.
Sensorineural loss: vibration noted in better ear.

   b. Rinne's test: hold fork at base and strike ends against palm of hand. Place base of vibrating fork against mastoid bone until sound is no longer audible. Then quickly hold ends of fork near auditory meatus (Fig. 13-22).

Normally client can hear sound twice as long over meatus after bone conduction is inaudible (positive Rinne's). In conduction deafness, sounds through air are no longer audible, indicating conduction problem through external and middle ears.

## Evaluation

1. Compare findings with normal assessment characteristics of ears.

Determines presence of abnormalities.

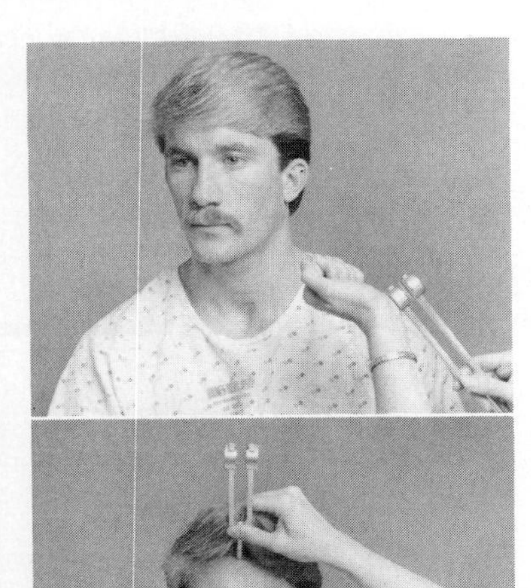

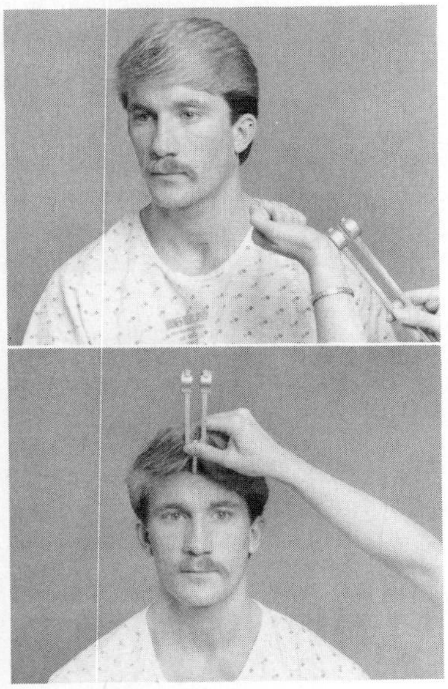

***Fig. 13-21***

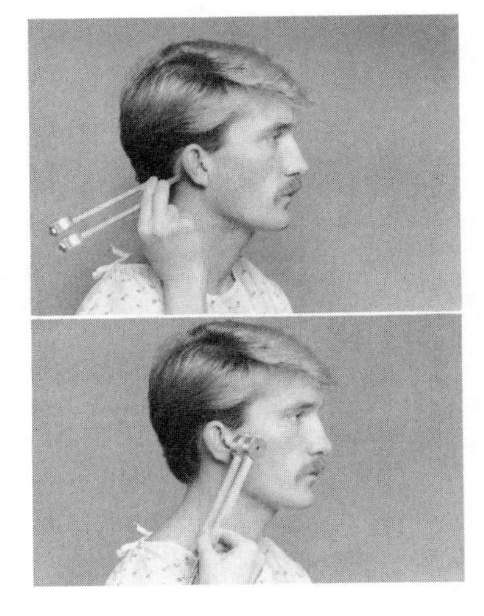

***Fig. 13-22***

| Steps | Rationale |
|---|---|
| ***Expected outcomes*** | |
| 1. Auricle and external ear canal are clear; color is normal. Cerumen may be present in canal. | Small amount of cerumen is normal. |
| 2. Eardrum is translucent; light reflex is present. | Eardrum intact. |
| 3. Hearing acuity is normal; client can identify spoken word. | Normal sound conduction and reception. |
| 4. Tuning fork tests are normal. | |
| ***Unexpected outcomes*** | |
| 1. Auricle or ear canal is swollen, inflamed, and tender to palpation. Drainage or lesions may be detected. | Usually indicates infection. |
| 2. Hearing acuity reduced, client cannot identify spoken word. | Indicates conduction or nerve deafness. |
| 3. Tuning fork tests reveal hearing loss. | Indicates conduction or nerve deafness. |
| ***Potential nursing diagnoses*** | |
| ▪ Pain: related to auditory canal inflammation. | Lining of ear is very sensitive. |
| ▪ Sensory alteration: related to hearing impairment. | Alters client's ability to communicate and react to environment. |
| ▪ Potential for injury: related to hearing impairment. | Nurse must provide safe environment. |
| **Recording and Reporting** | |
| 1. Record observations from inspection and palpation in nurses' notes. | Documentation of assessment data provides baseline for future assessments and records client's response to specific therapies. |
| 2. Record results of Weber's test and note if Rinne's test is positive or negative. | Allows nurse to plan for consistently effective communication techniques if hearing loss is present. |
| 3. Report hearing loss to charge nurse or physician. | Hearing loss may require further assessment. |
| **Follow-up Activities** | |
| 1. Obtain information about community resources for the hearing impaired. | Enables clients with hearing impairments the necessary resources to obtain special telephone, television, and emergency services. |

### Special Considerations

- For client with obvious hearing impairment speak clearly and concisely, stand so client can see your face, stand toward client's good ear, speak in low pitch, do not yell.
- Teachers of children may be good resource to report unusual behaviors in classroom.

### Teaching Considerations

- Instruct client about the proper way to clean outer ear (see Chapter 6), avoiding use of cotton-tipped applicators and sharp objects such as hairpins.
- Tell client to avoid inserting pointed objects into the ear canal.
- Encourage clients over age 65 to have regular hearing checks.
- Instruct family members of clients with hearing losses to avoid shouting and speak instead in low tones.

# *SKILL 13-7 Assessing the Nose and Sinuses*

Assessment of a client's nose and sinuses takes little time, and procedures are relatively simple. If clients have nasogastric or nasotracheal tubes inserted, however, the nurse should take care to inspect the nasal mucosa thoroughly. Such tubes can cause considerable trauma and discomfort.

### Purposes

1. Determine presence of allergies or infection.
2. Assess condition of nasal mucosa.

## Procedure 13-7

| Steps | Rationale |
|---|---|
| **Assessment** | |
| 1. Determine if client has experienced any trauma to nose. | Can result in deviation of septum and asymmetry of external nose. |
| 2. Assess if client has history of allergies, nasal discharge, epistaxis (nosebleeds), or postnasal drip. | Useful in determining source or nature of nasal and sinus drainage. |
| 3. Ask if client uses nasal spray or drops. | Overuse of over-the-counter nasal preparations can cause physical change in mucosa. |
| 4. Ask if client snores at night or has difficulty breathing. | Difficulty in breathing or snoring may indicate septal deviation or obstruction. |
| **Planning** | |
| 1. Develop individualized goals for assessment, including: | |
| a. Minimize client's discomfort. | Nasal mucosa can become very sensitive when inflamed. |
| b. Identify presence of abnormalities. | Findings may initiate therapeutic care measures. |
| 2. Prepare needed equipment and supplies: | Allows visualization of nasal mucosa, septum, and turbinates. |
| a. Penlight | |
| b. Nasal speculum | |
| 3. Prepare client: | |
| a. Explain steps of procedure and assure client that examination will not be painful or interfere with breathing. | Minimizes client's anxiety. |
| b. Have client assume sitting position with head tilted backward. | Provides for visualization of internal nasal structures. |
| **Implementation** | |
| 1. Inspect nose externally for placement, alignment, and symmetry. | Asymmetry may indicate trauma. |
| 2. Inspect nasal mucosa and position of septum at anterior end of nose. Note color of mucosa and any lesions, discharge, swelling, inflammation, or deformity. Use penlight for better illumination. | Reveals any nasal obstruction that may interfere with breathing. Character of discharge and inflammation indicate allergy or infection. Pale, swollen mucosa and clear, watery drainage indicate allergy. Red, swollen mucosa and yellowish or greenish discharge indicate infection. |
| 3. In clients with nasogastric or nasotracheal tubes, inspect nares for excoriation, inflammation, or sloughing of skin. | Swallowing or coughing reflex causes movement of tubes against nares. Failure to anchor tube properly causes pressure against nares and mucosa. |
| 4. Gently insert nasal speculum into nares and advance approximately 1 cm. Hold handle at 90° angle to side of nose. | Provides clearer view of septum and turbinates. |
| 5. Inspect septum for deviation, lesions, and superficial blood vessels. Repeat for opposite nostril. | Deviated septum obstructs air flow and interferes with passage of nasogastric tube. |
| 6. Palpate frontal sinus by placing thumb over ridge of upper orbit of each eye and pressing gently upward. | Pressure elicits tenderness if sinus is swollen or inflamed. |
| 7. Palpate maxillary sinuses by placing tips of middle three fingers over maxillary sinus, just to each side of nose, and apply upward pressure (Fig. 13-23). | Elicits tenderness in presence of inflammation. |

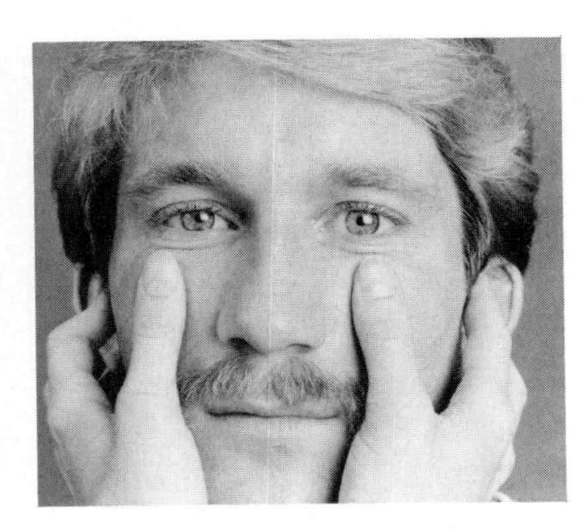

***Fig. 13-23***

| Steps | Rationale |
|---|---|
| **Evaluation** | |
| 1. Compare findings with normal assessment characteristics of nose and sinuses. | Determines presence of abnormalities. |
| ***Expected outcomes*** | |
| 1. Nose is aligned, symmetric, without obvious lesions. | Normal findings. |
| 2. Nasal mucosa is pink, clear, and dry. | |
| 3. Septum is in midline. | Deviated septum is relatively common. |
| 4. Sinuses are nontender. | Absence of local irritation. |
| ***Unexpected outcomes*** | |
| 1. Nose is asymmetric. | Frequently results from trauma. |
| 2. Nasal mucosa inflamed or swollen with drainage. | Indicates local irritation from tubing, infection, or allergy. |
| 3. Nasal airway obstructed by lesions, swelling, deviated septum, or drainage. | Alters client's ease in breathing. |
| 4. Sinuses are tender. | Indicates infection or allergy. |
| ***Potential nursing diagnoses*** | |
| ■ Ineffective breathing pattern: related to nasal obstruction. | Interferes with full ventilation. |
| ■ Pain: related to sinus tenderness. | Sinus tissues are extremely sensitive. |
| **Recording and Reporting** | |
| 1. Record observations in nurses' notes. | Documents baseline findings and changes in client's condition. |
| 2. Report abnormalities to nurse in charge. | Client may require specific therapies. |

## Special Considerations

- In children, speculum usually is unnecessary.

## Teaching Considerations

- Caution clients against overuse of over-the-counter nasal sprays. Overuse of such sprays can cause a rebound effect, and essentially worsens nasal irritation.
- Instruct parents on care of children with nose bleeds: have child sit up and lean forward to avoid aspiration of blood, apply pressure to anterior of nose with thumb and forefinger as child breathes through mouth, apply ice or a cold cloth to bridge of nose if pressure fails to stop bleeding.
- The elderly lose the sense of smell and thus should have smoke detectors in their homes.

# *SKILL 13-8 Assessing the Mouth and Pharynx*

Condition of the oral cavity can reveal significant information about a client's health, such as state of hydration, nutritional status, hygiene practices, and any specific pathologic conditions. Too frequently the nurse hurries through an assessment of the mouth and pharynx; yet it is important to perform the procedure thoroughly. The nurse can easily miss a lesion or local area of inflammation under or around the tongue and along the mucosal surfaces. A convenient time to perform the assessment is while administering oral hygiene.

## Purposes

1. Determine condition of structures within the mouth.
2. Assess client's oral hygiene practices.
3. Determine the fit of partial or complete dentures.

## *Procedure 13-8*

| Steps | Rationale |
|---|---|
| **Assessment** | |
| 1. Determine if client wears dentures and if they are comfortable. | Dentures must be removed to visualize and palpate gums. Ill-fitting dentures cause irritation to mucosa and gums. |
| 2. Determine if client has had recent change in appetite or weight. | Symptoms may result from painful conditions of mouth. |
| 3. Assess client's dental hygiene practices, e.g., frequency of brushing, flossing, and use of other aids. | Provides nurse opportunity for health education during examination. |
| 4. Determine if client smokes or chews tobacco. | Tobacco users have 4-15 times greater risk for mouth and throat cancers (Mahboub and Sayed, 1982). |
| 5. Review history for alcohol consumption. | Heavy drinkers appear to have a greater risk for oral cancer. |
| **Planning** | |
| 1. Develop individualized goals for assessment, including: | |
| a. Promote client's comfort. | Oral mucosa can become sensitive when inflamed. |
| b. Increase client's knowledge of hygiene practices. | Assessment is excellent time to discuss oral hygiene techniques. |
| c. Determine presence of abnormalities. | Poses implications for many areas of care, e.g., diet therapy, hygiene, preventive health care education. |
| 2. Prepare equipment and supplies: | |
| a. Tongue depressor | Retracts cheek and tongue. |
| b. Penlight | Illuminates all internal structures. |
| c. Disposable gloves | Can be used to palpate lesions. |
| 3. Prepare client: | |
| a. Have client sit facing nurse at eye level. | Allows nurse to easily visualize internal structures. |
| b. Explain need to open mouth fully during examination. | Client's cooperation reduces examination time, improves visibility of mouth structures, and eliminates need to use tongue depressor. |
| **Implementation** | |
| 1. Have client open mouth halfway and inspect lips for color, texture, hydration, contour, symmetry, and lesions. | Provides full view of lips, which should be pink, moist, smooth, and symmetric. Asymmetry may be caused by facial nerve paralysis. Herpes simplex virus causes "cold sores," singular or clustered vesicular eruptions. Dry, cracked lips may result from dehydration, constant licking, exposure to cold, fever, or mouth breathing. |
| 2. Inspect oral mucosa under upper and lower lips by asking client to open mouth slightly and gently pulling lower, then upper, lip from teeth (Fig. 13-24). Note color, texture, hydration, and any ulcers, abrasions, or cysts. | Client's ability to relax and open mouth prevents pulling or tension on mucosa. Mucosa should be pink, moist, and smooth. Child may participate by taking fingers and retracting lips for nurse to examine mucosa. |
| 3. Ask client to open mouth wide and inspect buccal mucosa (lining of cheeks) by gently retracting lips and cheeks with tongue depressor. Use penlight to view more posterior mucosa. Observe color, texture, and hydration (Fig. 13-25). | Full retraction is needed to see all mucosal surfaces. Hyperpigmentation is seen in 10% of whites and up to 90% of blacks over age 50. Thick, white patches (leukoplakia) resulting from excessive drinking and smoking can be precursors to cancer. In children, white curdy patches that bleed when scraped are signs of candidal (monilial) infection (thrush). |

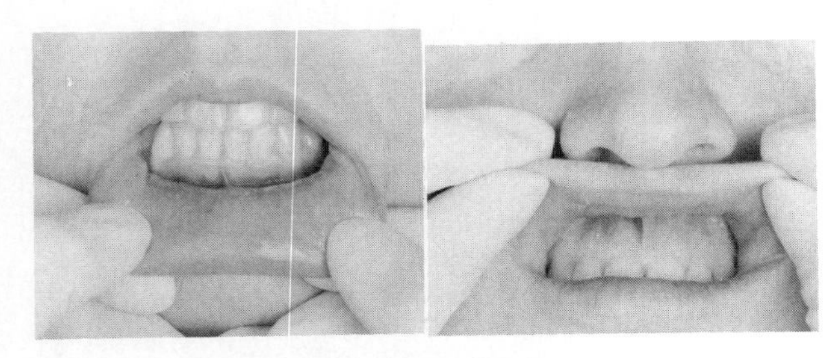

*Fig. 13-24*

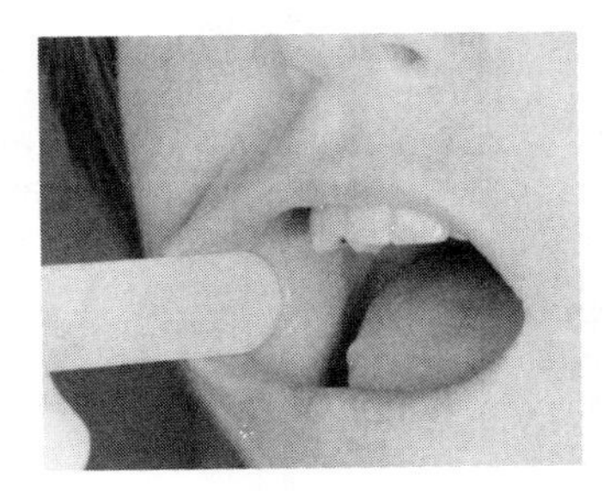

*Fig. 13-25*

| Steps | Rationale |
|---|---|

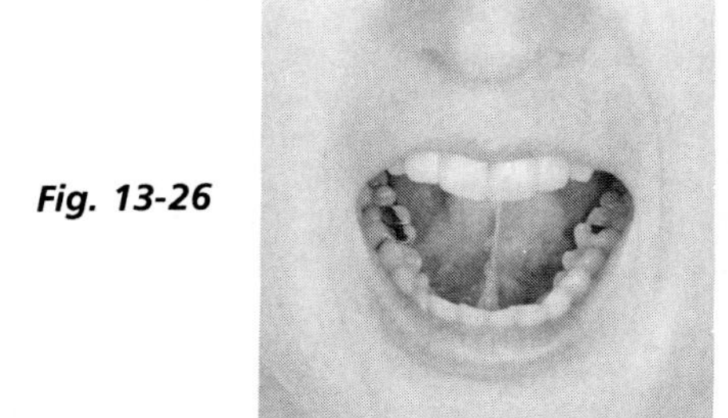

*Fig. 13-26*

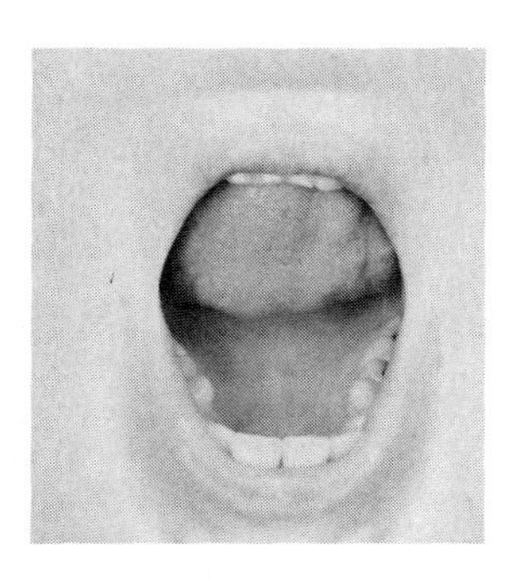

*Fig. 13-27*

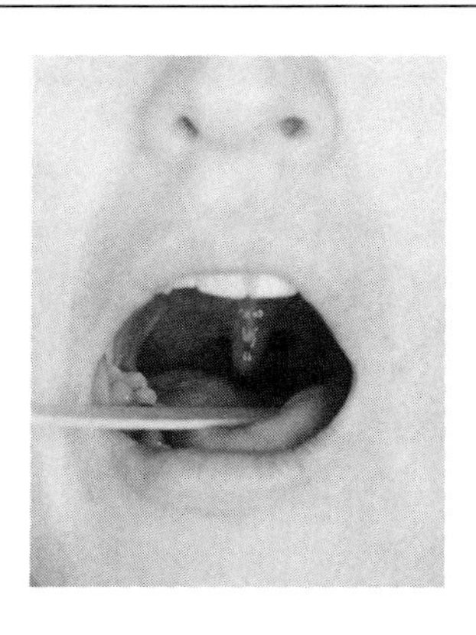

*Fig. 13-28*

4. Inspect gums for color, edema, retraction, bleeding, and lesions. Ask client if areas of tenderness exist.

   Gingivitis (inflammation of gums) is common periodontal disease of adults. Gum recession occurs in elderly from loss of tissue elasticity or periodontal tissue. Ill-fitting dentures cause inflammation of gums.

5. To examine teeth, ask client to open lips and clench teeth.

   Allows nurse to inspect position and alignment of teeth.

6. Count number of teeth in each dental arch.

   Provides measure of temporary and permanent teeth.

7. Inspect anterior, posterior, and chewing surfaces of teeth. Tongue depressor may be needed to retract cheeks and view molars. Observe color and any caries or extraction sites.

   Dental caries form along gum lines and between teeth where food particles accumulate. Chalky white discoloration is early sign of dental caries. Brown or black discoloration indicates advanced caries. Dark surface stains may be caused by tea, coffee, or tobacco.

8. Inspect tongue by asking client to relax mouth and protrude tongue halfway, then elevate it. Inspect all sides of tongue and floor of mouth. Note color, size, position, and texture of tongue and any lesions (Fig. 13-26).

   If client is forced to protrude tongue too far, gag reflex is elicited. Tongue mobility and function are essential for normal swallowing, chewing, and taste. Oral cancer frequently develops in floor of mouth.

9. With client extending head backward and holding mouth open, inspect hard and soft palates (Fig. 13-27). Penlight may be needed. Note color, shape, and extra bony prominences or defects.

   Infants may have congenitally formed clefts in soft palate, which require careful inspection to detect.

10. Ask client to say "ah." Tongue blade may be needed to visualize uvula and palate. Place tongue blade on middle third of tongue (Fig. 13-28). Tongue depressor placed anteriorly may cause posterior tongue to mound up and obstruct view.

    Assesses tenth cranial (vagus) nerve function. Uvula and soft palate should rise.

11. With penlight, inspect posterior pharynx, including anterior and posterior tonsillar pillars. Observe color, hydration, drainage, and any lesions.

    Common sites for infection or inflammation.

## Evaluation

1. Compare findings with normal assessment characteristics of mouth and pharynx.

   Determines presence of abnormalities. Findings document client's response to hygiene measures.

### *Expected outcomes*

1. Mucosal surfaces are pink or light red, well hydrated, and smooth.
2. Teeth are white, smooth, and shiny.
3. Gums are pink, moist, and attached to teeth.
4. Palate and pharynx are pink to red, well hydrated, and smooth.

Normal findings.

Adequate hydration and nutrition.

### *Unexpected outcomes*

1. Mucosa is dry, inflamed, and has lesions.

   Result of dehydration, trauma, or possibly infection.

2. Teeth are dull and have caries.

   Result of poor oral hygiene and reduced hydration.

3. Tongue is coated and edematous.

   Result of dehydration, poor hygiene, or inflammation.

4. Gums are inflamed and tender.

   Result of poor oral hygiene or poor nutrition.

5. Client complains of oral pain.

   May be caused by denture rubbing on tissues or actual lesion.

| Steps | Rationale |
|---|---|
| ***Potential nursing diagnosis*** | |
| ▪ Altered oral mucous membrane: related to poor oral hygiene, dehydration, trauma, or mouth breathing. | All diagnoses indicate need for vigorous hygiene measures. Client may also benefit from diet counseling. |
| **Recording and Reporting** | |
| 1. Record condition of oral cavity structures in nurses' notes. | Establishes baseline data for future comparisons after therapies. |
| 2. Report any lesions or bleeding to nurse in charge or physician. | Conditions indicate need for follow-up care. |

## Special Considerations

- Child may benefit from parent demonstrating how to say "ah." Most older children can be examined without tongue blade. Since infants and toddlers usually resist keeping mouth open, nurse may perform assessment near end of examination.
- Thick white coating is sign of poor hygiene. Patches of leukoplakia are not easily removed and may be precancerous lesions.
- Malocclusion can interfere with chewing.
- Helpful rule in estimating number of temporary teeth in children age 2 yr or younger: teeth expected equals child's age in mo minus 6 mo. Full set of teeth is 20 in children and 32 in adult.

## Teaching Considerations

- Discuss proper techniques for oral hygiene, including brushing and flossing.
- Explain early warning signs of oral cancer, including a sore that bleeds easily and does not heal, a lump or thickening, and a persistent red or white patch on the mucosa.
- Encourage yearly dental exams for children and adults. The elderly should visit a dentist every 6 mo.
- Elderly clients may need to eat soft foods and cut food into small pieces because of difficulty in chewing and changes in the teeth.

# *SKILL 13-9 Assessing the Structures of the Neck*

Primary structures within the neck that the nurse assesses include the cervical lymph node chains, thyroid gland, trachea, and carotid arteries and jugular veins. The nurse usually defers assessment of carotid arteries and jugular veins until the cardiovascular assessment (Skill 13-11). Generally the nurse assesses for similar characteristics of all neck structures, including symmetry, size, shape, and any lesions. The assessment techniques are normally painless.

## Purposes

1. Detect enlarged lymph nodes.
2. Assess condition of the thyroid gland.
3. Determine position of the trachea.

## *Procedure 13-9*

| Steps | Rationale |
|---|---|
| **Assessment** | |
| 1. Ask if client has had recent infection or cold. | Can cause temporary or permanent lymph node enlargement. |
| 2. Question client about type of table salt used. | Clients with goiter (enlarged thyroid gland) may not be ingesting adequate amounts of iodine. Iodized table salt has sufficient amounts of iodine. |
| 3. Determine if client takes thyroid medications. | Medications may influence tissue growth in thyroid gland. |
| 4. Ask if client has had a history of neck pain. | Neck pain may be indicative of muscle strain, local nerve injury, or an enlarged or swollen lymph node. |
| 5. Determine if client's medical condition indicates pneumothorax (collapsed lung) or bronchial tumor. | These preexisting conditions place client at increased risk for tracheal displacement. |

| Steps | Rationale |
|---|---|
| **Planning** | |
| 1. Develop individualized goals for assessment, including: | |
| a. Determine presence of abnormalities. | May pose implications for education or respiratory care. |
| b. Educate client regarding signs of lymph node or thyroid gland tumors. | Client can learn how to detect neck masses. |
| 2. Prepare equipment: | |
| a. Stethoscope | Used only if auscultating thyroid gland. |
| 3. Prepare client: | |
| a. Have client assume sitting position. | Provides easy access. Nurse examines all neck structures behind, to sides, and in front of client. |
| b. Explain that client will not experience choking sensation while trachea is palpated. | Client may be anxious about palpation of airway. |
| **Implementation** | |
| 1. Ask client to raise chin and tilt head backward, without tensing neck muscles. Inspect neck for symmetry, masses, or scars. | Neck extension improves exposure of underlying structures. Tensing muscles prevents access to lymph nodes for palpation. |
| 2. Palpate any apparent masses to determine size, shape, tenderness, consistency, and mobility. | Character of mass aids in determining presence of benign or malignant lesion or hypertrophy of underlying organs. |
| 3. Stand either behind or to side of client and palpate lymph nodes. Use middle three fingers and gently palpate in rotary fashion over regions where nodes are normally located. (Fig. 13-29). Palpate systematically along all lymph node chains. (Fig. 13-30). | Improves access for node preparation. Methodic palpation over each lymphatic chain prevents nurse from omitting any nodes. Vigorous palpation may obliterate small nodes and cause stimulation of carotid sinus. |
| 4. Inspect area of lower neck overlying thyroid gland for symmetry and masses (Fig. 13-31). | Gross inspection may reveal area of gland enlargement. |
| 5. Ask client to extend neck slightly and swallow. | Causes enlarged gland to bulge. |
| 6. To palpate thyroid gland, use posterior or anterior approach: | |
| a. To palpate posteriorly, ask client to lower chin. Place both hands gently around client's neck, with fingertips overlying lower trachea. Palpate thyroid isthmus and ask client to swallow (Fig. 13-32). Note any enlargement, nodules, or irregularities. To examine each lobe, ask client to turn head and flex neck slightly toward right. Using fingers of left hand, displace gland to right and palpate lobe with right hand. Repeat procedure for left lobe. | Relaxes neck muscles. Isthmus is usually only portion of gland ever palpable, since both lobes lie slightly behind sternocleidomastoid muscle. |
| b. To palpate anteriorly, stand in front of client. With second and third fingers of dominant hand, palpate for thyroid isthmus. Move fingers to each side and deep to edge of sternocleidomastoid muscle. Palpate each lobe. | |
| 7. If thyroid is enlarged, auscultate with bell of stethoscope for bruit. | Hypertrophy of thyroid gland increases vascular flow to area. |
| 8. Place thumb and index finger on each side of trachea, just above suprasternal notch (Fig. 13-33). Trachea is normally in midline above suprasternal notch. Avoid forceful pressure. | Gentle palpation prevents eliciting cough reflex. |

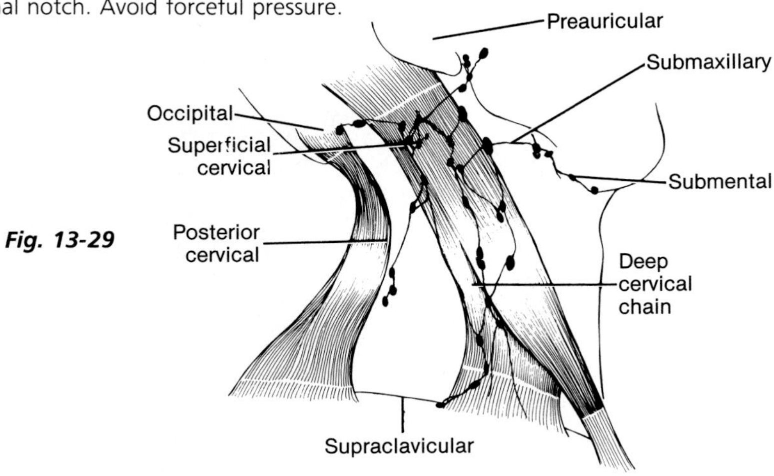


*Fig. 13-29*

**Steps** | **Rationale**

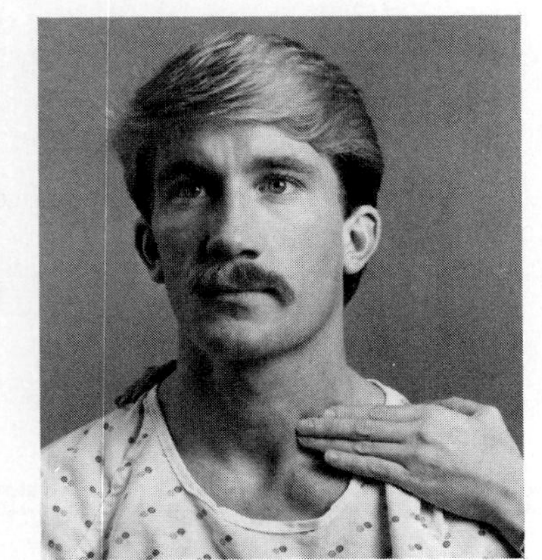

*Fig. 13-30*

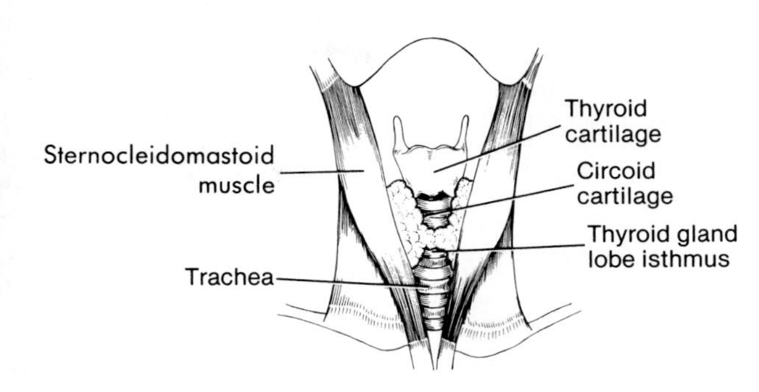


*Fig. 13-31*

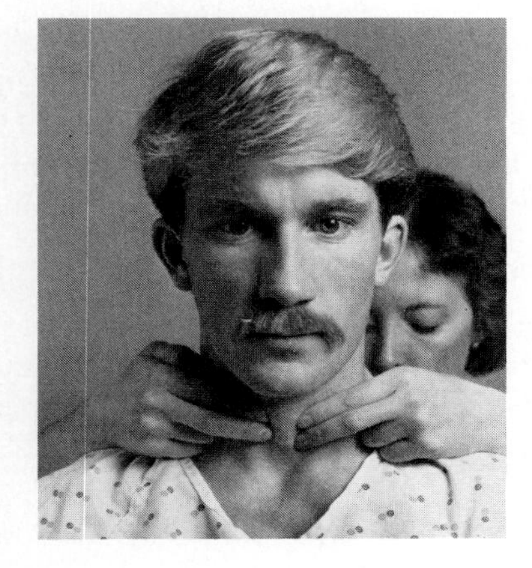

*Fig. 13-32*

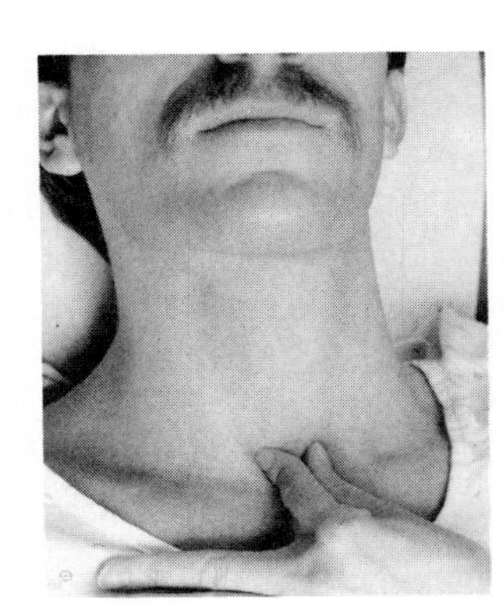

*Fig. 13-33*

## Evaluation

1. Compare findings with normal assessment characteristics of neck structures. — Determines presence of abnormalities.

### *Expected outcomes*

1. Lymph nodes are nonpalpable.
2. Thyroid gland is nonpalpable.
3. Trachea is in midline.

Normal findings.

### *Unexpected outcomes*

1. Lymph nodes are palpable, tender or nontender, fixed or movable, soft or hard. — Indicates benign or malignant lesion.
2. Thyroid gland is palpable and has nodules. — Indicates enlargement from hyperthyroidism or reveals benign or malignant lesions.
3. Trachea deviated to right or left. — Bronchial mass or pneumothorax is probable cause.

### *Potential nursing diagnosis*

- Assessment findings do not indicate specific nursing diagnosis. If client becomes aware of mass in neck, potential diagnosis might be anxiety related to impending diagnosis.

## Recording and Reporting

1. Record observations in nurses' notes. — Provides baseline findings for comparison.
2. Report abnormalities to physician immediately. — Potential nature of problems may necessitate further diagnosis or treatment.

### Special Considerations

- Goiter is relatively rare. However, client may benefit from education about normal dietary sources of iodine, e.g., green leafy vegetables, seafood.
- Any palpable mass involving neck structures must be reported immediately.
- Normally lymph nodes are not palpable. Tender, enlarged nodes indicate infection or inflammation. Malignant neck tumors are hard, immobile, irregularly shaped, and often nontender. In children, small nontender immovable nodes are normal.
- Normal gland is not palpable. Nurse may feel layer of tissue that rises as client swallows. Right lobe is normally larger than left. Enlarged gland results from thyroid dysfunction. Masses or nodules may indicate cancerous lesions.

### Teaching Considerations

- Stress importance of regular compliance with medication schedule to clients with thyroid disease.
- Instruct client to call physician when an enlarged lump or mass is noted in the neck.

# *SKILL 13-10 Assessing the Thorax and Lungs*

Physical assessment of the thorax and lungs requires consideration of vital ventilatory and respiratory roles of the lungs. Any alteration in pulmonary function usually affects other body systems. Thus the nurse must carefully assess findings from all body systems when determining the nature of pulmonary problems. For example, if a client's ventilation is impaired, the nurse should also assess skin color and the client's level of orientation to determine if oxygenation to tissues is adequate.

A convenient time to assess the thorax and lungs is when the client is sitting in a chair. To perform an assessment accurately, the nurse should be familiar with anatomic landmarks of the chest (Figs. 13-34 to 13-36). By keeping a mental image of the location of lung lobes, the nurse can better localize assessment findings.

### Purposes

1. Determine client's ability to ventilate lungs.
2. Assess for potential alterations in oxygenation.
3. Provide early screening for pulmonary disorders.

## *Procedure 13-10*

| Steps | Rationale |
|---|---|
| **Assessment** | |
| 1. Assess if client has smoking history: length of time smoked, number of cigarettes per day, cigar or pipe smoking. | Cigarette smoking is risk factor linked with incidence of lung cancer, heart disease, and chronic lung disease (emphysema, bronchitis). |
| 2. Ask if client experiences any of the following: cough (productive or nonproductive), sputum production, shortness of breath, orthopnea, poor activity tolerance. | Symptoms indicative of respiratory alterations may help nurse localize any objective findings. |
| 3. Determine if client works in environment containing pollutants, e.g., asbestos, coal dust, chemical irritants. | Environmental pollutants are risk factors for various lung diseases. |
| 4. Assess if client has history of allergies to pollens, dust, or other airborne irritants, as well as to any foods, drugs, or chemical substances. | Symptoms client demonstrates may be caused by allergic response to allergen: choking feeling, bronchospasm with respiratory stridor, wheezes on auscultation, dyspnea, cyanosis, diaphoresis. |
| 5. Review family history for cancer, tuberculosis, allergies, or chronic obstructive pulmonary disease (COPD). | Increases client's risk for lung disease. |
| **Planning** | |
| 1. Develop individualized goals for assessment, including: | |
| a. Determine presence of abnormalities. | May pose implications for education and respiratory care. |
| b. Educate client about risk factors for pulmonary disease. | Examination lends itself to discussing issues such as smoking and pollution. |
| c. Educate client about effects of posture on ventilation. | Clients can learn about benefits of good posture while performing maneuvers in examination. |
| 2. Prepare equipment: | |
| a. Stethoscope | Used to ausculate lung sounds. |

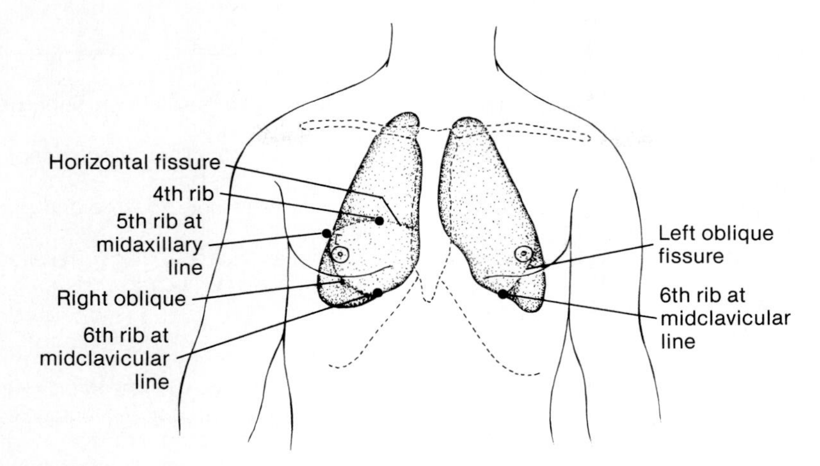


***Fig. 13-34*** Anterior position of lung lobes in relation to anatomic landmarks.

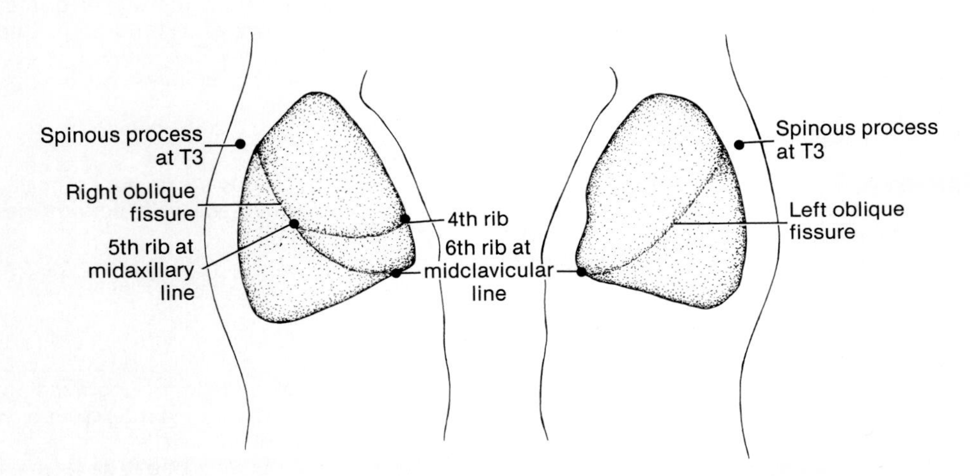


***Fig. 13-35*** Lateral position of lung lobes in relation to anatomic landmarks.

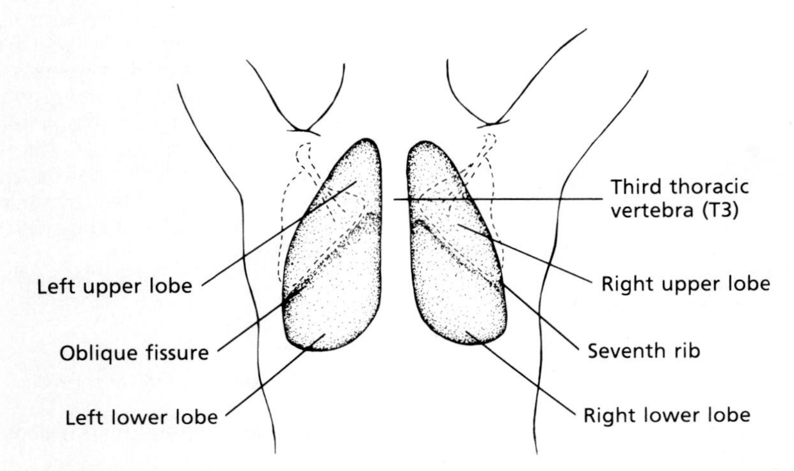


***Fig. 13-36*** Posterior position of lung lobes in relation to anatomic landmarks.

| Steps | Rationale |
|---|---|
| 3. Prepare client. | |
| a. Have client sit upright or elevate head of bed 45-90° for bedridden client. | Promotes full lung expansion during examination. |
| b. Allow client to lie supine or in Sims' position, with position changes necessary during examination. | Positions used for clients who cannot tolerate sitting. |
| c. Remove gown or drape from chest, keeping legs covered. | Avoids unnecessary exposure and provides full visibility of thorax. |
| d. Explain all steps of procedure, encouraging client to relax and breathe normally. | Anxiety may increase client's respiratory rate, thus interfering with analysis of findings. |

## Implementation

| Steps | Rationale |
|---|---|
| 1. Describe observations or findings made during examination regarding imaginary lines formed from anatomic landmarks of sternum, intercostal spaces, clavicle, spine, and scapula. Begin with posterior thorax. | Location of findings by common reference point helps successive examiners to confirm findings, locate abnormalities, and deliver appropriate therapies. |
| ***Posterior thorax*** | |
| 1. Standing at midline position behind client, inspect thorax for shape, posture, deformities, retraction or bulging of intercostal spaces, slope of ribs, and alignment of scapula. | Allows for identification of any factors that may impair chest expansion and any symptoms of respiratory distress. Chest contour is normally symmetric. In child, shape of chest is almost circular, with anteroposterior diameter in 1:1 ratio. In adult, chest is twice as wide as deep, with 1:2 anteroposterior diameter. Chronic lung disease results in 1:1 ratio. |
| 2. Palpate intercostal spaces, noting any masses or areas of localized tenderness. If suspicious mass or swollen area is detected, palpate for size, shape, and typical qualities of lesion. | Localized swelling or tenderness may indicate trauma to ribs or underlying cartilage. |
| 3. Palpate for chest excursion (Fig. 13-37). Standing behind client, place hand on lower third of each rib cage, with hands parallel and thumbs approximately 5 cm (2 in) apart, pointing toward spine. Fingers point out laterally. Press hands toward client's spine to form small skinfold between thumbs. After exhalation, client takes deep breath. Note movements of thumbs. Normally thumbs separate 3-5 cm (1.5-2 in) during chest excursion. | Assess depth of client's breathing. Technique is good measure to evaluate client's ability to perform deep-breathing exercises (Chapter 40). |
| 4. While palpating chest excursion, note symmetry of chest wall movement. | Assess equality of underlying lung expansion. Limited movement on one side may indicate client is voluntarily splinting ventilation because of pain. |
| 5. Palpate posterior chest wall for fremitus by first placing ball or lower palm of dominant hand on area of thorax over an intercostal space, then ask client to say "99" in voice of uniform intensity. Place hand over symmetric areas of thorax. | Vibrations created by movement of vocal cords travel through lung tissue to chest wall. Failure to palpate vibration indicates airway obstruction caused by mucus plug, tumor, or collapsed lung tissue. Palm of hand is most sensitive to vibrations. Symmetric placement of hands allows for comparison of fremitus on both sides of thorax, top to bottom. |
| 6. Moving from side to side and top to bottom percuss posterior chest wall. Ask client to fold arms forward across chest. Using indirect percussion, percuss intercostal spaces over symmetric areas of lung. Compare percussion notes for all lung lobes (Fig. 13-38). | Determines density of underlying lung tissue. Position separates scapulae to expose more lung tissue to assessment. Normal resonance indicates lung is air-filled. Dull percussion note is created by fluid or nurse percussing over bone. Flat percussion note is created by underlying lung mass. Chest is usually more resonant in child than adult. |
| 7. Auscultate breath sounds. For adult, place diaphragm of stethoscope on chest wall over intercostal spaces (Fig. 13-39). Ask client to take slow, deep breaths, with mouth slightly open. Listen to entire inspiration and expiration at each stethoscope position. Systematically compare breath sounds over right and left sides. If sounds are faint, ask client to temporarily breathe harder and faster. | Assesses movement of air through tracheobronchial tree. Nurse's recognition of normal airflow sounds allows detection of sounds caused by mucus or airway obstruction. Sounds are characterized by length of inspiratory and expiratory phases. |
| ***Lateral thorax*** | |
| 1. Instruct client to raise arms straight into air and inspect chest wall. | Improves access to lateral thoracic structures. |
| 2. Extend palpation, percussion, and auscultation of posterior thorax to lateral sides of chest, except for excursion measurement (Fig. 13-40). | Allows for location of abnormalities in lateral lung fields. |

| Steps | Rationale |
|---|---|

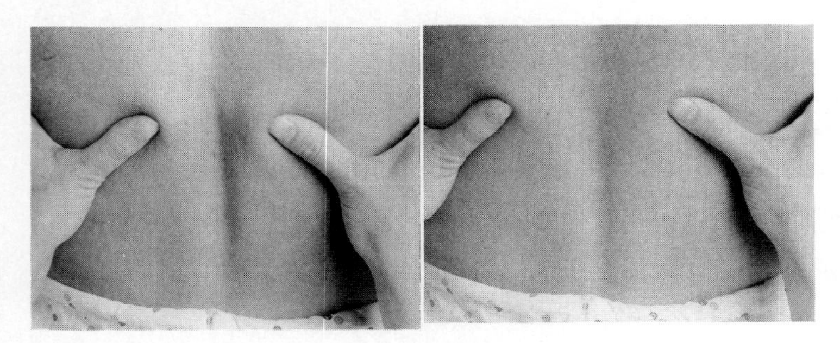

Fig. 13-37

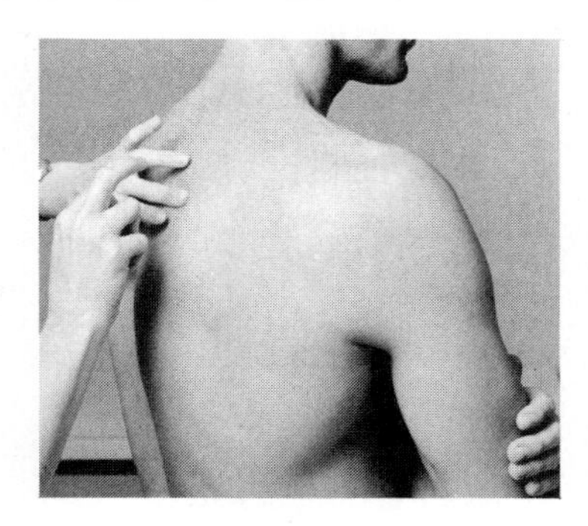

Fig. 13-38

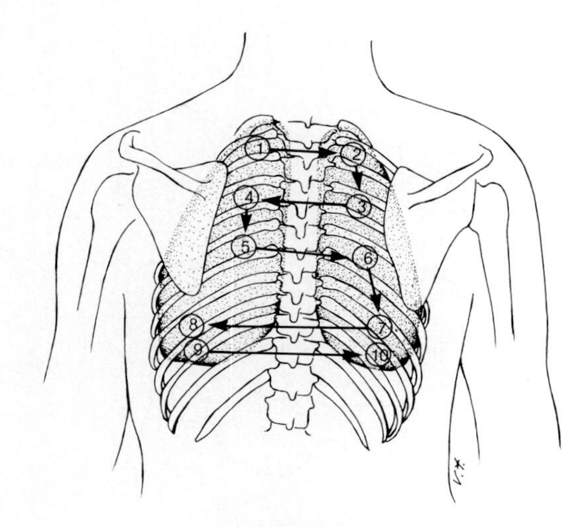


Fig. 13-39

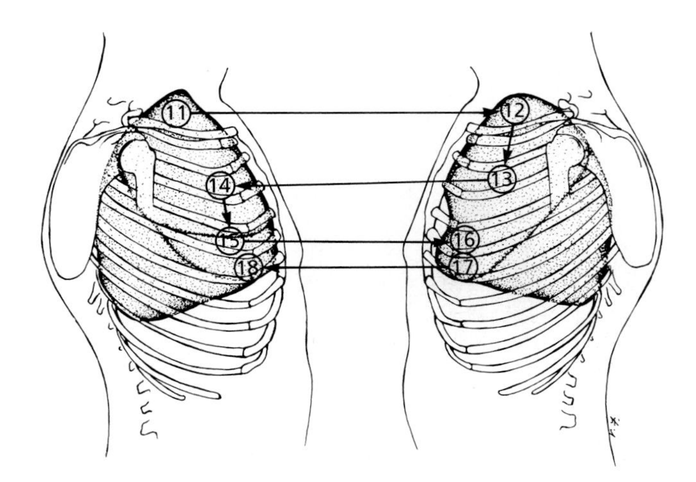


Fig. 13-40

***Anterior thorax***

1. Inspect width or spread of angle made by costal margins and tip of sternum.

   Indicates congenital, acquired, or traumatic alterations that may influence client's chest expansion.

2. Measure client's respiratory character, observing symmetry and degree of chest wall and abdominal movement (Chapter 12).

   Assesses client's effort to ventilate; symmetric, passive movement indicates no respiratory distress.

3. Palpate for areas of swelling or tenderness.

   Localized swelling or tenderness may indicate trauma to underlying ribs or cartilage.

4. Palpate anterior chest excursion. Place hands on lateral rib cage, with thumbs approximately 5 cm (2 in) apart and angled along each costal margin. Thumbs are pushed toward client's midline to create skinfold between thumbs (Fig. 13-41). During inspiration, thumbs normally separate approximately 3-5 cm (1.5-2 in), with each side expanding equally.

   Assesses depth of client's breathing and ability to perform deep-breathing exercises.

5. With palm of hand, palpate over anterior chest for tactile fremitus. In female, retract breasts gently to palpate chest wall.

   Reduced or absent fremitus indicates airway obstruction by mucus, tumor, or collapsed tissue. Sounds will not transmit through breast tissue.

6. Percuss thorax between intercostal spaces with client lying or sitting. Begin above clavicles (Fig. 13-42) and move across and then down.

   Lying position facilitates ability to deliver sharp blow to chest wall to elicit clear sound. Percussion over anterior thorax enables nurse to locate position of liver, heart, and lung. Normal lung is resonant. Underlying liver, heart, and stomach create different percussion notes from that of lung (Fig. 13-43).

| Steps | Rationale |
|---|---|

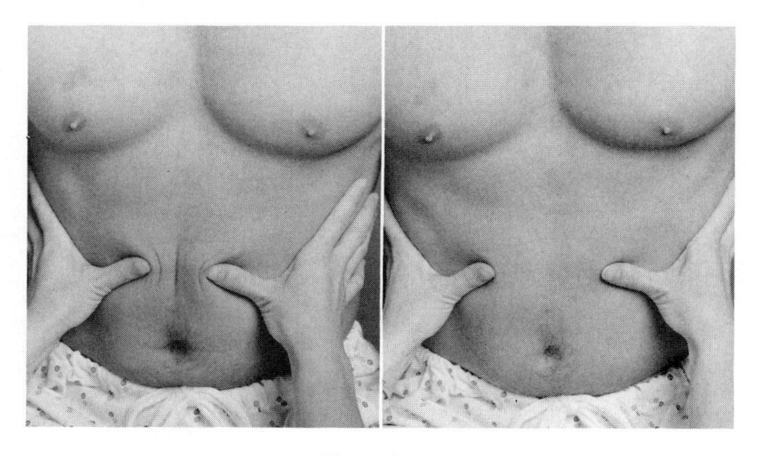

*Fig. 13-41*

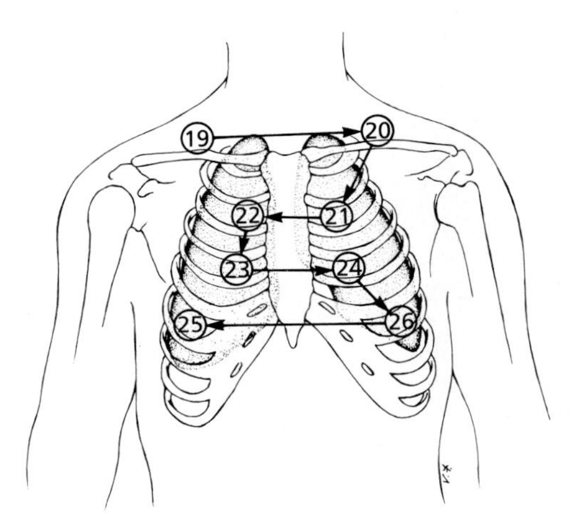


*Fig. 13-42*

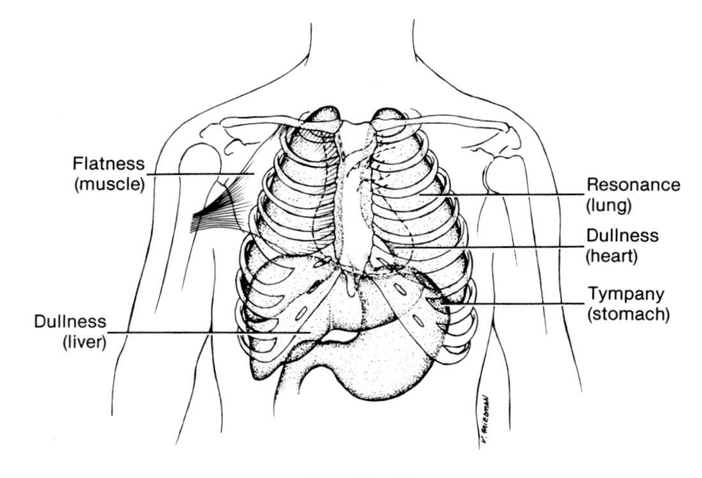


*Fig. 13-43*

| Steps | Rationale |
|---|---|
| 7. With client sitting, auscultate anterior thorax following same pattern as percussion. To encourage child to breathe deeply, demonstrate how to take deep breath by breathing in through nose and out through mouth. Child can pretend to blow out candle. If adventitious sounds are auscultated, have client cough. Listen with stethoscope to determine if sound has disappeared (Table 13-8). | Sitting position maximizes chest expansion and airflow through tracheobronchial tree. Expiration lasts longer than inspiration (3:2 ratio). Coughing can clear airways and remove adventitious sounds. |

## Evaluation

| Steps | Rationale |
|---|---|
| 1. Compare findings with normal assessment characteristics for thorax and lungs. | Determines presence of abnormalities. |

### *Expected outcomes*

| Steps | Rationale |
|---|---|
| 1. Thorax is symmetric, with normal anteroposterior diameter. | Normal findings. |
| 2. Respirations are passive, diaphragmatic or costal, and regular. | |
| 3. Percussion is resonant over all lung fields. | Air uniformly present in lung. |
| 4. Chest excursion is symmetric and full. | Normal ventilatory movement. |
| 5. Fremitus is symmetric over all lung fields. | |
| 6. Breath sounds are clear. | Without mucus or fluid in airways. |

### *Unexpected outcomes*

| Steps | Rationale |
|---|---|
| 1. Retraction or bulging of intercostal spaces is present. | Indicates increased ventilatory effort. |
| 2. Postural abnormality exists. | Results from fatigue, congenital defect, or aging. |

**TABLE 13-8** Adventitious Sounds

| Sound | Site Auscultated | Cause | Character |
|---|---|---|---|
| **Crackles (rales)** 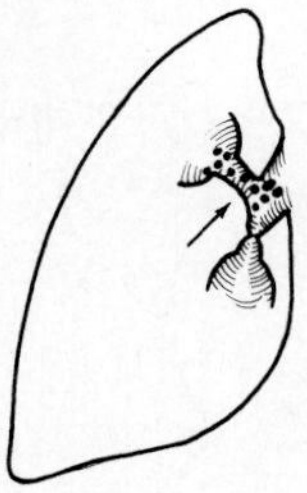 | Most common in dependent lobes: right and left lung bases. | Random, sudden reinflation of groups of alveoli. | Crackling sounds heard during inspiration, expiration, or both; vary in pitch: high, medium, or low; often clear when client coughs. |
| **Rhonchi** 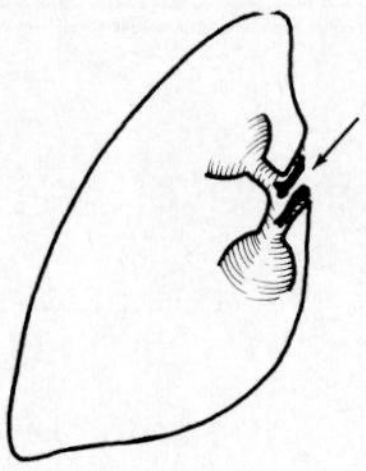 | Primarily over trachea and bronchi; if loud enough, can be heard over most lung fields. | Fluid or mucus located in larger airways, causing turbulence. | Coarse, rattling sounds heard more during expiration; louder and lower pitched than rales; may be cleared by coughing. |
| **Pleural friction rub** 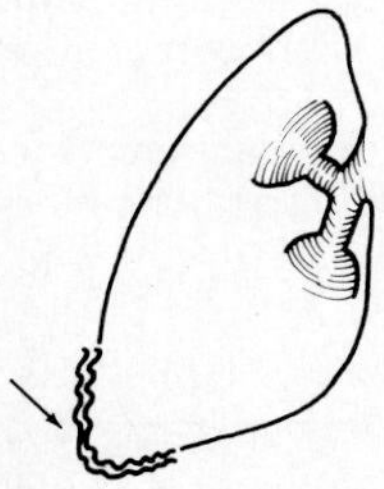 | Anterior lateral lung field (if client sitting upright). | Pleura becomes inflamed; parietal pleura rubs against visceral pleura. | Has grating quality, heard best on inspiration, does not clear with coughing. |
| **Wheezes** 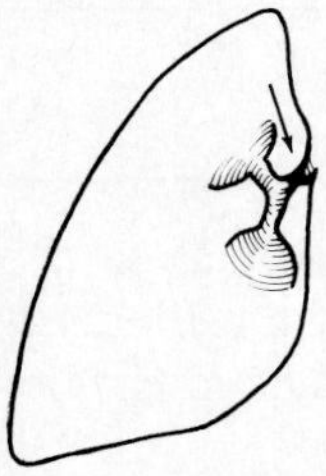 | Can be heard over all lung fields. | Narrowed airways (bronchospasm). | Groaning, creaking, musical sounds heard during inspiration or expiration; high or low pitched; do not clear with coughing. |

| Steps | Rationale |
|---|---|
| 3. Client uses accessory chest and neck muscles on inspiration and expiration. | Increased ventilatory effort. |
| 4. Respirations are shallow and irregular. | Indicates alteration in ventilation (e.g., pain, position) or alteration in respiratory status. |
| 5. Percussion note is full or flat over localized lung field. | Indicates fluid or mass in localized area of lobe. |

| Steps | Rationale |
|---|---|
| 6. Chest excursion is reduced. | Results from position, pain, fatigue, or aging. |
| 7. Fremitus may be reduced. | Indicates interference with airflow in airways. |
| 8. Adventitious sounds are heard on auscultation. | Results from secretions in airways, bronchial airway closure, or fremitus. |
| ***Potential nursing diagnoses*** | |
| ▪ Ineffective airway clearance: related to pain, increased secretions, etc.<br>▪ Ineffective breathing pattern: related to fatigue, pain, etc.<br>▪ Impaired gas exchange: related to altered oxygen supply, decreased chest-wall movements, etc. | Diagnoses may indicate need for aggressive respiratory therapy to improve oxygenation. |
| **Recording and Reporting** | |
| 1. Record observations and findings in nurses' notes. | Documents baseline findings. Data provide means to evaluate client's ongoing status and response to therapies. |
| 2. Record respiratory rate and character in vital signs flow sheet. | Provides simple means to compare trends and changes. |
| 3. Report abnormalities to nurse in charge or physician. | Findings may indicate need for therapy. |

## Special Considerations

- Determine if recently stopped smoking and how long client previously smoked.
- Clients with asthma have symptoms aggravated by change in temperature and humidity, irritating fumes or smoke, emotional stress, and physical exertion.
- Pain, postural deformity, and fatigue are conditions that can reduce chest excursion.
- In elderly clients, chest expansion is reduced because of calcification of rib cartilage and partial contraction of inspiratory muscles.
- Do not palpate deeply when pain or tenderness is elicited. Deep palpation of fractured rib segment could displace bone inward.
- Fremitus is normally symmetric but decreased over heart and breast tissue.
- Children under age 6 exhibit more abdominal or diaphragmatic movement. Older children and adults exhibit more costal or thoracic movement. Male adults may be more diaphragmatic than females.
- Use bell to auscultate breath sounds in children. Breath sounds are louder in children because of their thin chest wall.

## Teaching Considerations

- Explain risk factors for chronic lung disease and lung cancer, including cigarette smoking, history of smoking for over 20 yr, and exposure to environmental pollution.
- Discuss warning signs of lung cancer or chronic pulmonary disease, such as persistent cough, sputum streaked with blood, chest pains, and recurrent attacks of pneumonia or bronchitis.
- Elderly client may benefit from influenza and pneumonia vaccinations because of greater susceptibility to respiratory infection.

# *SKILL 13-11 Assessing the Heart and Vascular System*

The heart and vascular system are assessed together because the two systems work together in delivering blood to organs, tissues, and cells. An alteration in cardiac function frequently results in changes of the vascular system. Assessment provides an excellent opportunity for the nurse to educate clients about risk factors for heart disease and the importance of regular exercise, stress reduction, and good eating habits. Clients tend to seek information about heart disease because it remains the leading cause of death in the United States.

The nurse may begin assessment of the heart and then move peripherally to the vascular system, or vice versa. The assessment should be organized. It is usually convenient to progress from an examination of the thorax to the heart, since the client is already in a suitable position with chest exposed.

## Purposes

1. Assess cardiac function.
2. Assess adequacy of blood flow through the peripheral vascular system.
3. Determine cardiovascular response to exercise.
4. Screen for risk factors for cardiovascular disease.

## *Procedure 13-11*

| Steps | Rationale |
|---|---|
| **Assessment** | |
| 1. Assess client for history of smoking, exercise habits, and dietary patterns and intake. | Smoking, absent or reduced regular exercise, and intake of foods high in carbohydrates and cholesterol are risk factors for heart and vascular disease. |
| 2. Determine if client is taking medications for cardiovascular function, e.g., antiarrhythmics, antihypertensives. | Allows nurse to assess client's compliance with and understanding of drug therapies. Medications for cardiovascular function cannot be taken intermittently. |
| 3. Ask if client has experienced dyspnea, chest pain or discomfort, palpitations, excess fatigue, fainting spells, or edema. Ask if symptoms occur at rest or during exercise. | Cardinal symptoms of heart disease. Cardiovascular function may be adequate during rest but not during exercise. |
| 4. Determine if client has a stressful life-style. | Repeated exposure to stress may increase risk for heart disease. |
| 5. Assess client and family history for heart problems (e.g., heart attack, murmurs, or rheumatic heart disease). | Family history of heart problems increases risk for heart disease. |
| 6. Ask client about a history of heart trouble (e.g., congestive heart failure, congenital heart disease, coronary artery disease, dysrhythmias). | Knowledge reveals client's level of understanding of condition. A preexisting condition will influence examination techniques used by nurse. |
| 7. Ask if client has experienced leg cramps, numbness or tingling in extremities, or sensation of cold appendages. Also determine if client has noted swelling of feet, ankles, or hands. | Common signs and symptoms in peripheral vascular disease. |
| 8. If client experiences pain or cramping in the lower extremities ask if it is relieved or aggravated by walking. | Relationship of symptoms to exercise can clarify whether problem is vascular or musculoskeletal. Pain caused by vascular condition tends to increase with activity. |
| 9. Ask female clients if they wear tight-fitting garters or knee-length nylons. | Tight clothing around lower extremities can impair venous return. |
| 10. Assess medical history for heart disease, hypertension, phlebitis, diabetes, or varicose veins. | Circulatory and vascular disorders influence findings gathered during examination. |
| **Planning** | |
| 1. Develop individualized goals for assessment, including: | |
| a. Determine presence of abnormalities. | May reveal acute or long-term alterations. |
| b. Educate client about risk factors for heart and vascular disease. | Nurse can discuss effect of various factors during assessment. |
| c. Educate client about means to improve cardiovascular function. | Client can learn about exercise, diet, and stress reduction. |
| d. Discuss compliance with drug therapy. | Clients requiring medications for cardiovascular function often must take drugs daily. Nurse can discuss ways to maintain drug regimens (Chapter 18). |
| 2. Prepare equipment: | |
| a. Stethoscope | Used to auscultate heart sounds. |
| 3. Prepare client. | |
| a. Have client assume semi-Fowler's or supine position. | Provides adequate visibility and access to left thorax and mediastinum. |
| b. Explain procedure and avoid facial gestures reflecting concern while assessing heart function. | Client with previously normal cardiac history may become anxious if nurse shows concern. |
| **Implementation** | |
| ***Heart*** | |
| 1. Locate anatomic landmarks used to assess cardiac function (Fig. 13-44). Heart is located behind and to left of sternum, with base at top and apex at bottom. Find angle of Louis just below suprasternal notch between sternal body and manubrium; can be felt as bony prominence. Slip fingers down each side of angle to find second intercostal space; space on client's right is (1) *aortic area,* space on left is (2) *pulmonic area.* Carefully move fingers down left side of sternum until you palpate fourth intercostal space, the (3) *tricuspid area.* Move fingers laterally to client's left to locate fifth intercostal space at left midclavicular line, the (4) *apical area.* (5) *Epigastric area* is at tip of sternum. | Familiarity with landmarks allows nurse to describe findings more clearly and ultimately may improve diagnosis. |

| Steps | Rationale |
|---|---|

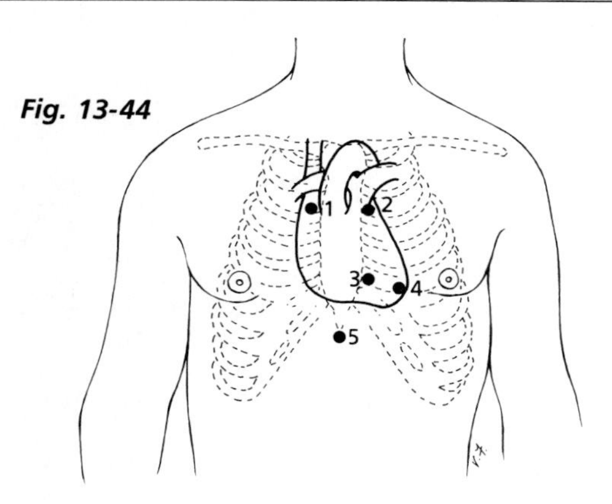


*Fig. 13-44*

| Steps | Rationale |
|---|---|
| 2. Inspect client's mediastinum and chest, along five landmarks, for any pulsations or lifts. Look at an angle or to side of client's chest wall. | Looking at chest wall from an angle improves ability to see movement of tissue between intercostal spaces. Pulsation below left intercostal space along midclavicular line is likely point of maximal impulse (PMI), where ventricles push against chest wall during systole. PMI in adult is normally at left fifth intercostal space along midclavicular line. Pulsations in any other area may indicate abnormalities in major vessels or improper valve closure. |
| 3. With ball of hand, palpate aortic, pulmonic, tricuspid, apical, and epigastric areas for vibrations. Use fingertips to palpate same site for pulsations. | Certain portions of hand are more sensitive to vibrations or pulsations. Deep palpation may be necessary in obese clients or those who have well-developed chest muscles. |
| 4. Locate PMI by palpating apical area along fourth or fifth intercostal space in midclavicular line (Fig. 13-45). | Locates apex of heart. PMI is light tap felt in area 1-2 cm (0.5 in) in diameter during systole. |
| 5. If palpating PMI is difficult, have client turn onto left side. | Moves heart closer to chest wall. |
| 6. If pulsation or vibration is located, time its occurrence in relation to the systole or diastole by auscultating heart sounds simultaneously. | Timing any pulsation or vibration may aid in diagnosing its source. |
| 7. Percuss chest wall beginning at fourth or fifth intercostal space along anterior axillary line and slowly move toward sternum. | Assesses heart size by percussion note changing from lung resonance to cardiac dullness. Cardiac dullness below fifth intercostal space, beyond left midclavicular line, or to right of sternum indicates heart enlargement. |
| 8. Instruct client not to speak, and with diaphragm of stethoscope, auscultate heart sounds (Fig. 13-46). | Heart sounds have low intensity and are difficult to hear. |
| a. Identify first ($S_1$) and second ($S_2$) heart sounds at apex. | Allows nurse to recognize normal heart sounds so that additional sounds can be identified later. |
| b. To hear $S_2$ more clearly, slowly move diaphragm of stethoscope toward aortic site until sound is clear. | $S_2$ is heard loudest at aortic area. |
| c. Use bell of stethoscope at apex to hear $S_1$ and $S_2$. | Bell picks up lower-pitched sounds, such as heart sounds and murmurs. |
| d. When $S_1$ and $S_2$ are recognized, systematically auscultate at aortic, pulmonic, tricuspid, and apical areas. At each site, alternately use both diaphragm and bell and auscultate for rate, rhythm, intensity, pitch of sounds; $S_1$; $S_2$; extra heart sounds during systole; extra heart sounds during diastole; murmurs, (blowing sounds over normal heart sounds). Note timing in relation to $S_1$ or $S_2$ (systolic is between $S_1$ and $S_2$, diastolic between $S_2$ and $S_1$. | Systematic assessment prevents nurse from missing any unusual or abnormal sounds. Assessing character of heart sounds helps detect nature of any abnormalities. Failure of heart to beat at regular interval is a dysrhythmia, which interferes with heart's ability to pump effectively. (Table 13-9). Extra heart sounds may indicate impaired heart or vascular function. Extra heart sounds, $S_3$ and $S_4$, are low pitched and heard best with bell. Both occur during diastole. $S_3$, heard best at apex, occurs just after $S_2$ to create "lub-dub-ee" or "ken-*tuc*-ky" sound. $S_3$ is normal in children but sign of heart failure in adults. $S_4$, heard best at apex, occurs just before $S_1$ to create "dee-lub- dub" or "Ten-nes-see" sound. $S_4$ is common in elderly clients but is also sign of hypertension. Murmurs result from changes in blood flow through heart or abnormalities in valve closure. Murmur is heard best over valve of heart structure responsible for turbulent blood flow. Murmurs may be asymptomatic and are typical in children. |
| e. At apical site, assess heart rate and rhythm for one min. Each combination of "lub-dub" counts as one heartbeat. | Determines apical pulse, effective measure of cardiac function and response of heart to activity or therapies. |
| 9. If apical pulse is irregular, auscultate apical pulse first and then immediately palpate radial pulse. Compare two rates. | Allows detection of pulse deficit, or inequality between apical and radial rates. With deficit, radial pulse is usually slower be- |

**TABLE 13-9** Common Types of Dysrhythmias

| Definition | Cause |
|---|---|
| **Sinus dysrhythmia** | |
| Pulse rate changes during respiration, increasing at peak of inspiration and declining during expiration. | Blood is momentarily trapped in lungs during inspiration, causing a fall in the heart's stroke volume. This is a normal condition for children. |
| **Sinus tachycardia** | |
| Pulse rhythm is regular, but the rate is accelerated to more than 100 beats/minute. | Exercise, emotional stress, and caffeine or alcohol ingestion are common factors that cause increased firing of the sinoatrial node. |
| **Sinus bradycardia** | |
| Pulse rhythm is regular, but the rate is slower than normal at 40-60 beats/minute. | The sinoatrial node fires less frequently. This is common in well-conditioned athletes. |
| **Premature ventricular contraction** | |
| Premature beat occurs before regularly expected heart contraction. | The ventricle contracts prematurely because of electrical impulse bypassing the normal conduction pathway. It may occur so early that it is difficult to detect as a second beat. It may be followed by a pause. |
| **Atrial fibrillation** | |
| Rapid, random contractions of the atria cause irregular ventricular beats at 130-150 beats/minute. | Atria discharge very rapidly with some impulses not reaching ventricles. This condition occurs in rheumatic heart disease and mitral stenosis. It causes reduced cardiac output. |

**TABLE 13-10** Signs of Venous and Arterial Insufficiency

| Assessment Criterion | Venous | Arterial |
|---|---|---|
| Color | Normal or cyanotic | Pale, worsened by elevation of extremity, dusky red when extremity lowered |
| Temperature | Normal | Cool (blood flow blocked to extremity) |
| Pulse | Normal | Decreased or absent |
| Edema | Often marked | Absent or mild |
| Skin changes | Brown pigmentation around ankles | Thin, shiny skin; decreased hair growth; nails thickened |

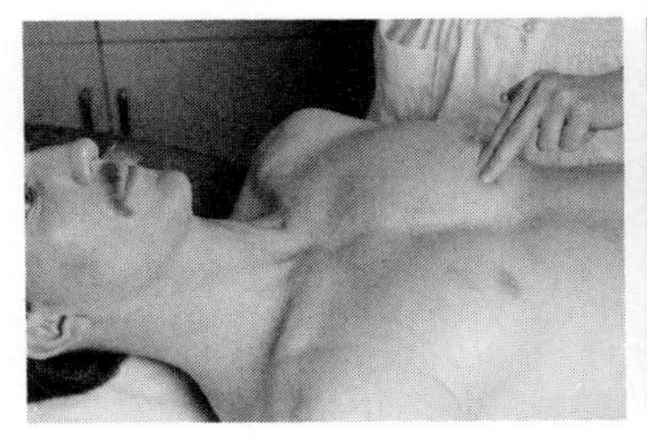

*Fig. 13-45*

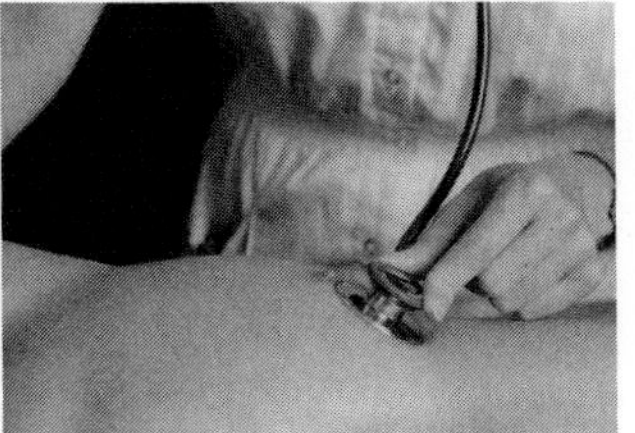

*Fig. 13-46*

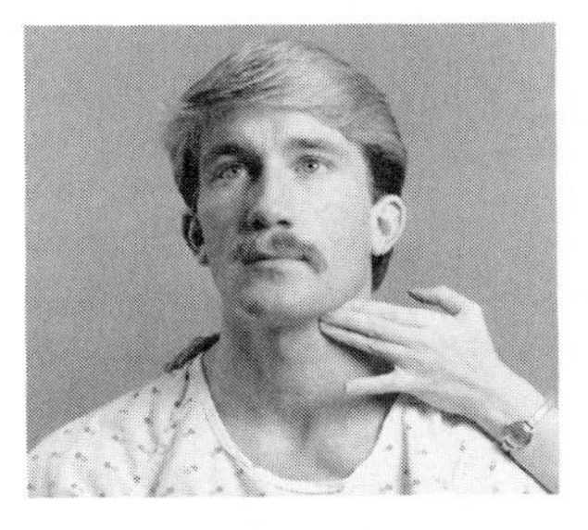

*Fig. 13-47*

| Steps | Rationale |
|---|---|
| Two nurses may work together, one assessing apical while other assesses radial. | cause ineffective heart contractions fail to transmit pulse waves to periphery. |
| ***Vascular system*** | |
| 1. Inspect color of client's skin and mucous membranes (data may have been gathered previously during assessment of oral cavity and integument). Focus on base of tongue, buccal cavity, lips, fingers, toes, and nail beds. | Color of skin or mucous membranes reveals status of blood flow and arterial oxygen saturation. |
| 2. Inspect extremities, noting edema of hands or feet and any changes: reduced hair growth; thick nails; thin, shiny skin; pigmentation changes (Table 13-10). | Edema may indicate venous pooling, resulting from poor cardiac output, or increased fluid overload. Nutrition deficiencies from reduced tissue perfusion cause changes in integument. Degree of pitting indicates severity of edema. |
| 3. If edema is present, assess for pitting by gently applying pressure to area for 5 sec with finger and checking for in- | Depth of pitting (indentation) determines degree of edema. |

| Steps | Rationale |
|---|---|
| dentation. Edema is measured by the following scale:<br>1 cm depth, 1+ edema<br>2 cm depth, 2+ edema<br>3 cm depth, 3+ edema<br>4 cm depth, 4+ edema | |
| 1. Palpate temperature of extremities with dorsum (back) of hand. | Temperature measures degree of blood flow to body part. |
| 2. Inspect jugular veins in neck. Place client in sitting position and note if veins are distended or collapsed. (Normally veins are collapsed or flat when person sits. Veins usually fill and distend when person is supine.) Then lower head of bed to 45° angle and reassess for vein distention. | Status of jugular veins aids in assessing venous pressure, venous tone, and blood volume. Distended veins in semisitting position reflect increased venous pressure possibly caused by right-sided heart failure or increased circulatory volume. |
| ***Arterial system*** | |
| 1. Assess carotid arteries: | |
| a. Ask client to assume sitting position. | Allows easier mobility of neck to expose artery for inspection and palpation. |
| b. Inspect neck on both sides for obvious pulsations of artery. Sometimes pulse wave can be seen. | Carotids are only sites to assess quality of pulse wave. Experience is required to evaluate wave in relation to events of cardiac cycle. |
| c. Palpate each carotid artery separately. Slide index and middle fingers around medial edge of sternocleidomastoid muscle. Ask client to turn head slightly away from side being examined (Fig. 13-47). Note rate and rhythm, strength, and elasticity of artery. | If both arteries were occluded simultaneously, client could lose consciousness from reduced circulation to brain. Turning head improves access to artery. |
| d. Repeat assessment for other artery. | |
| e. Place bell of stethoscope over each carotid, auscultating for blowing sound, or bruit. Bruits are common in elderly clients and those with arteriosclerosis. | Narrowing of carotid artery's lumen by arteriosclerotic plaques causes disturbance in blood flow. Blood passing through narrowed section creates turbulence and emits blowing or swishing sound. |
| 2. Assess each peripheral artery for following characteristics: | Palpation of peripheral arteries determines adequacy of blood flow to extremities. |
| a. Elasticity of vessel wall. | Determines integrity of vessel. Artery should be easily palpable and should return to shape after pressure is released. |
| b. Rate and rhythm of pulse. | Radial pulse is chosen to assess heart rate. Other peripheral pulses are assessed only to determine condition of local blood flow. |
| c. Strength. | Measure of force ejecting blood against arterial wall. Rating scale for strength:<br>▪ 0 No pulse is palpable.<br>▪ 1+ Pulse is difficult to palpate, weak and thready in character, easy to obliterate.<br>▪ 2+ Pulse less difficult to palpate, light pressure usually locates it, discriminating touch senses it is stronger than 1+.<br>▪ 3+ Normal pulse, easy to palpate, not easily obliterated.<br>▪ 4+ Strong pulse, easily palpated, bounds against fingertips, cannot be obliterated. |
| d. Type of pulse. | Useful in describing nature of pulse wave. Requires experience. |
| e. Equality of pulses. | Comparison of both sites allows nurse to determine any localized obstruction or disturbance in blood flow. |
| 3. Palpate radial pulse by lightly placing tips of first and second fingers in groove formed along radial side of forearm, lateral to flexor tendon of wrist (Fig. 13-48). | Pulse is relatively superficial and should not require deep palpation. |
| 4. Palpate ulnar pulse by placing fingertips along ulnar side of forearm (Fig. 13-49). | Palpated when arterial insufficiency to hand is expected or when nurse assesses effects radial occlusion might have on circulation to hand (Chapter 46). |
| 5. Palpate brachial pulse by locating groove between biceps and triceps muscles above elbow at antecubital fossa (Fig. 13-50). Place tips of first three fingers in muscle groove. | Artery runs along medial side of extended arm, requiring moderate palpation. |
| 6. With client supine, palpate femoral pulse by placing first three fingers over inguinal area below inguinal ligament, midway between pubic symphysis and anterosuperior iliac spine (Fig. 13-51). | Supine position prevents flexion in groin area, which interferes with artery access. |

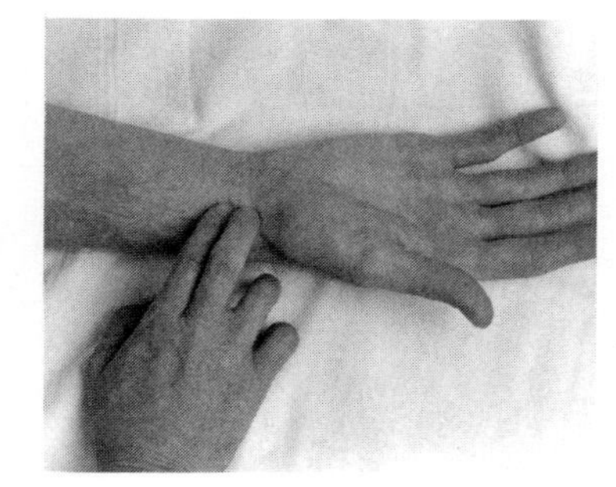

***Fig. 13-48***

| Steps | Rationale |
|---|---|

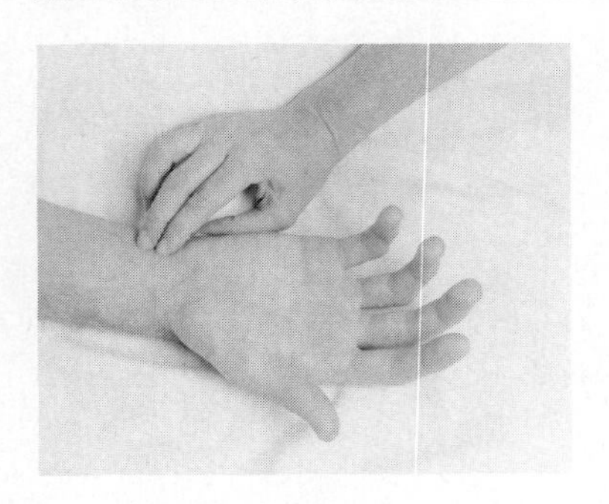

*Fig. 13-49*

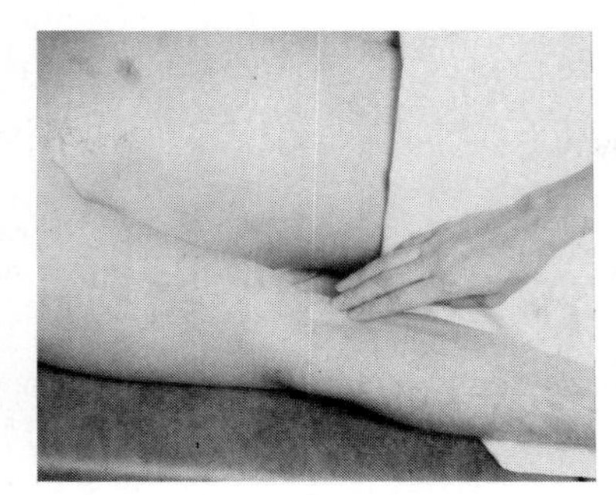

*Fig. 13-50*

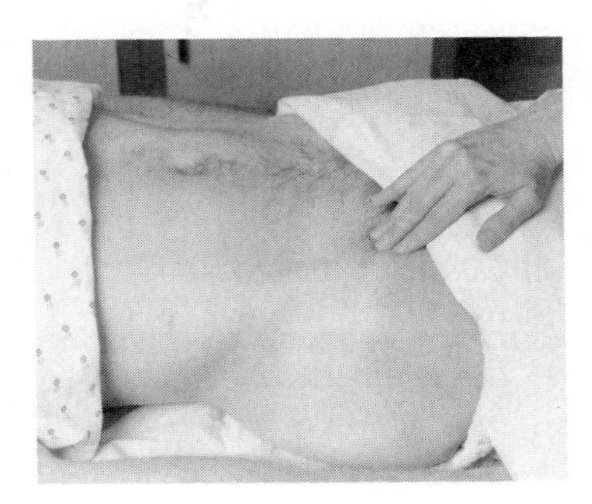

*Fig. 13-51*

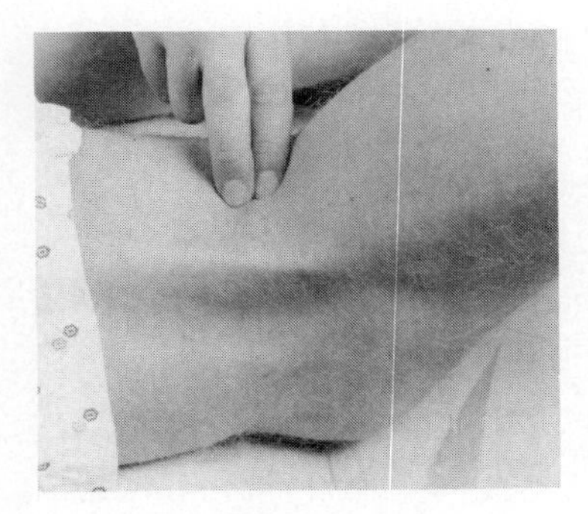

*Fig. 13-52*

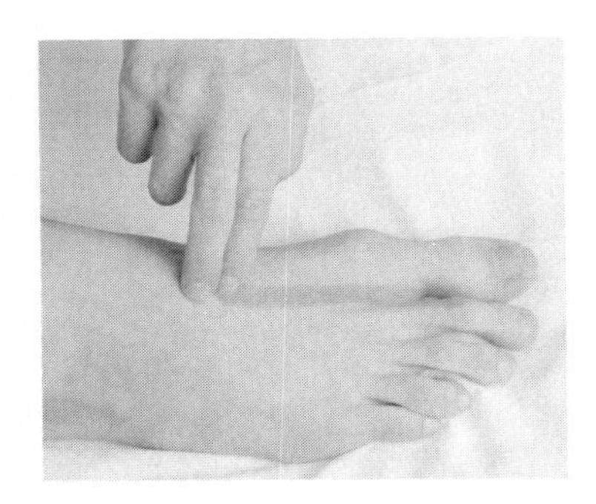

*Fig. 13-53*

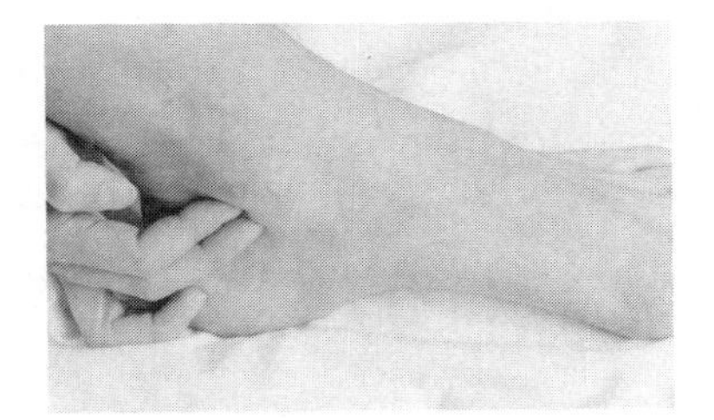

*Fig. 13-54*

7. Palpate popliteal pulse by having client slightly flex knee with foot resting on table or bed. Instruct client to keep leg muscles relaxed. Palpate deeply into popliteal fossa with fingers of both hands placed just lateral to midline. Client may also lie prone to achieve exposure of artery (Fig. 13-52).

   Flexion of knee and muscle relaxation improve accessibility of artery. Popliteal pulse is one of the more difficult pulses to palpate.

8. Have client lie supine with feet relaxed, and palpate dorsalis pedis pulse. Gently place fingertips between great and first toe and slowly move along groove between extensor tendons of great and first toe, until pulse is palpable (Fig. 13-53).

   Artery lies superficially and does not require deep palpation. Pulse may be congenitally absent.

9. Palpate posterior tibial pulse by having client relax and slightly extend feet. Place fingertips behind and below medial malleolus (ankle bone) (Fig. 13-54).

   Artery easily palpable with foot relaxed.

## Evaluation

1. Compare findings with normal assessment characteristics of heart and vascular system.

   Determines presence of abnormalities.

2. If pulses are not palpable, ask another nurse to assess client's pulses.

   Abnormal assessment findings can be caused by examiner's error.

3. If pulse still not palpable, obtain ultrasonic stethoscope with lubricant:
   a. Apply thin layer of lubricant over pulse site.
   b. Turn on stethoscope's volume.
   c. Place diaphragm gently over pulse site.
   d. Listen for intermittent "swooshing" or "blowing" sound.

   Specially designed stethoscope detects blood flow through arteries by producing amplified sound waves as vessel wall pulsates against stethoscope's diaphragm.

| Steps | Rationale |
|---|---|
| ***Expected Outcomes—heart assessment*** | |
| 1. Heart is in normal sinus rhythm (NSR) with rate from 60-100 beats per min (adolescent through adult). | Normal findings. |
| 2. $S_1$ and $S_2$ are normal, without extra sounds or murmurs. | |
| 3. PMI is at fifth intercostal space at left midclavicular line in adult. PMI at third or fourth intercostal space at left midclavicular line in infant or child. | |
| ***Expected outcomes—vascular assessment*** | |
| 1. Extremities are warm and pink, with normal hair growth and nail thickness. | Indicators of good tissue perfusion. |
| 2. All pulses are equal, elastic, and +3. | |
| 3. No carotid bruit is present. | Vessel patent. |
| 4. Jugular veins are flat when client's head is elevated. | Normal venous pressure. |
| ***Unexpected outcomes—heart and vascular system*** | |
| 1. Heart rate is irregular, with rate less than 60 beats/min or greater than 100 beats/min. | Indicates potential for inadequate pumping action of heart. |
| 2. $S_3$ auscultated. | Client's combined symptoms suggest heart failure. |
| 3. Jugular veins are distended when client's head is elevated. | Increased venous pressure. |
| 4. Skin is cool, clammy, pale, or cyanotic; and edema is noted in extremities. | Poor pumping action of heart fails to deliver blood flow peripherally. |
| 5. Peripheral pulses +1 or +2 and equal. | Impaired pumping action reduces pulse strength. |
| ***Potential nursing diagnosis—heart and vascular system*** | |
| ▪ Decreased cardiac output: related to dysrhythmia. | Inadequate blood volume reaches tissues. |
| ***Unexpected outcomes—vascular system*** | |
| 1. Peripheral pulses are 0 to +2. | Indicates inadequate arterial blood flow to tissues. |
| 2. Skin is pale, cool, thin, and shiny. | Result of chronic arterial insufficiency. |
| 3. Reduced hair growth present, with thickening of nails. | Result of chronic arterial insufficiency. |
| 4. Peripheral pulses are +2 or +3. | Arterial flow adequate but venous return altered. |
| 5. Skin is warm but cyanotic: dependent edema present in ankles, brown pigmentation is noted around ankles. | Venous stasis. |
| ***Potential nursing diagnoses—vascular system*** | |
| ▪ Altered tissue perfusion: related to arterial insufficiency. | Inadequate nutrients delivered to tissue increases chance of breakdown. Result of hypoxia. |
| ▪ Potential impaired skin integrity: related to arterial insufficiency. | |
| ▪ Pain: related to poor arterial perfusion. | Inadequate oxygen delivered to tissues during exercise can result in pain. |

## Recording and Reporting

| Steps | Rationale |
|---|---|
| 1. Record all findings for heart and vascular assessment in nurses' notes. | Documents baseline findings. Data also measure client's response to various therapies. |
| 2. Report any irregularities in heart function and indications of impaired arterial blood flow immediately to physician. | Any abnormalities can threaten client's health. |

## Special Considerations

- Clients with heart disease may have shortness of breath and may benefit from elevating upper body.
- In serious heart disease, cardiac muscle enlarges and PMI moves to left of midclavicular line.
- $S_1$ corresponds with almost simultaneous closure of mitral and tricuspid valves, is low pitched, resembles "lub," and is loudest at apex.
- $S_2$ corresponds with closure of aortic and pulmonic valves, is higher pitched, and resembles "dub."
- Do not press bell too firmly against chest wall, since transmission of sound is destroyed.
- Children have louder, higher-pitched heart sounds because of their thin chest walls.
- Central cyanosis is evident from bluish discoloration of mucosa at base of tongue. This indicates poor oxygen saturation, seen in lung disease and congenital heart defects of children.
- Peripheral cyanosis is evident from bluish discoloration of lips, appendages, and nail beds. This condition results from low cardiac output or local vasoconstriction.
- Avoid massaging carotid artery vigorously; this could stimulate carotid sinus, (located in upper third of neck), which causes reflex lowering of heart rate and blood pressure.
- Increased cardiac output (e.g., following fever, exercise) results in strong pulse.

### Teaching Considerations

- Explain risk factors for heart disease: high dietary intake of cholesterol, lack of regular aerobic exercise, smoking, stressful life-style, and family history of heart disease.
- Refer client (if appropriate) to resources available for controlling or reducing risks (e.g., nutritional counseling, exercise class, and stress-reduction programs).
- For clients with heart disease, explain importance of compliance with complete treatment plan.
- Tell clients their blood pressure reading. Explain normal reading for the clients' ages. Discuss implications of abnormalities.
- Instruct clients with risk or evidence of vascular insufficiency in the lower extremities to avoid tight clothing over the lower body or legs, to avoid sitting or standing for long periods of time, to walk regularly, and to elevate feet when sitting.
- Elderly clients with hypertension may benefit from regular monitoring of blood pressure (daily, weekly, or monthly). Home monitoring kits are available (see chapter 12). Teach clients how to use them.

## *SKILL 13-12 Assessing the Breasts*

It is important that the nurse assess the breasts of female clients and male clients alike. Even though the examination of the female is more detailed, the nurse should assess the male's breasts carefully to rule out possible growth of cancerous tumors.

Breast cancer is the leading cause of death among all forms of cancer for women of all ages (Silverberg, 1984). Examination should be a routine part of any female client's health screening. The nurse should also assume the responsibility of educating female clients about the importance of performing monthly self-breast examinations and the techniques for performing the examination correctly. Most breast masses are found by clients themselves; thus a female client should be familiar with the physical characteristics of her breasts.

### Purpose

1. Determine condition of breast tissue and neighboring lymph nodes.
2. Demonstrate techniques used in self-examination of breasts.
3. Educate female clients about signs of breast cancer.

## *Procedure 13-12*

| Steps | Rationale |
|---|---|
| **Assessment** | |
| 1. Determine if female client is over age 50, has a family history of breast cancer, had previous breast cancer, never had children, or had a first child after age 30 or did not breastfeed children. | High risk factors for occurrence of breast cancer. |
| 2. Ask if client (either sex) has noticed pain or tenderness of breast, discharge from nipple, change in size of breast, or presence of lump or mass. Have client point out any masses. | Potential signs and symptoms of breast cancer. Allows nurse to focus on specific areas of breast during assessment. |
| 3. Determine if female client performs monthly self-examination of breasts. If so, ask what time of month she performs examination in relation to menstrual cycle and ask her to describe method she uses. | One of primary roles of nurse during assessment of breast is to educate client about breast cancer and technique for self-examination. Early detection of cancerous lesion increases possibility of cure. |
| 4. Determine if client is taking oral contraceptives, digitalis, diuretics, steroids, or estrogen hormones. | Medications may cause nipple discharge. Hormones may cause fibrocystic changes in the breast. |
| **Planning** | |
| 1. Develop individualized goals for assessment, including: | |
| a. Maintain client comfort and self-esteem. | Female client in particular can be very self-conscious and anxious about examination. Nurse should maintain client's privacy and be gentle in approach. |
| b. Determine abnormalities of breast and lymph node tissue. | Certain findings may dictate immediate medical intervention. |

| Steps | Rationale |
|---|---|
| c. Educate client about signs of breast cancer. | Assessment offers nurse opportunity to describe signs to observe for in each portion of assessment. Client learns how to assess for each sign. |
| d. Educate client on techniques of breast self-examination. | Self-assessment can be practiced during the examination. |
| e. Improve client's familiarity with characteristics of breast tissue. | Female client must know what her own breasts normally feel like during palpation in order to recognize signs of abnormalities. |
| 2. Prepare equipment: | |
| a. Disposable gloves (optional). | Used only when there are draining lesions of breast. |
| 3. Prepare client for examination: | |
| a. Have client remove top gown or expose breasts fully. | Allows simultaneous viewing of both breasts. |
| b. Client initially assumes standing or sitting position with arms at side. | Inspection performed with breasts in normal position. |
| c. If mirror is available place it in front of client during examination. | Client can learn what to look for when performing self-examination. |
| d. Explain: (1) each step of examination clearly, describing what signs or features to observe for, (2) normal findings and deviations, and (3) proper techniques for thorough assessment. | During examination nurse's explanations serve to educate client about how to perform self-examination and what to observe for. To recognize abnormalities client must be familiar with normal appearance of breasts. |
| e. Allow client opportunities to ask questions and discuss concerns. | Breasts are linked to female's reproductive capacity and sexuality. Threat of abnormalities can cause severe anxiety. |

## Implementation

### *Female client*

| Steps | Rationale |
|---|---|
| 1. Describe observations or findings made during examination in relation to imaginary lines that divide breast into four quadrants and tail (Fig. 13-55). | Location of finding by common reference point helps successive examiners to confirm findings and locate abnormalities. |
| 2. Inspect breasts for size and symmetry. Note position of nipple in relation to underlying intercostal space. Observe area of chest over which breast extends. | Change in size or shape may indicate underlying mass or presence of inflammation. |
| 3. Observe contour or shape of breast, noting any masses, retraction of tissue, or flattening. If retraction is suspected, ask client to raise arms above head or press hands against hips. | Underlying mass, swelling, or inflammation may cause bulging or retraction of breast tissue. Maneuver causes contraction of pectoral muscles, which accentuates presence of retraction. |
| 4. Inspect overlying skin for color and venous pattern. If breasts are large, carefully lift breasts to inspect underlying skin surfaces. Normal breasts are same color as surrounding skin surfaces. Venous patterns are more easily seen in thin or pregnant women. | Vascular changes, edema, or inflammation may cause skin color changes. Undersurface of breast is common site for redness and excoriation caused by rubbing of breast against chest wall. |
| 5. Inspect areola and nipples for color, size, and shape. Note direction in which nipples point, presence of rashes or ulcerations. If there is discharge from nipple, note its color. | Hormonal changes cause changes in color and size of areola and nipples throughout woman's life span. Presence of underlying lesions may cause change in size, shape, and position of nipples. Underlying lesions may extend to skin's surface, causing ulcerations. Lesions or infection may cause discharge from nipples to range from bloody red to green or brown. |
| 6. With client sitting, palpate supraclavicular and infraclavicular lymph nodes. Use pads of finger tips of dominant hand to gently palpate in rotary motion along the distribution of lymph node chain. Stand on client's right side to palpate nodes on right; stand on left side to palpate nodes on left. | Lymphatic drainage from breast tissue drains into supraclavicular, infraclavicular, and axillary nodes. Normally lymph nodes are not palpable. Infection, inflammation, and cancerous cell growth can cause nodes to enlarge and become palpable. |
| 7. If a node is palpable, note its consistency, mobility, and presence of tenderness. | Characteristics of node help determine cause of enlargement. |
| 8. Have client sit with arms relaxed at sides to palpate axillary nodes. Gently abduct client's arm, supporting it with your nondominant hand (Fig. 13-56). | Abduction allows access of nodes located deep along chest muscle walls and upper arm. |
| 9. With fingertips of dominant hand palpate gently in circular motion the following areas: edge of pectoralis major muscle along anterior axillary line, chest wall in midaxilla, upper end of humerus, anterior edge of latissimus dorsi muscle along posterior axillary line. | Distribution of axillary lymph chain. |
| 10. Have client lie supine with right arm abducted and hand placed under head (Fig. 13-57). A small pillow or towel can be placed under client's right shoulder blade. | Position allows breast tissue to flatten evenly against client's chest wall. |

| Steps | Rationale |
|---|---|

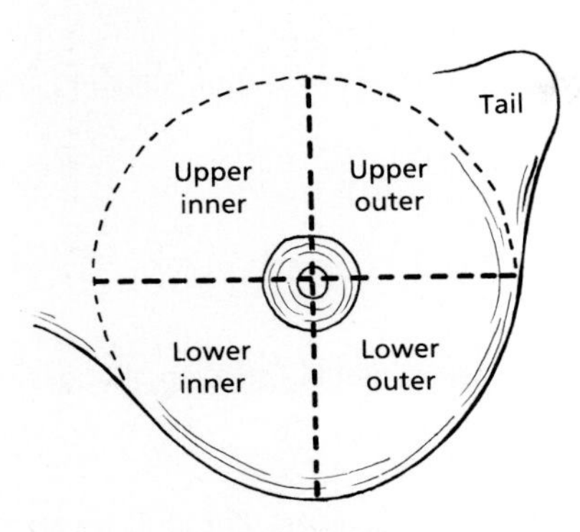


*Fig. 13-55*

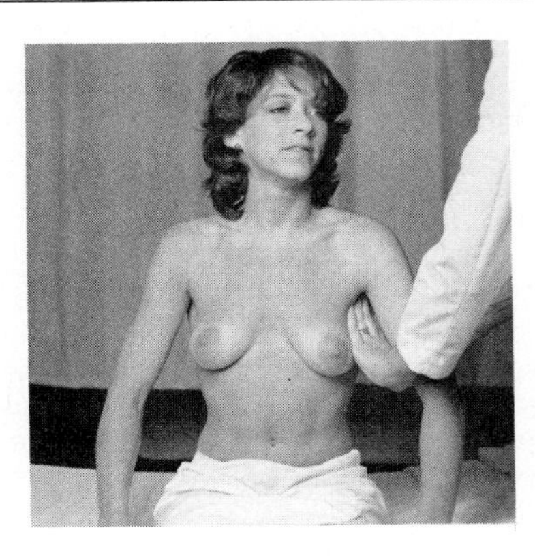

*Fig. 13-56*

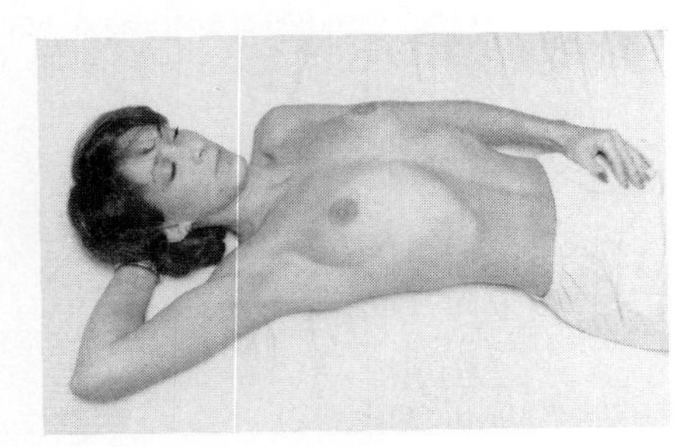

*Fig. 13-57*

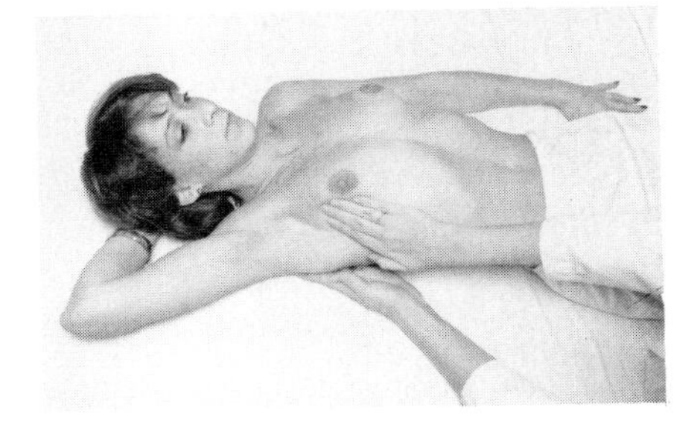

*Fig. 13-58*

| Steps | Rationale |
|---|---|
| 11. Stand at client's right side. Using systematic approach, gently palpate breast tissue with first three fingers of right hand moving in rotary fashion and compressing breast tissue against chest wall. Begin in one quadrant and thoroughly examine all surfaces before moving to other three quadrants and tail. You may also examine each quadrant by moving from nipple outward, like spokes of a wheel (Fig. 13-58). | Entire breast tissue must be thoroughly palpated to rule out presence of mass. |
| 12. If client complains of a mass, begin examination with opposite breast. | Allows more objective comparison of apparent normal tissue with abnormal tissue. |
| 13. Palpate breasts noting consistency of tissue. Take client's fingertips and move them gently over breast tissue. | Consistency of underlying tissue changes with age, pathologic conditions, and hormonal variations. Client must learn to feel normal variations of own breast tissue to be able to recognize abnormal masses. |
| 14. If a mass is found, palpate for following characteristics: location in relation to quadrants, size in centimeters, shape (e.g., round or discoid); consistency (soft, firm, or hard), tenderness, mobility, discreteness (are boundaries of mass easily detected?). | Data allow for definitive identification of type of mass. |
| 15. Use finger to gently compress the areola. Then with thumb and index finger gently compress nipple, observing for discharge. | Involvement of glandular tissue may cause discharge from nipple. |
| 16. Repeat procedure for opposite breast. | |
| 17. After palpation is completed have client demonstrate self-palpation. | Return demonstration provides feed-back to measure client's learning and to determine need for further instruction. |
| ***Male client*** | |
| 1. Inspect nipple and areola of male clients for nodules, edema, and ulceration. Note any swelling of breasts. Palpate breast tissue in same systematic pattern as for females. | Signs of breast cancer are same for male client. |

| Steps | Rationale |
|---|---|
| **Evaluation** | |
| 1. Compare findings with normal assessment characteristics. | Determines presence of abnormalities. |
| 2. Have female client describe findings of self-examination. | Feedback demonstrates client's understanding of signs to observe for. |
| ***Expected outcomes*** | |
| 1. Young to middle-aged adult: breasts are smooth, symmetric, without retraction flattening. Tissue is firm, elastic, with presence of soft, lobular underlying tissue. Areola are smooth with nipples symmetric and without discharge. | Normal findings. |
| 2. Older adult: breasts are smaller than middle age, evidenced by shrunken, wrinkled appearance of skin. Breasts sag. Tissue may feel stringy and nodular. Nipples point downward. | Changes in elasticity of tissue. Estrogen changes reduce size of glandular tissue. |
| 3. Lymph nodes nonpalpable. | Normal findings. |
| 4. Client able to perform self-breast examination correctly. | Learning a skill is best measured through demonstration feedback. |
| ***Unexpected outcomes—small mass*** | |
| 1. Breasts are smooth, symmetric without retraction or flattening. Localized mass is palpable on one side. Mass may be hard or soft, tender or nontender, mobile or fixed, and well differentiated. There is no discharge from nipples. Lymph nodes are nonpalpable. Client is unable to detect mass. | Symptoms indicative of small discrete breast mass. Repeated experience necessary for client to become familiar with own breasts. |
| ***Potential nursing diagnoses—small mass*** | |
| Related nursing diagnoses: | |
| ▪ Anxiety: related to unknown. | Without definitive diagnosis, client will be apprehensive. |
| ▪ Fear: related to unknown. | |
| ▪ Knowledge deficit regarding preventive health care: related to inexperience. | Client will require further instruction. |
| ***Unexpected outcomes—advanced lesion*** | |
| 1. Breast reveals dimpling or retraction unilaterally. Skin over area is inflamed with increased vascularity. Contour of involved breast is irregular; nipple is distorted with serous or bloody discharge. Palpable mass that is hard, fixed, nontender, and irregular in shape. | Symptoms indicate more advanced, invasive lesion. Immediate referral to physician is required. |
| 2. Lymph nodes are palpable. | |
| ***Potential nursing diagnoses—advanced lesion*** | |
| ▪ Fear: related to unknown. | Findings suggest severe type of problem. |
| ▪ Anxiety: related to unknown. | |
| ▪ Pain: related to inflammation of breast. | |
| ▪ Body image disturbance: related to breast mass. | Client fears loss of sexuality. |
| **Recording and Reporting** | |
| 1. Record all findings in nurses' notes. | Documents abnormalities or changes. Provides baseline data. |
| 2. Report abnormalities to nurse in charge or physician. | Further diagnosis will be required. |

## Special Considerations

- Breasts of young women normally extend in area from third to sixth ribs. Nipple usually at level of fourth intercostal space. Normal for one breast to be larger. Pregnancy causes breasts to enlarge two to three times previous size; nipples enlarge and may become erect; areola darkens; superficial veins become prominent. Menopause causes breasts to shrink and tissue becomes soft. In elderly, ligaments supporting breast tissue weakens, causing breasts to sag and nipples to lower.
- Cancerous nodes are hard, fixed, and nontender. Lymph nodes enlarged because of inflammation are usually tender.
- For larger pendulous breasts nurse may use bimanual palpation. Support inferior portion of breast in one hand while palpating breast tissue against supporting hand.
- Fibrocystic disease, a common disorder, is characterized by thickened nodular areas, located bilaterally, that usually become tender during or before menstrual period.

- Male breast cancer is rare. Routine self-examinations are unnecessary. Swelling of male breasts may result from obesity or glandular enlargement.

### Teaching Considerations

- Women at high school age and over should perform monthly self-examination of breasts. Best time for self-examination is on last day of menstrual period when breasts are no longer swollen or tender. Postmenopausal women should examine breasts same time each month. Pregnant women should examine breasts routinely each month.
- Women with fibrocystic disease must become familiar with character of cystic masses.
- Client may have difficulty learning to palpate own nodes because of awkward positioning. Have client lie supine with arm abducted, using right hand to palpate left axillary and clavicular areas and left hand to palpate right-sided nodes. Nurse takes client's hand and moves fingers in rotary fashion so client can feel proper technique.
- If client finds a mass during self-examination, caution her against rubbing or touching areas excessively. Pressure against cancerous or infected mass can disrupt cells and cause spread.
- Explain recommended frequency of mammography (performed yearly for women age 50 or over and for women age 40 or over with a family history of breast cancer) and breast self-examinations (every 3 yr from ages 20-40 and yearly after age 40) by a health care provider.
- Discuss signs and symptoms of breast cancer.

## *SKILL 13-13 Assessing the Abdomen*

Because there are multiple organs within the abdominal cavity the nurse must perform a thorough assessment in order to interpret all findings accurately. For example, if the client has abdominal pain, the symptom could be caused by alterations in any number of organs, such as the stomach, gallbladder, pancreas, or intestines. The nurse gathers specific historical data so that signs and symptoms can be localized to specific organ involvement.

When performing the assessment the nurse should maintain a mental image of the anatomic location of each organ. This practice ensures that the nurse is using assessment skills correctly. The nurse should remember to include assessment of organs that lie posteriorly, such as the kidneys.

An abdominal assessment is routine following abdominal surgery and for any client who has undergone invasive diagnostic tests of the gastrointestinal tract (Chapter 46). The order of an abdominal assessment differs from previous assessments. The nurse begins with inspection and then follows with auscultation. It is important to auscultate before palpation and percussion; otherwise these later maneuvers may alter the frequency and character of bowel sounds.

### Purposes

1. Assess gastrointestinal peristalsis.
2. Determine condition of underlying intestinal organs.

## *Procedure 13-13*

| Steps | Rationale |
|---|---|
| **Assessment** | |
| 1. If client has abdominal or low back pain, assess the character of pain in detail (location, onset, frequency, precipitating factors, aggravating factors, type of pain, severity, etc.) | Pattern of characteristics of pain help determine its source. |
| 2. Carefully observe client's movement and position such as:<br>a. Lying still with knees updrawn.<br>b. Moving restlessly to find a comfortable position.<br>c. Lying on one side or sitting with knees drawn up to chest. | Positions assumed by client may reveal nature and source of pain: peritonitis, renal stone, and pancreatitis. |
| 3. Assess client's normal bowel habits: frequency of stools; character of stools; recent changes in character of stools; measures used to promote elimination, e.g., laxatives, enemas, dietary intake; eating and drinking habits. | This data compared with information from physical assessment may help to identify cause and nature of elimination problems (Chapter 31). |
| 4. Determine if client has had abdominal surgery or trauma. | Surgical or traumatic alterations of abdominal organs may cause changes in expected findings, e.g., position of underlying organs. |
| 5. Assess if client has had any recent changes in weight or intolerance to diet, e.g. nausea, vomiting, cramping. | May be indicative of alterations in upper gastrointestinal tract, e.g., stomach or gallbladder, as well as lower intestinal tract. |

| Steps | Rationale |
|---|---|
| 6. Ask client to locate tender areas. | Painful areas are assessed last. Manipulation of body part can increase pain and client's anxiety and make remainder of assessment difficult to complete. |
| 7. Assess for difficulty in swallowing, belching, or flatulence, bloody emesis (hematemesis), black or tarry stools (melena), or heartburn. | These characteristic signs and symptoms indicate abdominal alterations. |

## Planning

| Steps | Rationale |
|---|---|
| 1. Develop individualized goals for assessment, including: | |
| a. Promote client's comfort. | Nurse techniques help client relax during palpation of organs. |
| b. Determine presence of abnormalities. | Can pose implications for a variety of nursing care measures. |
| 2. Prepare following equipment: | |
| a. Stethoscope | Used to auscultate bowel sounds. |
| b. Tape measure | Used to measure abdominal girth. |
| 3. Prepare client: | |
| a. Ask if client needs to empty bladder. | Palpation of full bladder can cause discomfort and feeling of urgency, and can make it difficult for client to relax. |
| b. Keep upper chest and legs draped. | Maintains client's warmth during examination, promoting relaxation. |
| c. Have client lie supine with arms down at sides. A small pillow under client's knees may be desired. | Position promotes optimal relaxation of abdominal muscles. Tightening of muscles prevents adequate palpation of underlying muscles. |
| d. Maintain conversation during assessment except during auscultation. Explain steps calmly and slowly. | Client's ability to relax during assessment improves accuracy of findings. |

## Implementation

| Steps | Rationale |
|---|---|
| 1. Describe observations or findings in relation to system of landmarks that map out abdominal region (Fig. 13-59): by quadrants—line extending from tip of xiphoid process to symphysis pubis crosses line intersecting umbilicus; by dividing abdomen into four equal sections (Fig. 13-59, *A*). Some clinicians may also divide the abdomen into nine equal sections for the abdominal examinations (Fig. 13-59, *B*). | Location of findings by common reference point helps successive examiners to confirm findings and locate abnormalities. |
| 2. While inspecting client's abdomen, first stand on client's right side, then sit to look across abdomen's surface. | Standing position helps to detect shadows and movement. Sitting position allows examiner to detect abnormal protuberances. |
| 3. Inspect skin of abdomen's surface for scars, venous patterns, lesions, silvery white striae (stretch marks), and artificial openings. Observe lesions for characteristics previously described in Skill 13-2. | Scars or artificial openings reveal evidence client has had past trauma or surgery. Striae indicate stretching of tissue by growth, obesity, pregnancy, ascites, or edema. Venous patterns may reflect liver disease (portal hypertension). |

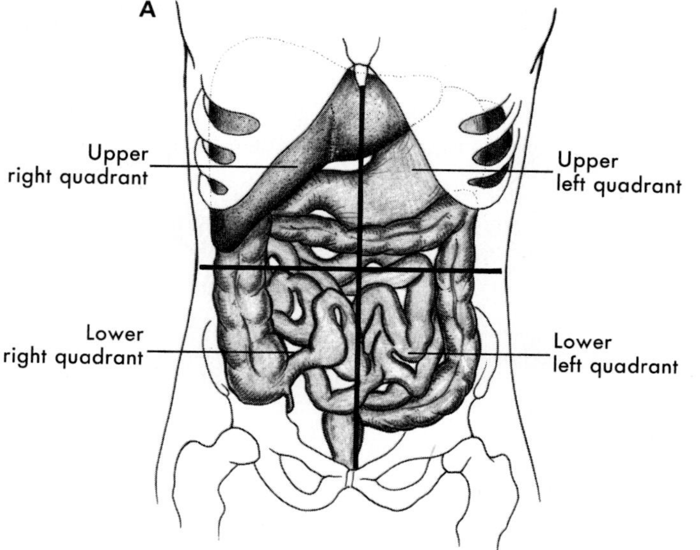


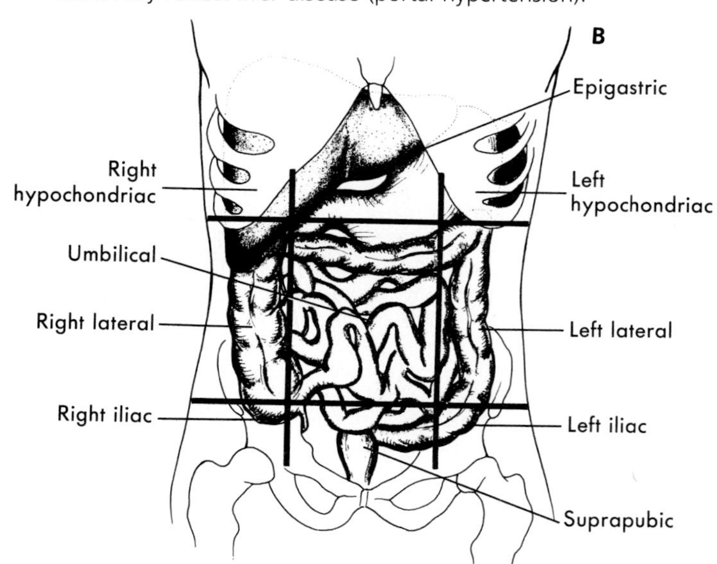


***Fig. 13-59*** Division of abdomen into quadrants.

| Steps | Rationale |
|---|---|
| 4. Inspect shape and symmetry of abdomen. Note presence of any masses or protrusions. (Have a child stand erect and then lie supine). | Changes in symmetry or contour may reflect presence of underlying masses, fluid collection, or gaseous distention. Normal abdomen of infants and young children is cylindric in erect position and flat in supine position. |
| 5. Have client roll onto side if distention is present. | Detects source of distention. Distention results from accumulation of intestinal gas, tumor, or fluid in abdominal cavity. If generalized, entire abdomen protrudes. Skin appears taut and stretched. If gas causes distention, flanks do not bulge. If fluid is source of distention, flanks bulge. When client rolls onto side protuberance forms on dependent side when fluid is present. |
| 6. Ask client if abdomen feels unusually tight. | Continued sensation of fullness helps to detect distention. Feeling of fullness after a heavy meal causes only temporary distention. |
| 7. Ask client to cough if visible mass is present. | Abdominal wall hernias will protrude or bulge out when client coughs because of increased abdominal pressure forcing loop of intestine through abdominal wall defect. |
| 8. Measure size of abdominal girth by placing tape measure around abdomen at level of umbilicus and note measurement. | Assesses increase or decrease in abdominal size caused by distention. |
| 9. Observe for movement or pulsations of abdominal surface by looking across abdomen from side. Observe for 1-2 min. Inspect epigastric area, midline above umbilicus, for aortic pulsation. | The presence of aortic pulsation, respiratory, or peristaltic movements, and any muscular contraction, can be visible on the abdominal surface. |
| 10. Observe position, shape, and color of umbilicus. Note presence of discharge or protruding mass. | Normal umbilicus is flat or concave hemisphere positioned midway between xiphoid and symphysis pubis. Assesses for presence of underlying pathologic conditions. Hernias cause upward protrusion of umbilicus during coughing, straining, or crying. |
| 11. Place diaphragm of stethoscope over one of four abdominal quadrants. Listen until you hear repeated gurgling or bubbling sounds. Repeat procedure for each quadrant. Describe sounds as normal or audible, absent, hyperactive, or hypoactive. Listen 3-5 min before deciding bowel sounds are absent. | Determines presence or absence of peristalsis. Sounds occur irregularly normally every 5-20 sec. Best time to auscultate is between meals. Performed before percussion and palpation, which may alter frequency and character of bowel sounds. Absent sounds indicate cessation of gastric motility. |
| 12. Place bell of stethoscope over midline of abdomen and auscultate for vascular sounds. If aortic bruit is auscultated. Stop assessment and notify physician. | Determines presence of turbulent blood flow (bruits) through thoracic or abdominal aorta. Percussion or palpation over abdominal bruit can cause damage if bruit is result of an abdominal aneurysm. Palpation can cause rupture of already weakened vessel wall. |
| 13. Have client roll to side and place bell of stethoscope posteriorly over costovertebral angle (CVA) (Fig. 13-60). | Determines presence of renal artery bruits. |
| 14. Have client return to supine position. Gently percuss each of four abdominal quadrants systematically. | Reveals presence of air or fluid in stomach and intestines. Normal percussion is tympanic because of swallowed air in gastrointestinal tract. Presence of fluid or underlying organs is revealed by dull or flat percussion. |

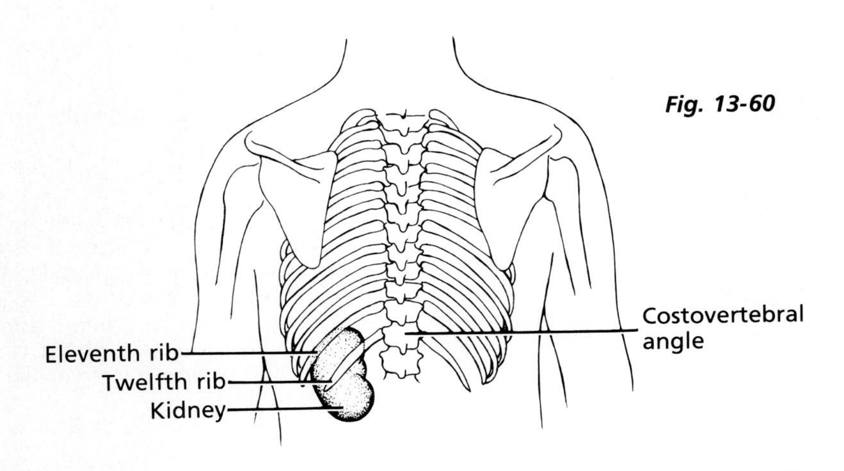


***Fig. 13-60***

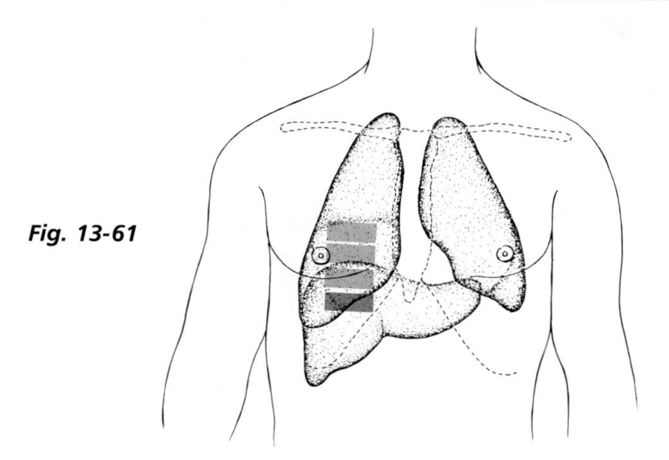

*Fig. 13-61*

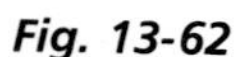

*Fig. 13-62*

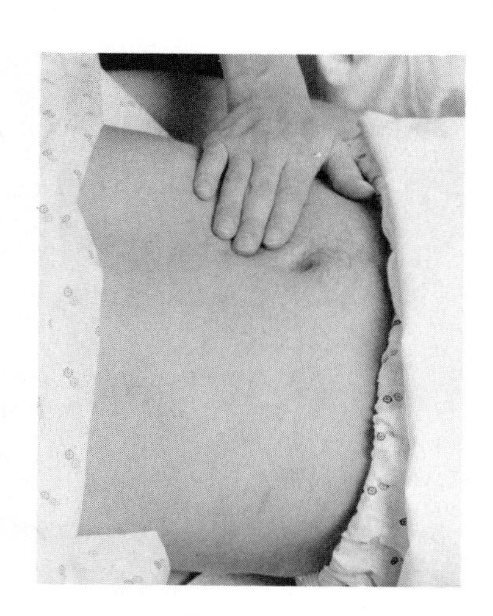

*Fig. 13-63*

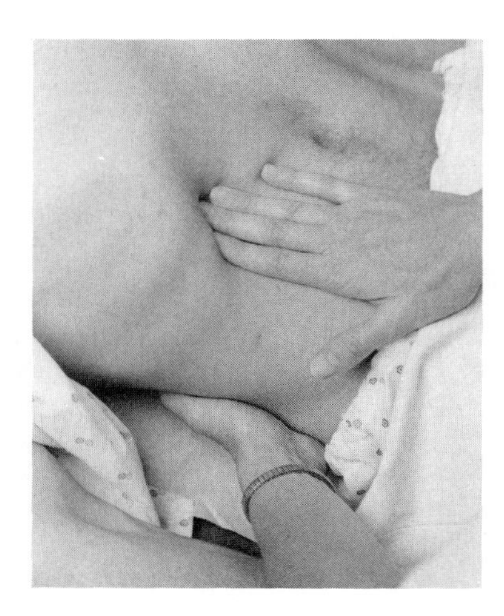

*Fig. 13-64*

| Steps | Rationale |
|---|---|
| 15. To locate liver percuss at intersection of the right iliac crest and right midclavicular line. Slowly inch pleximeter finger upward and percuss toward right costal margin until note becomes dull. | Detects position of liver's lower border. Percussion note changes from tympanic to dull at liver's lower border, usually found at right costal margin. |
| 16. Percuss at right midclavicular line below clavicle. Slowly inch pleximeter finger downward toward right costal margin until note becomes dull. Be sure pleximeter finger is in intercostal space during percussion (Fig. 13-61). Distance between liver's upper and lower border is normally 6-12 cm (2.5-5 in). | Detects position of liver's upper border. Percussion note changes from resonant to dull at liver's upper border, usually found in fifth, sixth, or seventh intercostal space. |
| 17. Ask client to sit and gently but firmly percuss over each CVA along scapular lines (Fig. 13-62). Use ulnar surface of fist to percuss directly or indirectly. Note if client experiences pain. | Determines presence of kidney inflammation. |
| 18. Lightly palpate over each abdominal quadrant, using palm and pads of fingertips in smooth, coordinated movement. Depress skin approximately 1 cm or 0.5 in. Note muscle tone, abdominal stiffness, presence of masses, and tenderness. Observe client's face. Note if abdomen is firm or soft to touch (Fig. 13-63). | Detects areas of localized tenderness, degree of tenderness, and presence and character of underlying masses. Palpation of sensitive area causes guarding, voluntary tightening of underlying abdominal muscles. Client's verbal and nonverbal cues may indicate discomfort from tenderness. Firm abdomen may indicate active obstruction with fluid or gas building up. Soft abdomen is normal or reveals obstruction is resolving. |
| 19. Just below umbilicus and above symphysis pubis palpate for smooth, rounded mass. | Detects presence of dome of distended bladder. |

| Steps | Rationale |
|---|---|
| 20. Systematically over each quadrant perform deep palpation. Be sure client is relaxed. Gently depress hands 2.5- 7.5 cm (1-3 in) into abdomen. *Do not use* deep palpation over surgical incision, tender organs, or abnormal masses. | Allows for assessment of characteristics of deep masses: size, shape, mobility, consistency, distribution, and presence of tenderness. |
| 21. If client experiences tenderness, assess for rebound tenderness by pressing hand deeply into involved area and then releasing quickly. | Indicates inflammation of peritoneal lining of abdomen. If pain is aggravated by release of hand, test is positive. |
| 22. Locate liver's lower border by placing left hand under client's right posterior thorax (just under small of back). Apply gentle upward pressure with left hand. With fingers pointing toward client's right costal margin, place right hand on client's right upper quadrant below costal margin. Ask client to take deep breath and gently palpate right hand in and up. As client inhales, liver's edge may be felt (Fig. 13-64). | Allows for location of liver and determination if organ is enlarged or disease is present. Upward pressure of left hand along with deep breathing maneuver causes liver to descend and be entrapped briefly for palpation. Liver's edge cannot usually be palpated in normal adult. Normal liver is nontender and has regular contour and sharp edge. |

## Evaluation

| | |
|---|---|
| 1. Compare assessment findings with normal assessment characteristics of abdomen. | Determines presence of abnormalities. |
| ***Expected outcomes*** | |
| 1. Abdomen is soft and symmetric with even contour. No mass or tenderness is palpable. | Normal findings. |
| 2. Bowel sounds are active and audible in all four quadrants. | Normal peristalsis. |
| 3. Abdomen is tympanic on percussion. | Normal air found in intestines. |
| 4. No CVA tenderness is present. | Kidney is normal. |
| 5. Liver is nonpalpable; location of borders is normal. | Liver is normal. |
| ***Unexpected outcomes*** | |
| 1. Abdomen is distended on palpation. Bowel sounds are hypoactive. Client complains of generalized cramping pain with rectal fullness. No localized mass or tenderness. | Intestinal peristalsis decreased or absent with retention of fecal material. |
| ***Potential nursing diagnoses*** | |
| ▪ Constipation: related to bedrest. | May be result of poor diet or reduced activity. |
| ▪ Pain: related to gastric distention. | Intestinal distention causes discomfort. |
| ***Unexpected outcomes*** | |
| 1. Abdomen distended, soft, or tight to palpation. Bowel sounds are absent. No tenderness or masses are palpable. Percussion note is tympanic. Client may have sense of abdominal fullness. | Peristalsis is absent. |
| ***Potential nursing diagnoses*** | |
| ▪ Constipation: related to decreased peristalsis. | Common diagnosis of postoperative clients who have had abdominal surgery or general anesthetic. Also appropriate for clients with paralytic ileus. |
| ***Unexpected outcomes*** | |
| 1. Abdomen tender to palpation with guarding. Client may grimace during assessment. Bowel sounds may be hypoactive or hyperactive. If area of obstruction developing, percussion note may be flat. | Symptoms indicative of potential obstruction requiring physician intervention. |
| ***Potential nursing diagnoses*** | |
| ▪ Pain: related to potential bowel obstruction. | Intestinal walls become distended. |
| ***Unexpected outcomes*** | |
| 1. Abdomen tender to palpation with client experiencing cramping. Bowel sounds hyperactive. Stools liquid or increased in frequency. | Symptoms of increased peristalsis. |
| ***Potential nursing diagnoses*** | |
| ▪ Diarrhea: related to stress, dietary intake. | Bowel habits change and lead to frequent loose stools. |

| Steps | Rationale |
|---|---|
| **Recording and Reporting** | |
| 1. Record results of assessment in nurses' notes. | Documents baseline data and any change in client's condition. Also serves to document tolerance to any diagnostic testing. |
| 2. Report serious abnormalities, e.g., absent bowel sounds, presence of mass, or acute pain to nurse in charge and physician. | Signs and symptoms indicate potentially serious alterations requiring further diagnosis or treatment. |

## Special Considerations

- Placement of arms under head or raising of knees during examination causes muscular contraction.
- Normal venous patterns are faint except in very thin clients. In infants and children skin is usually taut and without wrinkles or creases.
- All subsequent measurements of abdominal girth should be taken at same level of umbilicus to provide objective means to evaluate changes.
- Normal ventilation involves rhythmic movement of abdomen as diaphragm descends and rises. Normally there is slight pulsation of aorta with each beat of systole.
- Most common palpable mass in child is feces, usually felt in right lower quadrant.
- Normally bladder lies below symphysis pubis.
- Only skilled clinician should perform deep palpation. Qualified examiner should assist beginning student.

## Teaching Considerations

- Long-term progressive weight loss is sign of cancer.
- Explain factors such as diet, regular exercise, and fluid intake that promote normal bowel elimination (see Chapter 30).
- Caution clients about dangers of excessive use of laxatives or enemas.
- If client has chronic pain, explain measures for pain relief (e.g., relaxation exercises (see Chapter 5).
- If client notices change in bowel habits, blood in feces, or hematemeses, instruct to contact physician.
- Explain to clients the need to have a controlled weight reduction program when attempting to lose weight.

# *SKILL 13-14 Assessing the Female Genitalia and Rectum*

The nurse combines examination of the female genitalia and rectum because of the close proximity of the anatomic structures. Typically, the client will feel somewhat self-conscious and anxious during this portion of a physical assessment. Often the woman's cultural background contributes to any uneasiness she feels. The position the client must assume is also often cause for embarrassment. The nurse's rapport with the client and calm technique will help the client relax during the examination. If a male nurse performs the examination, a female nurse should be in attendance to protect the client's and male nurse's welfare. A vaginal examination and pap smear are relatively simple procedures and should be a part of each woman's preventive health care.

## Purposes

1. Assess condition of external genitalia and reproductive organs.
2. Assess condition of the rectal canal.
3. Educate female clients about risks related to vaginal and uterine cancer and sexually transmitted diseases.
4. Educate clients about the importance of regular vaginal examinations and Pap smear.

## *Procedure 13-14*

| Steps | Rationale |
|---|---|
| **Assessment** | |
| 1. Determine if client has previous illness or surgery involving reproductive organs, including history of sexually transmitted disease. | Can influence appearance and position of organs being examined. |
| 2. Review client's menstrual history including age at menarche; frequency and duration of menstrual cycle; character of flow, e.g., amount, presence of clots; presence of pain; dates of last two menstrual periods. | Information helps to reveal level of female's reproductive health including normalcy of menstrual cycle. |

| Steps | Rationale |
|---|---|
| 3. Ask client to describe obstetric history including description of each pregnancy and history of abortions or miscarriages. | Physical findings made during assessment of genitalia and reproductive organs vary depending on client's history of pregnancy. |
| 4. Ask client to describe current and past contraceptive practices and any problems encountered. | Use of certain types of contraceptives may influence reproductive health. |
| 5. Determine if client has symptoms or history of genitourinary problems. Symptoms might include burning during urination, frequency, urgency, nocturia, hematuria, or incontinence. | Urinary problems may be associated with gynecologic disorders. |
| 6. Assess client's sexual history. May be deferred if client is apparently symptom free. | Reveals client's risk for and understanding of sexually transmitted disease. |
| 7. Assess if client has signs and symptoms of vaginal discharge, painful or swollen perianal tissues, or lesions of the genitalia. | These signs and symptoms indicate sexually transmitted disease. |
| 8. Determine if client has experienced bleeding from the rectum, black or tarry stools (melena), rectal pain, or change in bowel habits (constipation or diarrhea). | Warning signs of colorectal cancer or other gastrointestinal alterations. |
| 9. Determine if client has personal or family history of colorectal cancer, polyps, or inflammatory bowel disease. | Risk factors for colorectal cancer. |
| 10. Assess dietary habits for high-fat intake or deficient fiber content. | Bowel cancer may be linked to dietary intake of fat or insufficient fiber intake. |
| 11. Determine if client has undergone screening for colorectal cancer (digital exam, stool blood slide test, proctoscopy). | Undergoing this screening reflects understanding and compliance with preventive health care measures. |
| 12. Assess medication history for use of laxatives or cathartic medications. | Repeated use can cause diarrhea and eventual loss of intestinal muscle tone. |
| 13. Assess use of codeine or iron preparations. | Codeine causes constipation. Iron turns color of feces black and tarry. |

## Planning

| Steps | Rationale |
|---|---|
| 1. Develop individualized goals for assessment, including: | |
| a. Maintain client's comfort. | Client's position, anxiety, and use of speculum can cause physical discomfort. |
| b. Control or relieve anxiety. | Many clients are apprehensive and embarrassed about procedure. |
| c. Maintain client's self-esteem. | Nurse's techniques can demonstrate respect for client's privacy and well-being. |
| d. Determine presence of abnormalities. | Dictates type of nursing care required, e.g., thorough hygiene or education. |
| e. Increase client's knowledge about risks for vaginal or uterine cancer and related preventive health care measures. | Nurse can use examination as time to discuss preventive care. Do not present information to frighten client into thinking signs of cancer are present. |
| 2. Prepare following equipment and supplies: | |
| a. Disposable gloves | |
| b. Vaginal speculum | |
| c. Gooseneck lamp | |
| d. Lubricant | |
| e. Sponge or cotton tipped swabs | |
| f. Wooden spatula | |
| g. Specimen bottle with fixative solution | Used for pap smear. |
| h. Glass microscopic slides | |
| 3. Prepare client for examination: | |
| a. Ask client to empty her bladder. | Frequently physician wishes to collect urine specimen. Empty bladder allows client to relax during examination. |
| b. Assist client to lithotomy position: | |
| ▪ Client lies supine on bed or table, flexes knees perpendicular to bed, relaxes thighs and allows each leg to abduct to the side. | Position used to examine only external genitalia. |
| ▪ Elevate client's head on pillow. | Provides comfort. |
| ▪ Client lies supine with thighs flexed and abducted, knees flexed, and feet in stirrups. | Optimal position to allow full visualization and access to genital area for speculum examination. |
| c. Place rectangular sheet with corner of drape over sternum; adjacent corners fall over each knee and fourth corner covers perineum. | Prevents unnecessary exposure of body parts. Clients often are embarrassed by exposure of external genitalia. |

| Steps | Rationale |
|---|---|
| d. Explain each step of procedure thoroughly with client. | Genital examination can cause anticipatory anxiety. Thorough explanation relieves client's fears and promotes cooperation. |
| 4. Have a female in attendance if a male is performing assessment. | Provides client with feeling of security during examination. |

## Implementation

### *External genitalia*

| Steps | Rationale |
|---|---|
| 1. Wash hands. | Reduces transmission of infection. |
| 2. Apply clean disposable gloves on both hands. | Gloves make it easier to manipulate perineal structures and prevent spread of infection. |
| 3. With perineum well illuminated, inspect quantity and distribution of hair growth, color of skin, and size and contour of labia. Note any areas of inflammation, edema, lacerations, lesions, or discharge. If structures appear distorted or if vaginal orifice is asymmetric, palpate tissues later in examination. | Assesses for gross abnormalities. Hormonal alterations can cause changes in pattern of hair growth. Irregularities may be result of lesions, scars, or inflammation of underlying tissue. |
| 4. Before touching perineum, first touch neighboring thigh. Explain that it is necessary to inspect deeper perineal structures. | Perineum is very sensitive and tender and should not be touched suddenly without warning. |
| 5. With nondominant hand gently place thumb and index finger inside labia minora and retract tissues outward (Fig. 13-65). Be sure to have firm hold during retraction. | Allows for inspection of structures and tissues within the labial folds. Firm hold prevents repeated retractions against sensitive tissues. |
| 6. Inspect clitoris for size and color. Note any drainage, inflammation, edema, ulcerations, or lesions. | Assesses for presence of malignant lesions (clitoris is common site in older women) or syphilitic lesions (common site in younger women). Inflammation causes clitoris to become bright cherry red. Syphilitic chancres are small, open ulcers that drain serous fluid. |

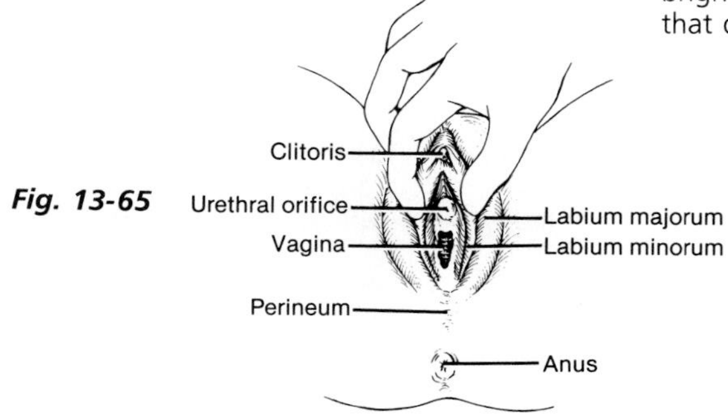


*Fig. 13-65*

| Steps | Rationale |
|---|---|
| 7. Observe urethral orifice, a small slit or pinhole opening just above vaginal canal. Note any inflammation, discharge, or masses. | Allows examiner to rule out any abnormality of lower urinary tract. |
| 8. If inflammation from orifice is present, place index finger in vaginal orifice approximately half finger's length. Bend finger to touch anterior wall of vagina in midline behind urethra. Gently milk urethra by exerting pressure from inside out toward orifice. Obtain a culture of purulent discharge (Chapter 45). | Maneuver causes discharge within urethral orifice to be expressed without causing client discomfort. |
| 9. If drainage is found, nurse changes gloves. | Prevents transfer of infectious material. |
| 10. Inspect labia minora for symmetry, size, color, lesions, and exudate. | Labia can be enlarged because of infection, underlying lesions, or trauma. Labia may also be site for venereal lesions. |
| 11. Inspect Bartholin's and Skene's glands located near vaginal opening and urethral orifice. Normally glands are not visible. Note any obvious swelling, inflammation, or discharge from sites. | Common sites of venereal infection. |
| 12. Palpate Bartholin's gland by placing index finger inside base of vagina and thumb on outside of labia majora, and compress fingers together gently. | Maneuver allows examiner to feel size of gland and detect any tenderness or presence of discharge. |
| 13. Palpate Skene's gland by placing index finger over site of gland near urethra and apply gentle inward pressure. | Detects enlargement of gland and presence of discharge. |
| 14. Inspect vaginal opening or orifice. Note condition of hymen just inside orifice. Hymen is thin strip of tissue that in virgin may restrict opening of vagina. | Determines symmetry of opening. |

| Steps | Rationale |
|---|---|

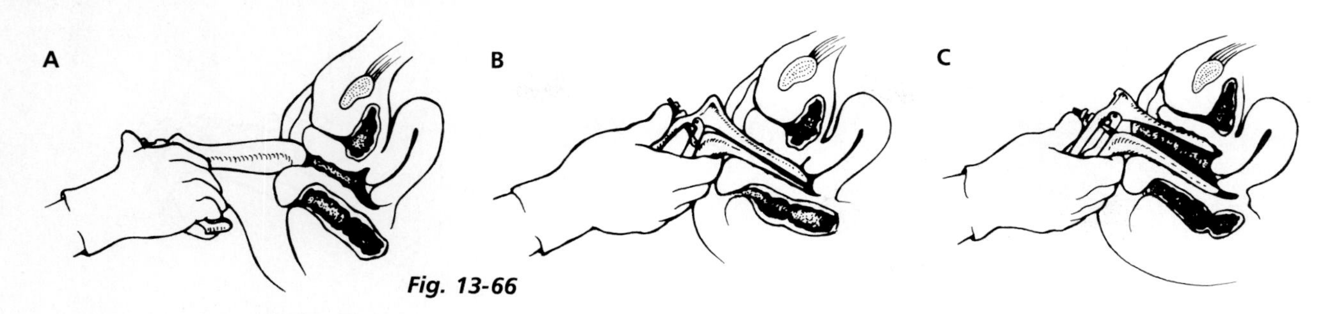

*Fig. 13-66*

| Steps | Rationale |
|---|---|
| 15. Ask client to bear down or strain as if she were voiding, observe vaginal opening for sudden appearance of tissue or gaping of vaginal walls. Normally there should only be slight bulging of entire perineum. | Assesses integrity of muscle tone of vaginal canal. Detects prolapse or fall of surrounding tissues, e.g., bladder or rectum into vaginal canal. |
| 16. Inspect anus for presence of lesions or hemorrhoids (enlarged blood vessels). | Area can be easily inspected with client in lithotomy position. |
| ***Internal genitalia*** | |
| 1. Nurse performs speculum examination only after special training under supervision. | Procedure can cause serious injury to client if performed incorrectly. |
| 2. Select proper-sized speculum. | Prevents trauma to vaginal wall. |
| 3. Place speculum blades under warm running water. Commercially prepared lubricants alter results of Pap smear. | Warming of blades minimizes discomfort. Water is ideal lubricant for insertion of blades. |
| 4. With nurse sitting on stool and facing client's perineum, light is adjusted over nurse's shoulder. | Illuminates perineum and vaginal orifice. |
| 5. Explain that speculum is about to be inserted and that client will feel pressure and some pulling. | Reduces client's anxiety. |
| 6. Gently insert first two fingers of nondominant hand into vaginal opening. | Allows nurse to palpate for abnormalities such as masses or swelling that may interfere with passage of speculum. |
| 7. With same two fingers, press down on perineal body just inside the intruitus. With vaginal blades in closed position gently introduce speculum obliquely (rotated 50° counterclockwise from vertical position) past fingers (Fig. 13-66, *A*). | Angle of insertion fits contour of vagina. Blades kept closed to prevent pinching of tissues. |
| 8. Insert speculum downward at 45° angle close to rectal wall. | Blades follow normal downward slope of vaginal canal (Fig. 13-66, *B*). |
| 9. After wide portions of blades (approximately three fourths length of blades) pass vaginal orifice, rotate speculum so blades are horizontal, with handle down in palm of hand. | Speculum should be positioned straight so that blades can fully retract tissue. |
| 10. Press on lever to open blades slowly after full insertion. Attempt to see cervix. Once cervix is in full view lock blades in open position (Fig. 13-66, *C*). | Cervix is located at posterior end of vaginal canal. View of cervix indicates speculum properly positioned. |
| 11. Inspect cervix and its opening (os). Note color, size, contour, symmetry, presence of discharge, lacerations, or lesions. Cancerous lesions bleed easily and margins of cervix are difficult to identify. Bluish appearance of cervix (Chadwick's sign) is early sign of pregnancy. Pale cervix is indicative of menopause. | Cervix is a common primary site for cancerous growths. Uterine cancer is fourth leading type of cancer among women (American Cancer Society, 1989). |
| 12. Obtain Pap smear: | Screening test for cervical cancer collects cells from three sites. Never perform smear during menstruation since menstrual flow may obscure any abnormal cells. |
| a. Gently insert cotton-tipped swab into cervical os. Smear specimen on glass slide labeled endocervical (Fig. 13-67, *A*). | Collection of endocervical cells. |
| b. With molded end of wooden spatula gently scrape a specimen from surface of cervix. Smear specimen on glass slide labeled cervical (Fig. 13-67, *B*). | Collection of outer cervical cells. |
| c. With opposite end of spatula collect secretions at base of cervix along floor of vagina. Smear specimen on glass slide labeled vaginal (Fig. 13-67, *C*). | Collection of cells from vaginal pool. |
| 13. Prepare each slide with fixative solution. | Prevents breakdown and drying of cells before microscopic examination. |

| Steps | Rationale |
|---|---|

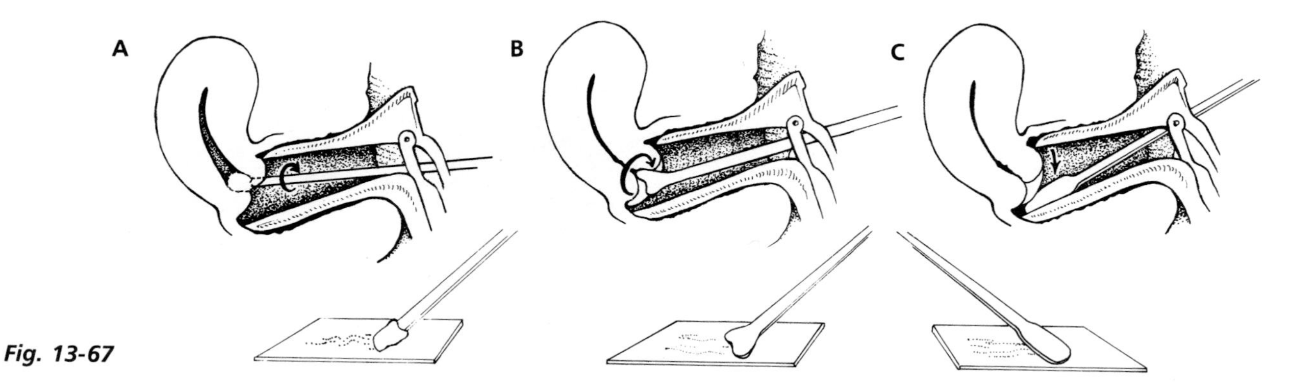


***Fig. 13-67***

| Steps | Rationale |
|---|---|
| 14. Note if there is bleeding of cervix after specimen collection. | Scraping of cervix commonly can cause spotting. Continuous bleeding suggests possible presence of cancerous lesion. |
| 15. Inspect vaginal walls while slowly withdrawing speculum. As speculum leaves cervix, loosen thumbscrew but keep blades retracted. Note vaginal wall's color, texture, presence of lesions, masses, discharge, and odor. | Assesses presence of infection or inflammation. Yeast infections, which are common, cause thick, white, patchy, curd-like discharge that clings to vaginal walls. |
| 16. Be sure speculum blades are closed completely before withdrawing speculum from vaginal orifice. | Prevents stretching and trauma to tissues. |
| 17. Assist client to lower legs from stirrups and return to supine position. Offer her opportunity to clean perineal area. | Lithotomy position can cause muscular strain. Secretions from vaginal canal can be source of discomfort. |
| 18. Remove gloves and wash hands. | Reduces transmission of microorganisms. |

***Rectal examination***

| Steps | Rationale |
|---|---|
| 1. Wash hands and don gloves. | Reduces transmission of infection. |
| 2. Have adult client assume dorsal recumbent or Sim's position. | Provides access to anal area. |
| 3. Child is placed on abdomen. | Provides access to anus and allows examiner to view gluteal folds. |
| 4. For child client, inspect symmetry of gluteal folds. | Asymmetry may indicate dislocation of hip. |
| 5. For child client, gently scratch skin around anus and note response. | Assesses for presence of anal reflex. |
| 6. For adult clients, apply lubricant to gloved index finger of dominant hand. | Minimizes friction during palpation of rectal walls. |
| 7. Ask client to bear down as though having a bowel movement. | Relaxes external anal sphincter. |
| 8. Warn client that it is normal to have sensation of having bowel movement during palpation. | Insertion of examiner's finger causes rectal fullness that normally elicits defecation. |
| 9. As anal sphincter relaxes insert fingertip into anus and direct it along rectal canal toward client's umbilicus. | Angle toward umbilicus follows contour of rectum. |
| 10. Palpate each side of rectal wall systematically for contour and consistency, noting any nodules or irregularities. Ask client if tenderness is felt. | Assesses for presence of rectal wall lesions. Cancerous tumors of rectum and colon were third in incidence for men and second in incidence for women (American Cancer Society '89). |
| 11. With finger advanced to full extent, ask client to again bear down. | Higher lesions will descend down against fingertips. |
| 12. Then ask client to tighten anal muscles around examining finger. | Assesses for sphincter tone. |
| 13. Withdraw finger and test any stool on glove for microscopic evidence of blood (Skill 46-7). | High lesions in colon or rectum may cause erosion of rectal wall that results in blood loss of very small proportions. Blood can only be identified through laboratory analysis. |
| 14. Clean any moisture or drainage from rectal area and assist client to sitting position. Drape lower torso. | Client should feel comfortable before next portion of examination begins. |
| 15. Dispose of gloves properly and wash hands. | Reduces transmission of microorganisms. |

## Evaluation

| Steps | Rationale |
|---|---|
| 1. Compare findings with normal assessment characteristics for genitalia and rectum. | Determines presence of abnormalities. |

| Steps | Rationale |
|---|---|
| 2. Evaluate client's emotional response toward examination noting voice tone, facial expression, body position, or movement. | Measures level of anxiety. |
| 3. Ask client to discuss importance of routine vaginal examinations. | Measures understanding of risks related to vaginal and uterine cancer. |
| ***Expected outcomes*** | |
| 1. Labia majora are symmetric, hair growth distributed in triangular pattern, and there are no lesions or discharge. | Normal findings. |
| 2. Clitoris is pink without lesions. | |
| 3. Urethral orifice intact and without exudate. | |
| 4. Labia minora are symmetric, pink, and without exudate. | |
| 5. Bartholin's and Skene's gland nonpalpable. | |
| 6. Vaginal orifice is symmetric without prolapse of tissue. | |
| 7. Anal area is clear. | |
| 8. Client able to discuss importance of routine vaginal examinations. | Demonstrates knowledge of preventive health care. |
| ***Unexpected outcomes*** | |
| 1. White chalky discharge noted within labial folds over clitoris. | |
| 2. Malodorous odor noted. | |
| 3. No inflammation or lesions noted. | |
| ***Potential nursing diagnoses*** | |
| ▪ Knowledge deficit regarding perineal hygiene techniques: related to misinformation. | May be caused by poor technique, misunderstanding of importance, or low motivation. |
| ▪ Potential for infection: related to poor hygiene. | Accumulation of secretions can harbor microorganism growth. |
| ***Unexpected outcomes*** | |
| 1. Clitoris inflamed. | Symptoms 1-6 are indicative of inflammation and infection of genitalia and lower urinary tract. |
| 2. Bartholin's and Skene's glands palpable and tender, with discharge expressed upon palpation. | |
| 3. Purulent discharge noted from vaginal orifice and within labial folds. | |
| 4. Client may complain of burning, frequency, and urgency during urination. | |
| 5. Client may have abdominal or pelvic discomfort. | |
| 6. Ulcers may be present involving external genitalia, cervix, and vaginal walls. | |
| ***Potential nursing diagnoses*** | |
| Symptoms are indicative of sexually transmitted infections. Related nursing diagnoses may include: | |
| ▪ Pain: related to inflamed tissue. | Inflammation of tissue is very painful. |
| ▪ Body image disturbance: related to threat to sexuality. | Alters person's sexuality. |
| ▪ Knowledge deficit regarding epidemiology of sexually transmitted diseases: related to misinformation. | May require instruction related to preventive health care. |
| ▪ Sexual dysfunction: related to infectious disease process. | May fear loss of sexual function. |
| ***Unexpected outcomes*** | |
| 1. Cervix is asymmetric and may have lesions or nodules involving surface. | Symptoms indicate cervical cancer. |
| 2. Tissue bleeds easily when scraped. | |
| 3. Pap smear positive. | |
| 4. Cervix appears normal, without lesions or discharge. | |
| ***Potential nursing diagnoses*** | |
| Symptoms are indicative of cervical cancer. Clients with early cervical carcinoma may only be detected by Pap smear results. Related nursing diagnoses: | |
| ▪ Fear: related to diagnosis, anticipated treatment, etc. | Client can be very apprehensive about findings. |
| ▪ Anxiety: related to possibility of death. | Client's prognosis depends on severity of disease. |
| ▪ Sexual dysfunction: related to anxiety. | Client unable to achieve desired satisfaction. |

| Steps | Rationale |
|---|---|
| **Recording and Reporting** | |
| 1. Record all assessment findings and describe client's reaction toward examination. | Documents baseline data and any change in client's condition. Evaluates response to procedure. |
| 2. Record size of speculum used. | Helpful information if further examinations are to be done. |
| 3. Report any abnormalities observed to nurse in charge or physician. | Abnormalities may indicate need for further diagnostic study or treatment. |

## Special Considerations

- Women suffering pain or deformity of hips or knees may not be able to assume lithotomy position. Client may abduct only one leg or have nurse assist in gently separating thighs.
- Evaluation of external genitalia in preschoolers, school-age girls, and adolescents causes anxiety because of their modesty and concern for privacy.
- Pubic hair growth begins with onset of puberty. Hair grows normally in triangle over female perineum with base near upper border of pubic bone and sides of triangle covering outer surfaces of labia majora. Soft, downy hair is early sign of sexual maturation. No hair growth after age 16 is abnormal.
- Labia majora are plump and well formed in normal adult. After childbirth, labia majora separate, causing labia minora to become more prominent.
- Menopause causes labia major to thin. Advancing age causes atrophy of labia majora.
- Children's rectal walls are not palpated because of danger of causing trauma.
- Common palpable rectal mass is hardened stool that is usually penetrable with finger and leaves brown discoloration on glove's tip.

## Teaching Considerations

- The American Cancer Society recommends that women over age 20 and/or who are sexually active but have low risk for cancer have annual Pap smears until two smears are negative, and then every 3 years until age 65.
- Women at risk for cervical cancer should have annual checkups. Best time to collect smear is 5-6 days after menstruation.
- Instruct client about recommended frequency of Pap smears and gynecologic examinations.
- Counsel clients with sexually transmitted disease about diagnosis and treatment. Teach preventive measures (e.g., male partner's use of condoms, restricting number of sexual partners, avoiding sex with persons who have several other partners, and perineal hygiene measures).
- Tell clients with sexually transmitted diseases that they must inform sexual partners of the need for an examination.
- Reinforce importance of perineal hygiene (as appropriate).
- Discuss the American Cancer Society's guidelines for early detection of colorectal cancer:
  1. Digital rectal examination performed yearly after age 40.
  2. Stool blood slide test (guaiac test) performed yearly after age 50.
  3. Proctosigmoidoscopy, involving visual inspection of the rectum and lower colon with a hollow, lighted tube. The test, performed by a physician, should be performed every 3-5 years after age 50, after two annual examinations with negative results.
- Discuss dietary planning to reduce fat and increase fiber content.
- Warn clients against problems caused by overuse of laxatives, cathartic medications, codeine, or enemas.

# *SKILL 13-15 Assessing the Male Genitalia and Rectum*

As in the case of the female examination, assessment of genitalia and rectum can be just as uncomfortable or embarrassing for the client. In performing assessment a nurse should feel comfortable about his or her own sexuality. If the nurse is embarrassed, this feeling will easily be transmitted to the client, causing him considerable discomfort at times. The female nurse should have a male nurse in attendance when possible.

Because the incidence of sexually transmitted disease is high in adolescents and young adults, assessment of the genitalia should be a routine part of health screening for these age-groups. The nurse should not discuss the client's sexual activity during the examination, since the client may perceive this as evaluative or judgmental.

## Purposes

1. Determine condition of external genitalia.
2. Assess condition of the rectal canal and prostate.
3. Educate client on techniques for performing testicular self-examination.
4. Educate client about risks for contracting sexually transmitted diseases.
5. Educate client about preventive health care.

## *Procedure 13-15*

| Steps | Rationale |
|---|---|
| **Assessment** | |
| 1. Review client's normal urinary elimination pattern: frequency of voiding; history of nocturia; character and volume of urine; fluid intake daily; symptoms of burning, urgency, frequency; difficulty starting stream; hematuria. | Urinary problems can be directly associated with gynecologic problems particularly because of anatomy of males' reproductive and urinary systems. |
| 2. Assess client's sexual history. | Reveals client's risk for and understanding of sexually transmitted disease. |
| 3. Determine if client has had previous surgery or illness involving urinary or reproductive organs. | Alterations resulting from disease or surgery may be responsible for client's presenting symptoms and changes in organ structure or function. |
| 4. Ask if client has noted penile pain or swelling, lesions of the genitalia, urethral discharge. | Signs and symptoms commonly associated with sexually transmitted diseases. |
| 5. Assess if client has signs and symptoms of penile discharge, painful or swollen perianal tissues, or lesions of the genitalia. | These signs and symptoms indicate sexually transmitted disease. |
| 6. Determine if client has experienced bleeding from the rectum, black or tarry stools (melena), rectal pain, or change in bowel habits (constipation or diarrhea). | Warning signs of colorectal cancer or other gastrointestinal alterations. |
| 7. Determine if client has personal or family history of colorectal cancer, polyps, or inflammatory bowel disease. | Risk factors for colorectal cancer. |
| 8. Assess dietary habits for high-fat intake or deficient fiber content. | Bowel cancer may be linked to dietary intake of fat or insufficient fiber intake. |
| 9. Determine if client has undergone screening for colorectal cancer (digital exam, stool blood slide test, proctoscopy). | Undergoing this screening reflects understanding and compliance with preventive health care measures. |
| 10. Assess medication history for use of laxatives or cathartic medications. | Repeated use can cause diarrhea and eventual loss of intestinal muscle tone. |
| 11. Assess use of codeine or iron preparations. | Codeine causes constipation. Iron turns color of feces black and tarry. |
| **Planning** | |
| 1. Develop individualized goals for assessment, including: | |
| a. Promote client's comfort. | Manipulation of external genitalia, if done incorrectly, can be uncomfortable. |
| b. Relieve client's anxiety. | Procedure can be embarrassing for nurse and client. Nurse must use calm, confident approach. |
| c. Maintain client's self-esteem. | Client's privacy is respected at all times. |
| d. Increase client's knowledge of signs and symptoms and risks for sexually transmitted diseases. | Before or after examination nurse can provide useful information. |
| e. Provide client with knowledge and skills for performing testicular self-examination. | Client can demonstrate techniques for nurse to observe. |
| 2. Prepare equipment and supplies: | |
| a. Disposable gloves | Minimize skin contact during manipulation of genitalia and prevent spread of infection if lesions or exudate are present. |
| 3. Prepare client: | |
| a. In preparation for examination, female nurse should feel comfortable about her own sexuality before performing assessment. | Nurse's anxiety can cause difficulty in helping client explore health-related problems. |
| b. Female nurse may wish to have male attendant present or request male nurse to perform examination. | Minimizes anxiety on part of nurse and client. |
| c. Explain each step of assessment procedure and results of findings. | Reduces client's apprehension and promotes cooperation and understanding. |
| d. Ask client to empty bladder. | Promotes relaxation during procedure. |
| e. Have adult client lie supine with chest, abdomen, and lower legs draped. | Prevents unnecessary exposure of body parts. |
| f. Throughout examination manipulate genitalia gently and move through assessment as quickly as possible. | Minimizes client's discomfort and preserves modesty. |

| Steps | Rationale |
|---|---|
| **Implementation** | |
| ***Genitalia*** | |
| 1. Wash hands and apply disposable gloves. | Reduces transmission of microorganisms. |
| 2. Inspect structures of penis: | Assesses for presence of infections, congenital anomalies, or lesions. |
| a. In uncircumcised males retract foreskin to reveal glans and urethral meatus. Note position of meatus and observe for discharge, edema, inflammation, and lesions of glans. | |
| b. If discharge is present from meatus, acquire specimen by gently milking penis from base to urethra. | Obtain for culture to determine if discharge is infectious and type of causative organism (Chapter 45). |
| c. Check entire circumference of glans. Glans is normally pink and smooth. | Lesions may develop along undersurface. |
| d. Carefully inspect area between foreskin and glans. | Common site for venereal lesions. Small amount of thick white secretion between glans and foreskin is normal. |
| e. Palpate any lesions for tenderness, size, consistency, and shape. | Character of lesion indicates type of lesion. |
| f. After inspection of glans pull foreskin down to original position. | Foreskin may act as a constricting band around penis, reducing blood flow and causing edema and pain. |
| g. Inspect entire shaft of penis, note color of skin and presence of lesions, scars, or areas of edema. | Abnormalities may develop at any point along shaft. Clients who have been lying in bed for prolonged period may develop edema. |
| 3. Inspect scrotum's size, shape, symmetry, skin color, and presence of lesions on surface. Normally left testis is lower than right. Scrotum should hang freely from perineum behind penis. | Allows nurse to rule out presence of infection, lesions, and structural abnormalities. |
| 4. Gently lift scrotal sac to view posterior surface. | Structures within scrotal sac are very sensitive. |
| 5. Warm hands and gently palpate each testis and epididymis using thumb and first two fingers. Palpate organs for size, shape, and consistency. Ask client if there is sensation of tenderness. | Cold stimulus can initiate cremasteric reflex. In infants, determine if testes descended into scrotal sac. In adult assessment reveals presence of infection and benign or malignant masses. |
| 6. Instruct client on method for performing testicular self-examination: | Technique can detect testicular cancer in its early stages. |
| a. Have client perform examination after bath or shower. | Scrotum will be warm and dartos muscle relaxed. |
| b. Have client use both hands, placing the index and middle fingers under the testicles and thumbs on top. | Allows for correct palpation of any lesions. |
| c. Have client gently roll the testicle, feeling for lumps, thickening, or a change in consistency. | Client who knows what is normal for him can more easily identify any abnormalities. |
| d. Have client feel for pea-sized lumps on front and side of testicle. | |
| 7. Palpate each spermatic cord as it ascends toward inguinal ring. Note edema or nodules. | Spermatic cord can be site of infection and it can become involved with testicular or pathologic states of epididymis. |
| 8. Ask client to stand and inspect both inguinal areas for signs of obvious bulging. Ask client to hold breath and bear down. | Assesses for presence of hernia through inguinal wall or canal. |
| 9. Palpate inguinal ring and canal (Fig. 13-68) by taking left index finger and gently invaginating loose scrotal tissue on right side. Start at a point low on scrotum so that finger moves freely. Follow spermatic cord up to inguinal ring. Tip of finger may enter inguinal canal but do not force it. Once finger reaches farthest point have client again bear down. | Technique allows nurse to palpate hernia high within inguinal ring. Excess stretching of scrotal tissue can cause client discomfort. |
| 10. Palpate lymph nodes in inguinal area for size, shape, consistency, and tenderness. | Indicates presence of local or systemic infection or metastatic disease. |
| 11. Remove gloves and wash hands. | Reduces transmission of infection. |
| ***Rectum*** | |
| 1. Wash hands and apply disposable gloves. | Reduces transmission of infection. |
| 2. Ask client to bend over forward with hips flexed and upper body resting across bed, or lie in Sims' position on bed or table. | Positions provide access to anus and rectal canal. Sims' position may cause least embarrassment for client. |
| 3. Inspect anus for any lesions, hemorrhoids, or breaks in skin. | Anal tissues are usually moist and intact. |
| 4. Apply lubricant to gloved index finger: | Lubricant reduces friction against tissues. |
| a. Ask client to breath slowly and deeply. As client exhales gently insert finger into rectal canal and advance toward client's umbilicus. | Maneuver relaxes anal sphincter. |

| Steps | Rationale |
|---|---|

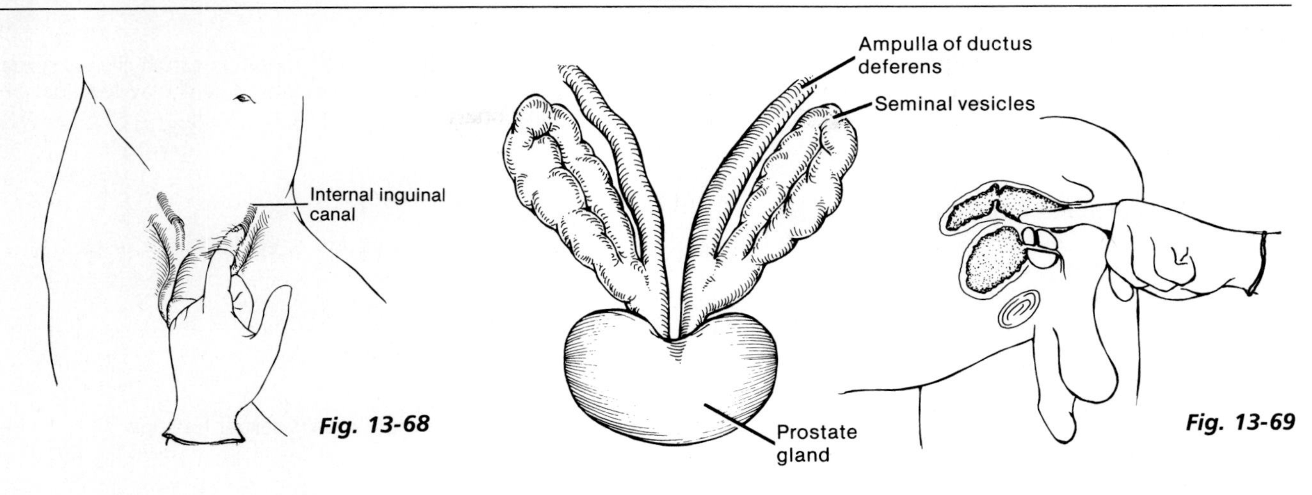


Fig. 13-68

Fig. 13-69

5. Palpate all rectal walls for masses or irregularities.

Assesses for presence of lesions. Rectal and colon cancer is third most common form of cancer among men (American Cancer Society). Hardened stool is common palpable mass.

6. Palpate prostate gland (situated a few centimeters from anterior rectal wall at base of bladder and surrounding urethra) (Fig. 13-69) by gently inserting finger toward client's umbilicus and against rectal wall. Note presence of tenderness or nodules.

Prostate cancer is second most common form of cancer in males (American Cancer Society). Normal gland is rounded, smooth, firm, and heart shaped. Small groove divides gland into two lobes. Normal size varies from 2.5-4 cm (1-1.5 in).

7. Remove finger and test any stool present on glove for microscopic evidence of blood.

Guaiac test indicates presence of minute quantities of blood that may result from bleeding high up in gastrointestinal tract.

8. Assist client in washing perineal area.

Promotes client's comfort before continuation of examination.

9. Remove gloves and wash hands.

Reduces transmission of infection.

## Evaluation

1. Compare findings with normal assessment characteristics for genitalia and rectum.

Determines presence of abnormalities.

2. Evaluate client's level of anxiety after examination, noting tone of voice, facial expression, and behaviors.

Client's response to examination may require further discussion with nurse to relieve anxiety.

3. Have client perform testicular examination independently.

Demonstration is most effective way to evaluate learning of a skill.

### *Expected outcomes—genital examination*

1. Glans is pink and smooth with meatus at tip.

Normal findings.

2. There is small amount of white secretion between glans and foreskin.

Normal secretion; amount varies depending on level of hygiene.

3. Shaft is without swelling or lesions.

Normal findings.

4. Scrotum hangs freely with both testes descended.
5. Scrotal skin is loose and without lesions.
6. Testes are smooth, ovoid, and nontender.
7. Spermatic cord is palpable without tenderness.
8. No bulging or protrusion is observed or palpated in scrotal or inguinal area.
9. Lymph nodes are nonpalpable.
10. Client performs testicular examination correctly.

Demonstrates client's understanding.

### *Unexpected outcomes—genital examination*

1. There is purulent discharge from urethra with swelling along penile shaft.
2. Epididymis is very tender to palpation with swelling of scrotal sac.
3. Papular lesions or ulcers may be present on glans or shaft.
4. Inguinal lymph nodes are enlarged and tender to palpation.

Signs and symptoms indicative of sexually transmitted infection.

| Steps | Rationale |
|---|---|
| ***Potential nursing diagnoses*** | |
| ▪ Sexual dysfunction: related to genital infection.<br>▪ Knowledge deficit regarding preventive health care: related to misinformation.<br>▪ Pain: related to inflamed tissues.<br>▪ Anxiety: related to threat to sexuality. | Presence of infection and discomfort curtail client's sexual activities. Health education is vital. Client may fear loss of sexual function. |
| ***Unexpected outcomes—genital examination*** | |
| 1. Severe pain, tenderness, and swelling of scrotum.<br>2. Skin of scrotum feels warm to touch.<br>3. There may be discharge from urethra.<br>4. Lymph nodes may become enlarged. | Symptoms reveal infection of epididymis or testis. |
| ***Potential nursing diagnoses*** | |
| ▪ Pain: related to tissue swelling. | |
| ▪ Sexual dysfunction: related to altered function. | Presence of infection impairs sexual function. |
| ▪ Anxiety: related to threat to sexuality. | |
| ***Expected outcomes—rectal examination*** | |
| 1. Anal area clear without lesions or irregularities.<br>2. Rectal walls smooth and without nodules.<br>3. No evidence of bleeding.<br>4. Prostate gland palpable, smooth, firm, of normal size. | Normal findings. |
| ***Unexpected outcomes—rectal examination*** | |
| 1. Anal area tender with hemorrhoids visible.<br>2. There may be visible oozing of bloody drainage. | Symptomatic of external hemorrhoids. |
| ***Potential nursing diagnoses*** | |
| ▪ Constipation: related to pain during defecation.<br>▪ Pain: related to inflamed tissues. | Client avoids defecation due to discomfort. |
| ***Unexpected outcomes*** | |
| 1. Lesion or irregularity in mucosa palpated along rectal wall or prostate gland may be enlarged with presence of hard nodule.<br>2. Client often has difficulty starting urinary stream. | Symptoms may indicate rectal or prostatic tumor. |
| ***Potential nursing diagnoses*** | |
| Further diagnostic testing is necessary. Nursing diagnoses may include: | |
| ▪ Fear: related to unknown diagnosis.<br>▪ Anxiety: related to unknown diagnosis. | Client will be apprehensive about findings. |

## Recording and Reporting

| Steps | Rationale |
|---|---|
| 1. Describe all assessment findings in nurses' notes and note client's reaction to examination. | Documents baseline data and any change in client's condition. |
| 2. Report abnormalities to charge nurse or physician. | May indicate further diagnosis or treatment. |

## Special Considerations

- In infants do not try to retract foreskin until child is several months of age. Skin is usually too tight.
- Phimosis is condition in which foreskin cannot be retracted. May interfere with hygiene. Also increases risk of cancer.
- Cancerous lesions of penis may first appear as small bump or wart. Nonhealing ulcer may also be first sign. Phimosis occurs in large percentage of penile cancer.
- Herpes lesions begin as single or multiple reddish papules that eventually become clear, fluid-filled vesicles. Later large ulcers form.

## Teaching Considerations

- If male adolescent has erection during examination, assure him that it is normal involuntary response to touch.
- Whether male infants are circumcised or not mothers should learn how to clean glans and manipulate foreskin correctly.
- Instruct client to routinely examine testicles. A majority of testicular cancers are found by the client or his sexual partner.
- All males 15 yr and older should perform testicular self-examination monthly. If a lump is found, a physician should be notified.

- Counsel clients with sexually transmitted diseases about diagnosis and treatment. Teach preventive measures (e.g., use condoms, restrict number of sexual partners, avoid sex with persons who have several other partners, and use perineal hygiene).
- Tell clients with sexually transmitted disease that they must inform sexual partners of the need for an examination.
- Discuss the American Cancer Society's guidelines for early detection of colorectal cancer:
  1. Digital rectal examination performed yearly after age 40.
  2. Stool blood slide test (guaiac test) performed yearly after age 50.
  3. Proctosigmoidoscopy, involving visual inspection of the rectum and lower colon with a hollow, lighted tube. The test, performed by a physician, should be performed every 3-5 years after age 50, after two annual examinations with negative results.
- Discuss dietary planning to reduce fat and increase fiber content.
- Warn clients against problems caused by overuse of laxatives, cathartic medications, codeine, or enemas.

# SKILL 13-16 Assessing the Musculoskeletal System

The nurse's assessment of the musculoskeletal system includes a general inspection of gait, posture, and body position, as well as a more thorough assessment of major bone, joint, and muscle groups. Much of the assessment can be performed while the nurse examines other body systems; for example, while assessing neck structures, the nurse can also assess neck range of motion (ROM). It is easy for the nurse to integrate musculoskeletal assessment into routine activities of care, for example, while bathing or positioning clients.

Information from the assessment can be valuable in determining a client's ability to perform activities of daily living or to tolerate exercise. The client's condition often may require use of assistive devices to maintain mobility and self-care function. Because musculoskeletal disorders are frequently manifestations of neurologic disease, a complete neurologic assessment should follow.

## Purposes

1. Determine condition of bones, joints, and muscles.
2. Assess client's mobility.
3. Determine client's ability to perform self-care activities.
4. Determine potential for neurologic alterations.

## Procedure 13-16

| Steps | Rationale |
|---|---|
| **Assessment** | |
| 1. Ask client to describe history of alteration in bone, muscle, or joint function, e.g., recent fall, trauma, lifting heavy objects, history of bone or joint disease with sudden or gradual onset, and location of alteration. | Assists in assessing nature of musculoskeletal problem. |
| 2. Assess nature and extent of client's pain (Chapter 5): location, duration, severity, predisposing and aggravating factors, relieving factors, type of pain. | Alterations in bone, joints, or muscle are frequently accompanied by pain, which has implications not only for comfort but also ability to perform activities of daily living (ADL). |
| 3. Determine how client's alteration influences ability to perform: | Level of nursing care will be determined by extent to which client is able to perform self-care. |
| a. ADL, e.g., bathing, feeding, dressing, toileting, ambulation. | |
| b. Household chores, work, social functions, e.g., recreation, sexual activities. | Type and degree of restriction in continuing social activities influences topics for client education and ability of nurse to identify alternative ways to maintain function. |
| **Planning** | |
| 1. Develop individualized goals for assessment, including: | |
| a. Minimize client's discomfort. | Many disorders of musculoskeletal structures can be painful. Nurse should not aggravate pain during examination maneuvers. |
| b. Determine presence of abnormalities. | Dictates type of nursing care required. |

| Steps | Rationale |
|---|---|
| c. Promote client's mobility. | While discussing findings, nurse often can offer suggestions for alternative ways to maintain mobility. |
| d. Encourage ROM exercises | Assessment provides excellent means for exercising client's joints and muscles. |
| 2. Prepare following equipment: | |
| a. Goniometer | Measures degree of motion in a joint. |
| b. Tape measure | Measures muscle size. |
| 3. Prepare client: | |
| a. Integrate musculoskeletal assessment during other portions of physical assessment or during nursing care. | As in case of assessment of integument, nurse can conduct assessment of musculoskeletal system as client moves in bed, rises from chair, walks, or goes through movements required during complete physical examination. Integration saves time for both nurse and client. |
| b. Plan time for short rest periods during assessment. | Movement of body parts and various maneuvers may fatigue client. |
| c. Instruct client on proper position for each portion of assessment, i.e., sitting, supine, prone, or standing. | Muscles and joints should be exposed and free to move to allow for accurate measurement. Each joint or muscle group may require different position for measurement. |
| d. Explain steps of procedures. | Elicits client's cooperation. |

## Implementation

| Steps | Rationale |
|---|---|
| 1. Inspect gait as client walks into examination room and stands. Observe for foot dragging, shuffling or limping, balance, presence of obvious deformity in lower extremities. | Gait is more natural if client is unaware of nurse's observation. Nature of gait may indicate type of alteration. Ambulation can accentuate presence of deformity. |
| 2. Stand behind client and observe postural alignment—position of hips relative to shoulders. Look sideways at cervical, thoracic, and lumbar curves (Fig. 13-70). | Postural changes may indicate muscular, bone, or joint deformity, pain, or muscular fatigue. Normal posture is an upright stance. Hips and shoulders should align in parallel. Head should be held erect. Abnormal curves of posture (Fig. 13-71) include lordosis (swayback, increased lumbar curvature), kyphosis (hunchback, exaggerated posterior curvature of thoracic spine), and scoliosis (lateral spinal curvature). Elderly may develop a degree of kyphosis because of osteoporosis. |
| 3. Ask client to walk in straight line and return to original standing position. | More formal assessment of gait and balance. |
| 4. Assist client in putting each joint through its full ROM (Table 13-11). Observe equality of motion in same body parts: | Detects presence of deformities, reduced mobility or fixation of joints. Assessment of client's normal ROM provides baseline for assessing later changes after surgery or inactivity. |
| a. Active motion: client needs no support or assistance and is able to move joint independently. | |
| b. Passive motion: nurse supports extremity and moves joints through full ROM. | |

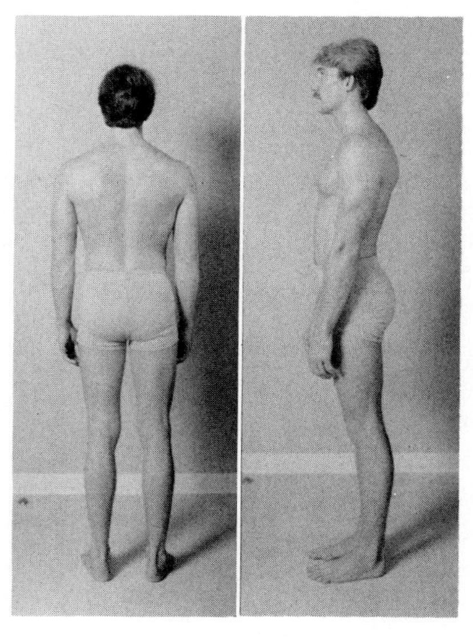

*Fig. 13-70*

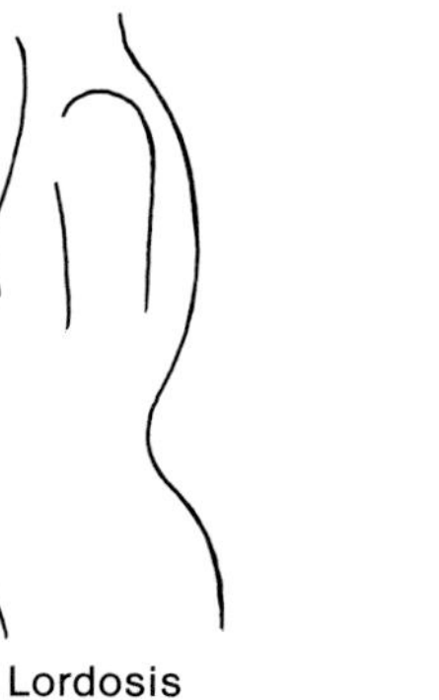


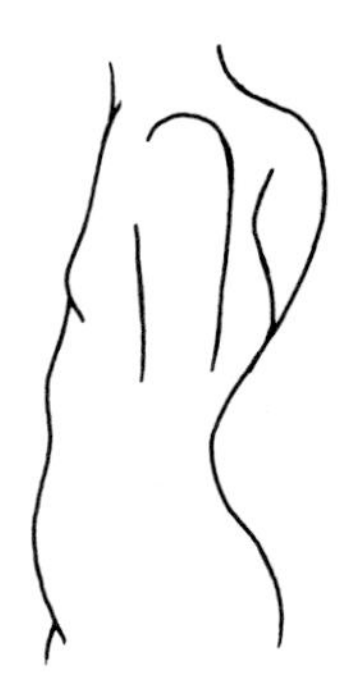


*Fig. 13-71*

**TABLE 13-11** Normal Range of Motion

| Body Part | Motion | Measurement |
|---|---|---|
| **Jaw** | Open and close jaw<br>Move jaw side to side<br>Move jaw forward | Able to insert three fingers<br>Bottom side teeth overlapping top side teeth<br>Top teeth behind lower teeth |
| **Neck** | Touch chin to sternum<br>Extend neck with chin pointing toward ceiling<br>Bend neck laterally, ear toward shoulder<br>Rotate neck with ear toward chest | Flexion 70°-90°<br>Hyperextension 55°<br>Lateral bending 35°<br>Rotation 70° to left and right |
| **Spine** | Bend forward at the waist<br>Bend backward<br>Bend to each side | Flexion 75°<br>Extension 30°<br>Lateral bending 35° |
| **Shoulder** | Abduct arm straight up<br>Adduct arm toward midline of trunk<br>Abduct arm straight horizontally to floor; bring arm backward toward spine and forward across chest<br>Flex or elevate forward with arm straight<br>Extend backward with arm straight | Abduction 180°<br>Adduction 45°<br>Horizontal extension 45°<br>Horizontal flexion 130°<br>Flexion 180°<br>Extension 60° |
| **Elbow** | Extend lower arm to normal extreme<br>Flex lower arm towards biceps<br>Hyperextend arm beyond normal resting point<br>Supinate lower arm<br>Pronate lower arm | Extension 150°<br>Flexion 150°<br>Hyperextension up to 10°<br>Supination 90°<br>Pronation 90° |
| **Wrist** | Flex wrist toward lower arm<br>Extend wrist backward<br>Deviate wrist laterally toward radius<br>Deviate wrist laterally toward ulna | Flexion 80°-90°<br>Extension 70°<br>Radial deviation 20°<br>Ulnar deviation 30°-50° |
| **Fingers** | Flex fingers into fist and then extend them flat<br>Spread fingers apart<br>Cross fingers together<br>Oppose fingers: touch each fingertip with thumb | Flexion 80°-100° (varies with joint)<br>Extension up to 45°<br>Abduction 20° between fingers<br>Adduction (fingers will touch)<br>Includes abduction and flexion |
| **Hip** | Raise leg with knee straight<br>Raise leg with knee flexed<br>Lying prone, extend leg straight back<br>Abduct partially flexed leg outward<br>Adduct partially flexed leg inward<br>Flex knee and swing foot away from midline<br>Flex knee and swing foot toward midline | Flexion 90°<br>Flexion 110°-120°<br>Extension 30°<br>Abduction 45°-50°<br>Adduction 20°-30°<br>Internal rotation 35°-40°<br>External rotation 45° |
| **Knee** | Flex knee with calf touching thigh<br>Extend knee beyond normal point of extension<br>Rotate knee and lower leg toward midline | Flexion 130°<br>Hyperextension 15°<br>Internal rotation 10° |
| **Ankle** | Dorsiflex foot with toes pointing toward head<br>Plantar flex foot with toes pointing down<br>Turn foot away from midline<br>Turn foot toward midline | Dorsiflexion 20°<br>Plantar flexion 45°<br>Eversion 20°<br>Inversion 30° |
| **Toes** | Curl toes under foot<br>Raise toes to point upward<br>Spread toes apart | Flexion 35°-60° (varies with joints)<br>Extension up to 90° (varies with joints)<br>Varies |

| Steps | Rationale |
|---|---|

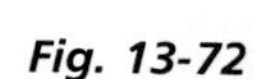
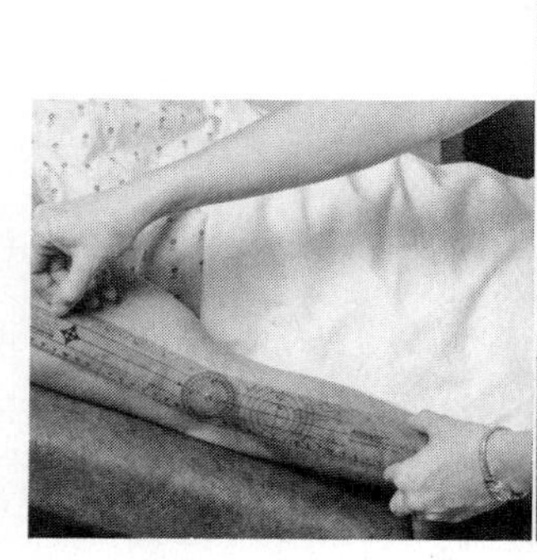
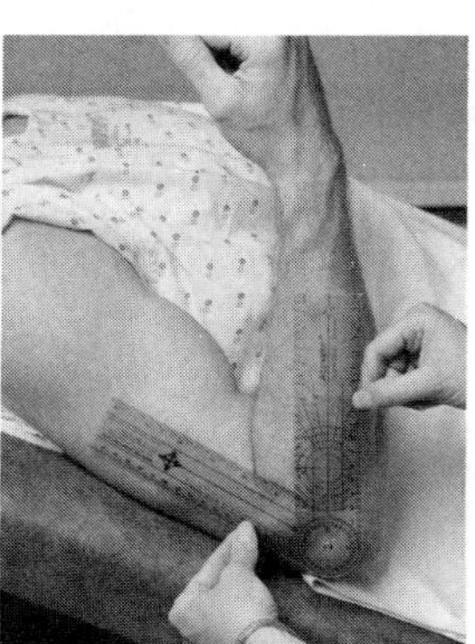

5. Measure precise degree of motion with goniometer: — Obtains precise measurement in clients with suspected reduction in ROM.
   a. Position center of protractor at center of joint being measured (Fig. 13-72).
   b. Extend each arm of goniometer along body parts extending from joint.
   c. Measure joint angle before moving joint.
   d. Take joint through its full ROM and measure angle again. — Determines degree of movement in each joint.
   e. Compare reading with normal degree of joint movement. — Determines abnormalities.
6. While measuring ROM note any instability of joint: — Crepitus is crunching or grating that occurs when joint is moved. It indicates pathologic condition of joint.
   a. Palpate for unusual movement of joint during its movement. — Signs of injury to supportive tissues.
   b. Palpate joint for swelling, tenderness, and heat and note any redness. — Signs of inflamed joint.
7. While assessing ROM ask client to allow extremity to relax or hang limp. Support extremity and move limb through ROM to detect muscular resistance. It may be helpful to palpate muscle mass being tested also. — Detects muscle tone in major muscle groups. Normal tone causes mild, even resistance to movement through entire ROM. If muscle has increased tone (hypertonicity), any sudden movement of joint is met with considerable resistance. Hypotonic muscle moves without resistance. Muscle feels flabby.
8. Be sure client is in stable position, one that will allow active contraction of muscle groups. Assess muscle strength by applying gradual increase in pressure to muscle group (i.e., attempting to extend client's elbow). Have client resist pressure applied by attempting to move against resistance (i.e., flex elbow). Have client maintain resistance until told to stop. Compare symmetric muscle groups. — Assesses strength of major muscle groups. Client's position should not be one that would easily cause a loss of balance or a fall.
9. If muscle weakness is identified, measure muscle size with tape measure placed around body of muscle. Compare with same muscle on opposite side of body. — Indicates degree of atrophy.

## Evaluation

1. Compare findings with normal assessment characteristics of musculoskeletal structures. — Determines presence of abnormalities.

### *Expected outcomes*

1. Gait is normal with arms swinging freely at side, balance good, posture erect with hips and shoulders aligned. — Normal findings.
2. Normal thoracic and lumbar curves present.
3. Full active ROM present in all joints with good muscle tone.
4. No deformities or crepitus.
5. Muscle groups strong, without atrophy.

### *Unexpected outcomes*

1. Reduced ROM in one or more major joints, i.e., shoulder, elbow, wrist, fingers, knee, hip. — Signs and symptoms of muscle or joint alterations.

| Steps | Rationale |
|---|---|
| 2. Client may have pain during movement. | |
| 3. Joints may be unstable, stiff, painful, swollen, or with obvious deformity. | |
| ***Potential nursing diagnoses*** | |
| ▪ Self-care deficit: related to immobility. | With musculoskeletal defect client may not be able to perform routine activities. |
| ▪ Pain: related to muscle strain. | |
| ▪ Potential for injury: related to reduced mobility. | Nurse must maintain safe environment. |
| ***Unexpected outcomes*** | |
| 1. Client demonstrates weakness in one or more major muscle groups or gait demonstrates poor balance with shuffling or stumbling of feet. | Can be musculoskeletal or neurologic in origin. |
| ***Potential nursing diagnosis*** | |
| ▪ Potential for injury: related to unsteady gait. | Nurse must maintain safe environment. |
| ***Unexpected outcomes*** | |
| 1. Postural abnormalities noted, i.e., lordosis, kyphosis, scoliosis. Reduced ROM in spine. | Alteration caused by congenital or traumatic conditions. |
| ***Potential nursing diagnoses*** | |
| ▪ Body image disturbance: related to postural abnormalities. | Alteration impairs client's appearance. |
| ▪ Alteration in breathing pattern: related to reduced chest wall movement. | Ventilatory movement is reduced. |
| **Recording and Reporting** | |
| 1. Record all findings in nurses' notes. | Documents baseline status and any change in client's condition. |
| 2. Report acute pain or sudden muscle weakness to nurse in charge or physician. | May be indicative of condition requiring immediate treatment. |

## Special Considerations

- Neurologic assessment is often conducted simultaneously because muscles may be weakened as result of nerve innervation loss.
- Normally a person walks with arms swinging freely at the sides, and head and face lead body.
- Never attempt to move joint when fracture is suspected. Clients weakened by illness will usually require passive motion assessment. With aging, ROM decreases in all joints because of reduction in muscle fiber size and tightening of joints.
- Clients who have been immobilized for several days, or those who have bone or joint disease, surgical correction of joint or bone, or pain, are at risk for reduced ROM. Joint that cannot be moved beyond a certain point within its range has a contracture.
- Upper and lower extremity on client's dominant side is normally stronger than nondominant side.
- Pain rather than weakness may cause reduced muscle strength. Likewise, long-term pain can lead to muscle weakening.

## Teaching Considerations

- Instruct client about correct postural alignment. Consult with physical therapist to provide client with exercises for improving posture.
- To reduce bone demineralization, instruct elderly client on a proper exercise program (e.g., walking) to be followed three or more times a week. Also encourage intake of calcium to meet recommended daily allowance. Increased vitamin D will aid calcium absorption.
- Instruct on use of assistive devices (e.g., zippers on clothing instead of buttons and elevation of chairs to minimize bending of knees and hips) when client is unable to perform activities of daily living.
- Instruct elderly to pace activities to compensate for loss in muscle strength.

# *SKILL 13-17 Assessing the Neurologic System*

Numerous factors have potential for influencing a client's neurologic status. Medications, fatigue, metabolic disturbances, and alterations in oxygenation are just a few examples. The neurologic system is responsible for many functions such as the initiation of movement, maintenance of coordination, and the reception of sensory impulses. Thus an assessment of neurologic function can be quite complex depending on a client's condition, and signs and symptoms.

An efficient nurse can integrate neurologic measurements with other parts of the physical examination. Cranial nerve function can be assessed in part during examination of the eyes. The nurse might measure coordination while assessing musculoskeletal function.

The nurse often decides how extensive the assessment should be. A client's level of consciousness influences the ability to follow directions and participate in a complete examination. If a client is physically disabled it becomes necessary to defer assessment of motor function. A client's chief complaint often determines whether a neurologic assessment is necessary. If a client has a headache, a neurologic assessment is important. However, if the client has nausea and vomiting, the neurologic review is not as critical.

## Purposes

1. Assess client's orientation to the environment.
2. Determine client's ability to make judgments or decisions.
3. Assess condition of motor and sensory nerve pathways.
4. Determine client's ability to ambulate safely.

## *Procedure 13-17*

| Steps | Rationale |
|---|---|
| **Assessment** | |
| 1. Determine if client is taking analgesics, sedatives, hypnotics, anti-psychotics, antidepressants, or nervous system stimulants as medication. | Forms of drugs that can alter level of consciousness or cause behavioral changes. |
| 2. Screen client for presence of the following symptoms: headache, seizures, dizziness, vertigo, numbness or tingling of body part, visual changes, weakness, and pain. | Symptoms that frequently originate from alterations in central nervous system or peripheral nervous system function. Identification of specific patterns of these symptoms may aid in diagnosis of pathologic condition. |
| 3. Discuss with spouse, family members, or friends any recent changes in client's behavior, e.g., increased irritability, mood swings, or memory loss. | Behavioral changes may result from intracranial pathologic states. |
| 4. Assess client for history of visual, hearing, olfactory, taste, or tactile changes. | Major sensory nerves originate from the brainstem. These symptoms may help to localize nature of the problem. |
| **Planning** | |
| 1. Develop individualized goals for assessment, including: | |
| a. Maintain client's safety. | Clients confused or who have poor coordination must be protected from injury. |
| b. Promote client's orientation. | Nurse's explanations and instructions can help promote client's orientation. |
| c. Determine presence of abnormalities. | Dictates level of nursing care required. |
| 2. Prepare needed equipment and supplies: | |
| a. Cotton applicator | Assesses client's sensation to light touch. |
| b. Safety pin | Assesses client's sensation to pain. |
| c. Vial containing hot or cold water | Assesses temperature sensation. |
| d. Reflex hammer | Assesses reflexes. |
| e. Vials containing coffee or vanilla extract | Assesses olfactory cranial nerve. |
| f. Sugar and salt | |
| g. Tongue blade | |
| h. Penlight | |
| i. Snellen chart | |
| j. Tuning fork | Measures vibrating sense. |
| 3. Prepare client: | |
| a. Explain procedure to client. | Minimizes client's anxiety. |

| Steps | Rationale |
|---|---|
| b. Integrate portions of neurologic assessment with other part of examination, i.e., cranial nerve function with survey of head and neck, mental and emotional status during nursing history, and reflexes while assessing musculoskeletal system. | Integration saves time and prevents client's fatigue. |
| c. Client may sit, lie, or stand depending on portion of assessment. | Sitting or lying provides position of comfort during mental and emotional assessment. Cranial nerve, cerebellar, sensory, and reflex function are assessed with client sitting. Nurse assesses balance with client standing. |
| d. Screen neurologic function when client presents no major symptomatology or has no recent history of head or spinal cord injury or disease. (Nurse assesses level of consciousness, orientation, pupillary reflexes, movement of extremities, and sensations). | Eliminates need for complete neurologic examination that can be time consuming. |

## Implementation

### *Mental and emotional status*

| Steps | Rationale |
|---|---|
| 1. Assess client's level of consciousness by directing questions and giving instructions that require response. Be sure client is as fully awake as possible before testing alertness. Note appropriateness of emotions, responses, and ideas expressed. To avoid confusion in the assessment of level of consciousness, the Glasgow Coma Scale (GCS) uses an objective numeric scale to measure consciousness (Table 13-12). | Alteration in mental status may reflect disturbances in cerebral functioning resulting from brain disorders, drug effects, or electrolyte and metabolic changes. Nurse can assess client's optimal level of alertness only by being assured client is fully responsive before testing. |
| 2. Rephrase or ask similar question if it is uncertain whether client understands. | Client's inappropriate response may be caused by a communication or language problem rather than deterioration of mental status. |
| 3. If client's responses are inappropriate, ask questions related to person, place, and time, e.g., "Tell me your name." "Tell me who I am." "What is the name of this place?" "Tell me where you live?" "What day is this?" "What month is this?" | Measures client's orientation to person, place, and time within environment. |
| 4. If client is unable to respond to questions of orientation, offer simple commands, e.g., "Squeeze my fingers" or "Move your toes." | Levels of consciousness exist along a continuum: from fully alert and responsive, to inability to consciously initiate meaningful behaviors, to unresponsiveness to external stimuli. |
| 5. When client fails to respond to verbal command, test response to painful stimuli: | The more reduced level of consciousness the greater the impairment of cerebral function. |
| a. Apply firm pressure with thumb on client's sternum or root of fingernail. | |
| b. Avoid pinching skin to elicit response. | Causes bruising and disfigurement. |

***TABLE 13-12*** Glasgow Coma Scale

| Action | Response | Score |
|---|---|---|
| Eyes open | Spontaneously | (4) |
| | To speech | 3 |
| | To pain | 2 |
| | None | 1 |
| Best verbal response | Oriented | (5) |
| | Confused | 4 |
| | Inappropriate words | 3 |
| | Incomprehensible sounds | 2 |
| | None | 1 |
| Best motor response | Obeys commands | (6) |
| | Localized pain | 5 |
| | Flexion withdrawal | 4 |
| | Abnormal flexion | 3 |
| | Abnormal extension | 2 |
| | Flaccid | 1 |
| | Total Score | (15) |

| Steps | Rationale |
|---|---|
| ***Behavior and appearance*** | |
| 1. During general survey and throughout assessment, observe client's mannerisms and actions. Note if client responds appropriately to directions and what type of mood client displays. Does client participate cooperatively with examination? | Client's mood or behavioral responses may be indicative of specific disease process. Client normally is anxious or concerned about findings during physical examination. Euphoria or lack of concern is inappropriate in presence of threatening events. |
| 2. Observe manner of client's speech. | Tone and pitch of voice and speed of spoken word may help to further reveal client's mood and behavioral status. |
| 3. Observe client's appearance: personal hygiene, cleanliness, fit and state of repair of clothes, choice of clothing and appropriateness to setting and type of weather, use and appropriateness of makeup. | Appearance can reflect client's self-image. Deterioration in one's appearance may result from poor self-image or inability to attend to process of grooming. |
| ***Intellectual function*** | |
| 1. Test memory of past events by asking client to recall previous medical history, family history, birthday, or anniversary. If seen on a previous day, ask if client remembers conversation that took place. | Type and extent of memory loss can indicate nature of brain disorder. |
| 2. Ask client to repeat series of numbers, i.e., "Repeat these numbers after me: 7, 4, 1, 8, 6" or "Repeat the following set of numbers backwards: 6, 1, 4, 3." | Tests immediate recall. |
| 3. Ask client to recall instructions given earlier during assessment or relate what physician explained previously. | Recent memory measures ability of person to remember events occurring on same day. |
| 4. Ask what client knows about illness or reason for hospitalization. Ask about knowledge of current events. | Assesses client's knowledge level, which determines ability to learn and understand. |
| 5. Have client explain meaning of simple proverb, e.g., "A stitch in time saves nine" or "Don't count your chickens before they're hatched." Note if explanations are literal or abstract. | Determine client's ability to interpret abstract ideas or concepts. Higher level of intellectual functioning is needed for abstract thinking. Client with altered mentation interprets phrase literally or merely rephrases words. |
| 6. Ask client to identify similarities or associations between terms or simple concepts, e.g., "A dog is to a beagle as a cat is to a ______." or "What do a tree and a rose have in common?" | Association is a higher intellectual function. |
| ***Cranial nerve function*** | |
| 1. Assess function of each of the 12 cranial nerves (Table 13-13). | Detects presence of motor and sensory impairment of nerves whose pathways extend from various intracranial sites. |
| ***Sensory function*** | |
| 1. Assess client's sensation to: pain, temperature, light touch, vibration, position, and two-point discrimination (Table 13-14). | Indicates presence of lesion or alteration along sensory pathways from periphery through spinal cord to brain. Each type of sensation follows different nerve pathway. |
| 2. Perform all sensory testing with client's eyes closed. | Client should not be able to see when or where stimulus strikes skin. |
| 3. Apply sensory stimuli in random, unpredictable order. Note anatomic area where sensation is reduced. | Maintains client's attention. Orderly sequence of stimulation makes it easy for client to outguess examiner and anticipate where stimulus is, even though client's sensation may be reduced. |
| 4. Compare symmetric areas of body while applying stimuli to face, arms, legs, and trunk. | Sensations along body's surface are felt equally on both sides. |
| 5. Ask client to say when particular stimulus is perceived. | Validates actual perception of sensation. Altered area of sensation allows examiner to pinpoint sensory nerve or affected spinal cord segment. |
| ***Motor function*** | |
| 1. Assess gait, stance, muscle strength and tone following procedures described in musculoskeletal assessment (Skill 13-16). | Changes in gait may be characteristic of specific neurologic disease. Assessment of muscle strength can reveal presence of partial or complete motor paralysis. Extent of muscle involvement indicates whether lesion involves peripheral motor nerves, spinal cord, or cerebral cortex. |
| 2. Ask client to assume sitting position. Demonstrate for client method for rapidly striking thigh with palm of hand, evenly, without hesitation. Then have client repeat maneuver. Note smoothness of movement. | Assesses client's coordination of upper extremity in performing rapid, rhythmic movement. Demonstration is easiest method for explaining how to perform rapidly alternating movements. |

**TABLE 13-13** Cranial Nerve Function and Assessment

| Nerve | | | | |
|---|---|---|---|---|
| **Number** | **Name** | **Function** | **Function** | **Method of Assessment** |
| I | Olfactory | Sensory | Sense of smell | Ask client to identify different nonirritating aromas such as coffee, vanilla |
| II | Optic | Sensory | Vision | Use Snellen chart; ask client to read printed material |
| III | Oculomotor | Motor | Extraocular eye movement | Assess directions of gaze |
| | | | Pupil constriction and dilation | Measure pupil reaction to light reflex. |
| IV | Trochlear | Motor | Upward and downward movement of eyeball | Assess directions of gaze |
| V | Trigeminal | Sensory and motor | Sensory nerve to skin of face | Assess corneal reflex; measure sensation of light, pain, and touch across skin of face |
| | | | Motor nerve to muscles of jaw | Assess client's ability to clench teeth |
| VI | Abducens | Motor | Lateral movement of eyeballs | Assess directions of gaze |
| VII | Facial | Sensory and motor | Facial expression | Ask client to smile, frown, puff out cheeks, raise and lower eyebrows |
| | | | Taste | Have client identify salty or sweet tastes on front of tongue |
| VIII | Auditory | Sensory | Hearing | Assess client's ability to hear spoken word |
| IX | Glossopharyngeal | Sensory and motor | Taste | Ask client to identify sour, salty, or sweet taste on back of tongue |
| | | | Ability to swallow | Use tongue blade to elicit gag reflex |
| | | | Movement of tongue | Ask client to move tongue |
| X | Vagus | Sensory and motor | Sensation of pharynx | Ask client to say "ah"; observe movement of palate and pharynx |
| | | | Ability to swallow | Use tongue blade to elicit gag reflex |
| | | | Movement of vocal cords | Assess client's speech for hoarseness |
| XI | Spinal accessory | Motor | Movement of head and shoulders | Ask client to shrug shoulders and turn head against examiner's passive resistance |
| XII | Hypoglossal | Motor | Position of tongue | Ask client to stick out tongue to midline |

***TABLE 13-14*** Assessment of Sensory Nerve Function

| Sensory Function | Equipment | Method | Precautions |
|---|---|---|---|
| **Pain** | Safety pin. | Ask client to tell you when dull or sharp sensation is felt. Alternately apply pointed and blunt ends of pin to skin's surface. Note areas of numbness or increased sensitivity. | Areas where skin is thickened, such as heel or sole of foot, may be less sensitive to pain. |
| **Temperature** | Two test tubes, one filled with hot water, other with cold. | Touch client's skin with tube. Ask client to identify hot vs cold sensation. | May omit test if pain sensation is normal. |
| **Light touch** | Cotton ball or cotton-tip applicator. | Apply light wisp of cotton to different points along skin surface. Ask client to tell you when sensation is felt. | Apply along areas where client's skin is thin or more sensitive, i.e., face, neck, inner aspect arms, or top of feet and hands. |
| **Vibration** | Tuning fork. | Apply vibrating fork to distal interphalangeal joint of fingers and interphalangeal joint of great toe. | Be sure client feels vibration and not merely pressure. Have client tell you when vibration stops. |
| **Position** | | Grasp client's finger, holding it by its sides with your thumb and index finger. Alternate moving finger up and down. Ask client to tell you whether finger is up or down. Repeat procedure with toes. | Avoid rubbing adjacent appendages as finger or toe is moved. |
| **Two-point discrimination** | Two safety pins. | Lightly apply points of two safety pins simultaneously to skin's surface. Ask if client feels one or two pinpricks. | Apply pins to same anatomic site by fingertips, palm of hand, or upper arms. Minimal distance at which client can discriminate two points varies (normally 2 or 3 mm on fingertips). |

| Steps | Rationale |
|---|---|
| 3. Demonstrate and have client alternately strike thigh with hand supinated and then pronated. Note speed and symmetry of movement. | Ability to perform skilled motor act will be disturbed by cerebellar dysfunction. |
| 4. Stand in front of client, holding index finger 2 ft stationary in front of client's face. Ask client to touch your finger with the index finger and then to touch nose alternately. Client moves finger back and forth repeatedly. Observe for tremor of hand or awkward movement. | Further assesses upper extremity coordination. |
| 5. Have client assume supine position. Place hand at ball of client's foot. Ask client to tap your hand with foot as quickly as possible. Note speed and smoothness of movement. | Assesses lower extremity coordination. |

**TABLE 13-15** Assessment of Common Reflexes

| Type | Procedure | Normal Reflex |
|---|---|---|
| **Deep tendon reflexes** | | |
| Biceps | Flex client's arm at the elbow with palms down. Place your thumb in the antecubical foxxa at base of the biceps tendon. Strike thumb with the reflex hammer. | Flexion of arm at elbow. |
| Triceps | Flex client's elbow, holding arm across the chest, or hold upper arm horizontally and allow lower arm to go limp. Strike the triceps tendon just above the elbow. | Extension at elbow. |
| Patellar | Have client sit with legs hanging freely over side of the bed or chair or have client lie supine and support the knee in a flexed position. Briskly tap the patellar tendon just below the patella. | Extension of lower leg at knee. |
| Plantar | Have client lie supine with legs straight and feet relaxed. Take handle end of the reflex hammer and stroke the lateral aspect of the sole from the heel to the ball of the foot, curving across the ball. | Flexion of toes. |
| **Cutaneous reflexes** | | |
| Gluteal | Have client assume a side-lying position. Spread apart client's buttocks and lightly stimulate perineal area with a cotton applicator. | Contraction of anal sphincter. |
| Abdominal | Have client stand or lie supine. Stroke abdominal skin with the base of a cotton applicator over the lateral borders of the rectus abdominis muscles toward midline. Repeat test in each abdominal quadrant. | Contraction of rectus abdominis muscles with pulling of umbilicus toward stimulated side. |

| Steps | Rationale |
|---|---|
| 6. Ask client to sit with eyes closed and place heel of one foot just below knee of opposite leg. Then instruct client to slide heel down shin toward foot. | Presence of involuntary movements or difficulty in controlling heel may indicate cerebellar problem. Normally maneuver is performed evenly without heel sliding off leg. |
| 7. Have client stand with feet close together and eyes open. Then have client close eyes. Note presence of swaying. | Romberg test assesses balance. Clients with proprioception problems have difficulty keeping balance with eyes closed. Cerebellar disease causes imbalance even with eyes open. |
| ***Reflexes*** | |
| 1. Assess deep tendon reflexes (Table 13-15). Reflexes should be symmetric on both sides of body. Reflexes are graded on scale:<br>0 No response.<br>1+ Low normal or diminished.<br>2+ Normal.<br>3+ Brisker than normal but may not indicate disease.<br>4+ Hyperactive, very brisk. Spinal cord disorder suspected. Deep tendon reflexes (DTRs) are still brisk in healthy aged. | Assesses integrity of sensory and motor pathways along reflex arc for specific spinal cord segments. |
| a. Ask client to relax extremity to be tested. | Relaxation of extremity prevents voluntary movement or muscle tensing that interferes with reflex response. |
| b. Position limb to slightly stretch muscle being tested. | Improves ability to initiate reflex. |
| c. Hold reflex hammer loosely between thumb and fingers. | Reflex hammer should swing freely to tap tendon briskly to elicit clean response. |
| d. Tap tendon briskly (Fig. 13-73). | |
| e. Compare symmetry of reflex from one side of body to the other. | Asymmetry of reflex response indicates alteration in reflex pathway. |

## Evaluation

| | |
|---|---|
| 1. Compare findings with normal assessment characteristics. | Determines presence of abnormalities. |

**Steps** **Rationale**

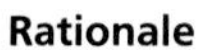

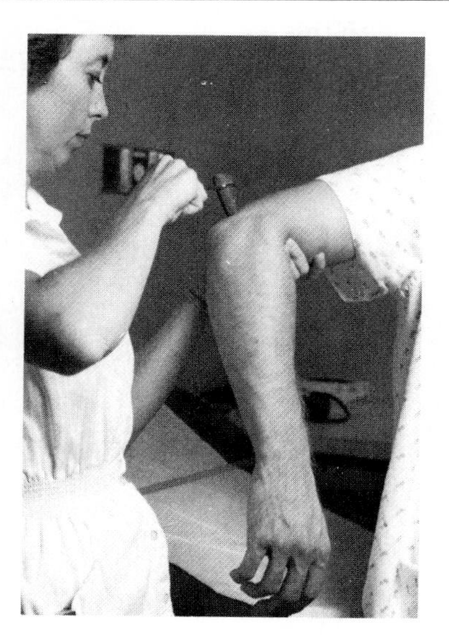

*Fig. 13-73*

### *Expected outcomes*

1. Client is alert, oriented, and responds appropriately to all questions.

   Alert to surroundings.
2. Appearance is well kept.
3. Demonstrates immediate recall of recent and past events.

   Memory intact.
4. Able to interpret abstract ideas and make associations of related concepts.

   Thought processes are normal.
5. Sensation intact for pain, temperature, light touch, and position.

   Normal sensation.
6. Cranial nerves intact.
7. Gait even and balance steady.

   Normal coordination and brainstem function.
8. Muscle strength normal and symmetric.
9. Reflexes symmetric and 2+.

   Intact spinal cord pathways.

### *Unexpected outcomes*

1. Client is confused, at times difficult to arouse by verbal stimulus.

   Reveals alteration in consciousness and thought processes.
2. Not consistently oriented to person, place, or time.
3. Speech slow and slurred.
4. Able to recall past events but unable to repeat series of five numbers.
5. Unable to interpret proverbs or associate related concepts.
6. Sensory and motor function intact, except client slow to respond to instructions.

### *Potential nursing diagnoses*

Client's level of consciousness and disturbed mental function may be associated with any number of medical problems. Related nursing diagnoses might include:

- Potential for injury: related to poor coordination.
- Self-care deficit: related to impaired thought processes.
- Altered thought processes: related to reduced consciousness.

Client's safety is chief concern. Alterations impair ability to carry out normal activities.

### *Unexpected outcomes*

1. Client alert and oriented.
2. Has reduced sensation to temperature, touch, and painful stimuli.

   May be caused by peripheral nerve or spinal cord injury.

### *Potential nursing diagnoses*

- Potential for injury: related to reduced sensation.
- Potential for impaired skin integrity: related to reduced sensation.

Nurse must institute preventive care.

| Steps | Rationale |
|---|---|
| ***Unexpected outcomes*** | |
| 1. Client alert and oriented.<br>2. Gait demonstrates dragging of left leg.<br>3. Reduced muscle strength in left lower and upper extremities.<br>4. Sensation to light touch, pain, temperature, and position decreased on left side.<br>5. Cranial nerve test demonstrates drooping of facial muscles on left. | Medically client demonstrates symptoms of cerebrovascular accident (stroke). |
| ***Potential nursing diagnoses*** | |
| ▪ Potential for injury: related to impaired mobility and sensation.<br>▪ Impaired physical mobility: related to neurologic injury.<br>▪ Potential impaired skin integrity: related to immobility.<br>▪ Body image disturbance: related to paralysis or speech impairment. | Poses implications for extensive rehabilitation. |
| **Recording and Reporting** | |
| 1. Record all assessment findings in nurses' notes. | Documents baseline data and change in client's condition. |
| 2. Report abnormalities to nurse in charge or physician. | Further diagnosis or treatment may be required. |

### Special Considerations

- Clients mental and emotional function can easily be assessed as nurse poses questions and gives instructions throughout the examination.
- Fully conscious client responds to questions quickly and perceives events occurring around him. As consciousness deteriorates, client may demonstrate irritability, shortened attention span, reduced perception of environment, and unwillingness to cooperate.
- Comatose state is one in which client fails to respond to verbal and painful stimuli. Fever and pain commonly cause confusion, disorientation, and irritability, depending on severity.
- Unkept hair, dirty body, and broken, dirty fingernails are good indicators of grooming habits. Poorly fitting clothes may be a symptom of poverty rather than inappropriate apparel.
- To maintain client's safety from falling, stand by side during test. Normally client does not break stance. Slight swaying is normal in elderly client.
- Cerebellar disease causes wide-based, staggering gait. Parkinson's disease causes slow, shuffling gait but as client walks there is increased rapidity or propulsive nature to gait as though person is about to fall. Paraplegia is paralysis of lower extremities. Quadriplegia is paralysis of upper and lower extremities. Hemiplegia is paralysis of one half of body (arm and leg).

### Teaching Considerations

- Client's cultural and educational backgrounds influence ability to answer test questions. Do not ask questions related to concepts or ideas with which client is unfamiliar.
- Explain to family or friends the implications of any mental impairment shown by the client.
- If client has sensory or motor impairments, explain measures to ensure safety (e.g., use of ambulation aids or use of safety bars in bathrooms or stairways).
- Teach elderly clients to plan enough time to complete tasks because reaction time is slowed.
- Teach elderly clients to observe skin surfaces for areas of trauma because their perception of pain is reduced.

## COMPLETING THE EXAMINATION

After the nurse completes the assessment the client dresses and is given the opportunity to perform necessary hygiene measures. The hospitalized client may need help in returning to bed and a comfortable position. When the client is comfortable, the nurse shares a summary of the assessment findings. This is an excellent time to reinforce client teaching and to request feedback from the client to evaluate understanding of information shared.

If assessment findings reveal serious abnormalities, such as a mass or a highly irregular heart rate, the client's physician should be consulted to validate findings before specific results are revealed. Delay in discussing assessment findings can cause the client anxiety, especially if the client senses something is abnormal. The nurse must remain supportive without attempting to make a diagnosis. It is the physician's responsibility to make definitive medical diagnoses. The nurse can explain that she has found a "growth" or noted "an irregularity in the heart beat," which the physician will examine.

The nurse is responsible for cleaning the examination area. The examination table should be washed and a new paper sheet applied (if available). If the client's bedside was the site for the examination, the nurse clears away soiled items from the bedside table and makes sure bed linen is clean and dry. The nurse stores all reusable equipment, disposes of supplies and equipment that cannot be reused, and makes sure there is a sufficient stock of supplies for the next examination.

After completing the examination, the nurse finishes recording of the assessment. If making entries on the assessment form, the nurse was delayed, the nurse does so at this time to avoid forgetting important information. It is also important to use an institution's recommended abbreviations so that all health team members can understand the nurse's assessment findings. If entries were made periodically during the examination, they are reviewed for accuracy and thoroughness. Significant findings are communicated to appropriate medical and nursing personnel either verbally or in the client's written care plan.

## BIBLIOGRAPHY


American Cancer Society: 1989 Cancer facts and figures, New York, 1989, The Society.

American Cancer Society: Guidelines for the cancer-related checkup: recommendations and rationale, New York, 1980, The Society.

Assessing your patients, 1982 Nursing Photobook, Springhouse, Pa, 1982, Intermed Communications, Inc.

Bates B: A guide to physical examination, ed 4, Philadelphia, 1987, JB Lippincott Co.

Becker KL, Stevens SA: Performing in-depth abdominal assessment, Nursing 18(6):59, 1988.

Bergstrom L, et al.: A high risk registry to find congenital deafness, Otolaryngol Clin North Am 4:369, 1971.

Berliner H: Aging skin, I, Am J Nurs 86:1138, 1986.

Berliner H: Aging skin, II, Am J Nurs 86:1259, 1986.

Blair JD: A quick, high-yield mouth exam, Patient Care 19:33, Oct. 30, 1985.

Block G, et al.: Health assessment for professional nursing, New York, 1981, Appleton-Century- Crofts.

Bowers A, Thompson J: Clinical manual of health assessment, St. Louis, 1984, The C.V. Mosby Co.

Brown MC, Brown JD, Boyer MM: Changing nursing practice through continuing education in physical assessment: perceived barriers to implementation, J Contin Educ Nurs 18(4):111, 1987.

Bulau J: Clinical policies and procedures for home health care, Rockville, Md, 1986, Aspen Publishers, Inc.

Burger D: Breast self-examination, Am J Nurs 79:1088, 1979.

Burggraf V, Donlon B: Assessing the elderly, system by system, Am J Nurs 85:974, 1985.

Calvani D: Assessing the elderly, II, Am J Nurs 85:1103, 1985.

Casey MP: Testicular cancer: the worst disease at the worst time, RN 50:36, 1987.

Church JC, Baer KJ: Examination of the adolescent: a practical guide. J Pediatr Health Care. 1(2):65, 1987.

Corrigan JD: Functional health pattern assessment in the emergency department. J Emerg Nurs 12(3):163, 1986.

Dennison, R: Cardiopulmonary assessment, Nurs 86, 16:34, April 1986.

Ebersole P, Hess P: Toward healthy aging, ed 3, St. Louis, 1989, The CV Mosby Co.

Erickson BA: Detecting abnormal heart sounds, Nurs 86 16:58, 1986.

Forgacs P: The functional basis of pulmonary sounds, Chest 73:399, 1978.

Fraser MC, McGuire DB: Skin cancer's early warning system, Am J Nurs 84:1232, 1984.

Hays AM, Borger F: Assessing the elderly: a test in-time, Am J Nurs 85:1107, 1985.

Henderson ML: Assessing the elderly: altered perception, Am J Nurs 85:1104, 1985.

Hurst JW, et al.: Noises in the neck, N Engl J Med 302:862, 1980.

Jacobs R: Physical changes in the aged. In Devereaux M, et al., eds: Elder care: a guide to clinical geriatrics, New York, 1981, Grune & Stratton, Inc.

Jones D: Health assessment manual, New York, 1986, McGraw-Hill Book Co.

Larson E: Evaluating validity of screening tests, Nurs Res 35:186, 1986.

Mahboub E, Sayed GM: oral cavity and pharynx. In Schottenfeld D, Fraumeni JF Jr., eds: Cancer epidemiology and prevention, Philadelphia, 1982, WB Saunders Co.

Malkiewicz J: A pragmatic approach to musculoskeletal assessment, RN 45:56, 1982.

Merry JA: Take your assessment all the way down to the toes, RN 51(11):60, 1988.

Miracle VA: Anatomy of a murmur, Nurs 86 16:26, 1986.

Miracle VA: Get in touch and in tune with cardiac assessment Nursing 1988 18(4):41, 1988.

Norman S: The pupil check, Am J Nurs 82:588, 1982.

Phipps W, et al.: Medical-surgical nursing: concepts and clinical practice, ed 3, St. Louis, 1987, The CV Mosby Co.

Potter PA, Perry AG: Fundamentals of nursing: concepts, process and practice, ed 2, St. Louis, 1989, The CV Mosby Co.

Reynolds JI, Logsdon JB: Assessing your patients' mental status, Nurs 79 9:26, 1979.

Rossman I: Anatomy of aging. In Rossman I, ed: Clinical geriatrics, ed. 2, Philadelphia, 1979, JB Lippincott Co.

Rutledge DN: Factors related to women's practice of breast self-examination, Nurs Res 36:117, 1987.

Sana JM, Judge RD: Physical assessment skills for nursing practice, ed. 2, Boston, 1982, Little, Brown, & Co.

Schweiger JL, et al.: Oral assessment: how to do it, Am J Nurs 80:654, 1980.

Seidel HM, et al.: Mosby's guide to physical examination, St. Louis, 1987, the CV Mosby Co.

Silverberg E: Cancer statistics, 1984, New York, 1984, American Cancer Society.

Smith C: Abdominal assessment: a blending of science and art, Nurs 81 11:42, 1981.

Smith CE: With good assessment skills you can construct a solid framework for patient care, Nursing 14(12):26, 1984.

Stark J: Urinary tract assessment, Nursing '88, 18(7):57, 1988.

Stevens SA, Becker KL: How to perform picture-perfect respiratory assessment, Nursing 18(1):57, 1988.

Stevens S, Becker K: Neurologic Assessment, I, Nursing 88, 18(9):53, 1988.

Tanner JM: Growth of adolescence, ed. 2, Oxford, 1962, Blackwell Scientific Publications.

Tishknobf MK: Breast cancer, the treatment evolution, Am J Nurs 84:1110, 1984.

U.S. Department of Health and Human Services, Cancer Rates and Risks, ed 3, 1985, National Institute of Health.

Visich MA: Breath and heart sounds, Nurs 81 11:64, 1981.

Whaley LF, Wong DL: Nursing care of infants and children, ed 3, St. Louis, 1987, The CV Mosby Co.

Wilkins RL: Lung sounds, St. Louis, 1987, The CV Mosby Co.

Yacone LA: Cardiac assessment: what to do, how to do it, RN 50:42, May 1987.

# UNIT V
# OXYGENATION

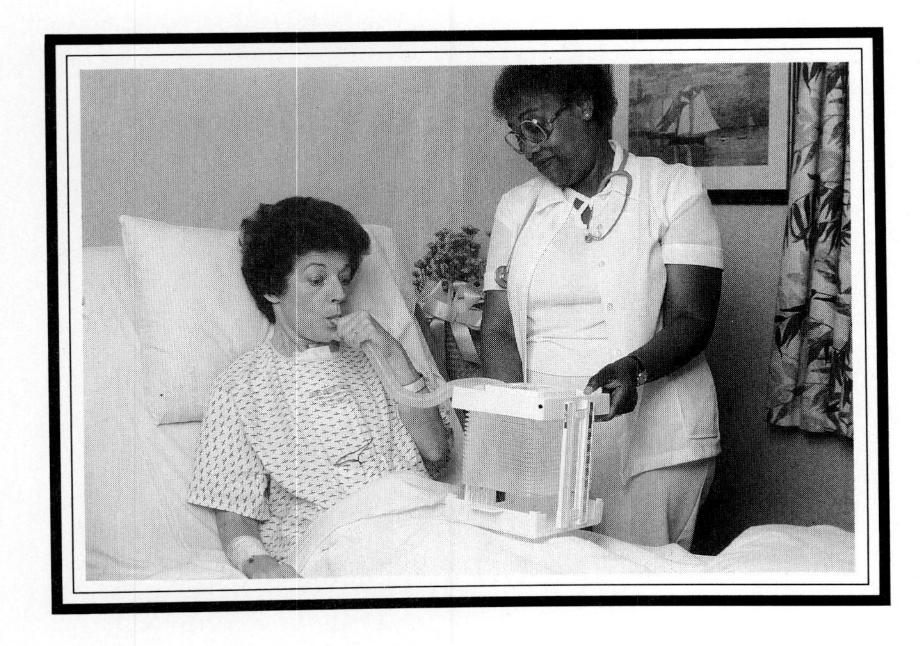

Oxygen is a basic human need and is required for life. Nurses frequently encounter clients who are unable to meet their oxygen needs. When oxygen needs remain unmet, hyperventilation, hypoventilation, or hypoxemia can result. Consequently, the client is unable to meet the oxygen demands of body organs and tissues, and, when severe, life-threatening situations and death occur.

The client's level of health, age, life-style, and environment affect the ability to meet tissue oxygen requirements. The nurse is responsible for assessing the client's ability to meet oxygen needs and determining when and which type of intervention are appropriate.

This unit explores nursing measures designed to improve oxygenation. Chapter 14, "Oxygen Therapy," teaches the student about various types of oxygen equipment currently used in clinical situations, as well as the advantages and disadvantages of each type of equipment. Chapter 15, "Chest Physiotherapy," describes techniques of postural drainage, percussion, vibration, and rib shaking and their impact on improving oxygenation. Chapter 16, "Airway Maintenance," presents specific invasive measures designed to maintain a patent natural or artificial airway. Chapter 17, "Emergency Measures for Life Support," presents essential skills necessary to restore optimal oxygenation in a life-threatening situation.

# 14
# OXYGEN THERAPY

## OBJECTIVES

*Mastery of content in this chapter will enable the nurse to:*

- Define key terms.
- Discuss indications for oxygen therapy.
- Discuss methods of oxygen therapy.
- Demonstrate the following skills on selected clients: applying nasal cannula, inserting nasal catheter, applying oxygen masks, administering oxygen therapy to a client with artificial airway, administering oxygen therapy to a pediatric client, using incentive spirometry, and using intermittent positive-pressure breathing (IPPB).
- Develop teaching plans for selected clients on use of home oxygen equipment.

## KEY TERMS

*Croupette*
*Hypoxemia*
*Hypoxia*
*Incentive spirometry*
*Intermittent positive-pressure breathing (IPPB)*
*Nasal cannula*
*Nasal catheter*
*Oxygen hood*
*Oxygen mask*
*Oxygen therapy*
*T-tube*
*Tracheostomy collar*

## SKILLS

**14-1** Applying a Nasal Cannula
**14-2** Inserting a Nasal Catheter
**14-3** Applying Oxygen Masks
**14-4** Administering Oxygen Therapy to a Client with an Artificial Airway
**14-5** Administering Oxygen Therapy to the Pediatric Client
**14-6** Using Incentive Spirometry
**14-7** Using Continuous Positive Airway Pressure
**14-8** Using Intermittent Positive-Pressure Breathing
**14-9** Using Home Oxygen Equipment
**14-10** Administering Mechanical Ventilation

Oxygen therapy is the administration of oxygen by any route to a client to prevent or relieve hypoxia. Hypoxia is a condition in which insufficient oxygen is available to meet the metabolic needs of tissues and cells. Hypoxia results from hypoxemia, which is a deficiency of oxygen in the arterial blood. For example, a client with pneumonia has decreased oxygen diffusion from the lungs to the arterial blood supply, and thus is hypoxic; oxygen is administered to reduce the hypoxia. Another client has chronic bronchitis, which is a chronic obstructive pulmonary disease (COPD). Blood oxygen levels remain within normal limits, except during sleep. The client is instructed to use oxygen at night to prevent hypoxia.

When hypoxia exists, the nursing assessment can reveal many findings, including change in blood pressure, cardiac arrhythmias, tachypnea, dyspnea, drowsiness, headaches, disorientation, nausea, and anxiety (Glover and Glover, 1978). Symptoms depend on client's age, level of health, and present disease process; and the presence of chronic illnesses. Another symptom of hypoxia is cyanosis, a bluish discoloration of the skin. Cyanosis is a late sign, and the nurse should never assume that because there is no cyanosis the client is not hypoxic.

The oxygen delivery system selected depends on the client's age, level of health, and orientation level; the presence of an artificial airway; and whether the setting is in the hospital or the home. An infant or young child may benefit from an oxygen tent as opposed to an oxygen mask, whereas an alert adult may prefer the mask. The influences of these variables are detailed in the special considerations section for each skill.

## OXYGEN SYSTEMS

Several oxygen systems presently are available in health care settings. Oxygen is delivered to a hospital or institutional setting through a bulk liquid oxygen system that is designed to store oxygen at −34° C (−29° F) and deliver it as a gas. Once the gas enters the hospital, it is

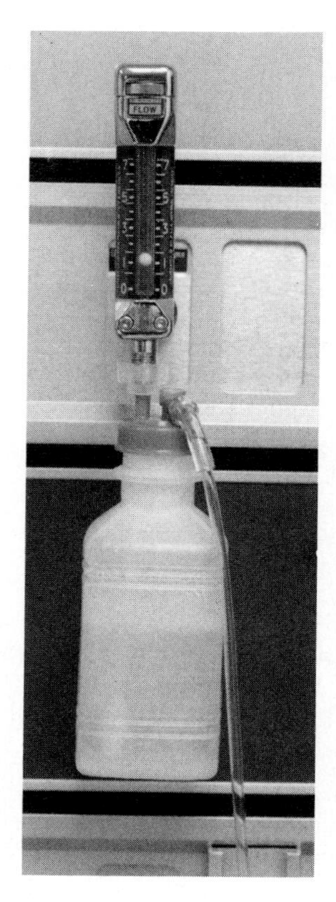

***Fig. 14-1*** Oxygen flowmeter.

controlled at a pressure of 50 psi (pounds per square inch) (Glover and Glover, 1978). Institutions using liquid oxygen systems have wall outlets in every client's room, and a flowmeter regulates the amount of oxygen delivered at any time (Fig. 14-1).

If a health care agency does not have a liquid oxygen system or only uses such a system in specified geographic areas of the agency, a gas cylinder may be substituted. Compressed oxygen in the gas cylinder usually exists as a nonliquified gas at 1800 to 2400 psi at 21° C (70° F). Oxygen cylinders used in hospitals are the "H" size and hold about 6600 L of oxygen (Glover and Glover, 1978). An oxygen regulator controls the amount of oxygen supplied from a cylinder.

Home oxygen systems usually include a portable oxygen system, which allows the client freedom to leave the home. Portable oxygen delivery systems use liquid oxygen and include an easy method for refill.

Skills presented in this chapter focus on respiratory therapies for improving the client's level of oxygenation. Some skills focus on administration of oxygen therapy. Other skills include those respiratory maneuvers designed to improve oxygenation by the promotion of lung expansion. Whatever nursing measures are utilized, the nurse bases care on specific assessment findings.

## GUIDELINES

1. Know client's normal range of vital signs. Hypoxia can affect the client's vital signs. Heart rate can become rapid and irregular because of the presence of cardiac arrhythmias. Initially blood pressure is elevated, but if hypoxemia remains uncorrected hypotension may develop. Respiratory rate and depth are elevated.
2. Know client's usual behavioral pattern. Hypoxia causes anxiety, apprehension, and inability to concentrate. As hypoxia worsens, the client's activity tolerance decreases, and friends and family may notice behavioral changes. Last, worsening of a hypoxic state results in a decreased level of consciousness.
3. Know client's medical history and present medications or therapies. This is of prime importance in the client with COPD. It is important that the nurse be aware of this disease because high inspired oxygen concentrations can result in severe side effects.
4. Be aware of environmental conditions that can affect the client's level of oxygenation or safety if oxygen therapy is administered. Clients with chronic respiratory diseases have difficulty maintaining optimal oxygen levels in polluted environments. Second, if a client is to receive home oxygen therapy, an environmental assessment is completed to determine hazards from smoke in the home, the use of gas stoves, or kerosene space heaters.
5. Assess for a temporary or permanent abnormal chest wall configuration. Temporary abnormalities that can affect oxygenation include obesity, pregnancy, and trauma. Congenital musculoskeletal abnormalities such as kyphosis affect oxygenation because of the decreased ability of the lungs to fully expand.
6. Document client's past or present smoking history. Smoking damages the ciliary clearance mechanism within the lungs and paralyzes the cilia. As a result, the cilia are unable to clear mucus from the airways; accumulation of mucus leads to the development of chronic bronchitis (Potter and Perry, 1989). Long-term chronic bronchitis ultimately results in hypoxia.
7. Know client's most recent hemoglobin values. Hemoglobin is the carrier of respiratory gases to and from the cells. Decreased hemoglobin levels decrease the ability of the body to transport oxygen to the cells and carbon dioxide away from the cells.
8. Know client's present and most recent arterial blood gas analysis. A state of acidemia can increase oxygen delivery to the tissue, whereas alkalemia has the opposite effect on the transfer of oxygen to the tissues.

Clients should be taught to regard oxygen as a medication. Increasing oxygen liter flow for shortness of breath is similar to doubling heart medication. It is important that the client receiving oxygen therapy understands proper use of the equipment. Safety measures for oxygen use are very important (see box). Oxygen will support combustion, however, it will not explode.

### PREREQUISITE KNOWLEDGE

1. Normal respiratory anatomy and physiology.
2. Factors affecting oxygenation and ventilation.
3. Pathophysiology of atelectasis, pneumonia, respiratory failure, and sleep apnea.
4. Effects of surgery or immobilization on oxygenation.

### PREREQUISITE SKILLS

1. Physical assessment (Chapter 13).
2. Proper handwashing techniques (Chapter 37).
3. Endotracheal or tracheostomy care (Chapter 18).
4. Endotracheal or tracheostomy tube care (Chapter 18).
5. Cough control exercises (Chapter 15).

### *OXYGEN SAFETY GUIDELINES*

- Keep oxygen delivery system 10 feet from any open flames.
- No smoking.
- If using cylinders, ensure that they will not fall over if stored upright.
- Do not adjust oxygen level without physician direction.
- Oxygen should be regarded as a medication.
- Oxygen will not explode, but it does support combustion.

# *SKILL 14-1* *Applying a Nasal Cannula*

A nasal cannula is a simple, comfortable device for delivering oxygen to a client. The two cannulas, about 1.5 cm (0.5 in) long, protrude from the center of a disposable tube and are inserted into the nostrils. Oxygen is delivered via the cannulas with a flow rate up to 5 to 6 L/min. Higher flow rates dry airway mucosa and do not increase inspired oxygen concentration ($FIO_2$) (Luce, Tyler, and Pierson, 1984). The nurse must know what flow rate produces a given percentage of $FIO_2$ (Table 14-1).

A nasal cannula is an effective mechanism for oxygen delivery. It allows the client to breathe through the mouth or nose, is available for all age groups, and is adequate for short-term or long-term use. Cannulas are inexpensive, disposable, generally comfortable, and easily accepted by most clients.

***TABLE 14-1*** Flow rate and inspired oxygen concentration

| Flow (liters/minute) | Concentration ($FIO_2$) |
|---|---|
| 1 | 24% |
| 2 | 28% |
| 4-6 | 35%-40% |

### Purposes

1. Deliver low flow oxygen concentration.
2. Relieve hypoxia.

## *Procedure 14-1*

| Steps | Rationale |
|---|---|
| **Assessment** | |
| 1. Observe for signs and symptoms associated with hypoxia: apprehension, anxiety, decreased ability to concentrate, decreased level of consciousness, increased fatigue, dizziness, behavioral changes, increased pulse rate, increased rate and depth of respiration, elevated blood pressure, cardiac dysrhythmias, pallor, cyanosis, clubbing, dyspnea. | Hypoxia is insufficient amount of oxygen available to tissues and cells to meet their metabolic needs. Left untreated, hypoxia is life-threatening and can produce cardiac dysrhythmias and death. |
| 2. Observe for patent airway and remove airway secretions. | Airway secretions can decrease delivery of oxygen via nasal cannula. |
| 3. If available, note client's most recent arterial blood gas (ABG) results. | ABGs objectively document hypoxemia and need for supplemental oxygen and measure effect of oxygen therapy (Chapter 47). |
| 4. Review client's medical record for medical order for oxygen. Note method of delivery, flow rate, and duration of oxygen therapy. | Oxygen is a drug and requires physician's order. |
| 5. Complete total respiratory system assessment (Chapter 13). | Determines presence of respiratory abnormalities that could impede oxygenation. |

| Steps | Rationale |
|---|---|
| **Nursing Diagnosis** | |
| 1. Cluster data to reveal actual or potential nursing diagnosis: | |
| a. Impaired gas exchange: related to altered oxygen supply. | Oxygen supply can be altered due to reduced rate and depth of respiration. |
| b. Impaired gas exchange: related to altered oxygen carrying capacity. | Postoperative clients may experience a decreased oxygen carrying capacity due to intraoperative bleeding, replacement of large amounts of blood products, or large amounts of IV fluid administration. |
| c. Impaired gas exchange: related to retained airway secretions. | Airway secretions decrease surface area available for transfer of oxygen from alveoli to arterial blood supply. In addition, airway secretions provide excellent medium for bacterial growth and subsequent respiratory tract infection. |
| **Planning** | |
| 1. Develop individualized goals for client based on nursing diagnoses: | |
| a. Increase lung expansion. | Increases amount of available oxygen to blood and improves clearance of pulmonary secretions. |
| b. Improve level of consciousness. | As more oxygen is available to bloodstream, cerebral tissues are less hypoxic. Unless decreased oxygen levels have caused cerebral ischemia, level of consciousness should improve. |
| c. Improve oxygenation. | Results from improved oxygen delivery to arterial blood. |
| 2. Obtain and place necessary equipment at client's bedside: a. Nasal cannula; b. Oxygen tubing; c. Humidifier; d. Sterile distilled water; e. Oxygen source; f. Flowmeter; g. "No smoking" sign | Allows nurse to attach nasal cannula quickly and efficiently. |
| 3. Explain to client and family what procedure entails and purpose of oxygen therapy. | Decreases client's anxiety and oxygen consumption; increases cooperation. |
| **Implementation** | |
| 1. Wash hands. | Reduces transmission of microorganisms. |
| 2. Attach nasal cannula to oxygen tubing. | Oxygen tubing has extension length so that client has some mobility. |
| 3. Attach nasal cannula and oxygen tubing to humidified oxygen source. | Humidification prevents drying of nasal and oral mucous membranes and airway secretions. |
| 4. Adjust oxygen flow rate to prescribed dosage, usually between 1-6 L/min. Observe that water in humidifier is bubbling. | Oxygen flow rates >6 L/min do not increase oxygen concentration but do irritate nasal mucosa and cause swallowing of gas and abdominal distention (Glover and Glover, 1978). |

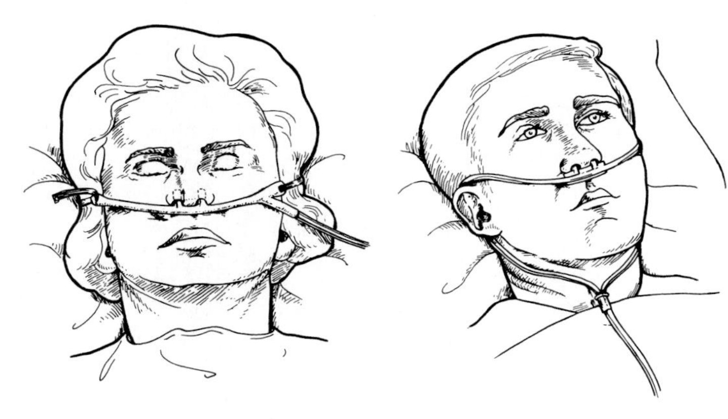

***Fig. 14-2***

From Wade JF: Comprehensive respiratory care: physiology and technique, ed 4, St Louis, 1986, The CV Mosby Co.

| Steps | Rationale |
|---|---|
| 5. Place tips of cannula into client's nares. | Directs flow of oxygen into client's upper respiratory tract. |
| 6. Adjust elastic headband or plastic slide until cannula fits snugly and comfortably (Fig. 14-2). | Client is more likely to keep cannula in place if apparatus fits comfortably. |
| 7. Allow sufficient slack on oxygen tubing and secure to client's clothes. | Allows client to turn head without dislodging cannula and reduces pressure on tips of nostrils. |
| 8. Check cannula every 8 hr. | Ensures patency of cannula and oxygen flow. |
| 9. Keep humidification jar filled at all times. | Prevents inhalation of dehumidified oxygen. |
| 10. Assess client's nares and external nose for skin breakdown every 6-8 hr. | Because of drying effects, prolonged use of nasal oxygen can increase risk of skin breakdown in client's nares and external nose. |
| 11. Encourage physician to obtain ABGs 20 min after initiating oxygen therapy or changing oxygen flow rate. | ABGs provide objective data regarding blood oxygenation (Chapter 46). |
| 12. Check physician's orders and flow of oxygen through cannula at least every 8 hr. | Identifies changes in physician's orders and documents patent nasal cannula. |
| 13. Wash hands. | Reduces transmission of microorganisms. |

## Evaluation

| | |
|---|---|
| 1. Reassess to determine client's response to administration of oxygen by nasal cannula. Observe for decreased anxiety; improved level of consciousness and cognitive abilities; decreased fatigue; absence of dizziness; decreased pulse, regular rhythm; decreased respiratory rate; return to normal blood pressure; improved color. | Hypoxia is corrected or reduced. |
| 2. Observe client's nares and superior surface of both ears for skin breakdown. | Oxygen therapy can cause drying of nasal mucosa. Pressure on ears from cannula tubing or elastic can cause skin irritation. |

### *Expected outcomes*

| | |
|---|---|
| 1. Increased lung expansion. | Reduced secretions and improved oxygenation assist in increasing lung expansion. |
| 2. Improved level of consciousness. | Improved arterial oxygen increases level of consciousness. |
| 3. Respiration, color, and ABGs return to normal. | Increased oxygen delivery improves oxygenation. |

### *Unexpected outcomes*

| | |
|---|---|
| 1. Client experiences nasal irritation, irritation to posterior surfaces of ear, drying of nasal mucosa, sinus pain, epistaxis. | One or more of these signs indicates adverse response to *method* of oxygen delivery. |
| 2. Client experiences occipital headache on awakening, depressed respiratory rate, somnolence, coma. | Signs and symptoms of oxygen side effects. Physician should be notified at once, and oxygen flow rate should be cut back to 1 L/min. |
| 3. Continued hypoxia can result in anxiety related to worsening hypoxia, ineffective breathing patterns related to hypoxia or excessive oxygen administration, ineffective airway clearance related to decreased level of consciousness or increased airway secretions, decreased cardiac output related to effect of hypoxia or cardiopulmonary function. | Uncorrected hypoxia can result in cardiac arrhythmias and death. As hypoxia worsens, work load of myocardium increases, but amount of oxygen available to myocardium decreases. Myocardial hypoxia can produce cardiac arrhythmias and ischemia. Cardiac contractility decreases amount of cardiac output and delivery of oxygen to brain, resulting in confusion, decreased level of consciousness, or coma. |

## Recording and Reporting

| | |
|---|---|
| 1. Record in nurse's notes at beginning and end of nursing shift and include in change-of-shift report the following: oxygen therapy; respiratory assessment findings; method of oxygen delivery, flow rate, patency of cannula, client's response; any adverse reactions or side effects; change in physician's orders. | Documents correct oxygen therapy for client when nurse begins and concludes care. Provides immediate validation with nursing care plan and next nursing shift of exact method of oxygen delivery and client's response to therapy. |

## Follow-up Activities

| | |
|---|---|
| 1. Begin discharge planning if client is to be discharged on home oxygen (Skill 14-8). | Assists smooth transition from oxygen use in hospital to home. |
| 2. If possible, obtain portable home oxygen equipment while client is still hospitalized. | Gives client opportunity to use new equipment while in structured environment. |
| 3. Teach postural drainage; percussion, vibration, and rib shaking; and cough control exercises (Chapter 15). | Provides measures for use in institution or home care setting to maintain airway clearance. |

### Special Considerations

- In clients with COPD, supplemental oxygen should be used cautiously, at flow rates of 1-2 L/min. Excessive oxygen can suppress respiratory drive in these clients.
- Clients at risk for oxygen side effects include those with COPD. Oxygen toxicity is not a risk with most nasal cannulas because of relatively low flow and low $FIO_2$.
- Oxygen tubings vary in length; in hospital or institutional setting, they are usually 120-240 cm (4-8 ft). In home setting extension tubing may be 15 m (50 ft).
- Physician may order warm humidification, which increases relative humidity of inspired air to 100% at body temperature (Blodgett, 1980). This in turn increases mobilization of airway secretions.
- If skin breakdown around nose or ear is observed, nurse can reduce pressure by loosening the elastic or applying 4 × 4 dressings over pressure site. When skin breakdown occurs, however, nurse also institutes hygiene measures to promote healing.

### Teaching Considerations

- Client should be able to apply nasal cannula.
- Discuss safety precautions for oxygen usage (see Oxygen Safety Guidelines, p. 317) with client and family.
- Discuss signs of oxygen toxicity and carbon dioxide retention, e.g., confusion, headache, decreased level of consciousness, somnolence.
- Instruct client's family on safety measures for home oxygen therapy.

### Home Care Considerations

- Client must know how to use the oxygen delivery system at home, e.g., cylinders, concentration, liquid oxygen.
- Client must know how to determine oxygen levels in cylinders and liquid systems.
- Assess client's respiratory status including breath sounds, respiratory effort, and skin color during each visit.
- Assess client's home for appropriate storage, checking that electrical equipment is properly grounded.
- Assess family's willingness to assist client with a home oxygen program.
- Determine whether oxygen and equipment will be paid for by client's health insurance program.

## *SKILL 14-2* *Inserting a Nasal Catheter*

Nasal catheters (Fig. 14-3) are used less frequently than nasal cannulas. The procedure involves insertion of an oxygen catheter through the nose into the nasopharynx. The oxygen catheter is a smooth, flexible tube approximately 40 cm (16 inches) in length. The distal tip of the catheter has many well-spaced openings from which oxygen is delivered.

The usual rate of flow of oxygen through the nasal catheter is 1 to 6 L/min. The $FIO_2$ ranges from 24% to 40%.

The advantage of a nasal catheter is that the client can breathe through the mouth or nose. It is available for clients of any age, and is inexpensive and disposable. The catheter sizes vary for children and adults and correlate to the sizes used for nasopharyngeal or nasotracheal suctioning (Chapter 16).

Nasal catheters have limited use because they are uncomfortable, can become lodged in the nasal cavity, and may cause excessive oropharyngeal drying. Also, the therapy is time consuming and frequently difficult to initiate.

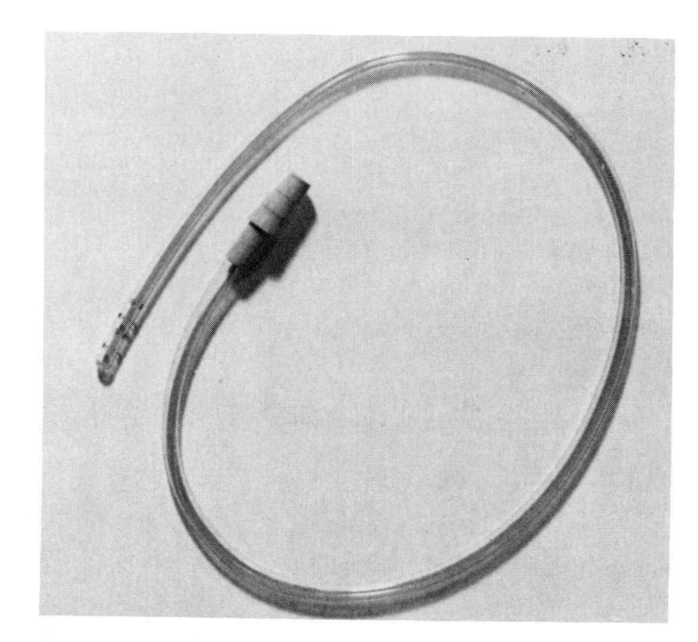

***Fig. 14-3*** Nasal catheter.
Courtesy Puritan-Bennett Corp, Overland Park, Kan.

### Purposes

1. Relieve short-term hypoxia.
2. Deliver low to moderate oxygen concentrations.

## *Procedure 14-2*

| Steps | Rationale |
|---|---|
| **Assessment** | |
| 1. Observe for signs and symptoms associated with hypoxia: apprehension, anxiety, decreased ability to concentrate, decreased level of consciousness, increased fatigue, dizziness, behavioral changes, increased pulse rate, increased rate and depth of respiration, elevated blood pressure, cardiac arrhythmias, pallor, cyanosis, clubbing, dyspnea. | Hypoxia is insufficient amount of oxygen available to tissues and cells to meet their metabolic needs. Left untreated, hypoxia is life-threatening and can produce cardiac dysrhythmias, hypotension, and death. |
| 2. Observe for patent airway and remove airway secretions. | Airway secretions can decrease delivery of oxygen via nasal cannula. |
| 3. If available, note client's most recent arterial blood gas (ABG) results. | ABGs objectively document hypoxemia and need for supplemental oxygen and measure effect of oxygen therapy (Chapter 47). |
| 4. Review medical order for oxygen. Note method of delivery, flow rate, and duration of oxygen therapy. | Oxygen is a drug and requires physician's order. |
| 5. Complete total respiratory system assessment (Chapter 13). | Determines presence of respiratory abnormalities that could impede oxygenation. |
| 6. Determine patency of nares. | Enables catheter to easily pass through client's nares. |
| **Nursing Diagnosis** | |
| 1. Cluster data to reveal actual or potential nursing diagnosis: | |
| a. Impaired gas exchange: related to altered oxygen supply. | Oxygen supply can be altered due to reduced rate and depth of respiration. |
| b. Impaired gas exchange: related to altered oxygen carrying capacity. | Postoperative clients may experience a decreased oxygen carrying capacity due to intraoperative bleeding, replacement of large amounts of blood products, or large amounts of IV fluid administration. |
| c. Impaired gas exchange: related to retained airway secretions. | Airway secretions decrease surface area available for transfer of oxygen from alveoli to arterial blood supply, and also provide excellent medium for bacterial growth and subsequent respiratory tract infection. |
| **Planning** | |
| 1. Develop individualized goals for client based on nursing diagnoses: | |
| a. Increase lung expansion. | Increases amount of available oxygen to blood and improves clearance of pulmonary secretions. |
| b. Improve level of consciousness. | As more oxygen is available to bloodstream, cerebral tissues are less hypoxic. Unless decreased oxygen levels have caused cerebral ischemia, level of consciousness should improve. |
| c. Decrease or halt airway secretions. | Results in improved oxygen delivery to arterial blood. |
| 2. Obtain necessary equipment and place at client's bedside: | Allows nurse to attach nasal catheter quickly and efficiently. |
| a. Correct size of nasal catheter | |
| b. Oxygen tubing | |
| c. Water-soluble lubricant | |
| d. Humidifier | |
| e. Sterile distilled water | |
| f. Oxygen source | |
| g. Oxygen flowmeter | |
| h. Tongue depressor | Used to locate position of catheter tip. |
| i. Flashlight | |
| 3. Explain to client and family what procedure entails and purpose of oxygen therapy. | Decreases anxiety and oxygen consumption and increases cooperation. |
| 4. Place "oxygen in use" and "no smoking" signs at entrance of client's room and at head of bed. | Provides client and staff safety while oxygen is in use. Oxygen is combustible and can fuel fire, even from cigarette sparks. |
| **Implementation** | |
| 1. Wash hands. | Reduces transmission of microorganisms. |
| 2. Attach nasal catheter to oxygen tubing. | Extension length of oxygen tubing gives client some mobility. |

| Steps | Rationale |
|---|---|

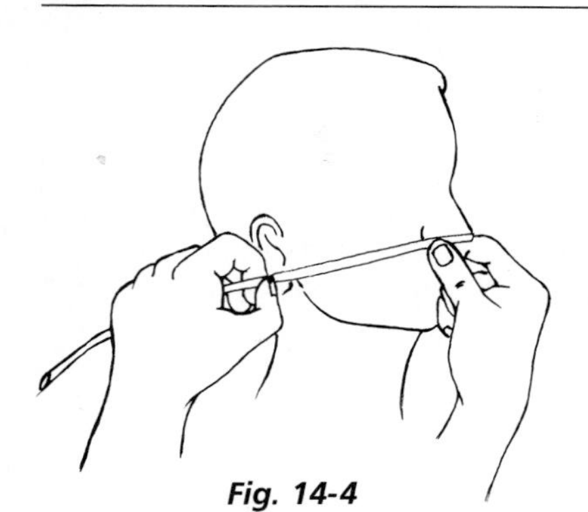
Fig. 14-4

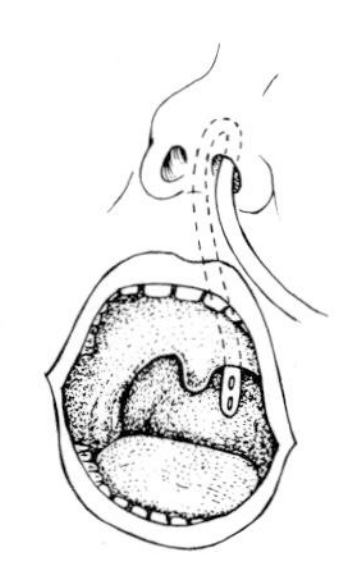
Fig. 14-5

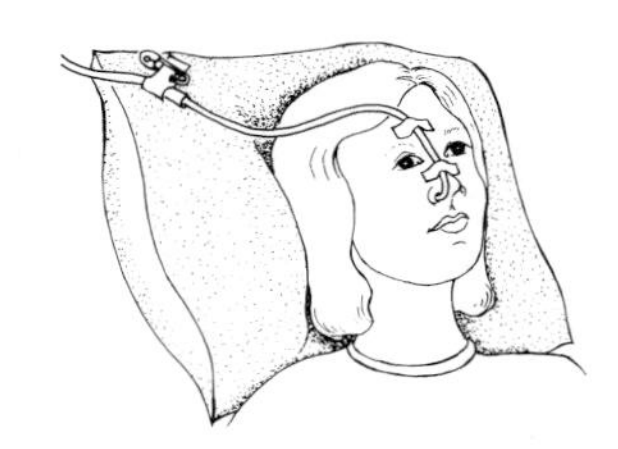
Fig. 14-6

| Steps | Rationale |
|---|---|
| 3. Attach nasal catheter and oxygen tubing to humidified oxygen source. Water in humidifier should be bubbling. | Humidification prevents drying of nasal and oral mucous membranes and airway secretions. |
| 4. Measure proper length of catheter to be inserted: measure distance from client's nose to earlobe (Fig. 14-4) and mark correct point with piece of tape. | Approximate distance from tip of nose to oropharynx. |
| 5. Lubricate tip of catheter with water-soluble jelly. | Decreases friction and promotes smooth insertion. |
| 6. Set flow rate to 2-3 L/min before inserting catheter. | Prevents occlusion of catheter by secretions during insertion. |
| 7. Gently place catheter into one nostril. Glide catheter medially along floor of nasal cavity. Stop at premarked point. | Promotes smooth passage of catheter past nasal turbinates and into oropharynx. |
| 8. Inspect oral cavity using tongue depressor and flashlight. Tip of catheter should be visible on either side of uvula (Fig. 14-5). | Verifies that catheter is in oropharynx. |
| 9. Withdraw catheter tip 0.6 cm (0.25 in) so that it is no longer visible. | Reduces amount of air swallowed by client. |
| 10. Secure catheter to client's nose (Fig. 14-6). | Prevents displacement of catheter. |
| 11. Adjust flow rate to prescribed setting, usually 1-6 L/min. | Ensures that correct amount of oxygen is being delivered to client. Flow rates greater than 6 L/min irritate nasal mucosa and can cause severe gastric distention. |
| 12. Secure connective tubing to client's gown or bedding, allow slack in tube. | Allows client to move and change positions without displacing catheter. |
| 13. Encourage physician to obtain ABGs 20 min after initiation of oxygen therapy. | ABGs provide objective data on blood oxygenation. |
| 14. Review physician's orders at least every 4 hr. | Nasal catheters are usually for short-term administration of oxygen, and physician may write new orders more frequently than when another form of oxygen therapy is used. |
| 15. Change catheter at least once daily or every 8 hr at most. Reinsert into opposite naris. | Catheter can become occluded with secretions and will no longer supply prescribed oxygen. Placing catheter into opposite naris reduces trauma to external nares secondary to pressure. |
| 16. Wash hands. | Reduces transmission of microorganisms. |

## Evaluation

| | |
|---|---|
| 1. Reassess to determine client's response to administration of oxygen by nasal cannula. Observe for decreased anxiety; improved level of consciousness and cognitive abilities; decreased fatigue; absence of dizziness; decreased pulse, regular rhythm; decreased respiratory rate; return to normal blood pressure; improved color. | Hypoxia is corrected or reduced. |
| 2. Observe client's nares. | Oxygen therapy can cause drying of nasal mucosa. Nasal catheters can press on mucous membranes of the nares, resulting in tissue damage. |

### *Expected outcomes*

| | |
|---|---|
| 1. Increased lung expansion. | Reduced secretions and improved oxygenation assist in increasing lung capacity. |
| 2. Improved level of consciousness. | Improved arterial oxygen increases level of consciousness. |
| 3. ABGs return to normal. | Increased oxygen delivery improves oxygenation. |

| Steps | Rationale |
|---|---|
| ***Unexpected outcomes*** | |
| 1. Client experiences nasal irritation, drying of nasal mucosa, sinus pain, epistaxis. | One or more of these signs indicates adverse response to *method* of oxygen delivery. |
| 2. Client experiences occipital headache on awakening, depressed respiratory rate, somnolence, coma. | Signs and symptoms of oxygen side effects. Physician should be notified at once and oxygen flow rate should be cut back to 1 L/min. |
| 3. Continued hypoxia can result in anxiety related to worsening hypoxia; ineffective breathing patterns related to hypoxia or excessive oxygen administration; ineffective airway clearance related to decreased level of consciousness or increased airway secretions; decreased cardiac output related to effect of hypoxia or cardiopulmonary function. | Uncorrected hypoxia can result in cardiac arrhythmias and death. As hypoxia worsens, work load of myocardium increases, but amount of oxygen available to myocardium decreases. Myocardial hypoxia can produce cardiac arrhythmias and ischemia. Cardiac contractility decreases amount of cardiac output and delivery of oxygen to brain, resulting in confusion, decreased level of consciousness, or coma. |
| **Recording and Reporting** | |
| 1. Record in nurse's notes at beginning and end of nursing shift and include in change-of-shift report the following: oxygen therapy; respiratory assessment findings; method of oxygen delivery, flow rate, patency of cannula, client's response; any adverse reactions or side effects; change in physician's orders. | Documents correct oxygen therapy for client when nurse begins and concludes care. Provides immediate validation with nursing care plan and next nursing shift or exact method of oxygen delivery and client's response to therapy. |
| **Follow-up Activities** | |
| 1. Notify physician or emergency personnel for worsening hypoxia. | Decreasing levels of oxygen have severe and occasionally fatal outcomes. Prompt nursing and medical actions can reduce effects of worsening hypoxia. |
| 2. Teach client's family about purpose of nasal catheter. | Clients with nasal catheters are usually too ill to respond to teaching. Teaching family members can help reduce anxiety. |

## Special Considerations

- Warming of inspired oxygen increases relative humidity to 100% and improves mobilization of airway secretions.
- Because measurements are anatomic, distance needed for children or adults is always determined by size of the client.
- Lipid-based lubricants (e.g., Vaseline) should never be used: if aspirated, they can cause severe lung irritation and pneumonia.
- If nostril is obstructed, do not force catheter.
- If catheter becomes stuck and is difficult to pull out, twist and pull it gently at same time.
- If skin breakdown is observed, nurse can reduce pressure by loosening the elastic or applying 4 × 4″ dressings over pressure site. When skin breakdown occurs, nurse also institutes hygiene measures to promote healing. Skin breakdown associated with nasal catheters are usually inside the nares.
- Clients at risk for oxygen side effects include those with COPD. Oxygen toxicity is not a risk with most nasal cannulas because of relatively low flow and low $FiO_2$.

## Teaching Considerations

- Discuss safety precautions for oxygen usage (see Oxygen Safety Guidelines, p. 317).
- Discuss signs of oxygen toxicity and carbon dioxide retention, e.g., confusion, headache, decreased level of consciousness.

## Home Care Considerations

- Nasal catheters are not used in home settings; they are used in environments that have oxygen available at client's bedside.
- Home oxygen when needed, is usually supplied via cannula (Skill 14-1) or mask (Skill 14-3).

# SKILL 14-3 Applying Oxygen Masks

An oxygen mask, used to administer oxygen, is shaped to fit snugly over the client's mouth and nose and is secured in place with a strap. The two primary types are high- and low-concentration oxygen masks. This skill module reviews oxygen masks presently used in the health care system.

A simple face mask is a flexible, cone-shaped device with a metal strip to mold the mask to the nose, an adjustable head strap, and multiple exhalation ports (Fig. 14-7). The mask is contraindicated for clients who retain carbon dioxide, such as clients with COPD.

A nonrebreathing mask is a flexible, cone-shaped device with a reservoir bag attached. A one-way flap valve is between the bag and the mask, and one-way flap valves cover the exhalation ports (Figure 14-8). A nonrebreathing bag is used for severe hypoxia because high oxygen concentrations with a high flow rate are obtainable. When a flow rate of 10 L/min or more is used, the $Fio_2$ is 90% to 95%. The reservoir bag should not collapse on inspiration (Glover and Glover, 1978).

A partial rebreathing mask is a flexible, cone-shaped device with a reservoir bag attached (Figure 14-9). This mask differs from the nonrebreathing mask in that there are no one-way flap valves between the bag and the exhalation ports (Blodgett, 1980). The partial rebreathing bag delivers medium to medium-high concentrations. An $Fio_2$ of 60% to 90% can be delivered. As with the other reservoir bag, its use is indicated in clients with severe hypoxia.

A Venturi mask is a cone-shaped device with entrainment ports of various sizes at the base of the mask (Fig. 14-10). The entrainment ports are adjustable to permit regulation of $Fio_2$ from 24% to 40%. However, the nurse also must regulate the oxygen flowmeter to correspond with the desired $Fio_2$ (Table 14-1, p. 317). This mask is useful because it delivers a known concentration of oxygen to the client.

The face tent is a shieldlike device that fits under the client's chin and sweeps around the face (Fig. 14-11). Oxygen concentrations of 21% to 50% may be delivered; a concentration of 21% is delivered if the device is used with compressed air for aerosol purposes only, since atmospheric air contains 21% oxygen. When higher oxygen concentrations are desired, the flow rate should be set at 10 L/min. Clients with retained airway secretions respond well to this type of oxygen therapy (Glover and Glover, 1978).

### Purposes

1. Deliver medium concentrations of oxygen ranging from 30% to 60%.
2. Deliver high humidity to the upper respiratory tract.

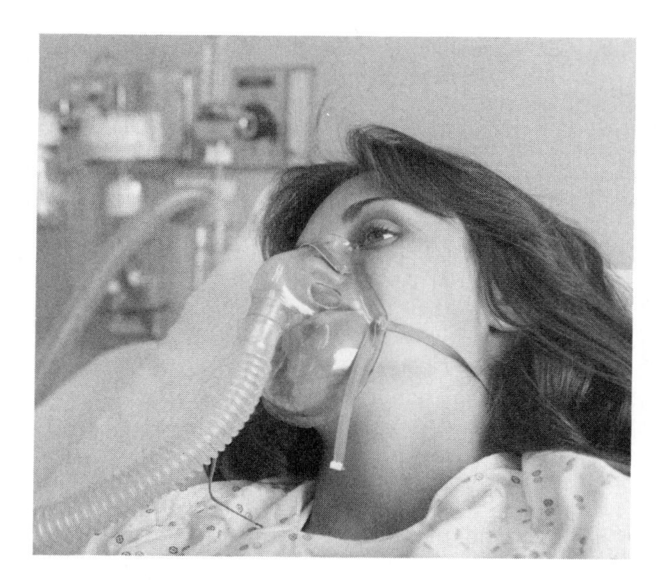

*Fig. 14-7* Simple face mask.

## Procedure 14-3

| Steps | Rationale |
|---|---|
| **Assessment** | |
| 1. Observe for signs and symptoms associated with hypoxia: apprehension, anxiety, decreased ability to concentrate, decreased level of consciousness, increased fatigue, dizziness, behavioral changes, increased pulse rate, increased rate and depth of respiration, elevated blood pressure, cardiac arrhythmias, pallor, cyanosis, clubbing, dyspnea. | Hypoxia is an insufficient amount of oxygen available to tissues and cells to meet their metabolic needs. Left untreated, hypoxia is life-threatening and can produce cardiac dysrhythmias, hypotension, and death. |
| 2. Observe for patent airway and remove airway secretions. | Airway secretions can decrease delivery of oxygen via nasal cannula. |
| 3. If available, note client's most recent arterial blood gas (ABG) results. | ABGs objectively document hypoxemia and need for supplemental oxygen and measure effect of oxygen therapy (Chapter 47). |

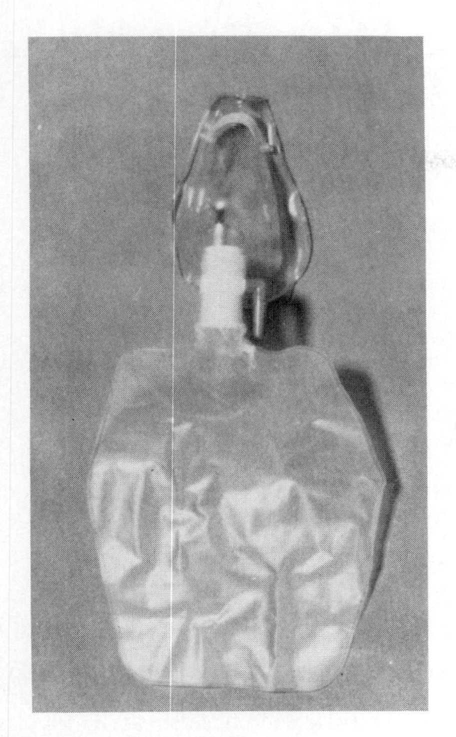

*Fig. 14-8* Nonrebreathing mask.
Courtesy Puritan-Bennett Corp, Overland Park, Kan.

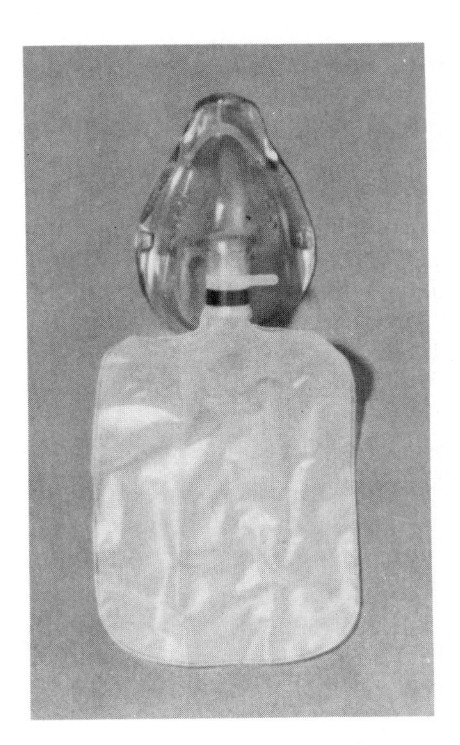

*Fig. 14-9* Partial rebreathing mask.
Courtesy Puritan-Bennett Corp, Overland Park, Kan.

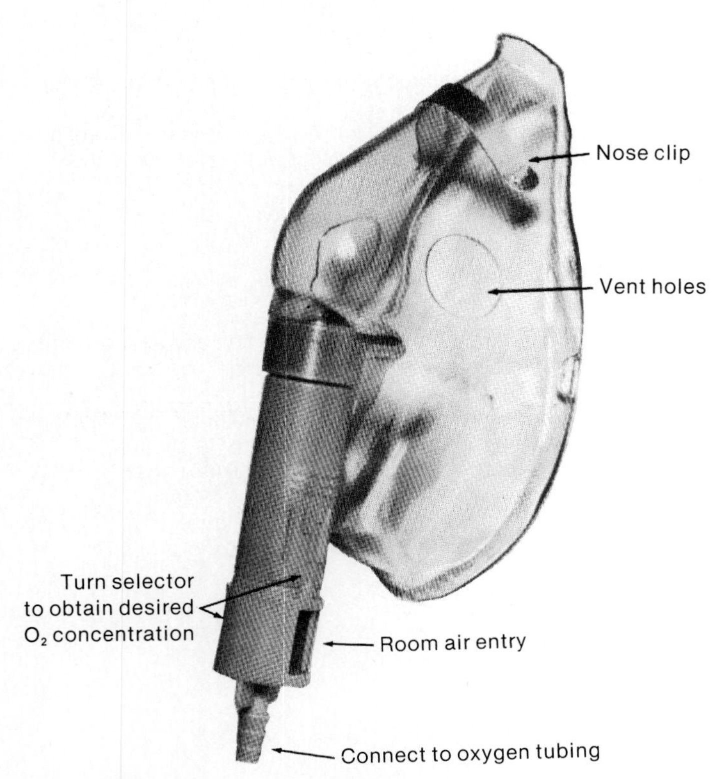


*Fig. 14-10* Venturi mask.
Courtesy Puritan-Bennett Corp, Overland Park, Kan.

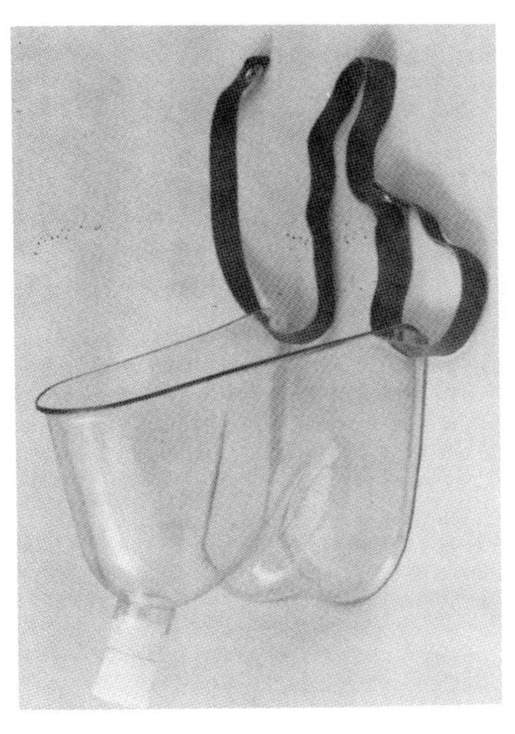

*Fig. 14-11* Face tent.
Courtesy Puritan-Bennett Corp, Overland Park, Kan.

| Steps | Rationale |
|---|---|
| 4. Review medical order for oxygen. Note method of delivery, flow rate, and duration of oxygen therapy. | Oxygen is a drug and requires physician's order. |
| 5. Complete total respiratory system assessment (Chapter 13). | Determines presence of respiratory abnormalities that could impede oxygenation. |

## Nursing Diagnosis

| Steps | Rationale |
|---|---|
| 1. Cluster data to reveal actual or potential nursing diagnoses: | |
| a. Impaired gas exchange: related to altered oxygen supply. | Oxygen supply can be altered due to reduced rate and depth of respiration. |
| b. Impaired gas exchange: related to altered oxygen carrying capacity. | Postoperative clients may experience decreased oxygen carrying capacity due to intraoperative bleeding, replacement of large amounts of blood products, or large amounts of IV fluid administration. |
| c. Impaired gas exchange: related to retained airway secretions. | Airway secretions decrease surface area available for transfer of oxygen from alveoli to arterial blood supply. In addition, airway secretions provide excellent medium for bacterial growth and subsequent respiratory tract infection. |

## Planning

| Steps | Rationale |
|---|---|
| 1. Develop individualized goals for client based on nursing diagnoses: | |
| a. Increase lung expansion. | Increases amount of available oxygen to blood and improves clearance of pulmonary secretions. |
| b. Improve level of consciousness. | As more oxygen is available to bloodstream, cerebral tissues are less hypoxic. Unless decreased oxygen levels have caused cerebral ischemia, level of consciousness should improve. |
| c. Decrease or halt airway secretions. | Results in improved oxygen delivery to arterial blood. |
| 2. Obtain necessary equipment and place at client's bedside: a. Face mask or face tent; b. Small-bore oxygen tubing*; c. Humidifier; d. Sterile water; e. Oxygen source; f. Flowmeter | Allows nurse to attach oxygen mask or face tent quickly and efficiently. |
| 3. Explain to client purpose of oxygen mask and show how mask fits. | Decreases anxiety and oxygen consumption and increases cooperation. |
| 4. Place "oxygen in use" and "no smoking" signs at entrance to client's room and over head of bed. | Provides client and staff safety while oxygen is in use. Oxygen is combustible and can fuel fire, even from cigarette sparks. |

## Implementation

| Steps | Rationale |
|---|---|
| 1. Wash hands. | Reduces transmission of microorganisms. |
| 2. Attach face mask or tent to appropriately sized oxygen tubing. | Connects mask or tent to oxygen source. |
| 3. Attach face mask or tent and oxygen tubing to humidified oxygen or gas source. | Prevents drying of oral and nasal mucosa and airway secretions. When compressed gas is used for room air, air should be humidified. |
| 4. Adjust oxygen flow rate to prescribed dosage. Verify that water in humidifier is bubbling. | Presence of bubbling distilled water in humidifier indicates that oxygen is being moistened before delivery to client. |
| 5. Place face mask or tent on client and adjust to snug but comfortable fit. | Maintains prescribed concentration of inhaled oxygen. If mask is too loose, oxygen escapes. |
| 6. Observe for proper function of face mask or tent: | |
| a. Nonrebreathing mask: reservoir bag will fill on exhalation and almost collapse on exhalation. | Ensures that specialized face masks are working properly. |
| b. Partial rebreathing mask: reservoir should fill on exhalation and almost collapse on inhalation. | |
| c. Venturi mask: percentage of $Fio_2$ should correlate with flow rate (Table 14-1). | |
| d. Face tent: mist should always be present. | |

*If face tent is used, substitute large-bore aerosol tubing.

| Steps | Rationale |
|---|---|
| 7. Observe for moisture in reservoir bags or large-bore oxygen tubing when face tent is used. Remove water from bag or tubing and discard. *Do not* drain reservoir bag or tubing into humidifying device. | Water is a medium for bacterial growth. Draining contaminated water into sterile distilled water contaminates entire humidifying unit. |
| 8. Humidity source should be checked every 4 hr. Container should be changed every 24 hr. | Ensures that humidity doesn't run dry. Reduces transmission of microorganisms. |
| 9. Observe for pressure necrosis with tightly fitting mask every 2 hr. | Reduces risk of skin breakdown around nose, mouth, and superior surfaces of ears. |
| 10. Encourage physician to obtain ABGs 20 min after initiation of therapy or change in oxygen concentration. | ABGs provide objective data regarding blood oxygenation (Chapter 47). |
| 11. Check physician orders every 2-4 hr. | Notes changes in oxygen therapy. |
| 12. Observe for gagging, retching, or vomiting; remove mask if one of these occurs. | Reduces risk of aspiration. |
| 13. Wash hands. | Reduces transmission of microorganisms. |

## Evaluation

| Steps | Rationale |
|---|---|
| 1. Reassess client to determine response to administration of oxygen by nasal cannula. Observe for decreased anxiety; improved level of consciousness and cognitive abilities; decreased fatigue; absence of dizziness; decreaed pulse, regular rhythm; decreased respiratory rate; return to normal blood pressure; improved color. | Hypoxia is corrected or reduced. |
| 2. Observe client's nares and superior surface of both ears for skin breakdown. | Oxygen therapy can cause drying of nasal mucosa. Pressure on ears from cannula tubing or elastic can cause skin irritation. |

### *Expected outcomes*

| Steps | Rationale |
|---|---|
| 1. Increased lung expansion. | Reduced secretions and improved oxygenation assist in increasing lung expansion. |
| 2. Increased level of consciousness. | Increased oxygenation improves level of consciousness. |
| 3. Respirations, color, and ABGs return to normal. | Increased oxygen delivery improves oxygenation. |

### *Unexpected outcomes*

| Steps | Rationale |
|---|---|
| 1. Client experiences irritation to nasal and oral mucosa, pressure areas from the mask, epistaxis, subcutaneous emphysema into ocular tissues at high flows. | One or more of these signs indicates adverse response to *method* of oxygen delivery. |
| 2. Client experiences occipital headache on awakening, depressed respiratory rate, somnolence, coma. | Signs and symptoms of oxygen *side effects.* Physician should be notified at once and oxygen flow rate should be cut back to 1 L/min. |
| 3. Client experiences stiff, noncompliant lung, alveolar edema, pulmonary congestion, chest pain, intra-alveolar hemorrhage, substernal chest pain. | Signs and symptoms of *oxygen toxicity.* Physicians should be notified at once. |
| 4. Continued hypoxia can result in anxiety related to worsening hypoxia, ineffective breathing patterns related to hypoxia or excessive oxygen administration, ineffective airway clearance related to decreased level of consciousness or increased airway secretions, decreased cardiac output related to effect of hypoxia or cardiopulmonary function. | Uncorrected hypoxia can result in cardiac arrhythmias and death. As hypoxia worsens, work load of myocardium increases, but amount of oxygen available to myocardium decreases. Myocardial hypoxia can produce cardiac arrhythmias and ischemia. Cardiac contractility decreases amount of cardiac output and delivery of oxygen to brain, resulting in confusion, decreased level of consciousness, or coma. |

## Recording and Reporting

| Steps | Rationale |
|---|---|
| 1. Record in nurse's notes at beginning and end of nursing shift and include in the change-of-shift report the following: oxygen therapy; respiratory assessment findings; method of oxygen delivery, flow rate, client's response; any adverse reactions or side effects; change in physician's orders. | Documents correct oxygen therapy for client when nurse begins and concludes care. Provides immediate validation with nursing care plan and next nursing shift of exact method of oxygen delivery and client's response to therapy. |

## Follow-up Activities

| Steps | Rationale |
|---|---|
| 1. Turn clients at risk of vomiting on their sides. If vomiting does occur, remove oxygen mask, notify physician, and request new order for oxygen delivery. | Promotes airway clearance of vomitus and reduces risk of aspiration. |
| 2. See Skill 14-1, Steps 1 and 3. | |

## Special Considerations

- Client's medical record should be reviewed at least every shift for changes in physician's orders. Clients whose health status is unstable, i.e., premature infants, clients with acute illnesses, and postoperative clients, may require frequent changes in oxygen therapy.
- Warm humidification may be ordered, particularly with face tents. This increases relative humidity and helps to mobilize airway secretions.
- Accumulation of water occurs more frequently with face tents and when humidified air is warmed.
- Partial rebreathing and nonrebreathing masks deliver medium to high concentrations of oxygen (90%-95%) and are not recommended for client with COPD, since spontaneous respirations could be suppressed. High concentrations of oxygen by mask can produce signs and symptoms of oxygen toxicity (Skill 14-1).
- Some clients may feel "closed in." Nurse frequently can relieve this sensation by remaining with and reassuring client. As hypoxia improves, this sensation frequently subsides. Febrile or diaphoretic clients need frequent mouth and skin care because of oxygen's drying effect. Clients unable to tolerate masks will remove them and may require some restraint (Chapter 4).
- When high concentrations of oxygen are used, as with rebreathing and nonrebreathing masks, nurse must objectively document improving or worsening hypoxia to evaluate medical therapy.
- Face mask should not be used in clients who are vomiting.
- If skin breakdown on ear or nose is observed, nurse can reduce pressure by loosening the elastic or applying 4 × 4 dressings over pressure site. When skin breakdown occurs, however, nurse also institutes hygiene measures to promote healing.
- Have suction equipment at bedside and be prepared to suction client's airway (Chapter 16).
- Pediatric client may wish to play with samples of face mask before and during oxygen therapy.

## Teaching Considerations

- If client's oxygen level is low enough to produce symptoms of confusion and decreased level of consciousness, teaching should be delayed until client can understand what is taught.
- Discuss safety precautions for oxygen use (see Oxygen Safety Guidelines, p. 317).
- Discuss signs of oxygen toxicity and carbon dioxide retention, e.g., confusion, headache, decreased level of consciousness, somnolence.

## Home Care Considerations

- Oxygen masks or face tents can readily be used at home; however, oxygen source frequently is gas cylinder.
- Client must be able to demonstrate use of oxygen delivery system, including determining level of oxygen available, safety precautions, and cleaning of airway equipment.

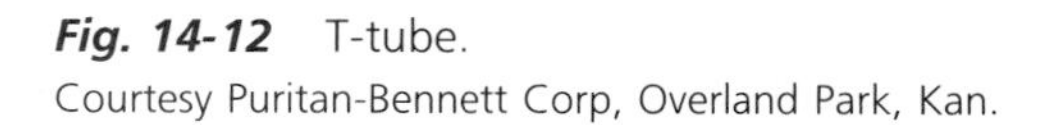

*Fig. 14-12* T-tube.
Courtesy Puritan-Bennett Corp, Overland Park, Kan.

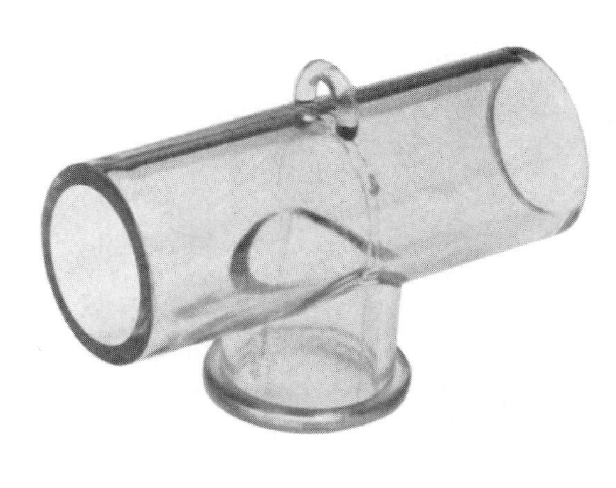

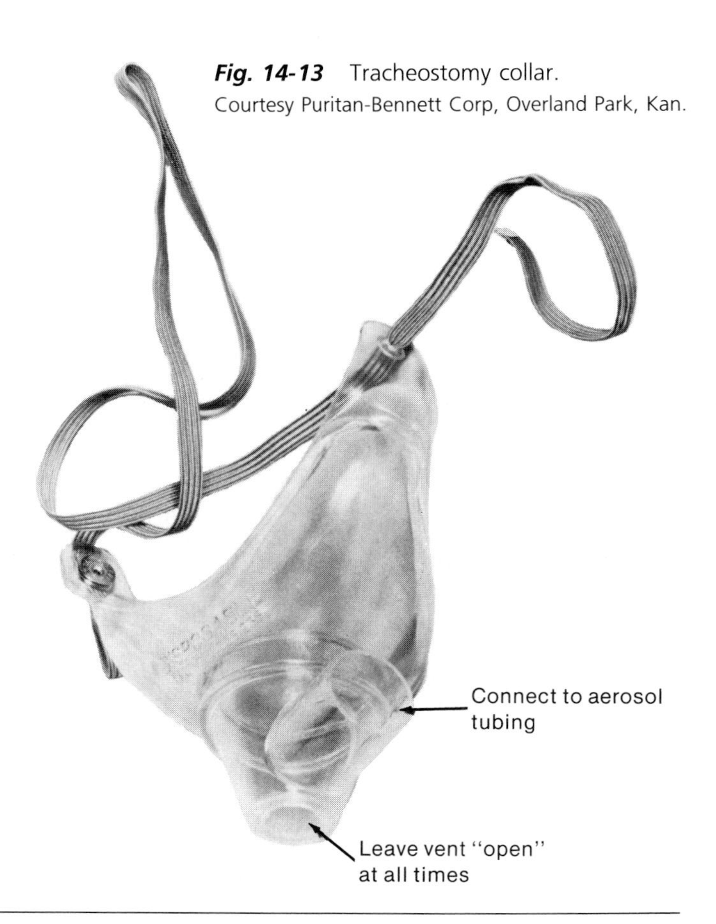


*Fig. 14-13* Tracheostomy collar.
Courtesy Puritan-Bennett Corp, Overland Park, Kan.

# SKILL 14-4 Administering Oxygen Therapy to a Client with an Artificial Airway

Clients with an artificial airway require constant humidification to the airway because the insertion of the airway bypasses the normal filtering and humidification process of the nose and mouth.

The two devices that supply humidified gas to an artificial airway are a T-tube, also called a Briggs adapter, and a tracheostomy collar. Both supply humidified oxygen or room air to the airway.

The T-tube is a T-shaped device attached to an endotracheal or tracheostomy tube with a 15 mm (3⁄5 in) connection (Fig. 14-12). The recommended flow rate is 10 L/min, with a nebulizer setting determining the $FiO_2$ (Glover and Glover, 1978).

A tracheostomy collar is a curved device with an adjustable strap that fits around the client's neck. An exhalation port remains patent at all times, and another connects large-bore oxygen tubing (Fig. 14-13). The collar provides humidification to the lower airways via the tracheostomy tube opening. As with the T-tube, the flow rate should be set at 10 L/min, with a nebulizer setting the appropriate $FiO_2$.

## Purposes

1. Deliver humidified gas to the lower airway.
2. Prevent hypoxia.

## Procedure 14-4

| Steps | Rationale |
|---|---|
| **Assessment** | |
| 1. Observe for signs and symptoms associated with hypoxia: apprehension, anxiety, decreased ability to concentrate, decreased level of consciousness, increased fatigue, dizziness, behavioral changes, increased pulse rate, increased rate and depth of respiration, elevated blood pressure, cardiac arrhythmias, pallor, cyanosis, clubbing, dyspnea. | Hypoxia is insufficient amount of oxygen available to tissues and cells to meet their metabolic needs. Left untreated, hypoxia is life-threatening and can produce cardiac dysrhythmias and death. |
| 2. Observe for patent airway and remove airway secretions. | Airway secretions can decrease the delivery of oxygen via T-tube or tracheostomy collar. |
| 3. If available, note client's most recent arterial blood gas (ABG) results. | ABGs objectively document hypoxemia and need for supplemental oxygen and measure effect of oxygen therapy (Chapter 47). |
| 4. Review client's medical record for medical order for oxygen. Note method of delivery, flow rate, and duration of oxygen therapy. | Oxygen is a drug and requires physician's order. |
| 5. Complete total respiratory system assessment (Chapter 13). | Determines presence of respiratory abnormalities that could impede oxygenation. |
| **Nursing Diagnosis** | |
| 1. Cluster data to reveal actual or potential nursing diagnoses: | |
| a. Impaired gas exchange: related to altered oxygen supply. | Oxygen supply can be altered due to reduced rate and depth of respiration. |
| b. Impaired gas exchange: related to altered oxygen carrying capacity. | Postoperative clients may experience decreased oxygen carrying capacity due to intraoperative bleeding, replacement of large amounts of blood products, or large amounts of IV fluid administration. |
| c. Impaired gas exchange: related to retained airway secretions. | Airway secretions decrease surface area available for transfer of oxygen from alveoli to arterial blood supply, and also provide excellent medium for bacterial growth and subsequent respiratory tract infection. |
| d. Impaired verbal communication: related to endotracheal (ET) tube and tracheostomy. | Artificial airways alter normal airway anatomy and pressures. Client is unable to speak (Chapter 18). |

| Steps | Rationale |
|---|---|
| **Planning** | |
| 1. Develop individualized goals for client based on nursing diagnoses: | |
| a. Increase lung expansion. | Increases amount of available oxygen to blood and improves clearance of pulmonary secretions. |
| b. Improve level of consciousness. | As more oxygen is available to bloodstream, cerebral tissues are less hypoxic. Unless decreased oxygen levels have caused cerebral ischemia, level of consciousness should improve. |
| c. Decrease or halt airway secretions. | Results in improved oxygen delivery to arterial blood. |
| 2. Obtain necessary equipment and place at client's bedside:<br>a. T-tube or tracheostomy collar<br>b. Large-bore oxygen tubing<br>c. Nebulizer<br>d. Sterile water<br>e. Oxygen or gas source<br>f. Flowmeter | Allows nurse to attach T-tube or tracheostomy collar quickly and efficiently. |
| 3. Explain purpose of T-tube or tracheostomy collar to client (or parent) and family. | Explanation decreases anxiety and reduces oxygen consumption. |
| 4. If humidified gas to T-tube or tracheostomy collar is oxygen, place "oxygen in use" and "no smoking" signs at entrance to client's room and over head of bed. | Provides client and staff safety while oxygen is in use. Oxygen is combustible and can fuel fire, even from cigarette sparks. |
| **Implementation** | |
| 1. Wash hands. | Reduces transmission of microorganisms. |
| 2. Attach T-tube or tracheostomy collar to large-bore oxygen tubing. | Provides connection to humidified gas. |
| 3. Attach oxygen tubing to humidified oxygen source. | Artificial airways bypass normal humidification function of nose and mouth. Thus, supplemental humidification must *always* be supplied. |
| 4. Adjust oxygen flow rate to 10 L/min and adjust nebulizer to proper $FIO_2$ setting. | Flow rate ensures humidification; nebulizer regulates $FIO_2$. |
| 5. Attach T-tube or tracheostomy collar to endotracheal or tracheostomy tube. | Provides humidified source to artificial airway. |
| 6. Observe for secretions within T-tube or tracheostomy collar and suction them out (Chapter 16). | Maintains patent airway. |
| 7. Obtain ABGs 20 min after initiating T-tube. | ABGs provide objective data regarding blood oxygenation (Chapter 47). |
| 8. Check physician orders every 2 hr initially. | Provides mechanism for identifying new orders for oxygen adjustment. |
| 9. Observe that T-tube does not pull on endotracheal or tracheostomy tube. | Pulling effect can increase client's discomfort and cause pressure to side of client's mouth or tracheal stoma. |
| 10. Observe oxygen tubing every 2 hr for accumulation of fluid. If fluid is present, drain tube away from client and discard fluid. | Excess water is medium for bacterial growth. Draining contaminated water into sterile distilled water contaminates entire humidifying unit. |
| 11. Place suction equipment at client's bedside. | Client usually experiences increased airway secretions. |
| 12. Wash hands. | Reduces transmission of microorganisms. |
| **Evaluation** | |
| 1. Assess to determine client's response to administration of oxygen by nasal cannula. Observe for decreased anxiety; improved level of consciousness and cognitive abilities; decreased fatigue; absence of dizziness; decreased pulse, regular rhythm; decreased respiratory rate; return to normal blood pressure; improved color. | Hypoxia is corrected or reduced. |
| 2. Observe client's nares and superior surface of both ears for skin breakdown. | Oxygen therapy can cause drying of nasal mucosa. Pressure on ears from cannula tubing or elastic can cause skin irritation. |
| ***Expected outcomes*** | |
| 1. Stoma remains pink, nontender, and free of secretions. | Absence of mechanical or bacterial irritation to stoma. |
| 2. No pressure areas noted on neck. | Absence of mechanical friction on client's neck due to oxygen delivery system. |

| Steps | Rationale |
|---|---|
| 3. Respiratory rate is regular; client alert and oriented. | Oxygen delivery to artificial airway increases oxygenation. |
| ***Unexpected outcomes*** | |
| 1. Client experiences stoma irritation; thick, tenacious secretions; pressure areas on neck or near stoma site. | One or more of these indicates adverse response to *method* of oxygen delivery. |
| 2. Client experiences occipital headache on awakening, depressed respiratory rate, somnolence, coma. | Signs and symptoms of oxygen *side effects.* Physician should be notified at once and oxygen flow rate should be cut back to 1 L/min. |
| 3. Continued hypoxia can result in anxiety related to worsening hypoxia, ineffective breathing patterns related to hypoxia or excessive oxygen administration, ineffective airway clearance related to decreased level of consciousness or increased airway secretions, decreased cardiac output related to effect of hypoxia or cardiopulmonary function. | Uncorrected hypoxia can result in cardiac dysrhythmias and death. As hypoxia worsens, work load of myocardium increases, but amount of oxygen available to myocardium decreases. Myocardial hypoxia can produce cardiac dysrhythmias and ischemia. Cardiac contractility decreases amount of cardiac output and delivery of oxygen to brain, resulting in confusion, decreased level of consciousness, or coma. |
| **Recording and Reporting** | |
| 1. Record in nurse's notes at beginning and end of nursing shift and include in change-of-shift report the following: oxygen therapy; respiratory assessment findings; method of oxygen delivery, flow rate, patency of cannula, client's response; any adverse reactions or side effects; change in physician's orders. | Documents correct oxygen therapy for client when nurse begins and concludes care. Provides immediate validation with nursing care plan and next nursing shift of exact method of oxygen delivery and client's response to therapy. |
| **Follow-up Activities** | |
| 1. Suction secretions from artificial airway. | Maintains patency of airway and promotes oxygen delivery. |
| 2. Begin discharge planning if client is to be discharged on home oxygen (Skill 14-8). | Assists smooth transition from oxygen use in hospital to home. |

## Special Considerations

- Clients at risk for oxygen side effects include those with COPD.
- Make sure oxygen tubing is long enough to provide some mobility for client.
- Frequently, humidified air is warmed to increase relative humidity of inspired air to 100% at body temperature (Blodgett, 1980), which increases mobilization of airway secretions.
- Mist should *always* be visible.
- Excessive water accumulation occurs more frequently at higher humidities.
- Client being weaned from mechanical ventilator is more likely to be anxious while breathing without ventilator's aid. Nurse can help reduce anxiety by remaining with client. However, nurse must complete serial respiratory assessments to evaluate whether anxiety is caused by psychologic dependency to ventilator or related hypoxia.
- T-tube is designed to fit 15 mm tracheostomy tube. Adapters are used to connect smaller tracheostomy tube to T-tube.
- Humidity level and amount of airway secretion determine frequency of suctioning airways.
- When client is being weaned from mechanical ventilator to T-tube, ABGs must always be obtained 20 min after initiation of T-tube or change in $Fio_2$.
- If skin breakdown is observed, nurse can reduce pressure by loosening the elastic or applying 4 × 4″ dressings over pressure site. When skin breakdown occurs, nurse also institutes hygiene measures to promote healing.

## Teaching Considerations

- Client demonstrates proper placement of oxygen device to tracheostomy tube.
- Discuss safety precautions for oxygen usage (see Oxygen Safety Guidelines, p. 317).
- Teach client signs and symptoms of oxygen toxicity and carbon dioxide retention, e.g., confusion, headache, decreased level of consciousness, somnolence.
- Instruct client on frequent ambulation or movement in bed to assist in mobilizing secretions.
- Encourage client in deep breathing and coughing techniques and to maintain adequate fluid intake to assist in liquefying secretions to cleanse the airway more easily.

## Home Care Considerations

- Client with artificial airway who is at home may have permanent tracheostomy as well as T-tube or tracheostomy collar.
- Client should be able to perform tracheostomy care and suctioning techniques (see Chapter 18).
- Assess client's home environment for presence of respiratory irritants, cleanliness, and location in which to clean suctioning equipment and hang it up to drain.

# *SKILL 14-5 Administering Oxygen Therapy to the Pediatric Client*

As in the adult, hypoxemia indicates the need for administration of oxygen in the pediatric client. In a child cyanosis is a late sign but remains the best criterion for supplemental oxygen. Dyspnea is not always relieved by oxygen. (Whaley and Wong, 1987). In children, oxygen can be administered by mask (Skill 14-3), nasal cannula (Skill 14-1), intermittent positive-pressure breathing (IPPB) (Skill 14-7), Croupette, oxygen hood, and oxygen tent. The last three are designed more specifically for the pediatric client, although the oxygen tent also can be used for the adult.

The mode of oxygen delivery is based on the required concentration of inspired air needed and the child's degree of cooperation. For most children requiring oxygen, an ambient oxygen concentration of 40% to 50% is satisfactory and should be analyzed periodically for percentage of concentration (Whaley and Wong, 1987). Oxygen for children may cause complications and should always be humidified.

A severe toxic effect of excessive oxygen concentration in the infant is retrolental fibroplasia, a disease of the eyes related to hypoxemia. It occurs almost exclusively in the premature infant, with incidence correlating with level of maturity: the shorter the gestational age, the greater is the likelihood of its development (Whaley and Wong, 1987). To date, no documented safety level of oxygen concentration or length of application is available. Thus careful monitoring of the infant and arterial oxygen concentration, through blood gas analysis (Chapter 47), is essential. The goal of therapy is to reduce the oxygen concentration, minimizing amount and duration of exposure (Hazinski, 1984).

The Croupette or oxygen tent provides an oxygen concentration of approximately 21% to 60%. Pediatric clients from 1 month to 10 years of age are candidates for the Croupette; older clients should be placed under an oxygen tent.

The oxygen hood delivers a controlled, high $FiO_2$ to an infant in respiratory distress. It also has the capacity to warm and humidify inspired gas to loosen airway secretions.

The skills presented here focus on the different types of oxygen apparatus designed specifically for the pediatric client: Croupette, hood, and oxygen tent.

## Purposes

1. Provide warm or cool humidification.
2. Reduce hypoxia.

## *Procedure 14-5*

| Steps | Rationale |
|---|---|
| **Assessment** | |
| 1. Observe for signs and symptoms of hypoxia usually associated with pediatric client. a. Infant or toddler: sternal retractions nasal flaring, lethargy, cyanosis, changes in vital signs. b. Older child: anxiety, lethargy, behavioral changes, sternal retractions, nasal flaring, cyanosis. | Hypoxia is insufficient amount of oxygen available to tissues and cells to meet their metabolic needs. Left untreated, hypoxia is life-threatening and can produce cardiac dysrhythmias and death. |
| 2. Observe for patent airway and remove airway secretions. | Airway secretions can decrease delivery of oxygen via nasal cannula. |
| 3. If available, note client's most recent arterial blood gas (ABG) results. | ABGs objectively document hypoxemia and need for supplemental oxygen and measure effect of oxygen therapy (Chapter 47). |
| 4. Review client's medical record for medical order for oxygen. Note method of delivery, flow rate, and duration of oxygen therapy. | Oxygen is a drug and requires physician's order. |
| 5. Complete total respiratory system assessment. | Determines presence of respiratory abnormalities that could impede oxygenation. |
| **Nursing Diagnosis** | |
| 1. Cluster data to reveal actual or potential nursing diagnoses: | |
| a. Impaired gas exchange: related to decreased lung expansion. | Decreased lung expansion reduces amount of oxygen delivered to lungs and ultimately transferred to arterial blood. |
| b. Impaired gas exchange: related to decreased level of consciousness. | Decreased level of consciousness decreases rate and depth of respiration, diminishing amount of oxygen inspired and transported to tissues and cells. |

| Steps | Rationale |
|---|---|
| c. Impaired gas exchange: related to retained airway secretions. | Airway secretions decrease surface area available for transfer of oxygen from alveoli to arterial blood supply, and also provide excellent medium for bacterial growth and subsequent respiratory tract infection. |

## Planning

| Steps | Rationale |
|---|---|
| 1. Develop individualized goals for client based on nursing diagnoses: | |
| a. Increase lung expansion. | Increases amount of available oxygen to blood and improves clearance of pulmonary secretions. |
| b. Improve level of consciousness. | As more oxygen is available to bloodstream, cerebral tissues are less hypoxic. Unless decreased oxygen levels have caused cerebral ischemia, level of consciousness should improve. |
| c. Decrease or halt airway secretions. | Results in improved oxygen delivery to arterial blood. |
| 2. Obtain necessary equipment and place at child's bedside. | Allows nurse to attach oxygen delivery system quickly and efficiently. |

a. Croupette (Fig. 14-14):
- Croupette
- Humidifier
- Sterile water
- Oxygen source
- Flowmeter
- Ice or refrigeration unit

b. Infant oxygen hood (Fig. 14-15):
- Oxygen hood
- Humidifier
- Temperature regulator to warm humidified oxygen
- Oxygen source
- Flowmeter

c. Oxygen tent (Fig. 14-16):
- Tent
- Oxygen tubing
- Oxygen source
- Oxygen flow regulator
- Oxygen analyzer
- Humidifier
- Sterile distilled water

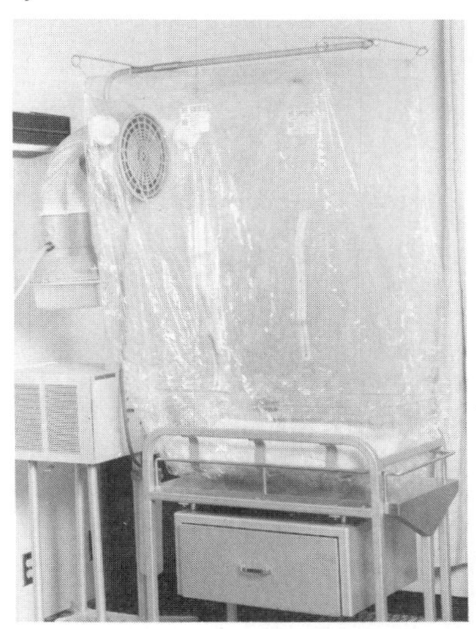

*Fig. 14-14*

| Steps | Rationale |
|---|---|
| 3. Explain to child and family what procedure entails and purpose of oxygen therapy. | Decreases parental and child anxiety and increases child's cooperation. |
| 4. Place "oxygen in use" and "no smoking" signs at entrance to client's room and over head of bed. | Provides client and staff safety while oxygen is in use. Oxygen is combustible and can fuel fire, even from cigarette sparks. |

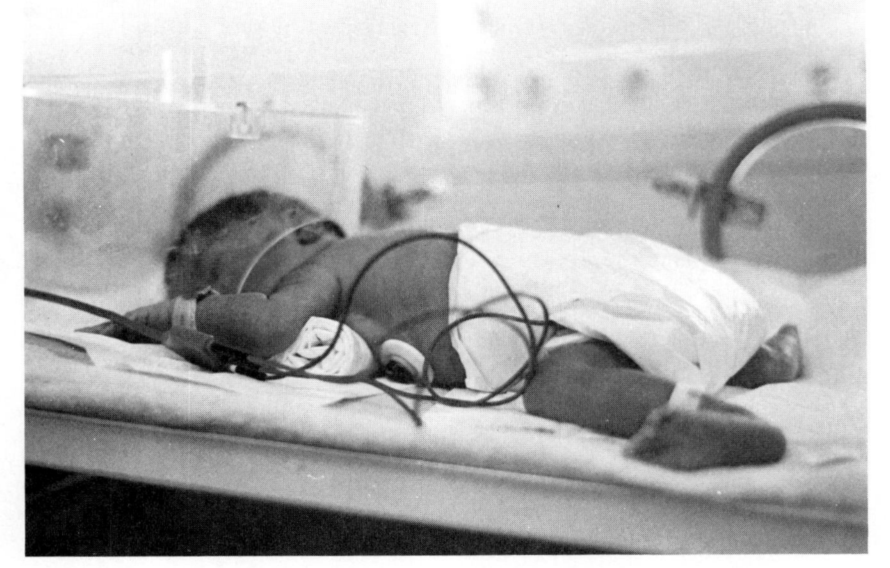

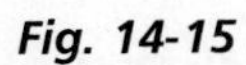

*Fig. 14-15*

From Whaley LF, Wong DL: Nursing care of infants and children, ed 2, St Louis, 1987, The CV Mosby Co.

| Steps | Rationale |
|---|---|

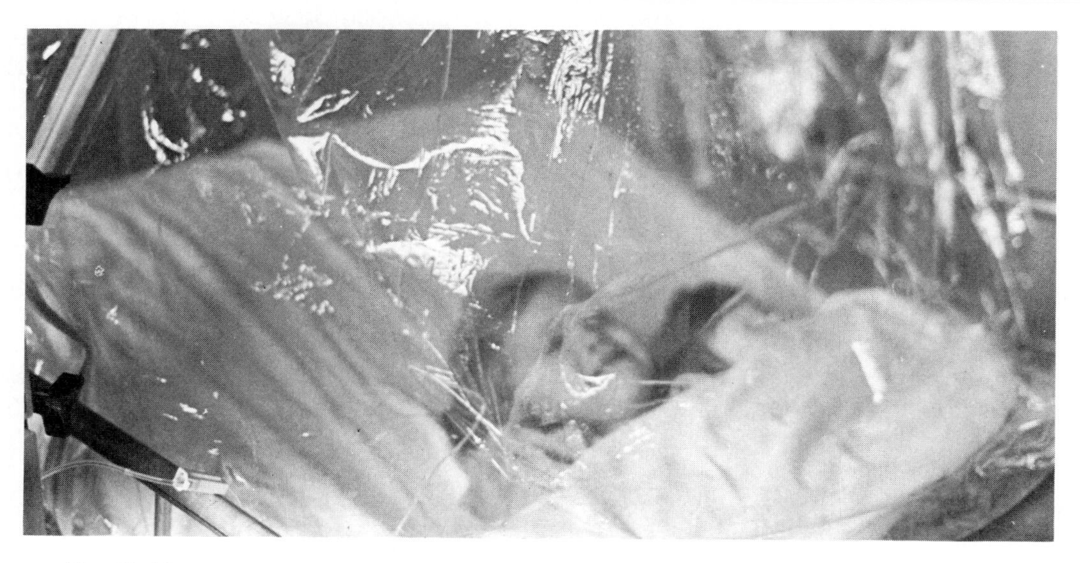

***Fig. 14-16***
From Whaley LF, Wong DL: Nursing care of infants and children, ed 2, St Louis, 1987, The CV Mosby Co.

## Implementation

### *Croupette or oxygen tent*

| Steps | Rationale |
|---|---|
| 1. Position cooling nebulizer unit on bed or crib and attach canopy to unit and position over bed. | Maintains oxygen delivery within environment of tent. |
| 2. Fill ice chamber or start refrigeration unit. | Because enclosed tent becomes very warm, cooling mechanism is needed (Whaley and Wong, 1987). |
| 3. Fill nebulizer reservoir with sterile distilled water and set flowmeter to at least 10 L/min (Blodgett, 1980). | Oxygen flow rate forms mist and maintains humidity within tent. Gas source and nebulizer unit determine $FiO_2$. |
| 4. Place child in tent, and if toy or blanket is present, be sure it does not produce friction or static electricity. | Toy or security blanket can decrease anxiety and help child to cooperate. If toy produces friction or static electricity, it represents safety hazards because oxygen is combustible. |
| 5. Tuck sides of canopy or tent under mattress and fold sheet over front portion of tent. Check tent frequently to be sure its sides and front are secured. | Oxygen is heavier than air, and loss is greatest at bottom of tent. |
| 6. Check ice reservoir frequently, do not allow chamber to empty. | Empty ice chamber increases temperature within tent and results in administration of dry oxygen. |
| 7. Organize nursing care so that tent is opened as infrequently as possible, but maintain continuous assessment of child's respiratory status. | Frequent opening of tent decreases oxygen content within tent. |
| 8. After tent has remained open, flush with oxygen by increasing flowmeter setting. *Reset flowmeter* to prescribed setting. | Rapidly raises oxygen concentration and humidity within tent. |

### *Oxygen hood*

| Steps | Rationale |
|---|---|
| 1. Attach oxygen hood to gas source with heated humidification. | Maintains adequate humidification of inspired gas. |
| 2. Place hood over infant, making sure that gas does not blow directly into infant's face. | Air applied to face stimulates receptors that trigger diving reflex, which causes bradycardia and shunting of blood from peripheral to central circulation (Whaley and Wong, 1987). |
| 3. Monitor temperature inside hood. | Prevents excessive temperature buildup within hood and possible pulmonary or tracheal burns. |
| 4. Change bedding and clothing if moisture accumulates. | Prevents chilling and skin breakdown. |

### *Oxygen tent and hood*

| Steps | Rationale |
|---|---|
| 1. Encourage physician to obtain ABGs 20 min after initiating oxygen therapy or changing oxygen flow rate. | ABGs provide objective data regarding blood oxygenation (Chapter 47). |
| 2. Check physician's orders and flow of oxygen to tents or hood at least every 2 hr. | Provides mechanism for identifying physician's orders. |

| Steps | Rationale |
|---|---|
| 3. Monitor child's color and respiratory status frequently. If child is permitted to leave tent for feeding, bathing, and comfort, immediately return child to tent if change in color, increased respiratory effort, or restlessness occurs. | Children's respiratory status changes quickly. Three cardinal signs for decreased respiratory status are change in color; increased respiratory effort, (nasal flaring, sternal retractions, stridor), restlessness. |

## Evaluation

| Steps | Rationale |
|---|---|
| 1. Assess client's response to administration of oxygen. Observe for improved color; decreased respiratory effort, i.e., decreased retractions, absence of stridor, absence of nasal flaring; decreased restlessness. | Determines if hypoxia is corrected or reduced. |
| 2. Inspect condition of oral and nasal mucosa. | Oxygen can cause drying of mucosa. |

### *Expected outcomes*

| Steps | Rationale |
|---|---|
| 1. Respirations normal, skin and mucosa pink. | Oxygen delivery system improves arterial oxygen. |
| 2. Increased level of consciousness. | Increased oxygenation improves level of consciousness. |
| 3. Improved airway clearance. | High humidity of oxygen delivery device increases moisturization and removal of airway secretions. |

### *Unexpected outcomes*

| Steps | Rationale |
|---|---|
| 1. Pediatric client experiences chilling, skin irritation from high humidity, drying oral and nasal mucous membranes. | Indicates adverse response to *method* of oxygen delivery. |
| 2. Infant under oxygen hood experiences bradycardia; peripheral cyanosis, indicating shift of blood from peripheral to central circulation. | Occurs when air supplied from oxygen hood is applied directly to infant's face. |
| 3. Continued hypoxia can result in anxiety related to worsening hypoxia, ineffective breathing patterns related to hypoxia or excessive oxygen administration, ineffective airway clearance related to decreased level of consciousness or increased airway secretions, decreased cardiac output related to effect of hypoxia or cardiopulmonary function. | Uncorrected hypoxia can result in cardiac dysrhythmias and death. As hypoxia worsens, work load of myocardium increases, but amount of oxygen available to myocardium decreases. Myocardial hypoxia can produce cardiac dysrhythmias and ischemia. Cardiac contractility decreases amount of cardiac output and delivery of oxygen to brain, resulting in confusion, decreased level of consciousness, or coma. |

## Recording and Reporting

| Steps | Rationale |
|---|---|
| 1. Record in nurses' notes at beginning and end of the nursing shift and include in the change-of-shift report the following: oxygen therapy; respiratory assessment findings; method of oxygen delivery, flow rate, client's response; any adverse reactions or side effects; change in physician's orders. | Documents correct oxygen therapy for client when nurse begins and concludes care. Provides immediate validation with nursing care plan and next nursing shift of exact method of oxygen delivery and client's response to therapy. |

## Follow-Up Activities

| Steps | Rationale |
|---|---|
| 1. Suction oral and tracheal airway if child unable to clear secretions. | Maintaining patent, secretion-free airway promotes oxygenation. |
| 2. Reinforce parent teaching, explain when oxygen therapy is necessary; why child should not be removed from therapy. | Decreases anxiety and reinforces to parents why they should not remove their child constantly from oxygen tent. |
| 3. Initiate discharge planning, with referrals to home care agencies and oxygen equipment suppliers. | Promotes smooth transition from hospital to home setting. |

## Special Considerations

- Have suction equipment at child's bedside (Chapter 16).
- Premature infants may require frequent changes in oxygen therapy.
- Temperature in Croupette or tent must be checked periodically to be certain it is at desired temperature.
- Loss of body heat can be significant in small infants if cool aerosol is used (Hazinski, 1984).
- Children requiring oxygen therapy frequently have rapid changes in physiologic status and oxygen requirements.
- Mist within tent should always be visible but may make visualizing child difficult. Thus, nurse must open tent to assess respiratory status. Since high humidity dampens child's bedding and clothing, they should be changed to avoid chilling, which would increase child's oxygen requirements (Hazinski, 1984; Whaley and Wong, 1987).
- Child requiring oxygen therapy is in respiratory distress, which increases oxygen requirements. Anxiety further increases oxygen requirements. Severely anxious children may be less frightened if they can see someone nearby and be reassured that they will not be left alone (Whaley and Wong, 1987).

### Teaching Considerations

- Discuss safety precautions for oxygen use (see Oxygen Safety Guidelines, p. 317).
- Nurse should stress to child's family that method of oxygen delivery is determined by concentration needed and by child's cooperative ability.
- Some toddlers or preschoolers may find oxygen tent less frightening if parents are encouraged to bring favorite bedtime toy or blanket to hospital.
- Review instructions for oxygen use with child's primary care giver.

### Home Care Considerations

- Home oxygen tents or Croupettes are used primarily for children with cystic fibrosis.
- Parents should demonstrate proper use of equipment to be used in the home:
  a. Maintain humidity and oxygen levels in the croupette.
  b. Check that oxygen mask, if being used, is situated over child's face and nose and has not slipped to other parts of the face.
  c. Cover child with blanket in Croupette.
  d. Select toys that retard absorption of oxygen, are washable, and easily cleaned for inside of the tent.
  e. Assess for oxygen toxicity.
  f. Wean from oxygen slowly with physician's orders.
  g. Check for tears in tent and maintain positive pressure with mist.

## *SKILL 14-6 Using Incentive Spirometry*

Incentive spirometry is a method of encouraging voluntary deep breathing by providing visual feedback to clients concerning their inspiratory volume. The two general types are flow-oriented and volume-oriented incentive spirometers.

Flow-oriented incentive spirometers consist of one or more plastic chambers that house freely movable, colored balls. The client is instructed to inhale briskly to elevate the balls and to keep them floating as long as possible. Clients need to be instructed that the goal is to keep the balls elevated for as long as possible to ensure maximal sustained inhalation, not to snap the balls to the top of the chamber with a rapid, very brief, low-volume breath. Even if a very slow inspiration does not elevate the balls, this pattern may achieve greater lung expansion (Luce, Tyler, and Pierson, 1984). The advantage of flow-oriented inspiratory spirometry is its low cost, but it does not determine the volume of inspiration.

Volume-oriented incentive spirometry devices have a bellows that is raised to a predetermined volume by an inhaled breath (Fig. 14-17). An achievement light or counter is used instead of a bellows in some devices. Some are constructed so the light will not turn on unless the bellows is held at a minimal desired volume for a specified period to enhance lung expansion. The advantage of volume-oriented incentive spirometry is that a known volume of inspiration can be maintained.

Incentive spirometry encourages clients to breathe to their normal inspiratory capacity. When this method is used with a postoperative client, it is helpful to know the client's preoperative inspiratory capacity. Because of postoperative pain, a postoperative inspiratory capacity one half to three quarters of the preoperative volume is acceptable (Luce, Tyler, and Pierson, 1984).

### Purposes

1. Prevent or treat atelectasis.
2. Improve lung expansion.
3. Improve oxygenation.

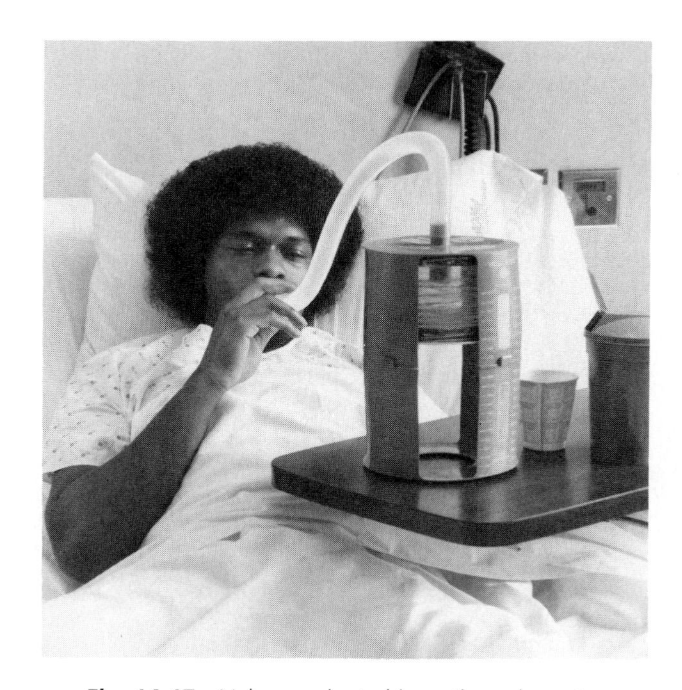

***Fig. 14-17*** Volume-oriented incentive spirometry.

## Procedure 14-6

| Steps | Rationale |
|---|---|
| **Assessment** | |
| 1. Identify clients who would benefit from incentive spirometry e.g., post-op clients, clients recovering from chest trauma, clients with pneumonia. | Alerts health care personnel to those clients at risk for respiratory complications during illness or postoperatively. |
| 2. Assess client's respiratory status: symmetry of chest wall expansion, respiratory rate and depth, production of sputum, lung sounds (Chapter 13). | Decreased symmetry in chest wall movement, increased respiratory rate, or increased sputum production can indicate need for incentive spirometry or other respiratory maneuvers to improve lung expansion. |
| 3. Review physician's order for incentive spirometry. | Health care institutions frequently require a medical order for incentive spirometry in order to receive third-party reimbursement. |
| **Nursing Diagnosis** | |
| 1. Cluster data to reveal actual or potential nursing diagnoses: | |
| a. Ineffective breathing pattern: related to pain. | Decreased lung expansion may be due to abdominal or thoracic incision. |
| b. Impaired gas exchange: related to retained secretions. | |
| c. Ineffective breathing pattern: related to decreased lung expansion. | Decreased lung expansion reduces amount of oxygen delivered to lungs and ultimately transferred to arterial blood. |
| **Planning** | |
| 1. Develop individualized goals for client based on nursing diagnoses: | |
| a. Increase lung expansion. | Increases amount of available oxygen to blood and improves clearance of pulmonary secretions. |
| b. Improve level of consciousness. | As more oxygen is available to bloodstream, cerebral tissues are less hypoxic. Unless decreased oxygen levels have caused cerebral ischemia, level of consciousness should improve. |
| c. Decrease or halt airway secretions. | Results in improved oxygen delivery to arterial blood. |
| 2. Obtain necessary equipment and place at bedside: | |
| a. Flow-oriented incentive spirometer | |
| b. Volume-oriented incentive spirometer | |
| 3. Identify learning objectives for preparing client to use incentive spirometer: correctly places mouthpiece; achieves satisfactory maximal inspiration; repeats maneuver the required number of times. | Successful incentive spirometry depends entirely on client's ability to learn how to use spirometer correctly. |
| **Implementation** | |
| 1. Wash hands. | Reduces transmission of microorganisms. |
| 2. Instruct client to assume semi-Fowler's or high Fowler's position. | Promotes optimal lung expansion during respiratory maneuver. |
| 3. Demonstrate to client how to place mouthpiece so that lips completely cover mouthpiece. | Demonstration is reliable technique for teaching psychomotor skill and enables client to ask questions. |
| 4. Instruct client to inhale slowly and maintain constant flow through unit. When maximal inspiration is reached, client should hold breath for 2-3 sec and then exhale slowly (Blodgett, 1980). | Maintains maximal inspiration and reduces risk of progressive collapse of individual alveoli. |
| 5. Instruct client to breathe normally for short period. | Prevents hyperventilation and fatigue (Blodgett, 1980). |
| 6. Have client repeat maneuver until goals are achieved. | Ensures correct use of spirometer. |
| 7. Wash hands. | Reduces transmission of microorganisms. |
| **Evaluation** | |
| 1. Assess respiratory status to determine client's response to incentive spirometry. | Determines client's ability to perform breathing exercise correctly. |

| Steps | Rationale |
|---|---|
| ***Expected outcomes*** | |
| 1. Client achieves target volume. | Promotes optimal lung expansion. |
| 2. Normal breath sounds and production of purulent sputum. | Alveoli open with clearance of airways. |
| 3. Client experiences absence of increased fatigue. | Client's tolerance should increase with continued use. |
| ***Unexpected outcomes*** | |
| 1. Inability to achieve incentive spirometry zone independently. | Client unable to achieve incentive spirometric volumes independently has decreased lung expansion and is at risk for retained pulmonary secretions. |
| 2. Abnormal breath sounds. | Indicates atelectasis and/or retained secretions. |
| **Recording and Reporting** | |
| 1. Record in nursing notes client's respiratory assessment before and after incentive spirometry, type of incentive spirometry used, any adverse effects. | Documents when and what type of treatment was received. Some agencies require such documentation for third-party reimbursements. |
| 2. Report to oncoming nursing personnel type of incentive spirometry, frequency ordered by physician, client's usual response to treatment. | Provides new nursing personnel with baseline information about therapy ordered and client's usual response. |
| **Follow-up Activities** | |
| 1. Consider use of IPPB (Skill 14-7) for clients who are unsuccessful at incentive spirometry. | IPPB therapy uses preset pressure to expand client's lungs. Client's inspiratory effort provides the stimulus for mechanical inflation of lungs. |
| 2. Reinforce incentive spirometry teaching in clients who are able to use this maneuver. | Reinforcement of prior learning assists client to perform activity correctly each time. |

### Special Considerations

- Clients benefiting from incentive spirometry include preoperative clients, especially before abdominal, cardiac, or orthopedic surgery; preoperative clients with history of smoking, pneumonia, or chronic respiratory disease; those with postoperative LeVeen Shunt to aid in removal of ascites; clients with atelectasis.
- Clients with flail chest require other respiratory maneuvers to correct asymmetric chest wall motion.
- Clients who may experience difficulty with incentive spirometry include those who are confused, malnourished, cognitively impaired, or who lack necessary motor skills.
- Use a nose clip if client is unable to breathe through the mouth piece.

### Teaching Considerations

- After incentive spirometer exercises, clients should practice cough control techniques (Chapter 15).
- Teach client to examine sputum for consistency, amount, and color changes.

### Home Care Considerations

- Have client return demonstrate correct procedure for use before discharge.
- Administer breathing treatments before client's meals to prevent occurrence of nausea and vomiting.

## *SKILL 14-7* ***Using Continuous Positive Airway Pressure***

Continuous positive airway pressure (CPAP) is the maintenance of a pressure above atmospheric pressure during the inspiratory and expiratory cycle in a client breathing spontaneously. CPAP prevents airway and alveolar collapse during the respiratory cycle and increases available surface area for oxygen transport, thus improving the client's level of oxygenation.

Clients with an adequate respiratory rate and tidal volume who are unable to adequately oxygenate as a result of some pathophysiologic problem can benefit from CPAP. Pathophysiologic problems include pneumonias, atelectases, respiratory failure, and sleep apnea. CPAP is also used in clients who are weaning by T-piece from mechanical ventilation as a means of preventing alveolar collapse and improving oxygenation during T-piece trials. CPAP can be administered via mask, endotracheal or tracheal tube, nasal mask, or nasal cannula (Fig. 14-18). CPAP via an endotracheal tube or tracheostomy tube is usually part of a weaning protocol and administered through the mechanical ventilator.

Clients may have a decreased venous return and subsequent fall in blood pressure as a result of increased intrathoracic pressure. Thus the cardiac output will decrease with a compensatory increase in heart rate. The nurse must be aware of the physiologic changes and monitor the client appropriately. After a few minutes on CPAP, thoracic pressures will equalize and the client's blood pressure and pulse will normalize.

CPAP is used in obesity hyperventilation syndrome via nasal mask or nasal cannula to prevent upper airway and soft palate collapse. Collapse of the soft palate results in periods of apnea, which may last from a few seconds to minutes. Low levels of CPAP (5 to 15 cm $H_2O$) act as a pneumatic splint holding the oropharyngeal airway open (Mims, 1988). CPAP is applied via a tight fitting nasal mask or nasal cannula, which is easily used and well tolerated by the client.

### Purposes

1. Prevent or treat atelectasis.
2. Improve oxygenation.
3. Improve lung expansion.
4. Prevent airway collapse.

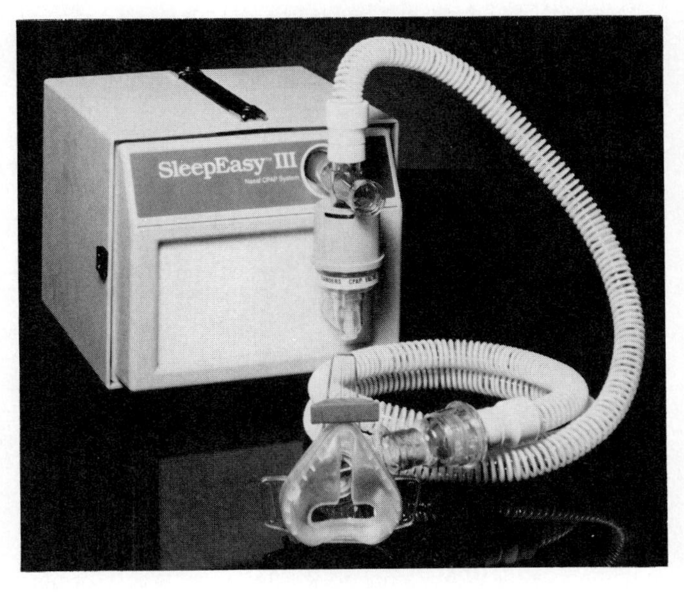


***Fig. 14-8***
Courtesy Puritan-Bennett Corp, Overland Park, Kan.

## *Procedure 14-7*

| Steps | Rationale |
|---|---|
| **Assessment** | |
| 1. Identify clients who would benefit from CPAP. | Alerts health personnel for respiration complications during illness. |
| 2. Assess client's respiratory status: chest wall expansion, spontaneous respiratory rate and tidal volume, lung sounds (Chapter 13). | Ensures client can tolerate CPAP adequately. Estimates baseline assessment data. |
| 3. Review physician's order for CPAP. | Medical order is required to administer CPAP to client. |
| **Nursing Diagnosis** | |
| 1. Cluster data to reveal actual or potential nursing diagnoses: | |
| a. Impaired gas exchange: related to alveolar hypoventilation. | Airway and alveolar collapse results in decreased surface area for gas exchange. |
| b. Impaired gas exchange: related to retained secretions. | |
| **Planning** | |
| 1. Develop individualized goals for client based on nursing diagnoses: | |
| a. Decrease or halt airway secretions. | Results in improved oxygen delivery to arterial blood. |
| b. Increase lung expansion. | Increases amount of available oxygen to blood and improves clearance of airway secretions. |
| 2. Obtain necessary equipment and place at bedside: a. Face mask b. CPAP valve c. Oxygen source d. CPAP generator (home use) | |
| 3. Identify learning objectives for preparing client for CPAP: correct application of mask, reason for CPAP, benefits of CPAP. | Assures client and family compliance. |

| Steps | Rationale |
|---|---|
| **Implementation** | |
| 1. Wash hands. | Reduces transmission of microorganisms. |
| 2. Position client in semi-Fowler's or high Fowler's position. | Promotes optimal lung expansion. |
| 3. Position face mask, nasal cannula, or nasal mask tightly. | Ensures maintenance of CPAP. |
| 4. Instruct client to breath normally. | Prevents hyperventilation and fatigue. |
| 5. Maintain CPAP for prescribed length of time. | |
| 6. Wash hands. | |
| **Evaluation** | |
| 1. Assess client's respiratory status to determine response to CPAP. | Determines oxygenation status and client's ventilatory capacity. |
| ***Expected outcomes*** | |
| 1. Client's arterial blood gases improve. | CPAP increases surface area for oxygen transport to alveoli. |
| 2. Client's periods of apnea while asleep are reduced. | |
| 3. Normal breath sounds, absence of abnormal breath sounds, production of purulent sputum. | CPAP prevents alveoli collapse. |
| ***Unexpected outcomes*** | |
| 1. Client has feeling of suffocation and shortness of breath. | Client may experience abnormal sensation from breathing against the CPAP valve. |
| 2. Client's arterial blood gases deteriorate. | Atelectasis or pneumonia worsen. |
| **Recording and Reporting** | |
| 1. Record in nurses' notes client's respiratory assessment before and after CPAP, amount of CPAP used, length of time on CPAP, any adverse effects. | Documents when and what type of treatment was received. |
| 2. Report to on-coming nursing personnel frequency of CPAP, client's tolerance for procedure, plan for continued CPAP. | Provides new nursing personnel with baseline information about therapy ordered and client's usual response. |
| **Follow Up Activities** | |
| 1. Reinforce proper use of CPAP setup. | Reinforces prior learning and assists client to perform activity correctly each time. |

## Special Considerations

- Client's initial feeling of breathlessness or suffocation from inspiring against the CPAP valve can be overcome with encouragement and client education.
- Teach client causes and treatment of obesity hypoventilation syndrome, if appropriate: weight loss, nutrition diet, effects on respiratory status.

## Teaching Considerations

- Teach client and family signs of hyperapnea: confusion, changes in level of consciousness (LOC), somnolence, headache.
- Teach signs and symptoms of respiratory infection: sputum color changes, fever, dyspnea.

## Home Care Considerations

- CPAP via nasal cannula and nasal mask is easily applied at home.
- Teach client and family members how to use home equipment.

# *SKILL 14-8 Using Intermittent Positive-Pressure Breathing*

Intermittent positive-pressure breathing (IPPB) devices assist lung hyperinflation by applying positive pressure to the airways. Hyperinflation depends on amount of pressure applied and on compliance of the chest wall. Clients with low compliance require higher IPPB pressures to achieve hyperinflation. Following the inspiration phase of the cycle, the machine automatically shuts off and passive exhalation occurs. The client's next inspiratory cycle triggers the machine to deliver the preset pressure.

Clients with respiratory muscle weakness, chest wall deformity, or thoracic or abdominal incisions are unable to take large inspiratory breaths voluntarily. These clients benefit from IPPB or incentive spirometry.

IPPB should not be used with semicomatose, restless, or confused clients. Because these clients are unable to cooperate fully, they are likely to swallow large volumes of air, leading to esophageal and gastric distention and often vomiting.

As with any procedure, potential complications with IPPB treatment exist. Nosocomial tracheobronchitis and pneumonia have been observed in some clients receiving IPPB therapy. The source of contamination in these cases was found to be the nebulizer, which adds humidification or medication to the inhaled gas (Luce, Tyler, and Pierson, 1984).

A second complication is barotrauma, a physical injury resulting from increased inhalation pressure. Barotrauma may occur with any procedure that distends the lung, but its incidence can be reduced if the pressure generated by an IPPB machine does not produce large volumes.

A third complication is respiratory alkalosis. This may occur if the IPPB machine is set to deliver rapid inspiration that is inappropriate for the client's normal breathing pattern.

Clients with COPD can develop psychologic dependence on IPPB. As a result, they do not use correct breathing exercises or coughing techniques but rely on IPPB to expand their lungs and mobilize secretions.

### Purposes

1. Improve lung expansion.
2. Improve oxygenation.
3. Prevent or relieve atelectasis.
4. Deliver aerosol medications to the lower airway.
5. Promote clearing of bronchial secretions.

## *Procedure 14-8*

| Steps | Rationale |
|---|---|
| **Assessment** | |
| 1. Identify clients who would benefit from IPPB therapy. | Alerts health personnel for respiratory complications during illness or postoperatively. |
| 2. Assess client's respiratory status: chest wall expansion, respiratory rate and depth, production of sputum, lung sounds. | May indicate need for IPPB therapy to improve lung expansion. |
| 3. Review client's medical record for physician's order for IPPB therapy. Typical order reads: frequency—qid; length of treatment—10-15 min; medication—saline 5 ml; pressure setting—10-20 cm $H_2O$. | Medical orders frequently are needed to receive third-party reimbursement. |
| **Nursing Diagnosis** | |
| 1. Cluster data to reveal actual or potential nursing diagnoses: | |
| a. Ineffective breathing pattern: related to pain. | Decreased lung expansion may be due to abdominal or thoracic incision. |
| b. Impaired gas exchange: related to retained secretions. | |
| c. Ineffective breathing pattern: related to decreased lung expansion. | Decreased lung expansion reduces amount of oxygen delivered to lungs and ultimately transferred to arterial blood. |
| **Planning** | |
| 1. Develop individualized goals for client based on nursing diagnoses: | |
| a. Increase lung expansion. | Increases amount of available oxygen to blood and improves clearance of pulmonary secretions. |
| b. Improve level of consciousness. | As more oxygen is available to bloodstream, cerebral tissues are less hypoxic. Unless decreased oxygen levels have caused cerebral ischemia, level of consciousness should improve. |
| c. Decrease or halt airway secretions. | Results in improved oxygen delivery to arterial blood. |
| 2. Obtain necessary equipment and place at client's bedside: | |
| a. Pressure-controlled ventilator | IPPB therapy requires that client achieve preset pressure to promote lung expansion. |
| b. Saline or prescribed inhalant medication | IPPB therapy should never be instituted without providing humidification, e.g., saline or medication to nebulizer; otherwise drying of airway secretions occurs. |

| Steps | Rationale |
|---|---|
| 3. Identify learning objectives for preparing client to use IPPB therapy: correctly places mouthpiece; achieves prescribed inspiratory pressure. | Success depends entirely on client's ability to learn use of IPPB correctly. |

## Implementation

| Steps | Rationale |
|---|---|
| 1. Wash hands. | Reduces transmission of microorganisms. |
| 2. Instruct client to assume semi-Fowler's or high Fowler's position. | Promotes optimal lung expansion during IPPB therapy. |
| 3. Demonstrate to client how to place mouthpiece so that lips entirely cover mouthpiece. | Demonstration is reliable technique for teaching psychomotor skill and enables client to ask questions. |
| 4. Determine that sensitivity is set at −1 or −2 cm water, and ensure that pressure setting is correct. | Very small respiratory effort should be needed to initiate ventilator cycle. |
| 5. Instruct that once ventilator inspiratory cycle has been initiated, client should cease inspiratory effort. | Allows pressure of ventilator to fill client's lungs to optimal volume. |
| 6. Encourage client to cough during and after treatment. | Removes airway secretions. |
| 7. Wash hands. | Reduces transmission of microorganisms. |

## Evaluation

| Steps | Rationale |
|---|---|
| 1. Assess client's respiratory status to determine response to IPPB therapy. Determine client's ability to participate actively in and to tolerate IPPB therapy. | Client participation and tolerance to therapy are essential to promote lung expansion. |

### *Expected outcomes*

| Steps | Rationale |
|---|---|
| 1. Client achieves target volume. | Promotes optimal lung expansion. |
| 2. Normal breath sounds, absence of abnormal lung sounds, production of purulent sputum. | IPPB prevents atelectasis. |

### *Unexpected outcomes*

| Steps | Rationale |
|---|---|
| 1. Sudden chest pain with tachypnea, tachycardia, hypotension, severe respiratory distress. | Signs and symptoms associated with barotrauma causing pneumothorax. Symptoms are result of atmospheric air entering pleural space, causing collapse of lung. |
| 2. Production of yellow, foul-smelling sputum frequently associated with fever and chills. | Associated with upper respiratory tract infection. If left untreated, can impair lung expansion and oxygenation. |

## Recording and Reporting

| Steps | Rationale |
|---|---|
| 1. Record in nurses' notes client's assessment before and after IPPB therapy, type of ventilator and medications used, any adverse effects. | Documents client's participation and tolerance to therapy. Documentation may be necessary for agencies to receive third-party reimbursement. |
| 2. Report to oncoming nursing personnel type of treatment, including medications; frequency of treatment; client's usual response. | Assists in providing oncoming nursing personnel with information to organize their care. |

## Follow-up Activities

| Steps | Rationale |
|---|---|
| 1. Prepare to assist with insertion of chest tube into pleural space if client has significant pneumothorax. | Allows air to be removed and promotes reexpansion of affected lung. |
| 2. Increase activities to mobilize secretions, e.g., postural drainage; percussion, vibration, and rib shaking; and controlled cough techniques (Chapter 15). | Removes media for bacterial growth from airways. |

## Special Considerations

- Clients benefiting from IPPB therapy include preoperative and postoperative clients; those with respiratory muscle weakness; those with congenital chest wall deformity; those requiring inhalation or aerosol medication.
- Clients with severe cognitive impairments may not be able to participate in IPPB therapy.
- Pressure-controlled ventilators include Bird Mark 7, Puritan-Bennett PR-2 (Fig. 14-19). Types of medication include saline, Bronchosol, Mucomyst.
- Mouthpiece is preferable to mask because clients feel less "closed in." These clients also may require nose clips to maintain proper airway pressures.
- Pressure initially is set low to allow client to adjust to ventilator.

- Some clients may require several practice sessions to complete IPPB therapy successfully.
- If client has abdominal or thoracic incision, splint incision with pillows during respiratory therapy and coughing exercises (Chapter 4).
- Presence of infection or barotrauma should be noted in nurses' notes at time they are observed and should be reported immediately to charge nurse and physician.

### Teaching Considerations

- Demonstrate proper assembly of equipment.
- Teach client proper care of equipment.
- Prevention of infection can be promoted by proper cleaning of IPPB equipment: rinsing nebulizer and mouthpiece after each use, cleansing tubing and humidifier daily.

### Home Care Considerations

- Evaluate client for side effects: dizziness, nausea and vomiting, rapid pulse rate, palpitations, or increased dyspnea.
- Evaluate use of hand-held nebulizers in conjunction with IPPB therapy to allow for documentation of volumes and delivery of medications.

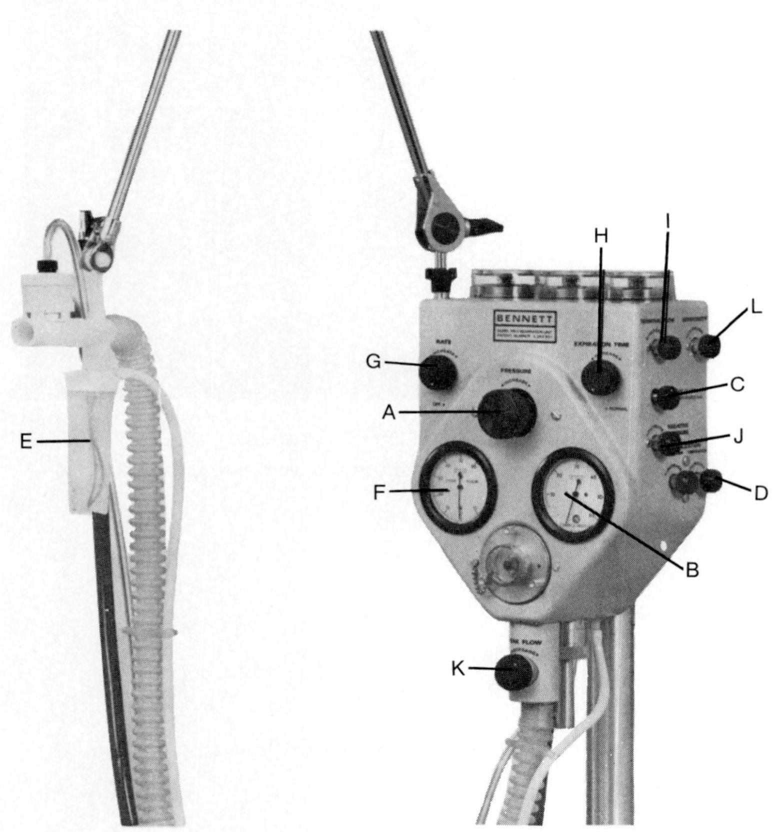


***Fig. 14-19*** Puritan-Bennett PR-2 ventilator. Turn knob *(A)* to adjust pressure recording on gauge *(B),* initially from 10 to 20 cm $H_2O$. Push knob *(C)* in for dilution; if 100% oxygen is desired, pull out. Turn inspiration nebulizer *(D)* slightly; adjust for proper mist. Add medication, if ordered, to nebulizer *(E).* Give IPPB treatment as instructed. On each inspiration, gauge *(F)* will rise to present pressure on gauge *(B).* For continuous operation on intubated patients, follow instructions for IPPB but use oxygen source to connect to ventilator. Turn on rate knob *(G),* and time cycle of ventilator. Be certain that expiration control *(H)* is at normal. Use spirometer and adjustable heated humidifier. Ensure that adequate ventilation is obtained when connected to patient.

From Glover DW, Glover MM: Respiratory therapy: basics for nursing and the allied health professions, St. Louis, 1978, The CV Mosby Co. Courtesy Puritan-Bennett Corp, Overland Park, Kan.

## *SKILL 14-9 Using Home Oxygen Equipment*

When home oxygen is required, it usually is delivered by a nasal cannula. When a client has a permanent tracheostomy, however, a T-tube or tracheostomy collar is necessary to deliver the oxygen. In the home the major consideration is the oxygen delivery source. Three types are used: compressed oxygen, liquid oxygen (Fig. 14-20), and oxygen concentrators (Fig. 14-21).

Compressed oxygen requires the delivery of several large oxygen tanks to the home. Each tank lasts approximately 50 hours at 2 L/min. Liquid systems use a small portable tank that is filled from a reservoir in the home. The oxygen concentrators extract oxygen from the room air and supply oxygen to the client at prescribed flow rates (Traver, 1982).

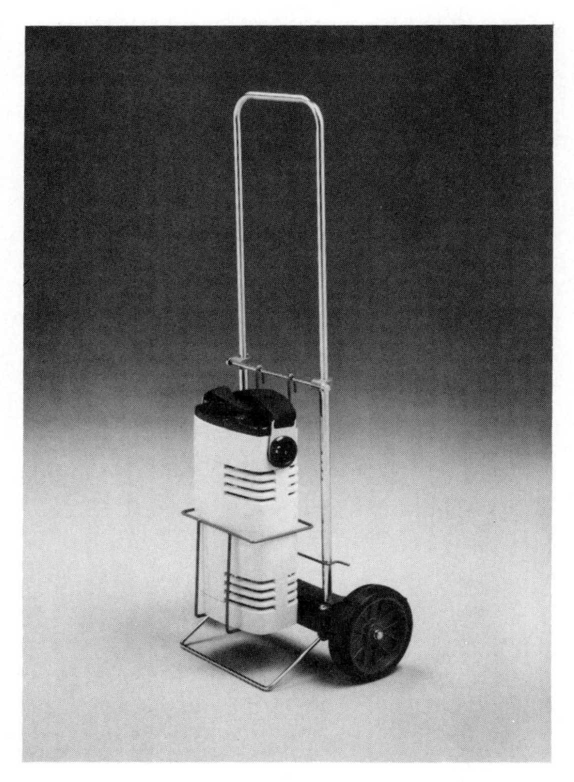

***Fig. 14-20*** Librator (Liquid oxygen).
Courtesy Cryogenic Associates, Indianapolis, Ind.

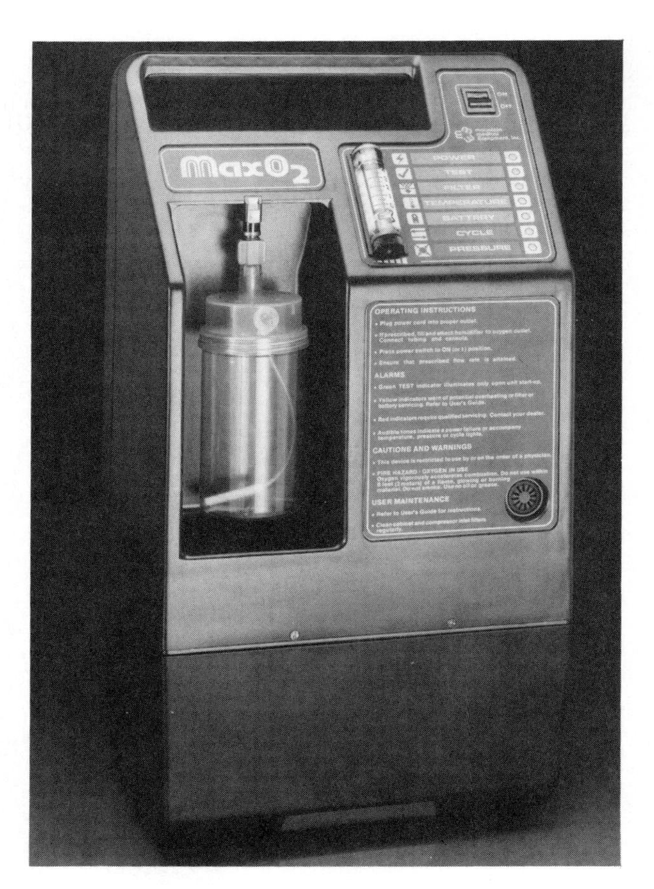


***Fig. 14-21*** Oxygen concentrator.
Courtesy Mountain Medical Equipment Inc, Littleton, Colo.

Clients requiring home oxygen need extensive teaching so that they can continue their oxygen therapy efficiently and safely. In preparation, the nurse must coordinate efforts between the client, primary nurse, visiting nurse, and home oxygen equipment vendor. Second, the nurse must set aside sufficient time for client and family teaching so that after discharge from the hospital, the client is confident in maintaining the oxygen delivery system.

## Purposes

1. Maintain tissue oxygenation.
2. Maintain independence.
3. Reduce cost of health care.
4. Allow client to return home.

## *Procedure 14-9*

| Steps | Rationale |
|---|---|
| **Assessment** | |
| 1. Determine client or family ability to use oxygen equipment correctly while in hospital, if possible, or assess for appropriate use of equipment in the home. | Physical or cognitive impairments may necessitate instructing family member or significant other how to operate home oxygen equipment. |
| 2. Assess client or family ability to observe for signs and symptoms of hypoxia: apprehension, anxiety, decreased ability to concentrate, decreased level of consciousness, increased fatigue, dizziness, behavioral changes, increased pulse, increased respiratory rate, pallor, cyanosis. | Hypoxia can occur at home when client uses oxygen. It can be caused by worsening of client's physical problem or another underlying condition, e.g., change in respiratory status. |

| Steps | Rationale |
|---|---|
| 3. Observe client or family use of prescribed oxygen therapy. | Enables nurse to determine specific components of skill that client or family can easily complete. |
| 4. Determine appropriate resource in the community for equipment and assistance. | Ensures repair service availability, readily available assistance, and additional equipment to clients with home oxygen. |
| **Nursing Diagnosis** | |
| 1. Cluster data to reveal actual or potential nursing diagnoses: | |
| a. Knowledge deficit regarding oxygen therapy: related to inexperience, lack of recall. | Nurse instructs client and family in home care techniques. |
| b. Knowledge deficit regarding oxygen therapy: related to cognitive limitation. | Special instructional methods may be needed. |
| **Planning** | |
| 1. Identify learning objectives for teaching plan. Client or family will be able to: state signs and symptoms of hypoxia and respiratory tract infections, state factors that affect oxygenation, correctly use prescribed oxygen delivery system, i.e., nasal cannula (Skill 14-1) or portable oxygen delivery system (Skill 14-8, Implementation). | Provides nurse with measurable criteria to determine client's or family's level of learning. |
| 2. Prepare needed equipment:<br>a. Nasal cannula (Skill 14-1)<br>b. Liberator and Stroller<br>▪ Nasal cannula<br>▪ Oxygen tubing<br>▪ In-home oxygen supply (Liberator)<br>▪ Portable system (Stroller) | Ensures that procedure is completed quickly and efficiently. |
| 3. Explain procedure to client and family. | Reinforces education received in the hospital. Enables client and family to ask questions. |
| **Implementation** | |
| 1. Wash hands. | Reduces transmission of microorganisms. |
| 2. Demonstrate steps for preparation and completion of oxygen therapy. | Demonstration is reliable technique for teaching psychomotor skill and enables client to ask questions. |
| 3. Prepare the Liberator Stroller for use: | |
| a. Place Liberator in a clutter-free environment (Fig. 14-22). | 30 L Liberator replaces 3.5 compressed oxygen cylinders. |
| b. Check oxygen levels of both Liberator and Stroller by depressing button at lower right corner and reading dial (Fig. 14-23). | Ensures timely and effective use of remaining oxygen supply and allows time for refill. |
| c. When necessary, refill Stroller: turn bayonet coupling lock on Stroller 45°. Insert female adapter (Liberator) to male adapter (Liberator) (Fig. 14-24). | Allows secure connection between Liberator and Stroller to prevent leakage of oxygen into room air. |
| d. Select prescribed rate. (Figure 14-25). | Ensures delivery of prescribed amount of oxygen. |
| e. Lock flowmeter. | Prevents client from changing oxygen flow rate. |

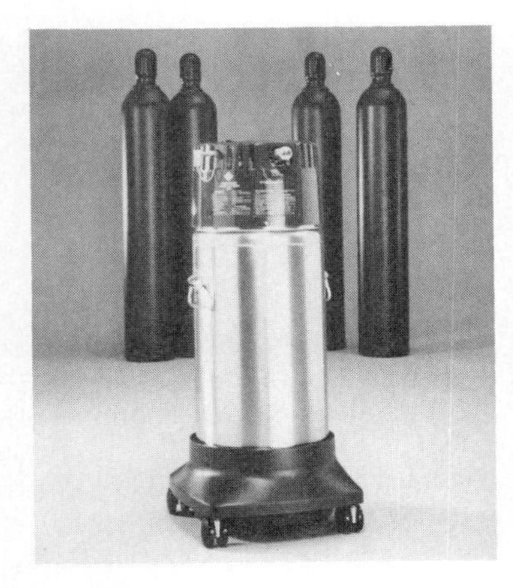

*Fig. 14-22*

Courtesy Cryogenic Associates, Indianapolis, Ind.

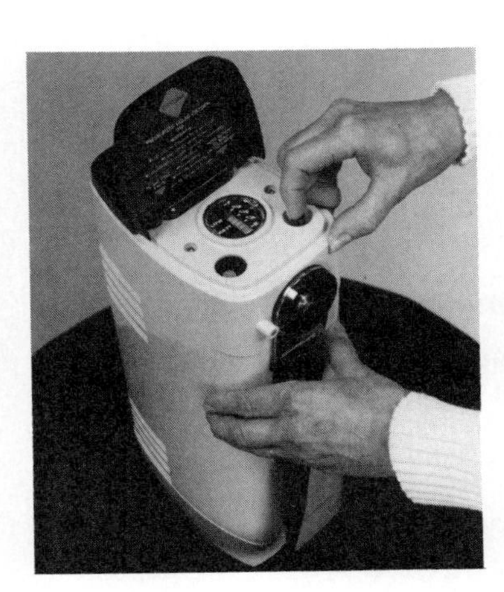

*Fig. 14-23*

Courtesy Cryogenic Associates, Indianapolis, Ind.

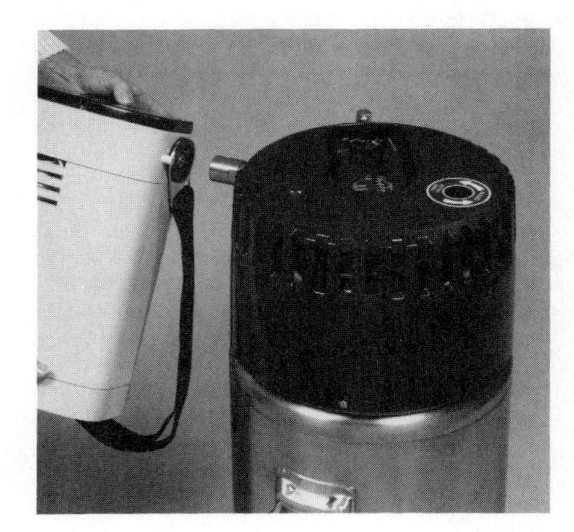

***Fig. 14-24***
Courtesy Cryogenic Associates, Indianapolis, Ind.

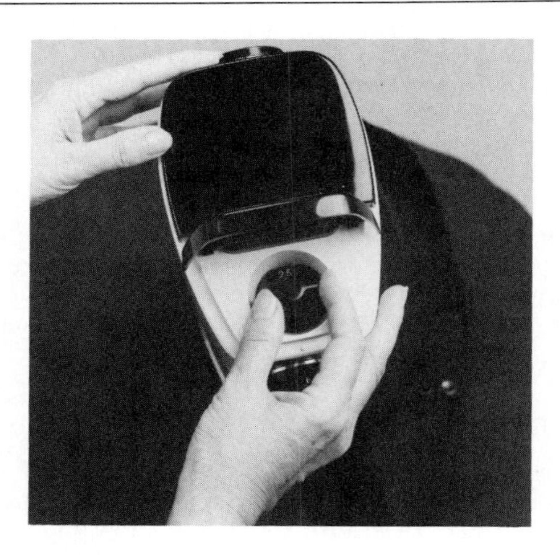

***Fig. 14-25***
Courtesy Cryogenic Associates, Indianapolis, Ind.

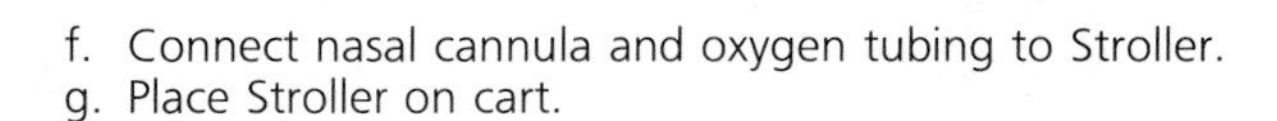

| Steps | Rationale |
|---|---|
| f. Connect nasal cannula and oxygen tubing to Stroller. | Connects oxygen source to delivery method. |
| g. Place Stroller on cart. | Allows client to ambulate freely without expending energy to carry Stroller. |
| 4. Have client or family perform each step with guidance from nurse. Provide written material for enforcement and review. | Allows nurse to correct any errors in technique and discuss their implications. |
| 5. Discuss signs and symptoms of respiratory tract infection: fever, increased sputum, change in color of sputum, foul sputum odor. | Respiratory tract infections increase oxygen demand and may affect oxygen transfer from lungs to blood. |
| 6. Instruct client or family to notify physician if signs or symptoms of hypoxia or respiratory tract infection occur. | Can prevent severe exacerbation of client's pulmonary disease. |
| 7. Wash hands. | Reduces transmission of microorganisms. |
| 8. Record teaching plan, information given to client, and validation of learning. | Provides written documentation of teaching plan for client and family. Documents client learning. |

## Evaluation

| Steps | Rationale |
|---|---|
| 1. Evaluate client's or family's ability to use oxygen at home. | Determines ability of client or family to deal with stressors associated with home oxygen use. Also indicates client's risk for inappropriate oxygen use. |

### *Expected outcomes*

| Steps | Rationale |
|---|---|
| 1. Client independently demonstrates oxygen therapy technique. | Feedback through independent demonstration of psychomotor skill is reliable method to evaluate learning. |
| 2. Client identifies signs and symptoms of hypoxia, factors affecting oxygenation, signs and symptoms of respiratory tract infection, when to notify physician. | Measures cognitive learning. |

### *Unexpected outcomes*

| Steps | Rationale |
|---|---|
| 1. Signs and symptoms associated with hypoxia (Assessment, Step 2). | Indicates inadequate oxygen delivery and can result from or lead to worsening of client's condition. |
| 2. Client uses unsafe practices with oxygen therapy, uses oxygen around fire, sets incorrect flow rate. | Indicates knowledge deficit regarding home oxygen. |

## Recording and Reporting

| Steps | Rationale |
|---|---|
| 1. Record in Kardex teaching plan preparations for teaching client to use home oxygen. | Provides written documentation for completing teaching plan for client or family. |
| 2. Record in nurses' notes information given to client or family and any validation of learning. | Documents client teaching in nurses' notes. |
| 3. Communicate client's or family's learning progress to other involved nursing personnel. | Provides continuing feedback to client regarding ability to independently use portable oxygen system. |

| Steps | Rationale |
|---|---|
| **Follow-up Activities** | |
| 1. Instruct client or family when to notify physician of signs of hypoxia. | Provides information to physician for changing oxygen prescription. |
| 2. Reinforce education, perform follow-up assessment when client returns home, make phone calls and health care referrals. | Provides opportunity to evaluate client's knowledge in home environment. |

## Special Considerations

- Equipment vendor and nurse should instruct client how frequently Liberator and Stroller must be filled. Small Liberator (Sprint) has 4 hr capacity, whereas 9.5 lb Stroller has 8 hr capacity. Refilling occurs automatically and takes a few sec to a min depending on amounts of oxygen required to fill stroller.
- Sprint has flow rate setting of 0.25, 0.5, 0.75, 1, 2, or 3 L/min. Standard Stroller has flow rate of 1, 1.5, 2, 2.5, 3, 4, or 6 L/min.
- Potential for oxygen desaturation and decreased oxygen delivery to brain impairs client's ability to remember previous learning. Thus nurse should provide more opportunity to reinforce previous learning into teaching plan.
- Some clients are able to manage portable oxygen system but are unable to fill their portable system and require assistance.
- Inform visiting nurse or home health agency of client's knowledge level at time of discharge.

## Teaching Considerations

- Instruct client to observe level of oxygen in cannister tanks and to use portable tanks when client is not at home.
- Instruct client to fill plastic humidity bottle with distilled water, every 24 hr. Tap water should *not* be used.
- Instruct client to test mask and tubing by placing hands or face over mask or cannula to feel air flow.
- Check to be sure mask is not too tight; it can leave marks on skin. Apply cotton or gauze sponge at pressure points.
- Instruct client to keep a bell handy for notifying primary care giver when help is needed.

## Home Care Considerations

- Provide two complete sets of tubing so that there is equipment for use while the other is being cleaned or repaired.
- Assess the home for availability of a three-pronged outlet for the compressor or the IPPB machine to prevent electric shock.
- Keep skin dry under mask, wash with soap and water. Nasal prongs can be cleaned by using moistened cotton applicator.
- Maintain constant flow rate, changing flow rate only with order of a physician.

# *SKILL 14-10 Administering Mechanical Ventilation*

Many clients require mechanical ventilation for support of respiration and oxygenation. Mechanical ventilation is used for clients with respiratory failure, chronic obstructive lung disease, neuromuscular diseases (such as Guillian-Barré), spinal cord trauma and respiratory muscle paralysis, as well as acute infectious processes such as pneumonia. The mechanical ventilator is a machine that applies positive pressure to the lungs to inflate them. Ventilators are available in pressure-cycled and volume-cycled types (Fig. 14-26). Pressure-cycled ventilators deliver a specified pressure to the client, achieving a tidal volume or amount of air per breath (see box). A volume-cycled ventilator delivers a specified tidal volume. Volume-cycled ventilators are most often used in the clinical setting. Clients using pressure-cycled ventilators are at more risk for development of pneumothorax, hypotension, and decreased cardiac output as a result of the ventilator's achieving the prescribed pressure without regard for lung compliance. Volume-cycled ventilators achieve tidal volume with pre-set pressure limits and are more sensitive to lung compliance.

| SYMBOL | | DEFINITION |
|---|---|---|
| $V_T$ | Tidal volume | Amount of air in ccs per breath |
| Rf or RR | Respiratory frequency<br>Respiratory rate | Number of breaths/min |
| $Fio_2$ | Fraction of inspired oxygen | Percent of inspired oxygen used |
| $V_E$ | Minute ventilation | Total amount of air moved per min, product of Rf × $V_T$ |
| A/C | Assist control | Mode of ventilation |
| IMV | Intermittent mandatory ventilation | Mode of ventilation |
| SIMV | Synchronized intermittent mandatory ventilation | Mode of ventilation |
| CMV | Continuous mechanical ventilation | Mode of ventilation |
| C | Control | Mode of ventilation |

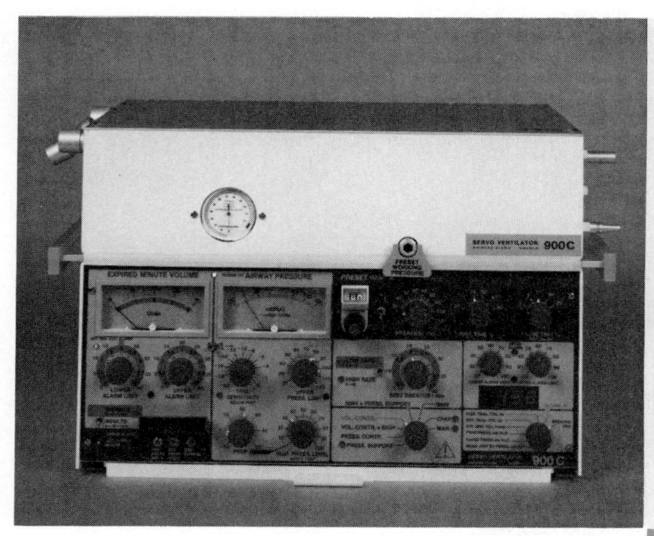


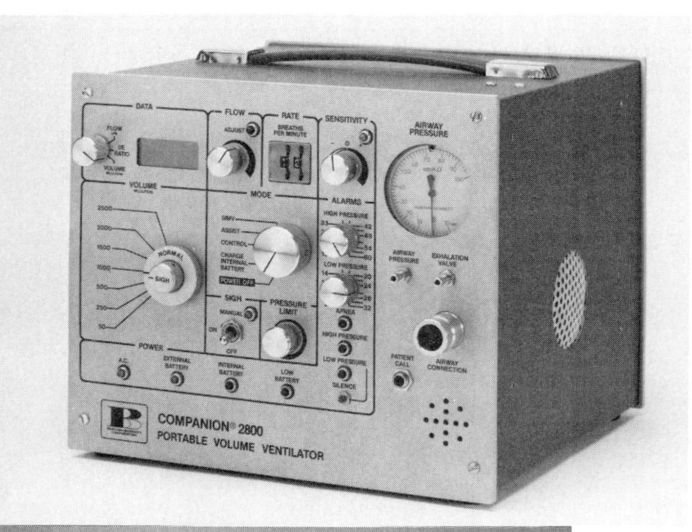


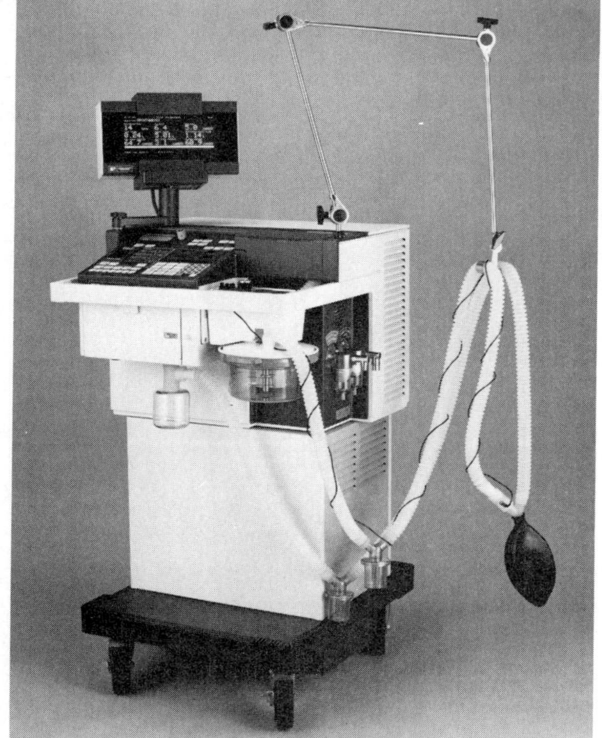

***Fig. 14-26***
Courtesy Puritan-Bennett Corp, Overland Park, Kan.

Mechanical ventilation provides the client with assistance in ventilation and precise levels of oxygenation. The client can be ventilated with assist/control (A/C) or continuous mechanical ventilation, control ventilation, intermittent mandatory (IMV) or synchronized intermittent mandatory (SIMV) ventilation, depending on the client's needs (see box).

Clients requiring acute mechanical ventilation are usually managed in the intensive care unit setting. The client will have an endotracheal tube or a tracheostomy tube. Many clients who are unable to wean from the mechanical ventilator are transferred to general nursing care divisions for their care or in preparation for home mechanical ventilation.

Mechanical ventilation for life support can be successfully managed in the home. Clients experiencing neuromuscular disease such as amyotrophic lateral sclerosis (ALS), muscular dystrophy, brain and spinal cord diseases, chest wall disease, central hypoventilation syndrome, and clients with advanced COPD are being managed at home on mechanical ventilators.

Many factors determine if a client and family are candi-

| VENTILATOR MODE | USES | VENTILATOR SETTINGS | ALARMS | CAUSES |
|---|---|---|---|---|
| Control | Pharmacologically paralyzed clients. Drug overdoses. | Preset tidal volume, preset respiratory rate. No spontaneous respirations. | High pressure alarm: indicates that high pressure limit has been exceeded. Low pressure alarm: indicates ventilator does not sense resistance to inspiration. | Pneumothorax, excessive secretions in airway, kink in ventilator tubing, client lying on ventilator tubing, decrease in client's lung compliance. Disconnection of ventilator from client, break in ventilator circuitry, Loose connection in circuit. |
| Assist/Control (A/C) | Allows clients to rest, improves minute ventilation, improves muscle fatigue. | Preset tidal volume, preset respiratory rate; spontaneous respiration at preset tidal volume. | | |
| Intermittent mandatory ventilation (IMV) or synchronized intermittent mandatory ventilation (SIMV) | Allows client to breath spontaneously between ventilator breaths, exercises respiratory muscles; used to wean from mechanical ventilator. | Preset tidal volume, preset respiratory rate; spontaneous respirations at client's own tidal volume. | | |

dates for home ventilation. Assessment criteria include: desire of the client and family, client's acceptance of ventilator dependence, client and family's ability to understand and perform daily care procedures, the home environment, personnel resources, monetary resources, and resources and technologies for support in the community (O'Donahue, 1986).

The goals of long-term ventilator care should include extension of life, enhancement of the quality of life, providing an environment that enhances individual potential, reduction of morbidity, improving physical and physiologic function and cost effectiveness (O'Donahue, 1986).

Clients and families who are candidates for home mechanical ventilation should be prepared for discharge by a multidisciplinary team including: nursing, medicine, dietary, social service, the home health nurse, and the home care durable medical equipment company. The nurse in the hospital must be familiar with the home ventilator to assist the client with discharge planning and education.

### Purposes

1. Improve oxygenation.
2. Improve ventilation.
3. Support respiration in clients unable to do so without assistance.
4. Protect and maintain an adequate airway.

## *Procedure 14-10*

| Steps | Rationale |
|---|---|
| **Assessment** | |
| 1. Observe for signs and symptoms associated with hypoxia: apprehension, anxiety, decreased ability to concentrate, decreased level of consciousness, increased fatigue, dizziness, behavioral changes, increased pulse rate, increased rate and depth of respiration, elevated blood pressure, cardiac dysrhythmias, pallor, cyanosis, clubbing, dyspnea. | Hypoxia is insufficient amount of oxygen available to tissues and cells to meet their metabolic needs. Left untreated, hypoxia is life-threatening and can produce cardiac dysrhythmias and death. |
| 2. Observe for patent airway and remove airway secretions. | Airway secretions can decrease the delivery of oxygen. |
| 3. If available, note client's most recent ABG results. | ABGs objectively document hypoxemia and need for supplemental oxygen and measure effect of therapy (Chapter 46). |

| Steps | Rationale |
|---|---|
| 4. Review medical order for mechanical ventilation and ventilator settings. | Oxygen is a drug and requires a physician's order. |
| 5. Complete total respiratory system assessment (Chapter 13). | Determines presence of respiratory abnormalities that could impede oxygenation. |

## Nursing Diagnosis

| Steps | Rationale |
|---|---|
| 1. Cluster data to reveal actual or potential nursing diagnoses: | |
| a. Impaired gas exchange: related to alveolar hypoventilation. | Decreased respiratory drive and decreased ventilatory effort lead to decreased gas exchange at the alveolar level. |
| b. Impaired gas exchange: related to decreased level of consciousness. | Decreased level of consciousness decreases rate and depth of respiration, diminishing amount of oxygen inspired and transported to tissues and cells. |
| c. Impaired gas exchange: related to retained airway secretions. | Airway secretions decrease surface area available for transfer of oxygen from alveoli to arterial blood supply. In addition, airway secretions provide excellent medium for bacterial growth and subsequent respiratory tract infection. |
| d. Ineffective breathing pattern: related to respiratory muscle fatigue and decreased respiratory mechanics. | Decreased ventilation leads to rising $Pa_{CO_2}$. Neuromuscular disease resulting in decreased ventilatory muscle function results in respiratory muscle fatigue. |

## Planning

| Steps | Rationale |
|---|---|
| 1. Develop individualized goals for client based on nursing diagnoses: | |
| a. Increase lung expansion, ventilation. | Increases amount of available oxygen to blood and improves clearance of pulmonary secretions. |
| b. Improve level of consciousness. | As more oxygen is available to bloodstream, cerebral tissues are less hypoxic. Unless decreased oxygen levels have caused cerebral ischemia, level of consciousness should improve. |
| c. Decrease or halt airway secretions. | Results in improved oxygen delivery to arterial blood. |
| 2. Obtain necessary equipment:<br>a. Appropriate mechanical ventilator<br>b. Oxygen source<br>c. Flow meter setup | Respiratory therapy may assist with the equipment and setup. |
| 3. Explain to client and others the purpose of mechanical ventilation. | Decreases anxiety and oxygen consumption and increases cooperation. |
| 4. Place "oxygen in use" and "no smoking" signs at entrance to client's room and over head of bed. | Provides client and staff safety while oxygen is in use. Oxygen is combustible and can fuel fire, even from cigarette sparks. |

## Implementation

| Steps | Rationale |
|---|---|
| 1. Wash hands. | Reduces transmission of microorganisms. |
| 2. Attach mechanical ventilator to endotracheal tube or tracheostomy tube. | Provides mechanical ventilation for client. |
| 3. Observe for proper functioning of mechanical ventilator. | Ensures equipment is working. |
| 4. Observe client for anxiety and respiration in synchronization with mechanical ventilation. | Ensures client is comfortable on ventilator. |
| 5. Monitor heart rate, blood pressure, and respiratory rate. | Implementation of mechanical ventilation can result in decreased venous return. |
| 6. Secure ventilator tubing to reduce pull on tracheostomy or endotracheal tube. | Prevents accidental dislodging of artificial airway. |
| 7. Encourage physician to obtain ABGs 20 min after initiation of therapy or change in ventilator setting. | ABGs provide objective data regarding oxygenation and ventilation. |
| 8. Check physician orders every 2-4 hr. | Provides mechanism for identifying new orders. |
| 9. Wash hands. | Reduces transmission of microorganisms. |

## Evaluation

| Steps | Rationale |
|---|---|
| 1. Evaluate client's response to mechanical ventilation. Observe for decreased anxiety; improved level of consciousness and cognitive abilities; decreased fatigue; absence of dizziness; decreased pulse, regular rhythm; decreased respiratory rate; return to normal blood pressure; improved color. | Hypoxia is corrected or reduced. |
| 2. Observe integrity of client ventilator system. | Ensures adequate delivery of mechanical ventilation. |

| Steps | Rationale |
|---|---|
| ***Expected outcomes*** | |
| 1. Client experiences reduction in feelings of dyspnea. | Ventilator providing adequate minute ventilation. |
| 2. Client experiences improved oxygenation and ventilation as evidenced by ABG results. | ABGs provide objective data to effectiveness of mechanical ventilation. |
| ***Unexpected outcomes*** | |
| 1. Client experiences stiff, noncompliant lung, alveolar edema, pulmonary congestion, chest pain, intra-alveolar hemorrhage, substernal chest pain. | Signs and symptoms of *oxygen toxicity.* Physician should be notified at once. |
| 2. Continued hypoxia can result in anxiety related to worsening hypoxia, ineffective breathing patterns related to hypoxia or excessive oxygen administration, ineffective airway clearance related to decreased level of consciousness or increased airway secretions, decreased cardiac output related to effect of hypoxia on cardiopulmonary function. | Uncorrected hypoxia can result in cardiac dysrhythmias and death. As hypoxia worsens, work load of myocardium increases, but amount of oxygen available to myocardium decreases. Myocardial hypoxia can produce cardiac dysrhythmias and ischemia. Cardiac contractility decreases amount of cardiac output and delivery of oxygen to brain, resulting in confusion, decreased level of consciousness, or coma. |
| **Recording and Reporting** | |
| 1. Record in nurses' notes at the beginning and end of the nursing shift and include in the change-of-shift report the following: oxygen therapy; respiratory assessment findings; method of oxygen delivery, flow rate, client's response; any adverse reactions or side effects; change in physician's orders. | Documents correct oxygen therapy for client when nurse begins and concludes care. Provides immediate validation with nursing care plan and next nursing shift of exact method of oxygen delivery and client's response to therapy. |
| **Follow Up Activities** | |
| 1. See Skills 16-5 and 16-6 ET Tube Care and Tracheostomy Care. | Promotes maintenance of adequate airway. |
| 2. See Skill 16-7, Managing Artificial Airway Cuff. | |

## Special Considerations

- Clients need a period of adjustment to be comfortable on mechanical ventilation.
- Frequent visits by the nurse and quick responses to call bells will help alleviate fears.
- Frequent airway care is necessary to prevent clogging of artificial airway with secretions.
- Before turning client, empty water that has accumulated in the ventilator tubing to prevent accidental dumping of water into airway. Empty water away from ventilator cascade.
- Secure ventilator tubing to prevent pulling and subsequent irritation to artificial airway.
- Frequent airway care is important especially when the endotracheal tube is in place.
- Repositioning may result in increased secretions and require more frequent suctioning.

## Teaching Considerations

- Client should understand rationale for mechanical ventilation.
- Client should be able to identify signs and symptoms of hypoxia.
- Teach client and primary care giver about equipment and how to use suction and oxygen if needed.
- Instruct client and primary care giver on what to do in case of respiratory distress or power failure. Check to determine availability of emergency batteries.
- Instruct on use of AMBU bag.
- Instruct on assessing airway, clean and suction tracheostomy tube.

## Home Care Considerations

- Clients requiring home mechanical ventilation need to be taught complete care of the mechanical ventilator system, suctioning, and artificial airway care.
- Skills should include how to assemble the ventilator circuit, cleaning of the circuit, and daily equipment maintenance.
- Client and family should have thorough knowledge of the operation of the home ventilator, the knobs and settings, and power sources.
- Use a checklist for ensuring consistency of care of client on ventilator.
- Evaluate the following areas during each visit: oxygen flow, alarm system, inspiratory pressure, high pressure alarm, tidal volume set, humidifier, respiratory rate, tubing, temperature, resusitation bag, tracheostomy care, breath sounds, suctioning, and tubing changes.
- The durable medical equipment provider, home health nurse, and primary care nurse should develop a teaching plan to ensure that client and family have a complete working knowledge of the ventilator before discharge.

## BIBLIOGRAPHY


Ayres SM, Schlichtig R, Sterling MJ: Care of the critically ill, Chicago, 1988, Yearbook Medical Publishers Inc.

Blodgett D: Manual of respiratory care procedures, Philadelphia, 1980, JB Lippincott Co.

Carroll P: Home care for the ventilator patient, Nursing '87 17(10):82, 1987.

Effland E: Teaching the ABC's of COPD, Nursing '87 17(1):61, 1987.

Fuchs P: Getting the best out of oxygen delivery systems, Nursing '80, 10(12):34, 1980.

Fireman P, et al.: Teaching self-management skills to asthmatic children and their parents in an ambulatory care setting, Pediatrics 68(3):341, 1981.

Glassanos MR: Infants who are oxygen dependent: sending them home, Am J Matern Child Nurs 5(1):42, 1980.

Glover DW, Glover MM: Respiratory therapy: basics for nursing and the allied health professions, St. Louis, 1978, The CV Mosby Co.

Golden S: Nursing a loved one at home, Philadelphia, 1988, Running Press Book Publishers.

Harper RA: A Guide to Respiratory Care: physiology and clinical applications, Philadelphia, 1981, JB Lippincott Co.

Hazinski MF: Nursing care of the critically ill child, St. Louis, 1984, The CV Mosby Co.

Kim MJ, McFarland GK, McLane AM: Pocket guide to nursing diagnosis, ed 2, 1987, St. Louis, The CV Mosby Co.

Luce JM, Tyler ML, Pierson DJ: Intensive respiratory care, Philadelphia, 1984, WB Saunders Co.

Mims BC: Advances in suctioning and airway care, Lewisville, Texas, 1988.

O'Donahue, WJ: Long-term mechanical ventilation, Chest 90(suppl 1): 1986.

Openbrier DR, et al.: Home oxygen therapy, Am J Nurs 192(7):198, 1988.

Potter PA, Perry AG: Fundamentals of nursing: concepts, process, and practice, ed 2, St. Louis, 1989, The CV Mosby Co.

Scipien G, et al.: Comprehensive pediatric nursing, New York, 1986, McGraw-Hill Book Co.

Shapiro BA, Harrison RA, Trent CA: Clinical application of respiratory care, Chicago, 1975, Yearbook Medical Publishers, Inc.

Traver GH, ed: Respiratory nursing, the science and the art, New York, 1982, John Wiley & Sons, Inc.

Wade JF: Respiratory nursing care: physiology and techniques, ed 3, St. Louis, 1981, The CV Mosby Co.

Walsh J, Persons C, Wieck L: Manual of Home Health Care Nursing, Philadelphia, 1987, JB Lippincott Co.

West JB: Respiratory physiology—the essentials, ed 2, Baltimore, 1979, Williams & Wilkins.

Whaley LF, Wong DL: Nursing care of infants and children, ed 3, St. Louis, 1987, The CV Mosby Co.

White KD, Perez PW: Your ventilator patient can go home again, Nursing '86 16:57, December, 1986.

Winters E: Monitoring ventilator patients for complications, Nursing '88, 18(6):38, 1988.

# 15

# PERFORMING CHEST PHYSIOTHERAPY

## OBJECTIVES

*Mastery of content in this chapter will enable the nurse to:*

- Define key terms.
- Assess the need to perform chest physiotherapy (CPT) maneuvers, including indications and physical assessment.
- Assess the need to modify or discontinue CPT maneuvers, including contraindications and individual variations.
- Explain how to prepare the client, family, nurse, and therapist for performance of each CPT maneuver.
- Identify goals for performing each CPT maneuver.
- Perform in a step-by-step method the outlined CPT maneuvers, including standard and modified versions.
- Describe expected and unexpected outcomes of each CPT maneuver.
- Document clearly and concisely assessment, planning, implementations, and evaluation of CPT maneuvers.
- Describe discharge teaching and planning related to use of each CPT maneuver in the home setting.

## KEY TERMS

*Chest physiotherapy*
*Cough*
*Mucociliary transport*
*Percussion*
*Postural drainage*
*Rib shaking*
*Rib vibration*

## SKILLS

**15-1** Performing Postural Drainage
**15-2** Performing Percussion, Vibration, and Rib Shaking
**15-3** Using Controlled Coughing Techniques

Chest physiotherapy (CPT) consists of physical maneuvers such as cough, chest wall percussion, vibration, rib shaking, and postural drainage. These maneuvers improve airway clearance of mucus in clients with retained tracheobronchial secretions. Diseases associated with accumulation of excessive mucus in the tracheobronchial tree include atelectasis, bronchitis, asthma, cystic fibrosis, and bronchiectasis. CPT is often used with other therapeutic modalities, including antibiotic therapy, avoidance of specific airway irritants, smoking cessation, bronchodilator treatment, aerosol therapy, and systemic hydration, to reduce mucus production and facilitate airway clearance. The goal is to reduce and prevent further airway obstruction and ventilatory dysfunction.

The precise mechanism by which CPT maneuvers enhance clearance of airway secretions is not fully understood. In general, they are designed to facilitate movement of secretions from smaller peripheral airways into larger central airways, where cough and suctioning are effective in removing them. Postural drainage involves placing the client in different positions to use gravitational forces for moving mucus from specific bronchi into the trachea. Exactly how externally applied forces of percussion, rib shaking, and vibration are transmitted to the airways to move secretions in a cephalad direction is unclear. Cough is a natural lung clearance mechanism that aids in removal of mobilized secretions. Coughing forcefully exhales air, providing clearance of mucus primarily from the large central airways, including the trachea and mainstem bronchi.

When disease causes excessive sputum production, therapeutic interventions are needed to help natural airway clearance mechanisms (cough and mucociliary transport) clear the airways of obstructing mucus. In the normal lung the mucociliary transport system is able to keep the airways clear of excessive mucus and inhaled particles. This system lines the internal lumen of the entire tracheobronchial tree and consists of a thin layer of mucus that is constantly being propelled toward the larynx by cells that have hairlike projections called cilia. Inhaled particles are trapped on the mucus, and the cilia act as a conveyor belt to sweep the mucus toward the throat, where it can be swallowed or removed by coughing. In this way, airways normally remain clear and mucus is constantly being cleared almost as fast as it is made. Normal mucus remains thin, white, and watery.

In various disease states, mucus clearance slows down or the cilia are overwhelmed by production of excessively large quantities of mucus. The lung can no longer clear the mucus as fast as it is made. Secretions stagnate in the airways, change color, and become thick, sticky, and tenacious. The cilia can not remove large amounts of thick mucus from the lungs. In addition, many people with lung disease cannot cough effectively to clear airways. Therefore it becomes important to employ systemic hydration and other maneuvers to aid in clearing lung secretions as fast as they are made. These therapeutic modalities prevent mucus from stagnating and allow secretions to return to their normal thin, white, and watery consistency.

Fluids are an important part of a lung clearance program. They make the mucus thin and watery so it can be mobilized, coughed up, and expectorated more easily. Unless contraindicated by other disease states, such as congestive heart failure or renal failure, fluids should be given along with CPT until mucus becomes thin and watery. During an acute exacerbation, it often takes three or four CPT treatments a day and 2.88 to 3.84 liters of fluid a day to mobilize and thin secretions. During more stable states, one to two CPT treatments and 1.92 to 3.84 liters of fluid a day can often keep secretions thin and watery, thereby preventing stagnation of mucus, which can lead to airway infection, airway obstruction, shortness of breath, increased work of breathing, and abnormal gas exchange.

This chapter presents three CPT skills as they are implemented in the clinical and home setting. Although they are separate skills, they must be thought of as different components of one CPT treatment. All must be mastered if treatment is to be effective.

## GUIDELINES

The nurse plans the client's care and subsequent selection of CPT skills on specific assessment findings. The following guidelines help the nurse in physical assessment and subsequent decision making:

1. Know client's normal range of vital signs. Conditions such as atelectasis and pneumonia requiring CPT can affect a client's vital signs. The degree of change is related to the level of hypoxia, overall cardiopulmonary status, and tolerance to activity.
2. Know client's present medications. Certain medications, particularly diuretics and antihypertensives, cause fluid and hemodynamic changes. These changes may decrease the client's tolerance to the positional changes of postural drainage. Steroid medications increase the client's risk of pathologic rib fractures and often contraindicate rib shaking.
3. Know client's medical history. Certain conditions, such as increased intracranial pressure, spinal cord injuries, or abdominal aneurysm resection, contraindicate the positional changes of postural drainage. Thoracic trauma or surgery also may contraindicate percussion, vibration, and rib shaking.
4. Know client's level of cognitive function. Participation in controlled cough techniques requires the client to understand and follow instructions. Congenital or acquired cognitive limitations may alter the client's ability to learn and to participate in these techniques.
5. Be aware of client's exercise tolerance. CPT maneuvers are fatiguing. When the client is not used to physical activity, initial tolerance to the maneuvers may be decreased. However, with gradual increases in activity and planned CPT, the client's tolerance to the procedure improves.

## PREREQUISITE KNOWLEDGE

1. Anatomy of the tracheobronchial tree (Fig. 15-1) and thoracic cage.
2. Postural drainage positions (Table 15-1).
3. Knowledge of body mechanics.
4. Teaching-learning process.

## PREREQUISITE SKILLS

1. Comfort measures (Chapter 5).
2. Physical assessment (Chapter 13).
3. Proper positioning techniques (Chapter 33).
4. Proper handwashing techniques (Chapter 37).

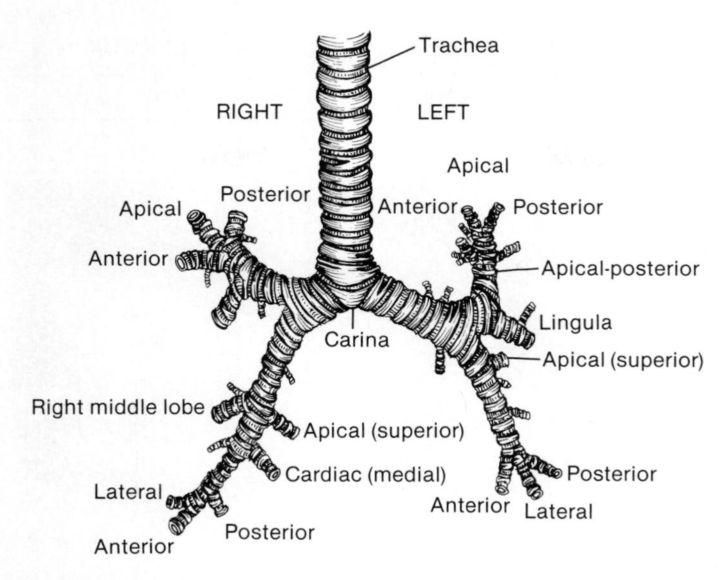


***Fig. 15-1*** Tracheobronchial tree.
Redrawn from Frownfelter DL, ed: Chest physical therapy and pulmonary rehabilitation, Chicago, 1978, Year Book Medical Publishers, Inc.

***TABLE 15-1*** Positions and Procedures for Drainage, Percussion, and Vibration

| Area and Procedure | Percussion | Vibration | Bronchial Lobe |
|---|---|---|---|
| **Left and Right Upper Lobe Anterior Apical Bronchi**<br>Have client sit in chair, leaning back. Percuss and vibrate with heel of hands at shoulders and fingers, over collarbones (clavicles) in front; can do both sides at same time. Note body posture and arm position of nurse. Nurse's back is kept straight, and elbows and knees are slightly flexed. | 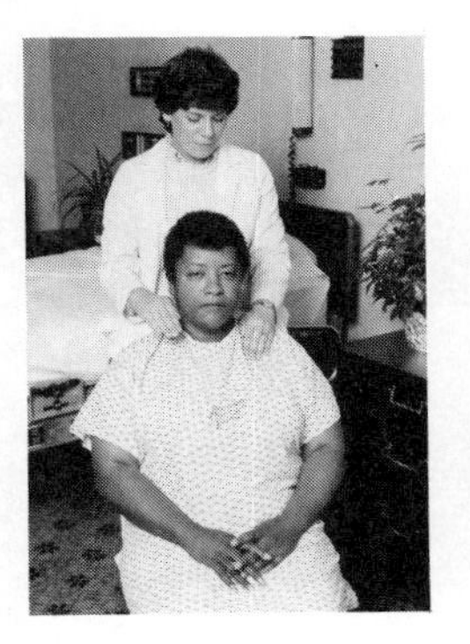 | 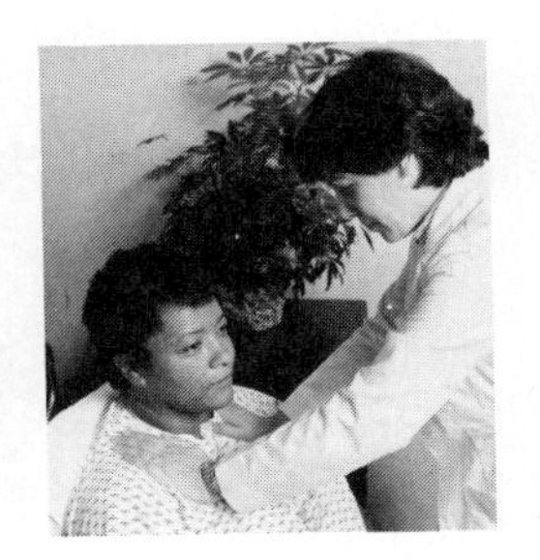 | 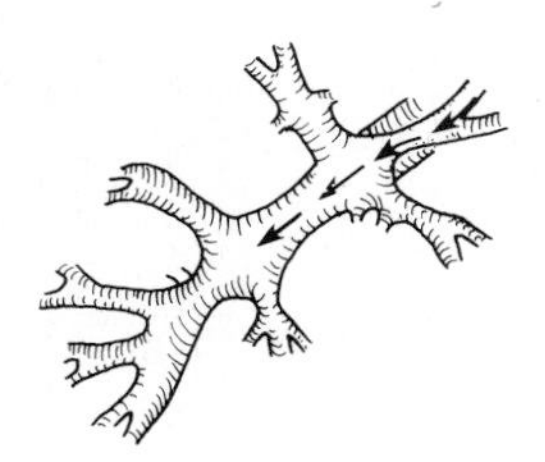 |
| **Left and Right Upper Lobe Posterior Apical Bronchi**<br>Have client sit in chair, leaning forward on pillow or table. Percuss and vibrate with hands on either side of upper spine. Can do both sides at same time. | 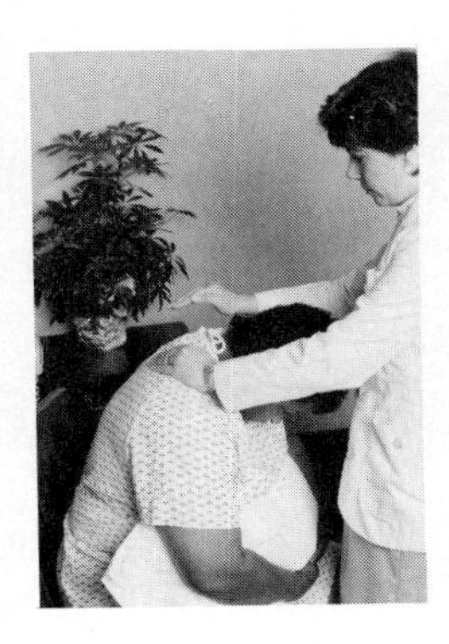 | 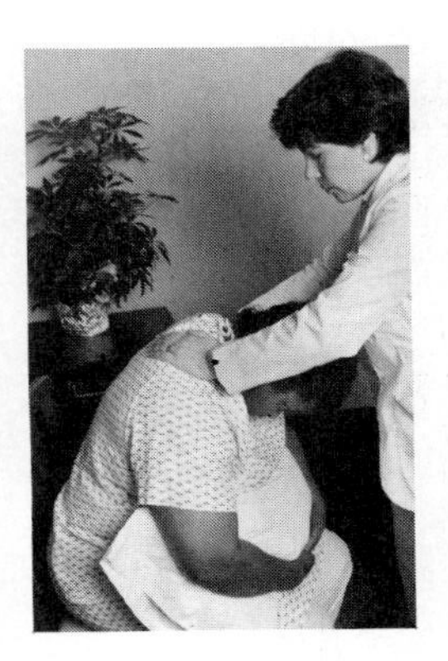 | 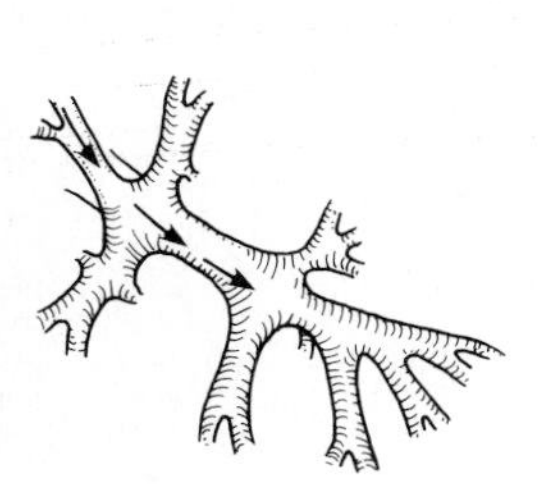 |

*Continued.*

***TABLE 15-1, cont'd*** Positions and Procedures for Drainage, Percussion, and Vibration

| Area and Procedure | Percussion | Vibration | Bronchial Lobe |
|---|---|---|---|
| **Right and Left Anterior Upper Lobe Bronchi** Have client lie flat on back with small pillow under knees. Percuss and vibrate just below clavicle on either side of sternum. | 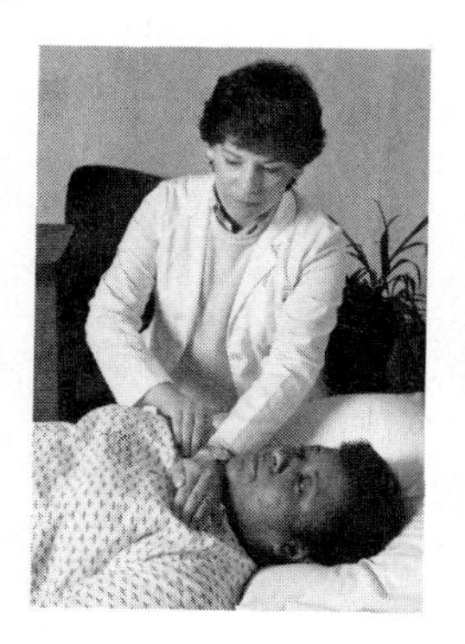 | 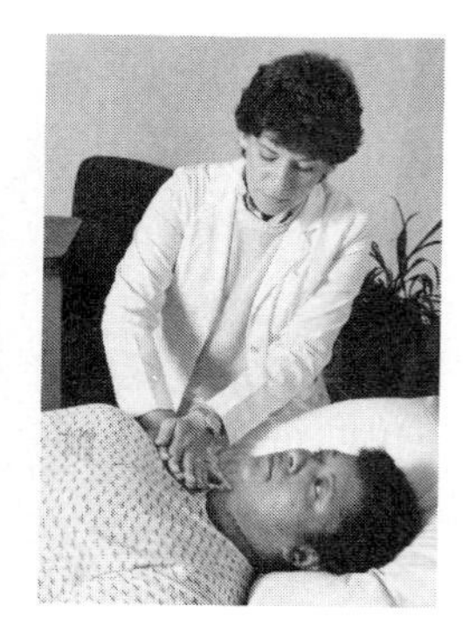 | 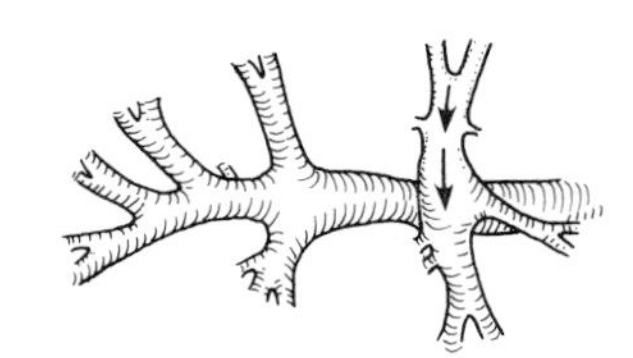 |
| **Left Upper Lobe Lingular Bronchus** Have client lie on right side with arm over head in Trendelenburg position, with foot of bed raised 30 cm (12 in). Place pillow behind back, and roll client one-fourth turn onto pillow. Percuss and vibrate lateral to left nipple below axilla. | 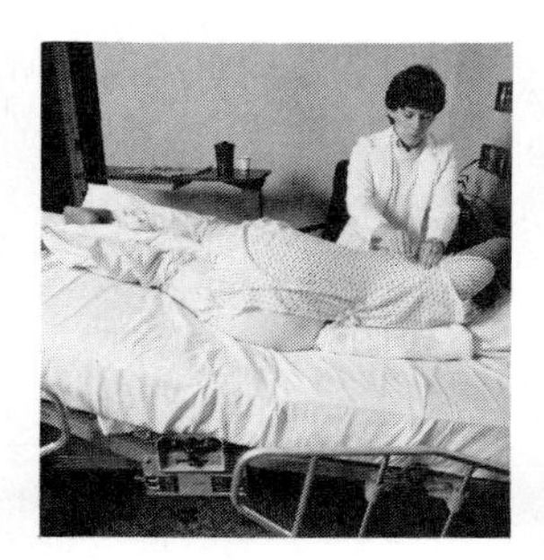 | 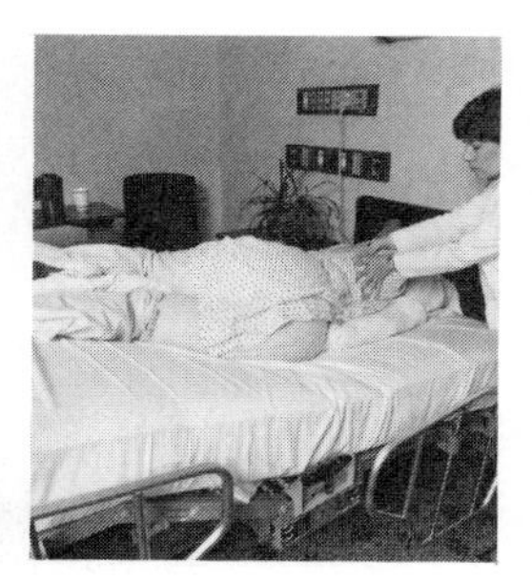 | 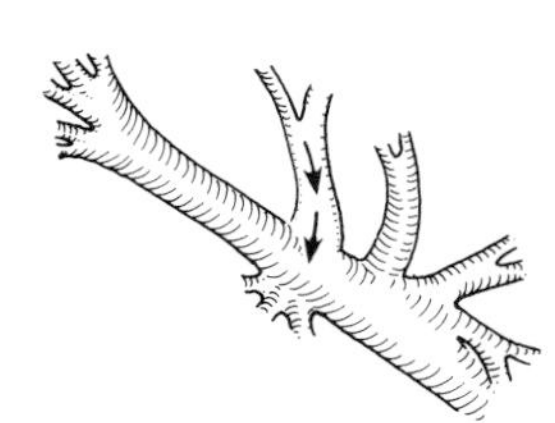 |
| **Right Middle Lobe Bronchus** Have client lie on left side and raise foot of bed 30 cm (12 in). Place pillow behind back and roll client one-fourth turn onto pillow. Percuss and vibrate lateral to right nipple below axilla. | 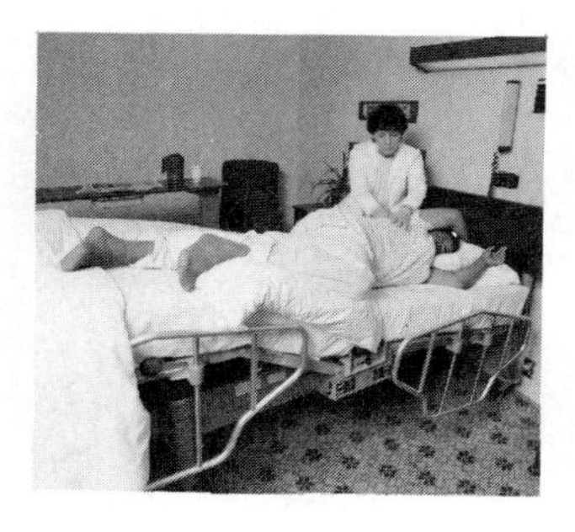 | 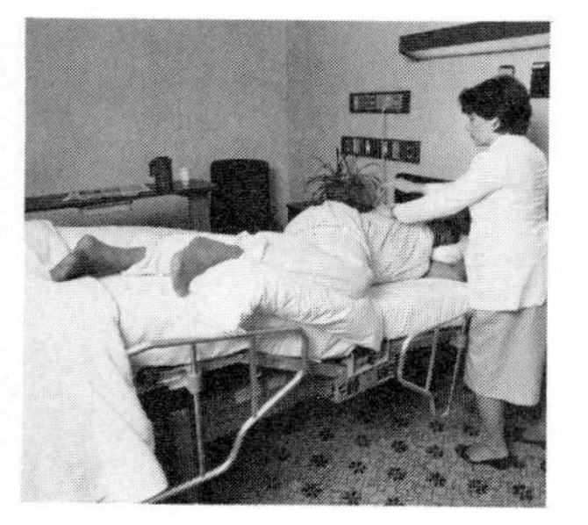 | 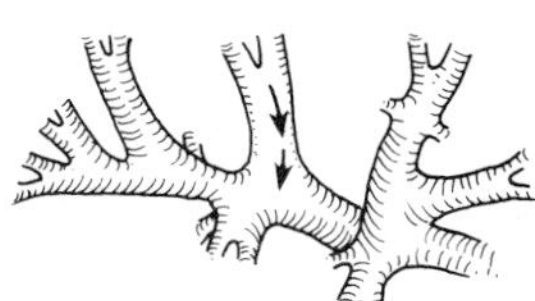 |
| **Left and Right Anterior Lower Lobe Bronchi** Have client lie on back in Trendelenburg position, with foot of bed elevated 45-50 cm (18-20 in). Have knees bent on pillow. Percuss and vibrate over lower anterior ribs on both sides. | 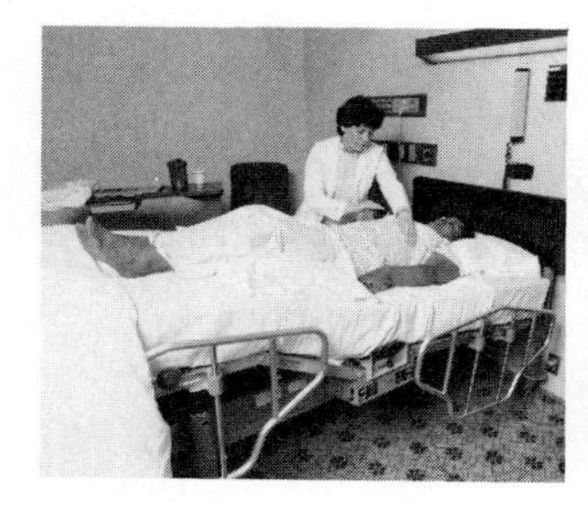 | 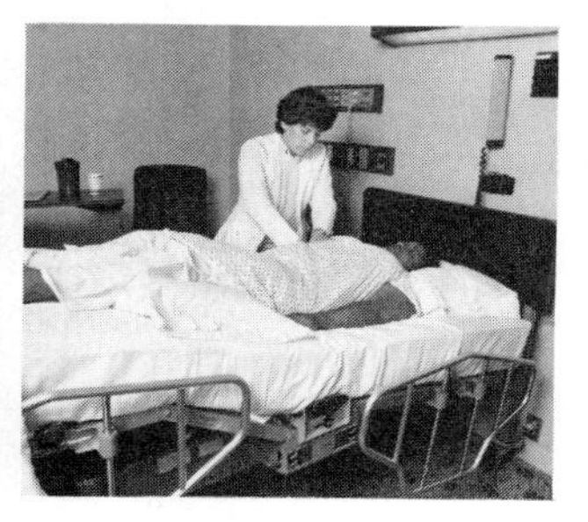 | 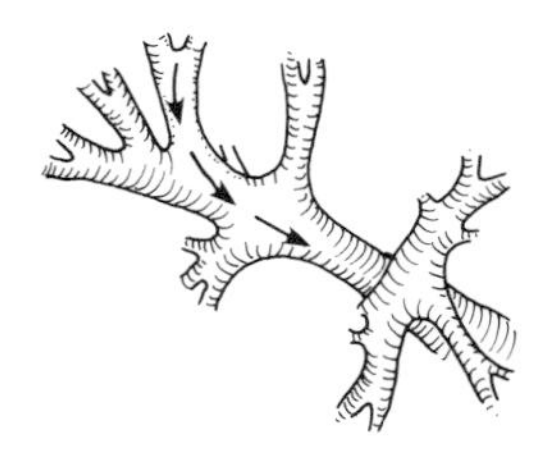 |

***TABLE 15-1, cont'd*** Positions and Procedures for Drainage, Percussion, and Vibration

| Area and Procedure | Percussion | Vibration | Bronchial Lobe |
|---|---|---|---|
| **Right Lower Lobe Lateral Bronchus**<br>Have client lie on left side in Trendelenburg position with foot of bed raised 45-50 cm (18-20 in). Percuss and vibrate on right side of chest below shoulder blades (scapulas) posterior to midaxillary line. | 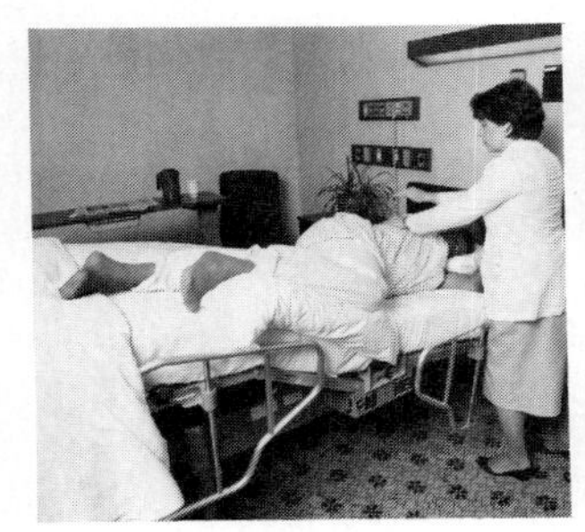 | 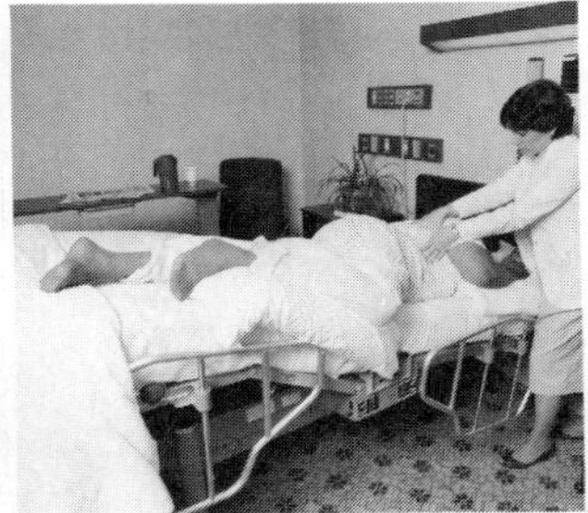 | 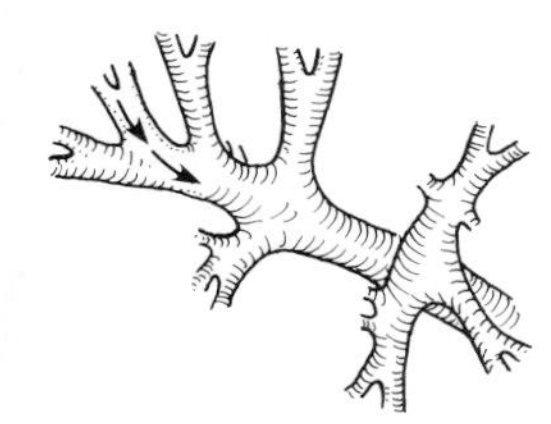 |
| **Left Lower Lobe Lateral Bronchus**<br>Have client lie on right side in Trendelenburg position with foot of bed raised 45-50 cm (18-20 in). Percuss and vibrate on left side of chest below scapulas posterior to midaxillary line. | 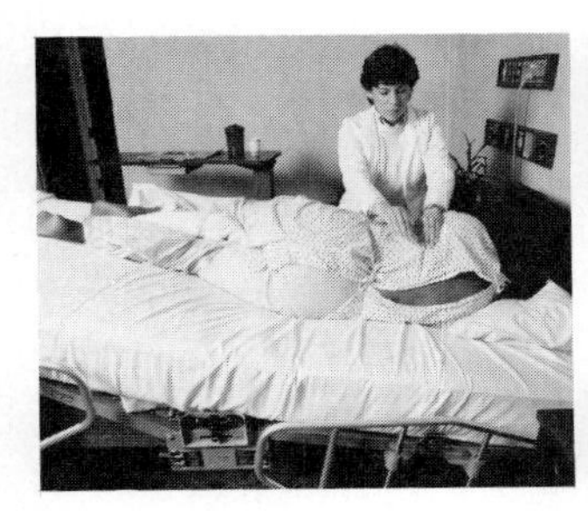 | 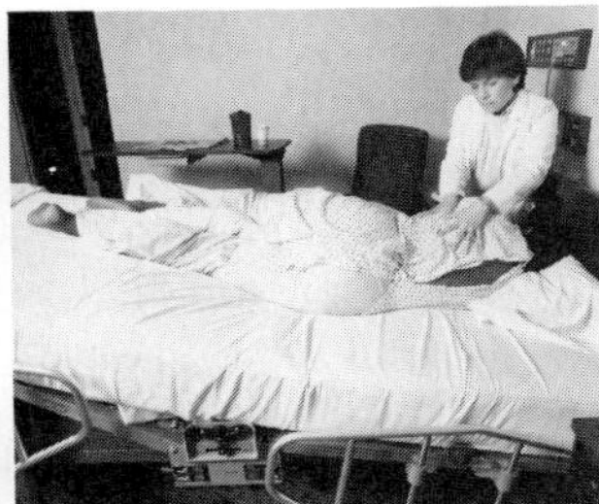 | 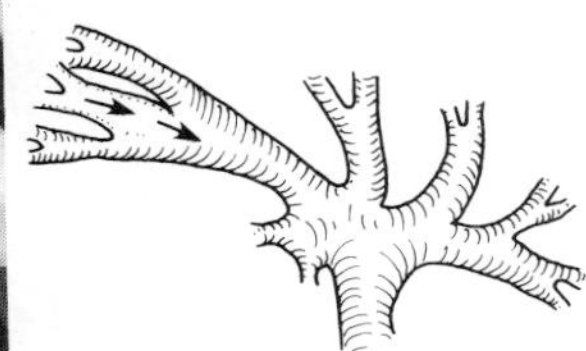 |
| **Right and Left Lower Lobe Superior Bronchi**<br>Have client lie flat on stomach with pillow under stomach. Percuss and vibrate below scapulas on either side of spine. | 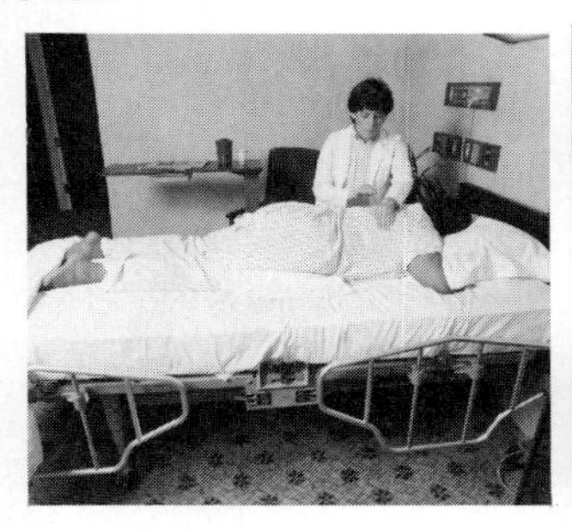 | 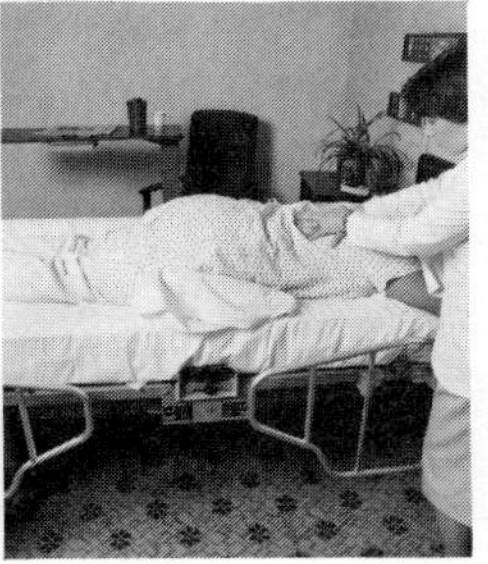 | 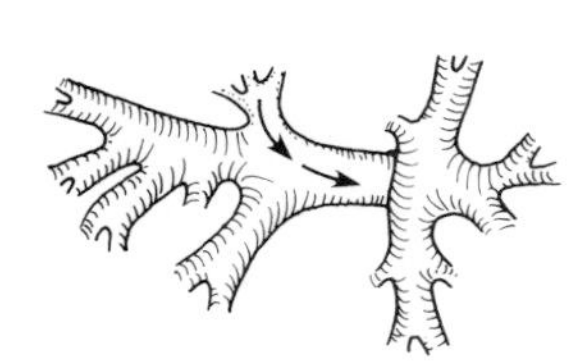 |
| **Left and Right Posterior Basal Bronchi**<br>Have client lie on stomach in Trendelenburg position with foot of bed elevated 45-50 cm (18-20 in). Percuss and vibrate over lower posterior ribs on either side of spine. | 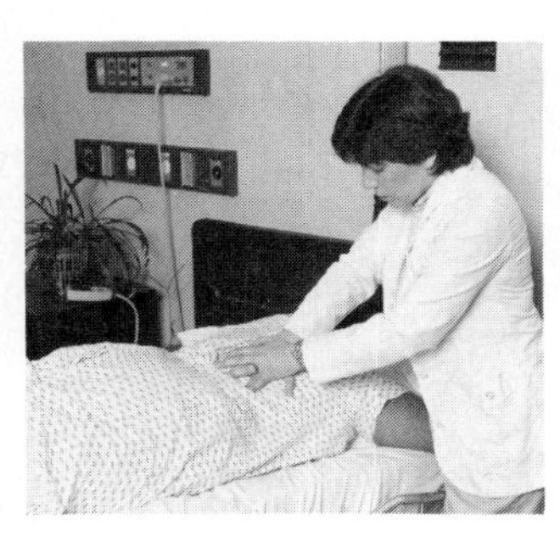 | 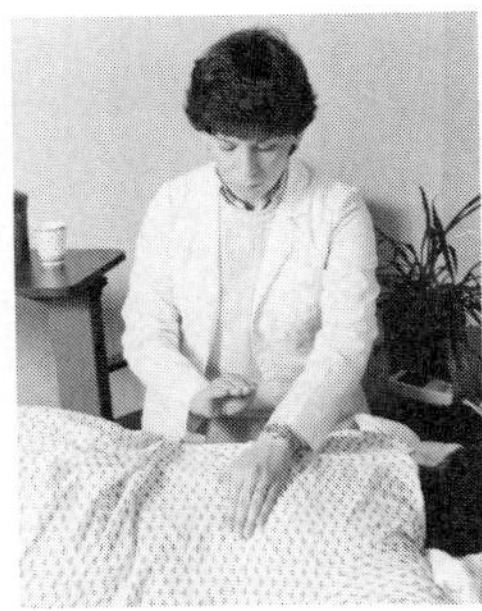 | 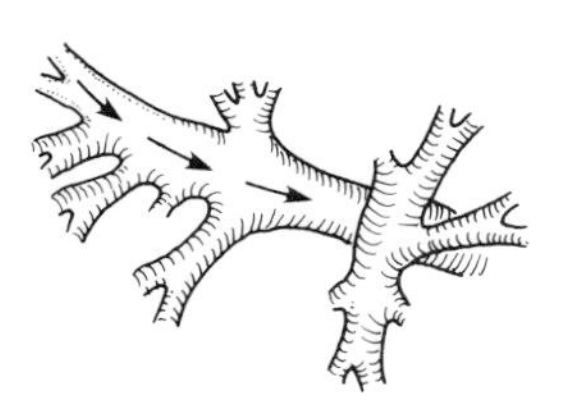 |

# SKILL 15-1 Performing Postural Drainage

In health, several factors provide for normal clearance of tracheobronchial secretions: normal functioning of the mucociliary escalator; adequate systemic hydration; absence of airway disease or infection; normal cough reflex; and normal ability to deep breathe, exercise moderately, and carry out activities of daily living. Loss or alterations in one or several of these factors can interfere with normal clearance of tracheobronchial secretions. A good example is the client with severe bronchitis who gets an airway infection, becomes dehydrated because of anorexia, and stays in bed for several days. These circumstances can lead to stagnation of mucus in the airways. A postoperative client who is on bed rest and cannot take deep breaths because of pain is also predisposed to abnormal clearance of tracheobronchial secretions.

Postural drainage is the gravitational clearance of airway secretions from specific bronchial segments by using one or more of 10 different body positions. Each position drains a specific corresponding section of the tracheobronchial tree, either from the upper, middle, or lower lung field, into the trachea. Coughing or suctioning can then remove secretions from the trachea. Fig. 15-1 on p. 355 shows the upper, middle, and lower lobe bronchi. The figures in Table 15-1 show how each bronchial lobe has a corresponding body posture for its drainage.

Various pathophysiologic conditions predispose the client to abnormal airway clearance and subsequent retention of lung secretions in peripheral airways. The location of these retained secretions may be localized or diffuse. For example, clients with tuberculosis frequently have involvement of their upper lung fields, and posturing would only be performed to drain these specific upper lobe areas. In contrast, clients with bronchiectasis, asthma, bronchitis, or cystic fibrosis frequently have more diffuse involvement of many lung fields, which may require postural drainage of several areas. Clients on bed rest who cannot turn may be placed in several or all drainage positions for several hours or a day to prevent atelectasis and stasis of lung secretions. Areas are selected for drainage based on (1) knowledge of client's condition and disease process, (2) physical assessment of the chest, and (3) chest x-ray results.

## Purposes

1. Help client with abnormal airway clearance to drain secretions from the more peripheral airways into the trachea so that they can be removed by coughing or suctioning.

## Procedure 15-1

| Steps | Rationale |
|---|---|
| **Assessment** | |
| 1. Assess for possible impairment of airway clearance. | Certain circumstances, disease processes, and conditions place client at risk for impaired airway clearance. Postural drainage and frequent repositioning can prevent or reduce associated complications. |
| 2. Identify signs and symptoms that indicate need to perform postural drainage: x-ray film changes consistent with atelectasis, pneumonia, or bronchiectasis; ineffective coughing; thick, sticky, tenacious, and discolored secretions that are difficult to cough up; abnormal breath sounds, such as wheezing, crackling, and gurgling; palpable crepitus; increased vocal fremitus; complete loss or decrease in fremitus and breath sounds. | X-ray film data and signs and symptoms indicate accumulation of pulmonary secretions. |
| 3. Identify which bronchial segments need to be drained by reviewing chest x-ray reports; auscultating over all lung fields for wheezes, crackles, and gurgles (Chapter 13); palpating over all lung fields for crepitus, fremitus, and chest expansion (Chapter 13). | Areas of lung congestion and postures for drainage will vary, depending on disease process, client condition, and clinical problems. Areas most in need of and responsive to postural drainage usually can be easily identified by presence of early inspiratory crackles, gurgles, and palpable crepitus, which indicate secretions in the airways. If airway is completely plugged, breath sounds and chest excursion decrease. |
| 4. Determine client's understanding of and ability to perform home postural drainage. | Allows nurse to identify potential need for instruction. Home drainage is indicated in clients with chronic inability to clear lung secretions adequately, such as those with cystic fibrosis, chronic bronchitis, asthma, or bronchiectasis. |

| Steps | Rationale |
|---|---|
| **Nursing Diagnosis** | |
| 1. Cluster data to reveal actual or potential nursing diagnoses: | |
| a. Ineffective airway clearance: related to impaired cough and mucociliary transport. | Postural drainage uses gravitational forces to assist in clearance of airway secretions. |
| b. Knowledge deficit regarding need for postural drainage and its implementation at home: related to inexperience. | Clients with chronic airway diseases need to understand purpose and procedure for home drainage. |
| **Planning** | |
| 1. Develop individualized goals for the client based on nursing diagnoses: | Provides guidelines for assessing outcomes of postural drainage and need for alterations in drainage program. |
| a. Achieve thin, white, watery secretions that are expectorated on first cough. | Improves client's ability to clear airways. |
| b. Decrease signs and symptoms of bronchial congestion, (decreased cough, diminished crackles, gurgles, clear breath sounds, etc.). | Goal assists in making airway function optimal in clients with airway disease. |
| c. Reexpand atelectatic area behind plugged bronchioles. | Goal frequently sought in postoperative or comatose client on bed rest. |
| 2. Assemble necessary equipment: | |
| a. Comfortable surface that can be slanted, such as Trendelenburg hospital bed or tilt table, and chair if draining upper lobe areas. | Trendelenburg hospital bed and tilt table are most convenient and comfortable for use in clinical setting. |
| b. One to four pillows, depending on client's posture and comfort. | Aids in securing client's position and promoting client's comfort and relaxation. |
| c. Water pitcher and glass; other fluids, as needed. | Sips of water during therapy help to keep mouth moist and sputum easier to expectorate. Client should be well hydrated to decrease tenacity of secretions and make them easier to drain out of lung. |
| d. Tissues and paper bag at bedside; clear, graduated screwtop container. | Use tissue for wiping mouth and dispose in paper bag. Have client expectorate all sputum in clear container, which is more sanitary and allows quantity and consistency to be examined. |
| 3. Prepare client: | |
| a. Explain purpose and rationale for procedure. Explain how it will be done, how long it will take, and any discomforts or side effects. | Helps promote cooperation. Well-prepared client is usually more relaxed and comfortable, which is essential for effective drainage. |
| b. Encourage high fluid intake program if not contraindicated by other diseases and if physician approves. Keep record of patient's fluid intake. | Fluids thin secretions and make them easier to cough up. Clients need close monitoring and encouragement when first starting high fluid intake program. |
| c. Plan treatments so they do not overlap with meals or tube feeding. Avoid postural drainage for 1-2 hr after meals. Stop all tube feedings for 30-45 min before postural drainage. Check for residual feeding in client's stomach; if greater than 100 ml, hold treatment. | Postural drainage should be done when client's stomach is empty to avoid vomiting and aspiration of stomach contents. |
| d. Schedule treatments at appropriate times during day. | Postural drainage should be scheduled to obtain best results and should not conflict with other activities. |
| e. Have client remove any tight or restrictive clothing. | Helps client relax and allows deep breathing. |
| **Implementation** | |
| 1. Wash hands. | Reduces transmission of microorganisms. |
| 2. Select congested areas to be drained based on assessment of all lung fields, clinical data, and chest x-ray data. | To be effective, treatment must be individualized to treat specific areas involved. |
| 3. Place client in position to drain congested areas; first area selected may vary from client to client. (Refer to Table 15-1 for correct positioning to drain upper, middle, and lower lobe bronchi.) Help client assume position as needed. Teach client correct posture and arm and leg positioning. Place pillows for support and comfort. | Specific positions are selected to drain each area involved. |
| 4. Have client maintain posture for 10-15 min. | In adults, draining each area takes time. |
| 5. During 10-15 min of drainage in this posture, perform chest percussion, vibration, or rib shaking (Skill 15-2) over area being drained. Table 15-1 shows all postures and hand placement for percussion, vibration, and rib shaking (P, V, and RS). | These maneuvers provide mechanical forces that aid in mobilization of airway secretions. |

| Steps | Rationale |
|---|---|
| 6. After 10-15 min of drainage in first posture, have client sit up and cough (Skill 15-3). Save expectorated secretions in clear container. If client cannot cough, suctioning may need to be performed. | Any secretions mobilized into central airways should be removed by cough or suctioning before placing client into next drainage position. Coughing is most effective when client is sitting up and leaning forward. |
| 7. Have client rest briefly if necessary. | Short rest periods between postures can prevent fatigue and help client better tolerate therapy. |
| 8. Have client take sips of water. | Keeping mouth moist aids in expectoration of secretions. |
| 9. Repeat Steps 3-8 until all congested areas selected have been drained. Each treatment should not exceed 30-60 min. | Postural drainage is used only to drain areas involved and is based on individual assessment. |
| 10. Wash hands. | Reduces transmission of microorganisms. |

## Evaluation

| Steps | Rationale |
|---|---|
| 1. Evaluate changes in chest assessment after drainage. | Clearance of secretions usually relieves gurgling, early inspiratory crackles, and palpable crepitus. |
| 2. Inspect character of sputum. | Determines if secretions are adequately thinned. |
| 3. Review diagnostic reports on client's pulmonary function. | Provides data on airway clearance and oxygenation status. |
| 4. Have client explain purpose and procedure for postural drainage. | Evaluates client's understanding of procedure. |

### *Expected outcomes*

| Steps | Rationale |
|---|---|
| 1. Airways are cleared of retained secretions. Chest assessment improves with successful postural drainage. Signs include absent or diminished early inspiratory crackles and gurgles; absent or diminished palpable crepitus; return of absent or diminished breath sounds; expansion of chest wall increases and is equal bilaterally; shortness of breath (dyspnea) decreases. | Careful postural drainage should reflect changes in lung congestion. |
| 2. After days, weeks, or months of therapy, expectorated secretions appear more normal: | Normal mucus is thin, clear, watery, and bubbly. |
| a. Sputum in jar settles into two layers (clear, serous layer with bubbly layer on top) instead of four layers (tiny plugs at bottom, cloudy discolored serous layer, large plugs, and bubbles at top). | Secretions appear normal if they are mobilized and coughed up as they are produced and do not stagnate in airways. |
| b. Sputum is coughed up more easily with one or two coughs. | Secretions are easier to cough up if they are thin, watery, and have been mobilized into trachea with drainage. |
| 3. Client subjectively notices less dyspnea, especially after several days of therapy, and can breathe deeper and more easily. | Removal of mucus relieves airway obstruction and decreases work of breathing. |
| 4. Patients who comply with long-term chest therapy for chronic lung disease usually notice decrease in frequency and severity of lung infections and exacerbations. | Retained secretions are excellent media for bacterial growth. If cleared regularly, airway infection is less likely to occur. |
| 5. Body temperature, white blood cell count, and chest x-ray films are normal. | Changes often seen in clients with lung infection such as postoperative atelectasis or with pneumonia caused by mucus plugging that have been successfully reversed with aggressive chest therapy. |
| 6. Pulmonary function studies and blood gases improve. | Relief of mucosal obstruction can result in improved lung volumes and flows and improved blood gases.Learning is achieved. |
| 7. Client able to explain purpose of postural drainage. | Learning is achieved. |

### *Unexpected outcomes*

| Steps | Rationale |
|---|---|
| 1. Client experiences severe dyspnea with bronchospasm, hypoxemia, and hypercarbia (hypercapnia). | In seriously ill clients with severe respiratory insufficiency, mobilization of secretions into large central airways can precipitate bronchospasm and increase work of breathing. These changes can worsen gas exchange and increase dyspnea. Clients at risk include those with (1) status asthmaticus and (2) severe exacerbation of bronchitis who are debilitated, tired, and whose blood gases are consistent with severe hypoxemia and hypercarbia. Chest therapy may have to be discontinued or modified for these clients. They may tolerate only 3-5 min of drainage per hr. Bronchodilator inhalation should be scheduled before postural drainage. |

| Steps | Rationale |
|---|---|
| 2. Hemoptysis occurs. | May be caused by infection, erosion of blood vessels, or other causes. |
| 3. No secretions are obtained. | May result from lack of secretions or secretions being too thick to mobilize. Continue therapy for several days to 1 wk in well-hydrated client before deciding on its efficacy. |
| 4. No change in crackles and gurgles, crepitus present, shortness of breath occurs, chest wall does not expand. | May result from excessive secretions or secretions too thick to mobilize on one treatment. Continue therapy. |
| 5. Client unable to explain purpose of postural drainage. | Secretions remain present in airways. Further instruction required. |

## Recording and Reporting

| | |
|---|---|
| 1. Record in nurses' notes pre- and post-assessment of chest; frequency and duration of treatment; postures used and bronchial segments drained; cough effectiveness; need for suctioning; color, amount, and consistency of sputum; hemoptysis or other unexpected outcomes; client's tolerance and reactions. | Helps evaluate outcomes and need for changes in therapy. |
| 2. If patient and family receive instruction in home care, chart instructions given; understanding of therapy; demonstration of skill; reactions to need for home care; barriers to learning and implementation; referral for follow-up, i.e., home care, rehabilitation, or pulmonary nurse specialist. | Provides continuity of client education among nursing staff. |

## Follow-up Activities

| | |
|---|---|
| 1. Use inhaled bronchodilators 20 min before postural drainage in client at risk for bronchospasm. | Provides optimal bronchodilation and reduces risk of bronchospasm, hypoxemia, and hypercarbia. |
| 2. In severe hemoptysis, stop therapy, remain calm, stay with client, request assistance, and keep client comfortable, warm, and quiet. | Postural changes and stimulation can increase hemoptysis and increase risk of hemorrhage. |

## Special Considerations

- Contraindications for therapy may include problems that preclude use of the Trendelenburg position or other postures, such as severe hypertension, severe hypoxemia, severe shortness of breath, head injuries, increased intracranial pressure, recent severe myocardial failure, lung hemorrhage, certain surgical procedures, pain, or traction. A physician's order for postural drainage may be necessary in some institutions.
- Have fluids available according to client's diet, likes, and dislikes. Teach client kinds and quantities of fluid to drink at home. Have client keep track of exact amount of fluid intake.
- Some clients are very sensitive and self-conscious about coughing up secretions. Be careful and nonjudgmental when observing their mucus.
- Discomforts and side effects are usually mild but may include increased shortness of breath; increased cough during and for 45-60 min after treatment; when in Trendelenburg position, client may experience nasal congestion and feeling of fullness in head, which will subside once client is upright. Reassure that client can sit up and rest at any time if necessary.
- Contraindications to high fluid intake are congestive heart failure and renal failure. When forcing fluids, build up daily intake gradually and strive toward 12-16 8-oz glasses or until mucus is thin, white, and watery.
- Review Table 15-1 for ideas on how to place pillows in each position. Note that in all flat and Trendelenburg positions, pillow can be placed under head to promote comfort. Rib cage will remain slanted as long as pillow is not under shoulder or upper back. To drain lingula and right middle lobe, as shown, roll client in one-quarter turn back from side-lying position and place pillow behind back for comfort and support.
- Best times for treatments are (1) in morning before breakfast, when client can clear secretions that accumulate overnight; and (2) about 1 hr before bedtime, so lungs are clear before sleeping and client has time after treatment to cough up any mobilized secretions. Frequency depends on need and client's tolerance and may vary from once daily to every 2-4 hr in acute situation. When client's condition is acute, short (10 min), frequent treatments are tolerated best. As condition stabilizes, one to four 30-45 min treatments work best. If client is receiving inhaled bronchodilators or aerosol treatment, postural drainage should be done 20 min after such therapy. Plan for rest period after postural drainage. Do not schedule major activities (exercise, bath, etc.) right after chest therapy treatment, especially in clients with severe obstructive lung disease.
- Sometimes client may experience transient dyspnea and fatigue because of irritation and bronchospasm from mobilizing secretions. Dyspnea usually subsides after sputum is coughed up.
- Small amounts of blood-streaked sputum usually clear with good drainage. Notify physician. If sputum is pure blood, stop all therapy and notify physician immediately. Keep client calm.
- Secretions are not always mobilized and coughed up after each posture. If, after two or three coughs, nothing is expectorated, proceed with next posture. Often secretions are coughed up 30-60 min after postural drainage.

- Immediately report severe dyspnea, hemoptysis, severe bronchospasm, or hypotension to physician.
- Postural drainage after various types of chest surgery has developed into a speciality. If specific posturing guidelines are used they can be very effective in preventing and treating atelectasis and pneumonia.

### Teaching Considerations

- Instruct client's family or primary care giver to recognize when the client's respiratory status requires breathing exercises or postural drainage.
- Encourage primary care giver or family member to encourage the client to participate in physical activities that will increase respiratory efficiency.
- Teach client and significant others how to assume postures at home. Some postures may need to be modified to meet individual needs, i.e., side-lying Trendelenburg position to drain lateral lower lobes may have to be done with client lying flat on side or in side-lying semi-Fowler's position if client is very short of breath.

### Home Care Considerations

- Assess home environment for ventilation. Determine client's access to clean, fresh air. Assess the home for air conditioning and client's reaction to air conditioning.
- Provide a basin or cup into which the client can expectorate secretions.
- Discuss need for home drainage with family. Assess if they perceive need for home care and if any barriers exist to learning and implementing home program. If specialized home or out-patient follow-up is needed, refer client to pulmonary nurse specialist, pulmonary rehabilitation team, or home health care personnel.
- In home setting, the Trendelenburg position can be achieved in several ways. Select most comfortable and practical method that best suits client:
  1. First choice is Trendelenburg hospital bed if client has insurance coverage or can afford it. Some clients, however, do not like hospital equipment in their home.
  2. Extra twin bed can be propped up at foot with 30-45 cm (12-18 in) blocks or bricks.
  3. Client can purchase slant board or make one out of old door or tabletop. Surface can be padded with foam or blankets.
  4. Client's hips can be elevated with stack of old newspapers and pillows or foam wedge. These props tend to be uncomfortable and often flatten out because of client's body weight.
  5. Wedge or stack of papers can be placed under bed board.

## *SKILL 15-2 Performing Percussion, Vibration, and Rib Shaking*

During postural drainage, physical maneuvers (percussion, vibration, and rib shaking [P, V, and RS]) can be performed on the rib cage by a trained nurse, therapist, or family member. The techniques are done on specific parts of the rib cage over each area being drained. Normally the mucociliary escalator and cough transport can effectively clear airway secretions. When airway clearance is impaired in certain disease states, however, these techniques are combined with postural drainage to help clear mucus.

Exactly why these physical maneuvers enhance clearance of mucus is not known. Several possible mechanisms have been suggested: (1) vibration alters mucus cross-linking; (2) vibratory forces enhance ciliary movement; (3) vibration and percussion stimulate reflexes in the chest wall that help clear mucus; and (4) vibration with rib shaking enhances peak expiratory flow to help dislodge mucus plugs.

These techniques are defined and explained in detail in this skill. Percussion involves clapping the chest wall with cupped hands. If done correctly, it painlessly sets up vibrations in the chest to dislodge retained secretions. Vibration is a downward vibrating pressure done only during exhalation with the flat part of the palm over the area being drained. Rib shaking is a constant downward rocking motion on the rib cage done with the flat part of the hand during exhalation. These last two maneuvers are performed only during prolonged exhalation through pursed lips. They augment the natural movement of the rib cage during exhalation.

The natural expiratory movement involves (1) a decrease in the lateral and anteroposterior diameter of the lower ribs as they move downward and closer together and (2) a decrease in the anteroposterior diameter of the upper chest as the sternum, clavicles, and upper rib cage move downward. Pressure during vibration and rib shaking is always directed toward these natural expiratory movements of the rib cage. They become even more effective if the client can relax the rib cage muscles during exhalation and blow out using abdominal muscles. This relaxation during vibration and rib shaking enhances the rocking motion of the rib cage, makes vibration optimal, and assists in dislodging mucus plugs.

In diseases associated with mucus plugging, the rib cage frequently becomes hyperinflated because air is trapped behind obstructed airways. The ribs can become somewhat fixed in their upward and outward position and lose their excursion and flexibility; rib shaking and vibration can improve both. They can also help to reduce air trapping by augmenting prolonged exhalation and relaxation of the chest wall muscles.

Before attempting to master these techniques, the nurse must know that each posture is associated with a general area of the rib cage to be percussed and vibrated. These postures and the specific areas are shown in Table 15-1. Generally, for any given posture, the area to be percussed and vibrated can be thought of as that portion of the rib cage at the greatest vertical height. Areas that are never percussed or vibrated regardless of their vertical height include the clavicles, breast tissue, spine, waist, and abdomen; the nurse must always stay over the ribs.

## Purposes

1. Clear airways of pulmonary secretions.
2. Promote a more effective cough.
3. Decrease atelectatic areas in the lungs.

## *Procedure 15-2*

| Steps | Rationale |
|---|---|
| **Assessment** | |
| 1. Assess breathing pattern, including muscles used for breathing, respiratory rate and depth, extent of excursion and chest wall movement. | Certain disease states place client at risk of developing ineffective breathing pattern. Rapid, shallow breathing with client using accessory muscles is seen in chronic obstructive lung disease, asthma, pain, hypoxemia, pneumonia, and atelectasis. |
| 2. Identify signs and symptoms and conditions that indicate need to perform these skills, such as use of postural drainage (Skill 15-1, Assessment); abnormal chest assessment indicating bronchial congestion; abnormal breathing pattern. | When tolerated and not contraindicated, these techniques are done during postural drainage. |
| 3. Identify and assess rib cage over bronchial segment being drained for pain, tenderness, abnormal configuration, excursion or chest wall movement during breathing, muscle tension. | Chest wall areas to be assessed and to receive P, V, and RS vary with each postural drainage posture (Table 15-1). When rib fracture or osteoporosis is expected, P, V, and RS are contraindicated. |
| 4. Assess client's understanding and ability to cooperate with therapy, both in hospital and at home. | Allows nurse to identify potential need for instruction of client, family, or significant others. |
| **Nursing Diagnosis** | |
| 1. Cluster data to reveal actual or potential nursing diagnoses: | |
| a. Ineffective breathing patterns: related to decreased chest wall excursion and air trapping. | V and RS improve breathing pattern, increase chest wall excursion, and decrease air trapping. |
| b. Ineffective airway clearance: related to impaired cough and mucociliary transport. | P, V, and RS help clear mucus and are integral part of chest physiotherapy. |
| c. Knowledge deficit regarding need for P, V, and RS at home during postural drainage: related to inexperience. | Clients with chronic lung diseases need to understand procedures and purposes to implement them at home. Family or significant others need to be involved as much as possible. |
| **Planning** | |
| 1. Develop individualized goals for client based on nursing diagnoses, including: | Provides guidelines for assessing effectiveness of P, V, and RS. |
| a. Achieve thin, white, watery secretions that are expectorated on first cough. | Goals a-h assist in making client's breathing pattern optimal. |
| b. Decrease signs and symptoms of bronchial congestion, (decreased cough, diminished crackles, gurgles, clear breath sounds, etc.). | |
| c. Reexpand atelectatic area behind plugged bronchioles. | Goals frequently sought in postoperative or comatose client on bed rest. |
| d. Improve chest wall excursion, movement, and flexibility. | |
| e. Slow respiratory rate. | |
| f. Induce relaxation. | |
| g. Decrease work of breathing. | |
| h. Reduce air trapping. | |
| 2. Assemble necessary equipment: | |
| a. Comfortable surface that can be slanted, such as Trendelenburg hospital bed or tilt table, and chair, if draining upper lobe areas. | Trendelenburg hospital bed and tilt table are most convenient and comfortable for use in clinical setting. |

| Steps | Rationale |
|---|---|
| b. One to four pillows, depending on client's posture and comfort. | Aid in securing client's position and promote client's comfort and relaxation. |
| c. Water pitcher and glass; other fluids, as needed. | Sips of water during therapy help to keep mouth moist and sputum easier to expectorate. Client should be well hydrated to decrease tenacity of secretions and make them easier to drain out of lung. |
| d. Tissues and paper bag at bedside; clear, graduated screwtop container. | Use tissue for wiping mouth and dispose in paper bag. Have client expectorate all sputum in clear container, which is more sanitary and allows quantity and consistency to be examined. |
| e. Mechanical vibrator or percussor (optional). | Used only as second choice to manual vibration and percussion. |
| f. Single layer of clothing or loose towel over chest wall. | Never percuss on bare skin, to avoid bruising. |
| 3. Prepare client: | |
| a. Explain procedure in detail: how it will be done, how long it will take, and any discomforts or side effects. | P, V, and RS cannot be done effectively without client's cooperation. |
| b. Encourage and help client to relax and deep breathe during P, V, and RS. Have client practice exhaling slowly through pursed lips while relaxing chest wall muscles. Client should blow out using abdominal muscles, not rib cage muscles. | P, V, and RS are most effective if client breathes properly and works well with therapist. If done properly these techniques should not cause pain or discomfort. |

## Implementation

| Steps | Rationale |
|---|---|
| 1. With client placed in appropriate drainage position (Skill 15-1, Implementation, Steps 1-3), assess and identify chest wall area to be percussed and vibrated. (See Table 15-1). | In general, for any given posture, rib cage area to be percussed and vibrated is in highest vertical position. Careful assessment of rib cage movement guides nurse in following natural movement during V and RS. |
| 2. Instruct client to relax; take slow, deep breaths, and exhale using abdominal, diaphragmatic, pursed lip breathing. | Client should not lie passively, but should relax and take deep breaths. |
| 3. Use good body mechanics when clapping: elevate bed to comfortable working height and stand close to bed with arms directly in front and knees slightly bent. Avoid bending over. | Avoids undue strain on therapist's back and legs. |
| 4. Begin percussion on appropriate part of chest wall over draining area (Table 15-1). Perform percussion for 5-7 min in each posture as tolerated. Always ask if client is experiencing any discomfort, such as undue pressure or stinging skin. | Percussion (P) helps clear mucus and should be painless, since air in hand acts as cushion. |
| a. Place hands side by side on chest wall over area to be drained. They may have to be molded slightly so that entire outer portion of hand makes contact with chest wall to avoid air leaks. | Chest percussion is performed with hands cupped and held rigid (see Table 15-1). No air spaces should exist between fingers or between thumb and forefinger. Wrists are slightly bent backward, and fingers are straight but bent slightly at joint most proximal to palm. When clapping, most of arm movement should come from the elbow and shoulder joint. Cupping can be done for 5-7 min without stopping or 2-3 min, alternating with V and RS. |
| b. Alternately clap chest with cupped hands to create rhythmic popping sound resembling galloping horse. Clapping can be done at moderate or fast speed, whichever is most comfortable and effective. | |
| 5. Perform chest wall vibration over each area being drained. See Table 15-1 for correct hand position to use in each posture: | Vibration (V) helps clear mucus. Vibrations are usually done in sets of three followed by coughing so that any mobilized mucus can be expectorated. |
| a. To perform vibration, gently place hands over area being drained, and have client take slow, deep breath through nose. | Coughing with V also aids in clearing mucus. Do not perform if rib cage is fractured or sore or if client is uncooperative. When applying pressure to ribs, always follow natural movement of rib cage. As client becomes comfortable and learns to relax rib cage during exhalation, chest wall movement and flexibility will increase. Allow client to sit up and cough as needed between vibrations. |
| b. Gently resist chest wall as it rises up during inhalation. | |
| c. Have client hold breath, and exhale through pursed lips, contracting abdominal muscles and relaxing chest wall muscles. Chest wall should relax and fall. | |
| d. While client is exhaling, gently push down and vibrate with flat part of hand. | |
| e. Repeat vibration three times, then have client cascade cough by taking deep breath and doing series of small coughs until end of breath. Client should not inhale between coughs. Vibrate chest wall as client coughs. | |
| 6. Assess client's tolerance of vibration and ability to relax chest wall and breathe properly as instructed. | May necessitate discontinuing procedure. |

| Steps | Rationale |
|---|---|
| 7. If client is able to achieve proper breathing and relaxation, perform rib shaking, which is usually done with vibration: | Rib shaking (RS) helps clear mucus. |
| a. Place flat part of hand over area being drained (Table 15-1). Maintain good body mechanics: lower bed so patient is about at your hip level; work with arms directly in front; maintain good leverage; do not lean over or strain your back. | Proper positioning of therapist prevents strain on back muscles. |
| b. Have client inhale slowly through nose. | |
| c. During inhalation, apply light pressure on ribs and stretch skin so it is tight. | |
| d. Have client hold breath for 2 sec. | |
| e. As client exhales, increase pressure. Maintain pressure while applying intermittent rocking motion on ribs. Pressure is directed toward following natural expiratory rib cage movement. | Optimizes vibration effect to dislodge mucus. |
| f. Client must exhale through pursed lips and relax chest wall muscles as much as possible. | Ribs can be rocked more vigorously in direction they naturally move, if rib cage is relaxed. |
| g. Repeat rib shaking three times, have patient inhale deeply, and then do rib shaking during cascade cough. | Coughing helps to clear mobilized secretions. |
| h. Perform total of three or four sets of three vibrations with rib shaking and coughing in each posture as tolerated. | Strength and frequency of V and RS will vary: V requires all muscles in arm and shoulder to contract and tremble; RS requires applying controlled pressure from shoulders and back while slightly leaning on chest; rocking motion is created by flexing and extending elbows using triceps. |
| i. Suction if client is unable to cough up mucus. | |
| 8. In each posture, complete vibrations and/or rib shaking. | |
| 9. If long-term therapy is needed, teach client and significant others P, V, and RS for home use. If they cannot learn or use, refer for out-patient or home health follow-up. | Long-term use of these techniques can make airway clearance optimal, reduce symptoms and infection, and improve chest mobility. |
| **Evaluation** | |
| 1. Evaluate changes in chest assessment after P, V, and RS. | These maneuvers usually relieve signs of congestion, slow respiratory rate, and improve chest mobility and expansion. |
| 2. Inspect character of mucus. | Determines if mucus is adequately thinned. |
| 3. Review diagnostic test results for pulmonary function. | Determines airway clearance and oxygenation status. |
| ***Expected outcomes*** | |
| 1. Airways are cleared of retained secretions. Chest assessment improves with successful postural drainage. Signs include absent or diminished early inspiratory crackles and gurgles; absent or diminished palpable crepitus; return of absent or diminished breath sounds; expansion of chest wall increases and is equal bilaterally; shortness of breath (dyspnea) decreases. | Careful postural drainage should reflect changes in lung congestion. |
| 2. After days, weeks, or months of therapy, expectorated secretions appear more normal: | Normal mucus is thin, clear, watery, and bubbly. |
| a. Sputum in jar settles into two layers (clear, serous layer with bubbly layer on top) instead of four layers (tiny plugs at bottom, cloudy discolored serous layer, large plugs, and bubbles at top). | Secretions appear normal if they are mobilized and coughed up as they are produced and do not stagnate in airways. |
| b. Sputum is coughed up more easily with one or two coughs. | Secretions are easier to cough up if they are thin and watery and have been mobilized into trachea with drainage. |
| 3. Client subjectively notices less dyspnea, especially after several days of therapy, and can breathe deeper and more easily. | Removal of mucus relieves airway obstruction and decreases work of breathing. |
| 4. Patients who comply with long-term chest therapy for chronic lung disease usually notice decrease in frequency and severity of lung infections and exacerbations. | Retained secretions are excellent media for bacterial growth. If cleared regularly, airway infection is less likely to occur. |
| 5. Body temperature, white blood cell count, and chest x-ray films are normal. | Changes often seen in clients with lung infection such as post-operative atelectasis or with pneumonia caused by mucus plugging that have been successfully reversed with aggressive chest therapy. |
| 6. Pulmonary function studies and blood gases improve. | Relief of mucosal obstruction can result in improved lung volumes and flows and improved blood gases. |
| 7. Client demonstrates decreased respiratory rate, increased | Signs of improved breathing pattern. |

| Steps | Rationale |
|---|---|
| depth of breathing, ability to exhale longer through pursed lips, ability to relax chest muscles and exhale only using abdominal muscles, increased relaxation and mobility of rib cage, improved excursion of rib cage. | |
| ***Unexpected outcomes*** | |
| 1. Client experiences severe dyspnea with bronchospasm, hypoxemia, and hypercarbia (hypercapnia). | In seriously ill clients with severe respiratory insufficiency, mobilization of secretions into large central airways can precipitate bronchospasm and increase work of breathing. These changes can worsen gas exchange and increase dyspnea. |
| 2. Hemoptysis occurs. | May be caused by infection, erosion of blood vessels, or other causes. |
| 3. No secretions are obtained. | May result from lack of secretions or secretions being too thick to mobilize. |
| 4. No change in crackles and gurgles; crepitus present; shortness of breath occurs; chest wall does not expand. | |
| 5. Client experiences rib fracture, rib pain, or tenderness of chest wall. | If techniques are not done properly rib pain and fractures can occur. |
| **Reporting and Recording** | |
| 1. For treatment given, along with postural drainage, record in nurses' notes pre- and post-assessment of chest mobility; client's cooperation with and tolerance of P, V, and RS; client's ability to relax and breathe properly; duration of percussion; number of V and RS series; cough effectiveness; suctioning. | Documents in client's record specific procedure and lung lobes involved. In addition, documentation will ensure third-party reimbursement. |
| 2. If client and significant others receive instruction in home use of P, V, and RS, chart instructions given; understanding of theory and skills; demonstration of P, V, and RS techniques; referral for follow-up. | Documentation of client teaching notes specifically what information client should know and what was taught. In some cases documentation and client teaching is necessary for accreditation. |
| **Follow-up Activities** | |
| 1. Use inhaled bronchodilators 30 min before P, V, and RS in clients at risk of bronchospasm. | Provides optimal bronchodilation and reduces risk of hypoxemia and hypercarbia. |
| 2. In severe hemoptysis, stop therapy, remain calm, stay with client, request assistance, and keep client comfortable, warm, and quiet. | Postural changes and stimulation can increase hemoptysis and increase risk of hemorrhage. |
| 3. If rib fracture is suspected, notify physician, obtain chest x-ray film, and curtail P, V, and RS. | Fractured rib increases client's risk for pneumothorax. Continued P, V, and RS further increase client's risk for lung puncture. |

## Special Considerations

- P, V, and RS may be contraindicated in certain situations, including rib fracture, fracture of other rib cage structures such as clavicle or sternum, pain, severe dyspnea, and severe osteoporosis, so nurse should obtain physician's order.
- Do not perform if client is uncooperative or if client has broken back or rib, rib pain or tenderness, bleeding in the lung, chest or back pain, upset stomach, or serious heart disease.
- After chest surgery, P and RS are contraindicated as they may increase pain and splinting and lead to more problems with atelectasis. Gentle vibration, deep breathing, and coughing are preferred along with postural drainage. Small mechanical vibrators used well above or well below the client's thoracotomy incision are effective and well tolerated.
- Never use P, V, or RS over spine, breast tissue, sternum or shoulder blades. Always stay over rib cage.
- If client is unresponsive, on mechanical ventilation or is uncooperative, breathing pattern usually cannot be altered. Vibrate during the exhalation phase between machine breaths.
- Students should learn RS under guidance of trained therapist.
- Sometimes client may experience transient dyspnea and fatigue because of irritation and bronchospasm from mobilizing secretions. Dyspnea usually subsides after sputum is coughed up.
- Clients at risk include those with (1) status asthmaticus and (2) severe exacerbation of bronchitis who are debilitated, tired, and whose blood gases are consistent with severe hypoxemia and hypercarbia. Chest therapy may have to be discontinued or modified for these clients. They may tolerate only 3-5 min of drainage per hr. Bronchodilator inhalation should be scheduled before postural drainage.
- Small amounts of blood-streaked sputum usually clear with good drainage. Notify physician. If sputum is pure blood, stop all therapy and notify physician immediately. Keep client calm.
- Continue therapy for several days to 1 wk in well-hydrated client before deciding on its efficacy.
- Thin, frail clients with osteoporosis are most susceptible to injury. To avoid injury during V and RS, apply pressure only during exhalation, follow natural movement of rib cage, encourage client to relax chest wall.

### Teaching Considerations

- Instruct client to tap on chest wall with finger tips to aid in loosening secretions.
- Instruct client to use frequent mouth washes.
- Instruct client to use tissues in expectorating and to assess sputum for blood, color, consistency, amount, odor.
- If home therapy is needed, instruct family member in techniques of P, V, and RS. Assess willingness to learn and follow through in home setting.
- Teach family members carefully and observe them closely as they demonstrate techniques for P, V, and RS.

### Home Care Considerations

- Mechanical devices are sometimes used (1) at home if trained therapist is not available or (2) if client does not tolerate manual therapy. They are available through most home equipment companies.

## *SKILL 15-3 Using Controlled Coughing Techniques*

Controlled coughing techniques (CCT) should be an integral part of every chest physiotherapy (CPT) treatment. They are also used in many other clinical situations, along with turning and deep breathing, to help clear mucus and prevent airway infections, atelectasis, and pneumonia. Cough is a natural defense mechanism that protects lungs from inhaled particles and accumulated secretions. The cough mechanism is weakened in the presence of severe obstructive lung disease, immobility, sedative and analgesic therapy, postoperative pain, anesthesia, severe restrictive lung disease, and an artificial airway. Use of controlled coughing techniques can enhance cough effectiveness, thereby mobilizing secretions and preventing mucus plugging.

The nurse must review the normal cough transport mechanism to understand how controlled coughing is most effective in disease states. Cough transport of mucus occurs by a sudden blast of expelled air in airway mucus. This mechanism is triggered by cough reflexes, which are present throughout the lung at tracheal and bronchial bifurcations. Irritation, inflammation, inhaled particles, and excessive mucus are some of the stimulants that normally trigger the cough reflex. Conditions that interfere with this reflex include central nervous system disease or its depression from pain medications, sedatives, and anesthesia. To compensate for loss in reflex sensitivity, clients with these conditions must be made to cough every 1 or 2 hours.

After cough is initiated, its effectiveness depends on how fast air can be expelled from the lung. During the cough, structural and mechanical forces allow air to flow with greater velocity through the central airways, the trachea, and mainstem bronchi and with less velocity through more distal bronchi. Cough, especially at high lung volumes, is more effective in clearing large central airways of secretions than smaller peripheral airways. Coughs at low lung volumes and with deep breathing provide a milking action within the smaller airways to help move secretions, whereas coughs at higher volumes primarily clear the proximal airways of secretions that have mobilized during postural drainage, percussion, vibration, and rib shaking.

The cascade cough described in this skill involves taking one deep breath and performing a series of little coughs from the top to the end of the breath. The client should not inhale between coughs. The coughs at the top of the breath are done at high lung volumes and help clear the trachea and mainstem bronchi; those toward the end are done at low lung volumes and help milk mucus out of the smaller peripheral airways. The effects of cascade cough are enhanced during vibration and rib shaking.

After the cough reflex is triggered, the next step is to take a slow, deep breath. Several problems can preclude the client's ability to do this, such as central nervous system disease, pain, restrictive lung disease, severe airway obstruction, immobility, supine or prone posturing, and presence of binders or restrictive dressings. In these situations, the nurse must assist the client in taking deep breaths.

The next step in the cough mechanism is breath holding with glottic closure. Laryngeal disease, laryngectomy, and an artificial airway prevent glottic closure. In these situations, cough can be ineffective, and the client may need tracheal suctioning.

During glottic closure the expiratory muscles in the chest wall and abdomen forcefully contract to build up a back pressure. Pain, muscle weakness, neuromuscular disease, and fatigue can reduce the contractile force of these muscles. Finally the glottis is suddenly and rapidly opened, and a blast of expelled air mobilizes mucus toward the throat. Providing pain medications and supporting an incision with a pillow can allow the postoperative client to breathe deeper and exhale more forcefully with less pain and discomfort. Pushing the abdomen toward the diaphragm during cough can help the client with neuromuscular disease generate a more forceful cough. This technique is called quad coughing.

This skill presents three controlled coughing techniques: the cascade, huff, and quad. Suggestions are provided for making each type most effective and for controlling the frequency of coughing. Ineffective coughing is exhausting and nonproductive. Emphasis is on teaching clients ways to control their cough so it does not control them.

### Purposes

1. Help clear mucus from airways.
2. Prevent airway infections, atelectasis, and pneumonia.

## *Procedure 15-3*

| Steps | Rationale |
|---|---|
| **Assessment** | |
| 1. Identify signs and symptoms that indicate need to perform controlled coughing techniques (CCT), including thick, sticky, tenacious secretions; weak, ineffective cough; fatigue of expiratory respiratory muscles; abnormal breath sounds, especially gurgling; inability to take deep breath. | Conditions that place a client at risk for impaired cough are: postoperative state, lung diseases, retained excessive lung secretions, central nervous system depression, neuromuscular disease, lung cancer, lung surgery, immobility, and artificial airway. CCT are always included as part of chest therapy. |
| 2. Identify reasons why cough is ineffective, take cough history, identify medical condition. | Cough therapy focuses on correcting specific problem. |
| 3. Assess client's understanding of and ability to perform CCT. | Client's cooperation and understanding allow nurse to assess need for instruction. |
| **Nursing Diagnosis** | |
| 1. Cluster data to reveal actual or potential nursing diagnoses: | |
| a. Ineffective airway clearance: related to severe airway disease or muscle paralysis. | Severe airway disease impedes cough by reducing expiratory airflow rates. Client unable to cough because of loss of muscle contraction and inability to take deep breath. |
| b. Ineffective airway clearance: related to incisional pain. | Client's cough impaired because of pain or use of anesthesia and analgesia. |
| c. Knowledge deficit regarding CCT: related to inexperience. | Client learns skill in order to perform regularly at home. |
| **Planning** | |
| 1. Develop individualized goals for client based on nursing diagnoses: | |
| a. Decrease fatigue associated with ineffective and uncontrolled coughing. | Coughing techniques conserve energy. |
| b. Relieve bronchial congestion and mucus stasis. | Effective coughing clears airways of mucus. |
| 2. Assemble necessary equipment: | |
| a. Pillows, depending on posture and individual comfort needs. | Aid in securing client's position and promoting comfort and relaxation. |
| b. Water pitcher and glass. | Fluids keep mouth moist and make expectoration easier. Forcing fluids helps make secretions thinner and easier to cough up. |
| c. Tissues and paper bag at bedside; clear, screw-top container. | Use tissues to wipe mouth. Collect sputum in clear jar for examination. |
| 3. Prepare client: | |
| a. Explain CCT to client: how it is done and any discomforts or side effects. | Clients must cooperate and understand CCT. Potential discomforts include mild transient dypsnea, pain in postoperative client, mild fatigue. Fatigue usually lessens after client learns to control cough with CCT. |
| b. Schedule CCT at appropriate times. | Best results obtained if CCT is properly scheduled. Best times are in morning when client first gets up, after chest therapy, after administration of pain medication, on empty stomach, every 1-2 hr in postoperative client. |
| c. Have client remove any tight or restrictive clothing. | Anything that binds chest wall or abdomen can interfere with CCT. |
| **Implementation** | |
| 1. Place client in best position possible to maximize cough effectiveness. Optimal posture is sitting up with feet on floor and leaning slightly forward. If confined to bed, have client lie on back or side and elevate head of bed. | Provides for maximal lung expansion and expiratory efforts. |

| Steps | Rationale |
|---|---|
| 2. Have client perform steps of CCT. | |
| a. Cascade coughing: | |
| ▪ Take slow, deep breath. | Building up air behind mucus helps to propel it toward mouth. Client should breathe in slowly so mucus is not sucked deeper into lung. |
| ▪ Hold breath for 2 sec and contract expiratory muscles. | Builds up pressure for an effective cough. |
| ▪ Open mouth and perform series of coughs from top of breath to end of breath. | Cascade cough helps clear large and small airways. |
| ▪ Pause. | Pausing is very important to help prevent paroxysms of coughing. |
| ▪ Breathe in slowly and gently. | Taking in fast breath after coughing can drive mucus back into lungs. |
| ▪ Rest. | Resting is extremely important. Helps client avoid coughing repeatedly. |
| b. Huff coughing: | |
| ▪ Use steps for cascade cough, however instead of a series of coughs, have client say "huff." | Huffing usually only clears central airways. Used in clients with lung disease who cannot perform cascade cough. Huff coughing can be very effective in stimulating natural cough reflex. |
| c. Quad coughing: | |
| ▪ Use same steps for cascade cough, except client or nurse presses inward and upward on abdominal muscles toward diaphragm while client performs maximal expiratory effort, thus causing cough. | External pressure applied to abdominal muscles simulates muscular activity of the cough. Quadriplegic clients may not have abdominal muscle control and need assistance while trying to cough. |

## Evaluation

| Steps | Rationale |
|---|---|
| 1. Evaluate changes in chest assessment before and after drainage. | Clearance of secretions usually relieves dypsnea and gurgling. |
| 2. Have client explain and demonstrate without assistance. | Determines client's learning of coughing techniques. |

### *Expected outcomes*

| Steps | Rationale |
|---|---|
| 1. Post-assessment shows clearance of secretions, more effective cough, cough controlled and less frequent, client less fatigued, client able to deep breathe easier, gurgling no longer present. | Documents that CCT have removed secretions from the airway. |
| 2. Client able to demonstrate CCT correctly. | Learning of skill achieved. |

### *Unexpected outcomes*

| Steps | Rationale |
|---|---|
| 1. Client experiences severe dyspnea with bronchospasm, hypoxemia, and hypercarbia (hypercapnia). | In seriously ill clients with severe respiratory insufficiency, mobilization of secretions into large central airways can precipitate bronchospasm and increase work of breathing. These changes can worsen gas exchange and increase dyspnea. |
| 2. Hemoptysis occurs. | May be caused by infection, erosion of blood vessels, or other causes. |
| 3. No secretions are obtained. | May result from lack of secretions or secretions being too thick to mobilize. |
| 4. No change in crackles and gurgles; crepitus present; shortness of breath occurs; chest wall does not expand. | Airways continue to contain mucus. |
| 5. Client unable to demonstrate CCT correctly | Further instruction required. |

## Recording and Reporting

| Steps | Rationale |
|---|---|
| 1. Record in nurses' notes type of CCT used; frequency of coughing, cough effectiveness, description of sputum expectorated, client's ability to perform proper cough, client's tolerance and reaction, teaching for home care, unexpected outcomes, pre- and post-assessment. | Provides proper documentation of CCT and client's tolerance of the procedure. If CCT is performed by a home health nurse, documentation of such therapy is necessary for third-party reimbursement. |

## Follow-up Activities

| Steps | Rationale |
|---|---|
| 1. Use inhaled bronchodilators 30 min before CCT in clients at risk for bronchospasm. | Provides optimal bronchodilation and reduces risk of hypoxemia and hypercarbia. |

## Special Considerations

- Huffing can be used after surgery because it can often be done effectively with less pain.
- In some airway diseases forceful cough can cause complete collapse of small airways, which makes cough ineffective. These clients are taught to cascade cough at low lung volumes and rely on chest therapy to help clear mucus.

## Teaching Considerations

- Teach controlled coughing to clients whenever possible. If done properly it can be very effective in easing the work of coughing and making the client more comfortable.
- Instruct client's family or primary care giver to recognize when the client's respiratory status requires controlled coughing to facilitate air exchange.
- Encourage primary care giver or family member to encourage client to participate in physical activities that will increase respiratory efficiency.

## Home Care Considerations

- In chronic disease states discuss importance of performing controlled coughing at home. Involve family in teaching whenever possible.
- Mechanical devices are sometimes used (1) at home if trained therapist is not available or (2) if client does not tolerate manual therapy. They are available through most home equipment companies.
- Assess home environment for ventilation; accessibility of clean, fresh air; presence of air conditioning; and client's reaction to each of these.
- Provide a basin into which the client can expectorate secretions.

---

### BIBLIOGRAPHY


Hogstel M: Home nursing care for elderly, Englewood Cliffs, NJ, 1985, Prentice Hall Publishing Company.

Judge RD, Zuidema GD: Methods of clinical examination: a physiologic approach, Boston, 1974, Little, Brown & Co.

King M, et al.: Tracheal mucus clearance in high frequency oscillation. II. chest wall versus mouth oscillation, Am Rev Respir Dis 103:703, 1984.

Long B, Phipps W: Medical-surgical nursing, ed 2, St. Louis, 1989, The CV Mosby Company.

McHugh J: Perfecting the three steps fo chest physiotherapy, Nursing '87, 17(11):54, 1987.

Meyers D: Client teaching guides for home health care, Rockville, Md, 1988, Aspen Publishers, Inc.

Potter PA, Perry AG: Fundamentals of nursing, ed 2, St. Louis, 1989, The CV Mosby Co.

Thompson J, et al.: Mosby's manual of clinical nursing, ed 2, St. Louis, 1989, The CV Mosby Co.

Walsh J, Persons C, Wieck L: Manual of home health care nursing, Philadelphia, 1987, JB Lippincott.

Wanner A: Does chest physical therapy move airway secretion? Am Rev Respir Dis 130:701, 1984.

# 16
# AIRWAY MAINTENANCE

### OBJECTIVES

*Mastery of content in this chapter will enable the nurse to:*

- Define key terms.
- Describe the methods of airway management.
- Discuss the indications for airway suctioning.
- Discuss the indications for tracheostomy care.
- Demonstrate the following skills on selected clients: bulb suctioning, pharyngeal suctioning, tracheal suctioning, endotracheal or tracheostomy tube suctioning, endotracheal tube care, tracheostomy tube care, cuff care.
- Develop teaching plans for selected home care clients for tracheostomy suctioning; tracheostomy tube care.

### KEY TERMS

| | |
|---|---|
| *Artificial airway* | *Intubation* |
| *Aspirant* | *Lower airway respiratory system* |
| *Aspirate* | *Nasal airway* |
| *Atelectasis* | *Oral airway* |
| *Bronchospasm* | *Sputum* |
| *Bronchus* | *Suction* |
| *Endotracheal tube* | *Suction catheter* |
| *Hemoptysis* | *Tracheal malacia* |
| *Hypoxemia* | *Tracheostomy* |
| *Hypoxia* | *Upper airway respiratory system* |

### SKILLS

**16-1** Performing Bulb Syringe Suctioning
**16-2** Performing Oral Pharyngeal (Yankauer) Suctioning
**16-3** Performing Nasal Pharyngeal and Nasal Tracheal Suctioning
**16-4** Performing Endotracheal or Tracheostomy Tube Suctioning
**16-5** Performing Endotracheal Tube Care
**16-6** Performing Tracheostomy Care
**16-7** Managing a Cuffed Endotracheal or Tracheostomy Tube
**16-8** Teaching Home Tracheostomy Care and Suctioning

Many courses of action are available to maintain a patent airway. Based on continual assessment of the client the nurse can include in the plan of care measures that aid in maintaining upper or lower airway patency and measures that have effects on both the upper and lower airways. Hydration, nutrition, postural drainage, percussion, vibration, rib shaking, deep breathing, coughing, and aerosol treatments are noninvasive techniques (Chapter 15) that are all helpful in maintaining a patent airway.

In some clients use of the above techniques is not sufficient to maintain a patent airway. More invasive measures may be necessary. This chapter presents nonemergent techniques designed to maintain patency of the anatomic and artificial airway. Techniques discussed include: bulb syringe, pharyngeal, tracheal, endotracheal tube, and tracheostomy tube suctioning; endotracheal tube, and tracheostomy tube care; artificial airway cuff inflation; and home care techniques for suctioning and tracheostomy tube care.

## GUIDELINES

1. Know client's normal range of vital signs. Baseline vital signs serve as a means to identify individual abnormalities. Normal vital signs for one client may be abnormal for another client.
2. Know client's medical history. Certain conditions such as chronic pulmonary diseases and abdominal surgery predictably place the client at risk for an obstructed airway.
3. Know client's baseline respiratory assessment. Baseline assessment has two meanings. First, know what is unusual or normal for the client. Second, know what client's condition has been for the last 8, 16, or 24 hours. These are relative baseline measurements, which assist the nurse in distinguishing between gradual and acute changes in the client's status.
4. Perform a systematic respiratory assessment. This includes upper and lower airways, identifying respiratory rate, respiratory pattern, respiratory muscles used, ability to cough effectively, and integrity of the rib cage (Chapter 13).

5. Determine the type and frequency of intervention, based on assessment findings. Care that is appropriate for one day or shift can change resulting in an increase or decrease in frequency of care or a change in the type of intervention.
6. Identify and become familiar with the application of equipment available at the institution. Many types of airways, suction catheters, and suction machines are available. Knowing how to operate the equipment before it is needed benefits both the nurse and the client.
7. Test all equipment before use. Equipment must work properly to provide safe nursing care. Determining that the suction machine is not generating adequate negative pressure when the client has a mucus plug or overwhelming secretions is not safe, competent nursing practice.
8. Know client's home care plan. Absence or interruption of certain therapies place the client at risk for an obstructed airway after discharge from the hospital.

Nurses can prevent or reduce both the amount of retained secretions and the amount of decreased ventilation by maintaining a patent airway, performing chest physiotherapy (Chapter 15), administering appropriate oxygen therapy (Chapter 14), using position changes, and using sedatives and narcotics judiciously.

### PREREQUISITE KNOWLEDGE

1. Airway anatomy of infants, children, and adults.
2. Mechanism of gas exchange.
3. Principles of medical and surgical asepsis.
4. Principles of cough.
5. Principles of airway resistance.
6. Indications for an artificial airway.
7. Complications of an artificial airway.

### PREREQUISITE SKILLS

1. Proper handwashing techniques (Chapter 37).
2. Physical assessment (Chapter 13).
3. Vital signs (Chapter 12).
4. Insertion of oral or nasal airway (Chapter 18).
5. Administration of oxygen (Chapter 14).
6. Opening sterile packages (Chapter 38).

## *SKILL 16-1 Performing Bulb Syringe Suctioning*

A bulb syringe is a soft, flexible, plastic device constructed with only one small opening through which air and mucus pass. The bulb syringe is traditionally used to suction infants and children; however, it can also be used in adults when nasal and oral secretions do not require use of the traditional suction catheter or the Yankauer suction. A bulb syringe is easy to use, requires minimal equipment, exerts gentle controlled pressure making it less traumatic than traditional suction catheters, does not require use of surgical asepsis, and can be performed rapidly. However, use of the bulb syringe is limited to the upper airway. The description of this procedure is geared to the infant; however, the principles and techniques are the same for an older child or adult.

A bulb syringe is standard equipment in most delivery rooms and newborn nurseries. The bulb syringe is initially used to aspirate amniotic fluid and mucus from the infant's oral and nasal passages immediately after delivery. Parents of a newborn are frequently given a bulb syringe as part of the mother's gift pack. The bulb syringe is useful when the child has congested nares from a cold or an allergy. Nurses can teach parents how to use the bulb syringe for suctioning.

### Purposes

1. Maintain a patent upper airway.
2. Relieve respiratory distress.

### *Procedure 16-1*

| Steps | Rationale |
|---|---|
| **Assessment** | |
| 1. Observe for signs and symptoms that indicate the presence of upper airway obstruction in neonate: increased respiratory rate, labored respirations, use of accessory muscles during breathing, increased or decreased pulse rate (hypoxia), fever, drooling, nasal flaring, obvious secretions in nares, mouth-breathing with or without ability to breathe through nares. | Newborn infants are obligate nose breathers for the first few months of life. They are unable to breathe when nares are obstructed. Physical signs and symptoms result from decreased oxygen (hypoxia) to tissues, as well as pooling of secretions in upper airways. |

| Steps | Rationale |
|---|---|
| 2. Determine factors that normally influence upper airway functioning. | Physiologic and environmental influences can impede gas exchange and result in need for bulb suctioning of infant. |
| 3. Assess parent's understanding of technique of bulb syringe suctioning. | Identifies potential educational needs of parents. |

## Nursing Diagnosis

| Steps | Rationale |
|---|---|
| 1. Cluster relevant data to reveal actual or potential nursing diagnoses: | |
| a. Impaired gas exchange: related to retained secretions. | Ventilation is altered because retained secretions inhibit normal air flow. |
| b. Ineffective airway clearance: related to thick secretions. | Retained secretions impede airway clearance. |
| c. Knowledge deficit: related to use of bulb syringe. | Parents and other care givers need instruction in use of bulb syringe. |

## Planning

| Steps | Rationale |
|---|---|
| 1. Develop individualized goals for client based on nursing diagnoses: | |
| a. Promote patent airway. | Removal of nasal and oral secretions in the infant improves comfort and oxygen delivery. |
| 2. Prepare needed equipment and supplies:<br>a. Bulb syringe<br>b. Soft tissue<br>c. Two soft cloths (washcloth, towel, or diaper)<br>d. Disposable gloves | Necessary equipment at bedside ensures that suctioning will be completed quickly and efficiently. In emergent situation nurse can immediately maintain patent airway without having to search for equipment. |
| 3. Prepare client for procedure: | |
| a. Explain reason for and technique of bulb syringe suction to care givers. | Relieves anxiety and encourages cooperation. |
| b. Position infant or small child. Use 1 of 3 methods: | Promotes easier removal of secretions. |
| ▪ Hold child in arms tucking arm closest to care giver around back and holding free arm with nurse's cradling arm. | Enables care giver to suction oral airway without interference from infant's hands. |
| ▪ Bundle child in blanket or large towel to restrain arms and hold child on nurse's lap. | Bundling is method of applying mummy restraint (Chapter 4). |
| ▪ Lay larger child on bed or couch face up with head slightly elevated and arms at sides. Sitting next to the child, care giver lays upper torso lightly across chest. If additional restraint is needed, child can be bundled in blanket or large towel. | Pressure from care giver's body on child's chest restrains arm movements while bulb suctioning is applied. |

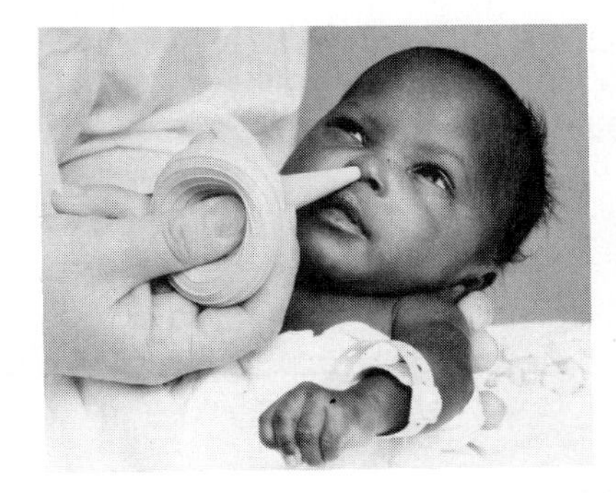

***Fig. 16-1***

## Implementation

| Steps | Rationale |
|---|---|
| 1. Wash hands and apply clean gloves. | Reduces transmission of microorganisms. |
| 2. Place soft cloth over chest biblike, and tissues within reach. | Prevents secretions from contaminating clothes. |
| 3. Holding bulb in free hand, firmly squeeze bulb end of syringe forcing air out of syringe. | Prevents forcing airway secretions into infant's bronchi. |
| 4. Insert small tip into client's airway (nose or mouth) while keeping pressure on bulb and gently release pressure from bulb to suction secretions (Fig. 16-1). | It is more effective to pull bulb tip away from airway, especially nose, as pressure is released. Rapid release of pressure can cause bulb tip to apply suction to mucosa in addition to applying suction to secretions. |
| 5. When all pressure is released from bulb, remove it from airway and rapidly squeeze bulb in and out several times over soft tissue. | Clears bulb tip of secretions and renders bulb syringe ready for subsequent suctioning. |
| 6. Reassess client's respiratory status. | Directs nurse to initiate intervention. |

| Steps | Rationale |
|---|---|
| 7. Repeat Steps 3-5 as needed to clear client's airway. | Maintains patent airway. |
| 8. Clean client's face and nares with soft tissue. | Promotes hygiene. Reduces transmission of microorganisms. |
| 9. Place client in comfortable position after soothing. | Positioning client on side promotes secretion drainage. Positioning client on back predisposes client to aspirate nasal or oral secretions into lungs. |
| 10. Discard tissue and bib into appropriate waste receptacles. | Reduces transmission of microorganisms. |
| 11. Rinse syringe under warm running water. Squeeze bulb several times to remove secretions. Hydrogen peroxide can be used to loosen resistant secretions. After rinsing, squeeze bulb in and out several times (in air) with tip pointed downward to remove excess water. | Prevents drying of secretions in the bulb syringe, which can make the syringe ineffective. |
| 12. Loosely wrap syringe in second cloth and store at client's bedside within easy reach. | Reduces transmission of microorganisms. |
| 13. Remove and discard gloves and wash hands. | Reduces transmission of microorganisms. |

## Evaluation

| | |
|---|---|
| 1. Compare client's respiratory status before and after bulb syringe suction. | Determines effectiveness of suction procedure. |

### *Expected outcomes*

| | |
|---|---|
| 1. Client's respiratory status improves as evidenced by decreased respiratory rate, decreased use of accessory muscles, and ability to breathe through nares. | Airway cleared of secretions. |

### *Unexpected outcomes*

| | |
|---|---|
| 1. Respiratory distress is increased, as evidenced by sternal retractions, flaring nares, and gurgling respirations. | Prolonged upper airway obstruction results in decreased oxygen delivery and cerebral hypoxia or cardiopulmonary arrest (Chapter 17) |

## Recording and Reporting

| | |
|---|---|
| 1. Record in nurses' notes: assessment findings for administering bulb syringe suctioning, frequency of administration of bulb syringe suctioning, infant tolerance of procedure, secretions obtained, notification and assistance of other medical personnel (e.g., physician). | Documents respiratory status and need for intervention, nursing care, expected and unexpected outcomes, and provides for future assessment parameters. |
| 2. Immediately report increasing respiratory distress to nurse in charge or physician. | Obtains necessary emergency personnel whose actions can reduce potential oxygen deficit to infant. |

## Follow-up Activities

| | |
|---|---|
| 1. Continued or increased respiratory distress (Assessment, Step 1): | |
| a. Repeat bulb syringe suctioning. | Removes additional secretions. |
| b. Notify physician. | Care needed is beyond scope of nursing practice. |

## Special Considerations

- Age: children have smaller nasal passages and proportionally larger tongue compared with adults. Younger client is more prone to total occlusion of air passages. It is difficult for very young children to clear upper air passages by blowing nose and coughing secretions from mouth. *Humidity:* secretions dry faster in nonmoist environment.
- Other therapies: antibiotics, decongestants, humidification, chest percussion, postural drainage, and oxygen may also enhance secretion removal.
- Positioning: if congenital anomaly is present, nurse's choice in positioning infant may be limited. Congenital anomalies include cleft palate, musculoskeletal defect, spinal bifida, birth injury (soft tissue injury, head trauma, fractured clavicle).
- Infection control: in newborn nursery each infant should have own waste receptacle attached to Isolette frame.

## Teaching Considerations

- Teach parents to assess for respiratory distress and need to suction airway.
- Demonstrate suction technique.
- Observe return demonstration for assessment and for suction technique.
- After demonstrating technique of bulb suctioning have care givers practice proper technique.
- Explain risks of squeezing air out of syringe into client's airway and improper cleaning.

### Home Care Considerations

- Discuss emergency procedures in event care givers are unable to clear airway with bulb syringe.
- Normal saline (1-2 drops) can be instilled in each naris to loosen secretions. Position child flat. Head may be kept midline or turned to side after drops have been instilled.
- Assess knowledge level of client, family, and primary care giver to determine the amount of instruction required and the frequency of visits necessary to reach the goals.
- Assess home for the presence of respiratory irritants including dust, pollen, or chemicals.

## *SKILL 16-2 Performing Oral Pharyngeal (Yankauer) Suctioning*

Nurses use a Yankauer or tonsillar tip suction to perform oral pharyngeal suctioning (Fig. 16-2). A Yankauer or tonsillar tip suction catheter is made of rigid, minimally flexible plastic. The tip of this suction catheter usually has one large and several small eyelets through which the mucus enters. The Yankauer suction catheter is angled to remove pharyngeal secretions through the mouth. This catheter is used instead of a standard suction catheter when oral secretions are extremely copius and thick. The Yankauer suctioning catheter is not used to suction the nares, except externally, because of its size.

The Yankauer suction apparatus is useful in the removal of secretions in clients after oral and maxillofacial surgery or after trauma to the mouth. Alert clients can be easily taught how to use this apparatus and control the secretions in the oral cavity.

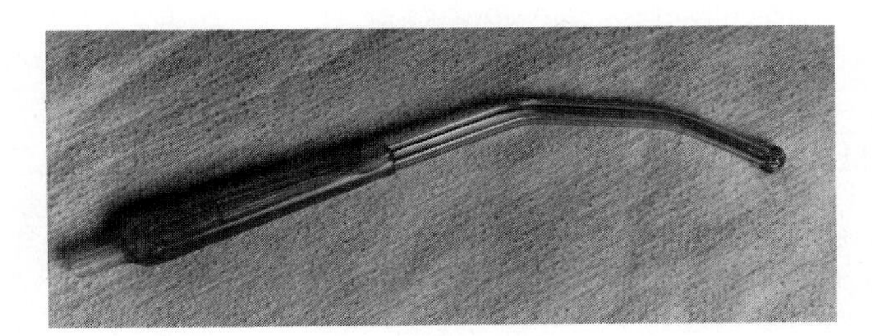

***Fig. 16-2***

### Purpose

1. Remove oral secretions that are too thick or copious for a standard suction catheter.
2. Maintain upper airway patency.

## *Procedure 16-2*

| Steps | Rationale |
|---|---|
| **Assessment** | |
| 1. Observe for signs and symptoms of upper and lower airway obstruction requiring Yankauer oral pharyngeal suctioning: gurgling on inspiration or expiration, restlessness, obvious excess oral secretions, drooling, gastric secretions or vomitus in mouth. | Physical signs and symptoms may indicate need to perform this procedure. |
| **Nursing Diagnosis** | |
| 1. Cluster data to reveal actual or potential nursing diagnoses: | |
| a. Ineffective airway clearance, related to: | |
| ▪ Decreased level of consciousness. | Cough reflex, gag reflex, or swallow may be impaired. |
| ▪ Upper airway secretion. | Client unable to remove secretions. |
| ▪ Inability to swallow or cough. | Stroke and other neurovascular injury can impair muscle function. |
| **Planning** | |
| 1. Develop individualized goals for client based on nursing diagnoses: | |
| a. Promote patent airway. | Partial airway obstruction reduces the amount of inhaled oxygen. |
| b. Mobilize airway secretions. | Removal of airway secretions reduces hazard of infection. |

| Steps | Rationale |
|---|---|
| 2. Prepare needed equipment and supplies:<br>a. Yankauer or tonsillar tip suction catheter<br>b. 2 nonsterile gloves<br>c. Disposable cup or nonsterile basin.<br>d. Water, approximately 100 ml<br>e. Towel<br>f. Portable or wall suction apparatus<br>g. 6 ft of connecting tubing<br>h. Oral airway, if indicated | Necessary equipment at bedside ensures that suctioning will be completed quickly and efficiently. In emergency situation, nurse can immediately maintain patent airway without having to search for equipment. |
| 3. Prepare client: | |
| a. Explain to client how the procedure will help clear the airway and relieve some of the breathing problems. Explain that coughing, sneezing, or gagging is normal. | Encourages cooperation, minimizes risks and associated anxiety. |
| b. Assist client to comfortable position for both nurse and client, usually semi-Fowler's or Sim's unless client is unconscious, then side-lying facing nurse. | Promotes client comfort, prevents nurse's back strain, promotes drainage, prevents aspiration. |
| c. Place towel across client's chest. | |

## Implementation

| Steps | Rationale |
|---|---|
| 1. Wash hands. | Reduces transmission of microorganisms. |
| 2. Fill cup or basin with approximately 100 ml of water. | For cleansing catheter after suctioning. |
| 3. Apply gloves. | Reduces transmission of microorganisms from client to nurse. |
| 4. Turn suction device on; set regulator to appropriate negative pressure:<br>*Wall suction*<br>Infants 60-100 mm Hg<br>Children 100-120 mm Hg<br>Adults 120-150 mm Hg<br>(Blodgett, 1980).<br>*Portable suction*<br>Infants 3-5 inches Hg<br>Children 5-10 inches Hg<br>Adults 7-15 inches Hg | Elevated pressure settings increase risk of trauma to the oral mucosa. |
| 5. Connect one end of connecting tubing to suction machine and other to Yankauer suction catheter. Fill cup with water. | Prepares suction apparatus. |
| 6. Check that equipment is functioning properly by suctioning small amount of water from cup or basin. | Ensures equipment function and lubricates catheter. |
| 7. Remove oxygen mask, if present. | |
| 8. Insert catheter into mouth along gum line to pharynx. Move catheter around mouth until secretions are cleared. Encourage client to cough. Replace oxygen mask. | Catheter provides continuous suction. Care must be taken not to allow suction tip to invaginate oral mucosal surfaces. Coughing moves secretions from lower airway into mouth and upper airway. |
| 9. Rinse catheter with water in cup or basin until connecting tubing is cleared of secretions. Turn off suction. | Rinses catheter and reduces probability of transmission of microorganisms. Clean suction tubing enhances delivery of set suction pressure. |
| 10. Reassess respiratory status. | Directs nurse to initiate or cease intervention. |
| 11. Remove towel, place in laundry. Remove gloves and dispose in receptacle. | Reduces transmission of microorganisms. |
| 12. Reposition client; Sims' position encourages drainage and should be used if client has decreased level of consciousness. | Facilitates drainage of oral secretions. |
| 13. Discard remainder of water into appropriate receptacle. Rinse basin in warm soapy water and dry with paper towels. Discard disposable cup into appropriate receptacle. Place catheter in clean dry area. | Reduces transmission of microorganisms and maintains medical asepsis. |
| 14. Wash hands. | Reduces transmission of microorganisms to other clients. |

## Evaluation

| Steps | Rationale |
|---|---|
| 1. Compare assessment findings before and after procedure. | Identifies physiologic effect of the suction procedure. |

| Steps | Rationale |
|---|---|
| ***Expected outcomes*** | |
| 1. Upper airway (oral pharynx) is cleared of secretions. | Suctioning was successful with cleared airway. |
| 2. No gurgling is heard in pharynx on inspiration and expiration. | Presence of secretions in large upper airway produces noisy respirations. |
| 3. Oral secretions are diminished or absent. | Excessive drooling indicates that client is unable to handle oral secretions. |
| 4. Vomitus and gastric secretions are absent from mouth. | Gastric secretions retained in oral cavity increase client's risk for aspiration pneumonia. |
| ***Unexpected Outcomes*** | |
| 1. Client becomes cyanotic, tachycardic or bradycardic, more restless, etc. | Client may have aspirated or developed cardiopulmonary compromise as result of tissue hypoxia. |
| 2. Bloody secretions are suctioned. | Bloody secretions can result from trauma to oral or pharyngeal mucosa, in excessively high suction procedure. |
| **Recording and Reporting** | |
| 1. Record in nurses' notes: respiratory assessments before and after suction; use of Yankauer suction catheter; duration of suctioning period; secretions obtained—odor, amount, color, consistency; frequency of suctioning; client's tolerance of procedure; amount of negative suction pressure used (unless standardized in institution). | Documents cardiopulmonary status, nursing care, expected and unexpected outcomes, and provides baseline future assessments. |
| **Follow-up Activities** | |
| 1. For client with worsening respiratory distress, evaluate need for: nasal or oral pharyngeal or tracheal suctioning, other means to protect airway (e.g., oral intubation, airway, positioning), supplemental oxygen (Chapter 14), manual breathing assistance after suctioning. | These measures maintain patency of airway and reduce airway obstruction. |
| 2. For return of bloody secretions evaluate amount of suction pressure used. Evaluate possibility of mucosal trauma from catheter tip. | Excessive suction pressure or trauma to oral mucosa produces bloody secretions. |

## Special Considerations

- Clients with following conditions are at risk for accumulation of oral secretions: decreased level of consciousness, impaired gag reflex, impaired cough, heavy sedation, oral surgery, oral trauma, head injury, spine injury.
- Clients at risk for bloody secretions include those with hemophilia, blood dyscrasias, chemotherapy. Lower suction pressure should be applied.
- Clients who bite the catheter preventing thorough suctioning may require insertion of an oral airway.
- If respiratory distress or signs of cardiopulmonary compromise occur, remain with client and complete serial cardiopulmonary nursing assessments (Chapter 13).
- If trauma to oral mucosa repeatedly occurs, incorporate frequent oral hygiene into nursing plan (Chapter 8).
- A Yankauer suction device is frequently given to clients with swallowing problems such as occur after stroke or post-intubation. Observe client when using to be sure that sutures, tubes, traumatized tissue, and dressings are undisturbed.
- If indicated, the nurse can leave a small disposable cup of tap water at the bedside for client rinsing. If the client is unable to independently rinse the suction device, the nurse should periodically rinse secretions from the tubing. Suction ability is reduced when secretions accumulate in the tubing.

## Home Care Considerations

- Yankauer suction devices can be soaked in hydrogen peroxide to remove encrusted secretions and then reused. Mouthwash mixed with hydrogen peroxide imparts a fresher smell and taste to the Yankauer suction device.
- Do not allow suction equipment to fall to the floor or become contaminated by excrement.
- Assess knowledge level of the client, family, and primary care giver to determine the amount of instruction required and the frequency of visits necessary to reach the goals.
- Assess home for the presence of respiratory irritants including dust, pollen, or chemicals.

# *SKILL 16-3 Performing Nasal Pharyngeal and Nasal Tracheal Suctioning*

Nasal pharyngeal and nasal tracheal suctioning are two techniques available to the nurse to maintain a patent airway. These techniques involve inserting a small rubber or plastic tube into the naris to the pharynx or trachea then applying negative pressure to withdraw mucus.

The major differences between pharyngeal and tracheal suctioning are the depth suctioned and the potential for complications. The nurse assesses the client to determine frequency and depth of suctioning. For an adult the catheter should be 20 cm long (Harper, 1981). The length of insertion of the suction catheter depends on the size of the infant or child. To determine the correct length of catheter, first determine the age of the child. Infants and young children can tolerate insertion of a catheter 8 to 14 cm, while the older child can tolerate a catheter depth of 14 to 20 cm. These lengths vary with each child. The nurse can verify the correct catheter length by measuring the distance from nose to ear and nose to midsternum for nasal tracheal suctioning or from the mouth to midsternum for oral tracheal suctioning. Proper suctioning technique promotes client safety and helps prevent suctioning-induced complications, including cardiopulmonary compromise, mucosal damage, and infection.

The nurse uses the techniques of suctioning primarily to remove accumulated nasal pharyngeal and tracheal secretions. Secretions should be suctioned from the pharynx as often as necessary. Secretions that are not removed are more likely to be aspirated into the lungs, increasing a risk for potential infection and respiratory failure. In addition, the nurse may need to remove other body fluids, primarily blood and gastric contents, from the oral and posterior pharynx to prevent their aspiration as well.

The carina, located at the bifurcation of the mainstem bronchi, has many cough receptors. Many times the nurse will be able to stimulate a client's decreased cough reflex by passing a suction catheter to the carina. Once the client coughs he is able to clear his lower airway more effectively.

### Purposes

1. Maintain upper and lower airway patency by removing secretions.
2. Prevent pulmonary aspiration of other body fluids, such as blood or vomitus.
3. Stimulate deep cough.

## *Procedure 16-3*

| Steps | Rationale |
|---|---|
| **Assessment** | |
| 1. Assess signs and symptoms of upper and lower airway obstruction requiring nasal or oral tracheal suctioning, including wheezes, crackles, or gurgling on inspiration or expiration; restlessness; ineffective coughing; unilateral or lobar absent or diminished breath sounds (in absence of pneumonectomy or lobectomy); tachypnea; hypertension or hypotension; cyanosis; acutely decreased level of consciousness; excess nasal secretions, drooling, gastric secretions or vomitus in mouth. | Physical signs and symptoms result from decreased oxygen to tissues, as well as pooling of secretions in upper and lower airways. |
| 2. Determine factors that normally influence lower airway functioning. | Physiologic and environmental influences can impede gas exchange and result in need for airway suctioning. |
| **Nursing Diagnosis** | |
| 1. Cluster data to reveal actual or potential nursing diagnoses: | |
| a. Ineffective airway clearance: related to impaired cough or retained secretions. | Client is unable to remove or to prevent aspiration of secretions. Retained secretions are ideal media for microorganism growth. |
| b. Impaired gas exchange: related to retained secretions. | Presence of lower airway secretions decreases transfer of respiratory gases across alveolar membrane. |

| Steps | Rationale |
|---|---|
| **Planning** | |
| 1. Develop individualized goals for client based on nursing diagnoses: | |
| a. Promote patent airway. | Partial airway obstruction from retained secretions reduces the amount of inhaled oxygen |
| b. Mobilize airway secretions. | Removal of airway secretions reduces hazard of pulmonary infection. |
| 2. Prepare needed equipment and supplies: | Necessary equipment at bedside ensures that suctioning will be completed quickly and efficiently. In emergency situation, nurse can immediately maintain patent airway without having to search for equipment. Catheter should not occlude airway by more than one half diameter (Luce, 1984). A larger catheter predisposes client to greater complications, especially hypoxemia and atelectasis. |
| a. Suction catheter with intermittent control port of appropriate size for client (Hazinski, 1984).<br>Newborn 6-8 Fr<br>Infant to 6 mo 6-8 Fr<br>18 mo 8-10 Fr<br>24 mo 10 Fr<br>2-4 years 10-12 Fr<br>4-7 years 12 Fr<br>7-10 years 12-14 Fr<br>10-12 years 14 Fr<br>Adults 12-16 Fr<br>If catheter does not have a suction control port, connect a small "y" adapter to the catheter. | |
| b. Water-soluble lubricant | Petroleum lubricant such as Vasoline should not be used because of hazard of chemical aspiration. |
| c. 2 sterile gloves or 1 sterile and 1 nonsterile glove | |
| d. Sterile basin | |
| e. Approximately 100 ml of sterile normal saline | |
| f. Clean towel or sterile drape from kit | |
| g. Portable or wall suction apparatus:<br>*Vacuum settings—Wall*<br>Infants 60-100 mm Hg<br>Children 100-120 mm Hg<br>Adults 120-150 mm Hg<br>(Blodgett, 1980)<br>*Vacuum setting—portable*<br>Infants 3-5 inches Hg<br>Children 5-10 inches Hg<br>Adults 7-15 inches Hg | |
| h. 6 ft of connecting tubing | |
| i. Nasal or oral airway, if indicated | |
| j. Sterile suction kit can be used (be sure all listed items not in kit are assembled) | |
| 3. Prepare client: | |
| a. Explain to client how procedure will help clear airway and relieve breathing problems. Explain that coughing sneezing, or gagging is normal. | Encourages cooperation and minimizes risks and anxiety. |
| b. Explain importance of and encourage coughing during procedure. | Facilitates secretion removal and may reduce frequency of future suctioning. |
| c. Assist client to assume position comfortable for nurse and client (usually semi-Fowler's or sitting upright with head hyperextended, unless contraindicated). If unconscious, lay client on side facing nurse. | Reduces stimulation of gag reflex, promotes client comfort and secretion drainage, prevents aspiration and nurse strain. |
| d. Place towel across client's chest. | Reduces transmission of microorganisms. |
| **Implementation** | |
| 1. Wash hands. | Reduces transmission of microorganisms. |
| 2. Turn suction device on and set vacuum regulator to appropriate negative pressure. | Excessive negative pressure damages nasal pharyngeal and tracheal mucosa and can induce greater hypoxia. |
| 3. If indicated, increase supplemental oxygen to 100% or as ordered by physician. | Reduces suction-induced hypoxemia. (The literature is inconclusive as to the necessity of hyperoxygenation.) |
| 4. Connect one end of connecting tubing to suction machine and place other end in convenient location. | Prepares for connection of suction catheter to suction apparatus. |

| Steps | Rationale |
|---|---|
| 5. If using suction kit: | |
| a. Open package. If sterile drape is available, place it across client's chest or use a towel. | Reduces transmission of microorganisms. |
| b. Open suction catheter package. Do not allow suction catheter to touch any surface other than inside of its package. | Prepares catheter and reduces transmission of microorganisms. Maintains medical asepsis. |
| c. Unwrap or open sterile basin and place on bedside table. Be careful not to touch inside of basin. Fill with about 100 ml sterile normal saline. | Saline is used to clean tubing after each suction pass. |
| 6. Open lubricant. Squeeze onto open sterile catheter package without touching package. | Prepares lubricant while maintaining sterility. Water soluble lubricant is used to avoid lipoid aspiration pneumonia. |
| 7. Apply sterile glove to each hand or apply nonsterile glove to nondominant hand and sterile glove to dominant hand. | Reduces transmission of microorganisms and allows nurse to maintain sterility of suction catheter. |
| 8. Pick up suction catheter with dominant hand without touching nonsterile surfaces. Pick up connecting tubing with nondominant hand. Secure catheter to tubing (Fig. 16-3). | Maintains catheter sterility. Connects catheter to suction. |
| 9. Check that equipment is functioning properly by suctioning small amount of normal saline from basin. | Ensures equipment function. Lubricates internal catheter and tubing. |
| 10. Coat distal 6-8 cm of catheter with water-soluble lubricant. | Lubricates catheter for easier insertion. |
| 11. Remove oxygen delivery device, if applicable, with nondominant hand. Without applying suction, gently but quickly insert catheter with dominant thumb and forefinger into naris using slight downward slant or through mouth when client breathes in. Do not force through naris (Fig. 16-4). | Application of suction pressure while introducing catheter into trachea increases risk of damage to mucosa, as well as increased risk of hypoxia due to removal of entrained oxygen present in airways. Epiglottis is open on inspiration and facilitates insertion into trachea. Client should cough. If client gags or becomes nauseated, catheter is most likely in esophagus. |
| a. Pharyngeal suctioning: in adults, insert catheter about 16 cm; in older children 8-12 cm; in infants and young children 4-8 cm. Rule of thumb is to insert catheter distance from tip of nose to base of ear lobe. | |
| b. Tracheal suctioning: in adults, insert catheter 20-24 cm; in older children, 14-20 cm; and in young children and infants 8-14 cm. | |
| c. Positioning: in some instances turning client's head to right helps nurse suction left mainstem bronchus; turning head to left helps nurse suction right mainstem bronchus. If resistance is felt after insertion of catheter for recommended distance, nurse has probably hit carina. Pull catheter back 1 cm before applying suction. | |
| 12. Apply intermittent suction for up to 10 sec by placing and releasing nondominant thumb over vent of catheter and slowly withdraw catheter while rotating it back and forth between dominant thumb and forefinger. Encourage client to cough. Replace oxygen device, if applicable. | Intermittent suction and rotation of catheter prevents injury to mucosa. If catheter "grabs" mucosa, remove thumb to release suction. Suctioning longer than 10 sec can cause cardiopulmonary compromise. |
| 13. Rinse catheter and connecting tubing with normal saline until cleared. | Removes secretions from catheter. |

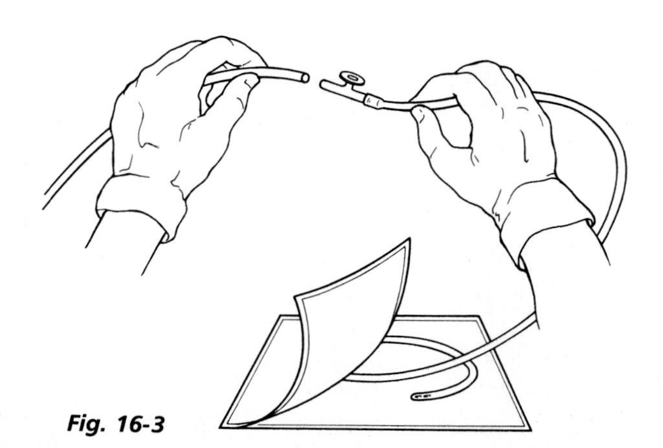

***Fig. 16-3***

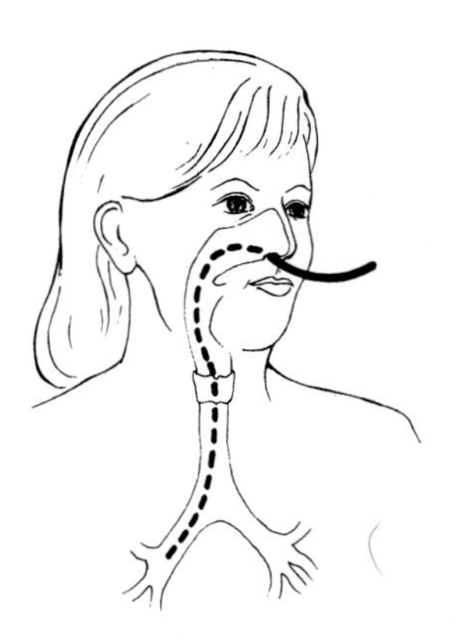

***Fig. 16-4***

| Steps | Rationale |
|---|---|
| 14. Repeat Steps 10-12 as needed to clear pharynx or trachea of secretions. Allow adequate time between suction passes for ventilation. | Repeated passes with the suction catheter clear the airway of excessive secretions and promote oxygenation. |
| 15. Monitor client's cardiopulmonary status between suction passes. Ask client to deep breath and cough. | Observe for alterations in cardiopulmonary status. Suctioning can induce hypoxia, dysrhythmias, and bronchospasm. Deep breathing reventilates and reoxygenates alveoli. |
| 16. When pharynx and trachea are sufficiently cleared of secretions, perform oral pharyngeal suctioning to clear mouth of secretions. | Removes upper airway secretions. |
| 17. When suctioning is completed, roll catheter around fingers of dominant hand. Pull glove off inside out so that catheter remains coiled in glove. Pull off other glove in same way. Discard in appropriate receptacle. Turn off suction device. | Reduces transmission of microorganisms. |
| 18. Remove towel, place in laundry. | Reduces transmission of microorganisms. |
| 19. Reposition client. | Promotes comfort. |
| 20. If indicated readjust oxygen to original level. | Prevents absorption atelectasis and oxygen toxicity. |
| 21. Discard remainder of normal saline into appropriate receptacle. If basin is disposable, discard into appropriate receptacle. If basin is reusable, rinse it out and place it in soiled utility room. | Reduces transmission of microorganisms. |
| 22. Wash hands. | Reduces transmission of microorganisms. |
| 23. Place unopened suction kit on suction machine or at head of bed. | Provides immediate access to suction catheter. |

## Evaluation

| | |
|---|---|
| 1. Compare client's respiratory assessments before and after suctioning. | Identifies physiologic effect of the suction procedure. |

### *Expected outcomes*

| | |
|---|---|
| 1. Lower and upper airways are cleared of secretions as evidenced by absent or diminished crackles, wheezes, and gurgles on inspiration and expiration; return of absent or diminished breath sounds; normalization of heart rate; absence of drooling, gastric secretions or vomitus in mouth, and nasal secretions. | Suctioning was successful; airways are cleared of secretions. |

### *Unexpected outcomes*

| | |
|---|---|
| 1. Client becomes cyanotic, tachycardic, bradycardic, more restless; less alert; suffers cardiac arrest; develops dysrhythmias. | Effect of prolonged hypoxia on client's cardiopulmonary and cerebral circulation. Client may have aspirated gastric secretions. |
| 2. Returned secretions are bloody. | Suctioning denuded cilia and mucosal lining. Bloody secretion may also indicate presence of infection. |
| 3. Nurse is unable to pass suction catheter through first naris attempted. | Obstruction present or catheter misplaced. |
| 4. Client has spasmodic episode of coughing. | Suctioning stimulates tracheal irritation. Bronchospasm may occur. Prolonged coughing episodes can disrupt ventilation and interfere with venous return to heart (Harper, 1981). |
| 5. No secretions are obtained. | When client is poorly hydrated and is not receiving humidified oxygen or room air, pulmonary secretions can consolidate in airways. |

## Recording and Reporting

| | |
|---|---|
| 1. Chart in nurses' notes respiratory assessments before and after suctioning; size of suction catheter used; duration of suctioning period; route(s) used to suction secretions obtained; odor, amount, color, consistency of secretions; frequency of suctioning; client's tolerance of procedure; amount of negative suction pressure used. | Documents cardiopulmonary status, nursing care, expected and unexpected outcomes, and provides baseline for future assessment. |

| Steps | Rationale |
|---|---|
| **Follow-up Activities** | |
| 1. Worsening respiratory assessment: | |
| a. Limit length of suctioning. | Steps a-d are measures to decrease effect of suction-induced hypoxia on client. |
| b. Evaluate need for more frequent suctioning, possibly of shorter duration. | |
| c. Evaluate need for supplemental oxygen. Supply oxygen between passes. | |
| d. Evaluate need for manual assistance with breathing after suctioning. | |
| e. Initiate resuscitation measures. | Steps e and f are emergency measures to restore client's cardiopulmonary status (Chapter 17). |
| f. Notify physician. | |
| 2. Return of bloody secretions: | |
| a. Evaluate amount of suction pressure used. May need to be decreased. | Decreases risk of damage to mucosa. |
| b. Evaluate nurse's use of intermittent suction and catheter rotation. | Continuous suction and lack of rotation of catheter pull at mucosal lining, causing hyperemia and ulcerations. |
| c. Evaluate suctioning frequency. | Suctioning in absence of secretions increase likelihood of mucosal damage. |
| 3. If unable to pass suction catheter through first naris attempted: | Methods used to bypass anatomic foreign obstructions. |
| a. Follow naris floor to avoid turbinates. | |
| b. Try other naris or oral route. | |
| c. If obstruction is mucus, apply suction to relieve obstruction. | |
| d. Increase lubrication. | |
| e. Insert nasal airway. | |
| 4. Period of spasmodic coughing: | |
| a. Allow client to use supplemental oxygen. | Prevents or reduces suction-induced hypoxia. |
| b. Unless emergent situation occurs, allow period of spasmodic coughing to subside before second catheter pass. | |
| c. Administer bronchodilator as prescribed by physician. | Relieves bronchospasm. |
| d. Instill topical anesthetic such as lidocaine, as prescribed by physician. | Anesthetizes cough receptors. |
| 5. No secretions obtained: | |
| a. Evaluate fluid status. | Dehydration results in thick, tenacious sputum that is difficult to remove with suction catheter. |
| b. Evaluate infection status. | Presence of infection increases likelihood of thick, tenacious sputum. |
| c. Evaluate humidity source for supplemental oxygen. | Insufficient humidity with supplemental oxygen results in thick sputum or consolidation of secretions. |

## Special Considerations

- Clients with following conditions are at greater risk: sinusitis, decreased level of consciousness, impaired gag reflex, impaired or absent cough, heavy sedation, neuromuscular disease, pneumonia, chronic obstructive pulmonary diseases (COPD), congestive heart failure, pulmonary edema; certain physical injuries contraindicate use of nasal pharyngeal suctioning: skull fractures, especially basillar; nasal fractures.
- *Age*: compared with adults infants and young children have smaller diameter airway and proportionally larger tongue. Glottis is higher; thorax is smaller with more horizontal ribs in soft rib cage. Diaphragm is higher and often impaired by abdominal size. Elderly have lost some properties of elastic recoil and gas exchange.
  - *Fluid status:* inadequately hydrated clients may have thick secretions.
  - *Nutrition:* inadequately nourished clients have impaired total lung function and ability to fight infection.
  - *Nasal structure:* septal deviations impair secretion drainage.
  - *Fluid status:* inadequately hydrated clients may have thick secretions.
- Positioning: Sims' position encourages drainage of oral and nasal secretions and should be used in clients who are comatose or semialert.
- Clients with history of deviated septum or facial trauma may require placement of nasal airway before nasal pharyngeal suctioning is attempted (Chapter 17).
- Clients with repeated nasal pharyngeal suctioning are at risk for return of bloody secretions and may require insertion of nasal or oral airway.

# SKILL 16-4 Performing Endotracheal or Tracheostomy Tube Suctioning

## CARE OF THE ENDOTRACHEAL AND TRACHEOSTOMY TUBES

Endotracheal (ET) and tracheostomy tubes (TT) are artificial airways inserted to relieve mechanical airway obstruction, provide mechanical ventilation, permit easy access for secretion removal, and protect the airway from aspiration due to impaired cough and gag reflexes.

Endotracheal intubation is a procedure performed by a physician or by specially trained personnel (e.g., nurse anesthetist, paramedic, critical care or emergency room nurse). An ET is inserted through the naris (nasal tracheal tube) or through the mouth (oral ET) past the epiglottis and vocal cords into the trachea.

ETs are usually left in place for up to 4 weeks after which time a TT is inserted directly into the trachea through a small incision made by the physician in the client's neck. Although ETs are temporary, a TT can be temporary or permanent. ETs are usually made of plastic; TTs are made of several different materials to meet a variety of client needs. Metal TTs are most frequently made of stainless steel or silver. Plastic TTs are also available in silastic. Some metal and plastic tubes have an inner, as well as an outer, cannula; others do not have an inner cannula.

ETs are cuffed, whereas TTs are available cuffed or uncuffed. Cuffs are made of plastic or plastic-covered foam. Plastic TTs have cuffs molded onto the main cannula. Metal tubes can frequently be adapted with a cuff. One of the hazards of using a nonpermanent cuff is that the attached cuff can be displaced from its proper position and occlude the airway.

ETs are not fenestrated. TTs can be fenestrated or nonfenestrated. A fenestration is a small hole in the outer cannula, which, when the cuff is deflated and the inner cannula is removed, permits the client to talk. Phonation is optimized when the outer cannula is plugged forcing all inhaled and exhaled air to travel by normal nasal and oral routes.

ET care is fairly well standardized. Tracheostomy care must be individualized to the client and the type of TT in place. For example, caring for a client with a TT with an inner cannula is different from caring for a client with a TT without an inner cannula. Care of a client with stomatitis differs from care of a client without localized tracheostomy stomal infection. These considerations must be addressed when planning nursing care.

On insertion of an ET or a TT the cuff is inflated. Preventing cuff-related problems is dependent on securing the tube properly, as well as properly inflating the cuff.

An inadequately secured ET or TT moves up and down the tracheobronchial tree. Allowing an ET to slip too far down into the lungs can prevent ventilation to one lung, usually the left lung because of anatomic differences. Allowing an ET to slide too far up the tracheobronchial tree can allow air to escape through the vocal cords and epiglottis or permit upper airway secretions to be aspirated. Proper securing of the ET or TT prevents loss of the artificial airway from coughing or pulling on the tube. In addition, an ET moving up and down the tracheobronchial tree can cause granulation tissue on the vocal cords, epiglottis, or trachea. Movement of either artificial airway places the client at risk for tracheal stenosis, tracheal malacia, erosion of the innominate artery, and tracheoesophageal fistula. Risks for each of these complications can be reduced by proper nursing care.

The goal in inflating the cuff on an ET or TT is to allow mechanical ventilation and prevent aspiration without impairing capillary circulation. The amount of air inserted into a cuff is based on several factors; the two most important factors are the size of the client's trachea and the size of the artificial airway. If two clients who are approximately the same size are intubated—one with a size 6 and one with a size 8—the client with the larger tube (size 8) will require less air in the cuff. This is because the larger tube occludes more of the airway than the smaller tube.

After the tube is inserted and secured and the cuff is inflated, the chief concern of the nurse is to maintain patency of the ET or TT. Patency of the ET or TT is achieved primarily by tracheal suctioning through the artificial airway. With a TT the nurse must also routinely clean the inner cannula, when one is present.

Suctioning is performed with a standard suction catheter. However, this skill is easier to perform than nasal tracheal suctioning because there is already direct access to the trachea by an artificial airway. Complications associated with ET or TT suctioning are the same as those associated with nasal or oral tracheal suctioning. However, the client with an artificial airway is at greater risk for developing complications because the client's physiologic status is so compromised that an artificial airway is required.

Applying the laws of physics enables the nurse to understand the effects of secretions in the airway. Increasing the diameter of a tube decreases airway resistance. Decreasing the diameter of a tube increases airway resistance and therefore the work of breathing. Removing these secretions maintains a patent airway, increases the diameter of the tube, and decreases the work of breathing. In addition, as stated before, a cough can be stimulated by suctioning. The client helps maintain airway patency with facilitation of the natural cough reflex.

All of the above skills are presented in this chapter. There are other needs of the intubated client which are not addressed in this chapter. Two important needs are communication and oral hygiene.

a. The intubated client is unable to speak. When caring for an intubated client, the nurse is encouraged to use verbal and nonverbal communication skills to communicate. Alphabet charts, pen and paper, and Magic Slates are three commonly used nonverbal client communication tools.
b. Placement of an oral ET tube affects oral hygiene. Excessive manipulation of the tube can dislodge it; toothbrushing and mouth rinsing are difficult, at best. Techniques are available to the nurse to provide or promote oral hygiene for the client. One technique is to rotate an oral ET tube from one side of the client's mouth to the other, thereby reducing pressure on the sides of the client's mouth as well.

A comprehensive plan and execution of care include properly securing the tube, inflating the cuff, and maintaining patency, as well as encouraging communication and oral hygiene. The next four Skills, 16-4, 16-5, 16-6, and 16-7 are components of ET and TT care.

### Purposes

1. Maintain airway patency.
2. Prevent infection.
3. Promote cleanliness.
4. Prevent skin breakdown around site of the tracheostomy stoma.
5. Decrease work of breathing.
6. Stimulate a deep cough.
7. Provide oral hygiene.
8. Prevent tracheal damage secondary to tube and cuff pressure.
9. Promote ventilation by maintaining the endotracheal tube in proper position.
10. Prevent endotracheal tube-related complications.

## *Procedure 16-4*

| Steps | Rationale |
|---|---|
| **Assessment** | |
| 1. Observe for signs and symptoms of lower airway obstruction requiring ET or TT suctioning: secretions in airway, wheezes or crackles on inspiration and/or expiration; restlessness; ineffective cough; unilateral (in absence of pneumonectomy or lobectomy) or bilateral absent or diminished breath sounds; tachypnea; acutely shallow respirations; tachycardia or bradycardia; hypertension or hypotension; cyanosis; acutely decreased level of consciousness. | Physical signs and symptoms result from lower airway obstruction and tissue hypoxia. |
| 2. Determine factors that influence normal airway function: impaired cough reflex, decreased level of consciousness, absent cough, heavy sedation, neuromuscular diseases, pneumonia, COPD, congestive heart failure, pulmonary edema, adult respiratory distress syndrome, hyaline membrane disease. | Allows nurse to accurately evaluate need to perform endotracheal tube or tracheostomy tube suctioning |
| **Nursing Diagnosis** | |
| 1. Cluster data to reveal actual or potential nursing diagnoses: | |
| a. Ineffective airway clearance: related to impaired cough. | Client is unable to increase intrathoracic pressure because of open epiglottis. |
| b. Potential for infection: related to retained secretions. | Retained secretions are ideal media for microorganism growth. Infected secretions are usually thicker and more difficult to expectorate. |
| c. Impaired gas exchange: related to retained secretions. | Presence of lower airway secretions decreases transfer of respiratory gases across alveolar membrane. |

| Steps | Rationale |
|---|---|
| **Planning** | |
| 1. Develop individualized goals for client based on nursing diagnoses: | |
| a. Promote patent airway. | Partial airway obstruction from retained secretions impedes air flow, which increases work of breathing and reduces amount of inhaled oxygen. |
| b. Mobilize airway secretions. | Removal of airway secretions reduces hazard of pulmonary infection. |
| 2. Prepare needed equipment and supplies: a. Bedside table; b. Suction catheter of appropriate size (see box); c. Water-soluble lubricant; d. 2 sterile gloves or 1 sterile and 1 nonsterile glove; e. Sterile basin; f. Approximately 100 ml sterile normal saline; g. Clean towel or sterile drape from kit; h. Portable or wall suction apparatus; i. 6 ft of connecting tubing; j. Sterile suction kit can be used, if available (be sure all listed items not in kit are assembled) | Necessary equipment at bedside ensures that suctioning will be completed quickly and efficiently. In emergent situation, nurse can immediately maintain patent airway without having to search for equipment. |
| 3. Prepare client: | |
| a. Explain procedure and client's participation. | Encourages cooperation, minimizes risks, reduces anxiety. |
| b. Explain importance of coughing during procedure. Practice now, if able. | Facilitates secretion removal and may reduce frequency of future suctioning. |
| c. Assist client to assume position comfortable for nurse and client, usually semi-Fowler's or Fowler's. If unconscious, place in side-lying position. | Promotes client comfort; prevents muscle strain. Promotes maximum lung expansion and deep breathing. Also reduces risk of aspiration. |
| d. Place towel across client's chest. | Reduces transmission of microorganisms. |
| **Implementation** | |
| 1. Wash hands. | Reduces transmission of microorganisms. |
| 2. Turn suction device on and set vacuum regulator to appropriate negative pressure (see box). | Excessive negative pressure damages tracheal mucosa and can induce greater hypoxia. |
| 3. Connect one end of connecting tubing to suction machine and place other end in convenient location. | Prepares suction apparatus. |
| 4. If using sterile suction kit: | |
| a. Open package. If sterile drape is available, place it across client's chest. | Prevents contamination of clothing. |
| b. Open suction catheter package. Do not allow suction catheter to touch any nonsterile surface. | Prepares catheter and prevents transmission of microorganisms. |
| c. Unwrap or open sterile basin and place on bedside table. Be careful not to touch inside basin. Fill with about 100 ml sterile normal saline. | Prepares catheter and prevents transmission of microorganisms. |
| 5. If indicated, open lubricant. Squeeze onto sterile catheter package without touching package. | Prepares lubricant for use while maintaining sterility. |

Appropriate catheter size for client:

| Client | Size |
|---|---|
| Newborn | 6-8 Fr |
| Infant to 18 mo | 6-8 Fr |
| 18 mo | 8-10 Fr |
| 24 mo | 10 Fr |
| 2-4 yr | 10-12 Fr |
| 4-7 yr | 12 Fr |
| 7-10 yr | 12-14 Fr |
| 10-12 yr | 14 Fr |
| Adults | 12-16 Fr |

Vacuum setting:

| | Wall: | Portable: |
|---|---|---|
| Infants | 60-100 mm Hg | 3-5 inches Hg |
| Children | 100-120 mm Hg | 5-10 inches Hg |
| Adults | 120-150 mm Hg | 7-15 inches Hg |

| Steps | Rationale |
|---|---|
| 6. Apply one sterile glove to each hand or apply nonsterile glove to nondominant hand and sterile glove to dominant hand. | Reduces transmission of microorganisms and allows nurse to maintain sterility of suction catheter. |
| 7. Pick up suction catheter with dominant hand without touching nonsterile surfaces. Pick up connecting tubing with nondominant hand. Secure catheter to tubing. | Maintains catheter sterility. |
| 8. Check that equipment is functioning properly by suctioning small amount of saline from basin. | Ensures equipment function; lubricates catheter and tubing. |
| 9. Coat distal 6-8 cm of catheter with water-soluble lubricant. In some situations catheter is lubricated only with normal saline. Nursing assessment indicates need for lubrication. | Promotes easier catheter insertion. If lubricant is needed, it must be water soluble to prevent petroleum-based aspiration pneumonia. Excessive lubricant can adhere to artificial airway. |
| 10. Remove oxygen or humidity delivery device with nondominant hand. | Exposes artificial airway. |
| 11. Hyperinflate and/or oxygenate client before suctioning, using manual resuscitation (AMBU) bag (Chapter 17) or sigh mechanism on mechanical ventilator. | Hyperinflation decreases atelectasis caused by negative pressure. Preoxygenation converts large proportion of resident lung gas to 100% $O_2$ to offset amount used in metabolic consumption while ventilator or oxygenation is interrupted, as well as to offset volume lost out of suction catheter (Luce, 1984). |
| 12. Without applying suction, gently but quickly insert catheter with dominant thumb and forefinger into artificial airway (best to time catheter insertion with inspiration). | Places catheter in tracheobronchial tree. Application of suction pressure while introducing catheter into trachea increases risk of damage to tracheal mucosa, as well as increased hypoxia due to removal of entrained oxygen present in airways. |
| 13. Insert catheter until resistance is met, then pull back 1 cm. | Stimulates cough and removes catheter from mucosal wall. |
| 14. Apply intermittent suction by placing and releasing nondominant thumb over vent of catheter and slowly withdraw catheter while rotating it back and forth between dominant thumb and forefinger. Encourage client to cough. | Intermittent suction and rotation of catheter prevents injury to tracheal mucosal lining. If catheter "grabs" mucosa, remove thumb to release suction. |
| 15. Replace oxygen delivery device. Encourage client to deep breathe. | Reoxygenates and reexpands alveoli. Suctioning can cause hypoxemia and atelectasis. |
| 16. Rinse catheter and connecting tubing with normal saline until clear. Use continuous suction. | Removes catheter secretions. Secretions left in tubing decrease suction and provide environment for microorganism growth. |
| 17. Repeat Steps 11-16 as needed to clear secretions. Allow adequate time (at least 1 full min) between suction passes for ventilation and reoxygenation. | Repeated passes with suction catheter clear airway of excessive secretions and promote improved oxygenation. |
| 18. Assess client's cardiopulmonary status between suction passes. | Suctioning can induce arrhythmias, hypoxia, and bronchospasm. |
| 19. When artificial airway and tracheobronchial tree are sufficiently cleared of secretions, perform nasal and oral pharyngeal suctioning to clear upper airway of secretions. After nasal and oral pharyngeal suctioning are performed, catheter is contaminated; do not reinsert into ET or TT. | Removes upper airway secretions. Upper airway is considered "clean" while lower airway is considered "sterile." Therefore, same catheter can be used to suction from sterile to clean areas, but not from clean to sterile areas. |
| 20. Disconnect catheter from connecting tubing. Roll catheter around fingers of dominant hand. Pull glove off inside out so that catheter remains in glove. Pull off other glove in same way. Discard into appropriate receptacle. Turn off suction device. | Reduces transmission of microorganisms. |
| 21. Remove towel and place in laundry, or remove drape and discard in appropriate receptacle. | Reduces transmission of microorganisms. |
| 22. Reposition client. | Promotes comfort. Sims' position encourages drainage and reduces risk of aspiration. |
| 23. Discard remainder of normal saline into appropriate receptacle. If basin is disposable, discard into appropriate receptacle. If basin is reusable, place it in soiled utility room. | Reduces transmission of microorganisms. |
| 24. Wash hands. | Reduces transmission of microorganisms. |
| 25. Place unopened suction kit on suction machine or at head of bed. | Provides immediate access to suction catheter. |

## Evaluation

| | |
|---|---|
| 1. Compare client's respiratory assessments before and after suctioning. | Identifies physiologic effects of suction procedures. |

| Steps | Rationale |
|---|---|
| ***Expected outcomes*** | |
| 1. Absent or diminished crackles and wheezes in large airways on inspiration and expiration, return of absent or diminished breath sounds, normalization of heart rate, normalization of respiratory rate, increased depth of respiration, normalization of blood pressure, absence of cyanosis. | Lower and upper airways are cleared of secretions. |
| ***Unexpected outcomes*** | |
| 1. Client becomes cyanotic, tachycardic, bradycardic, more restless, suffers cardiac arrest, develops arrhythmias. | Suctioning induced cardiopulmonary compromise. Suctioning removes oxygen in addition to tracheobronchial secretions. Hypoxia results. |
| 2. Bloody secretions are returned. | Suctioning denuded cilia and mucosal lining. Bloody secretions can also indicate presence of an infection. |
| 3. Client has paroxysms of coughing. | Suctioning induced airway spasm. Prolonged coughing episodes can disrupt ventilation and interfere with venous return to heart (Harper, 1981). |
| 4. No secretions are obtained. | When client is poorly hydrated or is not receiving humidified oxygen or room air, pulmonary secretions can consolidate in airways. |

## Recording and Reporting

| Steps | Rationale |
|---|---|
| 1. Chart in nurses' notes: respiratory assessments before and after suctioning; size of suction catheter used; amount of negative suction pressure used; duration of suctioning period; route(s) used to suction; secretions obtained and odor, amount, color, consistency; frequency of suctioning; client's tolerance of procedure. | Documents cardiopulmonary status, nursing care given, expected and unexpected outcomes, and provides baseline for future assessments. |

## Follow-up Activities

| Steps | Rationale |
|---|---|
| 1. Worsening respiratory status: | |
| a. See follow-up activities for Skill 16-3. | |
| b. Evaluate need for supplemental oxygen. Supply oxygen between catheter passes. | Reduces suction-induced hypoxia. |
| c. Evaluate size of suction catheter used to determine if it occluded lumen of tube by more than one half of tube diameter. | Occlusion of tube by suction catheter increases risk of suction-induced hypoxia. |
| 2. Bloody secretions: | |
| a. Evaluate amount of suction pressure used. May need to be decreased. | Reduces amount of trauma to respiratory mucosa. |
| b. Evaluate use of intermittent suction and catheter rotation. Continuous suction and lack of rotation of catheter cause pulling of mucosal tissue. | Reduces amount of trauma to respiratory mucosa. |
| c. Evaluate length of time between catheter insertion and removal of catheter. | Suctioning longer than 10 sec can cause increased cardiopulmonary compromise. |
| d. Evaluate need for suctioning frequency. | Suctioning in absence of secretions increases likelihood of mucosal damage. |
| 3. Paroxysms of coughing: | |
| a. Administer supplemental $O_2$. | Decreases hypoxia. |
| b. Allow client to rest between passes of suction catheter. | Reduces severity of suction-induced airway spasms. |
| 4. No secretions were obtained (See Skill 16-3, Follow-up Activities). | |

## Special Considerations

- With ET or TT there is loss of upper airway functions that include warming, filtering, humidifying. Any client with artificial airway must have humidification to airway.
- If client has thick, sticky secretions, assess hydration and infection. Inadequately hydrated clients may have thick secretions. Normal saline (5-10 ml) may be instilled before suctioning. Saline instillation has limited value, but it mechanically cleans artificial airway. Instilled saline solution should not remain in contact with secretions long enough to affect their consistency (Luce, 1984).
- Conditions increasing risk for adverse effects of suctioning include prematurity, shock, myocardial infarction, respiratory failure, sepsis.
- Spasmodic coughing may occur more frequently in clients with asthma, chronic pulmonary diseases, and congestive heart failure.

# SKILL 16-5 Performing Endotracheal Tube Care

## Procedure 16-5

| Steps | Rationale |
|---|---|
| **Assessment** | |
| 1. Observe for signs and symptoms of need to perform ET care: soiled tape; pressure sore on naris; pressure sore on lips or corner of mouth; excess nasal or oral secretions; client moving tube with tongue, biting tube or tongue; tube repositioned by physician or other specially trained personnel; foul-smelling mouth. | Presence of ET impairs ability of client to swallow oral secretions. Client is also at increased risk to develop pressure areas from impaired circulation as tube is pulled or pressed against nasal or oral mucosa. |
| 2. Observe for factors that increase risk of complications from endotracheal tubes: type of tube, duration of tube placement, amount of cuff inflation, presence of facial trauma. | Nasal tube cannot be rotated from side to side like oral tube. Pressure sores are more likely. Client can "tongue" oral tube easily and dislodge it. Longer duration of intubation is associated with increased risk of complications, as is facial trauma. |
| **Nursing Diagnosis** | |
| 1. Cluster data to reveal actual or potential nursing diagnoses: | |
| a. Impaired skin integrity: related to pressure from ET. | Continuous pressure of ET in one position impairs blood flow and promotes pressure sore formation. |
| b. Impaired gas exchange: related to improper ET placement. | Intubation of right mainstem bronchus impairs gas exchange to left lung. |
| c. Potential for infection: related to nasal ET placement. | Nasal ET impairs sinus drainage and can lead to sinus infections and otitis media. |
| **Planning** | |
| 1. Develop individualized goals for client based on nursing diagnoses:<br>a. Prevent breakdown of mucus membranes surrounding mouth.<br>b. Maintain correct placement of ET in bronchus. | Tube may exert pressure against capillaries, impede blood flow, and cause breakdown. Complications may result when ET moves up or down trachea. (Fig. 16-5 shows various stages of cuff inflation.) |

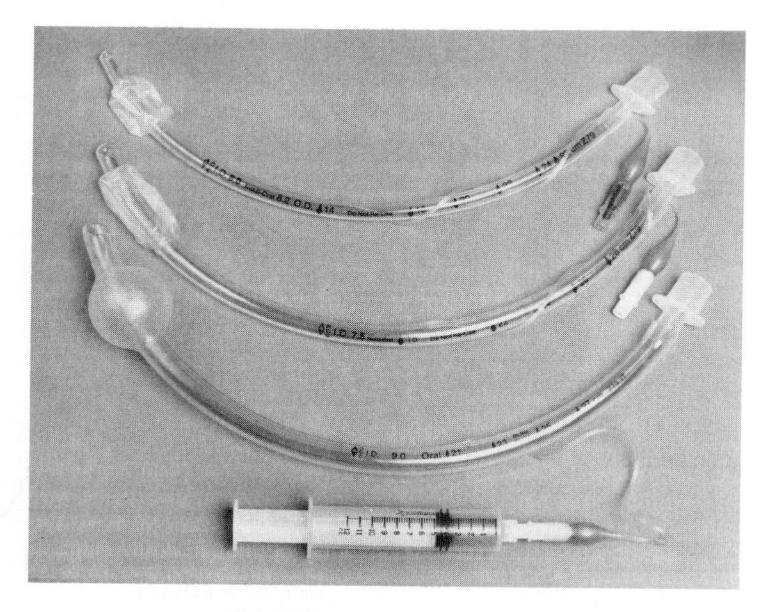

***Fig. 16-5*** Endotracheal tubes.

| Steps | Rationale |
|---|---|
| 2. Prepare needed equipment and supplies:<br>a. Bedside table<br>b. Towel<br>c. Endotracheal and oral pharyngeal suction equipment<br>d. 1 or 1.5 in adhesive or water proof tape (do not use paper tape) or commercial ET holder and mouthguard (follow manufacturer instructions for securing)<br>e. 2 pairs nonsterile gloves<br>f. Adhesive remover swab or acetone on cottonball<br>g. Mouthwash-soaked clean 4 × 4 gauze secured on tongue blade or sponge-tipped applicators<br>h. Toothbrush, toothpaste (optional), and shaving supplies<br>i. 1 wet and 1 soapy washcloth or paper towel<br>j. Clean 2 × 2<br>k. Tincture of benzoin liquid | Necessary equipment at bedside ensures that procedure will be completed quickly and efficiently. In addition, in emergency situation, nurse can immediately maintain patent airway without having to search for equipment. |
| 3. Obtain another nurse's assistance in this procedure (recommended) | Prevents accidental extubation of ET. |
| 4. Prepare client:<br>a. Explain procedure and client's participation, including importance of not biting or moving ET with tongue; removal of tape from face can be uncomfortable. | Encourages cooperation and minimizes risks. |
| b. Assist client to assume position comfortable for both nurse and client (usually supine or semi-Fowler's). | Promotes client comfort; prevents nurse muscle strain. |
| c. Place towel across chest. | Reduces transmission of microorganisms. |

## Implementation

| Steps | Rationale |
|---|---|
| 1. Wash hands. | Reduces transmission of microorganisms. |
| 2. Administer endotracheal, nasal and oral pharyngeal suction. | Removes secretions. Diminishes client's need to cough during procedure. |
| 3. Leave Yankauer suction catheter connected to suction source. | Prepares for oral pharyngeal suctioning. |
| 4. Prepare tape. Cut a piece of tape long enough to go completely around client's head from naris to naris plus 6 in, i.e., 24-48 cm (1-2 ft). Lay adhesive side up, on bedside table. Cut and lay 8-16 cm (4-8 in) of tape, adhesive side down, in center of long strip. Prevents tape from sticking to hair. | Allows nurse to have one hand positioned on ET throughout procedure. Adhesive tape must be placed around head from cheek to cheek below ears (Luce, 1984). |
| 5. Apply gloves. | Reduces transmission of microorganisms. |
| 6. Instruct assistant to apply pair of gloves and hold ET firmly at lips. | Maintains proper tube position and prevents accidental extubation. |
| 7. Carefully remove tape from ET and client's face. If tape is difficult to remove, moisten with water or adhesive tape remover. | Provides nurse with access to skin under tape for assessment and hygiene. |
| 8. Discard tape in appropriate receptacle if nearby. If not, place soiled tape on bedside table or on one end of towel. | Reduces transmission of microorganisms. |
| 9. Use adhesive remover swab to remove excess adhesive left on face after tape removal. | Promotes hygiene. Unremoved adhesive can cause damage to skin and prevent poor adhesion of new tape. |
| 10. Remove oral airway or bite block present and place on towel. | Provides access and complete observation of client's oral cavity. |
| 11. Clean mouth, gums, and teeth opposite ET with mouthwash solution and 4 × 4 gauze, sponge-tipped applicators, or lemon glycerine swabs. Brush teeth as indicated. | Promotes hygiene and reduces risk of infection to teeth and gums. |
| 12. *Oral ET only:* Note "cm" ET marking at lips or gums. With help of assistant, move ET to opposite side or center of mouth. Do not change tube depth at lips. | Prevents pressure sore formation at sides of client's mouth. |
| 13. Repeat oral cleaning as in Step 11 on opposite side of mouth. | Removes secretions from mouth and oral pharynx. |
| 14. If necessary, administer oral pharyngeal suctioning with Yankauer suction catheter. | Promotes hygiene. |
| 15. Clean face and neck with soapy washcloth or paper towel. Rinse with wet washcloth or paper towel. Dry with paper towel or with noncontaminated end of cloth or towel. Shave male client as necessary. | Moisture prevents adhesive tape adherence. |

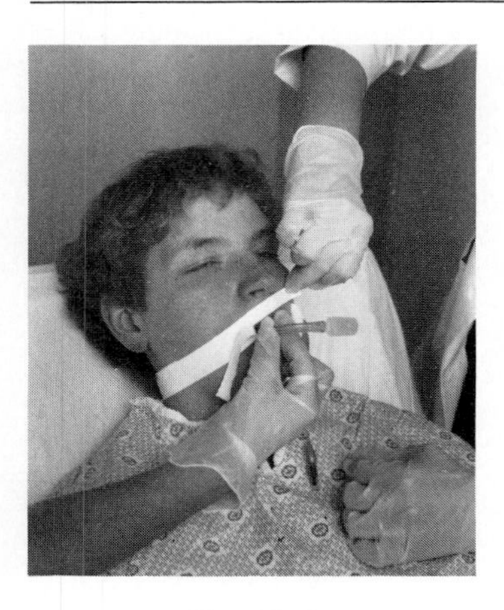

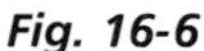

*Fig. 16-6*

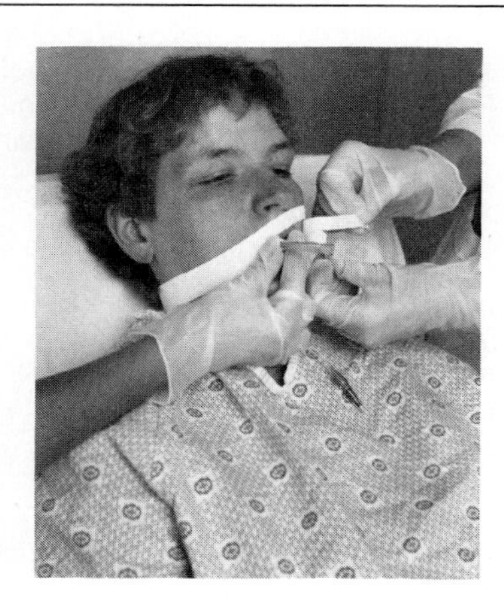

*Fig. 16-7*

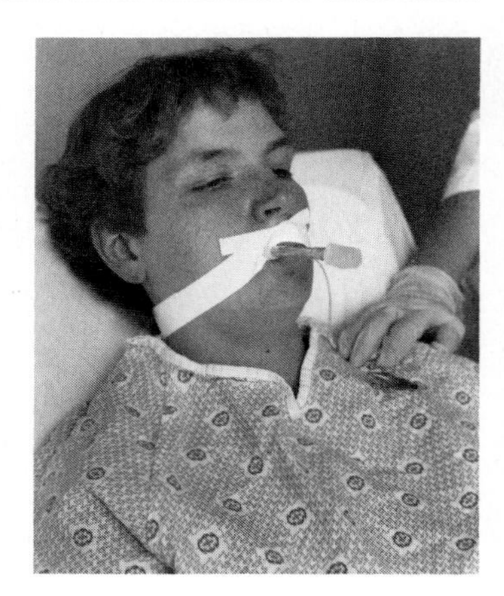

*Fig. 16-8*

| Steps | Rationale |
|---|---|
| 16. Pour small amount of tincture of benzoin on clean 2 × 2 and dot on upper lip (oral ET) or across nose (nasal ET) and cheeks to ear. Allow to dry completely. | Protects and makes skin more receptive to adhesive. |
| 17. Slip tape under client's head and neck, adhesive side up. Take care not to twist tape or catch hair. Do not allow tape to stick to itself. Center tape so that double-faced tape extends around back of head or neck from ear to ear. | Positions tape to secure ET in proper positioning. |
| 18. On one side of face, secure tape from ear to naris (nasal ET) or edge of mouth (oral ET). Tear remaining tape in half lengthwise forming 2 pieces that are 0.5-0.75 in wide. | Secures tape to face. |
| 19. Secure bottom half of tape across upper lip (oral ET) or across top of nose (nasal ET) (Fig. 16-6). Wrap top half of tape around tube and up from bottom. | Secures tape to face. Using top tape to wrap prevents downward drag on ET. |
| 20. Gently pull other side of tape firmly to pick up slack and secure to remaining side of face (Fig. 16-7). | Secures tape to face. |
| 21. Secure bottom half of tape across upper lip (oral ET) or nares (nasal ET). Wrap top half of tape around ET several times, bringing tape around tube from top to bottom (Fig. 16-8). *Note:* ET is secured. Assistant can release hold (nurse may want assistant to help reinsert oral airway, Step 22). | Secures tube. ET should be at same depth at the lips. Check Kardex or earlier assessment for verification of depth in centimeters. |
| 22. Clean oral airway in warm soapy water and rinse well. Hydrogen peroxide can aid in removal of crusted secretions. Shake excess water from oral airway. | Promotes hygiene. Reduces transmission of microorganisms. |
| 23. Reinsert oral airway upside down to prevent pushing tongue into oropharynx (Chapter 17) and rotate into position. | Prevents client from biting ET and allows access for oral pharyngeal suctioning. |
| 24. Discard soiled items in appropriate receptacle. Remove towel and place in laundry. Place clean items (i.e., tincture of benzoin, mouthwash, excess swabs) back in place of storage. | Reduces transmission of microorganisms. |
| 25. Reposition client. | Promotes comfort. |
| 26. Remove gloves and wash hands. Assistant is also to remove gloves and wash hands before leaving client's room. | Reduces transmission of microorganisms. |

## Evaluation

| Steps | Rationale |
|---|---|
| 1. Compare assessments before and after ET care. | Identifies any changes in presence and quality of breath sounds after procedure. |

### *Expected outcomes*

| Steps | Rationale |
|---|---|
| 1. ET is resecured at proper depth as evidenced by the following: clean tape is firmly secured to cheeks and tube only; | ET care was successful. |

| Steps | Rationale |
|---|---|
| tube is positioned on opposite side of mouth (oral ET only); oral airway, if used, is clean and reinserted; depth of tube is same as when started (same centimeter marking at lips); equal bilateral breath sounds. | |

***Unexpected outcomes***

| Steps | Rationale |
|---|---|
| 1. Tape is loose, ET is moving in or out. | Tape is improperly secured. |
| 2. Breath sounds are unequal. | Tube may have slipped into right mainstem bronchus if only right lung has adequate breath sounds. |
| 3. Pressure areas are present at corner of mouth or inner naris. | Pressure of tube impairs blood flow to skin and mucous membrane. |

## Recording and Reporting

| Steps | Rationale |
|---|---|
| 1. Chart in Kardex with pencil: appropriate depth of ET, frequency of ET care, pressure sore care needed and designated intervals. | Provides continuity of care and documents that oral hygiene was completed. |
| 2. Chart in nurses' notes: assessments before and after care, supplies used, client's tolerance of procedure, frequency and extent of ET care. | Documents cardiopulmonary status, nursing care delivered, and client's response. |

## Follow-up Activities

| Steps | Rationale |
|---|---|
| 1. ET moving in and out:<br>a. Repeat taping procedure. | Repetition of taping procedure tightens ET placement and decreases risk of accidental extubation. |
| 2. For unequal breath sounds evaluate ET for proper depth before and after ET care. If ET is deeper or shallower, reposition tube only if allowed by institution and nurse has received appropriate instructions. Notify physician, who may order chest x-ray film to verify placement and then reposition ET. Evaluate client for possible mucus plug in ET. | Unequal breath sounds indicate that there is decreased delivery of oxygen to one lung. To reduce risk of worsening hypoxia, tube must be properly repositioned. |
| 3. For pressure areas more frequent ET care is needed. Clean decubitus frequently with hydrogen peroxide and normal saline. Nasal ET only: if very painful for client, soak clean 2 × 2 in anesthetic solution (e.g., xylocaine solution or xylocaine jelly). Open soaked 2 × 2 and fold lengthwise 1-2 times (resulting in piece that is 0.5 by 4 in) and wrap around tube to center ET in naris and away from pressure area. Obtain physician's order, if necessary. Align oxygen and humidify supply tubings so that they do not pull ET, creating pressure areas. Monitor for infection. | Pressure areas have potential to cause systemic infections. Nurse should attempt to prevent such sores from occurring and to minimize degree of pressure placed on oral or nasal mucosa. |

## Special Considerations

- When ET is first placed, initial verification of its position is made by presence of equal bilateral breath sounds. Final position verification is made by chest x-ray film. Tip of ET should be midway between clavicles and carina. Documentation of depth of tube (in cm) at lips should be noted on Kardex. If tube is not at designated position, perform respiratory assessment, notify and follow physician's orders. If tube is at proper level, continue with procedure.
- If client has beard, it should be trimmed (with family or physician consent) to allow for proper securing of ET.
- To aid in tape removal, fold last half inch of tape back on itself, adhesive sides together.
- Clients who have had ET in place for 3 or more days may have reddened, tender skin.

## Home Care Considerations

- See Skill 16-8.

# SKILL 16-6 Performing Tracheostomy Care

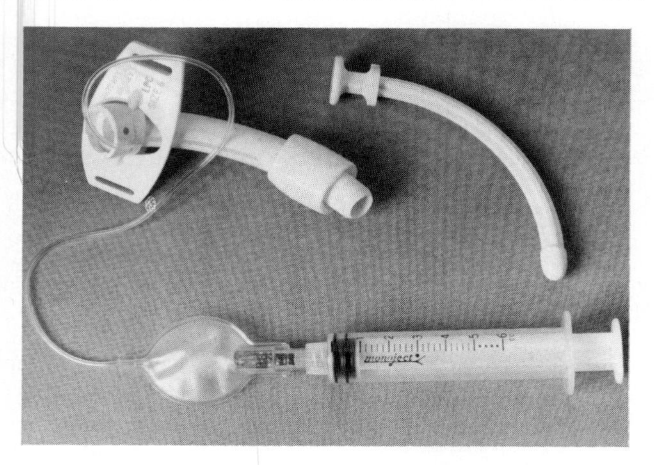

***Fig. 16-9*** Tracheostomy tube and inner cannula.

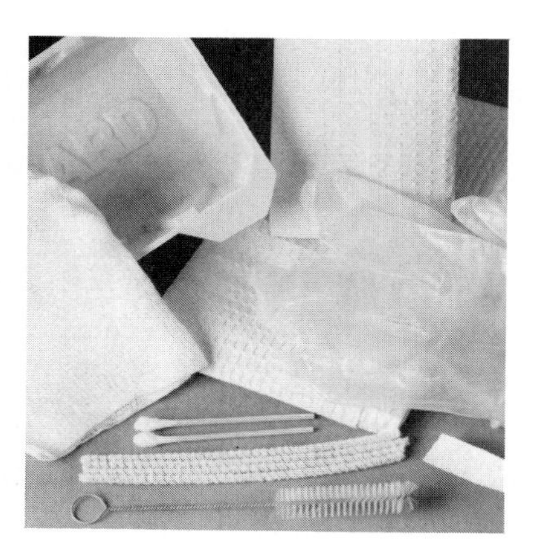

***Fig. 16-10*** Equipment and supplies.

## Procedure 16-6

| Steps | Rationale |
|---|---|
| **Assessment** | |
| 1. Observe for signs and symptoms of need to perform tracheostomy care: excess peristomal secretions, excess intratracheal secretions, soiled or damp tracheostomy ties, soiled or damp tracheostomy dressing, diminished air flow through TT, signs and symptoms of airway obstruction requiring TT suctioning. | Signs and symptoms are related to presence of secretions at stoma site or within tracheostomy tube. Fig. 16-9 shows a partially inflated cuff on an outer cannula, syringe used for cuff inflation, and an obturator that is used to insert outer cannula. |
| 2. Observe for factors, e.g., hydration, humidity, infection, nutrition, and ability to cough, that influence tracheostomy airway functioning. | Allows nurse to accurately assess need to perform tracheostomy care. |
| 3. Assess client's understanding of and ability to perform own tracheostomy care. | Allows nurse to identify potential need for instruction. |
| **Nursing Diagnosis** | |
| 1. Cluster data to reveal actual or potential nursing diagnoses: | |
| a. Altered gas exchange: related to tracheostomy. | Loss of normal pathway for airflow. |
| b. Impaired verbal communication: related to tracheostomy. | Loss of normal communication due to altered pathway of airflow. |
| c. Impaired skin integrity: related to tracheostomy incision. | Risk of infection exists in all surgical wounds. |
| d. Ineffective airway clearance: related to infection. | Retained secretions are ideal media for bacterial growth. |
| **Planning** | |
| 1. Develop individualized goals for client based on nursing diagnoses: | |
| a. Maintain patent airway. | Tracheostomy tube that is clear and free of secretion optimizes amount of oxygen delivered to client and limits risk of infection from retained secretions. |
| b. Maintain dry, clean tracheostomy stoma. | Dry, intact tracheostomy stoma reduces risk of subsequent systemic infection. |
| 2. Prepare needed equipment and supplies: (Fig. 16-10)<br>a. Bedside table<br>b. Towel<br>c. Tracheostomy suction supplies | Necessary equipment at bedside ensures that the procedure will be completed quickly and efficiently. In emergent situation, nurse can immediately maintain patent airway without having to search for equipment. |

| Steps | Rationale |
|---|---|
| d. Sterile tracheostomy care kit, if available (be sure all supplies listed that are not available in kit are collected) | |
| e. Sterile 4 × 4 gauze—3 pkg | |
| f. Hydrogen peroxide | |
| g. Normal saline | |
| h. Sterile cotton-tipped swabs | |
| i. Sterile tracheostomy dressing (precut and sewn surgical dressing) | |
| j. Sterile basin | |
| k. Small sterile brush | |
| l. Roll of twill tape or tracheostomy ties | |
| m. Scissors | |
| n. 2 sterile gloves | |
| 3. Have another nurse assist in this procedure (optional). | Prevents accidental extubation of tracheostomy tube. |
| 4. Prepare client: | |
| a. Explain procedure and client's participation. | Encourages cooperation, minimizes risks, and reduces anxiety. |
| b. Assist client to position comfortable for both nurse and client (usually supine or semi-Fowler's). | Promotes client comfort, prevents nurse muscle strain. |
| c. Place towel across client's chest. | Reduces transmission of microorganisms. |

## Implementation

| Steps | Rationale |
|---|---|
| 1. Wash hands and don gloves. | Reduces transmission of microorganisms. |
| 2. Administer tracheostomy suctioning. Before removing gloves, remove soiled tracheostomy dressing and discard in glove with coiled catheter. | Removes secretions so as not to occlude outer cannula while inner cannula is removed. |
| 3. While client is replenishing oxygen stores, prepare equipment on bedside table. Open sterile tracheostomy kit. Open three 4 × 4 gauze packages aseptically and pour normal saline on one package and hydrogen peroxide on another. Leave third package dry. Open two cotton-tipped swab packages and pour normal saline on one package and hydrogen peroxide on the other. Open sterile tracheostomy dressing package. Unwrap sterile basin and pour about 1.8 ml (0.75 in) in hydrogen peroxide into it. Open small sterile brush package and place aseptically into sterile basin. If using large roll of twill tape, cut appropriate length of tape and lay aside in dry area. Do not recap hydrogen peroxide and normal saline. | Prepares equipment and allows for smooth organized completion of tracheostomy care. |
| 4. Apply gloves. Keep dominant hand sterile throughout procedure. (For TT with inner cannula, complete Steps 5-17. For TT with no inner cannula or Kistner button, complete Steps 9-17). | Reduces transmission of microorganisms. |
| 5. Remove oxygen source and then inner cannula with nondominant hand. Drop inner cannula into hydrogen peroxide basin. | Removes inner cannula for cleaning. Hydrogen peroxide loosens secretions from inner cannula. |
| 6. Place tracheostomy collar oxygen source over outer cannula. Place T-tube (Briggs) and ventilator oxygen sources over or near outer cannula. *Note:* T-tube and ventilator oxygen devices cannot be attached to all outer cannulas when the inner cannula is removed. | Maintains supply of oxygen to client. |
| 7. To prevent oxygen desaturation in affected clients, quickly pick up inner cannula and use small brush to remove secretions inside and outside cannula. | Tracheostomy brush provides mechanical force to remove thick or dried secretions. |
| 8. Hold inner cannula over basin and rinse with normal saline, using nondominant hand to pour normal saline. | Removes secretions and hydrogen peroxide from inner cannula. |
| 9. Replace inner cannula and secure "locking" mechanism. Reapply T-tube (Briggs) and ventilator oxygen sources. | Secures inner cannula and reestablishes oxygen supply. |
| 10. Using hydrogen peroxide-prepared cotton-tipped swabs and 4 × 4 gauze, clean exposed outer cannula surfaces and stoma under faceplate extending 4-8 cm (2-4 in) in all directions from stoma. Clean in circular motion from stoma | Aseptically removes secretions from stoma site. |

| Steps | Rationale |
|---|---|
| site outward using dominant hand to handle sterile supplies. | |
| 11. Using normal saline-prepared cotton-tipped swabs and 4 × 4 gauze, rinse exposed outer cannula surfaces and stoma under faceplate extending 4-8 cm (2-4 in) in all directions from stoma. Rinse in circular motion from stoma site outward using dominant hand to handle sterile supplies. | Rinses hydrogen peroxide from surfaces. |
| 12. Using dry 4 × 4 gauze, pat lightly at skin and exposed outer cannula surfaces. | Dry surfaces prohibit formation of moist environment for microorganism growth and skin excoriation. |
| 13. Instruct assistant, if available, to securely hold TT in place. With assistant holding TT, cut ties. Assistant must *not* release hold on tracheostomy tube until new ties are firmly tied. If no assistant, do not cut old ties until new ties are in place and securely tied: | Promotes hygiene, reduces transmission of microorganisms. Secures TT. |
| a. Cut a length of twill tape long enough to go around client's neck 2 times; cut ends on diagonal. | Cutting ends of tie on diagonal aids in inserting tie through eyelet. |
| b. Insert one end of tie through faceplate eyelet and pull ends even. | |
| c. Slide both ends of tie behind head and around neck to other eyelet and insert one tie through second eyelet. | |
| d. Pull snugly. | 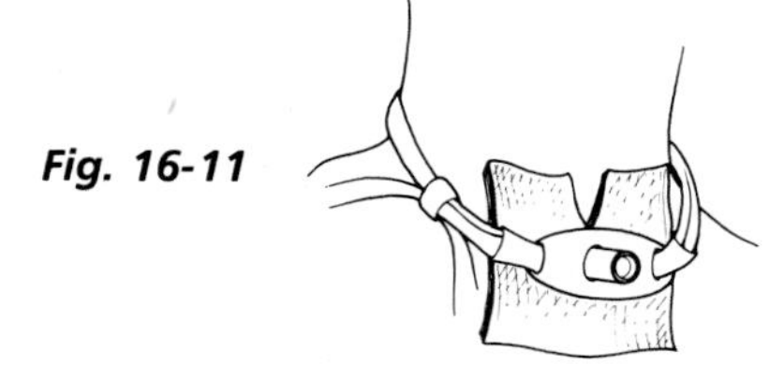 **Fig. 16-11** |
| e. Tie ends securely in double square knot allowing space for only one finger in tie. | One finger slack prevents ties from being too tight when tracheostomy dressing is in place. |
| 14. Insert fresh tracheostomy dressing under clean ties and faceplate (Fig. 16-11). | Absorbs drainage. |
| 15. Remove gloves and discard in appropriate receptacle with soiled tracheostomy ties. | Reduces transmission of microorganisms. |
| 16. Replace cap on hydrogen peroxide and normal saline bottles. Store reusable liquids and unused supplies in appropriate place. | Once opened, normal saline can be considered free of bacteria for 24 hr, after which it should be discarded. |
| 17. Position client comfortably and assess respiratory status. | Promotes comfort. Some clients may require posttracheostomy care suctioning. |
| 18. Wash hands. | Reduces transmission of microorganisms. |

## Evaluation

| | |
|---|---|
| 1. Compare assessments before and after tracheostomy care. | Determines effectiveness of tracheostomy care. |

### *Expected outcomes*

| | |
|---|---|
| 1. Successful tracheostomy care is indicated by the following: inner cannula and outer cannula of TT are free of secretions; ties are clean, secured snugly, and tied in double square knot. | TT is patent and secure. |
| 2. Stoma site is not reddened and hard, is free of mucoid secretions, and is free of foul-smelling, colored secretions. | Indicates absence of infection at stoma site. |

### *Unexpected outcomes*

| | |
|---|---|
| 1. Ties are looser than one finger snug. | Ties improperly secured. |
| 2. Stoma site is hard and reddened with or without excessive or foul-smelling secretions. | Stomatitis present. |
| 3. Pressure sore from faceplate or ties is present. | Pressure from faceplate or ties impairs blood flow to tissue. |
| 4. Client coughed out TT. | Improper technique used to change ties. |
| 5. Portion of inner cannula is exposed. | Inner cannula not secured properly in outer cannula. |

## Recording and Reporting

| | |
|---|---|
| 1. Chart in Kardex: type and size of TT, frequency of tracheostomy care, special care in event of stomatitis. | Provides continuity of care. |
| 2. Chart in nurses' notes: assessments, supplies used, frequency and extent of tracheostomy care, client's tolerance of procedure. | Documents cardiopulmonary and tracheostomy site status, nursing care, and client's response to procedure. |

| Steps | Rationale |
| --- | --- |
| **Follow-up Activities** | |
| 1. For excessively loose tracheostomy ties, apply new ties. | Excessively loose tracheostomy ties increase risk of accidental extubation. |
| 2. For stomatitis increase frequency of tracheostomy care, consider application of heat to increase blood flow and promote healing, consider topical application of antibacterial solution and allowing it to dry and provide bacterial barrier. | Cleansing of stoma aids in decreasing stomatitis. Ointments usually serve as moist reservoir for microorganism growth and are not recommended. |
| 3. For pressure sores increase frequency of tracheostomy care and keep dressing under faceplate at all times. May need to use double dressing. | Removing secretions from underlying skin reduces risk of pressure sore progression. |
| 4. For accidental extubation call for assistance and replace old tracheostomy tube with new tube. | Accidental tracheostomy extubation can result in occlusion of stoma. Generally after tracheostomy has been in place for 3 days stoma does not rapidly occlude. |

### Special Considerations

- There are alternate methods to apply tracheostomy ties. The one presented is considered the safest and easiest to master. Commercial products that use velcro and similar fastening devices are available in some institutions.
- Clients with new tracheostomy frequently have bloody secretions for 2-3 days after procedure or for 24 hr after each tracheostomy tube change.
- Tracheostomy obturator should be attached to head of bed of client with fresh tracheostomy. Obturators of different brands and sizes of tracheostomy tubes are not interchangeable. The obturator is used to reinsert the outer cannula if it is accidentally dislodged.
- Do not cut 4 × 4 gauze. Loose strings enter stoma and can cause infection and irritation.
- If long-term placement of tracheostomy tube is anticipated, nurse should plan to teach client and family tracheostomy care (Skill 16-8).
- Clients with following have greater need for tracheostomy care: tracheal stomatitis; pneumonia; bronchitis; tracheitis; short, fat neck.
- *Hydration:* inadequate hydration can cause thicker secretions. *Humidity:* inadequate inspired humidity predisposes client to drying, crusted secretions and dry infected mucous membranes. *Infection:* secretions increase in quantity in infected areas. *Nutrition:* inadequate nutrition predisposes client to poor healing and greater risk of infection. *Ability to cough:* coughing effectively removes airway secretions. Weak coughing ability promotes secretion accumulation. Coughing ability altered in tracheostomy clients.

### Home Care Considerations

- See Skill 16-8.

## *SKILL 16-7 Managing a Cuffed Endotracheal or Tracheostomy Tube*

### *Procedure 16-7*

| Steps | Rationale |
| --- | --- |
| **Assessment** | |
| 1. Observe for signs and symptoms of need to perform care including gurgling on expiration, decreased exhaled tidal volume (mechanically ventilated client), spasmodic coughing, tense test balloon on tube, flaccid test balloon on tube, phonation. | Partially deflated cuff allows secretions to enter trachea while high cuff pressure can result in necrosis, tracheal malacia, or tracheoesophageal fistula. |
| **Nursing Diagnosis** | |
| 1. Cluster data to reveal actual or potential nursing diagnoses: | |
| a. Potential for infection: related to retained secretions. | Retained secretions are ideal media for microorganisms growth. |
| b. Potential for injury: related to increased pressure on tracheal mucosa from over inflated cuff. | Excessive cuff pressure decreases blood supply. |

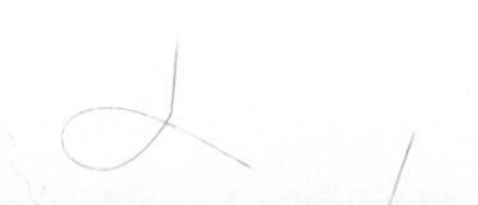

| Steps | Rationale |
|---|---|
| **Planning** | |
| 1. Develop individualized goals for client based on nursing diagnoses: | |
| a. Promote patent airway. | Patent airway improves oxygenation and removes retained secretions, which are ideal media for bacterial growth. |
| b. Prevent pressure to tracheal mucous membrane. | Pressure on tracheal mucosa can result in necrosis or tracheoesophageal fistula. |
| 2. Prepare needed equipment and supplies:<br>a. Endotracheal/tracheostomy suction apparatus (Skill 16-4)<br>b. Stethoscope<br>c. 6 cc syringe<br>d. Alcohol wipe | Necessary equipment at bedside ensures that procedure will be completed quickly and efficiently. In emergent situation, nurse can immediately maintain patent airway without having to search for equipment. |
| 3. Prepare client: | |
| a. Explain procedure and client's participation. | Encourages cooperation, minimizes risks, and reduces anxiety. |
| b. Assist client to position comfortable for nurse and client (usually semi-Fowler's). | Promotes client comfort, prevents nurse muscle strain, facilitates drainage. |
| **Implementation** | |
| 1. Wash hands. | Reduces transmission of microorganisms. |
| 2. Suction client. | Assures patent airway and facilitates hearing air flow with stethoscope. |
| 3. Connect syringe to pilot balloon. | Allows immediate access to equipment for adjusting cuff pressure. |
| 4. Place stethoscope in sternal notch or above TT and listen for minimal amount of air leak at end of inspiration (Fig. 16-12). | Assesses proper cuff inflation. |
| 5. If no air leak is heard, remove all air from cuff. | Releases excessive cuff pressure, which reduces capillary blood flow and increases risk of tissue necrosis. |
| 6. Slowly inflate cuff by adding 0.5-1 cc air at a time while listening with stethoscope. At point where no air leak is heard, stop instilling air and very slowly withdraw up to 0.5 cc air until point where air leak is audible with stethoscope. | Inflates cuff to minimal leak. |
| 7. If excessive air leak is heard, slowly add air as in Step 6. | Air leak may prevent adequate lung expansion and increase risk of aspiration. |
| 8. Remove stethoscope and wipe diaphragm with alcohol wipe. | Reduces transmission of microorganisms. |
| 9. Remove syringe and discard into appropriate receptacle or store per policy. Do not leave attached to pilot balloon valve. | Reduces transmission of microorganisms. Leaving syringe in pilot balloon can cause valve to break or "stick open" and when removed, air is lost from cuff. |
| 10. Reposition client. | Promotes comfort. |
| 11. Wash hands. | Reduces transmission of microorganisms. |

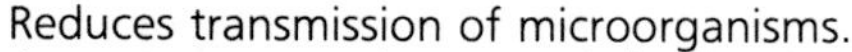

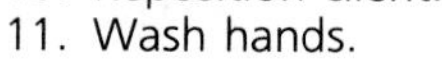

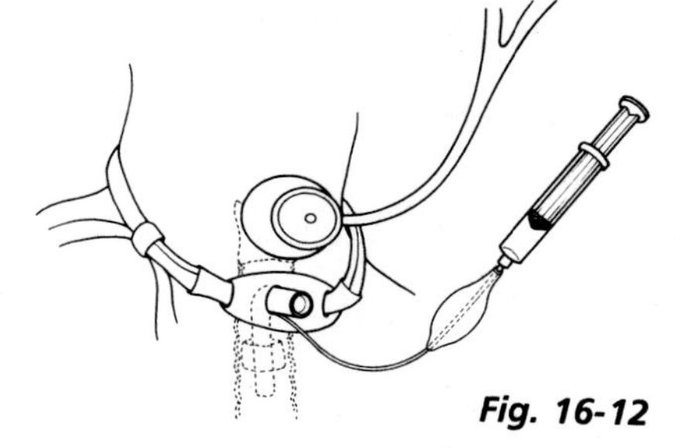

*Fig. 16-12*

| Steps | Rationale |
|---|---|
| **Evaluation** | |
| 1. Compare respiratory assessments before and after cuff care. | Determines effectiveness of cuff care procedure. |
| ***Expected outcomes*** | |
| 1. Minimal leak is heard at end inspiration. | Proper level of cuff inflation. |
| ***Unexpected outcomes*** | |
| 1. No air leak is heard at end inspiration. | Improper cuff inflation. |
| 2. Excessive air leak is heard through inspiration and expiration. | Cuff may have ruptured. |
| 3. Intratracheal bleeding is noted (bright red). | Erosion of blood vessel probably caused by high cuff pressure. |
| 4. Air leaks from cuff after syringe removed from pilot balloon. | Pilot balloon valve may be broken or "stuck open" allowing air to escape from cuff. |

| Steps | Rationale |
|---|---|
| **Recording and Reporting** | |
| 1. Chart in nurses' notes: presence of minimal leak at end inspiration, secretions obtained when suctioning, frequency of cuff care. | Documents safe cuff pressure levels. |
| **Follow-up Activities** | |
| 1. Excessive cuff pressure: a. Remove air from cuff and reassess minimal leak. | Excessive cuff pressure can lead to necrosis of tracheal mucosa and erosion of tracheal wall. |
| 2. Excessive volume required to inflate cuff: a. Notify physician. | Prepare to replace present tracheostomy tube with larger size if there is tracheal malacia or same size tube if ruptured cuff is present. |
| 3. Intratracheal bleeding: a. Notify physician. b. Hyperinflate cuff with several additional milliliters of air. | Hyperinflation of cuff can tamponade bleeding vessel. |
| 4. Broken or open pilot balloon valve: a. Insert 2- or 3-way stopcock into valve and turn off valve after cuff properly inflated. b. Clamp tubing between pilot balloon valve and ET or TT as close to balloon as possible. | Prevents loss of air from cuff until tube can be safely replaced. |

## Special Considerations

- Gloves should be worn when caring for clients with communicable diseases or contaminated secretions.
- When foam-cuffed tracheostomy tube is used there is no valve in the pilot balloon. Air port is left open to atmosphere and regulates the amount of air necessary to seal the cuff without exerting excessive pressure against capillaries and mucosal surfaces.
- In some institutions cuff pressure is measured with a manometer. Cuff pressure should not exceed 20-25 cm $H_2O$ or 14-17 mm Hg to maintain adequate capillary blood flow. Cuffs can be properly inflated with pressures well below these values. When elevated cuff pressures are necessary to ventilate a patient, the cuff should be temporarily deflated every 2-4 hr to reestablish capillary blood flow and drain secretions.
- Clients with endotracheal tubes do not commonly ingest food or medications orally.
- The volume of air required to properly inflate a cuff is dependent on size of the airway and size of the tube. If a large and a small tube are placed in clients with similar-sized airways, the client with the larger tube will need less air in the cuff than the client with the smaller tube.
- Clients who are alert and do not require mechanical ventilation may need their cuff inflated while eating, 30-60 min after meals, and after administration of medication to reduce risk of aspiration.
- Minimal leak technique allows secretions between the epiglottis and top of cuff to drain. In contrast, occlusive techniques allow secretions to collect in the subglottic area, which can result in conditions such as epiglottitis, pharyngitis, and tracheal stenosis.

# *SKILL 16-8 Teaching Home Tracheostomy Care and Suctioning*

The indications and procedure for performing tracheostomy care and suctioning in the home are similar to tracheostomy suctioning in the hospital except for one key variable: the use of principles of medical asepsis or "clean technique." In the hospital, principles of surgical asepsis are used because the client is more susceptible to infection and because more virulent or pathogenic microorganisms are usually present than in the home setting. In the home setting the majority of clients use the clean technique.

However, not all home care clients should use the clean technique. The nurse must use good nursing judgment in choosing clients who are candidates for using clean or aseptic technique. The immunocompromised client, who is at risk for severe infections, should continue to receive suctioning using principles of surgical asepsis. A client receiving care from visiting nurses or other care givers who have contact with other patients (or institutions) should be suctioned using sterile technique. Infected (not colonized) clients should be suctioned using sterile technique. Care givers who are infected with viral, bacterial, or fungal microorganisms should suction using principles of surgical asepsis. Clients living in nonhygienic (nonclean) conditions should be suctioned using sterile technique in hopes of preventing infection.

Caring for a tracheostomy at home begins in the hospital with teaching and return demonstration. The client usually learns better when less invasive techniques such as stoma care precede more invasive techniques such as inner cannula care and suctioning. The nurse continually develops, implements, and evaluates the teaching plan based on client performance. Some clients and their families learn quickly while others do not. Therefore, teaching should begin as soon as it is feasible.

### Purposes

1. Maintain airway patency.
2. Prevent infection.
3. Promote cleanliness.
4. Prevent skin breakdown around site of the tracheostomy stoma.
5. Allow client to return to the home setting earlier in convalescence.
6. Decrease work of breathing.
7. Stimulate a deep cough.

## *Procedure 16-8*

| Steps | Rationale |
|---|---|
| **Assessment** | |
| 1. Assess client's ability to properly perform tracheostomy care and suctioning while in the hospital setting. | Physical or cognitive impairments may necessitate instructing family member or significant other to perform tracheostomy care and suctioning. |
| 2. Assess client's or family member's knowledge and ability to observe for signs and symptoms of need to perform: | |
| a. Tracheostomy care including excess peristomal secretions, excess intratracheal secretions, soiled or damp tracheostomy ties, soiled or damp tracheostomy dressing, diminished airflow through TT. | Signs and symptoms are related to presence of secretions at stoma site or within tracheostomy tube. |
| b. Suctioning including wheezes or crackles on inspiration or expiration, restlessness, ineffective coughing, absent or diminished breath sounds, tachypnea, cyanosis, acutely decreased level of consciousness, hypertension or hypotension, tachycardia or bradycardia, acutely shallow respirations. | Physical signs and symptoms result from lower airway obstruction and tissue hypoxia. |
| 3. Assess client and family ability to observe for factors that normally influence tracheostomy airway functioning. | Allows client to accurately evaluate need to perform TT suctioning. |
| 4. Assess client understanding of and ability to perform own tracheostomy care and suctioning. | Allows nurse to identify potential need for instruction. |
| 5. Observe client or family member performing complete TT care and suctioning. | Enables nurse to determine which specific components of skill client or family member can easily complete and which are more difficult. |
| **Nursing Diagnosis** | |
| 1. Cluster data to reveal learning capabilities and needs and identify appropriate nursing diagnosis: | |
| a. Knowledge deficit: related to tracheostomy care and suctioning. | Lack of knowledge increases client and family anxiety and affects their independence. |
| b. Altered or impaired activity tolerance: related to decreased tissue oxygenation. | Oxygen deficit can decrease client's physical activity tolerance. |
| c. Impaired verbal communication: related to tracheostomy. | Presence of tracheostomy bypasses passage of air through vocal cords and speech is impaired. |
| d. Anxiety: related to newness of self-suctioning procedure. | Education increases client's exposure to self-suctioning procedure, and anxiety decreases. |
| e. Ineffective airway clearance: related to impaired cough. | Tracheostomy decreases effectiveness of client's cough. |
| **Planning** | |
| 1. Identify learning objectives for teaching plan: | Allows nurse to objectively measure client's learning and to modify teaching plan as necessary. |
| a. State signs and symptoms indicating need for TT care and for suctioning. | |

| Steps | Rationale |
|---|---|
| b. State factors that normally influence tracheostomy airway functioning. | Tracheostomy can impair normal airway clearance, humidification, and gas exchange. |
| c. Correctly demonstrate complete TT care and suctioning in controlled setting. | Provides documentation of client's ability to perform procedure. |
| 2. Select setting in home that client is most likely to use when completing TT care. | Practicing skill in same setting that skill will be routinely performed facilitates comprehension and learning. |
| 3. Demonstrate steps for preparing needed equipment and supplies:<br>a. Suction machine with connecting tubing<br>b. Nonsterile gloves<br>c. Small basin<br>d. Hydrogen peroxide, water (boiled preferred over tap) or normal saline, clean gauze 4 × 4s<br>e. Appropriate size of sterile or clean and disinfected catheter<br>f. Water-soluble lubricant<br>g. Small brush or clean pipe cleaner<br>h. Clean cotton-tipped swabs<br>i. Clean tracheostomy ties (twill tape, bias tape, shoe strings, nonelastic ribbon)<br>j. Mirror<br>k. Clean wet washcloth or paper towel<br>l. Clean dry cloth, towel, or paper towel | Necessary equipment in home ensures that procedure will be completed quickly and efficiently. In an emergency situation nurse, client, or family member can immediately maintain patent airway without having to search for equipment. Demonstration is best technique for teaching psychomotor skills. |
| 4. Discuss and demonstrate with client proper position for procedure (high Fowler's position in front of a mirror). | Promotes client's understanding of comfort and safety principles, as well as facilitating visibility. |

## Implementation

| Steps | Rationale |
|---|---|
| 1. Demonstrate steps for preparation and completion of tracheostomy tube suctioning: | Demonstration is reliable technique for teaching psychomotor skill, and also enables client to ask questions throughout procedure. |
| a. Wash hands. | Reduces transmission of microorganisms. |
| b. Prepare suction equipment according to manufacturer's direction. | Prepares suction. |
| c. Apply gloves. | Reduces transmission of microorganisms. |
| d. Fill basin with 0.5 cup water or normal saline. | Prepares catheter rinse. |
| e. Connect suction catheter to suction apparatus. | Prepares suction. |
| f. Check that equipment is functioning by suctioning small amount of fluid from basin. | Ensures proper equipment function before catheter insertion and lubricates internal catheter. |
| g. Coat distal ⅓ -½ of catheter with water-soluble lubricant. | Facilitates passage of catheter into tracheostomy tube. |
| h. In an adult insert catheter 12-16 cm (6-8 in) without applying suction. If resistance (carina) is met, pull catheter back 1 cm. | Places catheter in tracheobronchial tree. |
| i. Apply intermittent suction by placing and releasing thumb over catheter vent and slowly withdraw catheter while rotating it between thumb and forefinger. | Intermittent suction and rotation of catheter prevent injury to tracheal mucosa lining. |
| j. Using continuous suction, rinse catheter with basin fluid until clean. | Removes secretions from catheter. |
| k. Repeat Steps h-j as needed to remove secretions. | Promotes patent airway. |
| l. Suction nasal and oral pharynx if needed. | Removes secretions from upper airway. |
| m. Rinse catheter, as above. | Removes secretions from catheter. |
| n. Disconnect suction catheter, coil and discard. If catheter is to be cleaned and disinfected, set aside. | Reduces transmission of microorganisms. |
| o. Remove inner cannula, hold over basin, and pour hydrogen peroxide over and through inner cannula. Use brush or pipe cleaner to remove crusted or adhering secretions. | Removes secretions that have adhered to inner cannula. |
| p. Rinse inner cannula thoroughly with warm running tap water, boiled water, or normal saline. Let tap water flow freely for at least 15 sec before rinsing inner cannula. Shake excess water from cannula. Dry, if desired, with clean gauze. Replace inner cannula in proper position and lock. | Removes hydrogen peroxide from inner cannula. Remaining hydrogen peroxide could cause airway or stoma irritation. |
| q. Dip cotton-tipped swab into hydrogen peroxide and clean exposed outer cannula and stoma site. | Removes secretions that predispose client to localized infection. |

| Steps | Rationale |
|---|---|
| r. Rinse exposed outer cannula and skin sites with wet wash cloth or paper towel (boiled or freely running tap water or normal saline). | Removes hydrogen peroxide and cleans skin. |
| s. Dry exposed outer cannula and skin sites with dry towel. | Prevents moist environment for organism growth. |
| t. Change ties. | Secures tube and prevents accidental extubation. |
| u. Apply dressing. | Protects skin around stoma from pressure breakdown and collects secretions. |
| v. Clean reusable supplies in warm soapy water. Rinse thoroughly and dry between two layers of clean paper towels. Store supplies in loosely closed clear plastic bag. | Prevents transmission of microorganisms. |
| w. Remove and discard gloves. Wash hands. | Reduces transmission of microorganisms. |
| x. Reusable supplies should be disinfected at least weekly. To disinfect supplies use one of the methods described here: ▪ Method 1: Boil reusable (boilable) supplies for 15 min. Allow to cool and dry as in Step v. ▪ Method 2: Soak reusable supplies in equal parts of vinegar and water for 30 min. Remove, rinse thoroughly, and dry as in Step v. ▪ Method 3: Soak reusable supplies in prepared Control III or Instasan solution (quaternary ammonium chloride compounds) according to manufacturer's instructions. Rinse and dry as in Step v. | Reduces transmission of microorganisms. |
| 2. Have client or family member perform each step with guidance from nurse. | Nurse can correct any errors in technique as they occur and discuss their implications. |
| 3. Discuss signs and symptoms of: a. Stomal infection (redness, tenderness, drainage). b. Respiratory tract infection (fever, increased sputum, change in color of sputum, foul sputum odor, increased cough, chills, nightsweats). | Client must be able to recognize onset of inflammation or infection. |
| 4. Discuss importance of notifying physician when prolonged stoma inflammation or respiratory infection occurs. | Physician can prescribe medications to alleviate respiratory tract infection and inflammation. Clients must understand implication of upper respiratory tract infection. |

## Evaluation

| | |
|---|---|
| 1. Have client independently demonstrate technique for TT care and suctioning. | Feedback through independent demonstration of psychomotor skill is reliable method to evaluate learning. |

### *Expected outcomes*

| | |
|---|---|
| 1. Client is able to identify signs and symptoms indicating need for TT care and suctioning, signs and symptoms of stoma inflammation or respiratory tract infection, when to notify physician. | Measures cognitive learning. |
| 2. Lower and upper airways are cleared of secretions. Suctioning is successful as evidenced by absent or diminished crackles and wheezes in large airways, return of absent or diminished breath sounds, normalization of vital signs, increased depth of respirations, absence of cyanosis. | Successful suctioning. |
| 3. Stoma site is clean and free of infection; inner cannula is free of secretions. | Successful tracheostomy care. |

### *Unexpected outcomes*

| | |
|---|---|
| 1. Stoma site is reddened or hard, with or without drainage. | Contaminated tracheostomy site. |
| 2. Copious colored secretions are present around stoma or when client is suctioned. | Infection present. |
| 3. Client is unable to perform skill. | Increases risk of stomatitis and respiratory tract infection. |
| 4. Bloody secretions are suctioned. | Sign of denuded cilia and mucosal lining or infection. |
| 5. No secretions are suctioned. | No secretions present or secretions are too thick to suction. |
| 6. TT comes out. | TT improperly secured. |
| 7. Skin breakdown is present at stoma site. | Pressure areas have developed from faceplate of TT or area has not been kept clean and dry. |

| Steps | Rationale |
|---|---|
| **Recording and Reporting** | |
| 1. Record in nurses' notes: teaching done, accuracy of care delivered by client or family member. | Documents type and quality of self-care delivered by client and family. |
| **Follow-up Activities** | |
| 1. For bloody secretions evaluate suctioning technique, suctioning frequency, size of catheter used; identify other signs of infection. | Nursing measures are designed to reduce suction trauma to tracheal mucosa. |
| 2. In absence of secretions evaluate fluid status, need for increased humidity, size of suction catheter used, need for suctioning. | Absence of secretions can indicate that secretions have become thick and tenacious or have consolidated. |
| 3. For infected stoma site evaluate cleaning regimen for continued use of "clean technique." Evaluate other possible contaminants, including use of finger to occlude fenestrated TT for speech (encourage client to place clean facial tissue between finger and tube), scratching of dry skin (moisturize skin with lotion), environment. Increase tracheostomy care frequency. | Returning to sterile technique can resolve infection at stoma site. |
| 4. For copious, yellow secretions use sterile technique for suctioning and tracheostomy inner cannula care. Evaluate for adequate humidity (use room humidifier or tracheostomy collar humidity, if needed) (Chapter 14). Notify physician. | Sterile suctioning reduces entry of pathogens that would increase production of yellow secretions. |
| 5. For displaced TT initiate agency protocol for replacement or resuscitation as needed. | Client, care givers, and nurses need to be prepared for accidental extubation. |

## Special Considerations

- Physical limitation or weakness impairs client's motor coordination and prohibits client from being able to remove, clean, and reinsert inner cannula or change tracheostomy ties or suction. Cognitive impairments can result from primary disease or oxygen desaturation.
- Procedure must be performed at least daily in home setting. When tracheal secretions are copious, client or family member must complete procedure more frequently (e.g., q4h).
- *Hydration:* inadequate hydration can cause thicker secretions. *Humidity:* inadequate inspired humidity predisposes client to dry crusted secretions and dry, cracked, possibly infected mucous membranes. *Infection:* secretions increase in quality and quantity in infected areas. *Nutrition:* inadequate nutrition predisposes client to poor healing and greater risk of infection. *Ability to cough:* strong cough effectively removes secretions. Weak cough promotes secretion accumulation. Coughing ability is altered in tracheostomy clients.
- If client is able to complete suctioning and TT care, at least one other family member or significant other should be taught procedure. For child and for older client unable to perform independently, two members of household or one parent and significant other should be taught procedure.
- Clients with following are at greater risk: impaired or absent cough or gag reflex, decreased level of consciousness, neuromuscular diseases, pneumonia, chronic obstructive pulmonary disease, congestive heart failure, pulmonary edema. Families of tracheostomy clients must know how to obtain emergency assistance within their community.
- Caution against use of over-the-counter medications unless instructed by physician to use them.
- Loss of upper airway functions with tracheostomy can predispose client to greater secretions. Infants and young children have smaller diameter airway. Elderly have lost some properties of elastic recoil and gas exchange.
- Client is instructed that nose and mouth are considered "dirty" while tracheostomy is "clean." Client is instructed to suction clean areas first.
- Normal saline can be made at home by adding 2 tsp of table salt to 1 qt of boiled water. Store in jar that has been sterilized (i.e., boiled). Several quart or pint jars can be processed at one time if prepared with home canning equipment.

## BIBLIOGRAPHY

Ackerman MH: The use of bolus normal saline instillations in artificial airways: is it useful or necessary? Heart-Lung 14:505, 1985.

Amborn S: Clinical signs associated with the amount of tracheobronchial secretions, Nurs Res 25:(2):121, 1976.

Allan D: Patients with an endotracheal tube or tracheostomy, Nurs Times 80(13):36, 1984.

Barnes CA, Kirchhoff KT: Minimizing hypoxemia due to endotracheal suctioning: a review of the literature, Heart-Lung 15:164, 1986.

Birdsall C: What suction pressure should I use? Am J Nurs 85:866, 1985.

Blodgett D: Manual of respiratory care procedures, Philadelphia, 1980, JB Lippincott, Co.

Brown I: Trach care: take care—infection on the prowl, Nursing '82 12(5):45, 1982.

Bulau J: Clinical policies and procedures for home health care Rockville, Md, 1986 Aspen Publishers, Inc.

Burton GG, et al.: Respiratory care: a guide to clinical practice, Philadelphia, 1984, JB Lippincott Co.

Colaianni M, McNamara M: Teaching families to give trach care at home, Nursing '82 12(6):70, 1982.

Cosenza JJ, Norton LC: Secretion clearance: state of the art from a nursing perspective, Crit Care Nurs 6:23, 1986.

Feinstein D: What to teach the patient who's had a total laryngectomy, RN 50:53, 1987.

Fuchs P: Streamlining your suctioning techniques, Nursing '84, 14(7):39, 1984.

Glover DW, Glover MM: Respiratory therapy: basics for nursing and the allied health professions, St. Louis, 1978, The CV Mosby Co.

Harper RW: A guide to respiratory care: physiology and applications, Philadelphia, 1981, JB Lippincott Co.

Harris RB: National survey of aseptic tracheostomy care techniques in hospitals with head and neck/ENT surgical departments, Cancer Nurs Feb 1984.

Hazinski MF: Nursing care of the critically ill child, St. Louis, 1984, The CV Mosby Co.

Holloway NM: Nursing the critically ill adult, Menlo Park, Calif, 1979, Addison-Wesley Publishing Co.

Johanson BC, et al.: Standards for critical care, St. Louis, 1985, The CV Mosby Co.

Johnson DL, Giovanni RM, Driscoll SA: Ventilator-assisted patient care: planning for hospital discharge and home care, Rockville, Md, 1986, Aspen Publishers, Inc.

Jung RC, Gottlieb LS: Comparison of tracheobronchial suction catheters in human visualization by fiberoptic bronchoscopy, Chest 69(2):179, 1976.

Lockhart J, Griffin C: Occluded trach tube, Nursing '87 17(4):33, 1987.

Luce JM, et al.: Intensive respiratory care, Philadelphia, 1984, WB Saunders Co.

Mapp CS: Trach care: are you aware of all the dangers? Nurs 18:34, 1988.

McPherson SP: Respiratory therapy equipment, ed 3, St. Louis, 1981, The CV Mosby Co.

Pfaff S, Terry B: Discharge planning: infection prevention and control in the home, Nurs Clin North Am 15(4):893, 1980.

Riegel B, Forshee T: A review and critique of the literature on preoxygenation for endotracheal suctioning, Heart-Lung 14:507, 1985.

Rudy E, Baun M, Stone K, et al.: The relationship between endotracheal suctioning and changes in intracranial pressure: a review of the literature, Heart-Lung 15:488, 1986.

Traver GA, ed: Respiratory nursing: the science and the art, New York, 1982, John Wiley & Sons.

Walsh J, Persons C, Wieck L: Manual of home health care nursing, Philadelphia, 1987, JB Lippincott Co.

Woldum K, et al.: Patient education, Rockville, Md, 1985, Aspen Publishers, Inc.

# 17

# CLOSED CHEST DRAINAGE SYSTEMS

## OBJECTIVES

*Mastery of content in this chapter will enable the nurse to:*

- Define key terms.
- Explain the physiology of normal respiration.
- List three common sites for chest tube placement.
- List three conditions requiring chest tube insertion.
- Describe a closed chest drainage system.
- Describe chest tube suction.
- Describe methods of troubleshooting chest tube systems.
- Discuss the care for clients with chest tubes.

## KEY TERMS

*Atmospheric pressure*
*Chest tube*
*Client-centered air leak*
*External air leak*
*Hemothorax*
*Hemopneumothorax*
*Intrapleural*
*Intrapulmonic*
*Mediastinal shift*
*Negative pressure*
*Positive pressure*
*Parietal pleura*
*Pneumothorax*
*Tension pneumothorax*
*Visceral pleura*

## SKILLS

**17-1** Caring for clients with chest tube to water-seal drainage systems
**17-2** Obtaining specimen from chest tube drainage system
**17-3** Removing chest tubes

The chest cavity is a closed structure bound by muscle, bone, connective tissue, vascular structures, and the diaphragm. This cavity has three distinct sections, each one sealed from the other: one section for each lung and a third section for the mediastinum, which surrounds the heart, esophagus, trachea, aorta, etc.

The lungs are covered with a membrane called the visceral pleura. The interior chest wall is lined with another membrane, called the parietal pleura. The potential space between the visceral and parietal pleura is filled with approximately 4 milliliters of lubricating fluid and is called the intrapleural space.

To expand the lungs, intrapleural negative pressure must be maintained. During inspiration, the intercostal muscles pull outward and the diaphragm contracts and pulls down, thereby increasing the size of the chest cavity. This increase in size causes an increase in the amount of negative pressure (vacuum effect) that is being exerted in the intrapleural space.

Inspiration occurs when the increased negative pressure pulls the lungs against the enlarged chest cavity, expanding their size. The expanding lungs cause the intrapulmonic* pressure to fall lower than atmospheric pressure. Increased negative pressure within the lungs cause atmospheric air to rush into the lungs until the intrapulmonic pressure is equal to the pressure in the atmosphere.

When the chest cavity stops expanding and the lungs are full of air, the respiratory muscles and diaphragm relax, returning the chest cavity to its resting stage. At this time the intrapulmonic pressure is the same as the atmospheric pressure.

During expiration a passive relaxation of the respiratory muscles causes the chest cavity space to decrease. This decrease in space causes an increase in the intrapulmonic pressure, which forces the air in the lungs back into the atmosphere.

Trauma, disease, or surgery can result in air or fluid leaking into the intrapleural space. Small leaks are absorbed spontaneously (Shoemaker, et al., 1989). Occasionally, a flutter valve (Heimlich valve) is inserted through the chest wall to treat these leaks. A flutter valve

*Within the lung.

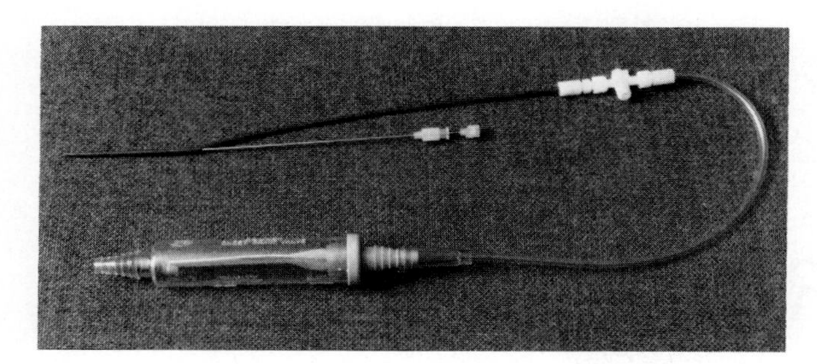

***Fig. 17-1*** Flutter (Heimlich) valve.

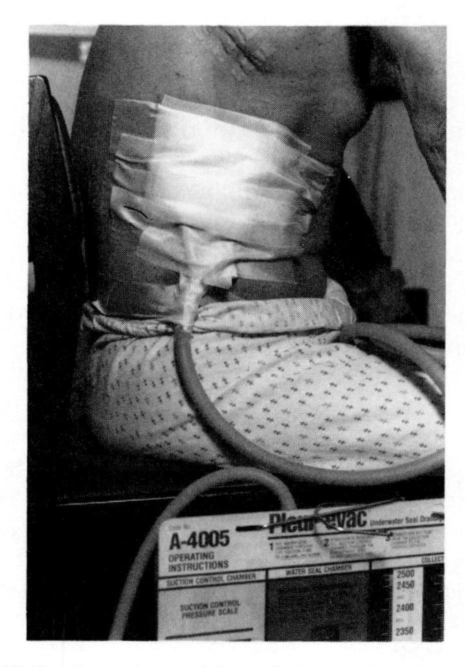


***Fig. 17-2*** Posterior and lateral chest tube placement.

(Fig. 17-1) is a disposable, one-way valve that allows air to exit from the intrapleural space on expiration, but prevents air from reentry during inspiration (Connor, 1987).

A chest tube is inserted after chest trauma, open chest surgery, or a large intrapleural leak. A closed chest drainage system and possibly suction is used to promote drainage of air and fluid. Lung reexpansion occurs as the fluid or air is removed by drainage or absorption.

The location of the chest tube indicates the type of drainage expected. Apical and anterior chest tube placement promotes removal of air, which occurs in a pneumothorax. Because air rises, these chest tubes are placed high, allowing evacuation of air from the intrapleural space and allowing the lung to reexpand.

Chest tubes are placed low and posterior or lateral to drain fluid (Fig. 17-2). Fluid in the intrapleural space is affected by gravity and localizes in the lower portion of the space. Tubes placed in these positions drain blood and fluid. Frequently this drainage is assisted by applying suction. Fluid drainage is expected with a hemothorax, after open chest surgery or with a chest trauma that causes a hemothorax.

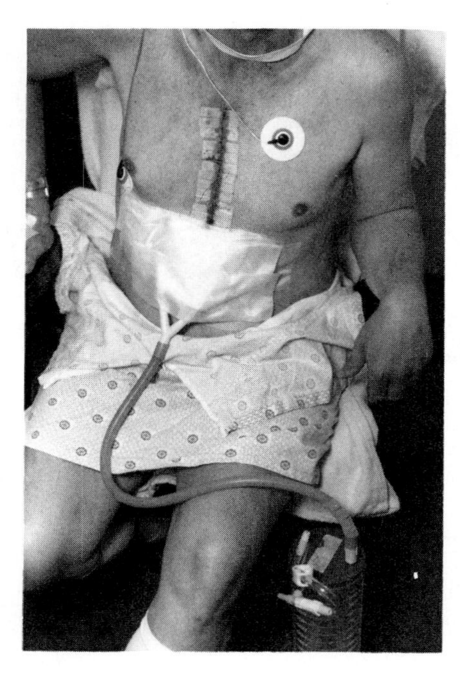

***Fig. 17-3*** Mediastinal chest tube placement.

A mediastinal chest tube is placed just below the sternum (Fig. 17-3). This tube drains blood or fluid, preventing accumulation around the heart. A mediastinal tube is commonly used after open heart surgery.

Four drainage systems are available: one-, two-, and three-bottle systems (Fig. 17-4), and a variety of disposable, commercial chest drainage systems (Fig. 17-5).

The single-bottle system is primarily used in the treatment of pneumothoraxes. It allows air from the pneumothorax to bubble out of the water-seal and escape through the air outlet while preventing air from reentering the intrapleural space. This system is used in emergency situations. However, it is not recommended for the evacuation of fluid because drainage would raise the level of the water-seal liquid. An increased height of fluid in the water-seal increases the resistance to drainage on expiration and will eventually stop the drainage entirely (Johanson, et al., 1988).

The two-bottle system provides a bottle for fluid or blood drainage and a second bottle for the water-seal. This system allows safe drainage of fluid without causing increased resistance.

The three-bottle system establishes a separate bottle for drainage, water-seal, and suction control. It is set up as a two-bottle system with the addition of a suction-control bottle, which is connected to a suction device (Johanson, et al., 1988).

Disposable commercial systems can function as a two-

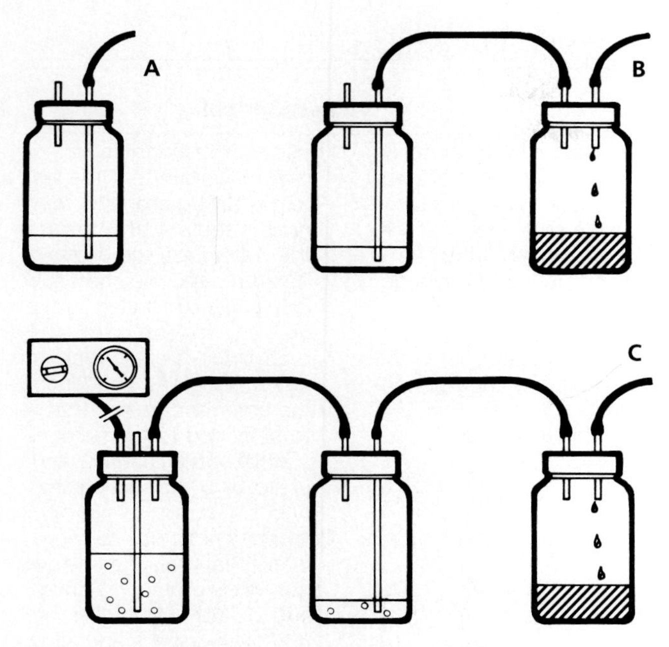


***Fig. 17-4*** Three types of chest tube bottle systems. **A,** One-bottle system. **B,** Two-bottle system. **C,** Three-bottle system with suction.

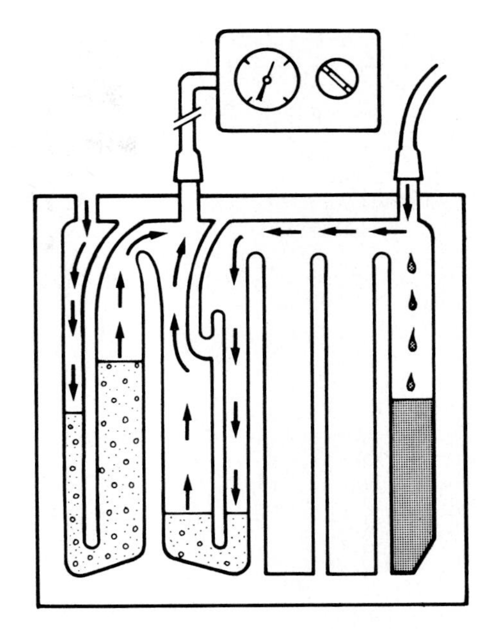

***Fig. 17-5*** Disposable, commercial chest drainage system.

bottle system without suction or as a three-bottle system with suction. These systems are more efficient, compact, and less prone to contamination due to fewer parts. In addition, they provide additional safety due to the ease in obtaining sterile specimens without disrupting the systems' negative pressure or sterility, and because the chambers are unbreakable.

This chapter focuses on chest tube drainage systems, suction, and the basic concerns and nursing care of the client with a chest tube or flutter valve.

## GUIDELINES

1. Document client's baseline for vital signs and respiratory sounds and movements, and monitor them closely. Changes in the vital signs or respiratory status can indicate a malfunctioning chest drainage system.
2. Observe the water-seal straw for intermittent bubbling from the tip or a rise and fall of fluid within the straw that is synchronous with respirations. These actions are considered normal and consistent with lung reexpansion. After 2 to 3 days, this activity is expected to stop, indicating that the lung has reexpanded (Luckmann and Sorensen, 1987). Constant bubbling in the water-seal and a sudden, unexpected stoppage of water-seal activity are considered to be abnormal.
3. Know the type and amount of expected chest tube drainage. A sudden decrease in the amount of chest tube drainage can indicate a possible clot or obstruction in the chest tube. A sudden increase in the amount of drainage can indicate fresh bleeding from the thorax. Any drainage from a pneumothorax is limited to the fluid caused by chest tube insertion trauma.
4. Know expected color of the drainage. Drainage from postoperative open-chest surgery is initially bright red and gradually becomes serous as the postoperative course continues. Pleural effusions usually drain straw-colored fluid.
5. Observe for constant, gentle bubbling in the suction-control chamber when the three-bottle system is connected to suction. No bubbling indicates that *no* suction is being exerted in the system. The suction source should be raised to the prescribed rate. Vigorous bubbling indicates that the suction source is set too high. The excessive suction is being dissipated through the bubbles in the water control chamber. The suction source needs to be lowered to the prescribed rate.

## PREREQUISITE KNOWLEDGE

1. Knowledge of respiratory physiology.
2. Principles of sterile asepsis.
3. Principles of pain management.

## PREREQUISITE SKILLS

1. Cardiopulmonary assessment (Chapter 13).
2. Measurement of vital signs (Chapter 12).
3. Proper handwashing techniques (Chapter 37).
4. Surgical aseptic techniques (Chapter 38).
5. Comfort measures (Chapter 5).

***TABLE 17-1*** Physician's Role and Responsibility in Chest Tube Placement

| Role | Responsibility |
|---|---|
| 1. Explain purpose, procedure, and possible complications to the client and have client sign consent form. | Provides informed consent. |
| 2. Wash hands. Cleanse chest wall with antiseptic. | Reduces transmission of microorganisms. |
| 3. Don mask and gloves. | Maintains surgical asepsis. |
| 4. Drape area of chest tube insertion with sterile towels. | Maintains surgical asepsis. |
| 5. Inject local anesthesia and allow time to take effect. | Decreases pain during procedure. |
| 6. Use blunt or sharp dissection to create incision in the skin and chest wall. | Opens chest for insertion of chest tube. A trochar is outdated and increases risk of tissue damage. |
| 7. Thread a clamped chest tube through the incision. Physician clamps chest tube until system is connected to water seal. | Inserts chest tube into the intrapleural space. Clamping prevents entry of atmospheric air into the chest and worsening of the pneumothorax. |
| 8. Suture chest tube in place, if suturing is policy or physician preference. | Secures chest tube in place. |
| 9. Cover the chest insertion site with a large, sterile occlusive pressure dressing. | Holds chest tube in place and prevents air leakage around the tube to prevent additional atmospheric air from entering the intrapleural space. |
| 10. Remove connector cover from client's end of chest drainage tubing, using sterile technique. Secure drainage tubing to the chest tube and drainage system. | Physician is responsible for making certain that the system is set up properly, the proper amount of water is in the water-seal, the dressing is secure, and the chest tube is securely connected to the drainage system. |
| 11. Connect system to suction or supervise a nurse connecting it to suction, if suction is to be used. | The physician is responsible for determining and checking the amount of water that is to be added to the suction-control bottle/chamber and prescribing the suction setting. |
| 12. Unclamp the chest tube. | Connects chest tube to the water-seal drainage and suction, thus promoting drainage of fluid or air from the intrapleural space and allowing the lung to reexpand. |
| 13. Order and review chest x-ray. | Verifies correct chest tube placement. |

# *SKILL 17-1 Caring for Clients with Chest Tube to Water-seal Drainage Systems*

## *Procedure 17-1*

| Steps | Rationale |
|---|---|
| **Assessment** | |
| 1. Obtain vital signs. | Baseline vital signs are essential for any invasive procedure. Clients requiring chest tube insertion frequently experience respiratory distress and vital signs are taken serially. A changing blood pressure and heart rate may indicate a tension pneumothorax. |
| 2. Observe for changes in heart rate, blood pressure, respiratory pattern, increased apprehension, and chest pain. | Changes in these parameters may indicate worsening of the initial condition. |
| 3. Assess client for known allergies. | Povidone-Iodine is an antiseptic used to cleanse the skin. Lidocaine is a local anesthetic administered to reduce pain. Also, clients should receive mild tranquilizers, sedation, or analgesics before the procedures. |
| 4. Review client's medication record for anticoagulant therapy. | Anticoagulation therapy can increase procedure-related blood loss. |

| Steps | Rationale |
|---|---|
| **Nursing Diagnosis** | |
| 1. Cluster data to reveal actual or potential nursing diagnoses: | |
| a. Potential knowledge deficit regarding chest tube insertion: related to inexperience. | Client education reduces anxiety and informs the client about the purpose and components of the procedure. |
| b. Anxiety related to: | |
| ▪ Procedure. | Client education can reduce anxiety and the dyspnea that results. |
| ▪ Respiratory distress. | Anxiety is frequent result of respiratory distress. This can add to increased oxygen demand. |
| c. Pain related to: ▪ Collapsed lung. ▪ Chest tube insertion. | Both a collapsed lung and chest tube insertion cause pain. Lidocaine's anesthetic effect is limited because it is difficult to anesthetize the pleura (Carroll, 1986). |
| d. Impaired gas exchange: related to limited lung expansion. | There is decreased intrapulmonic surface area for the transfer of respiratory gases due to pulmonary collapse. |
| **Planning** | |
| 1. Develop individualized goals for client based on nursing diagnoses: | |
| a. Anxiety is reduced. b. Respirations are nonlabored. | As hypoxia is resolved, the client is less anxious and respirations become nonlabored. |
| c. Reduction or absence of pain. | Reexpansion of the lung assists in resolving any chest pain that was associated with the collapsed lung. |
| d. Absence of hypoxia. e. Improved or full lung expansion. | Correction of a pneumothorax or hemothorax allows for complete lung expansion and the absence of hypoxia. |
| f. Absence of atelectasis. | Proper reexpansion is without atelectasis. |
| 2. Check agency policy and determine if informed consent was obtained. | Most institutions require informed and written permission for chest tube insertion. |
| 3. Review physician's role and responsibilities for chest tube placement (Table 17-1). | Helps differentiate doctor and nurse roles so that the nurse can function more effectively. |
| 4. Explain procedure to client. | Reduces anxiety and promotes patient cooperation. |
| 5. Gather the following equipment: a. Chest tube insertion tray b. Chest tube c. Povidone-Iodine (Betadine) d. Lidocaine | Equipment will vary from agency to agency. Be familiar with equipment that is available in the agency before assisting with any procedure. |
| e. Sutures | Secure chest tube to client's skin and reduce risk of accidental dislocation. |
| f. Requested drainage system (One-, two-, or three-bottle system or a disposable commercial system) | Physician's preference and client's condition will affect type of system used. |
| g. Sterile water or saline | Added to the water-seal bottle/chamber. Added to the suction-control bottle/chamber when appropriate. |
| h. Drainage tubing | Connects chest tube(s) to chest drainage systems. |
| i. Sterile gloves | Sterile procedure. |
| j. Adhesive tape (0.5-1") | Secures connections in the system. |
| k. Two shodded hemostats for each chest tube | Used *only* in emergency cases. Two shodded hemostats are used for each tube so that the maximum occlusion of the tube can be attained quickly without damaging tubing. Shodded hemostats have tubing covering the teeth of the hemostat blades. This prevents inadvertent puncture of the chest tube. |
| l. Dressing materials: sterile wick, noncotton-filled 4 × 4 gauze pads, petroleum gauze and ABDs or combination dressings, wide adhesive tape or elastoplast. | Occludes insertion site around chest tube to form an airtight seal around chest tube, helps stabilize chest tube, and holds dressing tightly in place. Aids in preventing bacteria entry into insertion site. |
| 6. Wash hands. | Reduces transmission of microorganisms. |
| 7. Set up the prescribed drainage system: | Provides prescribed closed-drainage system. |
| a. One-bottle system: | |
| ▪ Obtain a vented water-seal chest tube drainage bottle and remove cover from vent. | Vent allows air to be expressed from the intrapleural space during each expiration, until the lung is reexpanded (Erickson, 1981a). Prevents formation of positive pressure in the intrapleural space and drainage system, which would impede drainage. |

| Steps | Rationale |
|---|---|
| ▪ Pour sterile water or saline into bottle so that straw tip is submerged 2 cm (1 in). | Produces water seal and blocks air from reentering intrapleural space. Deeper submersion of the straw tip impedes drainage. |
| ▪ Assess system to ensure that all connections are airtight and the air vent is open. | Prevents atmospheric air from leaking into the system and the client's intrapleural space. Fluid and/or air will stop draining if negative pressure is not maintained in the system. |
| ▪ Tape all connections in a spiral manner. | Helps maintain an airtight seal. Allows visualization of drainage in the tubing. |
| ▪ If, during an emergency situation, a one-bottle system is used to drain fluid, place calibrated adhesive tape on side of the bottle. | Permits timely and efficient account of amount of drainage from the chest tube. Drainage is marked at specified periods of time and documented on the nurses' notes and I & O sheet. |
| ▪ Observe depth of the water-seal tip below the drainage level. | The deeper the water-seal straw tip is submerged beyond 2 cm, the greater the resistance to drainage. |
| b. Two-bottle system: | |
| ▪ Obtain a drainage collection bottle. | Collects intrapleural fluids drained by gravity into the first bottle without disturbing the water-seal. |
| ▪ Obtain a vented water-seal bottle. | Blocks air from entering the intrapleural space. Vent allows air to escape from the water-seal bottle into the atmosphere. |
| ▪ Pour sterile saline or water into water-seal bottle so the straw tip is submerged 2 cm (1 in). | Establishes water-seal, preventing air from reentering intrapleural space on inspiration. |
| ▪ Obtain connector tubing. Connect chest tube to the first (drainage) bottle rod. The second rod of this bottle is then connected to the water-seal straw. A final rod in the water-seal bottle is left open to air. | Tubing connects the chest tube to the drainage system. Drainage passes through tubing and into drainage bottle. Air, equal to the amount of drainage, passes from the drainage bottle through the water-seal bottle and into the atmosphere through the air vent. |
| ▪ Assess system to ensure that all connections are airtight. (Taping connections helps maintain an airtight seal.) | Prevents air from entering the system and clients intrapleural space. Thus, maintains negative pressure in the system. |
| c. Three-bottle system: | |
| ▪ Obtain drainage collection, water-seal, and suction-control bottles. | Suction increases the negative pressure gradient between the intrapleural space and the drainage system by evacuating air from the bottles, thus maintaining a constant, higher level of negative pressure. |
| ▪ Connect drainage and water-seal bottles as stated in the two-bottle system. | Maintains integrity of the water-seal by collecting drainage in the first bottle. |
| ▪ Pour sterile water or saline into water-seal bottle so the straw tip is submerged 2 cm (1 in). | Maintains water-seal, preventing air from reentering the intrapleural space. |
| ▪ Pour sterile water or saline into the suction control bottle. Physician is responsible for determining fluid level in the suction control bottle. It is usually set so that the suction control rod is submerged 20 cm (7.9 in) below the fluid surface. | Depth of rod below fluid level dictates the highest amount of negative pressure that can be present within the system, i.e., 20 cm of water is approximately −20 cm of water pressure. Any additional negative pressure applied to the system will be vented into the atmosphere through the suction-control rod. This safety device prevents damage to pleural tissues from an unexpected surge of negative pressure from the suction source. |
| ▪ Connect suction tubing from the suction-control bottle to the suction source. | While rod depth controls the maximum amount of negative pressure, the suction source establishes the minimum amount of effective negative pressure in the system. A constant, gentle bubbling in the suction-control bottle indicates that adequate negative pressure is being maintained (Erickson, 1981a). |
| ▪ Tape all connections in the system. | Maintains an airtight seal within the system. |
| ▪ Check system for patency by:<br>Clamping the drainage tubing that will connect the client to the system.<br>Connecting tubing from the suction-control bottle to the suction source.<br>Turning on the suction source to the prescribed level. | Provides a chance to ensure an airtight system before connecting it to the client. Allows correction or replacement of system if it is defective before connecting it to the client. *Note:* Bubbling will be seen from the water-seal at first because there is air in the tubing and system initially. This should stop after a few min unless there are other sources of air entering the system. If bubbling continues, check connections and locate source of the air leak as described in Table 17-2. |
| ▪ Turn off suction source and unclamp drainage tubing before connecting client to to the system. | Having the system connected to suction when it is initiated could cause damage to pleural tissues from sudden increase in negative pressure. The suction source is turned on again after the client is connected to the three-bottle system. |

| Steps | Rationale |
|---|---|
| d. Disposable commercial drainage system: | |
| ▪ Remove sterile wrapping. | Maintains sterility of the system. The system is packaged in this manner so it can be used under sterile operating room conditions (Carroll, 1986). |
| ▪ While maintaining sterility of the drainage tubing, stand the system upright and add sterile water or saline to the appropriate chambers: | The same system can be used as either a two- or three-bottle system depending upon the chambers used. |
| □ For a two-bottle system (without suction), add sterile solution to the water-seal chamber, (second chamber) bringing fluid to the required level as indicated. | Maintains water-seal, preventing air from reentering the intrapleural space. Fluid drains from the chest into the first chamber. |
| □ For a three-bottle system (with suction), add sterile solution to the water-seal chamber (second chamber) as described above and an amount of sterile solution (prescribed by physician) to the suction-control chamber, usually 20 cm (7.9 in). | Maintains water-seal and establishes maximum amount of negative pressure that can be exerted in the system. Turning up the suction source causes more vigorous bubbling in the suction-control chamber, but does not increase the amount of negative pressure exerted on the pleura (Carroll, 1986). Fluid drains from the chest into the first chamber. |
| ▪ If ordered, connect suction tubing to the suction source. | Maintains minimum amount of effective negative pressure in the system. This is indicated by a constant gentle bubbling in the suction control chamber (Erickson, 1981a). |
| ▪ Check system for patency (see Three-bottle system). | Provides a chance to ensure an airtight system before connecting it to the client. |
| ▪ Tape all connections in the system. | Provides an airtight seal within the system. |
| 8. Position the client: | Permits optimal drainage of fluid and/or air. |
| a. Semi-Fowler's to high Fowler's position to evacuate air (pneumothorax). | Air rises to the highest point in the chest. Pneumothorax tubes are usually placed on the anterior aspect at the midclavicular line, second or third intercostal space (Carroll, 1986). |
| b. High Fowler's position to drain fluid (hemothorax). | Permits optimal drainage of fluid. Posterior tubes are placed on the midaxillary line, eighth or ninth intercostal space. |

## Implementation

| Steps | Rationale |
|---|---|
| 1. Wash hands and don sterile gloves. | Reduces transmission of microorganisms. |
| 2. Administer parenteral premedications, such as sedatives, analgesics as ordered. | Reduces client anxiety and pain during procedure. |
| 3. Assist physician in providing psychologic support to the client. (See physician's responsibilities in Table 17-1, p. 406.) | Reduces client anxiety and assists in efficient completion of procedure. |
| a. Reinforce preprocedure explanation. | |
| b. Instruct client throughout procedure. | |
| 4. Show anesthetic to physician. | Allows physician to read label of drug before administering it to client. |
| 5. Hold anesthetic solution bottle upside down with label facing physician. Physician will withdraw solution. | Allows physician to withdraw solution properly while maintaining surgical asepsis. |
| a. Physician places chest tube. (A standard procedure is detailed in Table 17-1.) | |
| 6. Assist physician to attach drainage tube to chest tube. | Connects drainage system and suction (if ordered) to the chest tube. |
| 7. Tape the tube connection between the chest and drainage tubes. | Secures chest tube to drainage system and reduces risk of air leaks causing breaks in the airtight system. |
| 8. Check patency of air vents in system: | |
| a. Water-seal vent must be without occlusion. | Permits the displaced air to pass into the atmosphere. |
| b. Suction-control chamber vent must be without occlusion, when using suction. | Provides safety factor of releasing excess negative pressure into the atmosphere. |
| 9. Coil excess tubing on mattress next to the client. Secure with a rubber band and safety pin or the system's clamp. | Prevents excess tubing from hanging over the edge of the mattress in a dependent loop. Drainage could collect in the loop and occlude the drainage system. |
| 10. Adjust tubing to hang in a straight line from top of the mattress to the drainage chamber. | Promotes drainage. |
| 11. If the chest tube is draining fluid, indicate the time (e.g., 0900) that drainage was begun on the drainage bottle's adhesive tape of a bottle setup, or on the write-on surface of a disposable commercial system. | Provides a baseline for continuous assessment of the type and quantity of drainage. |
| 12. Strip or milk chest tube only if indicated: | Stripping is controversial and should be performed only if hospital policy permits and there is a physician's order (Krauss, 1985; Johanson, 1988). Stripping creates a high degree of negative pressure and has potential of pulling lung tissue or |
| a. Postoperative mediastinal chest tubes are manipulated if nursing assessment indicates an obstruction of drainage secondary to clots or debris in the tubing. | |

| Steps | Rationale |
|---|---|
| b. Postoperative assessment is done every 15 min for the first 2 hr. This assessment interval then changes *based on client's status.* | pleura into drainage holes of the chest tube (Duncan and Erickson, 1982; Duncan, Erickson, and Weigel, 1987). |
| 13. Provide 2 shodded hemostats for each chest tube. Shodded hemostats are usually attached to the top of the client's bed with adhesive tape or clamped to client's clothing during ambulation. | Chest tubes are only clamped under specific circumstances:<br>a. To assess for an air leak (see Table 17-2).<br>b. To empty or change the collection bottle or chamber (Farley, 1988). This procedure is performed only by physician or nurse who has received training in the procedure.<br>c. To change disposable systems (Erickson, 1981b). Have new system ready to be connected before clamping the tube, so that transfer can be rapid and the drainage system reestablished.<br>d. To change a broken water-seal bottle in the event that there is no sterile solution container available.<br>e. To assess if client is ready to have chest tube removed. This is done by physician's order (Farley, 1988). In this situation, nurse must monitor client for the recreation of a pneumothorax (see Table 17-2). |
| 14. Assist client to a comfortable position. | Reduces client anxiety and promotes cooperation. |
| 15. Remove gloves and dispose of used, soiled equipment. | Prevents accidents involving contaminated equipment. |
| 16. Wash hands. | Reduces spread of microorganisms. |

## Evaluation

| Steps | Rationale |
|---|---|
| 1. Assess client's physical and psychologic status. | Detects early signs and symptoms of complications:<br>a. Respiratory distress<br>b. Subcutaneous emphysema.<br>Ascertains client's emotional response to procedure. |
| 2. Assess client compliancy in activities of daily living related to care of the drainage system. | Detects educational needs and reinforces activities of care for the system. |
| 3. Observe: | |
| a. Chest tube dressing. | Ensure that dressing is patent and note any drainage. |
| b. Tubing. | Maintain tubing free of kinks and dependent loops. Note presence of clots or debris in tubing. |
| c. The Chest drainage system. System should be upright and below level of tube insertion. | System must be in this position to function properly. |
| d. Water-seal, for fluctuations with client's inspiration and expiration. | Fluid should rise in the water-seal with inspiration and fall with expiration. This indicates that the system is functioning properly (Erickson, 1981a; Carroll, 1986). |
| e. Bubbling in the water-seal bottle or chamber (see Table 17-2). | When system is initially connected to the client, bubbles are expected from the chamber. These are from air that was present in the system and in the client's intrapleural space (Farley, 1988). After a short period of time, the bubbling will stop. Fluid will continue to fluctuate in the water-seal on inspiration and expiration until the lung is reexpanded or the system becomes occluded. |
| f. Type and amount of fluid drainage: Nurse should note color and amount of drainage, client's vital signs, and skin color. | Sudden gush of drainage may be retained blood and not active bleeding. This increase in drainage can be result of client position change (Farley, 1988). |
| ▪ Less than 50-200 ml/hr immediately postoperative in a **mediastinal chest tube** (Johanson, 1988). Approximately 500 ml in the first 24 hr. Dark red drainage is expected early in the postoperative period, turning serous with time (Luckmann and Sorensen, 1987). | Reexpansion of lungs forces drainage into the tube. Coughing can also cause large gushes of drainage (Luckmann and Sorensen, 1987). |
| ▪ Between 100-300 ml of fluid may drain in a **posterior chest tube** during the first 2 hr after insertion. This rate will decrease after 2 hr, 500-1,000 ml can be expected in the first 24 hr. Drainage will be grossly bloody during the first several hours after surgery and then change to serous (Luckmann and Sorensen, 1987). | Excessive amounts and/or the continued presence of frankly bloody drainage after the first several hours of surgery should be reported to the physician, along with client's vital signs and respiratory status. |
| g. Bubbling in the suction control chamber (when suction is being used) (see Table 17-2). | Suction control chamber has constant, gentle bubbling. Tubing to the suction source should be free of obstruction and the suction source should be turned on to the appropriate setting. |

**TABLE 17-2** Problem Solving With Chest Tubes

| Problem | Solution |
|---|---|
| Air leak: | Locate leak. |
| Continuous bubbling in the water-seal bottle/chamber, indicating leak is between client and the water-seal. | Tighten loose connections between client and water-seal. Loose connections cause air to enter the system. Leaks are corrected when constant bubbling stops. |
| Bubbling continues, indicating the air leak has not been corrected. | Cross-clamp chest tube close to client's chest. If bubbling stops, the air leak is inside the client's thorax (client-centered) or at the chest tube insertion site (Palau and Jones, 1986). *Unclamp tube and notify physician immediately.* Reinforce chest dressing. Leaving chest tube clamped with a client-centered leak can cause collapse of the lung, mediastinal shift, and eventual collapse of the other lung from the buildup of air pressure within the pleural cavity. |
| Bubbling continues, indicating leak is not client-centered. | In an alternating fashion, gradually move clamps down the drainage tubing away from the client and toward the suction-control chamber, moving one clamp at a time. When bubbling stops, leak is in the section of tubing or connection that is in between the two clamps. Replace tubing or secure connection and release clamps (Erickson, 1981b). |
| Bubbling continues, indicating leak is not in the tubing. | Leak is in the drainage system. Change drainage system (Erickson, 1981b; Palau and Jones, 1986). |
| Tension pneumothorax:<br>Severe respiratory distress.<br>Chest pain.<br>Absence of breath sounds on affected side.<br>Hyperresonance on affected side.<br>Mediastinal shift to unaffected side.<br>Tracheal shift to unaffected side.<br>Hypotension.<br>Tachycardia. | Determine that chest tubes *are not clamped, kinked, or occluded.* Obstructed chest tubes trap air in the intrapleural space when there is a client-centered air leak.<br>Notify physician immediately.<br>Prepare immediately for another chest tube insertion; obtain a flutter (Heimlich) valve or large-gauge needle for short-term emergency release of air in the intrapleural space; have emergency equipment, e.g., oxygen and code cart, near the client. |
| Dependent loops of drainage tubing have trapped fluid. | Drain tubing contents into drainage bottle. Coil excess tubing on mattress and secure in place. |
| Water-seal is disconnected. | Connect water-seal and tape connection. |
| Water-seal bottle is broken. | Insert distal end of water-seal straw into sterile solution so that the tip is 2 cm below surface level (Carroll, 1986) and set up a new water-seal bottle. If no sterile solution is available, double clamp the chest tube while preparing a new bottle. |
| Water-seal straw is no longer submerged in sterile fluid. | Add sterile solution to the water-seal bottle until the distal tip is 2 cm under surface level (Erickson, 1981b); *or* set the water-seal bottle upright so that the tip is submerged. |

| Steps | Rationale |
|---|---|
| 4. Assess client for decreased respiratory distress and chest pain, breath sounds over affected lung area, and stable vital signs. | Increase in respiratory distress and/or chest pain, decrease in breath sounds over the affected and nonaffected lungs, marked cyanosis, asymmetric chest movements, presence of subcutaneous emphysema around tube insertion site or neck, hypotension, tachycardia, and/or mediastinal shift are critical and indicate a severe change in client status, such as excessive blood loss or tension pneumothorax. Notify physician immediately. |

***Expected outcomes***

| | |
|---|---|
| 1. Reduced anxiety. | Decreased hypoxia reduces anxiety. |
| 2. Breath sounds auscultated in all lobes, full symmetric lung expansion, absence of hypoxia, nonlabored respirations. | Reexpansion of the lung promotes normal respirations. |
| 3. Absence of chest pain. | Reexpansion of the lung reduces chest pain. |
| 4. Chest tube remains in place and chest drainage system remains airtight. | Ensures patency of the system. |

| Steps | Rationale |
|---|---|
| 5. After 2-3 days, drainage will decrease to less than 50 cc/day and fluctuations in the water-seal will cease. | Indicates that the lung has reexpanded. |
| ***Unexpected outcomes*** | |
| 1. Constant bubbling in water-seal chamber unrelated to respirations. | Indicates air leak between client and water-seal (see Table 17-2). |
| 2. Substantial increase in bright red drainage with tachycardia and hypotension. | Indicates client is actively bleeding. |
| 3. No drainage from a hemothorax and/or no fluctuation in water-seal within first 48 hr after tube insertion. | Indicates that tubing is occluded. Clots or kinks may have occluded the tubing, or the internal end of the chest tube may be against the pleural lining. |
| 4. No bubbling in suction-control bottle/chamber when suction is being used. | Indicates tubing to suction source is obstructed, kinked, or leaking, or the suction source is too low or off. |
| 5. Excessive bubbling in suction control bottle/chamber. | Indicates suction source is delivering too much negative pressure to the system. |
| 6. Water-seal straw is not submerged in water. | Indicates that the water-seal is not being maintained and air can reenter the intrapleural space. |
| 7. Water-seal bottle or disposable drainage system is turned on its side. | Indicates that the water-seal is not being maintained and air can reenter the intrapleural space. |
| 8. Water-seal bottle/chamber is broken. | Indicates that the water-seal is not being maintained and air can reenter the intrapleural space. This is an emergency situation. |
| 9. Drainage bottle/chamber is broken. | Indicates that the water-seal is not being maintained and air can reenter the intrapleural space. This is an emergency situation. |

## Follow-up Activities

| Steps | Rationale |
|---|---|
| 1. Locate source of the air leak; correct situation if it is in the tubing or drainage system, notify physician and document. A client-centered leak is an emergency situation requiring immediate reinforcement of the dressing and physician intervention. | External leaks can be corrected by the nurse. Documentation and physician notification are necessary to explain delayed progress.<br>Client-centered leaks progress to the reaccumulation of air in the intrapleural space, a tension pneumothorax, and eventually a mediastinal shift. |
| 2. Notify physician. Monitor vital signs and measure drainage at least every 15-30 min as indicated by client's condition (Carroll, 1986). | Immediate physician intervention is required to prevent patient from going into hypovolemic shock. |
| 3. Correct any visible occlusions caused by kinks and document. Milk or strip tubing to remove visible clots if approved and ordered, and document. Notify physician if no visible kinks or clots are found. | Removal of kinks should be documented to explain delayed progress. Milk tubing only if approved by hospital policy and ordered by physician. Document to explain delayed progress. Physician intervention will be needed to correct chest tube placement. |
| 4. Correct kink occlusions or leaks in tubing, remove occlusion to suction air vent or increase suction at the suction source and document. | Correct kinks or occlusions or set suction at proper suction setting to reestablish proper functioning of the system. Documentation explains delayed progress. |
| 5. Turn suction source to prescribed setting. | Documentation is not required because the suction control bottle fluid level is a safety control device that dissipates excessive negative pressure into the atmosphere. The suction setting is lowered to prevent loss of water from the suction control bottle through excessive bubbling. If water is lost from this chamber, the amount of negative pressure exerted in the system is decreased. |
| 6. Add sterile water or saline to the water-seal bottle/chamber, so that the straw is submerged 2 cm or 1 in below surface of the fluid. Document. | Reestablishes the water-seal. |
| 7. Set water-seal or disposable system upright. Encourage client to cough and deep breathe. Document. | Coughing and deep breathing helps expel air in the intrapleural space. Document to explain delayed progress. |
| 8. Double-clamp drainage tubing, connect tubing to new water-seal bottle/chamber and release clamps; *or* place water-seal straw so that the tip is 2 cm below the surface level in a container of sterile water, saline or IV solution while a new water-seal bottle/chamber is prepared. Then, double-clamp | Prevents air from reentering the intrapleural space.<br>Reestablishes the water-seal.<br>Establishes a quick, temporary water-seal thus preventing reentry of air into the intrapleural space (Carroll, 1986; Farley, 1988). |

| Steps | Rationale |
|---|---|
| drainage tubing while transferring to the new bottle/chamber and release the clamps. Have client cough and deep breathe. | |
| Document. | Document to explain delayed progress. |
| 9. Double-clamp drainage tubing, connect tubing to new drainage and water-seal bottles/chambers, and release the clamps. Have client cough and deep breathe. Document. | Prevents air from reentering the intrapleural space. Reestablishes the water-seal. Document to explain delayed progress. |

### Special Considerations

- Client with a hemothorax, who is also on anticoagulants, may need to have anticoagulant therapy reduced or discontinued until the hemothorax is resolved or controlled.
- Either chest tube clamps or shodded hemostats should be used to clamp chest tubes.
- When the chest tube must be clamped, cross clamp the chest tube close to the chest wall or the drainage tubing leading from the chest tube, whichever is appropriate.
- Three reasons for clamping chest tubes are: (1) to locate the source of an air leak, (2) to replace a drainage or water-seal bottle or commercial drainage system, and (3) to assess client tolerance to simulated tube removal. (These procedures are performed by physicians or experienced nurses.)
- Alternative to clamping for water-seal bottle replacement:
  1. Place distal end of the water-seal straw into a bottle of sterile water or saline so that the tip is 1 in below fluid surface.
  2. Tape water-seal straw to container in the proper position and stabilize the container.
  3. Prepare new bottle(s).
  4. Place water-seal straw in the new bottle.
- Make sure that the client is not lying on the drainage tubing and that it is not depressed or kinked.

### Teaching Considerations

Teach clients and families to:

- Inform the nurse of increased chest pain or difficult breathing.
- Never lift drainage system higher than the chest tube insertion site.
- Notify nurse immediately if a bottle breaks.
- Keep system upright at all times.
- Prevent pulling on the chest tube.
- Prevent accidental changes in the suction source setting.
- Notify the nurse immediately if there are changes in the way the system is functioning.

## *SKILL 17-2 Obtaining Specimen From Chest Tube Drainage System*

Specimens can be obtained from commercial drainage systems through a resealing diaphragm in the collection chamber or through the resealing drainage tubing.

### Purposes

1. Specimens are obtained from chest drainage systems for:
   a. Bacterial, viral, or fungal cultures.
   b. Cytology analysis.
   c. Assessment of cellular composition of the chest drainage.

## *Procedure 17-2*

| Steps | Rationale |
|---|---|
| **Assessment** | |
| 1. Determine that the water-seal system is patent and functioning properly. | Establishes baseline information regarding integrity of the system. |
| 2. Verify physician's order for specific specimen to be obtained. | Prevents obtaining inaccurate amount of drainage, placing the specimen in the wrong container, or sending the specimen to the wrong lab for analysis. |

| Steps | Rationale |
|---|---|
| **Nursing Diagnosis** | |
| 1. Cluster data to reveal actual or potential nursing diagnoses: | |
| a. Potential for infection, related to: | |
| ▪ Bacteria in the system.<br>▪ Break in sterile technique when obtaining a specimen or caring for equipment. | Infection can result from bacteria in the client's system or bacteria introduced by medical personnel while delivering care. |
| b. Fear related to: possible cytology report of cancer. | Cytology specimens are obtained to examine cell types for cancer. |
| **Planning** | |
| 1. Establish individualized goals for client based on nursing diagnoses: | |
| a. Absence of bacteria in the chest drainage system. | Asepsis reduces risk of contaminating system. |
| b. No increase in respiratory distress. | Chest drainage system functions properly. |
| 2. Explain procedure to client. | Reduces client anxiety and increases compliance. |
| 3. Obtain the following equipment: | |
| a. 10-20 ml syringe | Size of syringe varies with amount and type of specimen ordered. |
| b. 20-gauge needle | This gauge allows for aspiration of fluid or blood from the collection chamber or drainage tubing without damaging the resealing diaphragm or cells. |
| c. Specimen container | Containers vary according to the type of study ordered. |
| d. Addressograph label and requisition | Agencies require proper client labeling of all specimen containers and requisitions. |
| e. Antiseptic swab | To clean resealing diaphragm or tubing to reduce entry of microorganisms into the system. |
| f. Nonsterile gloves | Reduces risk of transmission of microorganisms. |
| **Implementation** | |
| 1. Wash hands. | Reduces transmission of microorganisms. |
| 2. Don gloves. | Reduces transmission of blood-borne organisms to the nurse. |
| 3. Attach needle to syringe. | |
| 4. Cleanse diaphragm or tubing with antiseptic swab. | Reduces entry of microorganisms into the chest drainage system. |
| 5. Insert needle into diaphragm or tubing so that bevel is in the drainage.<br>▪ Diaphragm aspirations obtain older specimens.<br>▪ Drainage tubing aspirations obtain fresh specimens. | Allows aspiration of chest drainage for specimen collection. |
| 6. Gently aspirate appropriate amount of fluid from the collection chamber or tubing and place into the appropriate specimen containers. | Some physicians may order multiple specimens, thus necessitating multiple specimen containers. |
| 7. Cleanse diaphragm with antiseptic swab. | Reduces blood-borne microorganisms on surface of the diaphragm. |
| 8. Dispose of needle and syringe in a protected container. | Current CDC guidelines recommend syringe and needle disposal into a protected container without recapping the needle. |
| 9. Label specimens and attach requisitions. | Provides client and test identification to specimen(s). |
| 10. Remove gloves and wash hands. | Reduces transmission of microorganisms. |
| 11. Arrange for delivery of specimen(s) to lab. | |
| **Evaluation** | |
| 1. Observe client and system for changes in status indicating an air leak. | If resealing diaphragm or tubing is ineffective, the client will have an increased respiratory rate and the water-seal will have constant bubbling. |
| 2. Observe client for symptoms of infection. | Any break in the system, such as obtaining a specimen for culture or cytology, increases risk for infection. |
| ***Expected outcomes*** | |
| 1. Drainage system remains patent. | Diaphragm or tubing resealed. |
| 2. Client is without signs of infection. | Aseptic technique and resealing diaphragm or tubing. |
| ***Unexpected outcomes*** | |
| 1. Air leak. | Diaphragm or tubing did not reseal. |

| Steps | Rationale |
|---|---|
| 2. Infection occurs. | Diaphragm or tubing did not reseal or improper technique was used. |

### Recording and Reporting

| | |
|---|---|
| 1. Record type and amount of specimen collected. | Documents what specimen was obtained and how much was collected. |
| 2. Record where specimen was sent. | Documents when and where specimen was sent. |

### Follow-Up Activities

| | |
|---|---|
| 1. Locate and correct air leak. | See Table 17-2. |
| 2. Notify physician of signs of infection. | Infections in the pleural cavity are serious and costly. They require immediate treatment. |

### Special Considerations

- Check resealing diaphragm for drainage, which could increase the risk of transfer of microorganisms.

## *SKILL 17-3 Removing Chest Tubes*

Actual removal of a chest tube is the function of physicians or nurses having advanced, specialized education. If nurses are to remove a chest tube, this procedure should be a written component of the agency's policy and procedures standards.

The nurse (1) prepares the client for chest tube removal by assessing the need for preremoval analgesia and obtaining the required medication orders and (2) instructs the client about the process and what will be requested of the client. During removal of the chest tube, it is important that the client takes a deep breath and holds it until the physician has removed the tube. This maneuver prevents air from being sucked into the chest as the tube is pulled out and before an occlusive dressing is applied.

This skill details for the nurse the actual nursing responsibilities and physician action for chest tube removal.

## *Procedure 17-3*

| Steps | Rationale |
|---|---|
| **Assessment** | |
| 1. Lung reexpansion is complete when: | |
| a. Chest x-ray reveals total lung reexpansion. | |
| b. Water-seal fluctuation has stopped for 24 hr. | Pleura of the expanded lung will seal holes on the internal tip of the chest tube, halting fluctuation in the water-seal. This can be expected 2-3 days after chest tube insertion. |
| c. Drainage is decreased to less than 50cc/day. | Drainage has been removed, allowing the lung to reexpand. |
| d. Percussion reveals tympany. | Normal percussion with reexpansion. |
| e. Auscultation reveals breath sounds are present throughout the chest cavity. | Normal breath sounds are heard with reexpansion. |
| 2. Clamp chest tube 12-24 hr before removal, or as ordered by the physician. | Physician orders tube clamping before removal to assess client's tolerance. |
| **Nursing Diagnosis** | |
| 1. Cluster data to reveal actual or potential nursing diagnoses: | |
| a. Potential for impaired gas exchange: related to reaccumulation of air or fluid in the intrapleural space. | Occasionally, a client experiences symptoms indicating a need to reinsert a chest tube. |

| Steps | Rationale |
|---|---|
| **Planning** | |
| 1. Develop individualized goals for client based on nursing diagnoses: | |
| a. Expansion of the lung is maintained. | Tubes are removed when lung has reexpanded and/or fluid has drained properly. |
| b. Client remains free of symptoms. | |
| c. Wound healing occurs. | |
| 2. Explain procedure to client. | Promotes cooperation and reduces anxiety. |
| 3. Assemble equipment. Check policy and procedure manual for list of supplies and equipment. | Facilitates removal of the chest tube. |
| **Implementation** | |
| 1. Administer prescribed medication for pain relief about 30 min before procedure. | Reduces discomfort and relaxes client. |
| 2. Assist client to sit on edge of bed or to lie on the side without chest tubes. | Physician prescribes client's position to facilitate tube removal. |
| 3. Support client physically and emotionally while physician removes dressing and clips sutures. | Reduces anxiety and promotes cooperation. |
| 4. Physician prepares an occlusive dressing of petroleum gauze on a pressure dressing and sets it aside on a sterile field. | Essential to prepare in advance for quick application to the wound upon tube withdrawal. |
| 5. Physician asks the client to take a deep breath and hold it or exhale completely and hold it. | Prevents air from being sucked into the chest as the tube is removed. |
| 6. Physician quickly pulls out the chest tube. | Prevents entry of air through the chest wound. |
| 7. Physician quickly applies prepared dressing over the wound and firmly secures it in position with elastoplast or wide tape. Physician sometimes uses skin clips or draws purse string sutures together before applying dressing. | Keeps wound aseptic. Prevents entry of air into the chest. Wound closure occurs spontaneously. Aids in skin closure. |
| 8. Assist client to a comfortable position. | Reassures client is comfortable. |
| 9. Remove used equipment from bedside. | Prevents spread of microorganisms. |
| 10. Wash hands. | Reduces transmission of microorganisms. |
| **Evaluation** | |
| 1. Observe client for subcutaneous emphysema or respiratory distress during the first few hours after removal. | Provides early notification of physician of adverse symptoms. Chest tubes may need reinsertion. |
| 2. Assess client's vital signs and psychologic status. | Detects early signs and symptoms of complications. Ascertains client's tolerance of procedure. |
| 3. Check chest dressing for drainage and patency. | Assures occlusion of chest wound. |
| ***Expected outcomes*** | |
| 1. Lung re-expansion occurs within 3 days. | Normal reexpansion time period. |
| 2. Client experiences no discomfort. | |
| 3. Spontaneous healing of chest tube insertion site after removal of tube without infection or other complications. | Large nonporous dressing seals puncture site. |
| ***Unexpected outcomes*** | |
| 1. Client reexperiences dyspnea, chest pain, labored respirations. | Recurrence of pneumothorax or hemothorax. |
| **Recording and Reporting** | |
| 1. Record removal of tube, the amount of drainage in the collection bottle, appearance of wound and of dressing, and client's response. Clients response should also include vital signs and respiratory assessment. | Documents procedure and status of wound and dressing. Documents client's response. |
| **Follow-Up Activities** | |
| 1. Notify physician immediately. | This is an emergency situation. |
| 2. Prepare for chest tube insertion. | Another chest tube will need to be inserted. Removes air from the intrapleural space. |

## Special Considerations

- When viewing chest x-ray immediately after tube removal, the chest tube tract may still be visible.
- Clients may still have a small pneumothorax, which will spontaneously absorb.

## Teaching Considerations

- Clients with histories of chronic obstructive pulmonary disease (COPD) should be encouraged to cough to clear their airways.

---

**BIBLIOGRAPHY**

Carroll PF: The ins and outs of chest drainage systems, Nurs '86 16(12):26, 1986.

Connor PA: When and how do you use a Heimlich flutter valve? Am J Nur 87:288, 1987.

Duncan C, Erickson R: Pressures associated with chest tube stripping, Heart-Lung 11(2):166, 1982.

Duncan C, Erickson R, Weigel RM: Effect of chest tube management on drainage after cardiac surgery, Heart-Lung 16(1):1, 1987.

Erickson R: Chest tubes: they're really not that complicated, Nurs '81 11(5):34, 1981a.

Erickson R: Solving chest tube problems, Nurs '81 11(6):62, 1981b.

Farley J: About chest tubes, Nurs '88 18(6):16, 1988.

Jackson EW: Providing respiratory care, Horsham, Pa, 1980, Intermed Communications, Inc.

Johanson BC, Wells SJ, Dungca CU, et al.: Standards for critical care, ed 3, St. Louis, CV Mosby Co, 1988.

Krauss PJ: Chest tube stripping: is it necessary? Focus on Critical Care, 12(6):41, 1985.

Luckmann J, Sorensen KC: Medical-surgical nursing: a psychophysiologic approach, ed 3, Philadelphia, 1987, WB Saunders Company.

Palau D, Jones S: Test your skill at trouble-shooting chest tubes, RN Oct:43, 1986.

Quinn A: Thora-Drain III: closed chest drainage made simpler and safer, Nurs '86, 16(9):46, 1986.

Shoemaker WC, Ayers S, Grenvik A, et al.: Textbook of critical care medicine, ed 2, Philadelphia, 1989, WB Saunders Company.

# 18

# EMERGENCY MEASURES FOR LIFE SUPPORT

### OBJECTIVES

*Mastery of content in this chapter will enable the nurse to:*

- Define key terms.
- Describe the population at risk for foreign body airway obstruction.
- State signs and symptoms associated with foreign body airway obstruction.
- Discuss indications for a nasal airway.
- Discuss indications for an oral airway.
- Discuss indications for an AMBU bag.
- State indications for cardiopulmonary resuscitation (CPR).
- State the goals for CPR.
- Demonstrate in a laboratory or clinical situation: removal of foreign body airway obstruction, insertion of a nasal and an oral airway, use of an AMBU manual ventilator, CPR.

### KEY TERMS

*Airway obstruction*
*AMBU*
*Cardiopulmonary arrest*
*Cardiopulmonary resuscitation*
*Foreign body airway maneuver*
*Nasal airway*
*Oral airway*
*Perfusion*
*Respiratory arrest*
*Ventilation*

### SKILLS

**18-1** Removing Foreign Body Airway Obstruction
**18-2** Inserting a Nasal Airway
**18-3** Inserting an Oral Airway
**18-4** Using an AMBU Manual Ventilator
**18-5** Performing Cardiopulmonary Resuscitation (CPR)

The oxygen transport system consists of the lungs and cardiovascular system. Adequacy of oxygen delivery depends on the amount of oxygen entering the lungs (ventilation), the blood flow to the lungs and to the tissues (perfusion), the adequacy of diffusion, and the capacity of the blood to carry oxygen. The blood's capacity to carry oxygen is influenced by the amount of dissolved oxygen in the plasma, the amount of hemoglobin, and the affinity of hemoglobin for oxygen.

Respiratory gases are exchanged in the alveoli and in the tissues. Oxygen is transferred from the lungs to the blood, and carbon dioxide is transferred from the blood to the lungs to be exhaled as a waste product. At the tissue level, oxygen is transferred from the blood to the tissues, and carbon dioxide is transferred from the tissues to the blood to return to the lungs and be exhaled. This transfer depends on the process of diffusion.

Only a relatively small amount of the required oxygen in the blood, approximately 3%, is dissolved in the plasma. Most of it is transported by hemoglobin. The hemoglobin molecule is the carrier for both oxygen and carbon dioxide; it combines with oxygen to form oxyhemoglobin.

Whenever the concentration of inspired oxygen declines, the oxygen-carrying capacity of the blood is decreased. Decreases in inspired oxygen concentration ($Fio_2$) can be caused by an upper or lower airway obstruction, decreased environmental oxygen (as occurs at high altitudes), or absence of respiration, as in respiratory or cardiopulmonary arrest.

An airway obstruction is a barrier that limits the amount of inspired oxygen delivered to the alveoli. As a result the amount of oxygen available for diffusion into the blood is decreased.

High altitudes lower the inspiratory oxygen concentration because the atmospheric oxygen is at a lower concentration. People who live at high altitudes adapt to the lowered atmospheric oxygen by increasing hemoglobin production.

A respiratory or cardiopulmonary arrest is an emergency situation that the nurse must be prepared to handle at any time. Clients at risk for either type of arrest include those with airway obstruction, cardiopulmonary illnesses, severe fluid and electrolyte disturbances, and excessive ingestion of chemical substances.

Cardiopulmonary resuscitation is intended for those clients who are not expected to die. It should not be used in clients in the terminal stages of illness (Guzzetta and Dossey, 1984).

Although the primary indication for initiating the skills in this chapter is an emergent situation, such as the presence of a foreign body or an arrest, the following guidelines can help the student identify clients at risk.

## GUIDELINES

1. Determine safety of an infants' or a toddlers' environment. These two age groups are at risk for foreign body aspiration of objects from their environment. A child frequently puts coins, buttons, or small objects from the floor or table top in his mouth. Also, table foods that are not cut into appropriate size can become lodged in the child's airway.
2. Counsel clients not to talk or laugh with food in their mouths. The inspiratory effort to initiate a cough or laugh can cause aspiration of food and thus airway obstruction.
3. Know the client's vital signs, noting any irregularities in cardiac rhythm. An irregular heartbeat in a client with cardiovascular disease can precipitate a cardiopulmonary arrest. Such cardiovascular conditions include coronary artery disease, myocardial infarctions, and open heart surgeries.
4. Obtain the most recent serum electrolyte values. Electrolyte imbalances (such as those involving potassium and calcium) can precipitate cardiopulmonary arrest.
5. When an overdose of a chemical substance is present, know the type and amount of the substance ingested. Certain chemicals such as alcohol, tranquilizers, and depressants depress the respiratory center and can result in a respiratory arrest. Some drug overdoses, such as heroin, can cause ventricular dysrhythmias and cardiopulmonary arrest.

## PREREQUISITE KNOWLEDGE

1. Principles of gas exchange.
2. Principles of circulation.
3. Normal cardiopulmonary anatomy.
4. Gross anatomy of head, neck, and abdomen.
5. Functions of the upper airway.
6. Principles of medical asepsis.
7. Indications for an artificial airway.

## PREREQUISITE SKILLS

1. Physical assessment (Chapter 13).
2. Obtaining vital signs (Chapter 12).
3. Oropharyngeal and tracheal suctioning (Chapter 16).
4. Proper handwashing technique (Chapter 37).
5. Endotracheal and tracheal tube suctioning (Chapter 16).

# *SKILL 18-1 Removing Foreign Body Airway Obstruction*

Airways obstructed by a foreign body can threaten life. In adults partially chewed food, especially meats and raw vegetables, and in children small toys or game pieces are the types of foreign bodies that most often result in partial or complete airway obstruction. Failure to remove a foreign body impairs gas exchange and can result in unconsciousness and cardiopulmonary arrest. Should cardiopulmonary arrest occur, the obstruction should be immediately removed and cardiopulmonary resuscitation initiated.

Prevention of foreign body aspiration is very important. In the alert adult and child aspiration of a foreign body can frequently be prevented by (1) chewing small pieces of food slowly and thoroughly, (2) avoiding excessive alcohol intake at mealtime, (3) choosing age-appropriate toys and restricting their use accordingly, (4) keeping children from placing small toys or game pieces in their mouths, and (5) avoiding excessive laughing and talking during chewing and swallowing.

In the unconscious client the tongue and other soft palate structures, as well as dentures and other nonpermanent dental work, can become dislodged and obstruct the airway. In addition, it is not uncommon for an unconscious client with diminished or absent cough and gag reflexes to vomit and then aspirate stomach contents.

In the unconscious client aspiration of a foreign body can frequently be prevented by (1) removing all nonpermanent dental work, (2) inserting an oral airway (Skill 18-3) to maintain tongue position, (3) insertion of a nasogastric tube (Chapter 27) to drain stomach contents, (4) placing the client in a side-lying position to prevent aspiration, and (5) when appropriate, insertion of an endotracheal tube by a physician to maintain a patent airway and prevent aspiration.

The key to successful management of a foreign body obstruction is (1) early recognition that an obstructed airway exists and (2) recognition of the extent to which the airway is obstructed. If the client is able to breathe in and out without difficulty and cough forcefully, no immediate intervention is necessary. If, however, the client who has difficulty breathing in and out or is not breathing, is cyanotic or is unable to speak, cough, or cough forcefully needs immediate assistance. *The universal distress signal for complete airway obstruction is clutching of the neck.*

There are two well-known procedures for removal of an airway obstruction caused by a foreign body: the Heimlich Maneuver and the Foreign Body Obstructed Airway Maneuver (FBOAM) recommended by the American Heart Association. The use of the Heimlich maneuver requires quick abdominal thrusts delivered in the region just below the rib cage and above the navel. This maneuver is beneficial to the choking victim; however, when performed by an inexperienced person, abdominal organ injury can result. The skill presented here is the American Heart Association Procedure, which does not have the associated risk of internal injuries.

### Purpose

1. Remove the foreign body from the airway to reestablish a normal breathing pattern and to prevent cardiopulmonary arrest (Skill 18-5).

## Procedure 18-1

| Steps | Rationale |
|---|---|
| **Assessment** | |
| 1. Identify signs and symptoms of foreign body airway obstruction needing immediate intervention: | Physical signs and symptoms may indicate need to perform FBOAM. |
| a. Cardiac: irregular pulse, rapid or slow pulse, cyanosis, absent pulse. | |
| b. Respiratory: irregular breathing pattern, rapid or slow, shallow breathing, apneic breathing periods, high-pitched inspiratory noises (crowing type), wheezing, inability to cough forcefully, inability to cough at all, inability to speak. | |
| c. Oral: vomitus in mouth or on face, partially chewed food in mouth, freely-floating dentures in mouth, tongue in posterior oropharynx. | |
| d. Signs and symptoms of foreign body airway obstruction *not needing immediate* intervention include ability to speak, to cough forcefully, to breath in and out, stable vital signs, alertness, wheezing between coughs. | |
| 2. Assess for factors that may influence use of FBOAM. | Allows nurse to assess for variations in FBOAM. |
| 3. Assess client's and family's understanding of FBOAMs and anticipated outcomes. Must be done quickly and in some situations the nurse omits this step. | Allows nurse to identify potential for teaching and crisis intervention. |
| **Nursing Diagnosis** | |
| 1. Cluster data to reveal actual or potential nursing diagnoses: | |
| a. Impaired gas exchange: related to airway obstruction. | Ventilation and oxygenation are impaired when air flow is limited or absent. |
| b. Ineffective individual coping: related to life crisis. | Client and relatives experience significant life stress because of obstructing event, intervention, or outcome (real or potential) of event. |
| c. Knowledge deficit regarding performance of FBOAM: related to inexperience, anxiety. | Potential for learning new skill is present, especially for families of clients at high risk. |
| **Planning** | |
| 1. Develop individualized goals for client based on nursing diagnoses: | |
| a. Maintain stable vital signs. | Comparison of vital signs directs nurse to intervene. |
| b. Promote patent airway. | Return of patent airway improves oxygen delivery to the tissues. |
| 2. Prepare needed equipment. | |
| a. In hospital setting: ▪ Emergency cart ▪ Suction equipment | |
| 3. If possible, explain FBOAMs to client, and emphasize importance of relaxation during maneuvers. | Clients are very anxious. Tense chest, arms, and abdomen muscles can limit effectiveness of maneuvers. |

| Steps | Rationale |
|---|---|

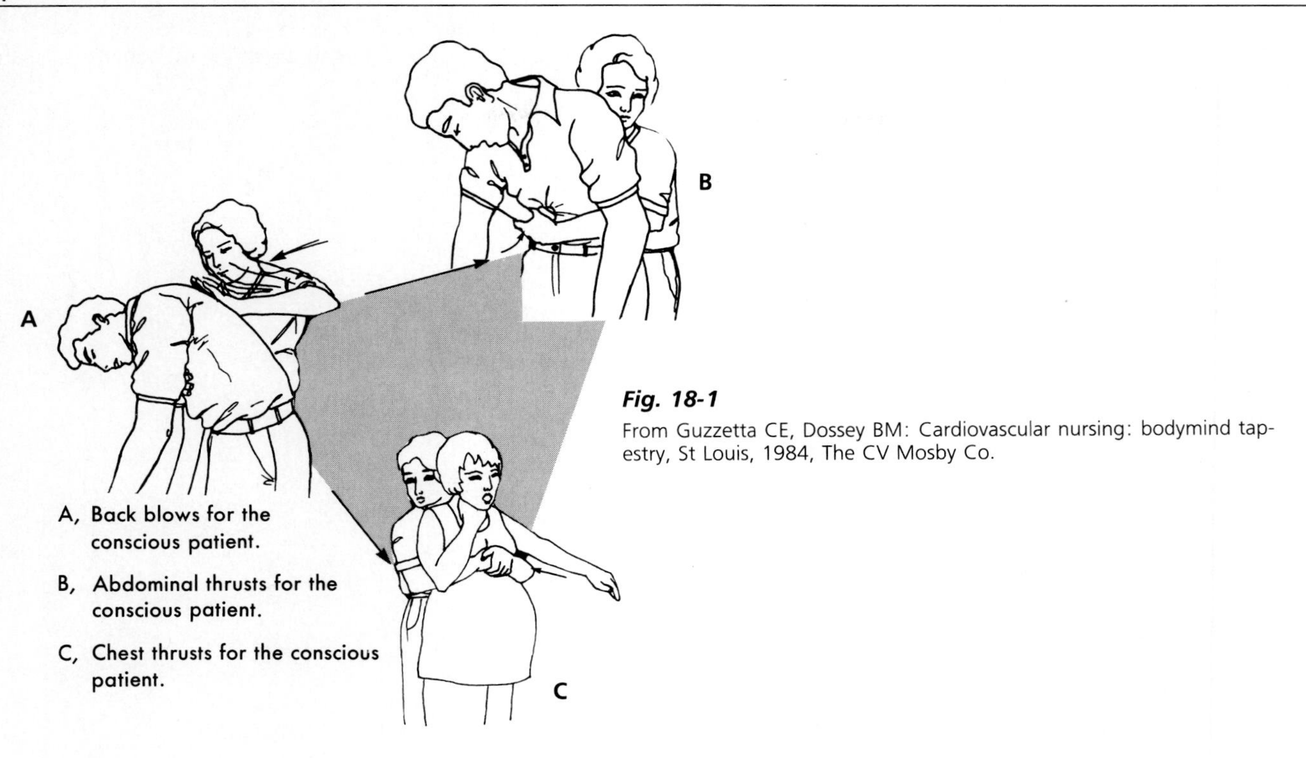


***Fig. 18-1***
From Guzzetta CE, Dossey BM: Cardiovascular nursing: bodymind tapestry, St Louis, 1984, The CV Mosby Co.

| Steps | Rationale |
|---|---|
| 4. Help client take position that allows nurse to perform maneuvers easily. Unconscious clients should be placed on floor. Alert clients may be seated in chair or allowed to stand. | Protects client and nurse from injury. |
| 5. Remove dentures or other nonpermanent dental work. | Prevents further airway obstruction from broken dentures or nonpermanent dental work. |

## Implementation

| Steps | Rationale |
|---|---|
| 1. Administer back blows (Fig. 18-1, *A*): | Dislodges foreign body from airway. (More effective in infant and child than adult). |
| a. Sit or stand at side and slightly behind victim. | Allows nurse access to client's back. |
| b. Place one hand firmly on client's chest. | Provides client support. |
| c. Deliver four sharp blows between client's shoulder blades, over spine, with heel of hand. | Dislodges foreign body. |
| 2. Administer abdominal thrusts (Fig. 18-1, *B*): | |
| a. Sit or stand behind client, and support client's back against your body and wrap your arms around client. | Allows nurse access to client's abdomen and provides support. |
| b. If client is in a supine position, kneel with knees next to client's hips *or* kneel over client's trunk by straddling one or both thighs and hyperextend client's neck to open the mouth. In clients with cervical spine injury, pull tongue up and out of mouth and lower jaw slightly without moving neck. | Allows nurse access to client's abdomen and opens airway. |
| c. Make fist and, covering fist with other hand, place thumb side of fisted hand against client's abdomen in midline between waist and xiphoid process on the sternum. | Provides correct position and coverage to administer manual thrusts. Hand covering fist guides thrusts and determines their impact. |
| d. Using quick inward and upward thrusts, press your fist into client's abdomen four times. | Dislodges foreign body. |
| 3. Administer chest thrusts (Fig. 18-1, *C*). | Chest thrusts are used with pregnant clients. |
| a. Standing directly behind bring your arms around under client's arms, or kneel and roll client on back if necessary. Open the mouth and hyperextend the neck, *or* in clients with cervical spine injury, pull tongue up and out of mouth and lower jaw slightly without moving neck. | Provides access to client's chest and opens airway. |

| Steps | Rationale |
|---|---|
| b. Allow client's body to rest against your body. | Provides support. |
| c. Make fist with one hand and cover it with other hand. Place thumb side of fisted hand against client's chest on sternum 1-2 cm above xiphoid process. *Or* if client is supine, with your shoulders directly over the chest, place heel of one hand 1-2 cm above the xiphoid process on sternum on midline. Place heel of other hand directly on top of first hand and interlock fingers. | Provides correct position and leverage to administer manual thrusts. |
| d. Using four quick inward thrusts or compressions, press covered fists into client's chest. | Dislodges foreign body. |
| 4. Administer finger sweep: | |
| a. Open client's mouth, grasping tongue and lower jaw with thumb and index finger and lift up, *or* in clients with a cervical spine injury pull tongue up and out of mouth and lower jaw slightly but do not move neck. If unable to open client's mouth easily, place thumb and index finger of one hand on upper and lower gumline and push teeth apart. | Opens client's airway. |
| b. Insert index finger of other hand along cheek to posterior pharynx and using a sweeping or hooking motion, dislodge foreign body and pull it up into and out of mouth. Be careful not to force foreign body deeper into client's airway. Thumb can be used to aid in removal of foreign body once located. In addition, it is often helpful to push foreign body against side of pharynx to help maneuver it up and out. | Removes foreign body. |
| 5. Take pulse and respiration measurements. | Determines cardiopulmonary status. |
| 6. Wash hands. | Reduces transmission of microorganisms. |

## Evaluation

| | |
|---|---|
| 1. Compare client's respiratory status before and after FBOAMs, if possible. | Provides information concerning changes in client's vital signs. |

### *Expected outcomes*

| | |
|---|---|
| 1. Foreign body is dislodged and removed. | Airway cleared of obstruction. |
| 2. Nurse is able to identify clients and families needing instruction in FBOAM. | Families need to know how to perform FBOAMs. |

### *Unexpected outcomes*

| | |
|---|---|
| 1. Foreign body is not dislodged or is partially dislodged but not removed: | |
| a. Call for immediate medical or surgical assistance. | Needed care beyond scope of nursing practice. |
| b. Repeat one or all maneuvers and stay with client. | Help is coming. Second attempt may be successful. |
| c. Monitor pulse and respiratory status. Begin CPR if client arrests (Skill 18-5). | Maintains cardiopulmonary function. |

## Recording and Reporting

| | |
|---|---|
| 1. Record nursing progress notes, including: | |
| a. Precipitating event, if known. | Alerts nurses to problem area (e.g., types of foods or toys that must be monitored closely). |
| b. Vital signs, if taken, and other assessments (color, ability to speak, breathe, talk) before and after FBOAMs. | Determines level of cardiopulmonary function. |
| c. Maneuver(s) performed. | Documents care given. |
| d. Result of maneuver(s) performed. | Documents effect of care given. |
| e. Any additional assistance requested or received and scope of assistance. | Documents additional care given and by whom (e.g., physician, tracheostomy). |

## Follow-up Activities

| | |
|---|---|
| 1. Take pulse and respirations. | Determines cardiopulmonary status. |
| 2. Reassess client and family and remain with client. | Reduces anxiety related to near-death experience. |

| Steps | Rationale |
|---|---|
| 3. After implementation of maneuvers, if foreign body is removed: | |
| a. Instruct client and family how to avoid obstruction by removing or avoiding offending agent. | Obstruction can possibly be prevented. |
| b. Instruct client and family in maneuvers should obstruction occur again. | Obstruction can be relieved before hospitalization. |
| 4. *After* implementation of maneuver if foreign body is *not* removed: | |
| a. State that you need additional help but that you will stay with client. | Patient will be reassured to know additional help is coming. |

## Special Considerations

- Clients at greater risk of foreign body aspiration include following conditions: neuromuscular diseases such as myasthenia gravis and amyotrophic lateral sclerosis; cerebral vascular accident (stroke) with hemiparesis; cleft palate; lesions of head, neck, esophagus, upper airway; seizure disorders; unconsciousness; heavy sedative or narcotic use; diminished or absent cough and gag reflexes.
  Not every child who gags or coughs while eating is truly choking. Child in distress cannot speak, becomes cyanotic, and collapses (Whaley and Wong, 1987).
- Factors that influence performance of FBOAM include: 1. Consciousness: in unconscious client, "lying" positions must be used for back blows and manual thrusts. In conscious client, nurse may experience difficulty in opening client's mouth and sweeping out contents. 2. Age: in all children and infants (and occasionally adults) be careful when using finger sweep *not* to force foreign body deeper into throat. 3. Abdominal girth: if nurse is unable to wrap arms around client's abdomen or if use of abdominal thrust can cause additional problems, use of chest thrust is better. 4. Client's in whom chest thrust should be used in place of abdominal thrust include infants, clients with gross obesity or liver failure with ascites, and pregnant women).
- Nurse should not strain muscles to reach client and perform maneuvers. Positioning for child depends on its age. Infant is placed over rescuer's arm with head lower than trunk (Fig. 18-2). Children too large to straddle rescuer's forearm can be draped across rescuer's thighs with rescuer kneeling on the floor (Fig. 18-3) (Whaley and Wong, 1987).

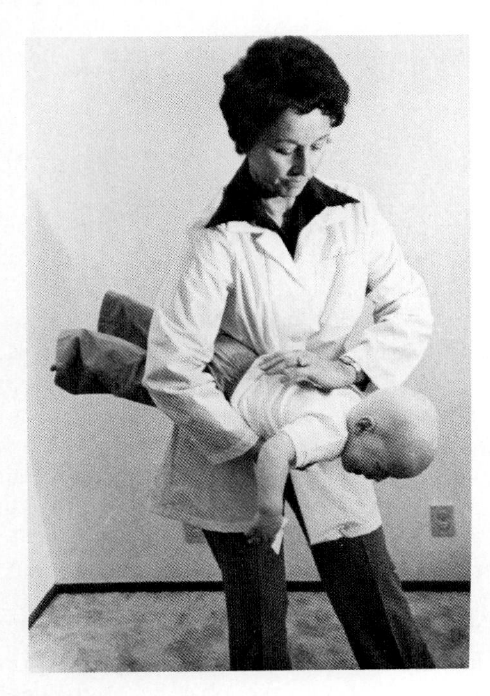

***Fig. 18-2***
From Whaley LF, Wong DL: Nursing care of infants and children, ed 3, St Louis, 1987, The CV Mosby Co.

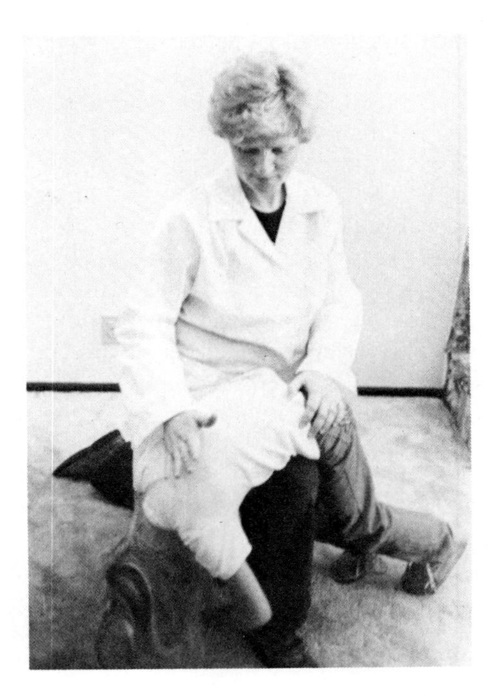

***Fig. 18-3***
From Whaley LF, Wong DL: Nursing care of infants and chidren, ed 3, St. Louis, 1987, The CV Mosby Co.

- If airway remains obstructed after performing FBOAM, nurse should be prepared with equipment for physician to perform intubation or tracheostomy. In event of cardipulmonary arrest, nurse must be prepared to initiate basic life support cardiopulmonary resuscitation (Skill 18-5).
- Combination of three maneuvers to remove a foreign body airway obstruction is more effective than each single maneuver. The back blows and manual thrusts maneuvers work by increasing intrathoracic pressure, forcing the patient to "cough" and expel foreign body.
- Each maneuver should be delivered as if it were the only one needed to dislodge foreign body. Use caution in delivering back blows over spine of client with healing back (spinal) wound or osteoporosis.
- While performing chest thrusts: if hands are too low, xiphoid process can be fractured. If hands are too high, intrathoracic pressure will not be sufficiently increased to expel foreign body. If client is supine, this is same position used when performing CPR. Placing hands over xiphoid process or over ribs can cause fractures and internal injuries.

### Teaching Considerations

- Instruct client and family how to avoid obstruction by removing, modifying, or avoiding offending agent; instruct client and family in maneuvers should obstruction occur again.
- Ask client and family to state signs and symptoms of foreign body obstruction.
- Have client and family perform techniques on doll or dummy. Observe for correct technique.

## *SKILL 18-2 Inserting a Nasal Airway*

A nasal airway is a flexible curved piece of rubber or plastic with one wide or trumpetlike end and one narrow end that, once inserted, extends from the nares (remains external to the nose) past the sinuses to the pharynx (Fig. 18-4).

The nasal airway varies in length (measured in centimeters or inches) and diameter (measured in millimeters). Some companies indicate nasal airway size by number (e.g., 5, 6, 7, 8, 9, 10), others by grouping two or more numeric sizes into one nasal airway (e.g., small, medium, large). In general, a small nasal airway corresponds to a 5 or 6 mm diameter nasal airway; a medium nasal airway corresponds to a 7 or 8 mm diameter nasal airway; and a large nasal airway corresponds to a 9 or 10 mm diameter nasal airway.

The nurse chooses the size of a nasal airway based on the size (ideal body weight), nasal structure, sex, and age of the client. In a client weighing less than 100 pounds with a small bone structure, the nurse will generally use a small nasal airway. Clients weighing up to 150 pounds with small bone structures can usually accept a medium size nasal airway. In clients weighing greater than 150 pounds, the nurse can usually place a large nasal airway without difficulty. In addition, in male clients who have large nares, and no history of chronic sinus problems, the next larger size nasal airway can frequently be inserted without difficulty.

Use of a nasal airway can frequently help keep the nasal passage open. However, the effectiveness of an airway in accomplishing this task is related to the cause of nasal air passage closure. For example, placement of a nasal airway can tamponade a small bleeding blood vessel by exerting gentle pressure against the mucosal wall. On the other hand, edema of the nasal passage secondary to trauma can cause complete closure; however, the amount of patency maintained depends on the rigidity of the airway and the amount of the edema.

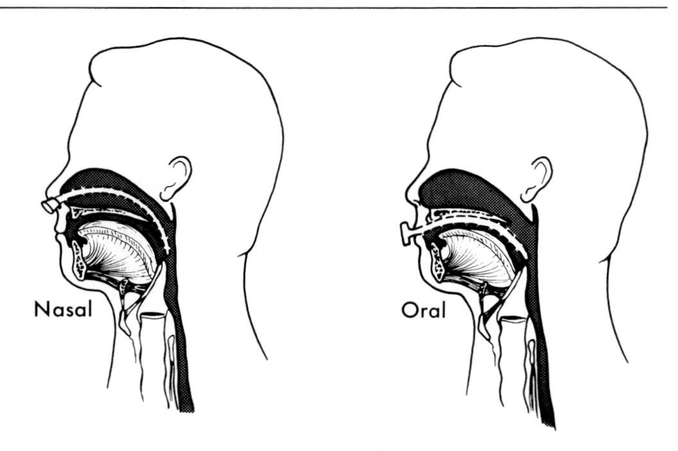

***Fig. 18-4*** Placement of nasal and oral airways.

In clients requiring nasal pharyngeal or nasal tracheal suctioning (Chapter 16), the nasal airway provides easy access to the pharynx. An added benefit of the nasal airway in clients who require frequent nasal pharyngeal or nasal tracheal suctioning is that nasal trauma is kept to a minimum. Clients who do not have a nasal airway inserted frequently experience edema and bleeding from irritation if secretions must be suctioned often. The nurse must evaluate each client for insertion of a nasal airway.

### Purposes

1. Aid in maintaining a patent nasal air passage.
2. Provide an access to the pharynx or trachea for suctioning.
3. Prevent nasal trauma from repeated suctioning.

## Procedure 18-2

| Steps | Rationale |
|---|---|
| **Assessment** | |
| 1. Identify signs and symptoms of need to insert a nasal airway: frequent nasal pharyngeal or nasal tracheal suctioning, edematous nasal mucosa, bleeding of nasal mucosa secondary to irritation from suctioning. | Certain conditions require a nasal airway to be in place. |
| 2. Determine size of nasal airway to use:<br>Weight: <100 lb — 5, 6, or small<br><150 lb — 7, 8, or medium<br>>150 lb — 9, 10, or large<br>Sex: Males may use next larger size. | Proper size ensures a patent airway and minimizes trauma to client. |
| **Nursing Diagnosis** | |
| 1. Cluster data to reveal actual or potential nursing diagnoses: | |
| a. Impaired gas exchange: related to nasal obstruction. | Nasal obstruction prevents normal functioning of upper airway. |
| b. Potential for infection: related to retained secretions. | Inability to remove secretions because of nasal obstructions predisposes client to infection. Insertion of nasal airway prevents normal sinus drainage; secretions not removed provide media for organism growth. |
| c. Impaired skin integrity: related to frequent nasal pharyngeal or nasal tracheal suctioning. | Repeated irritation of nasal mucosa by suctioning may cause edema, bleeding of nasal mucosa, and loss of ciliary function. |
| **Planning** | |
| 1. Develop individualized goals for client based on nursing diagnoses:<br>a. Improve oxygenation.<br>b. Promote patent airway.<br>c. Facilitate removal of secretions. | Patent airway improves oxygenation and eases removal of airway secretions. |
| 2. Prepare needed equipment:<br>a. Appropriate size nasal airway<br>b. Nonsterile gloves<br>c. Water-soluble lubricant<br>d. Soft tissues<br>e. Tape<br>f. Appropriate suction equipment, if needed. | Necessary equipment at bedside promotes safe, quick completion of procedure. |
| 3. Prepare client for procedure: | |
| a. Explain reason(s) for insertion of airway and client's participation. | Relieves anxiety and encourages cooperation. |
| b. Help client assume comfortable position, usually semi-Fowlers. | Promotes client comfort and prevents nurse straining. |
| **Implementation** | |
| 1. Wash hands, put on gloves. | Reduces transmission of microorganisms. |
| 2. Prepare nasal airway. Use principles of medical asepsis: | |
| a. Remove nasal airway from package, check for smooth edges. | Prevents insertion of traumatic product. |
| b. Open lubricant package, squeeze about 1 tablespoon on nasal airway package or soft tissue. | Provides large surface area of lubricant with which to coat nasal airway. |
| c. Lubricate entire nasal airway making sure narrow end is generously coated with lubricant. | Provides "slick" surface for insertion and prevents friction against dry mucus membranes, which causes trauma. |
| 3. Clean excess secretions from client's nares with tissues. If necessary, suction secretions (Chapter 16). | Provides largest possible diameter airway for ease of insertion. |
| 4. Holding nasal airway by wide end, insert it into naris using gentle inward and downward pressure. | Prevents trauma by following natural course of nasal structures. |
| 5. Clean excess lubricant from client's face and nares. | Excess lubricant will dry and act as obstruction if not removed. |
| 6. Secure airway if necessary (see Chapter 16 for taping endotracheal tube [ET]). | Prevents accidental removal and deeper penetration into nasal and pharyngeal structures. |
| 7. Place client in comfortable position. | Promotes client comfort. |

| Steps | Rationale |
|---|---|
| 8. Remove gloves and discard in appropriate receptacle. Wash hands. | Reduces transmission of microorganisms. |
| 9. At least daily, remove nasal airway, clean in warm soapy water, and reinsert. Hydrogen peroxide can be used to remove encrustations. Small brush is helpful to clean inner core of nasal airway. | Removes accumulated secretions and microorganisms. |

## Evaluation

| | |
|---|---|
| 1. Assess client's respiratory status and observe color and quantity of secretions. | Identifies client's response to insertion of nasal airway and/or removal of airway secretions. |

### *Expected outcomes*

| | |
|---|---|
| 1. Suctioning-induced nasal edema and bleeding diminishes immediately and ultimately stops. | Limited irritation results from insertion of nasal airway. |
| 2. Nasal air passage is patent. | Artificial airway maintains patency. |
| 3. Client is more cooperative to nasal pharyngeal or nasal tracheal suctioning. | Client will be more comfortable because of decreased pain in nares from repeated suctioning; promotes ability to breathe more easily. |
| 4. No pressure area on nares. | Prolonged use of nasal airway can result in pressure area around nares. |

### *Unexpected outcomes*

| | |
|---|---|
| 1. Nurse is unable to insert nasal airway. | Excessive edema or obstruction may be present. |
| a. Attempt to insert a smaller size airway. | Airway may be smaller than anticipated. |
| b. Notify physician. | Care exceeds scope of nursing practice. |
| 2. Client begins to have nasal bleeding. | Airway insertion can cause irritation or bleeding. |
| a. Apply pressure over nasal pressure points for at least 5-10 min. | Allows blood-clotting system to form clot. |
| b. If bleeding continues, notify physician and follow instructions. | Care exceeds scope of nursing practice. |
| c. Monitor vital signs. | Excessive bleeding predisposes client to develop shock. |
| 3. Client complains of severe pain in ear and has fever. | Otitis media can result from impaired sinus drainage secondary to nasal airway. |
| 4. Client complains of headache (over sinuses) with or without fever. | Sinusitis may be present. |

## Recording and Reporting

| | |
|---|---|
| 1. Record in nurses' progress notes: | |
| a. Assessment finding for nasal airway. | Documents degree and potential cause of obstruction. |
| b. Size of airway inserted. | Documents size for other care givers and for reimbursement. |
| c. Client's tolerance of procedure. | Documents expected and unexpected outcomes. |
| d. Secretions suctioned. | Documents nursing care and provides assessment parameters for future. |
| e. Method of securing (if done). | Documents nursing care. |

## Follow-up Activities

| | |
|---|---|
| 1. Report uncontrolled bleeding to physician. | Continual bleeding may occlude airway. |
| 2. Report presence of severe ear pain or headaches and monitor fever. | Presence of otitis media or sinusitis and associated fever can be alleviated promptly by antibiotics. |

## Special Considerations

- Clients with following conditions are at greater risk for complication when nasal airway is inserted: chronic sinus infections or drainage, nasal fractures, basilar skull fractures, spontaneous intranasal bleeding (unless ordered by a physician), deviated septum, postoperative reconstructive nasal and facial surgery.
- Excessive epistaxis is dangerous in clients with hemophilia, active leukemia, aplastic anemia.
- Petroleum-based lubricants (e.g., Vaseline) should not be used because of dangers of chemical aspiration pneumonia.

# *SKILL 18-3 Inserting an Oral Airway*

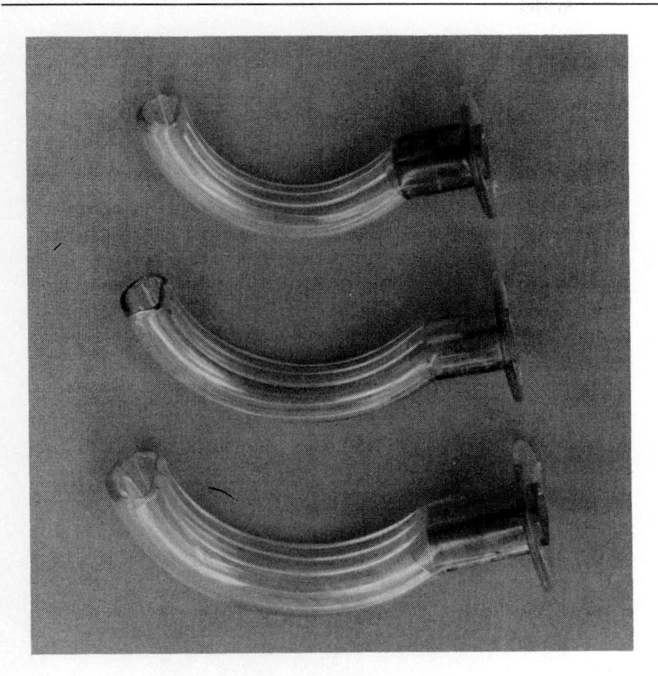

***Fig. 18-5*** Oral airways.

**TABLE 18-1** Oral Airways Guidelines for Size by Age

| Size | Age |
|---|---|
| 000 | Premature neonates |
| 00 | Newborn |
| 0 | Newborn to 1 yr |
| 1 | 1-2 yr |
| 2 | 2-6 yr |
| 3 | 6-18 yr |
| 4 and larger | ≥18 yr |

An oral airway is a minimally flexible curved piece of hard plastic (Fig. 18-5). When inserted, it extends from exterior to the lips over the tongue to the pharynx (see Fig. 18-4). Some oral airways enable the nurse to suction through a central core, whereas others facilitate resuscitation. The airways facilitating resuscitation do not have a central core for suctioning.

The oral airway is sized for adults and children. Its size varies by length and width. Pediatric sizes are 000, 00, 0, 1, 2, and 3. Adult sizes are 4 through 10 or small, medium, and large. The nurse chooses the size of an oral airway based on the width and length of the client's mouth and age. There are general size guidelines for choosing an oral airway (Table 18-1).

With clients who are not fully alert (for example, after anesthesia, multiple trauma, head injury, drug overdose, sepsis, shock), the nurse may insert an oral airway to prevent removal or damage to indwelling tubes. Clients can unknowingly bite an ET or oral gastric tube, severing the plastic. Loss of a supportive airway or a drainage tube can precipitate an emergency. Many of these clients can injure themselves by biting and lacerating their tongues or grinding their teeth. Aspiration of blood or tooth particles can cause airway damage or occlusion. In these two instances, the oral airway can function as a "biteblock."

Many oral airways have a separate central chamber that permits oral pharyngeal suctioning with a standard catheter. Insertion of an oral airway in clients who are unable to swallow or expectorate their own oral secretions enables the nurse to remove these secretions by suctioning and thus prevent occlusion of the lower airway by removing upper airway secretions.

## Purposes

1. Prevent client from biting tongue, grinding teeth, or biting ET or oral gastric tubes.
2. Facilitate airway secretions removal.
3. Promote client safety and maintain a patent airway before, during, and after a seizure.

## *Procedure 18-3*

| Steps | Rationale |
|---|---|
| **Assessment** | |
| 1. Identify need to insert an oral airway. Signs and symptoms include: upper airway "gurgling" with respiratory cycle, increased oral secretions or excretions, excessive drooling, grinding teeth, clenched teeth, biting of oral tracheal or gastric tubes, labored respirations, increased respiratory rate. | Certain conditions place clients at risk for obstruction of upper airway. |

| Steps | Rationale |
|---|---|
| 2. Determine factors that normally influence upper airway functioning, e.g., age (children have a proportionally larger tongue), presence of nasal and oral airway and drainage tubes (swallowing is more difficult with tubes in place). | Allows nurse to accurately assess need for an oral airway. |
| 3. Assess for presence of gag reflex. | Provides guide as to when oral airway can be safely removed in postoperative client. |

## Nursing Diagnosis

| Steps | Rationale |
|---|---|
| 1. Cluster data to reveal actual or potential nursing diagnoses: | |
| a. Ineffective airway clearance: related to decreased ability to clear oral secretions. | Secretions that accumulate above epiglottis can be aspirated into lungs on inspiration. |
| b. Potential for infection: related to retained secretions. | Retained secretions are ideal media for microorganism growth. |
| c. Potential for injury: related to decreased level of consciousness. | Partially alert clients can unintentionally harm themselves by biting mucous membranes, tongue, and indwelling tubes. |

## Planning

| Steps | Rationale |
|---|---|
| 1. Develop individualized goals for client based on nursing diagnoses: | |
| a. Maintain or promote patent airway. | Optimal airway allows for removal of secretions or prevents airway occlusion. |
| b. Facilitate removal of secretions. | |
| c. Prevent mucous membrane injury. | |
| 2. Prepare needed equipment: | Placing necessary equipment at client's bedside promotes safe, quick, procedure completion. |
| a. Choose appropriate oral airway size. Airway is sterile when first inserted in client; for successive insertions in same client, airway must be clean. Each client must have own oral airway. | |
| b. Nonsterile gloves | |
| c. Soft tissues or washcloth | |
| d. Suction equipment, if needed | |
| 3. Prepare client for procedure: | |
| a. Explain reason for oral airway insertion and technique for use. | Relieves anxiety and encourages cooperation. |
| b. Position client; semi-Fowler's position is preferred unless contraindicated. | Promotes nurse and client comfort. Provides easy access to oral cavity. |

## Implementation

| Steps | Rationale |
|---|---|
| 1. Wash hands and apply nonsterile gloves. | Reduces transmission of microorganisms. |
| 2. Ask client to open mouth *or* if unable, use thumb and fore finger of nondominant hand to pry jaws and teeth apart. | Provides access to oral cavity. |
| 3. Insert oral airway: | Provides patent airway and prevents displacement of client's tongue into posterior oropharynx. |
| a. Hold oral airway with curved end up, insert until end nurse is holding is parallel with client's nose (vertical), then turn airway over 180° and follow natural curve of tongue. | |
| 4. Secure with tape. | Prevents expulsion of airway. |
| 5. Suction secretions, if needed. | Removes secretions, maintains patent airway. |
| 6. Reassess client's respiratory status. | Directs nurse to initiate intervention. |
| 7. Clean client's face with soft tissue or washcloth. | Promotes hygiene. |
| 8. Discard soft tissue into appropriate receptacle, place washcloth in laundry, remove gloves and discard in appropriate receptacle, wash hands. | Reduces transmission of microorganisms. |

## Evaluation

| Steps | Rationale |
|---|---|
| 1. Compare client's respiratory assessments before and after insertion of oral airway. | Identifies client's response to insertion of airway. |

| Steps | Rationale |
|---|---|
| ***Expected outcomes*** | |
| 1. Client's respiratory status improves as evidenced by easier respirations with a normal rate, easier removal of secretions, and lack of gurgling noise in throat with respirations. | Airway cleared of secretions. |
| 2. Client is not able to grind teeth or bite tubes. | Oral airway prevents tooth contact with each other or with tubes. |
| 3. Client does not swallow tongue or otherwise obstruct airway. | Oral airway maintains tooth and tongue position. |
| ***Unexpected outcomes*** | |
| 1. Client continually coughs and gags when airway inserted. | Airway may be too large or long. |
| 2. Client pushes airway out of place or out of mouth. | Airway not secured. |
| 3. Nurse is unable to insert oral airway in client with decreased level of consciousness for various reasons including combative client; nurse unable to pry mouth open. | One nurse performing procedure insufficient to protect nurse or client, obtain additional assistance. |

## Recording and Reporting

| Steps | Rationale |
|---|---|
| 1. Record in nurses' progress notes: | |
| a. Assessment finding for inserting an oral airway. | Documents respiratory status and need for intervention. |
| b. Size of oral airway. | Documents size for other care givers. |
| c. Other procedures performed at same time, especially positioning, secretions obtained. | Documents nursing care. |
| d. Clients tolerance of procedure. | Documents expected and unexpected outcomes. |

## Follow-up Activities

| Steps | Rationale |
|---|---|
| 1. If client continually gags, remove oral airway and turn client on side. Attempt to replace with smaller size oral airway. | Reduces risk of aspiration pneumonia. |
| 2. If client continues to push oral airway out of mouth, this indicates: | |
| a. Airway not secured. | Secure airway to maintain patent airway. |
| b. Client is able to maintain patent airway without presence of artificial airway. | |
| 3. Assess need for airway. | Assessment allows nurse to recognize and intervene with presence of recurrent respiratory distress. |
| 4. Obtain additional assistance if nurse is unable to insert oral airway. | Provides additional personnel needed to maintain patent airway. |
| 5. Remove oral airway at least daily, clean in warm soapy water, reinsert. Hydrogen peroxide and small brush can be used to remove crusted secretions. Wear gloves. | Allows nurse to inspect oral cavity for ulceration. Gives nurse opportunity to provide complete oral hygiene. |
| 6. Administer mouth care q2-4h. | Oral airways increase drying of oral mucosa. |

## Special Considerations

- Clients at greater risk for upper airway obstruction are infants, children, and adults with: colds and flus, loss of consciousness, seizure disorders, neuromuscular diseases, increased oral secretions or excretions.
- If airway obstruction is not relieved and respiratory status is not improved or declines, obtain immediate assistance.
- Avoid causing trauma to gums or hard palate. Keep airway in midline. Client may cough initially. If this lasts more than few min or if client is gagging, airway may be too long. Try next smaller size. Some airways can be cut shorter; however, ends are usually rough. Cutting an oral airway is not recommended.

## Teaching Considerations

- Instruct family members of seizure prone clients to insert oral airway. Observe their technique on model to assess for proper technique.
- Instruct family members in proper cleaning techniques. Observe their technique for adequacy.

# SKILL 18-4 Using an AMBU Manual Ventilator

AMBU stands for Air Mask Bag Unit (Fig. 18-6). Many health professionals think of an AMBU bag as being used only in emergency situations such as cardiopulmonary arrest. However, the AMBU bag has many other uses. It is important in providing manual hyperinflation of the lungs when suctioning secretions. Its use is also necessary in the transportation of ventilator-dependent clients between hospital areas.

An AMBU bag has the following components: a mask, an endotracheal or tracheostomy tube adapter, a large reservoir or "bag," an oxygen adapter, and a valve or spring system to control air flow. Bags are available in infant, child, and adult models to deliver inhaled volumes of 240 to 2000 cc per breath, depending on the manufacturer.

AMBU bags are not difficult to use. The mask is firmly placed over the client's nose and mouth or it is connected to the endotracheal or tracheostomy tube with the adapter. The reservoir is squeezed with one or both hands, forcing air into the airways. When the bag is released, it self-inflates, ready for the next breath. If necessary, the bag can deliver supplemental oxygen.

The nurse often administers additional tidal volume or vital capacity breaths before suctioning to help expand the lungs and loosen secretions. She also may provide supplemental breaths after suctioning to more quickly restore depleted oxygen levels and to reestablish normal carbon dioxide levels.

The nurse may also supplement respirations of clients with acutely diminished minute ventilation (for example, apneic episodes) or acutely increased intracranial pressure. By increasing the client's minute ventilation, the nurse is able to correct elevated carbon dioxide levels. However, the nurse must be aware that, because of the decreased hypoxic drive, decreasing carbon dioxide levels, while desired in some clients, can be hazardous in other clients such as those with chronic obstructive pulmonary disease (COPD).

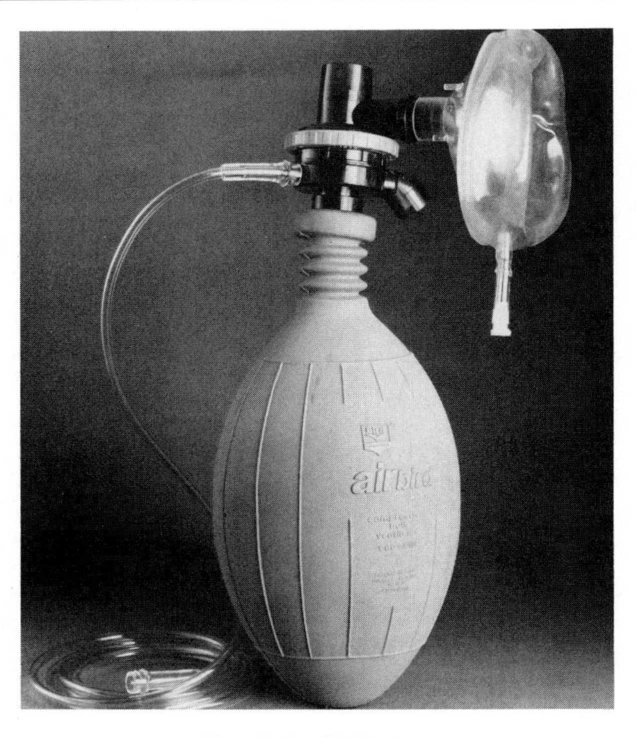

***Fig. 18-6*** AMBU bag.

### Purposes

1. Hyperinflate lungs.
2. Increase minute ventilation.

## Procedure 18-4

| Steps | Rationale |
|---|---|
| **Assessment** | |
| 1. Identify need to use AMBU manual ventilator. Signs and symptoms of need for AMBU manual ventilatory assistance include absent respirations or pulse; diminished respirations or pulse; apneic periods; cyanosis; acutely elevated $Paco_2$; acutely decreased $Pao_2$ "bucking" or fighting mechanical ventilator; elevated intracranial pressure; thick, tenacious sputum; suctioning mucus plugs; cardiopulmonary arrest. | Certain conditions place client at risk for needing AMBU manual ventilatory assistance. |
| 2. Factors that affect respiratory drive include: level of consciousness (LOC), neurologic injury or central nervous system tumor, rib cage function (suboptimal gas exchange), direct pulmonary injury, metabolic rate, psychosocial. | Nurse is able to accurately assess need to provide AMBU manual ventilation. |

| Steps | Rationale |
|---|---|
| **Nursing Diagnosis** | |
| 1. Cluster data to reveal actual or potential nursing diagnoses: | |
| a. Ineffective airway clearance: related to retained secretions. | Retained secretions are ideal media for microorganism growth. |
| b. Impaired gas exchange: related to hypoventilation. | Shallow breathing and slow respiratory rate can decrease amount of inspired oxygen. |
| **Planning** | |
| 1. Develop individualized goals, including: | |
| a. Improve oxygenation. | Use of AMBU bag allows large volume of oxygen to be inhaled by client. |
| b. Restore artificial respiration. | AMBU bag can supply sufficient oxygen during cardiopulmonary or respiratory arrests. |
| c. Decrease intracranial pressure (ICP). | Hyperventilation temporarily decreases cerebral blood flow and reduces increased ICP. |
| 2. Prepare needed equipment: | Placing necessary equipment at client's bedside promotes efficient use of manual ventilation. |
| a. AMBU bag with mask for nonintubated client *or* AMBU bag with ET or T-tube adapter for intubated clients. | |
| b. Oxygen supply tubing if needed. | |
| c. Oral and nasal tracheal or endotracheal and tracheostomy suctioning apparatus. | |
| 3. Prepare the client: | |
| a. Explain procedure and client's participation. | Encourages cooperation and minimizes risks. |
| b. Help client take position comfortable for him and nurse. | Promotes client comfort, prevents strain on nurse. |
| **Implementation** | |
| 1. If not emergency situation (e.g., cardiopulmonary arrest), wash hands. | Reduces transmission of microorganisms. |
| 2. Prepare suction apparatus. | Readies equipment for use. |
| 3. Connect oxygen supply tubing to AMBU bag and oxygen flowmeter. Adjust oxygen flowmeter to ordered $Fio_2$ or 100% $Fio_2$. | Provides supplemental oxygen. |
| 4. If client is intubated and normal saline lavage is ordered to facilitate secretion removal: | |
| a. Remove oxygen delivery device. | Prepares artificial airway for hyperinflation with AMBU bag. |
| b. Instill 5-10 ml normal saline during inspiration. | Normal saline loosen secretions. |
| c. Connect AMBU bag to artificial airway. | |
| d. Administer 1 breath every 3-5 sec to hyperventilate by compressing AMBU bag with 2 hands. | Increases $Pao_2$ and decreases $Paco_2$ before suctioning. |
| e. Suction client. | Removes secretions. |
| f. Repeat Steps c-e as needed. | |
| 5. If client is not intubated: | Correct placement of mask forms an occlusive seal for proper ventilation. |
| a. Place AMBU mask over client's nose and mouth. Proper placement is as follows: 1. Place mask under chin. 2. Pull mask up and over nose. | |
| b. Unless contraindicated, hyperextend client's neck. | Facilitates ventilation and reduces amount of air entering client's stomach. |
| c. Administer breaths according to CPR protocol. | Avoids hypocapnea (low $Paco_2$) and hypercapnea (elevated $Paco_2$) Provides adequate ventilation |
| d. Be prepared to suction client as indicated. Client may need nasogastric intubation. | Pulmonary secretions may be loosened. Client may vomit if too much air is swallowed. |
| 6. Continue to "bag" client until assessment indicates it is no longer necessary, such as: | Provides supplemental ventilation and oxygenation. |
| a. increased blood pressure, improved color, normalized vital signs, normalized level of consciousness. | |
| b. Presence of spontaneous respirations. | |
| c. Decreased ICP. | |
| 7. Repeat Steps 4-6 as needed. Then remove bag and replace oxygen delivery device. | Restores supplemental oxygen. |

| Steps | Rationale |
|---|---|
| 8. Assess client throughout procedure. | Assesses cardiopulmonary and neurologic status. |
| 9. Turn off oxygen flow to AMBU bag. Disconnect bag from oxygen tubing, if indicated. Some institutions leave bag connected to oxygen source at all times. | Discontinues oxygen supply to bag. |
| 10. Reposition client. | Promotes comfort. |
| 11. Remove "elbow" that connects bag to ET tube, T-tube, or mask; wash in warm soapy water. Shake off excess water and allow to dry undisturbed (paper towel can be used to facilitate drying). When dry, reconnect mask or elbow to AMBU bag. | Reduces transmission of microorganisms. |
| 12. Wash hands. | Reduces transmission of microorganisms. |

## Evaluation

| | |
|---|---|
| 1. Compare assessments before and after AMBU bag use. | Identifies client's response to AMBU bag procedure. |

### *Expected outcomes*

| | |
|---|---|
| 1. Secretions are loosened and easier to remove as evidenced by normalized respiratory rate, secretions or mucous plugs suctioned from large airways, improved breath sounds, less restlessness. | AMBU manual ventilatory assistance was successful. |
| 2. Intracranial pressure is decreased as evidenced by pressure waves and digital readout. | AMBU manual ventilatory assistance was successful. |
| 3. "Normal" arterial blood gases in cardiopulmonary arrest, during transportation, after seizures and apneic episodes. | AMBU manual ventilatory assistance was successful. |
| 4. Client ceases "bucking" ventilator. | AMBU manual ventilatory assistance was successful. |

### *Unexpected outcomes*

| | |
|---|---|
| 1. Client becomes acidotic/hypercapneic:<br>a. Intubation and continuous ventilation needed.<br>b. Ventilator rate/tidal volume needs increase. | Client needs additional supplemental breathing. |
| 2. Client becomes alkalotic/hypocapneic:<br>a. Decrease volume/rate of bagging. | Client needs less supplemental breathing |

## Recording and Reporting

| | |
|---|---|
| 1. Chart in nurses' progress notes: | |
| a. Assessments before and after bagging. | Documents cardiopulmonary status. |
| b. Rate and volume of bagging. | Documents nursing care. |
| c. Amount of normal saline lavage, if used. | Documents nursing care. |
| d. Amount of supplemental oxygen used. | |
| e. Client's tolerance of procedure. | Documents expected and unexpected outcomes. |
| f. Secretions suctioned (quality and quantity). | Documents nursing care. |

## Follow-up Activities

| | |
|---|---|
| 1. Inform physician of client's response to AMBU manual ventilatory assistance. | Readjustment of mechanical ventilation requires medical order; client should be evaluated by physician. |

## Special Considerations

- Clients at greater risk to need AMBU are those with pneumonia, seizure or sleep apnea disorders, multiple trauma, cardiopulmonary arrest, sudden infant death syndrome, drug overdose, neurologic injury. Also at risk is ventilator-dependent client needing transportation to another hospital area.
- 15 mm AMBU bag adapter must be obtained for most metal and Silastic T-tubes. Lavage is most effective if cuff is inflated throughout procedure.
- If client is infant, use three quick puffs with pediatric AMBU bag.
- Inflation can be held for a few sec by not allowing client to exhale into bag.

## Teaching Considerations

- Demonstrate techniques of bagging to care givers. Allow time for practice on dummy or client. Assess for proper technique in administering technique and cleaning equipment.

# SKILL 18-5 Performing Cardiopulmonary Resuscitation

Cardiopulmonary arrest is characterized by an absence of pulse and respiration and is frequently accompanied by dilated pupils. If the nurse determines that the client has experienced cardiac arrest, CPR must be initiated. CPR is a basic emergency procedure for life support, consisting of artificial respiration and manual external cardiac massage. CPR has three main goals, called the ABCs of cardiopulmonary resuscitation: establish an *A*irway, initiate *B*reathing, and maintain *C*irculation. A cardiac and pulmonary arrest is a sudden cessation of respirations, pulse, and circulation. When an arrest occurs, oxygen is not delivered to the tissues, carbon dioxide is not transported from the tissues, tissue metabolism becomes anaerobic, and metabolic and respiratory acidosis occurs. Tissue damage, including permanent heart and brain damage, occurs within 5 minutes. A respiratory arrest is the cessation of respirations; pulse is often present.

Once the nurse determines that a respiratory or cardiopulmonary arrest has happened, she must quickly provide a patent airway by removing any foreign body obstruction (Skill 18-1), removing secretions (Chapter 12), insert an oral airway (Skill 18-3), or hyperextending the neck as detailed in this skill.

The initiation of breathing is achieved by one of two methods. First, if immediately available, the nurse can use an AMBU manual ventilator (Skill 18-4). Second, the nurse can initiate mouth-to-mouth artificial ventilation as described in this skill.

The maintenance of circulation is achieved by external cardiac compression. Two elements must be present to ensure safe and efficient cardiac massage. First, the client's spine must be supported during compression by placing him on a hard surface such as a board or the floor. Second, sternal pressure must be forceful but not traumatic (Whaley and Wong, 1987).

## Purpose

1. Restore cardiopulmonary functioning.

## Procedure 18-5

| Steps | Rationale |
|---|---|
| **Assessment** | |
| 1. Determine if person is unconscious by shaking him or shouting at him: "Are you OK?" | Confirms that person is unconscious as opposed to intoxicated, sleeping, or hearing impaired (Guzzetta and Dossey, 1984). |
| 2. Determine presence of carotid pulse and respirations. | Presence of pulse *and* respiration contraindicates initiation of CPR. |
| **Nursing Diagnosis** | |
| 1. Cluster data to diagnose respiratory or cardiopulmonary arrest. | |
| a. Decreased cardiac output: related to absence of pulse. | Absence of pulse indicates cardiac standstill or fibrillation, both of which result in decreased cardiac output. |
| b. Impaired gas exchange: related to absence of spontaneous respirations. | Absence of respirations decreases amount of gas exchanged in alveoli and results in tissue hypoxia. |
| c. Ineffective breathing pattern: related to airway obstruction. | Airway obstructions prevent entry of oxygen to lungs and ultimately decreases oxygen exchange in alveoli. |
| **Planning** | |
| 1. Call for assistance, seek help from passerby, call for additional nurses. Goals of care: restore airway, breathing, circulation. | One person cannot maintain CPR indefinitely. Without relief, rescuer fatigues, chest compressions are ineffective, and volume of air ventilated into victim's lungs decreases. |
| 2. Place victim on hard surface such as floor, ground, or backboard. | External compression of heart is facilitated. Heart is compressed between sternum and hard surface. |
| 3. Place yourself in correct position, which is also somewhat comfortable: | You may be administering CPR for extended period, particularly in community setting. Correct comfortable position decreases skeletal muscle fatigue. |
| a. *One-person rescuer:* position yourself facing victim, on your knees, parallel to victim's sternum. | Allows rescuer to quickly move back and forth from victim's mouth to sternum. |

| Steps | Rationale |
|---|---|

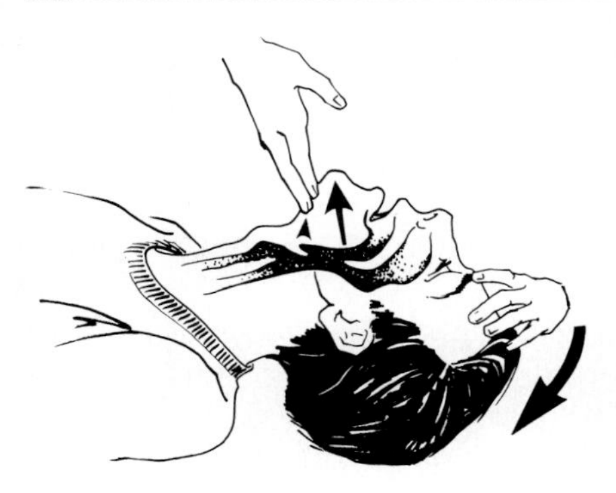
Fig. 18-7

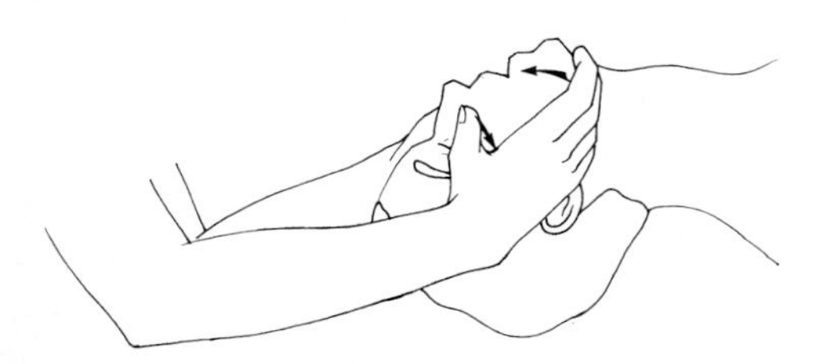
***Fig. 18-8***
From Guzzetta CE, Dossey BM: Cardiovascular nursing: bodymind tapestry, St Louis, 1984, The CV Mosby Co.

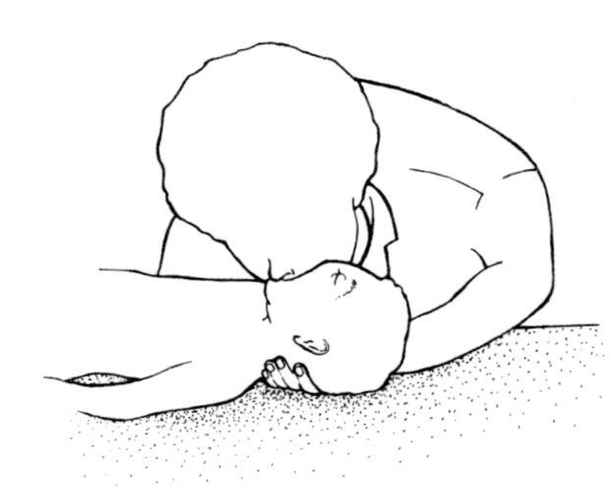
***Fig. 18-9***

| Steps | Rationale |
|---|---|
| b. *Two-person rescuer:* one person faces victim, kneeling parallel to victim's head. Second person moves to opposite side and faces victim, kneels parallel to victim's sternum. | Allows one rescuer to maintain breathing while other maintains circulation, without getting in each other's way. |

## Implementation

| Steps | Rationale |
|---|---|
| 1. Restore open airway: | |
| a. Head tilt-chin lift (Fig. 18-7): Elevate chin with one hand and apply downward pressure on forehead until teeth are almost together but mouth is still open. | Airway obstruction from tongue is relieved. If necessary, remove foreign body (see Skill 18-1). |
| b. Jaw thrust maneuver (Fig. 18-8) can be used by health professionals but is not taught to general public. Grasp angles of victim's lower jaw and lift with both hands, displacing the mandible forward while tilting the head backward. | |
| 2. If readily available, insert oral airway (Skill 18-3). | Maintains tongue on anterior floor of mouth and prevents obstruction of posterior airway by tongue. |
| 3. Administer artificial respiration: | |
| a. Mouth-to-mouth: | |
| ▪ Adult: pinch victim's nose and occlude mouth with yours. | Airtight seal is formed and air is prevented from escaping from nose. |
| Blow 2 full breaths into victim's mouth (each breath should take 1-1.5 sec); allow victim to exhale between breaths. | Hyperventilation is promoted and assists in maintaining adequate blood oxygen levels. In most adults this volume is 800 ml and is sufficient to make the chest rise. An excess of air volume and fast inspiratory flow rates are likely to cause pharyngeal pressures that exceed esophageal opening pressures, allowing air to enter the stomach and result in gastric distention, thereby increasing the risk of vomiting. |
| ▪ Child: Place your mouth over child's nose and mouth (Fig. 18-9). | Airtight seal is formed and air is prevented from escaping from nose. |
| For mouth-to-mouth resuscitation of child, administer two slow breaths lasting 1-1.5 sec. with a pause in between. | Because an infant's air passages are smaller with resistance to flow quite high, it is difficult to make recommendations about the force or volume of the rescue breaths. However, three factors should be remembered: (1) rescue breaths are the single most important maneuver in assisting a nonbreathing child, (2) an appropriate volume is one that makes the chest rise and fall, and (3) slow breaths provide an adequate volume at the lowest possible pressure, thereby reducing the risk of gastric distention. |
| b. AMBU: | |
| ▪ Adult and child: For AMBU bag resuscitation use proper size face mask and apply it under chin, up and over victim's mouth and nose (Fig. 18-10). | Airtight seal is formed as bag is compressed and oxygen enters client. |
| 4. Observe for rise and fall of chest wall with each respiration. If lungs do not inflate, reposition head and neck and check for visible airway obstruction, such as vomitus. | Ensures that artificial respirations are entering lungs. |

| Steps | Rationale |
|---|---|

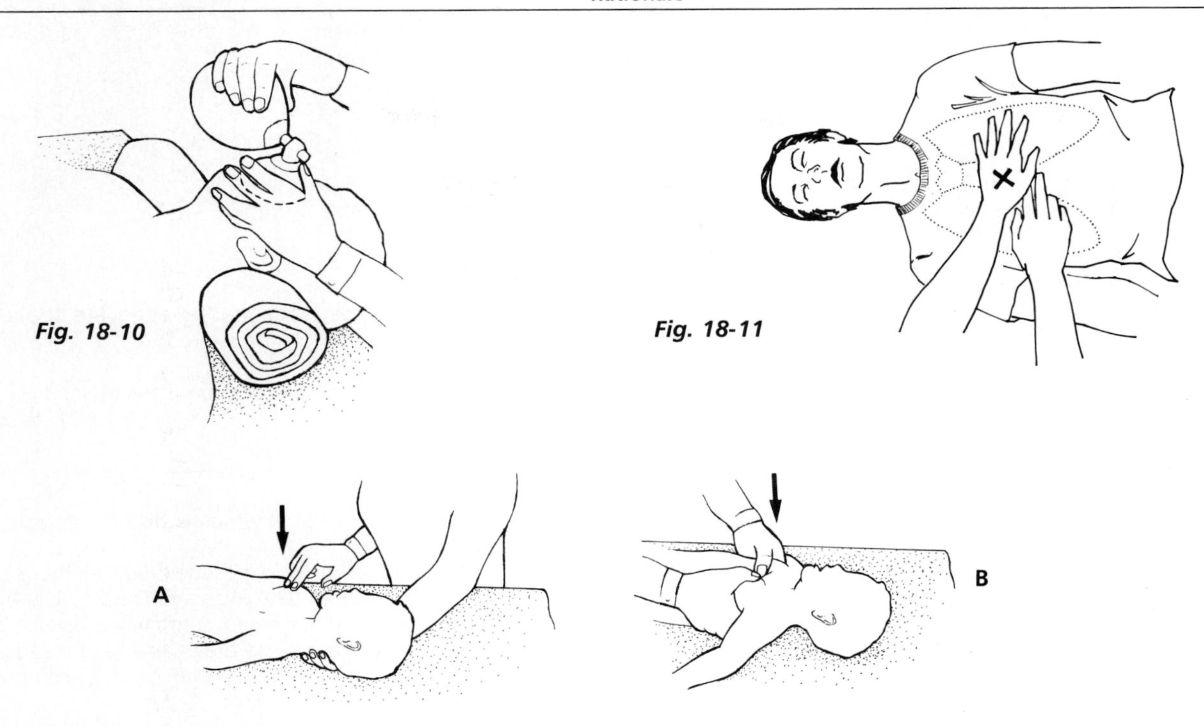

Fig. 18-10

Fig. 18-11

Fig. 18-12

| Steps | Rationale |
|---|---|
| 5. Suction secretions if necessary or turn victim's head to one side. | Suctioning prevents airway obstruction. Turning client's head to one side allows gravity to drain secretions. |
| 6. Assess for presence of carotid pulse (adults) or brachial pulse (infants). | Carotid artery pulse will persist when the more peripheral pulses are no longer palpable. Performing external cardiac compressions on a victim who has a pulse may result in serious medical complications. |
| 7. If pulse is absent, initiate chest compressions:<br>a. Assume correct hand position:<br>▪ Adult: place hands 1-2 cm above xiphoid process on sternum. Keep hands parallel to chest and fingers above chest. Interlocking fingers is helpful. Extend arms and lock elbows. Maintain arms straight and shoulders directly over victim's sternum (Fig. 18-11).<br>▪ Child: place finger tips of index and middle fingers of 1 hand 1-2 cm above xiphoid process. Fingers should be on the sternum at the level of the nipples (Fig. 18-12, *A*).<br>▪ Infant: Place thumbs together on sternum with fingers extending around ribs (Fig. 18-12, *B*). | Places hands and fingers over heart in proper position. Prevents xiphoid process and rib fracture, which can further compromise cardiopulmonary status. |

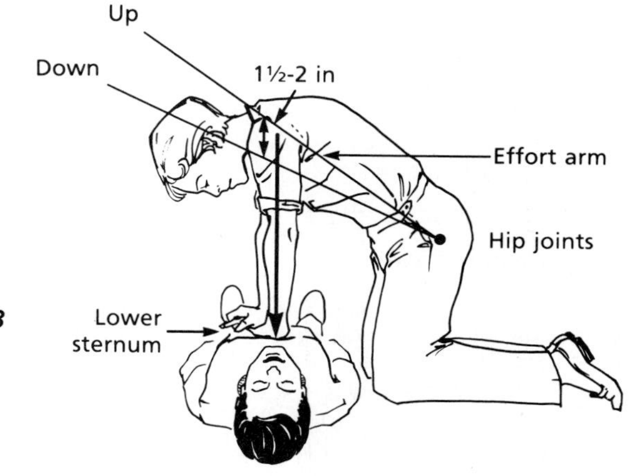

Fig. 18-13

| Steps | Rationale |
|---|---|
| b. Compress sternum to proper depth from shoulders. Do not rock.<br>▪ Adult and adolescent: 4-5 cm (1.5-2 in) (Fig. 18-13).<br>▪ Older child: 3-4 cm (1-1.5 in).<br>▪ Toddler and preschooler: 2-4 cm (0.75 - 1.5 in).<br>▪ Infant: 1-2 cm (0.5-1 in). | Compression occurs only on sternum. Pressure necessary for external compression is created by nurse's upper arm muscle strength. |

| Steps | Rationale |
|---|---|
| c. Maintain proper rate of compression: ratio of compressions to breaths for two rescuers is 5 to 1; for one rescuer, the ratio is 15 to 2.<br>▪ Adult and adolescent: 80/min (count one 1000; two 1000).<br>▪ Older child, 80-100/min.<br>▪ Toddler and infant: 100-200/min. | Proper number of compressions/min should be delivered to ensure adequate cardiac output. |
| d. Continue mouth-to-mouth or AMBU ventilations.<br>▪ Adult and adolescent: every 5 sec (12/min).<br>▪ Older child: every 4 sec (15/min).<br>▪ Infant and toddler: every 3 sec (20/min). | Adequate ventilations promoted. |
| 8. Palpate for carotid pulse with each external chest compression for first full minute. If carotid pulse is not palpable, compressions are not strong enough. | Assessment of pulse validates that adequate stroke volume is achieved with each compression. |
| 9. Continue CPR until relieved or until victim regains spontaneous pulse and respirations. | Artificial cardiopulmonary function is maintained. |
| **Evaluation** | |
| 1. Assess carotid pulse at 5 min intervals following first minute of CPR. | Documents adequacy of external cardiac compressions. |
| 2. Assess pupillary response to light. | Pupils will constrict when exposed to light if there is adequate oxygenation to brain (Guzzetta and Dossey, 1984); widely dilated pupils that respond to light may indicate cerebral hypoxia without serious cerebral damage. Persistently dilated nonreactive pupils may indicate serious cerebral damage (Guzzetta and Dossey, 1984). |
| 3. CPR is not interrupted for more than 5 secs. | Maintain adequacy of oxygenation and circulation. |
| **Recording and Reporting** | |
| 1. Immediately report arrest indicating exact location of victim:<br>a. In hospital setting, follow hospital policy.<br>b. In community setting, dial 911 or other emergency number. | Obtains immediate expert assistance for victim. |
| 2. Record in nurse's notes onset of arrest, medication given, procedures performed, and victim's response. | Documents medical care delivered. |
| **Follow-up Activities** | |
| 1. Notify victim's family and provide support:<br>a. Contact chaplain services.<br>b. Contact social worker. | Uncertainty of situation causes extreme anxiety in the family. Presence of supportive personnel can help family deal with anxiety and fears. |
| 2. Reassure successfully resuscitated victim:<br>a. Educate regarding presence of any equipment.<br>b. Help client work through fears of rearrest. | After CPR victims fear being alone because of potential of rearrest and feelings of helplessness. |
| 3. Complete postmortem care on victims for whom CPR was unsuccessful (Chapter 47). | |

## Special Considerations

- Oral airways are readily available in hospital and extended care and out-patient settings. However, they are not available in all community settings. *CPR can effectively be accomplished without an oral airway. Do not wait until an oral airway is found.*
- Spinal cord injury should be suspected with face or head injury or laceration, diving accident, or football or other contact sports injury.
- Unconsciousness can be caused by substance abuse, hypoglycemia, ketoacidosis, shock. If unconscious person has adequate respirations *and* pulse, remain until further assistance is present. Continue to determine presence of pulse and respiration because respiratory or cardiopulmonary arrest is still possible.
- In the community setting, instruct someone to call for emergency medical service (EMS). Dial 0 or 911, depending on community resources. Tell operator or dispatcher exact location of victim; in hospital setting, instruct someone to call a CODE by following agency procedure.
- Soft surface such as mattress, car seat, or grassy surface decreases efficiency of external cardiac compressions.
- Pupillary responses do not consistently reflect effectiveness of CPR and client's condition.
- CPR is interrupted when changing CPR personnel, during defibrillation, or when transporting the victim; during intubation, CPR may be interrupted for more than 5 secs, but should not exceed 30 secs. Nurse should remind rescue team of number of seconds elapsing during intubation.

- "Code status" should be determined on clients by the physician and documented in the client record. The rule in most institutions is to "code" all clients unless ordered otherwise.
- Lay learners are taught one-man CPR. With one person CPR the ratio of compressions to ventilations is:
  Infant and child to 8 years: 5:1
  8 years to adult: 15:2

## Teaching Considerations

- If a client is at high risk for cardiopulmonary arrest, the family or care givers should be instructed and certified in CPR by certified instructor from the institution, the American Red Cross, or the American Heart Association.
- The client and family should keep emergency numbers taped to the phone. These numbers may include fire department, ambulance, hospital, and physician. Instruct client and family who to call. The family may also need to know what to do when a client is found "deceased."

---

**BIBLIOGRAPHY**

Bulau J: Clinical policies and procedures for home health care, Rockville, Md, 1986, Aspen Publishers, Inc.

Burden N: Preparing for medical emergencies in the ambulatory setting, Current Reviews for Post Anesthesia Care Nurses 9(17):134, 1987.

Dennison RD: Managing the patient with upper airway obstruction, Nurs 17:34, 1987.

First aid for the choking child, Pediatrics 81(5):740, 1981.

Gatch G, Myre L, Black RE: Foreign body aspiration in children: causes, diagnosis, and prevention, AORN 46:850, 1987.

Goodwin BA: Pediatric resuscitation, Crit Care Nurs Quart 10:69, 1988.

Guzzetta CE, Dossey BM: Cardiovascular nursing, bodymind tapestry, St. Louis, 1984, The CV Mosby Co.

Heimlich HJ: A life-saving maneuver to prevent choking, JAMA 234:398, 1975.

Jacobs B, et al.: Prehospital resuscitation of the trauma patient, Top Emerg Med 9(3):1, 1987.

Martin DA, Redland AR: Legal and ethical issues in resuscitation and withholding of treatment, Crit Care Nurs Quart 10:25, 1988.

Middaugh RE, Middaugh DJ, Menk EJ: Current considerations in respiratory and acid-base management during cardiopulmonary resuscitation, Crit Care Nurs Quart 10:25, 1988.

Rosequist CC: Current standards and guidelines for cardiopulmonary resuscitation and emergency cardiac care, Heart-Lung 16:408, 1987.

Standards & guidelines for cardiopulmonary resuscitation (CPR) and emergency cardiac care (ECC), JAMA 255:2903, 1986.

Visintine RE, Baick CH: Ruptured stomach after Heimlich maneuver, JAMA 234:415, 1975.

Walsh J, Persons C, Wieck, L: Manual of home health care nursing, Philadelphia, 1987, JB Lippincott Co.

Whaley LF, Wong DL: Nursing care of infants and children, ed 3, St. Louis, 1987, The CV Mosby Co.

Willens J, Copel L: Performing CPR on adults, Nursing '89 19(1):34, 1989.

Willens J, Copel L: Performing CPR on children, Nursing '89 19(2):57, 1989.

# UNIT VI

# MEDICATIONS

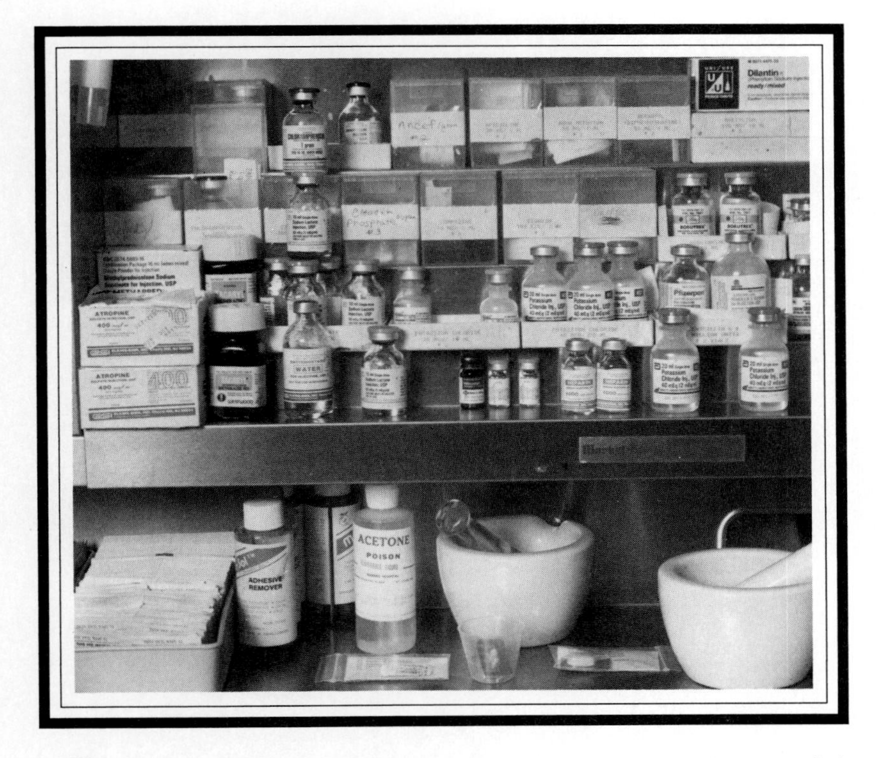


Safe and accurate administration of medications is one of the nurse's most important responsibilities. All drugs have potential for creating harmful effects and each client can react very differently to those effects. The nurse must have a good understanding of how drugs act, the desired and undesired effects of each medication, the proper method for administration, and the measures taken to monitor client response. The nurse's judgment is critical in determining when and how to administer medications. A client's condition can change quickly, indicating the need for drug therapy. Often clients receive more than one medication and the combined effects can cause unusual reactions. Timing of drug administration often must be coordinated with other therapies the client receives. The nurse is in the best position to administer medications and monitor their effects so that clients may benefit optimally from the therapy.

The nurse administers medications by oral and parenteral routes. Parenteral medications include those given by topical application, injection, and inhalation. The nurse must be knowledgeable in choosing the safest route for a client since each has specific advantages and disadvantages. This unit on medication administration provides nurses with skills needed to administer drugs by all routes.

# 19
# ORAL MEDICATIONS

## OBJECTIVES

*Mastery of content in this chapter will enable the nurse to:*

- Define key terms.
- Correctly administer a medication by the oral route.
- Identify guidelines for safe administration of medications.
- Discuss common types of drug actions.
- Identify the system of measurement for a given prescribed drug.
- Describe the five rights of drug administration.
- Describe factors to assess before administering oral medications.
- Identify conditions contraindicating the administration of oral medications.
- Identify aseptic techniques used in preparing and administering oral medications.
- Explain techniques to prevent clients from aspirating oral drug preparations.
- Prepare a teaching plan on drug therapy for a select client.

## KEY TERMS

*Anaphylaxis*
*Aspiration*
*Compliance*
*Drug abuse*
*Drug addiction*
*Drug dependence*
*Drug plateau*
*Enteric-coated*
*Idiosyncratic reaction*
*NPO*
*Onset of action*
*Over-the-counter drug*
*Peak action*
*Side effect*
*Synergistic reaction*
*Unit dose system*

## SKILLS

***19-1*** Administering Oral Medications
***19-2*** Helping Clients with Self-Medication

Safe and accurate administration of medications is one of the nurse's most important responsibilities. The nurse's judgment is critical for safe drug administration. The nurse must understand a drug's action and effects, administer it correctly, monitor the client's response, and help the client self-administer drugs correctly.

## DRUG FORMS

Drugs are available in a variety of forms or preparations. The form of the drug determines its route of administration. The composition of a drug is designed to enhance its absorption and metabolism within the body. Many drugs are available in several forms such as tablets, capsules, pediatric elixirs, and suppositories. When administering a medication, the nurse must be certain to give the medication in the proper form (Table 19-1).

## DRUG ACTIONS

Because of its chemical makeup and physiologic action, a drug may produce more than one effect.

### Therapeutic Effects

The therapeutic effect is the intended or predicted physiologic response a drug causes. Each drug has a desired or therapeutic effect for which it is prescribed. For example, the nurse administers codeine phosphate to create analgesia. A single medication may have many therapeutic effects. For example, aspirin creates analgesia and reduces inflammation of arthritis.

#### Side Effects

Predictably a drug will cause unintended, secondary effects. Side effects may be harmless or injurious. In the example of codeine phosphate, a client may also experience constipation. If the side effects are serious enough to negate the beneficial effects of a drug's therapeutic action, the physician may discontinue it. Clients often stop taking medications because of side effects.

***TABLE 19-1*** Forms of Medication

| Form | Description |
|---|---|
| **Capsule** | Solid dosage form for oral use; medication in a powder, liquid, or oil form and encased by a gelatin shell; capsule colored to aid in product identification. |
| **Elixir** | Clear fluid containing water and alcohol; designed for oral use; usually has a sweetener added. |
| **Extract** | Concentrated drug form made by removing the active portion of a drug from its other components; e.g., a fluid extract is a drug made into a solution from a vegetable source. |
| **Glycerite** | Solution of drug combined with glycerin for external use; contains at least 50% glycerin. |
| **Liniment** | Preparation usually containing alcohol, oil, or soapy emollient applied to the skin. |
| **Lotion** | Drug in liquid suspension applied externally to protect the skin. |
| **Ointment (salve)** | Semisolid, externally applied preparation, usually containing one or more drugs. |
| **Paste** | Semisolid preparation, thicker and stiffer than an ointment, absorbed through the skin more slowly than an ointment. |
| **Pill** | Solid dosage form containing one or more drugs, shaped into globules, ovoids, or oblong shapes; true pills rarely used, since they have been replaced by tablets. |
| **Solution** | Liquid preparation that may be used orally, parenterally, or externally; can also be instilled into a body organ or cavity (e.g., bladder irrigations), contains water with one or more dissolved compounds; must be sterile if for parenteral use. |
| **Suppository** | Solid dosage form mixed with gelatin and shaped in the form of a pellet for insertion into a body cavity (rectum or vagina); melts when it reaches body temperature, releasing the drug for absorption. |
| **Suspension** | Finely divided drug particles dispersed in a liquid medium; when suspension is left standing, particles settle to the bottom of the container; commonly an oral medication and is not to be given intravenously. |
| **Syrup** | Medication dissolved in a concentrated sugar solution; may contain flavoring to make drug more palatable. |
| **Tablet** | Powdered dosage form compressed into hard disks or cylinders; in addition to primary drug, contains binders (adhesive to allow powder to stick together), disintegrators (to promote tablet dissolution), lubricants (for ease of manufacturing), and fillers (for convenient tablet size). |
| **Enteric-coated** | Tablet for oral use coated with materials that do not dissolve in the stomach; coatings dissolve in the intestine where medication is absorbed. |
| **Tincture** | Alcohol or water-alcohol drug solution. |
| **Troche (lozenge)** | Flat, round dosage form containing drug, flavoring, sugar, and mucilage; dissolves in mouth to release drug. |

### Toxic Effects

After prolonged intake of high doses of medication, or use of drugs intended for external application or when a drug accumulates in the blood because of impaired metabolism or excretion, toxic effects develop. Excess amounts of a drug within the body may have lethal effects, depending on the drug's action. For example, morphine, a narcotic analgesic, relieves pain by depressing the central nervous system. However, toxic levels of morphine cause severe respiratory depression and death.

### Idiosyncratic Reactions

Medications may cause unpredictable effects, such as an idiosyncratic reaction in which a client overreacts or underreacts to a drug or has a reaction different from normal. It is impossible to predict which client will have an idiosyncratic response.

### Allergic Reactions

Allergic reaction is another unpredictable response to a drug. Exposure to an initial dose of a medication may cause an immunologic response. The drug acts as an antigen, which causes antibodies to be produced. With repeated administration the client develops an allergic response to the drug, its chemical preservatives, or a metabolite.

An allergic reaction may be mild or severe. Allergic symptoms vary, depending on the individual and the drug. Among the different classes of drugs, antibiotics cause a high incidence of allergic reactions. Common, mild allergy symptoms are summarized in Table 19-2. Severe or anaphylactic reactions are characterized by sudden constriction of bronchiolar muscles, edema of the pharynx and larynx, and severe wheezing and shortness of breath. The client may also become severely hypotensive, necessitating emergency resuscitation measures.

A client with a known history of an allergy to a medication should wear an identification bracelet or medal, which alerts nurses and physicians to the allergies if the client is unconscious when receiving medical care.

**TABLE 19-2** Mild Allergic Reactions

| Symptom | Description |
|---|---|
| **Urticaria (hives)** | Raised, irregularly shaped skin eruptions with varying sizes and shapes; eruptions have reddened margins and pale centers. |
| **Eczema (rash)** | Small, raised vesicles that are usually reddened; often distributed over the entire body. |
| **Pruritus** | Itching of the skin; accompanies most rashes. |
| **Rhinitis** | Inflammation of mucous membranes lining the nose, causing swelling and a clear watery discharge. |
| **Wheezing** | Constriction of smooth muscles surrounding bronchioles that decreases diameter of airways; occurs primarily on inspiration because of severely narrowed airways; development of edema in pharynx and larynx that further obstructs airflow. |

## Drug Tolerance

Some persons have an unusually low metabolism in response to a drug. An increase in dosage may be needed to cause a therapeutic effect. Opiates are a common form of drug that may cause drug tolerance.

## Drug Interactions

When one drug modifies the action of another drug, a drug interaction occurs. Drug interactions are common in individuals taking many medications. A drug may potentiate or diminish the action of other drugs and may alter the way in which another drug is absorbed, metabolized, or eliminated from the body.

When two drugs act synergistically, the effect of the two drugs combined is greater than the effect that would be expected if the individual effects of the two drugs acting alone were added together. Alcohol is a central nervous system depressant that has a synergistic effect on antihistamines, antidepressants, and narcotic analgesics.

A drug interaction is not always undesirable. Often a physician orders combination drug therapy to create a drug interaction for therapeutic benefit. For example, a client with moderate hypertension typically receives several drugs, such as diuretics and vasodilators, that act together to keep the blood pressure at a desirable level.

## Drug Dose Responses

After the nurse administers a drug, it undergoes absorption, distribution, metabolism, and excretion. The quantity and distribution of a drug in different body compartments change constantly.

When a medication is prescribed, the goal is to achieve a constant blood level within a safe therapeutic range. The client and nurse must follow regular dosage schedules and administer prescribed doses at correct dosage intervals. Knowledge of the following time intervals of drug action also helps to anticipate a drug's effect.

1. Onset of drug action—Period of time it takes after a drug is administered for it to produce a response.
2. Peak action—Time it takes for a drug to reach its highest effective concentration.
3. Duration of action—Length of time during which the drug is present in a concentration great enough to produce a response.
4. Plateau—Blood serum concentration reached and maintained after repeated, fixed doses.

***TABLE 19-3*** Factors Influencing Choice of Administration Routes

| Route | Advantages | Disadvantages/Contraindications |
|---|---|---|
| Oral, buccal, sublingual. | Easy and comfortable to administer, economical, may produce local or systemic effects, rarely causes anxiety. | Avoid giving to clients with alterations in gastrointestinal function (e.g., nausea and vomiting) reduced motility (after general anesthesia or inflammation of bowel), and surgical resection of portion of gastrointestinal tract. Some drugs are destroyed by gastric secretions. Oral administration is contraindicated in clients unable to swallow (e.g., clients with neuromuscular disorders, esophageal strictures, and lesions of the mouth). Oral medications cannot be given when client has gastric suction and are contraindicated in clients before some tests or surgery. An unconscious or confused client is unable or unwilling to swallow or hold medication under the tongue. Oral medications may irritate lining of gastrointestinal tract, discolor teeth, or have an unpleasant taste. |
| Subcutaneous, intramuscular, intravenous, intradermal. | Provides route of administration when oral drugs are contraindicated, more rapid absorption than with topical or oral drugs, intravenous infusion provides drug delivery when client is critically ill or peripheral perfusion is inadequate. | There is a risk of introducing infection, the drugs are expensive, and these routes are to be avoided in clients with bleeding tendencies. There is a risk of tissue damage with subcutaneous injections. Intramuscular and intravenous routes are dangerous because of rapid absorption. These routes cause considerable anxiety in many clients, especially children. |
| Skin. | Primarily provides local effect; painless, limited side effects. | Extensive applications may be bulky and cause difficulty in maneuvering. Clients with skin abrasions are at risk for rapid drug absorption and systemic effects. |
| Mucous membranes: buccal, sublingual, eye, ear, nose, vagina, rectum. | Therapeutic effects provided by local application to involved sites; aqueous solutions readily absorbed and capable of causing systemic effects; provides route of administration when oral drugs are contraindicated. | Mucous membranes are highly sensitive to some drug concentrations. Insertion of rectal and vaginal medications often causes the client embarrassment. Rectal suppositories are contraindicated if the client has had rectal surgery or if active rectal bleeding is present. Client with ruptured eardrum cannot receive irrigations. |
| Inhalation. | Provides rapid relief for local respiratory problems and easy access for introduction of general anesthetic gases; for seriously weakened or unconscious client, oxygen can still be delivered with appropriate respiratory therapy equipment. | Some local agents can cause serious systemic effects. Drugs developed to act on body systems other than the lungs cannot be administered by inhalation. |

### Routes of Administration

The route chosen for administering a drug depends on its properties and desired effect and on the client's physical and mental condition. The nurse is often the best person to judge the route most desirable for a client. Table 19-3 summarizes the common routes of drug administration and the factors influencing the choice of those routes.

## SYSTEMS OF DRUG MEASUREMENT

The proper administration of medication depends on the nurse's ability to compute drug dosages accurately and measure medications correctly. A careless mistake in placing a decimal point or adding a zero to a dosage can lead to a fatal error. The physician and client depend on the nurse to check the dosage before administering a drug. The nurse is also responsible for teaching clients the dosages prescribed for them. Three systems of measurement are used in drug therapy: metric, apothecary, and household.

### Metric System

As a decimal system, the metric system is the most logically organized of the measurement systems. Metric units can be easily converted and computed through simple multiplication and division. Each basic unit of measurement is organized into units of 10. Multiplying or dividing by 10 forms secondary units. In multiplication, the decimal point moves to the right; in division, the decimal moves to the left.

The basic units of measurement in the metric system are the meter (length), the liter (volume), and the gram

***TABLE 19-4*** Volume Equivalents of Measurement

| Metric | Apothecary | Household |
|---|---|---|
| 1 ml | 15 minims (m) | 15 drops (gtt) |
| 15 ml | 4 fluidrams (fʒ) | 1 tablespoon (tbsp) |
| 30 ml | 1 fluid ounce (f℥) | 2 tablespoons (tbsp) |
| 240 ml | 8 fluid ounces (f℥) | 1 cup (c) |
| 480 ml (approximately 500 ml) | 1 pint (pt) | 1 pint (pt) |
| 960 ml (approximately 1 L) | 1 quart (qt) | 1 quart (qt) |
| 3840 ml (approximately 4000 ml) | 1 gallon (gal) | 1 gallon (gal) |

(weight). For drug calculations the nurse uses primarily volume and weight units. In the metric system small or large letters are used to designate the basic units:

Gram = g or Gm

Liter = l or L

Small letters are abbreviations for subdivisions of major units:

Milligram = mg

Milliliter = ml

A system of Latin prefixes designates subdivision of the basic units: deci- (1/10 or 0.1), centi- (1/100 or 0.01), and milli- (1/1000 or 0.001). Greek prefixes designate multiples of the basic units: deka- (10), hecto- (100), and kilo- (1000). When writing drug dosages in metric units, physicians and nurses use either fractions or multiples of a unit. Fractions are always in decimal form, and a zero is always placed in front of the decimal to prevent error.

## Apothecary System

The apothecary system of measurement is familiar to most people in the United States and Canada. The standards for measurement can be easily seen in the home: milk is bottled in pints and quarts, a yardstick has inches and feet, and a bathroom scale weighs in pounds.

The basic unit of weight is a grain. Units of weight derived from the grain are the dram, ounce, and pound. The apothecary unit for volume or fluid measurement is the minim. The minim is the approximate quantity of water that weighs a grain. The fluidram, fluid ounce, pint, quart, and gallon are measures derived from the minim.

In the apothecary system, small letters or symbols are used for measurement units:

Grain = gr

Ounce = oz or ℥

Fluid ounce = f℥

Minim = m or min

Dram = ʒ

Lowercase Roman numerals designate the quantities of the apothecary units. The Roman numeral follows the unit of measure

3 grains = gr iii

***TABLE 19-5*** Weight Equivalents of Measurement

| Metric | Apothecary | Household |
|---|---|---|
| 1 mg | 1/60 gr | — |
| 60 mg | 1 gr | — |
| 1 g | 15 gr | — |
| 4 g | 1 ʒ | — |
| 30 g | 1 oz (℥) | 1 oz |
| 500 g | 1.1 lb | 1 lb |
| 1000 g (1 kg) | 2.2 lb | 2 lb |

Physicians often use fractions as well as symbols, with apothecary units:

$2\frac{1}{2}$ fluid ounces = f℥ iiss

$\frac{1}{2}$ fluid ounce = f℥ $\frac{1}{2}$ or ℥ ss

## Household Measurements

Household measures are familiar to most people and used when more accurate systems of measure are unnecessary. Included in household measures are drops, teaspoons, tablespoons, cups, and glasses for volume, and ounces and pounds for weight. Although pints and quarts are considered household measures, they are also used in the apothecary system.

## Conversions

Drugs are not always dispensed in the unit of measure in which they are ordered. Drug companies package and bottle certain standard equivalents. The nurse often must convert available units of volume and weight to desired dosages. The nurse must know approximate equivalents in all of the measurement systems (Tables 19-4 and 19-5).

## Dosage Calculations

The nurse can use a simple formula in many types of dosage calculations. The formula can be applied when preparing solid or liquid forms of medications.

$$\frac{\text{Dose ordered}}{\text{Dose on hand}} \times \text{Amount on hand} = \text{Amount to administer}$$

Where the dose ordered is the amount of pure drug the physician prescribes for a client, the dose on hand is the weight or volume of drug available in units supplied by

ALLERGIES: Codeine

RECOPIED BY INITIALS: L.T R.N. SIGNATURE: Ben Wilson, R.N.

| SIGNATURES | | | |
|---|---|---|---|
| NITES | Mary Doerrer, R.N. | Mary Doerrer, R.N. | Mary Doerrer, R.N. |
| DAYS | Pat Little, R.N. | Pat Little, R.N. | Tom Say, R.N. |
| EVES | Donna C. Gail, R.N. | Donna C. Gail, R.N. | |

BARNES HOSPITAL PATIENT ROUTINE MEDICATION RECORD

| ORDER DATE / EXP DATE | INIT | ROUTINE MEDICATION Name of drug strength and frequency | RTE | SCHEDULE | SHIFT | DATE 6/14/89 | DATE 6/15/89 | DATE 6/16/89 |
|---|---|---|---|---|---|---|---|---|
| 2/6 | PL | Lanoxin 0.25 mg q.d. | PO | | NITES | | | |
| | | | | 10 | DAYS | 0950 PL | 1000 PL | 1010 TS |
| | | | | | EVES | | | |
| 2/7 | DG | Lasix 40 mg b.i.d. | PO | | NITES | | | |
| | | | | 10 | DAYS | | | 1010 TS |
| | | | | 16 | EVES | | 1545 DG. | |
| 2/7 | DG | Ancef Gm i q6° | IVPB | 06 | NITES | | | 06 MD |
| | | | | 12 | DAYS | | 1215 PL | 1200 TS |
| | | | | 18-24 | EVES | | 18 DG 2345 DG | |
| 2/8 | TS | Nitro Paste 1 inch q8° | Top | 06 | NITES | | | |
| | | | | 14 | DAYS | | | 1410 TS |
| | | | | 22 | EVES | | | |
| 2/8 | TS | Neosporin Ophthalmic Oint. O.D. | Top | | NITES | | | |
| | | | | 10 | DAYS | | | 1010 TS |
| | | | | 22 | EVES | | | |
| | | | | | NITES | | | |
| | | | | | DAYS | | | |
| | | | | | EVES | | | |
| | | | | | NITES | | | |
| | | | | | DAYS | | | |
| | | | | | EVES | | | |
| | | | | | NITES | | | |
| | | | | | DAYS | | | |
| | | | | | EVES | | | |
| | | | | | NITES | | | |
| | | | | | DAYS | | | |
| | | | | | EVES | | | |
| | | | | | NITES | | | |
| | | | | | DAYS | | | |
| | | | | | EVES | | | |
| | | | | | NITES | | | |
| | | | | | DAYS | | | |
| | | | | | EVES | | | |
| | | | | | NITES | | | |
| | | | | | DAYS | | | |
| | | | | | EVES | | | |
| | | | | | NITES | | | |
| | | | | | DAYS | | | |
| | | | | | EVES | | | |
| | | | | | NITES | | | |
| | | | | | DAYS | | | |
| | | | | | EVES | | | |
| | | | | | NITES | | | |
| | | | | | DAYS | | | |
| | | | | | EVES | | | |
| | | | | | NITES | | | |
| | | | | | DAYS | | | |
| | | | | | EVES | | | |

FORM # 570 (REV 4/85)

***Fig. 19-1***

Courtesy Barnes Hospital, St Louis.

the pharmacy (the dose on hand may be listed on the drug label as the contents of a tablet or capsule or the amount of drug dissolved per unit volume of liquid). The amount on hand is the basic unit or quantity of the drug containing the dose on hand (for solid drugs the amount on hand may be 1 tablet or capsule). The amount of liquid on hand may be, for example, a milliliter or liter depending on the capacity of the container and the amount to administer is the actual amount of available medication the nurse will give to the client (always expressed in the same unit as the amount on hand).

### Pediatric Dosages

Calculating children's drug dosages requires caution. A child's metabolism and body size necessitate smaller dosages than adults. Physicians usually calculate safe dosages before ordering medications. When working on nursing units that care for children, the nurse should refer to the pharmacy or drug references to determine safe dosages.

### Older Adult Dosages

As yet there are not special formulas for calculating drug dosages for older adults. Most drug references do not list recommended older adult dosages. Because of changes in the older adult's metabolism and excretion of drugs, the nurse should be cautious when dosages are ordered on the high end of an adult dosage range. Consultation with the physician may help to ensure safe dosage administration.

### Medication Administration

Preparing and administering medications requires accuracy by the nurse. The nurse must pay full attention to the procedure and not try to do other tasks simultaneously. The "five rights" of drug administration include:

1. The *right* drug.
2. The *right* dose.
3. The *right* client.
4. The *right* route.
5. The *right* time.

#### Correct Transcription and Communication of Orders

The nurse or a designated unit secretary writes the physician's complete order on the appropriate medication forms or tickets. (Figs. 19-1 and 19-2). The transcribed order includes client's full name, room, and bed number; date order is written; drug name, dosage; and time and route of administration. Each time a drug dosage is prepared the nurse refers to the medication form or ticket. With unit-dose systems only one transcription is necessary, limiting the opportunity for errors. When transcribing orders, the nurse should be sure names, dosages, and symbols are legible. The nurse rewrites any smudged or illegible transcriptions.

In some institutions a computer printout lists all currently ordered medications with dosage information (Fig. 19-3). Orders are entered directly into the computer, preventing the need for transcription of orders. The same printout may be used to record medications given.

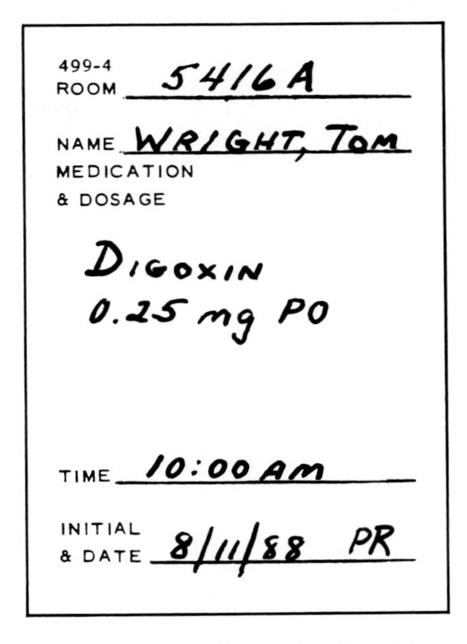


*Fig. 19-2* Sample medication ticket.

A registered nurse checks all transcribed orders against the original order for accuracy and thoroughness. If an order seems incorrect or inappropriate, the nurse consults the physician. The nurse who gives the wrong medication or an incorrect dosage is legally responsible for the error.

#### Accurate Dosage Calculation and Measurement

When measuring liquid drugs, the nurse uses standard measuring receptacles. The procedure for drug measurement is systematic to lessen the chance of error.

#### Correct Administration

To administer a medication safely, the nurse uses aseptic technique and proper procedures in handling and giving medications. Clients must be correctly identified by checking the identification band worn on their wrist. Certain drugs require the nurse to perform assessments at the time of administration, such as assessing heart rate before giving antidysrhythmic medications.

#### Recording

After administering a drug the nurse records it immediately in the appropriate record form (Fig. 19-1; see Fig. 19-3). Information to record includes:

Drug name.
Dosage.
Route of administration.
Time of administration.
Signature and title of nurse administering drug.

Usually this information is recorded on a special medi-

7300-4422-01 THE JEWISH HOSPITAL OF ST. LOUIS
09:00 AM SCHEDULED MEDICATIONS DUE 7300 05/05/89
ISSUED 08:02 AM 05/05/89

7301-1 GIV NGIV

ZANTAC RANITIDINE TAB 150MG,, PO, QD, (05/05/89 09 AM-..) ___ ___

ISORDIL ISOSORBIDE DINITRATE TAB 10MG,, PO, QID, (05/04/89 05PM-..) ___ ___

DIPYRIDAMOLE TAB 75MG,, PO, TID, (05/04/89 05PM-!!) ___ ___

SYNTHROID LEVOTHYROXINE SOD TAB 0'.15MG,, PO,, QD, (05/05/89 09AM-!!) ___ ___

CALCIUM 6 00MG (10 GR) TABLET,, PO, BID, (05/04/89 09PM-..) ___ ___

HYDRALAZINE HCL TAB 100MG,, PO, TID, (05/04/89 05PM-!!) ___ ___

7304-1 GIV NGIV

ZANTAC RANITIDINE TAB 150MG,, PO, BID, (05/01/89 09PM-!!) ___ ___

BEROCCA B-COMPLEX W/C TABLET, PO, QD, (05/02/89 09AM-..) ___ ___

7304-2 GIV NGIV

MULTIVITAMIN TAB 1, PO, QD, (05/02/89 09AM-!! ___ ___

7307-1 GIV NGIV

SYNTHROID LEVOTHYROXINE SOD TAB 0:1MG,, PO, QD, (05/02/89 09AM-!! ___ ___

ZANTAC RANITIDINE TAB 150MG,, PO, BID, (05/01/89 09PM-..) ___ ___

PERICOLACE DOCUSATE SODIUM 100MG & CASANTHRANOL 30MG CAP.. PO, BID, (05/01/89 09PM-!!) ___ ___

7308-1 GIV NGIV

DRUG:*PRINIVIL/LISINOPRIL 10MG TAB, 1 PO, DAILY - EQUIVALENT TO ZESTRIL 10MG., (04/26/89 09AM-!!) ___ ___

ASPIRIN TAB, ENTERIC COATED 300MG,, PO, QD, (04/26/89 09AM-..) ___ ___

COLCHICINE TAB 0.6MG,, PO, QD, (04/26/89 09AM-!!) ___ ___

LANOXIN DIGOXIN TAB 0.125MG,, PO, QD, (04/26/89 09AM-!! ___ ___

DIPYRIDAMOLE TAB 75MG,, PO, TID, (04/26/89 09AM-!!) ___ ___

***Fig. 19-3***

Courtesy Jewish Hospital, St. Louis.

cation flow sheet. In addition, any data pertinent to the client's response or assessment data collected at the time of administration should be recorded either on nurses' notes or appropriate flow sheets.

### Client and Family Teaching

A properly informed client is more likely to take drugs correctly. The nurse provides information about the purpose of medications, their actions, side effects, dosage schedules, and actions to take in case side or toxic effects develop. Special instructional booklets or leaflets are often available as teaching aids.

## ORAL MEDICATIONS

The easiest and most desirable way to administer medications is by mouth. Clients usually are able to self-administer oral drugs with a minimum of problems. The primary contraindications to giving oral medications include the presence of gastrointestinal alterations, the inability of a client to swallow food or fluids, and the use of gastric suction. An important precaution to take when administering any oral preparation is to protect clients from aspiration. Proper positioning prevents the accumulation of liquid or solid material in the back of the throat. A client who has difficulty swallowing should never be forced to take a large amount of liquid.

## GUIDELINES

1. A physician's order is required for all medications to be administered by the nurse (except in states where nurse practice acts allows certain nurses to prescribe in specific situations).
2. Assess client's need for and response to drug therapy. The assessment includes: medical history, history of drug allergies, medication history (including over-the-counter drugs), diet history, client's attitude about and understanding of drug therapy, and a review of client's current condition.
3. Be informed about each drug ordered including drug action and purpose, normal dosage and route, time interval for action, side effects, and nursing implications for administration and monitoring.
4. Check all transcribed orders carefully against the physician's order. Any smudged or illegible transcriptions must be rewritten.
5. Take time to calculate drug dosages accurately. Standard measuring receptacles should be used in preparing liquid medications. Calculate dosages while preparing the drug.
6. Use aseptic technique in preparing medications and handling all equipment.
7. Respect a client's right to refuse a medication.
8. Respect the client's right to be informed of the drug's name, purpose, action, and potential undesired effects.
9. When preparing a dosage always check the label of the drug container with the order form or medicine ticket three times: before removing medicine from drawer or shelf; as the amount of drug ordered is removed from the container; and before returning the container to storage.
10. Administer only medications you have prepared. Never administer a drug prepared by another nurse.
11. To avoid common errors (1) do not give medications from containers with labels that are unmarked or illegible; (2) do not give medications that are cloudy or have changed color; (3) discard a liquid medication if sediment can be seen in the bottom of the medication container; and (4) always check the expiration date of a drug.
12. Identify a client before administering a medication by checking the name on the medication ticket or form with the client's identification bracelet, and ask client to state name. Replace any smudged or illegible bracelets.
13. Always determine whether a medication should be given. The physician can make an error. The client's condition may change before the drug is given.
14. Give medications within 30 min of the time ordered to ensure that therapeutic blood levels are maintained. Stat and preoperative medications should be given at the specific times ordered. Insulin should be given at a precise interval before a meal.
15. Never record a medication before administering it.
16. Institute necessary observations and measures before drug administration (e.g., assessing blood pressure before giving an antihypertensive; withholding a cardiotonic drug if the pulse rate is below 60).
17. Never return an unused medication to a container; discard it.
18. Do not leave medications at a client's bedside without a physician's order.
19. After administering medications record the procedure immediately. Also note client's response including any undesired effects. Chart why a certain medication is refused.
20. Monitor the client during the period after drug administration for any serious side effects.
21. When an error is made, acknowledge it immediately. The nurse has an ethical and professional responsibility to report the error to the client's physician. Measures to counteract the effects of the error may be necessary.

# SKILL 19-1 Administering Oral Medications

The nurse usually prepares oral medications in the medication room or at the unit dose cart. When preparing medications for more than one client at a time, the nurse must be very careful about preparing the right dose for each client.

Oral medications come in two forms: solid and liquid. However, there are various types of solid and liquid preparations. The following tips ensure proper oral medication preparation:

1. Give an adequate amount of fluid with tablets and capsules.
2. If appropriate, instruct the client to chew the drug before swallowing.
3. Mix powdered medications with liquids just before administration.
4. Give effervescent powders and tablets to the client immediately after they are dissolved.
5. Never crush enteric-coated tablets or gelatin capsules.
6. Do not give fluids after a client takes a syrup. Fluids will wash the medication away.

## Purposes

1. Provide safe, effective drug therapy with minimal complications.
2. Administer medications with minimal discomfort.
3. Provide a simple route for drug administration that clients can easily learn.

### PREREQUISITE KNOWLEDGE

1. Principles of medical asepsis.
2. Principles of drug preparation.
3. Pharmacokinetics of drugs being administered.
4. Drug dosage calculation.
5. Principles of recording and reporting.

### PREREQUISITE SKILLS

1. Basic handwashing technique (Chapter 37).
2. Measurement of vital signs (Chapter 12).

## Procedure 19-1

| Steps | Rationale |
|---|---|
| **Assessment** | |
| 1. Gather information pertinent to the drug(s) ordered: action, purpose, normal dosage and route, common side effects, time of onset and peak action, nursing implications. | Allows nurse to anticipate effects of drug on client and to observe client's response. Also allows nurse to judge appropriateness of therapy as client's condition changes. |
| 2. Assess for any contraindications to client receiving oral medication: is client able to swallow? is client suffering from nausea/vomiting? is client diagnosed as having bowel inflammation or reduced peristalsis? has client had recent gastrointestinal surgery? does client have gastric suction? | Alterations in gastrointestinal function interfere with drug distribution, absorption, and excretion. Medication can be suctioned from gastrointestinal tract before it can be absorbed. |
| 3. Assess client's medical history, history of allergies, medication history, or diet history. | These factors can influence how certain drugs act. Information also reflects client's need for medications. |
| 4. Consider client's age. | Physiologic changes of aging influence how oral medications are distributed, absorbed, and excreted. Oral route is preferred in children. Solid preparations, however, are not recommended until child is 5 yr old and capable of chewing and swallowing safely. |
| 5. Assess client's knowledge regarding health and medications received. | Determines client's need for drug education. Also assists in identifying client's adherence to drug therapy at home. Assessment may reveal drug use problems (e.g., abuse, addiction, or dependence). |
| 6. Assess client's preferences for fluids. | Offering fluids during drug administration is excellent way to increase client's fluid intake. |
| **Nursing Diagnosis** | |
| 1. Cluster data to reveal actual or potential nursing diagnoses: | |
| a. Knowledge deficit regarding drug therapy: related to inexperience, cognitive impairment. | Nurse educates client or family member while administering medication. |
| b. Impaired physical mobility: related to upper extremity weakness. | Influences degree of assistance required by client in taking medication. |

| Steps | Rationale |
|---|---|
| c. Impaired swallowing: related to neuromuscular impairment. | May result in choice of different route of administration. Extra caution needed to prevent aspiration. |
| d. Noncompliance regarding drug regimen: related to client's health beliefs or limited resources. | Poses implications for client/family teaching and discharge planning. |
| **Planning** | |
| 1. Develop individualized goals for client based on nursing diagnoses: | |
| a. Prevent injury from aspiration. | Positioning client properly prevents aspiration. |
| b. Promote ease in swallowing. | Administration techniques can make swallowing easy for client. |
| c. Promote optimal absorption and distribution of medication. | Proper administration techniques ensures drug efficacy. |
| d. Client understands purpose of drug therapy. | Ultimately will help client learn to self-administer drugs correctly. |
| 2. Prepare needed supplies and equipment: | |
| a. Medication cards, computer printout, or record form | |
| b. Medication cart or tray | |
| c. Disposable medication cups | |
| d. Glass of water, juice or preferred liquid | |
| e. Drinking straw | |
| f. Mortar and pestle (optional) | Used to crush tablets for clients who have difficulty swallowing. |
| g. Paper towels | |
| 3. Gather medication cards or forms that list all drugs to be given to client at prescribed time. | Cards and forms contain transcribed orders listing drugs client should receive. |
| 4. Check accuracy and completeness of each card or form with physician's written medication order. Check client's name, drug name and dosage, route of administration, and time for administration. | Physician's order is most reliable source and only legal record of drugs client is to receive. (Orders should be checked at least every 24 hr.) |
| 5. Recopy any card or portion of form that is illegible. | Forms that are soiled or illegible can be source of drug error. |
| **Implementation** | |
| 1. Preparing medications: | |
| a. Wash hands. | Reduces transfer of microorganisms from nurse's hands to medications and equipment. |
| b. Arrange medication tray and cups in medicine room or move medication cart to position outside client's room. | Organization of equipment saves time and reduces error. |
| c. Unlock medicine drawer or cart. (Narcotics are stored in a double lockbox.) | Medications are safeguarded when locked in cabinet or cart. |
| d. Prepare medications for one client at a time. Keep medication tickets or forms for each client together. | Prevents preparation errors. |
| e. Select correct drug from stock supply or unit dose drawer. Compare label of medication with medication form, card, or printout (Fig. 19-4). | Reading label against transcribed order reduces error. |

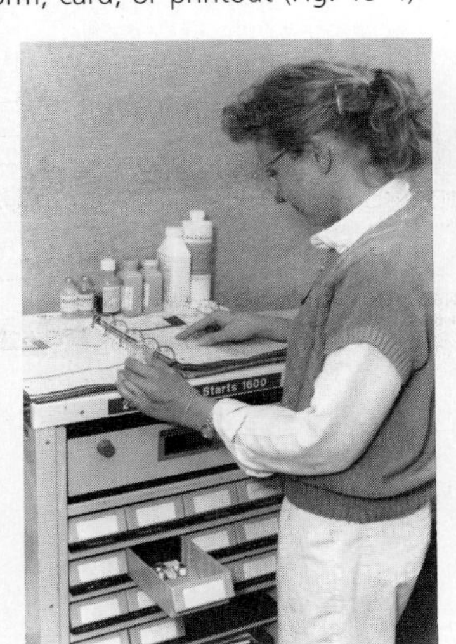


***Fig. 19-4***

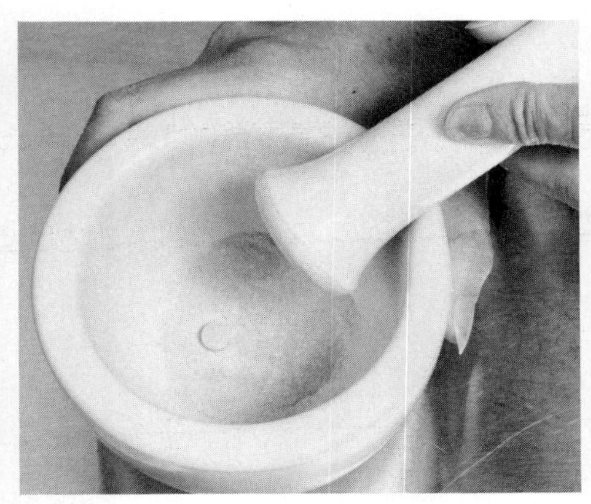

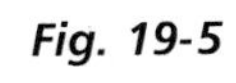

***Fig. 19-5***

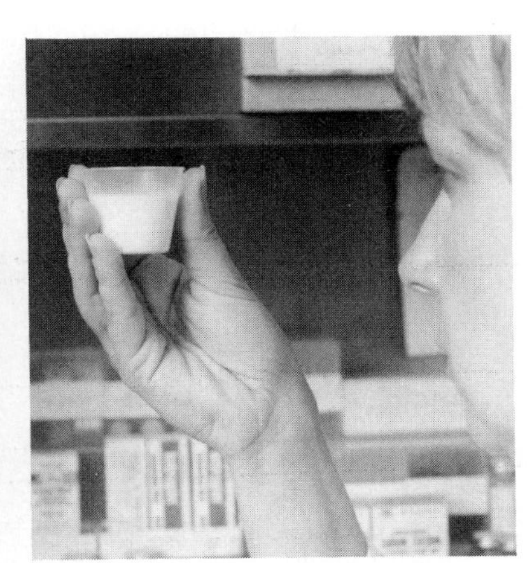

***Fig. 19-6***

| Steps | Rationale |
|---|---|
| f. Calculate correct drug dosage. Take time. Double check calculation. | Calculation is more accurate when information from drug label is at hand. |
| g. *To prepare tablet or capsules from bottle,* pour required number into bottle cap and transfer medications to medication cup. Do not touch medicines with fingers. Extra tablets or capsules may be returned to bottle. | Drugs are very expensive; avoid waste. |
| h. *To prepare unit dose tablets or capsules,* place packaged tablet or capsule directly into medicine cup. (Do not remove wrapper). | Wrapper maintains cleanliness of medications and identifies drug name and dosage. |
| i. All tablets or capsules given to client at same time may be placed in one cup except for those requiring preadministration assessments (e.g., pulse rate or blood pressure). | Keeping medications that require preadministration assessments separate from others makes it easier for the nurse to withold drugs as necessary. |
| j. If client has difficulty swallowing, grind tablets in mortar with pestle (Fig. 19-5). Place tablet in bottom of mortar and mix. Continue to crush fragments of tablet until smooth powder remains or place tablet between two medication cups and grind with a blunt instrument. Mix tablet in small amount of soft food, such as custard or applesauce. | Large tablets can be difficult to swallow. Ground tablet mixed with palatable soft food is usually easy to swallow. |
| k. Prepare liquids (Fig. 19-6). | |
| ▪ Remove bottle cap from container and place cap upside down. | Prevents contamination of inside of cap. |
| ▪ Hold bottle with label against palm of hand while pouring. | Spilled liquid will not soil or fade label. |
| ▪ Hold medication cup at eye level and fill to desired level on scale. (Scale should be even with fluid level at its surface or base of meniscus, not edges.) | Ensures accuracy of measurement. |
| ▪ Discard excess liquid in cup into sink. Wipe lip of bottle with paper towel. | Prevents contamination of bottle's contents and prevents bottle cap from sticking. |
| l. When preparing narcotic, check narcotic record for previous drug count and compare with supply available. | Controlled substance laws require careful monitoring of dispensed narcotics. |
| ▪ Narcotics are kept in specially designed plastic containers that are sectioned and numbered (Fig. 19-7). Remove the next available tablet and drop it in a cup. Complete necessary information on narcotic form and sign. | |
| m. Compare medication form, card, or printout with prepared drug and container. | Reading label second time reduces error. |
| n. Return stock containers or unused unit-dose medications to shelf or drawer and read label again. | Third check of label reduces administration errors. |
| o. Place medications and cards, form, or printout together on tray or cart. | Drugs are labeled at all times for identification. |
| p. Do not leave drugs unattended. | Nurse is responsible for safekeeping of drugs. |

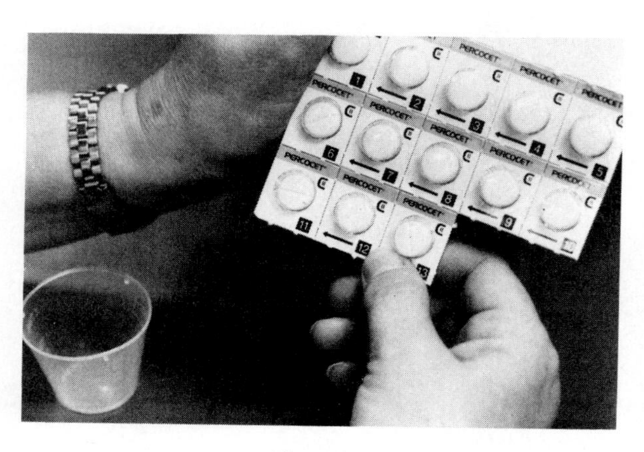

*Fig. 19-7*

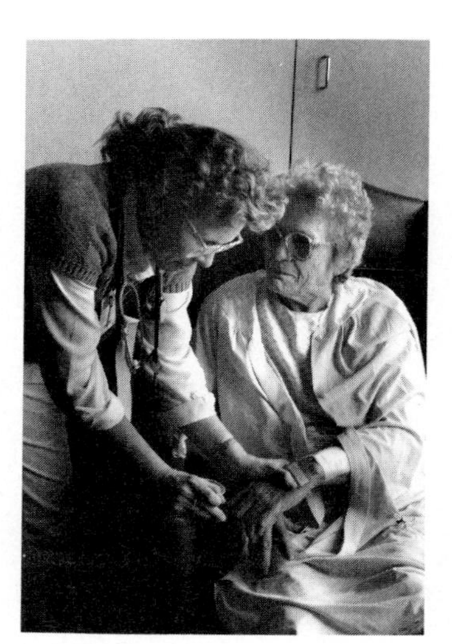

*Fig. 19-8*

| Steps | Rationale |
|---|---|
| 2. Administering medications: | |
| a. Take medications to client at correct time. | Medications are administered within 30 min before or after prescribed time to ensure intended therapeutic effect. Stat or single-order medications should be given at time ordered. |
| b. Identify client by comparing name on card, printout form, or with name on client's identification bracelet. Ask client to state name (Fig. 19-8). | Identification bracelets are made at time of client's admission and are most reliable source of identification. Replace any missing or faded identification bracelets. |
| c. Perform necessary preadministration assessment for specific medications (e.g., blood pressure or pulse). | Assessment data determine whether specific medications should be given at that time. |
| d. Explain purpose of each medication and its action to client. Allow client to ask any questions about drugs. | Client has right to be informed, and client's understanding of purpose of each medication will improve compliance with drug therapy. |
| e. Assist client to sitting or side-lying position. | Sitting position prevents aspiration during swallowing. |
| f. Administer drugs properly: | |
| ▪ Client may wish to hold solid medications in hand or cup before placing in mouth. | Client can become familiar with medications by seeing each drug. |
| ▪ Offer full glass of water or juice with drugs to be swallowed. Give cold carbonated water if available. | Choice of fluid promotes client's comfort and can improve fluid intake. Carbonated water helps passage of tablet through esophagus. |
| ▪ For sublingual administered drugs, have client place medication under tongue and allow it to dissolve completely. Caution client against swallowing. | Drug is absorbed through blood vessels of undersurface of tongue. If swallowed, drug is destroyed by gastric juices or so rapidly detoxified by liver that therapeutic blood levels are not attained. |
| ▪ For buccal administered drugs, have client place medication in mouth against mucous membranes of the cheek until it dissolves. | Buccal medications act locally on mucosa or systemically as they are swallowed in saliva. |
| ▪ Mix powdered medications with liquids at bedside and give to client to drink. | When prepared in advance, powdered drug forms may thicken and even harden, making swallowing difficult. |
| ▪ Caution client against chewing or swallowing lozenges. | Drug acts through slow absorption through oral mucosa, not gastric mucosa. |
| ▪ Give effervescent powders and tablets immediately after dissolving. | Effervescence helps improve unpleasant taste of drug and often has therapeutic value for gastrointestinal problems. |
| g. If client is unable to hold medications, place medication cup to the lips and gently introduce each drug into the mouth, one at a time. Do not rush. | Prevents contamination of medications. Administering single tablet or capsule eases swallowing and prevents aspiration. |
| h. If tablet or capsule falls to the floor, discard it and repeat preparation. | Drug is contaminated when it touches floor. |
| i. Stay until client has completely swallowed each medication. Ask client to open the mouth if uncertain whether client swallowed medication. | Nurse assumes responsibility for ensuring that client receives ordered dosage. If left unattended, client may not take dose or may save drugs, causing risk to health. |
| j. For highly acidic medications (e.g., aspirin) offer client nonfat snack (e.g., crackers). | Reduces gastric irritation. |
| k. Assist client in returning to comfortable position. | Maintains client's comfort |
| l. Dispose of soiled supplies and wash hands. | Reduces transmission of microorganisms. |
| m. Return medication cards, forms, or printouts to appropriate file for next administration time. | Cards, forms, and printouts are used as reference for when next dosage is due. Loss can lead to administration error. |
| n. Replenish stock such as cups and straws, return cart to medicine room, and clean work area. | Clean working space assists other staff in completing duties efficiently. |
| **Evaluation** | |
| 1. Return within 30 min to evaluate client's response to medications. | By monitoring client's response nurse assesses drug's therapeutic benefit and can detect onset of side effects or allergic reactions. |
| 2. Ask client or family member to explain purpose, action, dosage, and potential side effects of drug. | Determines level of knowledge gained by client and family. |
| ***Expected outcomes*** | |
| 1. Client may show improvement in condition (e.g., relief of pain, regular heart rate, stable blood pressure). | Drug has had time to exert therapeutic action. |
| 2. Client denies any gastrointestinal discomfort or symptoms of alterations. | Oral medications can irritate gastrointestinal mucosa. |
| 3. Client explains purpose of medication. | Demonstrates understanding of drug therapy. |

| Steps | Rationale |
|---|---|
| ***Unexpected outcomes*** | |
| 1. Client exhibits side effects common to medication. | Drugs cause secondary effects that can be harmful or injurious. |
| 2. Client exhibits toxic drug effects. | Result of prolonged intake of high doses of medications. |
| 3. Client exhibits allergic reaction to drug with symptoms such as urticaria, rash, pruritis, rhinitis, and wheezing. | Client sensitizes immunologically to constituents of drug. |
| ***Recording and Reporting*** | |
| 1. Record actual time each drug was administered on the medication record. Include your initials or signature (Fig. 19-1). | Prompt documentation prevents errors such as repeated doses. Nurse's signature establishes accountability for administering the drug. |
| 2. If drug is withheld, record reason in nurses' notes. Circle time the drug normally would have been given in the medication record. | Provides documented explanation for why routine order was not administered. |

## Follow-up Activities

| Steps | Rationale |
|---|---|
| 1. With onset of toxic effects or allergic reaction, hold further doses and notify physician. | Further administration of medication can be fatal to client. |
| 2. With onset of side effects notify physician. | Alerts physician to observe for more serious reactions should therapy continue. |
| 3. Assess further client's or family member's knowledge of medications and guidelines for drug safety. | Further education may be necessary to prepare client to self-administer medications at home. |

## Special Considerations

- Clients with neuromuscular disorders, esophageal strictures, lesions of mouth, and who are unresponsive or comatose cannot swallow. Clients with nasogastric tube or gastrostomy tubes to suction are generally NPO.
- Clients with drug allergies should wear special identification bracelet that is color coded and lists drugs to which client is allergic.
- Common physiologic changes of aging include: loss of elasticity in oral mucosa making clients susceptible to drugs that cause dry mouth; delayed esophageal clearance impairs swallowing; reduction in gastric acidity and stomach peristalsis, which increases client's susceptibility to highly acidic drugs; reduced colon motility slowing drug excretion. Rinse the client's oral cavity frequently with tepid water, floss daily, and brush gently. Administer a full glass of water with medications aids passage of the drug. Taking medications with a nonfat snack will reduce gastric distress.
- Be sure to give all of a drug.
- Liquid medications packaged in single-dose cups need not be poured into medicine cups.
- An accurate measuring technique is drawing small doses of liquids into a syringe.
- When administering oral medications to children follow these tips:
  a. Liquid forms are safer to swallow to avoid aspiration.
  b. Carbonated beverages poured over finely crushed ice reduce nausea.
  c. When mixing drugs with tasty flavorings, such as syrup, use only a small amount.
  d. When administering liquid drugs, a spoon, plastic cup, or oral syringe (without needle) is useful.
- When giving oral drugs through a nasogastric tube:
  a. Be sure a solid drug form can be crushed (compressed tablets can almost always be crushed).
  b. Crush any tablets or capsules into a fine powder for better absorption.
  c. Soft, gelatin capsules should be dissolved in a cup of water before administering.
  d. Place powdered drug in a cup and add 20-30 ml warm water. Administer following agency guidelines for bolus-tube feedings (Chapter 33).
  e. Follow medications with at least 60 cc $H_2O$ or Coca-Cola (Metheny and others, 1988).

## Teaching Considerations

- Instruct client on specific information pertaining to drug regimen (purpose, action, dosage, dosage intervals, side effects, foods to avoid or take with drugs).
- All clients should learn the basic guidelines for drug safety.
  1. Keep each drug in its original, labeled container.
  2. Be sure labels are legible.
  3. Discard any outdated medications.
  4. Always finish a prescribed drug unless otherwise instructed. Never save a drug for future illnesses.
  5. Dispose of drugs in a sink or toilet. Do not place drugs in the trash within reach of children.
  6. Do not give a family member a drug prescribed for another.
  7. Refrigerate medications that require it.
  8. Read labels carefully and follow all instructions.

## SKILL 19-2 Helping Clients with Self-Medication

Many clients who are on drug regimens at home fail to take medications correctly. Poor compliance with drug therapy exists for several reasons: clients stop taking medications once symptoms subside; regimens involving multiple drugs are confusing; the consequences of not taking medications are poorly understood; prescriptions are costly; and many clients fear addiction. Generally clients are poorly educated about their drug therapy. A large portion of clients who do not comply are the elderly who frequently suffer sensory and mobility problems that interfere with the ability to prepare and take medications correctly. In a survey conducted by the *American Journal of Nursing,* 25% of the 1,225 nurses who responded reported that 50% of their clients did not follow instructions in taking medications (Moree, 1985).

The following skill is actually an outline to help prepare clients for following drug regimens in the home.

### Purpose

1. Reduce complications resulting from poor adherence with drug dosage schedules.
2. Promote client understanding of the purpose of their medications.
3. Simplify drug regimens.
4. Provide a means by which clients can easily identify or recognize the medicines they take.

### PREREQUISITE KNOWLEDGE

1. Principles of teaching and learning
2. Principles of communication

### PREREQUISITE SKILLS

1. Perform physical assessment of sensory function and motor coordination (Chapter 13)

## Procedure 19-2

| Steps | Rationale |
|---|---|
| **Assessment** | |
| 1. Assess client's knowledge regarding drug therapy: names of drugs, purpose or action, daily dosages and times taken, side effects to expect, what to do if problems occur. | Reveals client's level of understanding and need for instruction. |
| 2. Assess family members' knowledge of drug therapy: why client takes drug, daily dosages, side effects, what to do if problems arise. | Family members or support persons are important resources to help clients comply with therapy. |
| 3. Assess client's sensory function: sight, hearing, touch, physical coordination. | Client's sensory impairments create need for specific types of teaching strategies so that nurse can be sure clients have capacity to learn. Sensory and coordination deficits may impair client's ability to see medications, open prescription bottles, and read labels. |
| 4. Assess client's ability to ambulate and tolerate exercise. | For clients living alone mobility problems may interfere with ability to get to pharmacy. |
| 5. Assess reading ability by having client read teaching pamphlet. | Nurse will get general impression of how easily client reads. |
| 6. Assess client's belief in need for drug therapy. Consider cultural values, religious beliefs, personal experiences with medications, significant others' values about drugs. | Factors that influence client's willingness to follow drug regimen. |
| 7. Check client's prescribed drugs: has more than one physician prescribed medications? are medications obviously inappropriate? are labels clearly marked? are time schedules confusing? do different drugs look alike? does client store several medications together? | Assists nurse in determining sources of confusion affecting client's compliance. |
| **Nursing Diagnosis** | |
| 1. Cluster data to reveal actual or potential nursing diagnoses: | |
| a. Knowledge deficit regarding drug regimen: related to incomplete or poor instruction. | Nurse can plan teaching strategies according to client's learning needs and capacity to learn. Methods can be instituted to make drug schedules easier to understand and follow. Instruction must also focus on implications on client's health when drug therapies are not followed. |

| Steps | Rationale |
|---|---|
| b. Sensory alteration (visual or tactile): related to altered status of sensory organs, neurologic impairment. | Nurse makes adjustments in instructions and techniques to help client prepare drugs correctly. |
| c. Impaired physical mobility: related to weakened grasp. | See above. |
| d. Noncompliance with drug therapy: related to conflicting values. | Client may be unwilling to comply unless value is seen in taking medications. |

## Planning

| Steps | Rationale |
|---|---|
| 1. Develop individualized goals for client based on nursing diagnoses. Client will be able to:<br>a. Explain purpose of each medication and why it is beneficial.<br>b. Explain common side effects and measures to alleviate them.<br>c. Discuss when it is important to notify physician about drug problems.<br>d. Discuss what to do when dosages are missed.<br>e. Demonstrate preparing a drug from prescription bottle.<br>f. Read each label and explain when each drug should be taken. | Teaching plan must provide content that will enable client to choose and follow drug regimen. |
| 2. Prepare environment for teaching session:<br>a. Select room that is well lit.<br>b. Provide comfortable seating.<br>c. Be sure client is close to and can see nurse clearly.<br>d. Control sources of noise and distractions. | Room environment should be designed to minimize existing sensory alterations. Comfortable environment free of distractions promotes client's attention. |
| 3. Prepare teaching materials:<br>a. Written materials printed in large bold letters.<br>b. Illustrations of safety guidelines.<br>c. Written schedules or individualized instruction sheets. | Teaching materials should be designed to meet client's learning needs as well as client's capacity to learn. |
| 4. Be sure clients who wear glasses or hearing aids do so during teaching session. | Use of glasses or hearing aids increases client's sensory perception and increases likelihood of attending to teaching session and understanding content. |
| 5. Consult with physician to review medications client is receiving and to simplify regimen if possible. | Review of medications can help minimize risk of drug interactions from multiple medications. Simplification of regimen can improve likelihood of compliance. |
| 6. Arrange teaching time so family members may participate. | Family can serve as positive resources to client. |

## Implementation

| Steps | Rationale |
|---|---|
| 1. Present information clearly and concisely:<br>a. Face learner, be sure nurse's face is illuminated.<br>b. Use short sentences and speak in slow, low-pitched voice. | Client with hearing or visual problem will be able to see nurse's expressions and hear voice more clearly. |
| c. Provide descriptions in understandable terms. | Prevents confusion of terminology. |
| 2. Provide frequent pauses so that client can ask questions and express understanding of content. | Increases client's participation in learning process. Ongoing feedback assures nurse that client is acquiring information. |
| 3. Discuss following content: purpose of drugs and their positive effects, how drug works and why it helps, dosage schedules and rationale, how dosage schedules can be made to fit client's daily routines, common side effects, what to do to relieve side effects, what to do if dose is missed, when to call for problems, who to call with problems, drug safety guidelines, implications when medications are not taken. | Content presented, if learned, will improve client's ability to self-medicate correctly. Individualizing dosage schedules makes it easier for client to comply. |
| 4. Provide frequent short teaching sessions. | Improves client's attention and retention of information discussed. |
| 5. Provide client with special charts, diagrams, or learning aids (Fig. 19-9). | Simplest mechanism for reminding clients of when to take medications will improve compliance. |
| 6. Offer assistance as client practices preparing medications: "Let's prepare the medications you will take with your meals." "Prepare the medicines you first take in the morning." | Nurse can observe client's ability to read labels correctly and prepare all medications for prescribed times. |
| 7. Have pharmacy provide clear, large-print labels for medication bottles if appropriate. | Improves client's ability to read and follow directions. |
| 8. Make arrangements for pharmacy to deliver medications at home if client unable to reach facility. | Availability of drugs influences compliance. |

| Steps | Rationale |
|---|---|

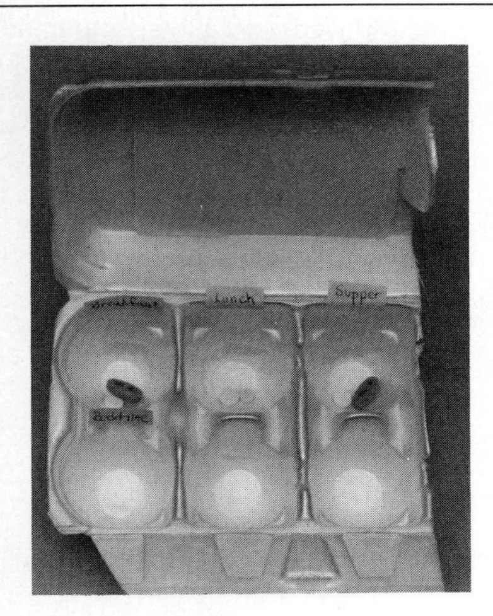

***Fig. 19-9***
Egg carton used to organize drug dosages.

## Evaluation

| Steps | Rationale |
|---|---|
| 1. Have client or family prepare dosages for all prescribed medications client is to take for day. | Measures client's understanding of dosages and schedules. |
| 2. Have client and family explain information pertinent to each drug, side effects, safety guidelines, etc. | Feedback measures client's cognitive learning. |
| 3. Offer opportunity for additional clarifying questions. | Minimizes any remaining confusion or misunderstanding. |

***Expected outcomes***

| Steps | Rationale |
|---|---|
| 1. Client is able to prepare dosages for all medications to be taken in 24-hr period. | Evaluation is based upon established learning objectives. |
| 2. Client correctly describes all information pertinent to each drug, drug safety, and preventive care. | |

***Unexpected outcomes***

| Steps | Rationale |
|---|---|
| 1. Client makes errors in preparing medications. | May be result of misunderstanding or sensory deficits. |
| 2. Client is unable to explain all information discussed in teaching session. | Requires additional instruction. |

## Recording and Reporting

| Steps | Rationale |
|---|---|
| 1. Document instruction provided to client in nurses' notes. | Documentation of teaching provides continuity of care when other nurses attempt to resume teaching or reinforce client's learning. |

## Follow-up Activities

| Steps | Rationale |
|---|---|
| 1. After client returns home, check if medication regimens are followed. In clinic or physician's office count pills remaining in bottles. | Once at home client is influenced by various factors that can interfere with self-medication routines (e.g., conflicting work or social schedules, irregular meal times). |

## Special Considerations

- Elderly commonly have decreased sensitivity to light and inability to adapt to glare. Visual and hearing acuity declines. Elderly client may have difficulty understanding language since high-frequency tones are often less perceptible. Elderly may have reduced sensation in extremities.
- Some clients are illiterate. Some commercially prepared booklets contain instructions that are too complex or contain medical jargon.
- Nurse should be sure client's glasses are well fitted and have current corrective lenses. Hearing aid should be fitted with working battery (Chapter 10).
- Teaching approach must be individualized for each client. Put physician's phone number on label placed on phone. Guidelines for drug safety include: keep each drug in original labeled container, be sure labels are legible, discard outdated drugs, discard unused portions of drugs prescribed for specific illness, dispose of medicines in sink or toilet, keep drugs away from children's reach, do not give family member drug prescribed for another person, refrigerate medications as required, read labels carefully and follow instructions.

- If difficult to plan separate teaching session instruct client while administering medications.
- If client wears glasses, instruct client to be sure to wear glasses while preparing medications at home.

## Teaching Considerations

- Examples of learning aids: homemade calendars for each week that contain plastic bags containing medications to take at specific times, egg cartons divided into color-coded sections with medications for day, clock faces for clients who cannot read or see clearly, color-coding for drug types, (e.g., blue for sedative, red for pain pill).

## Home Care Considerations

- Assess client's, family's, or primary care giver's knowledge of medication use as prescribed for the client only and of the need to provide proper storage of medications. Medications stored in the bathroom cabinet are at risk of damage from steam formed by tap water at the sink, bath tub, or shower.
- Recommend the use of devices for reminding the client to take medications as ordered by the physician. The devices may be purchased, e.g., specially marked one-day pill boxes, or may be made by the nurse, e.g., handmade wall charts.
- Establish a unified medication record, including prescribed drugs, over-the-counter drugs, and home or folk preparations.
- Assess presence of a language barrier and the availability of adequate translators.

---

**BIBLIOGRAPHY**

Allen MD: Drug therapy in the elderly, Am J Nurs 80:1474, 1980.

Bernal H: In-home medication checks with diabetics, Home health care nurses 6(5):14, 1988.

Birdsall C, Uretsky S: How do I administer medication by NG? Am J Nurs 84:1259, 1984.

Brock A: Self-administration of drugs in the elderly: nursing responsibilities, J Gerontol Nurs 6:402, 1980.

Bulau J: Clinical policies and procedures for home health care, Rockville, Md, 1986, Aspen Publishers, Inc.

Davis NM, Cohen MR: Learning from mistakes: 20 tips for avoiding medication errors, Nursing '82, 12:65, March, 1982.

Ebersole P, Hess P: Toward healthy aging, ed 3, St. Louis, 1989, The CV Mosby Co.

Giving medications, Nursing Photobook, Springhouse, Pa, 1983, Intermed Communications Inc.

Govoni L, Hayes J: Drugs and nursing implications, New York, 1980, Appleton-Century-Crofts.

Hayes JE: Normal changes in aging and nursing implications of drug therapy, Nurs Clin North Am 17:253, 1982.

Metheny N, et al.: Effect of feeding tube properties and three irrigants on clogging rates, Nurs Res 37(3):165, 1988.

Moree NA: Nurses speak out on patients and drug regimens, Am J Nurs 85:51, 1985.

Potter PA, Perry AG: Basic nursing, St Louis, 1987, The CV Mosby Co.

Potter PA, Perry AG: Fundamentals of nursing: concepts, process, and practice, ed 2, St. Louis, 1989, The CV Mosby Co.

Scipien G, et al.: Comprehensive pediatric nursing, New York, 1986, McGraw-Hill Book Co.

Shlafer M, Marieb E: The nurse, pharmacology, drug therapy, Menlo Park Calif, 1989, Addison-Wesley Publishing Co.

Simonson W: Medications and the elderly: a guide for promoting proper use, Rockville, Md, 1984, Aspen Publishers, Inc.

Smith S, Duell D: Clinical nursing skills, Los Altos, Calif, 1985, National Nursing Review.

Spencer RT, et al.: Clinical pharmacology and nursing management, Philadelphia, 1983, JB Lippincott Co.

Walsh J, Persons C, Wieck L: Manual of home health care nursing, Philadelphia, 1987, JB Lippincott Co.

Whaley LF, Wong DL: Nursing care of infants and children, ed 3, St. Louis, 1987, The CV Mosby Co.

# 20

# TOPICAL MEDICATIONS

## OBJECTIVES

*Mastery of content in this chapter will enable the nurse to:*

- Define key terms.
- Explain factors influencing the type of effects caused by topical medications.
- Identify safety precautions used in administering different topical medications.
- Identify guidelines for administering topical medications.
- Identify methods used to apply topical medications.
- Differentiate types of topical administrations that require sterile technique and those that require clean medical aseptic technique.
- Compare different methods used to administer skin applications.
- Apply skin applications, correctly.
- Administer eyedrops and ointment, eardrops, and nosedrops correctly.
- Instruct clients in proper use of metered dose inhalers.
- Administer vaginal suppository or cream and rectal suppositories correctly.
- Instruct clients on self-administration of topical medications.

## KEY TERMS

*Adrenergic drug*
*Anaphylaxis*
*Anesthesia*
*Antianginal drug*
*Cerumen*
*Compound*
*Cycloplegic*
*Dermatitis*
*Dermatologic*
*Eczema*
*Glaucoma*
*Lotion*
*Mydriasis*
*Nares*
*Nasal*
*Nitroglycerine*
*Overdose (OD)*
*Ointment*
*Ophthalmic*
*Orifice*
*O.S.*
*Otic*
*O.U.*
*Pruritis*
*Suppository*
*Suspension*
*Sympathomimetic*
*Topical*
*Transdermal*
*Vertigo*

## SKILLS

***20-1*** Administering Skin Applications
***20-2*** Administering Eyedrops and Ointment
***20-3*** Administering Eardrops
***20-4*** Administering Nasal Instillations
***20-5*** Using Metered Dose Inhalers
***20-6*** Administering Vaginal Instillations
***20-7*** Administering Rectal Suppositories
***20-8*** Administering Ear Irrigations

Topical administration of medications involves applying drugs locally to skin, mucous membranes, or tissue membranes. This method avoids puncturing skin and lessens the risk of infection and tissue injury, as compared to injections. The client experiences few gastrointestinal disturbances. The risk of serious side effects is generally low because topical agents primarily act locally. However, serious systemic effects can occur.

The nurse applies medications to the skin by painting, spraying, or spreading medication over an area, applying moist dressings, soaking body parts in solution, or giving medicated baths (Chapter 6). There are also adhesive-backed medicated discs that apply neatly to the skin to provide sustained continuous release of medication over several hours or days. Systemic effects from topical agents can occur if the skin is thin, if drug concentration is high, or if contact with the skin is prolonged.

Drugs applied to membranes such as the cornea or rectal mucosa are absorbed quickly because of the membrane's vascularity. When drug concentrations are high, there can be systemic effects, such as bradycardia following atropine instillation to the eye. Mucous and other tissue membranes differ in their sensitivity to medications. The cornea of the eye, for example, is extremely sensitive to any chemical. Clients commonly experience burning sensations during administration of eye and nose drops. Medications are generally less irritating to vaginal or rectal mucosa.

The nurse uses several methods for applying medications to mucous membranes and tissues:

1. Direct application of liquid—eye drops, gargling, swabbing the throat.
2. Inserting drug into body cavity—suppository insertion into rectum or vagina.
3. Instillation of fluid into body cavity—ear drops, nose drops, bladder and rectal instillation (fluid is retained).
4. Irrigation of body cavity—flushing eye, ear, vagina, bladder, or rectum with medicated fluid (fluid is not retained).
5. Spraying—instillation into nose or throat.
6. Inhalation of medicated aerosol spray—distributes medication throughout the tracheobronchial airways.

### GUIDELINES

1. Use aseptic technique when applying medications directly to skin surfaces or membranes.
2. Carefully inspect condition of skin or membranes over which medications are to be applied before administration.
3. Know client's allergies, particularly to preservatives or fragrances in topical drugs.
4. Know potential local and systemic effects of all topically applied medications.
5. If clients are mentally and physically able, instruct them on self-administration techniques.

### PREREQUISITE KNOWLEDGE

1. Principles of medical asepsis.
2. Principles of drug preparation.
3. Anatomy and physiology of body parts being treated.
4. Principles of teaching and learning.
5. Pharmacokinetics of drugs being administered.

### PREREQUISITE SKILLS

1. Proper handwashing techniques (Chapter 37).
2. Physical assessment of body part being treated (Chapter 13).
3. Application of sterile gloves (skin applications only) (Chapter 38).

## *SKILL 20-1* *Administering Skin Applications*

Because many locally applied drugs such as lotions, pastes, and ointments can create systemic and local effects, the nurse should apply these drugs using gloves and applicators. Sterile technique is important, especially if the client has an open wound.

Skin encrustations and dead tissues harbor microorganisms and block contact of medications with the tissues to be treated. Simply applying new medications over previously applied drugs does little to prevent infection or offer therapeutic benefit. The nurse cleans the skin thoroughly before applying medications by washing the area gently with soap and water, soaking an involved site, or locally debriding tissue.

Each type of medication, whether an ointment, lotion, or powder, should be applied a specific way to ensure proper penetration and absorption. For example, the nurse applies lotions and creams by smearing them lightly onto the skin's surface, whereas powders are dusted lightly over affected areas. Before and during any skin application the nurse assesses the skin thoroughly.

### Purposes

1. Maintain or improve hydration of skin layers.
2. Protect skin surfaces.
3. Reduce localized skin irritation.
4. Treat local skin infection.
5. Create local anesthesia over skin surfaces.
6. Reduce number of bacteria residing on skin surfaces.

### *Procedure 20-1*

| Steps | Rationale |
|---|---|
| **Assessment** | |
| 1. Determine whether client has known allergy to topical agent. Ask if client has had reaction to a cream or lotion applied to the skin. | Allergic contact dermatitis is relatively common and can worsen dermatologic condition. |
| 2. Assess condition of client's skin. (If topical agent is present, first wash site with mild, nondrying soap and warm water.) Note if client has symptoms of skin irritation, e.g., pruritis or burning. | Site should be clear for proper assessment of skin surface. Assessment provides baseline to determine change in condition of skin after therapy. Application of certain topical agents can lessen or aggravate these symptoms. |

| Steps | Rationale |
|---|---|
| 3. Review physician's order for client's name, name of drug, strength, time of administration, and site of application. | Ensures drug will be administered safely and accurately. |
| 4. Determine amount of topical agent required for application by assessing skin site and reviewing physician's order. | An excessive amount of topical agent can cause chemical irritation of skin or negate drug's effectiveness. A thin even layer is usually adequate. |
| 5. Review information pertinent to medication, e.g., action, side effects, normal strength, method of application, and nursing implications. | Provides nurse with knowledge to administer drug correctly and to monitor client's response. |
| 6. Assess client's knowledge of action and purpose of medication being given. | Reveals client's level of understanding and whether instruction is necessary. |
| 7. Determine if client is physically able to apply medication by assessing fine grasp, hand strength, coordination. | Necessary if client is to self-administer drug in the home. |

## Nursing Diagnosis

| Steps | Rationale |
|---|---|
| 1. Cluster data to reveal actual or potential nursing diagnoses: | |
| a. Impaired skin integrity: related to burn or allergic reaction. | Topical agents are applied to open or closed wounds and lesions. |
| b. Knowledge deficit regarding purpose of medication: related to inexperience. | Clients who are to self-administer drugs or who must be knowledgeable of side effects require instruction. |
| c. Pain: related to skin irritation. | Topical agents can relieve symptoms of discomfort. |
| d. Impaired physical mobility: related to neuromuscular alteration. | Prevents client from self-administering medication. Thus any instruction given must involve family. |

## Planning

| Steps | Rationale |
|---|---|
| 1. Develop individualized goals for client based on nursing diagnoses: | |
| a. Skin lesions or wound will show evidence of healing. | Proper drug application ensures therapeutic effect of drug. |
| b. Ensure proper drug application and absorption. | Topical agents must be applied evenly over skin surface for proper absorption. |
| c. Client acquires knowledge of drug and method of application. | Nurse explains procedure or application and purpose of medication during application. |
| 2. Wash hands. | Reduces transmission of microorganisms. |
| 3. Prepare following equipment and supplies: | |
| a. Ordered topical agent (e.g., cream, ointment, lotion, aerosol spray, powder, etc.) | |
| b. Medication ticket, form, or printout | |
| c. Small sterile gauze dressings | Use to apply suspension-based preparation. |
| d. Disposable or sterile gloves | Use of gloves depends on condition of skin lesions and risk of cross-contamination. |
| e. Cotton tipped applicator or tongue blade | Use for hard to reach areas. |
| f. Basin with warm water, washcloth, towel, and nondrying soap | Skin surface is cleansed before topical agent is applied. |
| g. Gauze dressings, plastic wrap, and tape | Use to protect client's clothes from discoloration or soiling. |
| 4. Compare medication ticket with label of topical agent. | Ensures client receives correct medication. |
| 5. Check client's identification bracelet and ask name. | Ensures correct client receives medication. |
| 6. Explain procedure to client, including description of skin area to be treated. | Makes client participant in care and minimizes anxiety. |

## Implementation

| Steps | Rationale |
|---|---|
| 1. Arrange supplies at client's bedside. | Topical agents are not usually premeasured in medication room. |
| 2. Close room curtain or door. | Provides client privacy. |
| 3. Position client comfortably. Remove gown or bed linen, keeping unaffected skin areas draped. | Provides easy access to area being treated. Promotes client's comfort. |
| 4. Wash affected area, removing all debris, crustations, and previous medication. | Removal of debris enhances penetration of topical drug through skin. Cleansing removes microorganisms resident in remaining debris. |
| 5. Pat skin dry or allow area to air dry. | Excess moisture can interfere with even application of topical agent. |
| 6. If skin is excessively dry and flaking, apply topical agent while skin is still damp. | Retains moisture within skin layers. |

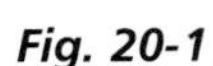

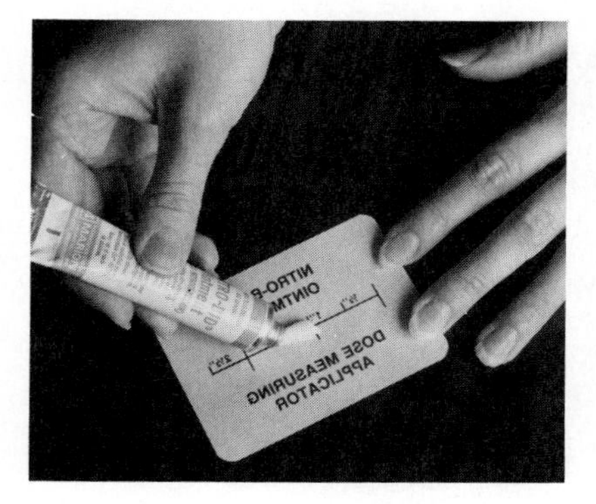

**Fig. 20-1**

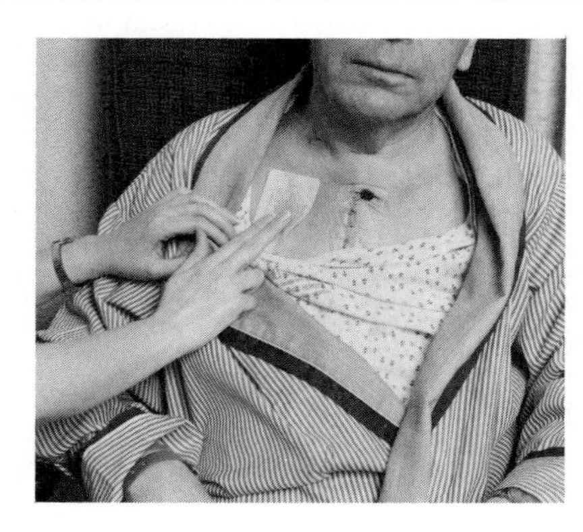

**Fig. 20-2**

| Steps | Rationale |
|---|---|
| 7. Don gloves. | Sterile gloves are used when applying agents to open, noninfected skin lesions. Disposable gloves prevent cross-contamination of infected or contagious lesions, and protects nurse from drug effects. |
| 8. Apply topical agent: | |
| a. Cream, ointment, and oil-based lotion: | |
| ▪ Place approximately 1-2 tsp of medication in palm of hand and soften by rubbing briskly between hands. | Softening of topical agent makes it easier to apply to skin. |
| ▪ Once medication is thin and smooth, smear it evenly over skin surface using long even strokes that follow direction of hair growth. | Ensures even distribution of medication. Technique prevents irritation of hair follicles. |
| ▪ Explain to client that skin may feel greasy after application. | Ointments often contain oils. |
| b. Antianginal (nitroglycerine) ointment: | |
| ▪ Apply desired number of inches of ointment over paper measuring guide (Fig. 20-1). | Ensures correct dosage of medication. |
| ▪ Apply ointment to skin surface by holding edge or back of the paper wrapper and placing ointment and wrapper directly on the skin. Do not rub or massage ointment into skin (Fig. 20-2). | Drug can absorb through nurse's fingertips, causing serious systemic effects. Medication is designed to absorb slowly over several hours and should not be massaged. |
| ▪ Cover ointment and paper with plastic wrap and tape securely (optional). | Prevents soiling of clothing. |
| c. Aerosol spray: | |
| ▪ Shake container vigorously. | Mixes contents and propellant to ensure distribution of fine even spray. |
| ▪ Read container's label for distance recommended to hold spray away from area (usually 6-12 in, 15-30 cm). | Proper distance ensures fine spray hits skin surface. Holding container too close results in thin watery distribution. |
| ▪ If neck or upper chest are to be sprayed, ask client to turn face away from spray or briefly cover face with towel. | Prevents inhalation of spray. |
| ▪ Spray medication evenly over affected site (in some cases spray is timed for select period of seconds). | Entire affected area of skin should be covered with thin spray. |
| d. Suspension-based lotion: | |
| ▪ Shake container vigorously. | Mixes powder throughout liquid to form well-mixed suspension. |
| ▪ Apply small amount of lotion to small gauze dressing or pad and apply to skin by stroking evenly in direction of hair growth. | Method of application leaves protective film of powder on skin after water base of suspension dries. Technique prevents irritation to hair follicles. |
| ▪ Explain to client that area will feel cool and dry. | Water evaporates to leave thin layer of powder. |
| e. Powder: | |
| ▪ Be sure skin surface is thoroughly dry. | Minimizes caking and crusting of powder. |
| ▪ Fully spread apart any skin folds such as between toes or under axilla. | Fully exposes skin surface for application. |
| ▪ Dust skin site lightly with dispenser so that area is covered with fine, thin layer of powder. | Thin layer of powder is more absorbent and reduces friction by increasing area of moisture evaporation (Anders, 1982). |
| 9. Cover skin area with dressing if ordered by physician. | May help prevent agent from being rubbed off skin. |

| Steps | Rationale |
|---|---|
| 10. Assist client to comfortable position, reapply gown, and cover with bed linen as desired. | Provides for client's sense of well-being. |
| 11. Remove gloves, dispose of soiled supplies in proper receptacle and wash hands. | Keeps client's environment neat and reduces transmission of infection. |

## Evaluation

| | |
|---|---|
| 1. Inspect condition of skin site between applications. | Application of agent will improve or worsen dermatologic condition. |
| 2. Evaluate client for symptoms of tenderness or pruritis. | Determines response to application. |
| 3. Ask client to discuss knowledge of drug. | Measures client's understanding of therapy. |

### *Expected outcomes*

| | |
|---|---|
| 1. Over repeated applications skin becomes clear, without inflammation or drainage from lesions. | Existing lesions heal and/or disappear. |
| 2. Client denies presence of pruritis or tenderness. | Result of reduced inflammation. With healing less histamine is released to site, causing less pruritis. |
| 3. Client is able to describe action, purpose and side effects of drug. | Demonstrates learning. |

### *Unexpected outcomes*

| | |
|---|---|
| 1. Skin site may appear inflamed and edematous with blistering and oozing of fluid from lesions. | Signs indicative of subacute inflammation or eczema that can develop from worsening of skin lesions. |
| 2. Client will continue to complain of pruritis and tenderness. | Indicates slow or impaired healing; alternate therapies may be needed. |
| 3. Client unable to explain information about drug. | Reinstruction necessary or client unable to learn. |

## Recording and Reporting

| | |
|---|---|
| 1. Describe condition of skin before topical agent application in nurses' notes. | Documents client's condition and helps evaluate progress and response to therapy. |
| 2. Record type of agent applied, strength, and site of application in nurses' notes and on medication record. | Prompt documentation prevents medication errors. |
| 3. Report any abnormalities in skin condition to nurse in charge or physician. | May indicate change in type of agent used or method of treatment. |

## Follow-Up Activities

| | |
|---|---|
| 1. Offer client opportunity to apply topical agent during next application and to ask questions. | Continued home care may be necessary. |

## Special Considerations

- Antianginal (nitroglycerine) ointments are usually ordered in inches and can be measured on small sheets of paper marked off in one-half inch markings.
- In some cases soaking may be needed to remove debris or crusting from skin.
- If skin is inflamed, use only warm water rinse without soap for cleansing.
- When applying creams or ointments do not pat or rub skin. This may cause irritation.
- Rotate site when applying nitroglycerine pastes. Also avoid markedly hairy areas that might alter drug absorption.
- Infants and small children are sensitive to topical antihistamines and the "caine" type of anesthetics (Whaley and Wong, 1987).

## Teaching Considerations

- It may be necessary for a family member or friend to learn skill of topical application.
- When instructing client be sure lighting is adequate and area to be treated is well exposed.

# SKILL 20-2 Administering Eyedrops and Ointment

Common medications used by clients are eye drops and ointments, including over-the-counter preparations such as artificial tears and vasoconstrictors (for example, Visine and Murine). However, many clients receive prescribed ophthalmic drugs for eye conditions such as glaucoma and postcataract extraction.

The eye is the most sensitive organ to which the nurse applies medications. The cornea is richly supplied with sensitive nerve fibers. Care must be taken to prevent instilling medication directly onto the cornea. The conjunctival sac is much less sensitive and thus a more appropriate site for medication instillation.

Any client receiving topical eye medication should learn correct self-administration of the medication, especially clients with glaucoma, for example, who often must receive medications permanently for control of their disease. Donnelly (1987) recommends instructing clients by breaking down drop instillation into a series of steps so that if problems occur their exact nature can be determined. Nurses can easily instruct clients while administering medications. At times it may become necessary for family members to learn how to administer eye drops or ointment. This is particularly true immediately after eye surgery when a client's vision is so impaired that it is difficult to assemble needed supplies and handle applicators correctly.

Eye medications come in a variety of concentrations. Instilling the wrong concentration may cause local irritation to eyes, as well as certain systemic effects. Certain ophthalmic medications, such as mydriatics and cycloplegics, temporarily blur a client's vision. Use of the wrong drug concentration can prolong these undesirable effects.

### Purposes

1. Dilate the pupil for measurement of lens refraction or visualization of internal eye structures.
2. Paralyze lens muscles for measurement of lens refraction.
3. Relieve local irritation of the eye.
4. Locally treat eye disorders such as infection or glaucoma.
5. Maintain lubrication of cornea and conjunctiva.

## Procedure 20-2

| Steps | Rationale |
|---|---|
| **Assessment** | |
| 1. Review physician's medication order including client's name; drug name, concentration, number of drops (if a liquid); time; and eye (right or left) to receive medication. | Ensures correct administration of medication. |
| 2. Review information pertinent to medication including action, purpose, side effects, nursing implications. | Allows nurse to administer drug properly and monitor client's response. |
| 3. Assess condition of external eye structures (Skill 13-5). (May also be done just before drug instillation.) | Provides baseline to later determine if local response to medications occurs. Also indicates need to clean eye before drug application. |
| 4. Determine whether client has any known allergies to eye medications. | Protects client from risk of allergic drug response. |
| 5. Determine whether client has any symptoms of visual alterations. | Certain eye medications act to either lessen or increase these symptoms. Nurse must be able to recognize change in client's condition. |
| 6. Assess client's level of consciousness and ability to follow directions. | If client becomes restless or combative during procedure there is greater risk of accidental eye injury. Client may require restraining. |
| 7. Assess client's knowledge regarding drug therapy. | Client's level of understanding may indicate need for health teaching. |
| 8. Assess client's ability to manipulate and hold dropper. | Reflects client's ability to learn to self-administer drug. |
| **Nursing Diagnosis** | |
| 1. Cluster data to reveal actual or potential nursing diagnoses: | |
| a. Sensory/perceptual alteration (visual): related to blurred vision or reduced acuity. | Preexisting eye condition indicates need for medication. Visual impairment will affect ability to self-administer drug. |
| b. Potential for injury: related to visual alteration. | Existing eye disorders can impair vision to threaten client's safety. Certain drugs such as anticholinergic eye drops cause blurred vision for several hours after administration. |

| Steps | Rationale |
|---|---|
| c. Knowledge deficit regarding drug action and purpose: related to newly prescribed medication. | Discussion of drug can be incorporated into procedure. |
| d. Pain: related to eye irritation. | Many disorders treated with eye medications can be painful. |
| e. Impaired physical mobility: related to reduced grasp. | Inability of client to position or hold dropper prevents learning self-administration. Thus any instruction given must involve family. |

## Planning

| Steps | Rationale |
|---|---|
| 1. Develop individualized goals for client based on nursing diagnoses: | |
| a. Prevent injury to eye. | Eyedropper or ointment tube should not be allowed to touch eye structures. |
| b. Client experiences minimal discomfort. | Nurse avoids instilling drops directly onto cornea. |
| c. Client acquires knowledge of drug action and effects and techniques of administration. | Client's understanding of medication therapy improves adherence to drug regimen. |
| d. Client's visual symptoms are reduced. | Certain eye medications can produce quick relief. |
| 2. Wash hands and don gloves. | Reduces transmission of microorganisms. |
| 3. Prepare following equipment and supplies: | |
| a. Medication bottle with sterile eye dropper or ointment tube | Ophthalmic drops come in plastic or glass bottles. Ointments are prepared in small tubes. |
| b. Medication card, form, or printout | |
| c. Cotton ball or tissue | |
| d. Wash basin filled with warm water and washcloth | |
| e. Eye patch and tape (optional) | |
| 4. Compare medication ticket with label of eye medication. | Ensures right drug is administered. |
| 5. Check client's identification bracelet and ask name. | Ensures correct client receives medication. |
| 6. Explain procedure to client. | Clients often become anxious about medication being instilled into eye because of potential discomfort. |

## Implementation

| Steps | Rationale |
|---|---|
| 1. Arrange supplies at bedside, don gloves. | Ensures a smooth orderly procedure. |
| 2. Ask client to lie supine or sit back in chair with head slightly hyperextended. | Position provides easy access to eye for medication instillation and minimizes drainage of medication through tear duct. |
| 3. If crusts or drainage are present along eyelid margins or inner canthus, gently wash away. Soak any crusts that are dried and difficult to remove by applying damp washcloth or cotton ball over eye for few min. Always wipe clean from inner to outer canthus (Fig. 20-3). | Crusts or drainage harbor microorganisms. Soaking allows easy removal and prevents pressure from being applied directly over eye. Cleansing from inner to outer canthus avoids entrance of microorganisms into lacrimal duct. |
| 4. Hold cotton ball or clean tissue in nondominant hand on client's cheekbone just below lower eyelid. | Cotton or tissue absorbs medication that escapes eye. |
| 5. With tissue or cotton resting below lower lid, gently press downward with thumb or forefinger against bony orbit (Fig. 20-4). | Technique exposes lower conjunctival sac. Retraction against bony orbit prevents pressure and trauma to eyeball and prevents fingers from touching eye. |
| 6. Ask client to look at ceiling. | Action retracts sensitive cornea up and away from conjunctival sac and reduces stimulation of blink reflex. |
| 7. Instill eyedrops: | |
| a. With dominant hand resting on client's forehead, hold filled medication eye dropper approximately 1-2 cm (0.5-0.75 in) above conjunctival sac (Fig. 20-5). | Helps prevent accidental contact of eyedropper with eye structures, thus reducing risk of injury to eye and transfer of infection to dropper. Ophthalmic medications are sterilized. |

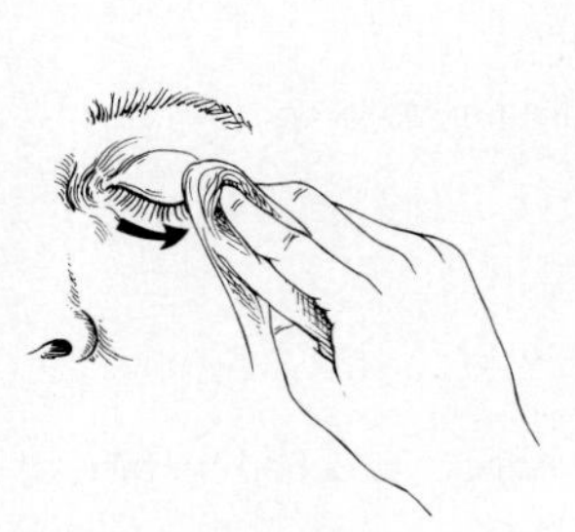

*Fig. 20-3*

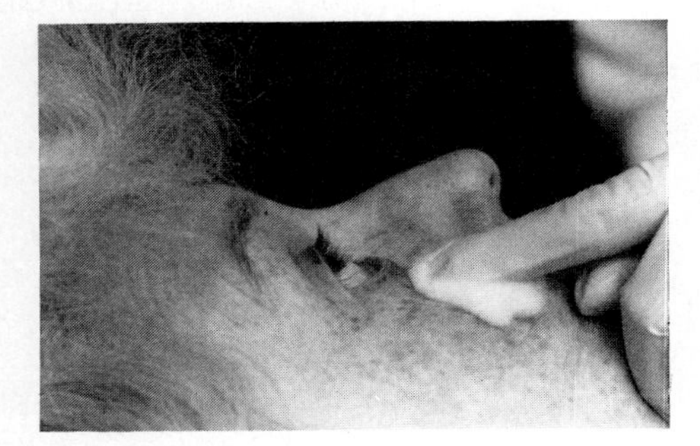

*Fig. 20-4*

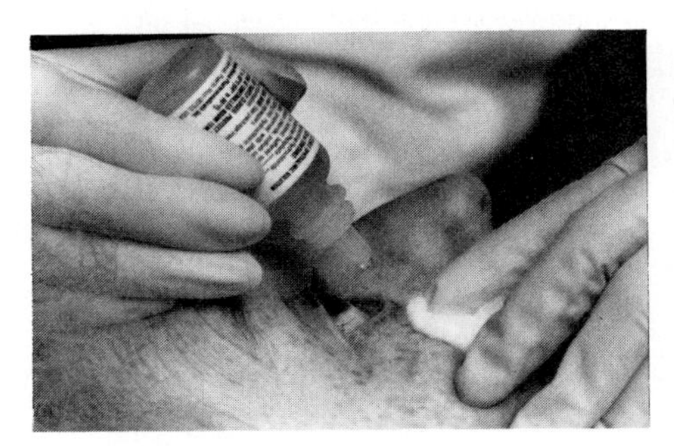

*Fig. 20-5*

| Steps | Rationale |
|---|---|

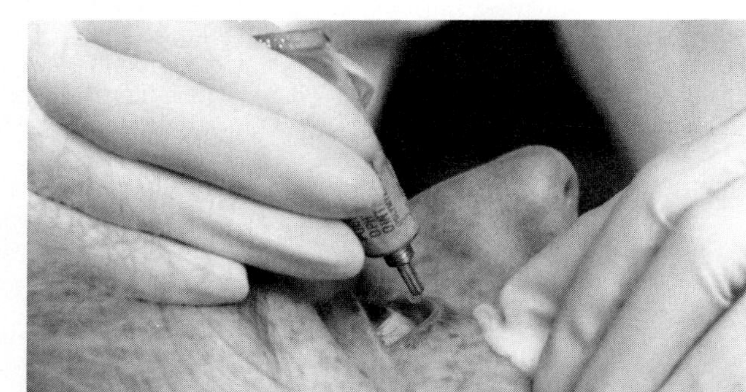

*Fig. 20-6*

| Steps | Rationale |
|---|---|
| b. Drop prescribed number of medication drops into conjunctival sac. | Conjunctival sac normally holds 1-2 drops. Applying drops to sac provides even distribution of medication across eye. |
| c. If client blinks or closes eye or if drops land on outer lid margins, repeat procedure. | Therapeutic effect of drug obtained only when drops enter conjunctival sac. |
| d. When administering drugs that cause systemic effects, protect your finger with clean tissue and apply gentle pressure to client's nasolacrimal duct for 30-60 sec. | Prevents overflow of medication into nasal and pharyngeal passages. Prevents absorption into systemic circulation. |
| e. After instilling drops, ask client to close eye gently. | Helps to distribute medication. Squinting or squeezing of eyelids forces medication from conjunctival sac. |
| 8. Instill eye ointment: | |
| a. Holding ointment applicator above lid margin, apply thin stream of ointment evenly along inside edge of lower eyelid on conjunctiva (Fig. 20-6). | Distributes medication evenly across eye and lid margin. |
| b. Ask client to look down. | Reduces blinking reflex during ointment application. |
| c. Apply thin stream of ointment along upper lid margin on inner conjunctiva. | Distributes medication evenly across eye and lid margin. |
| d. Have client close eye and rub lid lightly in circular motion with cotton ball. | Further distributes medication without traumatizing eye. |
| 9. If excess medication is on eyelid, gently wipe it from inner to outer canthus. | Promotes comfort and prevents trauma to eye. |
| 10. If client had eye patch, apply clean one by placing it over affected eye so entire eye is covered. Tape securely without applying pressure to eye. | Clean eye patch reduces chance of infection. |
| 11. Remove gloves, dispose of soiled supplies in proper receptacle and wash hands. | Maintains neat environment at bedside and reduces transmission of microorganisms. |

## Evaluation

| | |
|---|---|
| 1. Note client's response to instillation, ask if any discomfort was felt. | Determines if procedure was performed correctly and safely. |
| 2. Observe response to medication by assessing visual changes and noting any side effects. | Evaluates effects of medication. |
| 3. Ask client to discuss drug's purpose, action, side effects, and technique of administration. | Determines client's level of understanding. |

### *Expected outcomes*

| | |
|---|---|
| 1. Client denies discomfort. | Drug administered correctly without injury to client. |
| 2. Client experiences no side effects, and symptoms (e.g., irritation) are relieved. | Drug distributed and absorbed properly. |
| 3. Client is able to discuss information about medication and technique correctly. | Demonstrates learning. |

### *Unexpected outcomes*

| | |
|---|---|
| 1. Client complains of burning or pain. | Eye drops instilled onto cornea or dropper touched surface of eye. |
| 2. Client experiences local side effects, e.g., headache, bloodshot eyes, local eye irritation. | Drug concentration and client's sensitivity influences chances of side effects developing. |

| Steps | Rationale |
|---|---|
| 3. Client experiences systemic effects from drops, e.g., increased heart rate and blood pressure from epinephrine, decreased heart rate and blood pressure from timolol. | Systemic absorption through tear duct can cause potentially dangerous effects. |
| 4. Client unable to discuss information about medication correctly. | Reinstruction needed or client unable to learn. |

### Recording and Reporting

| | |
|---|---|
| 1. Record drug, concentration, number of drops, time of administration, and eye (left or right) that received medication in medication record. | Timely documentation prevents drug errors, e.g., repeated or missed doses. |
| 2. Record appearance of eye in nurses' notes. | Documents status or condition of eye. |
| 3. Report and record any undesirable side effects to nurse in charge or physician. | Nature of client's reaction may require additional therapy. |

### Follow-up Activities

| | |
|---|---|
| 1. Clients who will be administering drugs at home should demonstrate drop instillation. | Determines need for instruction. |

### Special Considerations

- Local anesthetics and antibiotics may cause anaphylaxis.
- If eye drops are stored in refrigerator rewarm to room temperature before administering.
- Clients experienced in self-instillation may be allowed to give drops under nurse's supervision (check agency policy).
- Never press directly against client's eyeball.
- When instilling drops in infant or young child, have parent gently restrain child's head with child in parent's lap.
- Note that clients with eye infections often have drainage along eyelid margins.
- Warn clients receiving mydriatics that vision will be temporarily blurred. Wearing sunglasses will reduce photophobia.
- Clients who receive cycloplegics should temporarily not drive or attempt to perform any activity that requires acute vision.

### Teaching Considerations

- Many clients lack confidence in their ability to instill drops without supervision, such as from a family member.
- There is room for individual variation in techniques provided the client suffers no injury (Donnelly, 1987).
- For clients who are unable to manipulate the dropper or are unable to see, instruct a family member on the technique.

## *SKILL 20-3* Administering Eardrops

Ear medications are easy to administer; however, to protect clients nurses should be aware of certain safety precautions. Internal ear structures are very sensitive to temperature extremes. Failure to instill a solution at room temperature can cause vertigo (severe dizziness) or nausea and debilitate a client for several minutes. Although structures of the outer ear are not sterile, it is wise to use sterile drops and solutions in case the eardrum is ruptured. Entrance of nonsterile solutions into the middle ear can cause serious infection. A final precaution is avoidance of forcing any solution into the ear. The nurse must not occlude the ear canal with a medicine dropper because this can cause pressure within the canal during instillation and subsequent injury to the eardrum. If these precautions are followed, instillation of eardrops is a safe and effective therapy.

### Purposes

1. Relieve inflammation and discomfort.
2. Soften cerumen for removal.
3. Treat localized disorders such as infection.

## *Procedure 20-3*

| Steps | Rationale |
|---|---|
| **Assessment** | |
| 1. Review physician's medication order for client's name; drug name, concentration, time of administration, number of drops to instill; and ear (right or left) to receive medication. | Ensures safe and correct administration of medication. |
| 2. Review pertinent information related to medication, e.g., action, purpose, side effects, and nursing implications. | Allows nurse to administer drug properly and monitor client's response. |
| 3. Assess condition of external ear structures and canal (Skill 13-6). (May also be done just before drug instillation.) | Provides baseline to determine later if local response to medication occurs, whether client's condition improves, or whether it will be necessary to clean ear before instilling medication. |
| 4. Determine whether client has symptoms of discomfort or hearing impairment. | Disorders of external ear can be painful. Occlusion of external ear canal by swelling, drainage, or cerumen can impair hearing acuity. These conditions may change after drug instillation. |
| 5. Assess client's level of consciousness and ability to follow instructions. | Client must lie still during drug administration. Sudden movements can cause injury from ear dropper. |
| 6. Assess client's level of knowledge regarding drug therapy. | Client's knowledge level will determine whether health teaching is required. |
| 7. Assess client's ability to grasp and manipulate dropper. | Determines client's ability to self-administer drug. |
| **Nursing Diagnosis** | |
| 1. Cluster data to reveal actual or potential nursing diagnoses: | |
| a. Sensory/perceptual alteration (hearing): related to impacted cerumen or swelling of ear canal. | Drops may relieve irritation or loosen cerumen that causes conduction deafness. |
| b. Pain: related to ear inflammation. | External ear canal is very sensitive when inflammed. |
| c. Knowledge deficit regarding drug therapy: related to inexperience. | Discussion of drug can be incorporated into procedure. |
| **Planning** | |
| 1. Develop individualized goals for client based on nursing diagnoses: | |
| a. Client experiences less pain. | Medications aimed at reducing inflammation will minimize pain. |
| b. Client gains improved hearing. | Clearance of external canal with medication will improve sound conduction. |
| c. Client acquires knowledge of drug action and effects and techniques of administration. | Client's understanding of medication therapy improves adherence to drug regimen. |
| 2. Wash hands. | Reduces transmission of microorganisms. |
| 3. Prepare following equipment and supplies: | |
| a. Medication bottle with dropper | |
| b. Medication card, form, or printout | |
| c. Cotton tipped applicator | To remove cerumen or drainage. |
| d. Tissue | |
| e. Cotton ball (optional) | |
| 4. Compare medication ticket with label of medication. | Ensures right drug is administered. |
| 5. Check client's identification bracelet and ask name. | Ensures right client receives drug. |
| 6. Explain procedure to client. | Reduces client anxiety. |
| **Implementation** | |
| 1. Arrange supplies at bedside. | Helps nurse perform procedure smoothly. |
| 2. Have client assume side-lying position with ear to be treated facing up. | Position provides easy access to ear for instillation of medication. Ear canal is in position to receive medication. |
| 3. If cerumen or drainage occludes outermost portion of ear canal, wipe out gently with cotton tipped applicator (Fig. 20-7). *Do not force wax inward to block or occlude canal.* | Cerumen and drainage habor microorganisms and can block distribution of medication into canal. Occlusion of canal interferes with normal sound conditions. |
| 4. Straighten ear canal by pulling auricle down and back (children) or upward and outward (adult). | Straightening of ear canal provides direct access to deeper external ear structures. |
| 5. Instill prescribed drops holding dropper 1 cm (0.5 in) above ear canal (Fig. 20-8). | Forcing drops into occluded canal can cause injury to eardrum. |

| Steps | Rationale |
|---|---|

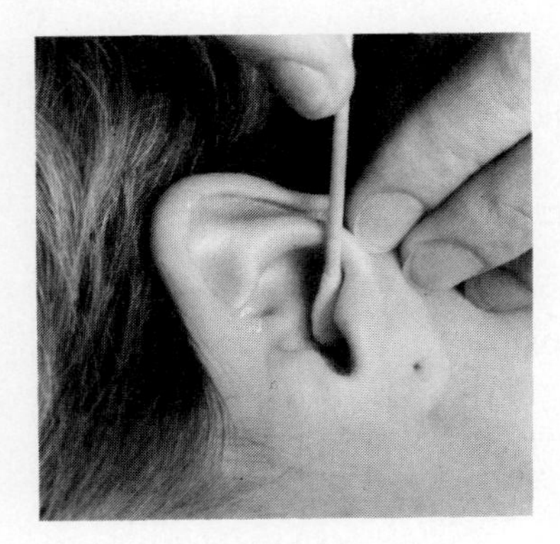

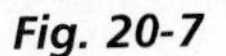

Fig. 20-7

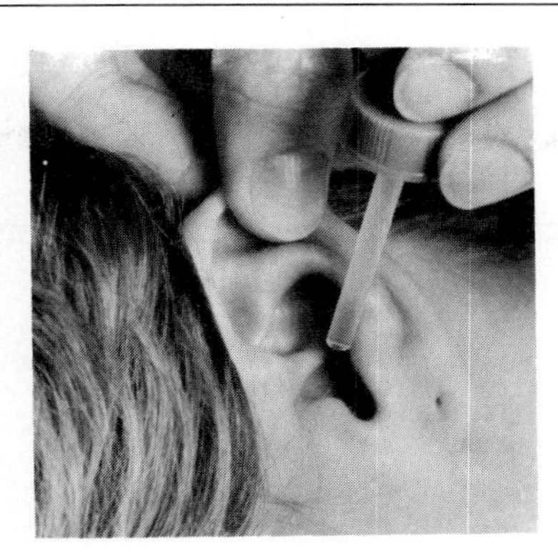

Fig. 20-8

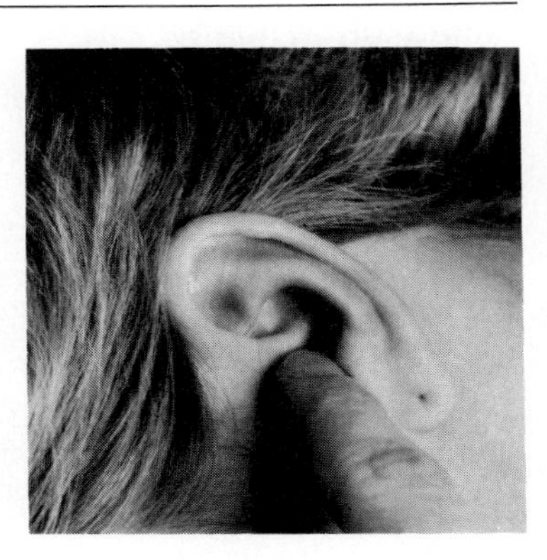

Fig. 20-9

| Steps | Rationale |
|---|---|
| 6. Ask client to remain in side-lying position 2-3 min. Apply gentle massage or pressure to tragus of ear with finger (Fig. 20-9). | Allows complete distribution of medication. Pressure and massage moves medication inward. |
| 7. At times physician orders insertion of portion of cotton ball into outermost part of canal. Do not press cotton into canal. | Inserting cotton into outer canal prevents escape of medication when client sits or stands. Cotton should not block canal to impair hearing. |
| 8. Remove cotton in 15 min. | Time period promotes drug distribution and absorption. |
| 9. Dispose of soiled supplies and wash hands. | Keeps bedside neat and orderly. Reduces transmission of infection. |
| 10. Assist client to comfortable position after drops are absorbed. | Restores comfort. |

## Evaluation

| Steps | Rationale |
|---|---|
| 1. Ask client during instillation if any discomfort is felt. | Determines if procedure is performed correctly and reveals severity of symptoms. |
| 2. Evaluate condition of external ear between drug instillations. | Determines response to medication. |
| 3. Evaluate client's hearing acuity. | Hearing may change after drug administration. |
| 4. Ask client to explain technique for instilling eardrops and purpose of medication. | Evaluates degree of learning. |

### *Expected outcomes*

| Steps | Rationale |
|---|---|
| 1. Client denies discomfort during administration. | Procedure performed correctly without injury to client. |
| 2. Ear canal becomes clear, without drainage, cerumen, or inflammation, as medication is repeatedly instilled. | Drug action is effective. |
| 3. Client's hearing acuity improves. | This response will occur only if hearing loss was caused by obstruction in external ear canal. |
| 4. Client is able to explain steps for instilling eardrops and technique for administration. | Cognitive learning occurs. |

### *Unexpected outcomes*

| Steps | Rationale |
|---|---|
| 1. Ear canal is inflamed, swollen, tender to palpation. Drainage is present. | Symptoms of continuing ear infection. |
| 2. Ear canal is occluded by cerumen. | Wax has become impacted in canal. |
| 3. Client is unable to explain drug information and steps for drug instillation. | Nurse must repeat instructions, or client is unable to learn. |
| 4. Client's hearing acuity continues to be reduced. | Obstruction within ear canal is unrelieved. |

## Recording and Reporting

| Steps | Rationale |
|---|---|
| 1. Record drug, concentration, number of drops, time administered, and ear into which drops instilled on medication form. | Timely documentation prevents drug errors, e.g., repeated doses. |
| 2. Record condition of ear canal in nurses' notes. | Documents client's status and response to therapy. |
| 3. Report any sudden change in client's hearing acuity. | May require further medical care. |

| Steps | Rationale |
|---|---|
| **Follow-up Activities** | |
| 1. Have client demonstrate instillation of eardrops during next administration. | Simple technique can usually be performed by client with minimal instruction. Client should know how to avoid injuring ear. |

### Special Considerations

- If client suffers hearing loss use communication techniques such as enunciating words, getting client's attention, speaking in normal tone of voice, talking toward client's best ear.
- Ear drops should be warmed to room temperature. Hold bottle in hands or place in warm water.
- Infant or young child may be restrained in supine position with head turned to expose affected ear. Hold child in this position until drug has time to absorb.
- Children with otitis media often have extensive drainage: position on side with affected ear in dependent position to facilitate drainage.
- Some elderly clients experience excessive accumulation of cerumen in the ear.

### Teaching Considerations

- This procedure is simple to teach clients and family members.
- Instruct client on proper way to cleanse ears, avoiding use of sharp objects in ear canal.
- Teach the signs of hearing loss and the need for frequent follow-up care to parents with children who have chronic otitis media.

# *SKILL 20-4 Administering Nasal Instillations*

Clients with nasal sinus alterations may receive drugs by spray, drops, or tampons. The most commonly administered form of nasal instillation is decongestant spray or drops used to relieve sinus congestion and cold symptoms. Many over-the-counter nose drops contain sympathomimetic drugs (such as Afrin or Neo-Synephrine) that are relatively safe because of small doses needed topically. However, the drugs can enter the systemic circulation by way of the nasal mucosa or gastrointestinal tract if an excess amount is swallowed. Repeated use of sprays can also worsen nasal congestion due to a rebound effect. Saline drops are considered safer as a decongestant for children than sympathomimetics.

It is easiest for a client to self-administer sprays. In the supine position with head tilted back, the client holds the tip of the container just inside the nares and inhales as the spray enters the nasal passages. In children, nasal sprays should be given with the head in an upright position so excess spray will drip anteriorly from the nostrils and not be swallowed (Nurses Drug Alert, 1984).

Nasal drops often contain antibiotics for the treatment of sinus infections. Proper positioning of clients during instillation is essential for medication to reach the affected sinus. Nasal tampons are used for severe nose bleeds to stop hemorrhaging. Tampons are usually inserted by a physician.

### Purposes

1. Relieve nasal congestion for improved breathing.
2. Treat nasal mucosa and sinus irritation from inflammation, infection, or allergy.

## *Procedure 20-4*

| Steps | Rationale |
|---|---|
| **Assessment** | |
| 1. Review physician's medication order for client's name, drug name, concentration of solution, number of drops, and time of administration. | Ensures safe and correct administration of medication. |
| 2. Review pertinent information related to medication including action, purpose, side effects, and nursing implications. | Allows nurse to administer drug properly and to monitor its response. |

| Steps | Rationale |
|---|---|
| 3. For nasal drops determine which sinus is affected by referring to medical record. | Will affect client's position during drug instillation. |
| 4. Assess client's history of hypertension, heart disease, diabetes, and hyperthyroidism. | These conditions can contraindicate use of decongestants that stimulate central nervous system and cause side effects of transient hypertension, tachycardia, palpitations, and headache. |
| 5. Inspect condition of nose and sinuses (Chapter 13). Palpate sinuses for tenderness. (May be done just before instillation.) | Findings provide baseline to monitor effect of medication. Presence of discharge will interfere with drug absorption. |
| 6. Assess client's knowledge regarding use of nasal instillations and technique for instillation. | May necessitate health teaching regarding use of drugs. |

## Nursing Diagnosis

| Steps | Rationale |
|---|---|
| 1. Cluster data to reveal actual or potential nursing diagnoses: | |
| a. Pain: related to nasal or sinus irritation. | Inflamed mucosa is tender. Congestion of sinuses can lead to severe headache. |
| b. Ineffective breathing pattern: related to nasal congestion. | Client adjusts to congestion by mouth breathing. |
| c. Knowledge deficit regarding drug therapy: related to information misinterpreted. | Nurse can instruct client about drug therapy during instillation. |

## Planning

| Steps | Rationale |
|---|---|
| 1. Develop individualized goals for client based on nursing diagnoses: | |
| a. Promote proper drug distribution and absorption. | Technique of administration involves clearing nasal passages before instillation and positioning client correctly. |
| b. Nasal mucosa becomes clear, nonswollen. | Nasal medications are designed to relieve congestion and irritation. |
| c. Client acquires knowledge of drug therapy and technique of instillation. | Client must understand how to safely self-administer medications. |
| 2. Wash hands. | Reduces transmission of microorganisms. |
| 3. Prepare following equipment and supplies: | |
| a. Prepared medication with clean dropper or spray container | Dropper or applicator need not be sterile but should be clean. |
| b. Medication card, form, or printout | |
| c. Facial tissue | |
| d. Small pillow (optional) | Used in positioning client. |
| e. Washcloth (optional) | Used to clean nares. |
| 4. Compare medication ticket with label of nasal medication. | Ensures right drug is administered. |
| 5. Check client's identification bracelet and ask name. | Ensures right client receives drug. |
| 6. Explain procedure to client regarding positioning and sensations to expect, such as burning or stinging of mucosa, or choking sensation as medication trickles into throat. | Helps client anticipate experience of procedure to reduce anxiety. |

## Implementation

| Steps | Rationale |
|---|---|
| 1. Arrange supplies and medications at bedside. | Ensures smooth, orderly procedure. |
| 2. Instruct client to clear or blow nose gently unless contraindicated (e.g., risk of increased intracranial pressure or nose bleeds). | Removes mucus and secretions that can block distribution of medication. |
| 3. Administer nasal drops: | |
| a. Assist client to supine position. | Position provides access to nasal passages. |
| b. Position head properly: | Position allows medication to drain into affected sinus. |
| ▪ Posterior pharynx—tilt client's head backward. | |
| ▪ Ethmoid or sphenoid sinus—tilt head back over edge of bed or place small pillow under client's shoulder and tilt head back (Fig. 20-10). | |
| ▪ Frontal and maxillary sinus—tilt head back over edge of bed or pillow with head turned toward side to be treated (Fig. 20-11). | |
| Support client's head with nondominant hand. | Prevents straining of neck muscles. |
| c. Instruct client to breathe through mouth. | Mouth breathing reduces chance of aspirating nasal drops into trachea and lungs. |

**Steps** | **Rationale**

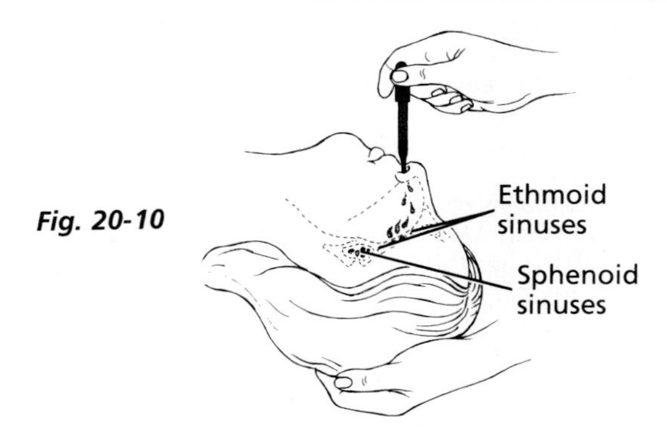

*Fig. 20-10*

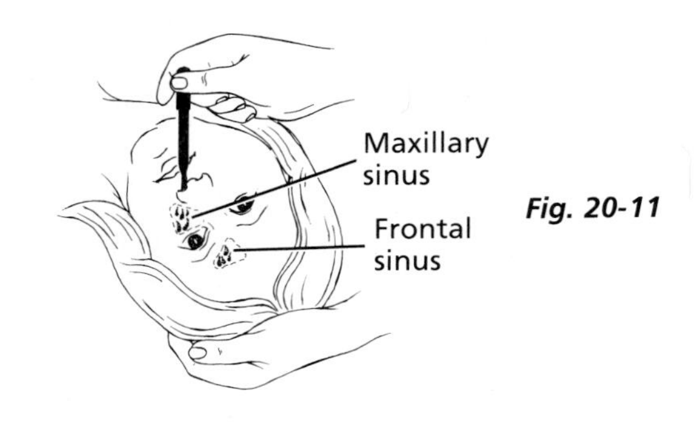

*Fig. 20-11*

| Steps | Rationale |
|---|---|
| d. Hold dropper 1 cm (0.5 in) above nares and instill prescribed number of drops toward midline of ethmoid bone. | Avoids contamination of dropper. Instilling toward ethmoid bone facilitates distribution of medication over nasal mucosa. |
| e. Have client remain in supine position 5 min. | Prevents premature loss of medication through nares. |
| f. Offer facial tissue to blot runny nose, but caution client against blowing nose for several min. | Allows maximum amount of medication to be absorbed. |
| 4. Assist client to a comfortable position after drug absorbed. | Restores comfort. |
| 5. Dispose of soiled supplies in proper container and wash hands. | Maintains neat, orderly environment. Reduces spread of microorganisms. |

## Evaluation

| Steps | Rationale |
|---|---|
| 1. Observe client for onset of side effects 15-30 min after administration. | Drugs absorbed through mucosa can cause systemic reaction. |
| 2. Ask if client is able to breathe through nose after decongestant administration. May be necessary to have client occlude one nostril at a time and breathe deeply. | Determines effectiveness of decongestant medication. |
| 3. Reinspect condition of nasal passages between instillations. | Condition of mucosa reveals response to medication. |
| 4. Ask client to review risks of overuse of decongestants and methods for administration. | Feedback assures that client can self-administer drugs properly. |

### *Expected outcomes*

| Steps | Rationale |
|---|---|
| 1. Client is able to breathe with ease through nose. | Nasal congestion relieved. |
| 2. Nasal sinuses become clear, moist, pink, without drainage after repeated instillations (applies to antiinfective medications). | Inflammation of mucosa relieved. |
| 3. Client is able to explain how to administer nasal instillations correctly. | Feedback reflects client's learning. |

### *Unexpected outcomes*

| Steps | Rationale |
|---|---|
| 1. Client is unable to breathe easily through nasal passages. Mucosa appears swollen. | Congestion unrelieved. Client may be experiencing rebound effect. |
| 2. Nasal mucosa remains inflamed and tender with discharge from nares. | Inflammatory or infective process remains. |
| 3. Client complains of sinus headache. | Sinuses remain congested. |
| 4. Client unable to explain technique and risks of drug therapy. | Further explanation is required. |

## Recording and Reporting

| Steps | Rationale |
|---|---|
| 1. Record medication administration including drug name, concentration, number of drops; nostril into which drug was instilled; and time of administration. | Timely documentation prevents drug errors. |
| 2. Record client's response in nurses' notes. | Documents response to therapy. |
| 3. Report any unusual systemic effects to nurse in charge or physician. | Response may require further treatment or monitoring. |

### Special Considerations

- Infant or small child should be restrained. Optimal positions include: hold in arms with football hold, supine with head extended and stabilized between nurse's arms and hands, supine with arms and hands restrained at sides and head extended over edge of bed or pillow.
- Clear nasal discharge indicates sinus problem. Yellow or greenish discharge indicates infection.
- Only use over-the-counter nasal sprays or nose drops for one illness; bottles become easily contaminated with bacteria.

### Teaching Considerations

- Instruct clients that each family member should have a different dropper or spray applicator. Applicators should be washed or rinsed after each use.

### Home Care Considerations

- Saline drops for children can be made by dissolving 1 tsp of salt in 1 pint of warm water.

## SKILL 20-5 *Using Metered Dose Inhalers*

The least common route of drug administration is by inhalation. Drugs administered with hand-held inhalers are dispersed through aerosol spray, mist, or fine powder to penetrate lung airways. The deeper passages of the respiratory tract provide a large surface area for drug absorption. The alveolar-capillary network absorbs medication rapidly.

Inhaled medications are usually designed to produce local effects; for example, bronchodilators open narrowed bronchioles, and mucolytic agents liquefy thick mucous secretions. However, since these medications are absorbed rapidly through the pulmonary circulation, some have potential for creating systemic side effects. Isoproterenol (Isuprel) dilates bronchioles but can also cause cardiac arrythmias.

Clients who receive drugs by inhalation frequently suffer chronic respiratory disease such as asthma or bronchitis. Drugs given by inhalation provide control of airway obstruction, and because clients depend on medications for disease control, they must learn about them and how to administer them safely.

A metered dose inhaler delivers a measured dose of drug with each push of a canister. Approximately 5 to 10 pounds of pressure must be used to activate the aerosol (Statz, 1984). However, hand strength diminishes with age and from chronic respiratory disease. Because use of a metered dose inhaler also requires coordination during the breathing cycle many clients only spray the back of their throats and fail to receive a full dose. Statz (1984) found that metered dose inhalers work best when clients use a three-point or lateral hand position to activate canisters. A new device called an *aerochamber* fits metered dose inhalers and improves a client's ability to deliver a proper dose of medication.

### Purposes

1. Provide rapid and sustained relief of bronchospasm.
2. Provide an alternate route of drug administration over that of parenteral injection.
3. Provide clients with capability of managing their own medication therapies.

## *Procedure 20-5*

| Steps | Rationale |
|---|---|
| **Assessment** | |
| 1. Assess client's ability to hold and manipulate inhaler. | Any impairment of grasp or presence of tremors of hands will interfere with client's ability to depress canister within inhaler. |
| 2. Assess client's readiness to learn: client asks questions about medication, disease, or complications; requests education in use of inhaler; is mentally alert; participates in own care. | Affects client's ability to understand explanations and actively participate in teaching process. |
| 3. Assess client's ability to learn: client should not be fatigued, in pain, or respiratory distress; assess level of understanding of technical vocabulary terms. | Mental or physical limitations will affect client's ability to learn and methods nurse uses for instruction. |
| 4. Assess client's knowledge and understanding of disease and purpose and action of prescribed medications. | Knowledge of disease is essential for client to realistically understand use of inhaler. |
| 5. Assess drug schedule and number of inhalations prescribed for each dose. | Influences explanations nurse provides for use of inhaler. |
| 6. If previously instructed in self-administration of inhaled medicine assess client's technique in using an inhaler. | Nurse's instruction may require only simple reinforcement depending on client's level of skill. |

| Steps | Rationale |
|---|---|

## Nursing Diagnosis

1. Cluster data to reveal actual or potential nursing diagnoses:
   a. Knowledge deficit regarding disease process or treatment: related to inexperience. — Nurse will include discussion of therapy and rationale while instructing client.
   b. Impaired physical mobility: related to weak hand grasp or tremors. — Client's inability to hold or depress inhaler will necessitate prescription of alternative drug form. Procedure need not be performed.
   c. Potential noncompliance with drug therapy: related to poor understanding. — Nurse must include specific instructions on frequency of inhaler use and avoidance of over-the-counter inhalers.

## Planning

1. Develop individualized learning objectives for teaching plan, including: — Provides organization for teaching plan and guidelines to evaluate client's success.
   a. Manipulate mouthpiece, canister, and inhaler correctly.
   b. Discuss proper time during respiratory cycle to inhale spray.
   c. Identify number of inhalations for each administration correctly.
   d. Discuss side effects of medications.
   e. Identify criteria for calling health care person if dyspnea develops.
   f. Self-administer inhalation correctly.
   g. Cleaning inhaler after use correctly.
2. Have client prepare following equipment and supplies:
   a. Metered dose inhaler with medication canister (Fig. 20-12).
   b. Aerochamber (optional)
   c. Facial tissues (optional)
   d. Wash basin or sink with warm water
   e. Paper towel

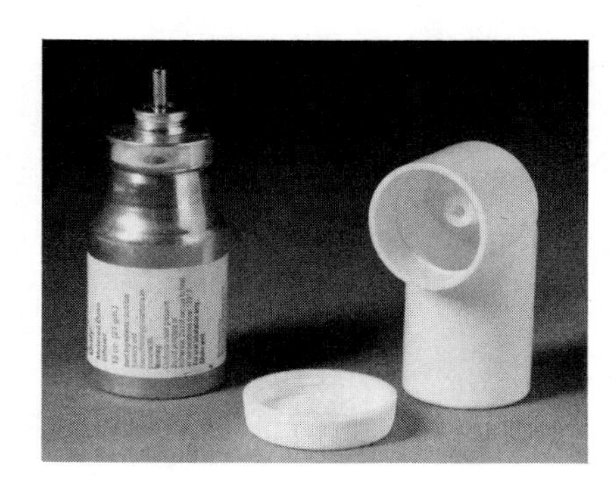

***Fig. 20-12***

3. Instruct client in comfortable environment by sitting in chair in hospital room, sitting at kitchen table in home. — Client will be more likely to remain perceptive of nurse's explanations.
4. Provide adequate time for teaching session. — Prevents interruptions. Instruction should occur when client is receptive.

## Implementation

1. Allow client opportunity to manipulate inhaler and canister. Explain and demonstrate how canister fits into inhaler. — Client must be familiar with how to use equipment.
2. Explain what metered dose is, and warn client about overuse of inhaler, including drug side effects. — Client must not arbitrarily decide to administer excessive inhalations because of risk of serious side effects. If given in recommended doses, side effects are uncommon.
3. Explain steps to administer inhaled dose of medication (demonstrate steps when possible): — Use of simple, step-by-step explanations allows client to ask questions at any point during procedure. Nurse demonstrates actual depression of canister without self-administering drug dose.
   a. Remove mouthpiece cover from inhaler.
   b. Shake inhaler well. — Ensures fine particles are aerosolized.
   c. Open lips and place inhaler in mouth with opening toward back of throat. — Directs aerosol spray toward airway.
   d. Exhale fully, then grasp mouthpiece with teeth and lips while holding inhaler with thumb at the mouthpiece and the index finger and middle finger at the top (Fig. 20-13). — Medication should not escape through mouth.
   e. While inhaling slowly and deeply through mouth, depress medication canister fully. — Medication is distributed to airways during inhalation. Inhalation through mouth rather than nose draws medication more effectively into airways.
   f. Hold breath for approximately 10 sec. — Allows tiny drops of aerosol spray to reach deeper branches of airways.
   g. Exhale through pursed lips. — Pursed lip breathing keeps small airways open during exhalation.
4. Explain steps to administer inhaled dose of medication using aerochamber (demonstrate when possible):
   a. Remove mouthpiece cover from metered dose inhaler and mouthpiece of aerochamber. — Inhaler fits into end of aerochamber.

| Steps | Rationale |
|---|---|

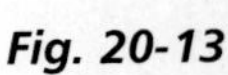
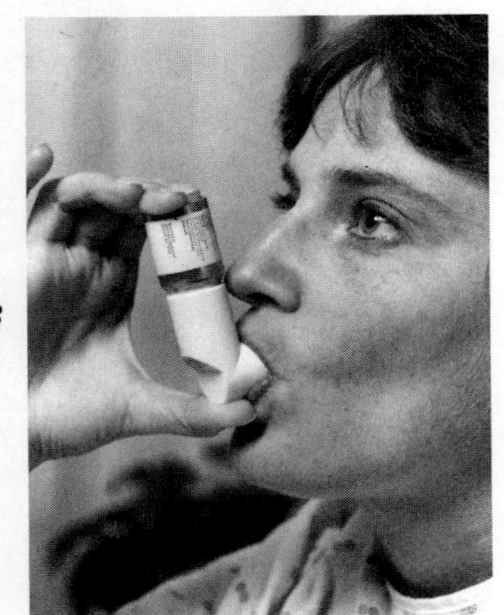

*Fig. 20-13*

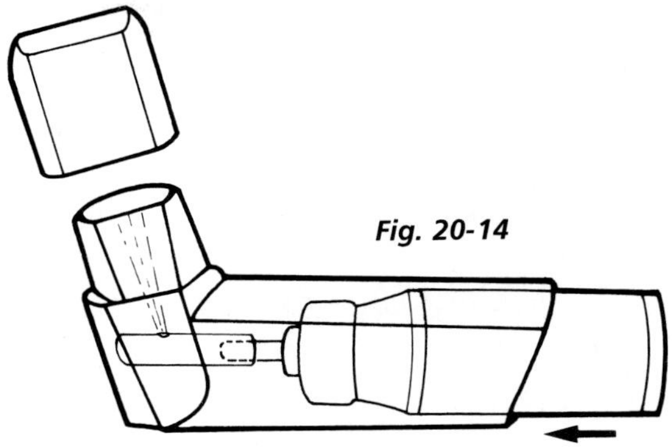

*Fig. 20-14*

| Steps | Rationale |
|---|---|
| b. Insert metered dose inhaler into end of aerochamber (Fig. 20-14). | Aerochamber is a spacer that extends the distance between the inhaler and the client's mouth. |
| c. Shake inhaler well. | Ensures fine particles are aerosolized. |
| d. Place aerochamber mouthpiece in mouth and close lips. Do not go beyond raised lip on mouthpiece. Avoid covering small exhalation slots with the lips. | Medication should not escape through mouth. |
| e. Breath normally through aerochamber mouthpiece. | Allows client to relax before delivering medication. |
| f. Depress medication canister, spraying one puff into aerochamber. | Emits spray that allows finer particles to be inhaled. Large droplets are retained in aerochamber. |
| g. Breathe in slowly and fully (+ 5 sec). | Ensures particles of medication are distributed to deeper airways. |
| h. Hold full breath for 5-10 sec. | Ensures full drug distribution. |
| 5. Instruct client to wait 5-10 min between inhalations or as ordered by physician. | Drugs must be inhaled sequentially. First inhalation opens airways and reduces inflammation. Second or third inhalations penetrate deeper airways. |
| 6. Instruct client against repeating inhalations before next scheduled dose. | Drugs are prescribed at intervals during day to provide constant bronchodilation and minimize side effects. |
| 7. Explain that client may feel gagging sensation in throat caused by droplets of medication on pharynx or tongue. | Results when inhalant is sprayed and inhaled incorrectly. |
| 8. Instruct client in removing medication canister and cleaning inhaler in warm water. | Accumulation of spray around mouthpiece can interfere with proper distribution during use. |
| 9. Ask if client has any questions. | Provides opportunity to clarify misconceptions or misunderstanding. |

## Evaluation

| Steps | Rationale |
|---|---|
| 1. Have client explain and demonstrate steps in use of inhaler. | Return demonstration provides feedback for measuring client's learning. |
| 2. Ask client to explain drug schedule. | Improves likelihood of compliance with therapy. |
| 3. Ask client to describe side effects of medication and criteria for calling physician. | Will allow client to recognize signs of overuse and need to seek medical support when drugs are ineffective. |

### *Expected outcomes*

| Steps | Rationale |
|---|---|
| 1. Client is able to successfully meet each previously identified objective. | Objectives provide guidelines for evaluation of client's knowledge and skills. |

### *Unexpected outcomes*

| Steps | Rationale |
|---|---|
| 1. Client is unable to meet one or more of established learning objectives. | Indicates need for further practice and instruction. |

## Recording and Reporting

| Steps | Rationale |
|---|---|
| 1. Describe in nurses' notes content on skills taught and client's ability to perform skill. | Information provides continuity to teaching plan so other members of nursing staff will not teach same material. |

| Steps | Rationale |
|---|---|
| **Follow-up Activities** | |
| 1. Client may need practice with assistance for several different steps of procedure before being able to perform each skill independently. | Several repetitions of practice of skill increases client's learning. |

## Special Considerations

- Signs and symptoms of overuse of xanthines and sympathomimetic drugs include: tachycardia, palpitations, headache, restlessness, and insomnia.
- Client may gag or swallow medication if unable to inhale while spray is administered. A child may need to hold nose shut during inhalation.
- Client's need for a bronchodilator more than every 4 hr can signal respiratory problems.

## Teaching Considerations

- Do not try to teach a client how to use an inhaler during an episode of shortness of breath. Client's attention span will be very poor.

# *SKILL 20-6 Administering Vaginal Instillations*

Female clients often develop vaginal infections requiring topical application of antiinfective agents. Medications are available in foam, jelly, cream, or suppository form. Medicated irrigations or douches can also be given. However, their excessive use can lead to vaginal irritation.

Suppositories come individually packaged in foil wrappers. Storage in a refrigerator prevents the solid, oval-shaped suppositories from melting. After a suppository is inserted into the vaginal cavity, body temperature causes the suppository to melt and be distributed. Foam, jellies, and creams are administered with an inserter or applicator (Procedure 15-10). A suppository is given with a gloved hand or applicator. Clients often prefer administering their own vaginal medications and should be given privacy. After instillation of the drug a client may wish to wear a perineal pad to collect excess drainage. Because vaginal medications are frequently given to treat infection, any discharge may be foul smelling. Good aseptic technique should be followed and the client should be offered frequent opportunities to maintain perineal hygiene (see Chapter 6).

## Purposes

1. Treat vaginal infections.
2. Relieve localized pruritis or irritation.

## *Procedure 20-6*

| Steps | Rationale |
|---|---|
| **Assessment** | |
| 1. Review physician's order including clients name, drug name, form (cream or suppository), route, dosage, and time of administration. | Ensures safe and correct administration of medication. |
| 2. Review pertinent information related to medication, including action, purpose, side effects, and nursing implications. | Allows nurse to administer drug properly and to monitor client's response. |
| 3. Inspect condition of external genitalia and vaginal canal (Chapter 13). (May be done just before insertion.) | Findings provide baseline to monitor effect of medication. |
| 4. Ask if client is experiencing any symptoms of pruritis, burning, or discomfort. | Assesses for symptoms of vaginal irritation. |
| 5. Assess client's ability to manipulate applicator or suppository and to position self to insert medication. (May be done just before insertion.) | Mobility restriction will indicate level of assistance required from nurse. |
| 6. Review client's knowledge of purpose of drug therapy. | May indicate need for health teaching. Understanding influences compliance with therapy. |

| Steps | Rationale |
|---|---|
| **Nursing Diagnosis** | |
| 1. Cluster data to reveal actual or potential nursing diagnoses: | |
| a. Pain: related to vaginal irritation. | Most common form of vaginal infection, monilial, can cause severe pruritis. |
| b. Knowledge deficit regarding purpose for drug therapy: related to misinterpreted information. | Limited understanding affects client's ability to follow drug regimen. |
| c. Impaired physical mobility: related to weakened hand coordination. | Client unable to self-administer drug; any instruction must involve family. |
| **Planning** | |
| 1. Develop individualized goals for client based on nursing diagnoses: | |
| a. Ensure proper drug distribution and absorption. | Medication must be properly instilled into vaginal canal. |
| b. Client attains sense of comfort. | Proper drug administration and perineal hygiene will relieve pruritis. |
| c. Client acquires knowledge of drug therapy. | During administration nurse explains therapy. |
| 2. Wash hands. | Reduces transfer of microorganisms. |
| 3. Prepare following supplies for suppository insertion: | |
| a. Vaginal suppository (Fig. 20-15) | These are stored in refrigerator to maintain solid shape. |
| b. Clean disposable gloves | Reduces transfer of microorganisms. |
| c. Lubricating jelly | Eases insertion of suppository. |
| d. Facial tissues | |
| e. Perineal pad (optional) | |
| f. Medication ticket, form, or printout | |
| 4. Prepare following supplies for cream instillation: | |
| a. Vaginal cream | Prepared in plastic tube. |
| b. Plastic applicator | |
| c. Clean disposable gloves | Reduces transfer of microorganisms. |
| d. Paper towel | |
| e. Perineal pad (optional) | |
| f. Medication ticket or form | |
| 5. Compare medication ticket with label of medication. | Ensures right medication is administered. |
| 6. Check client's identification bracelet and ask name. | Ensures right client receives medication. |
| 7. Explain procedure to client. Be specific if client plans on self-administering medication. | Promotes client's understanding. Will enable client to self-administer drug if physically able. |
| **Implementation** | |
| 1. Arrange supplies at bedside. | Helps nurse perform procedure smoothly. |
| 2. Close room curtain or door. | Provides privacy. |
| 3. Assist client to lie in dorsal recumbent position. | Position provides easy access to and good exposure of vaginal canal. Dependent position also allows suppository to dissolve in vagina without escaping through orifice. |
| 4. Keep abdomen and lower extremities draped. | Minimizes client's embarrassment. |
| 5. Don disposable gloves. | Prevents transmission of infection between nurse and client. |
| 6. Be sure vaginal orifice is well-illuminated by room light or gooseneck lamp. | Proper insertion requires visualization of external genitalia. |

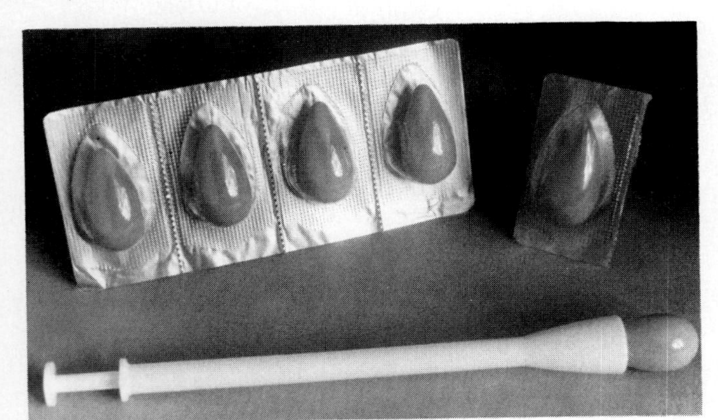

***Fig. 20-15*** Vaginal suppositories.

| Steps | Rationale |
|---|---|
| 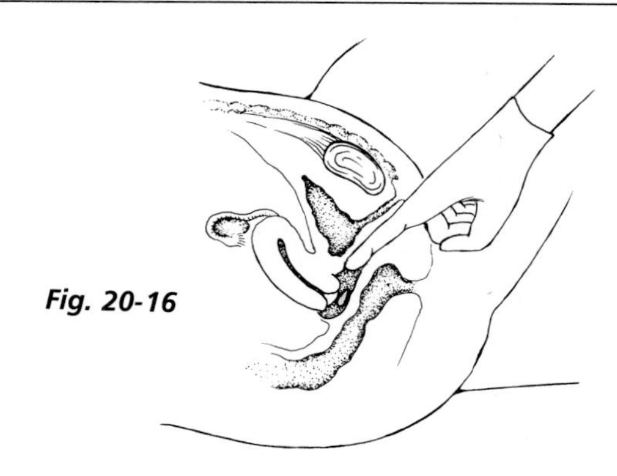 *Fig. 20-16* | 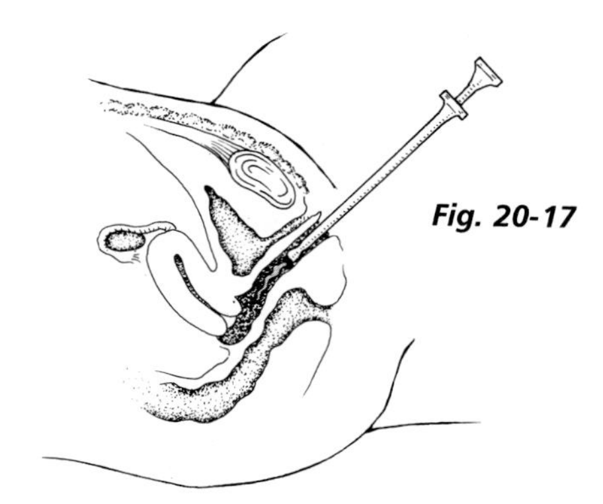 *Fig. 20-17* |
| 7. For suppository insertion: | |
| a. Remove suppository from foil wrapper and apply liberal amount of petroleum jelly to smooth or rounded end. Lubricate gloved index finger of dominant hand. | Lubrication reduces friction against mucosal surfaces during insertion. |
| b. With nondominant gloved hand, gently retract labial folds. | Exposes vaginal orifice. |
| c. Insert rounded end of suppository along posterior wall of vaginal canal entire length of finger (7.5-10 cm or 3-4 in) (Fig. 20-16). | Proper placement of suppository ensures equal distribution of medication along walls of vaginal cavity. |
| d. Withdraw finger and wipe away remaining lubricant from around orifice and labia. | Maintains comfort. |
| 8. For application of cream or foam: | |
| a. Fill cream or foam applicator following package directions. | Dosage is prescribed by volume in applicator. |
| b. With nondominant gloved hand, gently retract labial folds. | Exposes vaginal orifice. |
| c. With dominant gloved hand, insert applicator approximately 5-7.5 cm (2-3 in). Push applicator plunger to deposit medication into vagina (Fig. 20-17). | Allows equal distribution of medication along vaginal walls. |
| d. Withdraw applicator and place on paper towel. Wipe off residual cream from labia or vaginal orifice. | Residual cream on applicator may contain microorganisms. |
| 9. Remove gloves by pulling them inside out and discard in appropriate receptacle. | Reduces transfer of microorganisms. |
| 10. Instruct client to remain on her back for at least 10 min. | Medication will be distributed and absorbed evenly throughout vaginal cavity and not be lost through orifice. |
| 11. If applicator is used, wash with soap and warm water, rinse, and store for future use. | Vaginal cavity is not sterile. Soap and water assist in removal of bacteria and residual cream. |
| 12. Offer perineal pad when client resumes ambulation. | Provides client comfort. |

## Evaluation

| Steps | Rationale |
|---|---|
| 1. Inspect condition of vaginal canal and external genitalia between applications. | Determines whether vaginal medication effectively reduced irritation or inflammation of tissues. |
| 2. Question client regarding continued pruritis, burning, or discomfort. | Determines whether symptoms relieved. |
| 3. Note client's nonverbal reaction as drug is given. | May indicate client is embarrassed by procedure. |
| 4. Ask client to discuss purpose, action, side effects of medication. | Reflects client's understanding of drug therapy. |

### *Expected outcomes*

| Steps | Rationale |
|---|---|
| 1. Vaginal tissues are pink and smooth. Genitalia are clear and without discharge. | Normal characteristics of tissues. |
| 2. Client denies symptoms of discomfort. | Inflammation resolved. |
| 3. There may be a small amount of discharge that is the color of medication exiting from vaginal canal. | When suppository or cream becomes distributed, small amount may escape from orifice. |
| 4. Client appears relaxed. | Client free of embarrassment. |
| 5. Client is able to discuss information about prescribed drug. | Feedback reflects client's learning. |

| Steps | Rationale |
|---|---|
| ***Unexpected outcomes*** | |
| 1. There is thick, white, patchy, curdlike discharge clinging to vaginal walls. Vaginal walls appear bright pink or inflamed. | Signs of yeast infection, a common female disorder. |
| 2. Client reports localized pruritis and burning. | Result of infection or inflammation. |
| 3. Client exhibits restlessness, facial tension, movements of hands or feet. | Indicative of embarrassment of anxiety. |
| 4. Client unable to discuss drug therapy correctly. | Requires repeated instruction or client is unable to learn. |

## Recording and Reporting

| | |
|---|---|
| 1. Record drug name, dosage, route, and time of administration on medication record. | Timely recording prevents drug errors. |
| 2. Record appearance of vaginal canal and genitalia in nurses' notes and report any unusual findings. | Documented description provides guidelines to determine change in client's condition and records client's response to therapy. |

### Special Considerations

- Caution: rectal and vaginal suppositories may be stored together in a refrigerator. Vaginal suppositories are larger and more oval.
- Be sure perineal structures are well visualized during assessment and administration of medication.
- Clients with restricted mobility in knees or hips may lie supine with legs abducted.
- If suppository fails to dissolve and solid form is expelled, check expiration date on package (new supply may be needed).

### Teaching Considerations

- Teach client value of and technique for regular perineal hygiene.

# SKILL 20-7 Administering Rectal Suppositories

A variety of medications may be given rectally. Drugs administered rectally exert either a local effect on gastrointestinal mucosa, such as promoting defecation, or systemic effects, such as relieving nausea or providing analgesia. The rectal route is not as reliable as oral or parenteral routes in terms of drug absorption and distribution. However, the medications are relatively safe, since they rarely cause local irritation or side effects. Rectal medications are contraindicated in clients with rectal surgery or active rectal bleeding.

Rectal suppositories differ in shape from vaginal suppositories, being thinner and bullet-shaped (Fig. 20-18). The rounded end prevents anal trauma during insertion. When the nurse administers the suppository it is important to place it past the internal anal sphincter and against the rectal mucosa. Improper placement can result in expulsion of the suppository before the medication dissolves and is absorbed into the mucosa. Never force a suppository into a mass of fecal material. It may be necessary to administer a small cleansing enema before a suppository can be inserted. If a client prefers to self-administer a suppository, the nurse should give specific instructions so that the medication is deposited correctly.

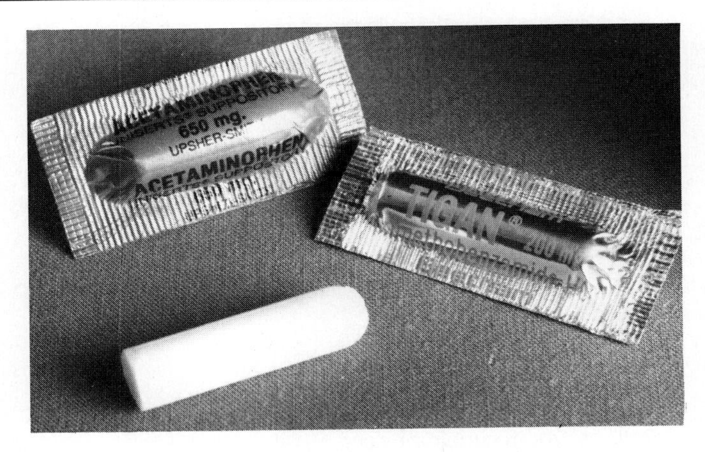


***Fig. 20-18*** Rectal suppositories.

### Purposes

1. Promote local effects on gastrointestinal mucosa.
2. Provide an alternate route for systemic-acting medications when the oral route is contraindicated.
3. Provide an alternate route to control vomiting when oral medications are unsuitable.

## Procedure 20-7

| Steps | Rationale |
|---|---|
| **Assessment** | |
| 1. Review physician's order, including client's name; drug name, form, route, and time of administration. | Ensures safe and correct administration of medication. |
| 2. Review pertinent information related to medication, including action, purpose, side effects, and nursing implications. | Allows nurse to administer drug properly and to monitor client's response. |
| 3. Review medical record for history of rectal surgery or bleeding. | Conditions contraindicate use of suppository. |
| 4. Review any presenting signs and symptoms of gastrointestinal alterations. | Conditions may indicate use of suppository. |
| 5. Assess client's ability to hold suppository and to position self to insert medication. | Mobility restriction indicates need for nurse to assist with drug administration. |
| 6. Review client's knowledge of purpose of drug therapy. | May indicate need for health teaching. |
| **Nursing Diagnosis** | |
| 1. Cluster data to reveal actual or potential nursing diagnoses: | |
| a. Constipation: related to imbalanced dietary intake. | A number of bowel alterations may indicate use of suppositories. |
| b. Knowledge deficit regarding purpose of medication: related to inexperience. | Limited understanding affects client's ability to follow drug regimen. |
| c. Pain: related to inflammation of anal tissues. | Insertion of suppository can aggravate irritated tissues. |
| d. Impaired physical mobility: related to reduced range of motion. | Can prohibit client from self-administering suppository. Thus any instruction must involve family. |
| **Planning** | |
| 1. Develop individualized goals for client based on nursing diagnoses: | |
| a. Client has soft, formed stools regularly. | Medication that softens stools and promotes defecation will ease constipation. |
| b. Client's pain is reduced or relieved. | Medications that reduce local inflammation will relieve pain. |
| c. Ensure proper drug distribution and absorption. | Correct placement of suppository ensures absorption of drugs with systemic effects. |
| d. Client acquires knowledge of drug therapy | During administration nurse explains therapy. |
| 2. Wash hands. | Reduces transfer of microorganisms. |
| 3. Prepare following equipment and supplies: | |
| a. Rectal suppository | |
| b. Lubricating jelly (water-soluble) | |
| c. Clean disposable gloves | Prevents contact with infected material. |
| d. Tissue | |
| e. Medication ticket, form, or printout | |
| 4. Compare medication form with label of medication. | Ensures right medication is administered. |
| 5. Check client's identification bracelet and ask name. | Ensures right client receives medication. |
| 6. Explain procedure to client. Be specific if client wishes to self-administer drug. | Promotes client's understanding and cooperation. Will enable client to self-administer drug if physically able. |
| **Implementation** | |
| 1. Arrange supplies at bedside. | Helps nurse perform procedure smoothly. |
| 2. Close room curtain or door. | Maintains privacy and minimizes embarrassment. |
| 3. Assist client in assuming a side-lying Sims' position with upper leg flexed upward. | Position exposes anus and helps client to relax external anal sphincter. |
| 4. Keep client draped with only anal area exposed. | Maintains privacy and facilitates relaxation. |
| 5. Apply disposable gloves. | Prevents contact with infected material. |
| 6. Examine condition of anus externally and palpate rectal walls as needed (see Chapter 13). Dispose of gloves by turning them inside out and placing them in proper receptacle if they become soiled. | Determines presence of active rectal bleeding. Palpation determines whether rectum filled with feces, which may interfere with suppository placement. Reduces transmission of infection. |
| 7. Apply disposable gloves (if previous gloves were soiled and discarded). | Minimizes contact with fecal material to reduce transmission of infection. |

| Steps | Rationale |
|---|---|

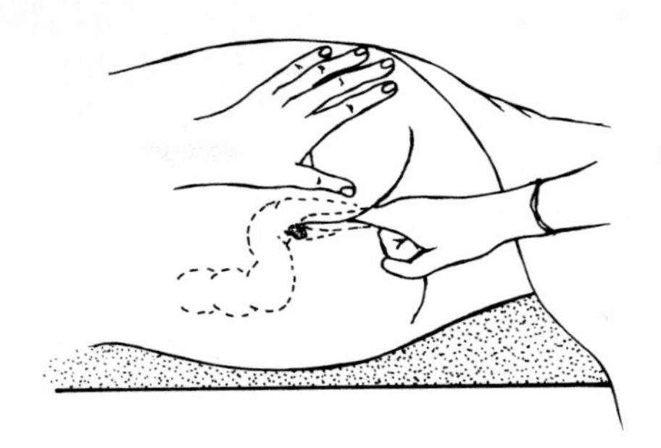

*Fig. 20-19*

| Steps | Rationale |
|---|---|
| 8. Remove suppository from foil wrapper and lubricate rounded end with jelly. Lubricate gloved index finger of dominant hand. | Lubrication reduces friction as suppository enters rectal canal. |
| 9. Ask client to take slow deep breaths through mouth and to relax anal sphincter. | Forcing suppository through constricted sphincter causes pain. |
| 10. Retract client's buttocks with nondominant hand. With gloved index finger of dominant hand, insert suppository gently through anus, past internal sphincter, and against rectal wall, 10 cm (4 in) in adults, 5 cm (2 in) in children and infants (Fig. 20-19). | Suppository must be placed against rectal mucosa for eventual absorption and therapeutic action. |
| 11. Withdraw your finger and wipe client's anal area. | Provides comfort. |
| 12. Discard gloves by turning them inside out, and dispose in appropriate receptacle. | Reduces transfer of microorganisms. |
| 13. Ask client to remain flat or on side for 5 min. | Prevents expulsion of suppository. |
| 14. If suppository contains laxative or fecal softener, place call light within reach so client can obtain assistance to reach bedpan or toilet. | Ability to call for assistance provides client with sense of control over elimination. |
| 15. Wash hands. | Reduces risk of transfer of infection. |

## Evaluation

| | |
|---|---|
| 1. Return within 5 min to determine if suppository expelled. (Evaluate client for 30-60 min.) | Determines if drug properly distributed. Reinsertion may be necessary. |
| 2. Ask if client experienced localized anal or rectal discomfort during insertion. | Determines whether insertion of suppository was irritating. |
| 3. Evaluate client for relief of symptoms medication was prescribed to relieve or eliminate. (Within time expected action of drug occurs.) | Determines medication's effectiveness. |
| 4. Ask client to explain purpose of medication. | Reflects client's understanding of drug therapy. |

### *Expected outcomes*

| | |
|---|---|
| 1. Suppository is retained. | Drug inserted properly. |
| 2. Client reports relief or reduction in symptoms for which medication is prescribed. | Drug acts effectively. |
| 3. Client has minimal or no rectal discomfort during insertion. | Insertion is nontraumatic. |
| 4. Client describes purpose of medication. | Feedback reflects client's learning. |

### *Unexpected outcomes*

| | |
|---|---|
| 1. Suppository expelled prematurely. | New suppository must be inserted. Suppository not inserted past internal sphincter. |
| 2. Side effects of specific medication develop. Symptoms previously reported are unrelieved. | Dependent on type of drug administered. May require alternate therapy. |
| 3. Client reports rectal pain during insertion. | Suppository may need to be better lubricated or rectal route may be contraindicated. |
| 4. Client unable to explain purpose of drug therapy. | Reinstruction necessary or client unwilling to learn. |

## Recording and Reporting

| | |
|---|---|
| 1. Record drug name, dosage, route, and time of administration on medication record. | Timely recording prevents drug errors. |
| 2. Record and report client's response to medication, including any unusual reactions. | Documents effect of medication. |

### Special Considerations

- Do not palpate client's rectum if client has had rectal surgery.
- If client has hemorrhoids use liberal amount of lubricant.
- With experience nurse is able to feel internal sphincter relax around finger after suppository passes up into rectum.
- It may be necessary to hold buttocks of an infant or small child together for several min until suppository is absorbed.
- Elderly clients with loss of sphincter control may have difficulty retaining suppository.

### Teaching Considerations

- If clients choose to self-administer suppositories teach principles and techniques of infection control to prevent contact with and spread of fecal material.

## *SKILL 20-8 Administering Ear Irrigations*

Medications may be used to irrigate or wash out a body cavity and are delivered through a stream of solution. In a health care setting sterile solutions of water, saline, or antiseptics are used on the eye, ear, throat, and vagina. This is especially important if there is a break in the skin or mucosa or if the tympanic membrane of the ear is ruptured. In the home setting sterile supplies are usually not necessary because cavities to be irrigated are not sterile and the risk of cross contamination is lessened.

The more common indications for irrigation of the external ear are presence of a foreign body, local inflammation of the canal, and accumulation of cerumen. Precautions must be taken to avoid instilling hot or cold fluid into the ear to lessen causing dizziness or vertigo in clients.

The greatest danger during administration of an ear irrigation is rupture of the tympanic membrane. Fluids must not be instilled under pressure or with the ear canal occluded by the irrigating device. Children are the most common clients for which the procedure is performed.

### Purposes

1. Relieve localized inflammation and irritation.
2. Loosen and remove impacted cerumen or foreign objects.

## *Procedure 20-8*

| Steps | Rationale |
|---|---|
| **Assessment** | |
| 1. Review physician's order including client's name, solution to be instilled, affected ear(s), time of administration. | Ensures safe and correct administration of medication. |
| 2. Review pertinent information related to ordered antiseptics including action, purpose, nursing implications. | Allows nurse to administer drug properly and monitor client's response. |
| 3. Review medical record for history of ruptured tympanic membrane. | Will contraindicate irrigation. |
| 4. Inspect the pinna and external auditory meatus for redness, swelling, drainage, abrasions, and presence of cerumen or foreign objects. (If indicated use an otoscope to inspect deeper portions of the auditory canal.) | Findings provide baseline to monitor effects of medication or solution. |
| 5. Ask if client is experiencing discomfort. Note client's ability to hear clearly. | Pain is symptomatic of external ear infection or inflammation. Occlusion of auditory canal by cerumen or foreign object can impair hearing. |
| 6. Review client's knowledge of purpose for irrigation and normal care of the ears. | May indicate need for instruction regarding hygiene. |
| **Nursing Diagnosis** | |
| 1. Cluster data to reveal actual or potential nursing diagnoses: | |
| a. Pain: related to inflammation of auditory canal. | Skin overlying canal is extremely sensitive when inflammed or irritated. |
| b. Sensory/perceptual alteration (auditory): related to external ear occlusion. | Conductive hearing loss results from obstruction in canal, which can be removed by irrigation. |
| c. Knowledge deficit regarding ear hygiene: related to inexperience. | Indicates need for instruction on care of ears and purpose of irrigation. |

| Steps | Rationale |
|---|---|
| **Planning** | |
| 1. Develop individualized goals for client based on nursing diagnoses: | |
| a. Ensure safe instillation of fluid into auditory canal. | Irrigating fluid must not be introduced under pressure. |
| b. Client gains relief from inflammation and discomfort. | Proper instillation will relieve swelling and irritation of tissues. |
| c. Client regains hearing acuity. | Cerumen or foreign object are effectively removed. |
| d. Client acquires knowledge of proper ear care. | During administration nurse explains proper techniques for ear care. |
| 2. Wash hands. | Reduces transfer of microorganisms. |
| 3. Prepare the following equipment and supplies: | |
| a. Container of sterile irrigating solution warmed to room temperature and sterile round basin. | Warmed solution minimizes chance of causing client to feel dizzy when solution comes in contact with tympanic membrane. |
| b. Irrigating syringe (rubber bulb or asepto) | Used to introduce solution under low pressure. |
| c. Kidney-shaped basin | Used to collect irrigating solution. |
| d. Towel or absorbent pad | |
| e. Applicator swab and cotton balls | Used to clean and dry ear canal. |
| 4. Check client's identification by reading identification bracelet and asking name. | Ensures correct client receives irrigation. |
| 5. Explain procedure. Warn that the irrigation may cause sensation of dizziness, fullness, and warmth. | Prepares client to anticipate effects of irrigation, and promotes cooperation. |
| **Implementation** | |
| 1. Arrange supplies at bedside. | Helps nurse to perform procedure smoothly. |
| 2. Close curtain or room door. | Maintains privacy. |
| 3. Assist client to a sitting or lying position with head turned toward the affected ear. Place towel under client's head and shoulder and have client hold basin under affected ear (Fig. 20-20). | Position minimizes leakage of fluids around neck and facial area. Solution will flow from ear canal to basin. |
| 4. Pour irrigating solution into sterile round basin. | |
| 5. Gently clean auricle and ear canal with moistened cotton applicator. Do *not* force drainage or cerumen into the ear canal. | Prevents infected material from reentering ear canal. |
| 6. Fill irrigating syringe with solution (approximately 50 cc). | Enough fluid is needed to provide a steady irrigating stream. |
| 7. Gently grasp the auricle of the ear and straighten the ear canal by pulling it down and back (children) or upward and outward (adult). | Allows fluid to flow length of the canal. |
| 8. Slowly instill irrigating solution by holding the tip of the syringe 1 cm (0.5 in) above the opening to the ear canal. Allow fluid to drain out during instillation. Continue until canal is cleansed or solution is used (Fig. 20-21). | Slow instillation prevents buildup of pressure in the ear canal and ensures contact of the solution with all canal surfaces. |
| 9. Do *not* occlude the canal with the tip of the syringe. | Buildup of fluid in canal under forced pressure could cause rupture of the tympanic membrane. |
| 10. Dry outer ear canal with cotton ball. Leave cotton loosely in place for 5-10 min. | Maintains comfort. Absorbs excess moisture in ear canal. |
| 11. Assist client to a sitting position. | Maintains comfort. |
| 12. Wash hands and dispose of supplies. | Reduces transmission of infection. |
| **Evaluation** | |
| 1. Ask client if discomfort is noted during instillation of solution. | Fluid instilled improperly under pressure causes discomfort. |

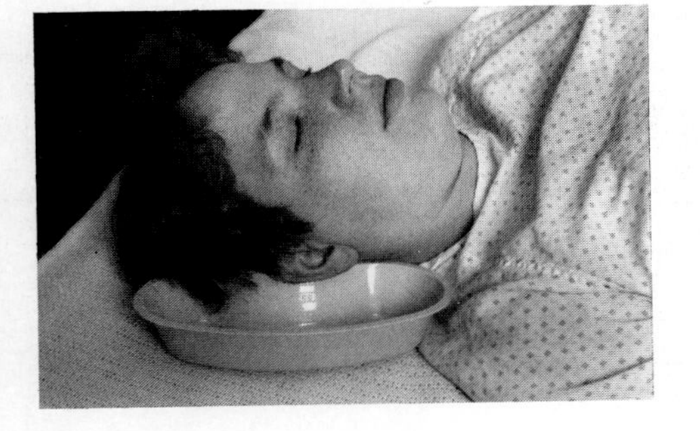

*Fig. 20-20*

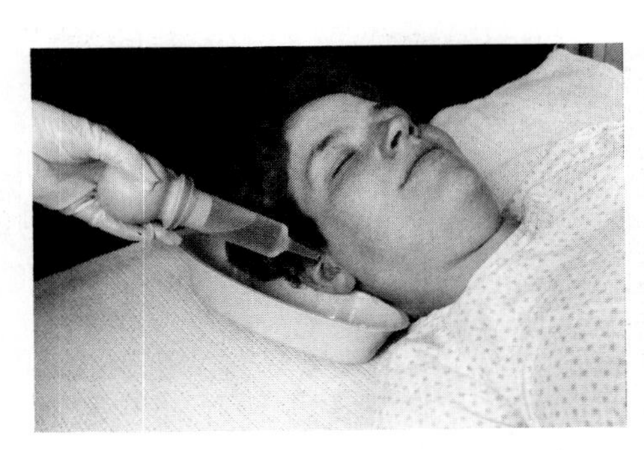

*Fig. 20-21*

| Steps | Rationale |
|---|---|
| 2. Reinspect condition of meatus and canal. | Determines if solution relieves symptoms and removes foreign materials. |
| 3. Measure client's hearing acuity. | Determines if conduction deafness relieved. |
| 4. Ask client to describe purpose of irrigation and proper techniques for ear care. | Reflects client's understanding of procedure and proper hygiene. |
| ***Expected outcomes*** | |
| 1. Client denies pain during instillation. | Fluid properly instilled. |
| 2. Skin overlying meatus and canal becomes clear, without redness, swelling, tenderness, or discharge. Canal is clear of cerumen and foreign material. | Inflammation, irritation, and occlusion of canal relieved. |
| 3. Client hears conversation clearly. | Obstruction in ear canal relieved. |
| 4. Client is able to discuss purpose of irrigation and describe correct ear care techniques. | Feedback reflects client's learning. |
| ***Unexpected outcomes*** | |
| 1. Client expresses pain during irrigation. | Fluid instilled under pressure or irrigating syringe contacts inflammed tissue. |
| 2. Auditory canal remains inflammed, irritated, or occluded. | Repeated irrigations may be needed. |
| 3. Client continues to have impaired hearing. | Auditory canal remains occluded. |
| 4. Client unable to discuss purpose of irrigation or ear hygiene. | Reinstruction is necessary or client unwilling to learn. |

## Recording and Reporting

| | |
|---|---|
| 1. Record in nurses' notes procedure, amount of solution instilled, time of administration, and ear receiving irrigation. | Timely documentation prevents treatment errors. |
| 2. Record appearance of external ear and client's hearing acuity in nurses' notes. | Documents status of ear. |
| 3. Report and record any undesirable side effects to nurse in charge or physician. | Nature of client's reaction may require additional therapy. |

## Special Considerations

- Always attempt to remove foreign objects in the ear first by simply straightening the ear canal.
- Never irrigate the ear if vegetable matter is occluded in the canal. The material can swell on contact with water.
- Refer clients to an otolaryngologist if a foreign object remains occluded after irrigation.

## Teaching Considerations

- Instruct clients to clean ears daily with a washcloth, soap, and warm water.
- Warn clients against placing sharp objects in the ears.
- Instruct parents of young children to check their ears for foreign objects.

### BIBLIOGRAPHY


Anders JE: Topical, a welter of options calls for refined application techniques, RN 45:33, 1982.

Bernal H: In-home medication checks with diabetics, Home Healthcare Nurse, 6(5):14, 1988.

Bulau J: Clinical policies and procedures for home health care, Rockville, Md, 1986, Aspen Publishers, Inc.

Clark JB, Queener SF, Karb VB: Pharmacological basis of nursing practice, ed 3, St. Louis, 1990, The CV Mosby Co.

Donnelly D: Instilling eye drops: difficulties experienced by patients following cataract surgery, J Adv Nurs 12:235, 1987.

Ebersole P, Hess P: Toward healthy aging, ed 3, St. Louis, 1989, The CV Mosby Co.

Gever LN: Administering drugs through the skin, Nursing '82, 12:88, 1982.

Giving Medications, Nursing Photobook, Springhouse, Pa, 1983, Intermed Communications, Inc.

Govoni L, Hayes J: Drugs and nursing implications, New York, 1980, Appleton-Century Crofts.

Helping asthmatics help themselves, Emerg. Med. 14:133, 1982.

Kim MJ, et al.: Pocket guide to nursing diagnoses, ed 2, St. Louis, 1989, The CV Mosby Co.

Kirilloff LH, Tibbals SC: Drugs for asthma, a complete guide, Am J Nurs 83:55, 1983.

Nurses drug alert: hazards of nasal decongestants in young children, Am J Nurs 84:1265, 1984.

Potter PA, Perry AG: Basic nursing, St. Louis, 1987, The CV Mosby Co.

Potter PA, Perry AG: Fundamentals of nursing: concepts, process, and practice, St. Louis, ed 2, 1989, The CV Mosby Co.

Rothstein MS: Guidelines for the use of topical medications, J Enterostomal Ther 10:203, 1983.

Scipien G, et al.: Comprehensive pediatric nursing New York, 1986, McGraw-Hill Book Co.

Shlafer M, Marieb E: The nurse, pharmacology, drug therapy, Menlo Park, Calif, 1989, Addison-Wesley Publishing Co.

Smith S, Duell D: Clinical nursing skills Los Altos, Calif, 1985, National Nursing Review.

Statz E: Hand strength and metered dose inhalers, Am J Nurs 84:800, 1984.

Todd B: Drugs and the elderly: using eye drops and ointments safely, Geriatr Nurs 4(1):55, 1983.

Walsh J, Persons C, Wieck L: Manual of home health care nursing, Philadelphia, 1987, JB Lippincott Co.

Whaley LF, Wong DL: Nursing care of infants and children, ed 3, St. Louis, 1987, The CV Mosby Co.

# 21
# PARENTERAL MEDICATIONS

## OBJECTIVES

*Mastery of content in this chapter will enable the nurse to:*

- Define key terms.
- Identify advantages and disadvantages of administering medications by each injection route.
- Discuss factors to consider when selecting injection sites.
- Explain the importance of selecting proper syringes and needles for an injection.
- Discuss ways to maintain client comfort while administering an injection.
- Explain risks associated with administering injections.
- Correctly prepare an injectable medication from a vial and an ampule.
- Correctly administer a subcutaneous, intramuscular, and intradermal injection.
- Correctly administer an intravenous infusion by intravenous bolus, piggyback, or large volume infusion.
- Compare the risks of three different intravenous routes.

## KEY TERMS

*Air embolus*
*Ampule*
*Anaphylactic reaction*
*Aqueous*
*Aspirate*
*Bolus*
*Diluent*
*Hematoma*
*Heparin lock*
*Incompatibility*
*Induration*
*Infiltration*
*Infusion*
*Injection*
*Intradermal injection*
*Intramuscular (IM) injection*
*Intravenous (IV) injection*
*Lipodystrophy*
*Parenteral*
*Phlebitis*
*Physician's Desk Reference (PDR)*
*Piggyback infusion*
*Subcutaneous (SQ, SC) injection*
*Vial*
*Z-track*

## SKILLS

**21-1** Preparing Injections from Ampules and Vials
**21-2** Mixing Medications from Two Vials
**21-3** Administering Subcutaneous Injections
**21-4** Teaching Clients How To Administer Self-Injections
**21-5** Administering Intramuscular Injections
**21-6** Administering Intradermal Injections
**21-7** Adding Medications to Intravenous Fluid Containers
**21-8** Administering Intravenous Medications by Intermittent Infusion Sets
**21-9** Administering Medications by Intravenous Bolus

Parenteral injections are used to instill medications into body tissues. The procedures are invasive and thus pose greater risk than administering oral medications. Injected drugs act more quickly than oral medications, and thus the client's condition can change rapidly. The nurse must monitor the client's response closely and be aware of potential side effects or allergic reactions. A risk of infection once a needle pierces the skin also exists. The nurse uses strict aseptic technique whenever preparing and administering injections. Infection can originate from a variety of sources (Table 21-1).

The four major sites for parenteral injection are:

1. *Subcutaneous*— injection into tissues just below the dermis of the skin.
2. *Intramuscular*— injection into the body of a muscle.
3. *Intradermal*— injection into the dermis just under the epidermis.
4. *Intravenous*— injection into a vein.

Each type of injection requires a certain set of skills to make certain the medication reaches the proper location. Failure to inject a medication correctly can result in complications such as rapid drug response, nerve injury with associated pain, localized bleeding, and sterile abscess. A variety of syringes and needles are available and designed to deliver a certain volume of medication into a specific tissue. The nurse uses informed judgment in determining which syringe or needle is most effective.

## SYRINGES

A syringe consists of a cylindrical barrel, a tip designed to fit the hub of a hypodermic needle, and a close-fitting

**TABLE 21-1** Preventing Infection during an Injection

| Goal | Actions |
|---|---|
| Prevent contamination of solution. | Draw medication from vial quickly. Do not allow vial to stand open. |
| Prevent needle contamination. | Avoid letting needle touch contaminated surface: outer edges of ampule or vial, outer surface of needle cap, nurse's hands, countertop, or table surface. |
| Prevent syringe contamination. | Avoid touching length of plunger or inner part of barrel. Keep tip of syringe covered with cap or needle. |
| Prepare skin. | Wash skin soiled with dirt, drainage, or feces with soap and water, and dry. Use friction and a circular motion while cleaning with an antiseptic swab. Swab from center of site and move outward in 5 cm (2 in) radius. |

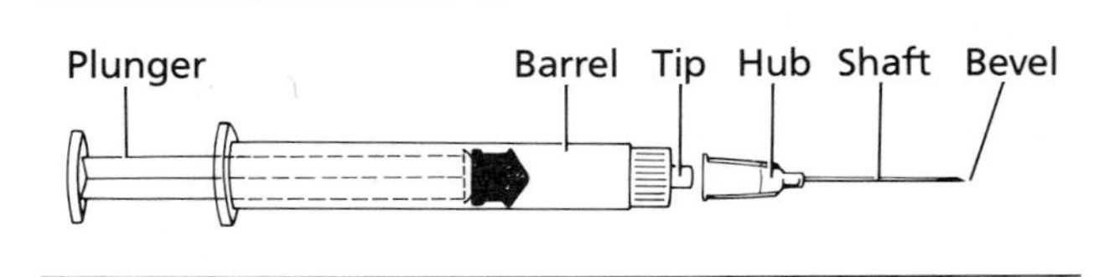


***Fig. 21-1*** Parts of a syringe and hypodermic needle.

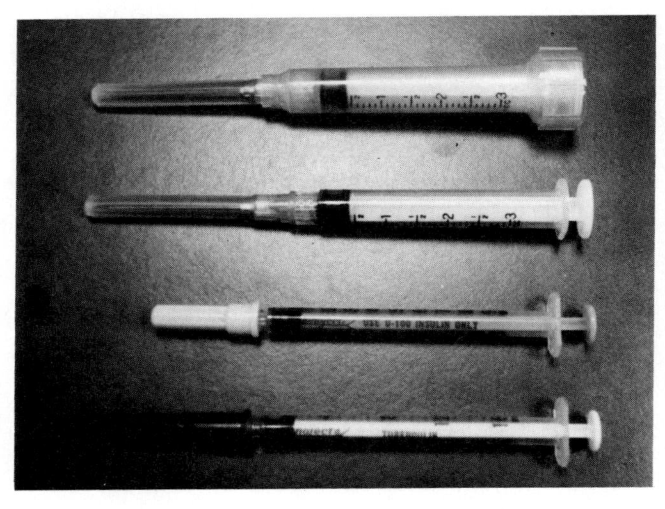

***Fig. 21-2*** Types of syringes. *Top to bottom,* Disposable plastic syringe and needle in case, 3 cc hypodermic syringe, insulin syringe, and tuberculin syringe.

plunger (Fig. 21-1). Syringes are made of glass or plastic. Most institutions use disposable, single-use plastic syringes, which are inexpensive and easy to manipulate. Syringes are packaged separately, with or without a sterile needle, in a paper wrapper or rigid plastic container. Glass syringes require sterilizing between uses and are expensive.

The nurse fills a syringe by aspiration, pulling the plunger outward while the attached needle tip remains immersed in the prepared solution. To prevent contamination and maintain sterility, the nurse holds only the outside of the syringe barrel and the plunger's handle. The nurse also avoids letting any unsterile object touch the tip or inside of the barrel, the shaft of the plunger, or the needle. Syringes come in various sizes, varying in capacity from 1 to 50 ml (Fig. 21-2).

It is unusual to use a syringe larger than 5 ml for an injection. A 2 to 3 ml syringe is adequate for intramuscular and subcutaneous injections. A larger volume causes discomfort. Hypodermic syringes have two scales along the barrel. One scale is divided into minims and the other into tenths of a milliliter.

## NEEDLES

Needles come packaged in individual sheaths to allow flexibility in choosing the right needle for a client. Some needles are preattached to standard size syringes. Most needles are made of stainless steel, although intravenous catheters are plastic. Needles are disposable, except for those made from surgical steel, which are attached to glass syringes.

A needle has three parts: the hub, which fits onto the tip of a syringe; the shaft, which connects to the hub; and the bevel or slanted tip (see Fig. 21-1). The nurse may handle the needle hub to ensure a tight fit on the syringe; however, the shaft and bevel must remain sterile at all times.

Each needle has three characteristic features: the bevel's slant, the shaft's length, and the needle gauge or diameter. The bevel creates a narrow slit that quickly closes to prevent leakage of medication, blood, or serum.

A short bevel is best for intravenous injections because it is not easily occluded against the inside of a blood vessel wall. Long bevels are sharper, which minimizes discomfort caused by subcutaneous and intramuscular injections.

Needles vary in length from ¼ to 5 inches, although 1½ inches is the maximum length for injections given by nurses. The nurse chooses needle length according to client size and weight and the type of tissue into which the drug is to be injected. A child or slender adult generally requires a shorter needle. The nurse uses longer needles

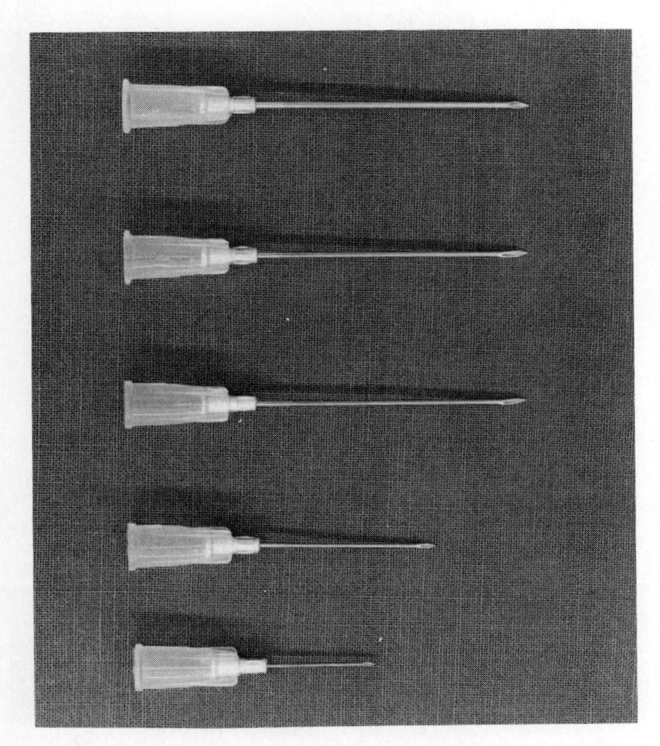

***Fig. 21-3*** Hypodermic needles arranged in order of gauge. *Top to bottom,* 16 gauge, 19 gauge, 20 gauge, 23 gauge, and 25 gauge.

(1 to 1½ inches) for intramuscular injections and a shorter needle (⅜ to ⅝ inch) for subcutaneous injections.

The smaller the needle gauge, the larger the needle diameter (Fig. 21-3). The selection of a gauge depends on the viscosity of fluid to be injected or infused. The rationale for needle selection is included in each skill.

## DISPOSABLE INJECTION UNITS

Disposable, single-dose, prefilled syringes are available for some medications. With these units the nurse does not have to prepare doses, except perhaps to expel portions of unneeded medications.

The Tubex and Carpujet injection systems include reusable plastic syringes that hold prefilled, disposable, sterile cartridge-needle units (Fig. 21-4). The nurse slips the cartridge into the syringe, secures it (following package directions) and checks for air bubbles in the syringe. The nurse advances the plunger to expel medication as in a regular syringe. A new type of injection system involves screwing a plunger-like device into the end of a prefilled vial containing a needle. After the medication is given the entire unit is disposed of in a receptacle.

## GUIDELINES

1. Know volume of medication to administer and the characteristics of medication (such as an irritating or

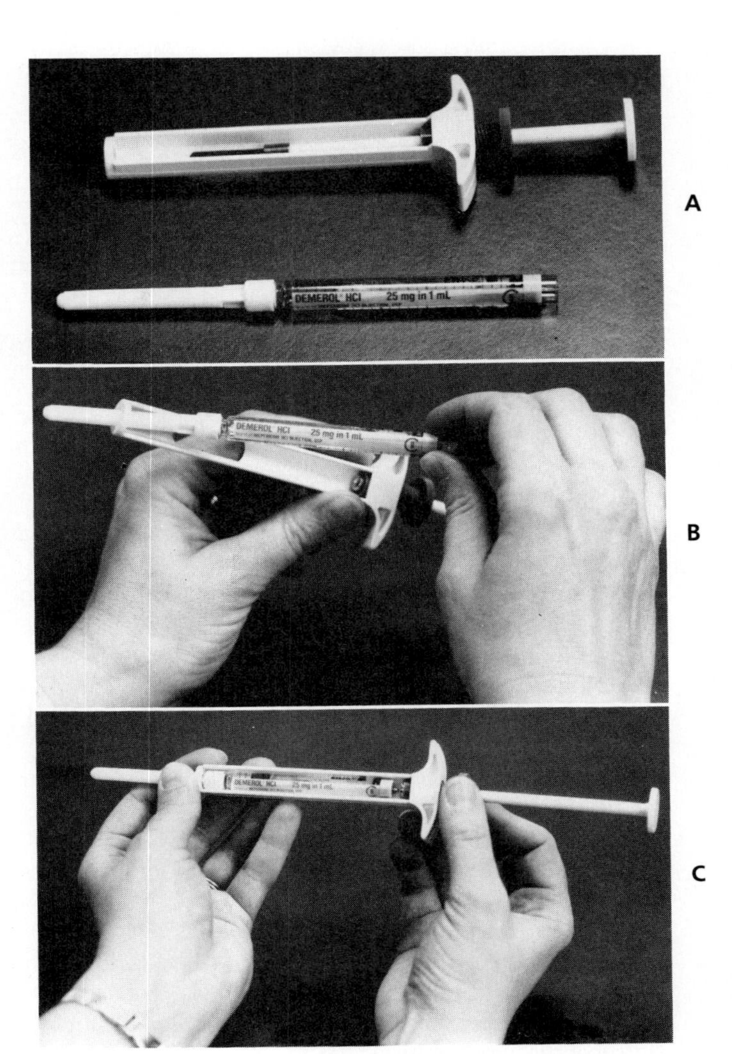


***Fig. 21-4*** **A,** Carpuject syringe and prefilled sterile cartridge with needle. **B,** Assembling the carpuject. **C,** Cartridge slides into syringe barrel, turns and locks at needle end. Plunger then screws into the cartridge end.

viscous substance). Injecting too large a volume of medication can cause extreme pain and local tissue damage.
2. Know location of anatomical structures underlying injection sites (major nerves, blood vessels) to prevent injury to the client.
3. Be sure to inject at the proper angle of insertion to deliver medications into the correct tissue (Fig. 21-5).
4. Aspirate a syringe before injecting medication to be sure the needle has not pierced a vein or artery. Injection directly into a blood vessel can cause a rapid drug response. (Exception: do not aspirate subcutaneous heparin.)
5. Attempt to minimize client's discomfort when giving an injection:
   a. Use sharp, beveled needles in smallest length and gauge possible.

Intramuscular
Subcutaneous
Intradermal
90°
45°
15°
Skin
Subcutaneous tissue
Muscle

***Fig. 21-5*** Comparison of angles of insertion for intramuscular (90°), subcutaneous (45°), and intradermal (15°) injections.

b. Apply ice to injection sites to create local anesthesia before needle insertion.
c. Insert needles smoothly and quickly to reduce push on tissue.
d. Hold syringe steady when needle is in tissues.
e. Hold an alcohol swab firmly against the skin around the needle when removing it to reduce tissue pulling.
f. Position clients comfortably to reduce muscular tension.
g. Divert client's attention from the injection.
h. Massage the injected area gently for several seconds unless contraindicated.
i. Rotate injection sites.
j. Increase the duration of injection time, which may reduce pain perception (Perez, 1984).

6. Use strict medical aseptic technique during all steps of preparation and administration.
7. Apply guidelines for administering medications listed in Chapter 19.
8. After administering injections, do not cap needles before disposal. Covering a needle may predispose the nurse to an accidental needle stick (Centers for Disease Control [CDC], 1983).

## PREREQUISITE KNOWLEDGE

1. Principles of medical asepsis.
2. Drug dosage calculation.
3. Pharmacokinetics of drug actions.
4. Anatomy and physiology of tissues to be injected.
5. Teaching and learning principles.

## PREREQUISITE SKILLS

1. Proper handwashing techniques (Chapter 37).
2. Assessment of integument and musculoskeletal system (Chapter 13).
3. Skills for maintaining IV lines (Chapter 23) (IV medications only).

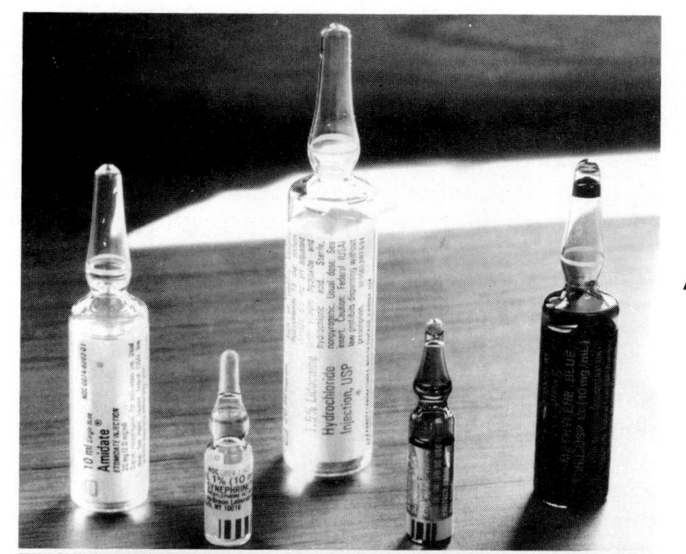


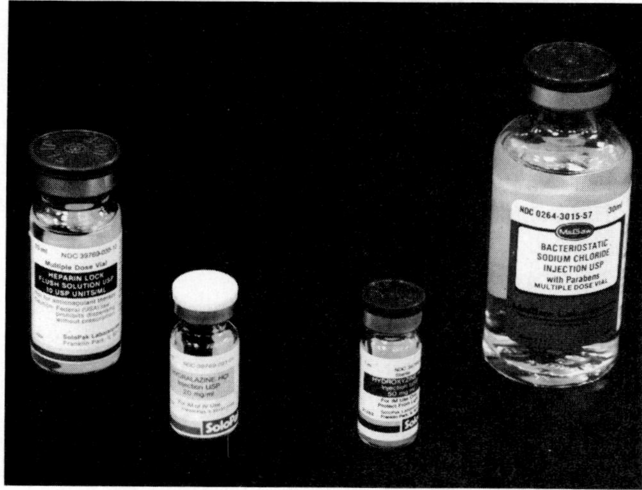


***Fig. 21-6*** **A,** Ampules. **B,** Vials

# *SKILL 21-1 Preparing Injections From Ampules and Vials*

Ampules contain single doses of injectable medication in a liquid form and are available in several sizes, from 1 to 10 ml or more (Fig. 21-6, *A*). An ampule is made of clear glass with a constricted neck that must be snapped off to allow access to the medication. A colored ring around the neck indicates where the ampule is prescored to be broken easily. Medications are easily drawn from ampules by simply aspirating the syringe plunger. The fluid enters the syringe because no vacuum exists within the ampule.

A vial is a single-dose or multidose glass container with a rubber seal at the top (Fig. 21-6, *B*). A metal cap protects the seal until it is ready for use. Vials contain liquid or dry forms of medications; drugs that are unstable in solution are packaged in dry form. The vial label specifies the solvent to use to dissolve the dry drug and the amount of solvent needed to prepare a desired drug concentration. Unlike the ampule, the vial is a closed system, and air must be injected into it to permit easy withdrawal of the solution.

**PURPOSES**

1. Prevent contamination of vial or ampule contents.
2. Maintain sterility of needle and syringe parts.
3. Prepare accurate dosages.

## *Procedure 21-1*

| Steps | Rationale |
|---|---|
| **Assessment** | |
| 1. Consider type of syringe and needles needed for injection. | Depends on type of injection to be administered and size and weight of client. |
| **Planning** | |
| 1. Wash hands. | Reduces transmission of infection. |
| 2. Prepare needed equipment and supplies: | |
| a. Ampules | |
| ▪ Ampule containing medication | |
| ▪ Syringe and needle | |
| ▪ Small gauze pad or alcohol swab | |
| ▪ Container for disposing of glass | |
| ▪ Small metal file (optional) | Used to score or etch cut into ampule's glass neck. |
| b. Vials | |
| ▪ Vial with medication | |
| ▪ Syringe and needle | |
| ▪ Alcohol swab | |
| ▪ Solvent, e.g., normal saline or sterile water (optional) | Used to dissolve drugs in dry form. |
| c. Medication card, form, or printout. | Verifies order. |
| **Implementation** | |
| 1. Assemble supplies at work area in medicine room. | Makes procedure orderly. |
| 2. Check medication card, form, or printout against label on the ampule or vial. | Ensures right drug and dosage to prepare. |
| 3. Ampule preparation: | |
| a. Tap top of ampule lightly and quickly with finger until fluid leaves neck (Fig. 21-7). | Dislodges any fluid that collects above the neck. All solution moves into lower chamber. |
| b. Partially file neck of ampule if it is not prescored. Place small gauze pad or dry alcohol swab around neck of ampule. | Filing ensures a clean break. Placing pad or swab around neck protects nurse's fingers from trauma as glass tip is broken off. |
| c. Snap neck of ampule quickly and firmly away from hands (Fig. 21-8). | Prevents shattering glass toward or in nurse's fingers or face. |
| d. Draw up medication quickly. Hold ampule upside down or set it on flat surface. Insert syringe needle into center of ampule opening (Fig. 21-9). Do not allow needle tip or shaft to touch rim of ampule. | System open to airborne contaminants. Broken rim of ampule is considered contaminated. As long as needle tip or shaft does not touch ampule's rim, solution does not dribble out. |
| e. Aspirate medication into syringe by gently pulling back on plunger (Fig. 21-10). | Withdrawal of plunger creates negative pressure within syringe barrel, which pulls fluid into syringe. |

| Steps | Rationale |
|---|---|

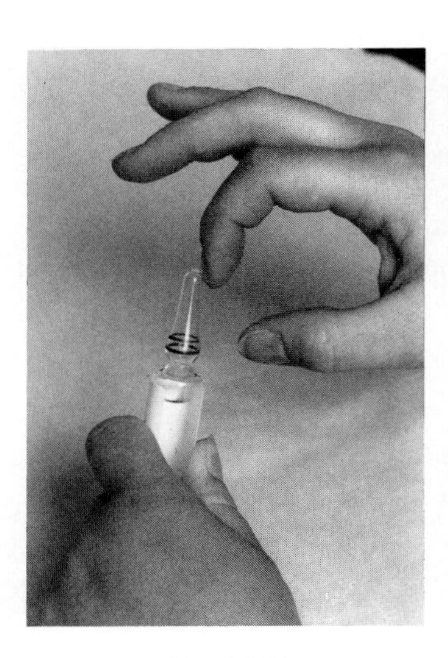

*Fig. 21-7*

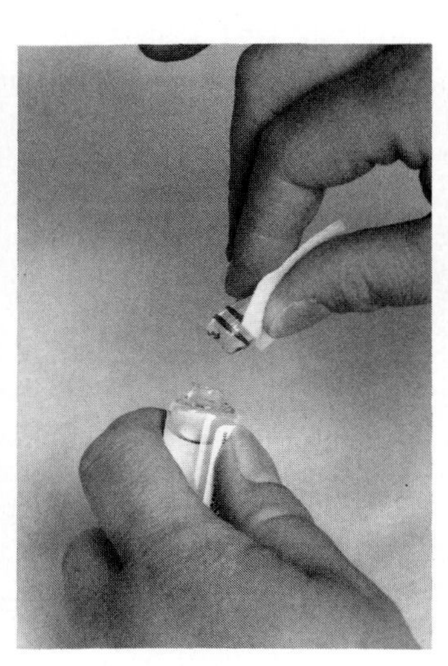

*Fig. 21-8*

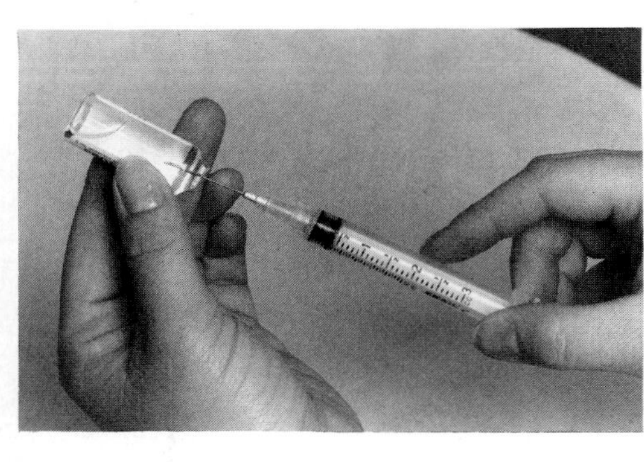

*Fig. 21-9*

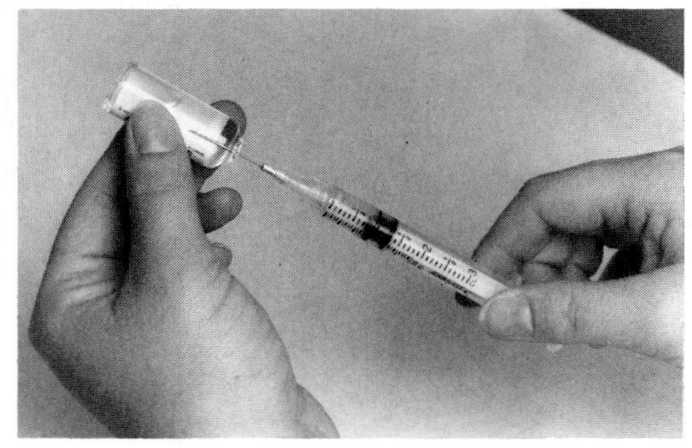

*Fig. 21-10*

| Steps | Rationale |
|---|---|
| f. Keep needle tip below surface of liquid. Tip ampule to bring all fluid within reach of needle. | Prevents aspiration of air bubbles. |
| g. If air bubbles are aspirated, do not expel air into ampule. | Air pressure may force fluid out of ampule, and medication will be lost. |
| h. To expel excess air bubbles, remove needle from ampule. Hold syringe with needle pointing up. Tap side of syringe to cause bubbles to rise toward needle. Draw back slightly on plunger, and then push the plunger upward to eject air. *Do not eject fluid.* | Withdrawing plunger too far will pull it from barrel. Holding syringe vertically allows fluid to settle in bottom of barrel. Pulling back on plunger allows fluid within needle to enter barrel so fluid is not expelled. Air at top of barrel and within needle is then expelled. |
| i. If syringe contains excess fluid, use sink for disposal. Hold syringe vertically with needle tip up and slanted slightly toward sink. Slowly eject excess fluid into sink. Recheck fluid level in syringe by holding it vertically. | Medication is safely dispersed into sink. Position of needle allows medication to be expelled without it flowing down needle shaft. Rechecking fluid level ensures proper dosage. |
| j. Cover needle with its sheath or cap. Change needle on syringe. | Prevents contamination of needle and protects nurse from needle stick. Changing needle is required if nurse suspects medication is on needle shaft. New needle prevents tracking medication through skin and subcutaneous tissues. |
| k. Dispose of soiled supplies. Place broken ampule in special container for glass. Clean work area. Wash hands. | Controls transmission of infection. Proper disposal of glass prevents accidental injury to personnel. |
| 4. Vial preparation: | |
| a. Remove metal cap covering top of unused vial. Expose rubber seal. | Vial comes packaged with cap to prevent contamination of rubber seal. |
| b. Wipe off surface of rubber seal with alcohol swab. | Removes dust or grease but does not sterilize surface. |
| c. Take syringe and remove needle cap. Pull back on plunger to draw amount of air into syringe equivalent to volume of medication to be aspirated from vial (Fig. 21-11). | To prevent buildup of negative pressure in vial when aspirating medication, air must first be injected into vial. |
| d. Insert tip of needle, with bevel pointing up, through center of rubber seal (Fig. 21-12). Apply pressure to tip of needle during insertion. | Center of seal is thinner and easier to penetrate. Keeping bevel up and using firm pressure prevents cutting rubber core from seal. |
| e. Inject air into vial, holding on to plunger. | Air must be injected before aspirating fluid. Plunger may be forced backward by air pressure within vial. |
| f. Invert vial while keeping firm hold on syringe and plunger (Fig. 21-13). Hold vial between thumb and middle fingers of nondominant hand. Grasp end of syringe barrel and plunger with thumb and forefinger of dominant hand. | Inverting vial allows fluid to settle in lower half of container. Position of hands prevents movement of plunger and permits easy manipulation of syringe. |

| **Steps** | **Rationale** |
|---|---|

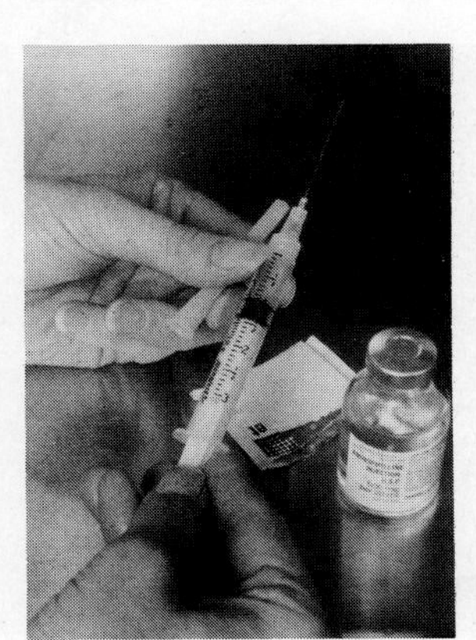

*Fig. 21-11*

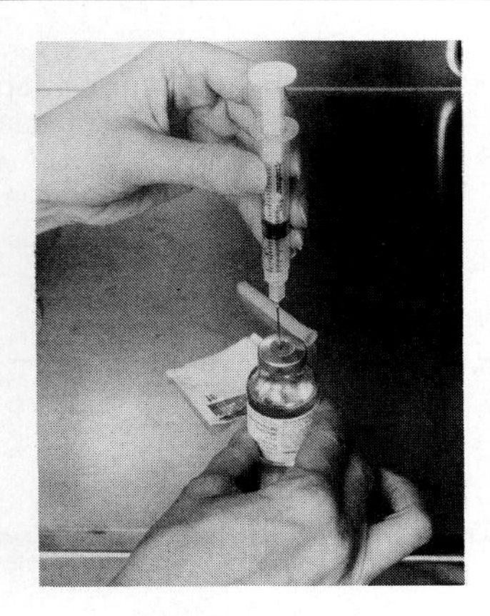

*Fig. 21-12*

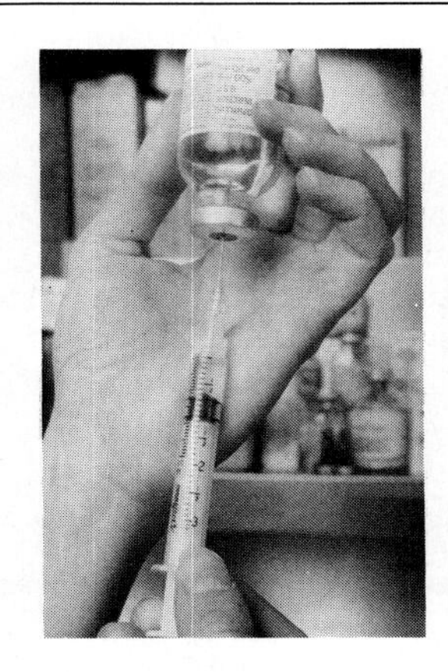

*Fig. 21-13*

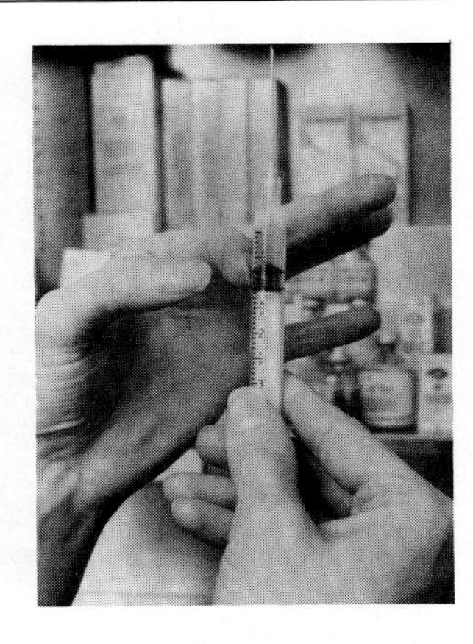

*Fig. 21-14*

| Steps | Rationale |
|---|---|
| g. Keep tip of needle below fluid level. | Prevents aspiration of air. |
| h. Allow air pressure to fill syringe gradually with medication. Pull back slightly on plunger if necessary. | Positive pressure within vial forces fluid into syringe. |
| i. Tap side of syringe barrel carefully to dislodge any air bubbles. Eject any air remaining at top of syringe into vial. | Forcefully striking barrel while needle is inserted in vial may bend needle. Accumulation of air displaces medication and causes dosage errors. |
| j. When correct volume is obtained, remove needle from vial by pulling back on barrel of syringe. | Pulling plunger rather than barrel causes separation from barrel and loss of medication. |
| k. Remove any remaining air from syringe by holding it and needle upright. Tap barrel to dislodge any air bubbles (Fig. 21-14). Draw back slightly on plunger, then push plunger upward to eject air. Do not eject fluid. | Holding syringe vertically allows fluid to settle in bottom of barrel. Pulling back on plunger allows fluid within needle to enter barrel so fluid is not expelled. Air at top of barrel and within needle is then expelled. |
| l. Change needle and cover. | Inserting needle through a rubber stopper may blunt bevel. New needle is sharper, and because no fluid is along shaft, it will not track medication through tissues. |
| m. For multidose vial, make label that includes date of mixing, concentration of drug per milliliter, and nurse's initials. | Ensures that future doses will be prepared correctly. Certain drugs should be discarded after set number of days after mixing of vial. |
| n. Dispose of soiled supplies in proper containers. Clean work area. | Reduces transmission of infection. |
| o. Wash hands. | Reduces transmission of infection. |

## Evaluation

| | |
|---|---|
| 1. Check fluid level in syringe and compare with desired dosage. | Ensures that accurate dosage has been prepared. |

***Expected outcome***

| | |
|---|---|
| 1. Proper dosage is prepared. No air bubbles exist within syringe barrel. | Indicates that medication is prepared correctly. |

***Unexpected outcome***

| | |
|---|---|
| 1. Air bubbles remain within syringe barrel. | Creates risk of incorrect dosage. |

## Special Considerations

- Be sure to select needle long enough to reach bottom of an ampule. If needle is longer than needed to administer medication choose new needle just before injection.
- Never use wet alcohol swab to wrap around top of ampule as alcohol may leak into ampule.
- If glass fragments are suspected in an ampule, discard it and begin again.
- Dispose of soiled needles in puncture and leak-proof container. Do not break needles.
- Dry, powdered drugs usually dissolve easily. It may be necessary to withdraw needle from vial and then mix contents thoroughly. Mix by gently shaking or rolling vial between hands.
- When preparing medication from single-dose vial, do not assume volume listed on label is total volume in vial. Some manufacturers provide small amount of extra liquid, expecting loss during preparation. Be sure to draw up only desired volume.

### Home Care Considerations

- Assess client's and primary care giver's ability and motivation to prepare medications. Identify a back-up person in the event of an emergency.
- Evaluate visual acuity of the client and primary care giver to determine their ability to accurately see markings on the syringe and label on the vials and ampules.
- Assess client's physical environment to identify an appropriate storage location for medication and equipment.
- Chart date of instruction and the individual responsible for preparation and administration of medication.
- Provide client and primary care giver with a medication documentation sheet to be kept with the client.
- Obtain a signed client consent acknowledging understanding of training, program risks, and family and home health agency responsibilities.

## *SKILL 21-2 Mixing Medications From Two Vials*

Occasionally the nurse must mix medications from two vials or from a vial and an ampule. This prevents having to give a client more than one injection at a time. It is essential that any medications mixed are compatible. When mixing medications, the nurse must simply remember the differences in how to correctly aspirate fluid from each type of container. When using multidose vials, the nurse must not contaminate the vials' contents with medication from another vial or ampule.

Mixing medications from a vial and ampule is simple, since adding air to withdraw medication from an ampule is unnecessary. The nurse prepares medications from the vial first and then, using the same syringe and needle, withdraws medication from the ampule. Mixing medications from two vials is somewhat more complicated, since air must be added to both vials.

Special consideration must be given to the proper preparation of insulin. Insulin is the hormone used to treat diabetes. Often clients with diabetes receive a combination of different types of insulin in order to effectively control their blood sugar levels. Regular, unmodified insulin is a clear solution that can be given subcutaneously or intravenously. The other types of insulin are cloudy solutions because of the addition of a protein, which slows absorption. There are simple guidelines for mixing two kinds of insulin in the same syringe:

1. Regular insulin can be mixed with any other type of insulin.
2. Lente insulins can be mixed with each other and regular insulin but should not be mixed with any other types of insulin.

### Purposes

1. Minimize number of injections a client receives.

## *Procedure 21-2*

| Steps | Rationale |
|---|---|
| **Assessment** | |
| 1. Consider type of syringe and needles needed for injection. | Depends on type of injection to be administered and weight and size of client. |
| **Planning** | |
| 1. Wash hands. | Reduces transmission of microorganisms. |
| 2. Prepare needed supplies and equipment: | |
| a. Single or multidose vials containing medications | |
| b. Syringe with needle | |
| c. Extra needles | New needle is applied to syringe after mixing is completed. |
| d. Alcohol swab | To clean top of vials. |
| e. Containers for disposing of syringes, needles, and glass | |
| f. Medication card, form, or printout | Verifies order. |
| **Implementation** | |
| 1. Assemble supplies at work area in medicine room. | Makes procedure orderly. |

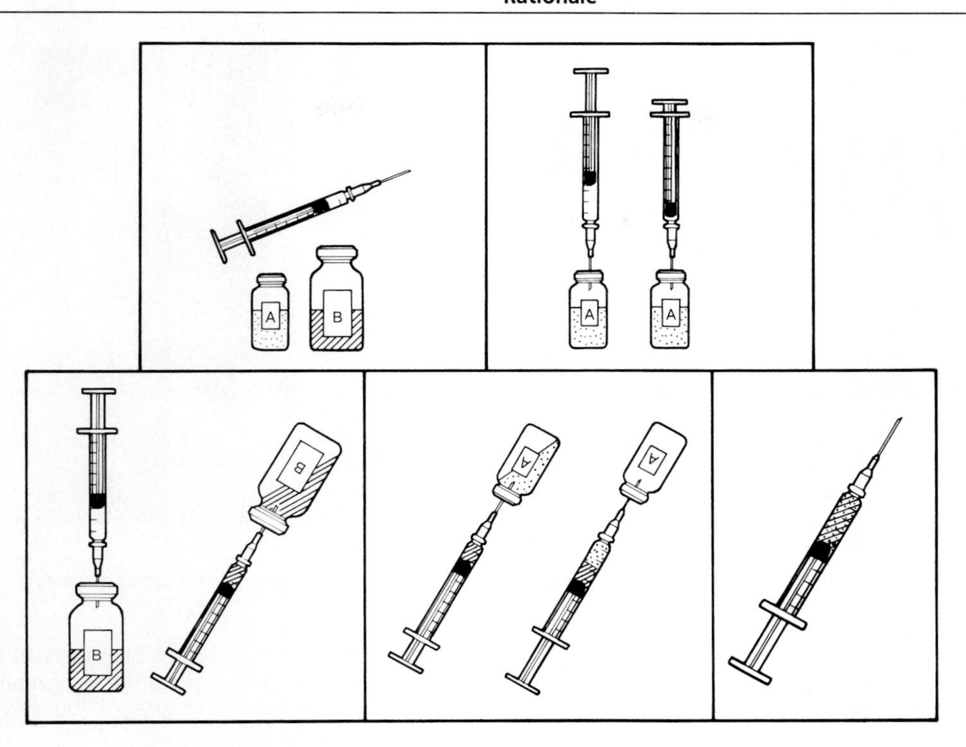


***Fig. 21-15*** Steps in mixing medications from two vials.

| Steps | Rationale |
|---|---|
| ***Mixing medications from vials*** | |
| 1. Take syringe and aspirate volume of air equivalent to first medication's dosage (vial A) (Fig. 21-15). | Air must be introduced into vial to create positive pressure needed to withdraw solution. |
| 2. Inject air into vial A, making sure needle does not touch solution (see Fig. 21-15). | Prevents cross-contamination. |
| 3. Withdraw needle and syringe and then aspirate air equivalent to second medication's dosage (vial B). | Air is injected into vial to withdraw desired dosage. |
| 4. Insert needle into vial B, inject air, and then fill syringe with proper volume of medication from vial (see Fig. 21-15). | First portion of dosage has been prepared. |
| 5. Withdraw needle and syringe from vial by pulling on barrel, check dosage. | Prevents accidental pulling of plunger, which may cause loss of medication. Ensures correct dosage prepared. |
| 6. Determine at which point on syringe scale combined volume of medications should measure. | Prevents accidental withdrawal of too much medication from second vial. |
| 7. Insert needle into vial A, being careful not to push plunger and expel medication into vial. Invert vial and carefully withdraw desired amount of medication into syringe (see Fig. 21-15). | Positive pressure within vial A allows fluid to fill syringe without need to aspirate. |
| 8. Withdraw needle and expel any excess air or fluid from syringe (see Fig. 21-15). | Air bubbles should not be injected into tissues. Excess fluid causes incorrect dosage. |
| 9. Change needle on syringe. | New needle prevents tracking of medication into tissues. |
| 10. Dispose of soiled needle and supplies in proper receptacles. | Controls spread of infection and prevents accidents. |
| 11. Wash hands. | Reduces transmission of infection. |
| ***Mixing insulin*** | |
| 1. Take insulin syringe and aspirate volume of air equivalent to dosage to be withdrawn from modified insulin (cloudy vial) (Fig. 21-16). | Air must be introduced into vial to create pressure needed to withdraw solution. |
| 2. Inject air into vial of modified insulin (cloudy vial). Be sure needle does not touch solution. | Prevents cross-contamination. |
| 3. Withdraw needle and syringe from vial and aspirate air equivalent to dosage to be withdrawn from unmodified regular insulin (clear vial). | Air is injected into vial to withdraw desired dosage. |

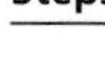

| Steps | Rationale |
|---|---|
| 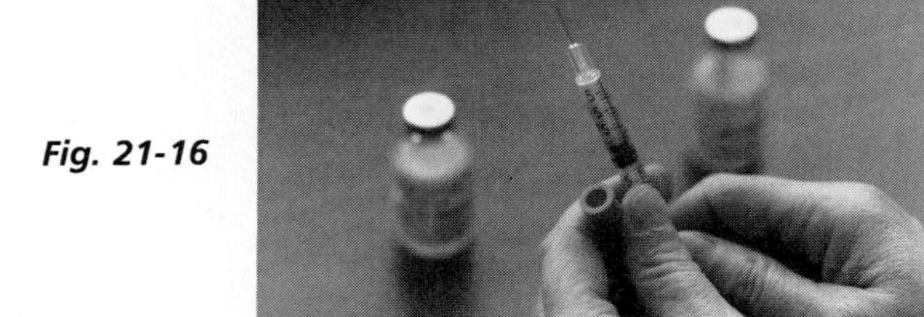 *Fig. 21-16* | 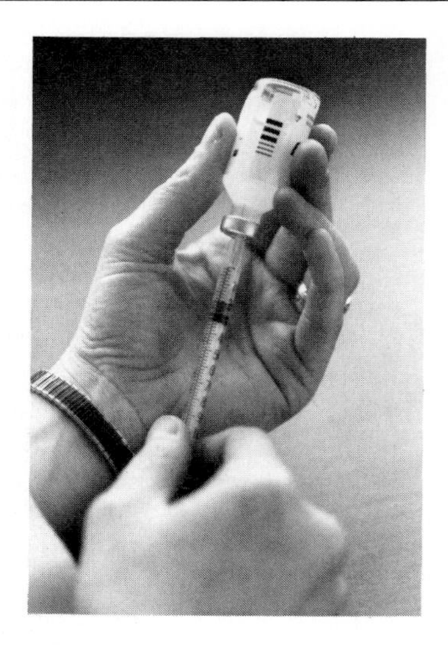 *Fig. 21-17* |
| 4. Insert needle into vial of unmodified regular insulin (clear vial), inject air and then fill syringe with proper insulin dosage. | First portion of dosage has been prepared. |
| 5. Withdraw needle and syringe from vial by pulling on barrel, check dosage. | Prevents accidental pulling of plunger, which may cause loss of medication. Ensures correct dosage prepared. |
| 6. Determine at which point on syringe scale combined units of insulin should measure. | Prevents accidental withdrawal of too much insulin from second vial. |
| 7. Insert needle into vial of modified insulin (cloudy vial). Be careful not to push plunger and expel medication into vial. Invert vial and carefully withdraw desired amount of insulin into syringe (Fig. 21-17). | Positive pressure within vial of modified insulin allows fluid to fill syringe without need to aspirate. |
| 8. Withdraw needle and check fluid level in syringe. | Ensures accurate dosage. |
| 9. Dispose of soiled supplies in proper receptacle. | Controls spread of infection. |
| 10. Wash hands. | Reduces transmission of infection. |

## Evaluation

| | |
|---|---|
| 1. Check syringe scale for dosage of combined medications. | Accurate dosage ensures safe medication administration. |

### *Expected outcomes*

| | |
|---|---|
| 1. Combined medications equal correct dosage. No air bubbles exist in syringe barrel. | Indicates that medication is prepared correctly. |

### *Unexpected outcomes*

| | |
|---|---|
| 1. Air bubbles remain in syringe barrel. | Creates risk of incorrect dosage. |

## Follow-Up Activities

| | |
|---|---|
| Administer mixture of insulins within 5 min of preparation. | Regular insulin binds with neutral protamine Hagedorn (NPH) and the action of regular insulin is reduced. |

## Special Considerations

- Always fill syringe with unmodified (regular) insulin first to prevent adding it to the modified (NPH or lente) vial.
- If two modified forms of insulin are mixed, it makes no difference which vial is prepared first.

## Home Care Considerations

- See Skill 21-1.
- Assess client's understanding of the treatment program, inherent risks, and financial requirements.

# SKILL 21-3 Administering Subcutaneous Injections

A subcutaneous injection involves depositing medication into the loose connective tissue underlying the dermis (see Fig. 21-5, p. 488). Subcutaneous tissue is not as richly supplied with blood vessels as muscles; thus drugs are not absorbed as quickly as those given intramuscularly. One exception is heparin, which is absorbed quickly by both subcutaneous and intramuscular routes. Anything affecting local blood flow to tissues, such as physical exercise or the local application of hot or cold compresses, will influence the rate of drug absorption. Conditions such as circulatory shock or occlusive vascular disease impair client's blood flow and thus contraindicate subcutaneous injections.

Drugs given subcutaneously are isotonic, nonirritating, nonviscous, and water soluble. Examples of drugs given by this route are epinephrine, insulin, tetanus toxoid, other vaccines, narcotics, and vitamin $B_{12}$. Only small doses of medications (0.5 to 1 ml) should be given subcutaneously. The tissue is sensitive to irritating solutions and large volumes of medications. Medications collecting within the tissues can cause sterile abscesses, which appear as hardened, painful lumps.

The best sites for subcutaneous injections include vascular areas around the outer aspect of the upper arms, the abdomen from below the costal margins to the iliac crests, and the anterior aspect of the thighs. These areas are easily accessible, especially for clients who must self-administer insulin. The site most frequently recommended for heparin injections is the abdominal wall. Other sites include the scapular areas of the upper back and the upper ventral or dorsal gluteal areas (Fig. 21-18). Injection sites should be free of infection, skin lesions, scars, bony prominences, and large underlying muscles or nerves. Clients with diabetes regularly rotate daily injection sites to prevent hypertrophy (thickening) of the skin and lipodystrophy (atrophy of tissues). No injection site should be used more than every 6 to 7 weeks (Fig. 21-19).

Body weight influences the depth of the subcutaneous layer; therefore, the nurse uses body weight as the criteria for selecting needle length and angle of insertion. Generally a 25-gauge, ⅝-inch needle with a medium bevel inserted at a 45° angle (see Fig. 21-5) deposits medication into subcutaneous tissue of a normal-sized client. A child may require only a 27-gauge, ½-inch needle. If a client is obese, the nurse often pinches the tissue and uses a needle long enough to insert through the fatty tissue at the base of the skinfold. The preferred needle length is one-half the width of the skinfold. A ⅞-inch needle is the longest needle for subcutaneous use. When injecting obese clients, the angle of insertion may be between 45° and 90°. Thin, cachectic clients may have insufficient tissue for subcutaneous injections. To ensure insulin reaches subcutaneous tissue, a simple rule can be followed: if 2 inches of tissue can be grasped, the needle should be inserted at a 90° angle; if 1 inch of tissue can

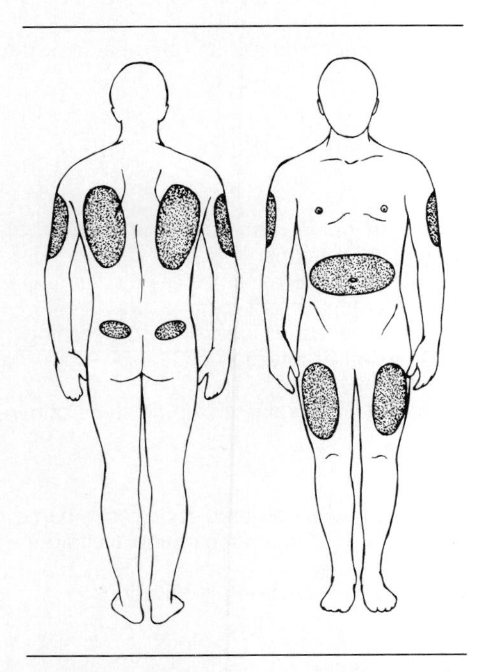

***Fig. 21-18*** Common sites for subcutaneous injections.

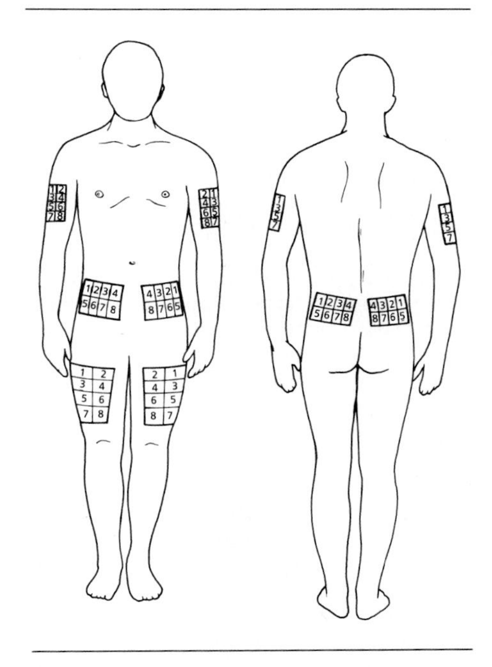

***Fig. 21-19*** Subcutaneous injection site diagram.

be grasped, the needle should be inserted at a 45° angle. The upper abdomen is the best injection site for clients with little peripheral subcutaneous tissue.

**Purposes**

1. Deposit medication into the subcutaneous tissue layers safely.
2. Avoid injury to the client.
3. Ensure proper drug absorption after injection.

## *Procedure 21-3*

| Steps | Rationale |
|---|---|
| **Assessment** | |
| 1. Review physician's medication order for client's name, drug name, dosage, time and route of administration. | Ensures safe and correct administration of medication. |
| 2. Gather information pertinent to drug(s) ordered: action, purpose, time of onset and peak action, normal dosage, common side effects, nursing implications. | Nurse must be able to anticipate drug's effects and observe client's response. Allows nurse to judge appropriateness of therapy as client's condition changes. |
| 3. Assess for factors that may contraindicate subcutaneous injections, such as circulatory shock or reduced local tissue perfusion. | Reduced tissue perfusion interferes with drug absorption and distribution. |
| 4. Assess indications for subcutaneous injections: unconscious or confused client; client who is unable to swallow, or has gastrointestinal disturbances; presence of gastric suction. | Contraindicates use of oral medications; parenteral route thus more desirable. |
| 5. Assess client's medical history, history of allergies, and medication history. | May influence how certain drug acts. Information also indicates client's need for medication. |
| 6. Consider client's age. | Physiologic changes of aging influence methods for administering injections. Medications are not administered subcutaneously to infants or younger children (except for insulin). |
| 7. Assess client's knowledge regarding medication to be received. | Information may pose implications for client education. Assessment may also reveal drug use problems at home. |
| 8. Observe client's verbal and nonverbal responses toward injection. | Injections can be painful. Clients may experience considerable anxiety, which can increase pain. |
| **Nursing Diagnosis** | |
| 1. Cluster data to reveal actual or potential nursing diagnoses: | |
| a. Anxiety: related to receiving injection. | Nurse must use techniques during administration that minimize client's anxiety. |
| b. Altered peripheral tissue perfusion: related to hypovolemia. | Diagnosis would contraindicate use of subcutaneous injection. |
| c. Knowledge deficit regarding medication: related to inexperience. | Indicates need for health education during administration. |
| **Planning** | |
| 1. Develop individualized goals for client based on nursing diagnoses: | |
| a. Minimize discomfort from injection. | Nurse follows basic guidelines in avoiding injury to client when administering all injections. |
| b. Client will feel less anxious. | Smooth, confident actions minimize client's fears. |
| c. Promote optimal drug absorption and distribution. | Ensures drug's therapeutic effect. |
| d. Client attains knowledge of drug therapy. | Discussion during injection is ideal time for teaching. |
| 2. Wash hands. | Reduces transmission of infection. |
| 3. Prepare needed equipment and supplies: | |
| a. Syringe (1- 2-ml) | Size chosen according to volume of drug to be administered. |
| b. Needle (27-25 gauge, ⅜-⅝ in) | |
| c. Antiseptic swabs, e.g., alcohol | |
| d. Medication ampule or vial | |
| e. Medication card, form, or printout | Identifies medication dose ordered and client's name. |
| 4. Prepare correct medication dosage from ampule or vial (Skill 20-1). Check dosage carefully. | Ensures medication is sterile. Preparation techniques differ for ampule and vial. |
| 5. Identify client by checking identification armband and asking client's name. Compare with medication ticket. | Ensures correct client is receiving medication. |
| 6. Explain procedure to client and proceed in calm, confident manner. | Helps client anticipate nurse's actions. Calm approach minimizes client's anxiety. |

| Steps | Rationale |
|---|---|
| **Implementation** | |
| 1. Close room curtains or door. | Provides privacy. |
| 2. Keep sheet or gown draped over body parts not requiring exposure. | Proper selection of injection site may require exposure of body parts. |
| 3. Select appropriate injection site. Inspect skin's surface over sites for bruises, inflammation, or edema. Palpate site for masses, edema, or tenderness. *NOTE:* When administering heparin subcutaneously, use abdominal injection sites. | Injection site should be free of lesions that might interfere with drug absorption. *NOTE:* Anticoagulant may cause local bleeding and bruising when injected into areas such as arms and legs, which are involved in muscular activity. |
| 4. In cases of repeated daily injections (e.g., insulin), rotate injection site daily within single anatomical region, then change site (Emergency Medicine, 1980). Do not reuse same site for 6 wk. | Rotation of site prevents subcutaneous scarring and lipodystrophy, which interfere with drug absorption. Studies by Koivisto and Felig (1980) suggest rotating within single anatomical region and making sure no one site is injected more than once every 6 wk. |
| 5. Be sure you have correct needle size by forming skinfold at site with thumb and forefinger. Measure skinfold from top to bottom, and be sure needle is approximately one-half this length. | Ensures that needle will be injected into subcutaneous tissue. |
| 6. Assist client to comfortable position and to relax arm, leg, or abdomen depending on site chosen for injection. Talk with client about subject of interest. | Relaxation of area minimizes discomfort during injection. Promoting client's comfort through positioning and distraction helps reduce anxiety. |
| 7. Relocate site using anatomic landmarks. | Accurate injection of medication requires insertion in correct site to avoid injury to underlying nerves, bone, or blood vessels. |
| 8. Cleanse site with an antiseptic swab (Fig. 21-20). Apply swab at center of site and rotate outward in circular direction for about 5 cm (2 in). | Mechanical action of swab removes secretions containing microorganisms. |
| 9. Hold swab between third and fourth fingers of nondominant hand. | Swab remains readily accessible when needle is withdrawn. |
| 10. Remove needle cap from needle by pulling it straight off. | Preventing needle from touching sides of cap prevents contamination. |
| 11. Hold syringe between thumb and forefinger of dominant hand as if grasping dart. Hold syringe with palm up for 45° angle of insertion and palm down for 90° angle (Fig. 21-21). | Quick, smooth injection requires proper manipulation of syringe parts. |
| 12. Administer injection: | |
| a. For average-sized client, spread skin tightly across injection site or pinch skin with nondominant hand. | Needle penetrates tight skin easier than loose skin. Pinching skin elevates subcutaneous tissue. |
| b. Inject needle quickly and firmly at 45°-90° angle (Fig. 21-22). (Then release skin, if pinched.) | Quick, firm insertion minimizes discomfort. (Injecting medication into compressed tissue irritates nerve fibers.) |
| c. For obese client, pinch skin at site and inject needle below tissue fold. | Obese clients have fatty layer of tissue above subcutaneous layer. |

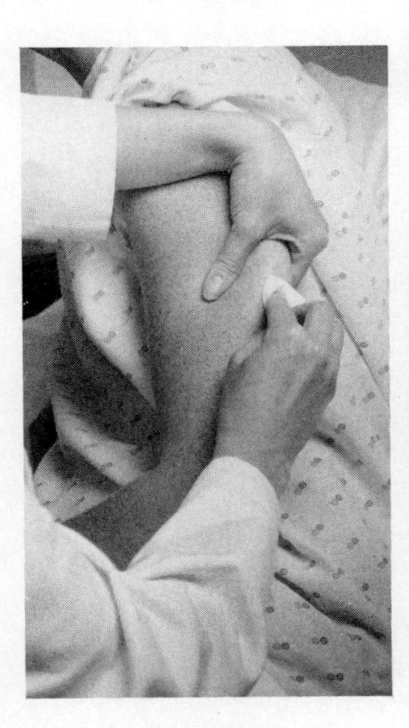

***Fig. 21-20***

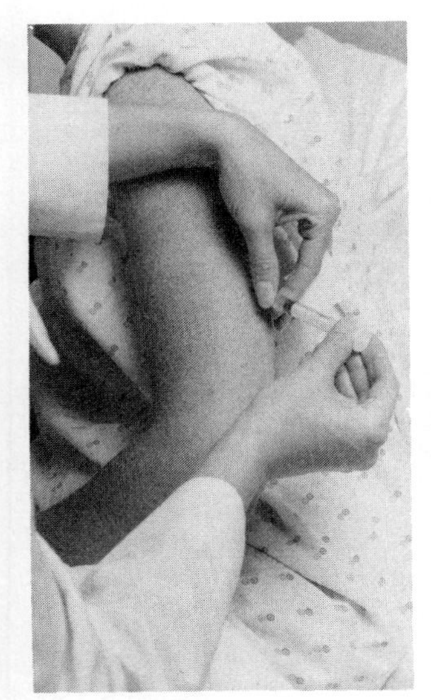

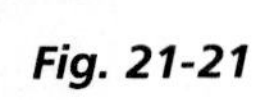

***Fig. 21-21***

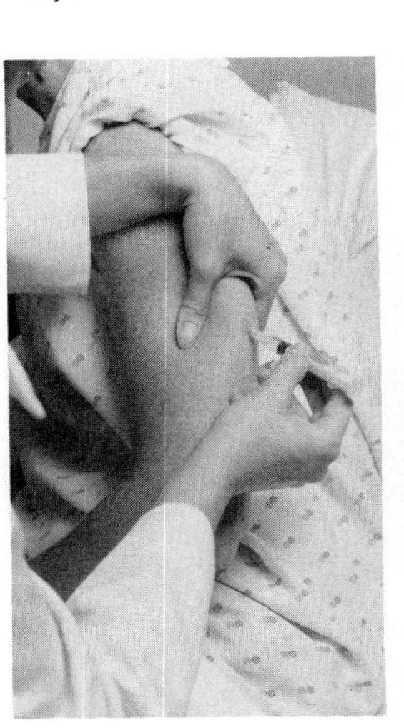

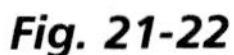

***Fig. 21-22***

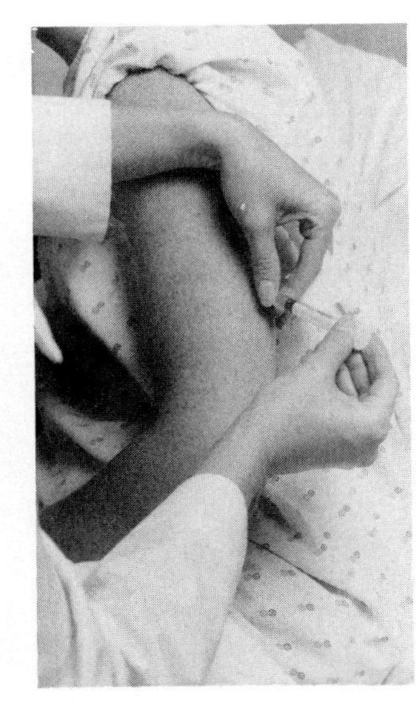

***Fig. 21-23***

| Steps | Rationale |
|---|---|
| 13. After needle enters site, grasp lower end of syringe barrel with nondominant hand. Move dominant hand to end of plunger. Avoid moving syringe (Fig. 21-23). | Properly performed injection requires smooth manipulation of syringe parts. Movement of syringe may displace needle and cause discomfort. |
| 14. Slowly pull back on plunger to aspirate medication. If blood appears in syringe, withdraw needle, discard medication and syringe properly, and repeat procedure. If no blood appears, inject medication slowly. NOTE: Some institutional policies recommend not aspirating subcutaneous heparin injections. | Aspiration of blood into syringe indicates intravenous placement of needle. Subcutaneous medications are generally not for intravenous absorption. Slow injection reduces pain and trauma. |
| 15. Withdraw needle quickly while placing antiseptic swab gently above or over site. | Supporting tissues around injection site minimizes discomfort during needle withdrawal. |
| 16. Massage site lightly. (If heparin is given, simply press alcohol pledget to site for few sec.) | Massage stimulates circulation and improves drug distribution and absorption. However, massage may cause bruising. |
| 17. Assist client to comfortable position. | Gives client sense of well-being. |
| 18. Discard unsheathed needle and attached syringe in appropriately labeled receptacle. | Prevents injury to client and health care personnel. CDC warns that capping needles increases risk of needle stick. |
| 19. Wash hands. | Reduces transmission of microorganisms. |

## Evaluation

| | |
|---|---|
| 1. Return to room and ask if client feels any acute pain, burning, numbness, or tingling at injection site. | Continued discomfort indicates injury to underlying bones or nerves. |
| 2. Observe client's response to medication 30 min after injection. | Determines efficacy of drug and allows evaluation of undesirable side effects. |
| 3. Ask client to explain purpose and effects of medication. | Evaluates client's understanding of information taught. |

### *Expected outcomes*

| | |
|---|---|
| 1. Client complains of mild burning at injection site. | Subcutaneous medications are nonirritating to tissues, but displacement of tissues causes mild burning. |
| 2. No allergies or undesired effects of medication occur. | Drug action is normal. |
| 3. Client explains purpose and effects of medication. | Demonstrates learning. |

### *Unexpected outcomes*

| | |
|---|---|
| 1. Client complains of localized pain or continued burning at injection site. | Indicates potential injury to nerve or tissues. |
| 2. Client displays signs of urticaria, eczema, pruritus, wheezing, and dypsnea. | Indicates allergic response to drug. |
| 3. Client unable to discuss information regarding medication. | Reinstruction necessary or client unable to learn at this time. |

## Recording and Reporting

| | |
|---|---|
| 1. Immediately after administration, chart medication dosage, route, site, time, and date given in medication record. Correctly sign according to institutional policy (Fig. 21-24). | Timely documentation prevents future drug administration errors. |
| 2. Report any undesirable effects from medication to nurse in charge or physician. | Client's response may indicate additional medical therapy. |
| 3. Record client's response to pain medications or similar drugs in nurses' notes. | Documents client's response to care. |

ALLERGIES: Codeine

RECOPIED BY INITIALS: L.T | R.N. SIGNATURE: Ben Wilson, R.N.

BARNES HOSPITAL — PATIENT ROUTINE MEDICATION RECORD

| SIGNATURES | | | |
|---|---|---|---|
| NITES | Mary Doerrer, R.N. | Mary Doerrer, R.N. | Mary Doerrer, R.N. |
| DAYS | Pat Little, R.N. | Pat Little, R.N. | Tom Say, R.N. |
| EVES | Donna C. Gail, R.N. | Donna C. Gail, R.N. | |

| ORDER DATE / EXP DATE | INIT | ROUTINE MEDICATION Name of drug, strength and frequency | RTE | SCHEDULE | SHIFT | DATE 6/14/89 | DATE 6/15/89 | DATE 6/16/89 |
|---|---|---|---|---|---|---|---|---|
| 2/6 | PL | Lanoxin 0.25 mg q.d. | PO | | NITES | | | |
| | | | | 10 | DAYS | 0950 PL | 1000 PL | 1010 TS |
| | | | | | EVES | | | |
| 2/7 | DG | Lasix 40 mg b.i.d. | PO | | NITES | | | |
| | | | | 10 | DAYS | | | 1010 TS |
| | | | | 16 | EVES | | 1545 DG. | |
| 2/7 | DG | Ancef Gm i q6° | IVPB | 06 | NITES | | | 06 MD |
| | | | | 12 | DAYS | | 1215 PL | 1200 TS |
| | | | | 18-24 | EVES | | 18DG 2345DG | |
| 2/8 | TS | Nitro Paste 1 inch q8° | Top | 06 | NITES | | | |
| | | | | 14 | DAYS | | | 1410 TS |
| | | | | 22 | EVES | | | |
| 2/8 | TS | Neosporin Ophthalmic Oint. O.D. | Top | | NITES | | | |
| | | | | 10 | DAYS | | | 1010 TS |
| | | | | 22 | EVES | | | |
| | | | | | NITES | | | |
| | | | | | DAYS | | | |
| | | | | | EVES | | | |
| | | | | | NITES | | | |
| | | | | | DAYS | | | |
| | | | | | EVES | | | |
| | | | | | NITES | | | |
| | | | | | DAYS | | | |
| | | | | | EVES | | | |
| | | | | | NITES | | | |
| | | | | | DAYS | | | |
| | | | | | EVES | | | |
| | | | | | NITES | | | |
| | | | | | DAYS | | | |
| | | | | | EVES | | | |

***Fig. 21-24***

Courtesy Barnes Hospital, St. Louis.

## Special Considerations

- Be sure client wears allergy bracelet indicating medications and substances to which client is allergic.
- Well-illuminated area is necessary to inspect injection site thoroughly.
- Anatomic chart may be kept in nursing Kardex or care plan to keep track of injection sites.
- Keeping syringe and needle out of client's line of vision often minimizes anxiety.
- Study by Vanbree (1984) compared techniques of aspiration and nonaspiration. As noted, results showed no significant difference in bruising with heparin administration. Heparin in low doses is safe, if absorbed intravenously.
- Aging clients have reduced subcutaneous skinfold thickness. Skin is less elastic.
- Considerable literature exists regarding the need to administer irritating subcutaneous medications via an air lock. An air lock is 0.1-0.2 ml of air drawn into a syringe after the medication is prepared. After a drug is given the air lock, which looks like an air bubble, clears the syringe needle of all medication and ensures that the drug is trapped in subcutaneous tissues. Syringes are made so that the prescribed dosage fills the barrel and not the needle. There is some risk that an air lock could deliver excess medication that is in the needle. Check agency policy for use of an air lock (Chaplin, et al., 1985).

## Teaching Considerations

- Clients who require daily injections will need to learn techniques of self-administration (Skill 21-4).

## Home Care Considerations

- See Skill 21-1.

# SKILL 21-4 Teaching Clients How to Administer Self-Injections

There are clients with diabetes who may require daily subcutaneous injections of insulin. The client or a friend or family member must learn to administer injections. Insulin is not available by the oral route, since the medication is destroyed within the gastrointestinal tract.

Education of diabetic clients includes many aspects of care: blood glucose monitoring, diet management, types and concentrations of insulin, the role of exercise in controlling blood glucose levels, how to prepare insulin in a syringe, and how to adjust dosages. This skill describes techniques the nurse may use to assist diabetic clients in administering injections safely and correctly. The nurse will be responsible not only for teaching clients how to give injections for the first time, but also for evaluating injection techniques used by clients previously placed on insulin.

The ability of diabetic clients to learn how to administer injections depends in part on the progress of their disease. Diabetes is a chronic condition that ultimately can cause visual loss and loss of peripheral nerve sensation. The nurse may need to adapt the equipment available to the client or educate only a family member. Special syringes with plunger locks ensure that only a specific dosage is prepared. Syringes with large, numbered scales or magnifying glass adaptors are available for clients with visual impairment.

## Purposes

1. Provide clients with capability to manage their own medication therapy.
2. Ensure safe effective administration of insulin.
3. Prevent injury to the client during insulin administration.

## Procedure 21-4

| Steps | Rationale |
|---|---|
| **Assessment** | |
| 1. Assess visual acuity by having client read numbers on insulin syringe or directions on vial of insulin. If acuity is reduced, ask client to read numbers on syringe with enlarged number scale or use magnifier with syringe. | Diabetic clients often experience swelling of the lens because of elevated blood glucose levels, causing reduction in visual acuity. For clients unable to see the syringe scale, a nurse must educate family member instead. |
| 2. Assess client's ability to hold and manipulate a syringe and hold insulin vial. | Peripheral neuropathy can alter diabetic client's sensation of touch and affect ability to handle syringe and vial safely. |
| 3. Assess client's readiness to learn: client asks questions about disease, treatment, or injections; requests to learn how to give injections; is mentally alert; is participating in own care. | Reflects client's ability to understand explanations and actively participate in teaching process. |
| 4. Assess client's ability to learn: determine if client can read; make sure client is not fatigued or in pain; assess level of understanding of technical terms. | Mental or physical limitations affect client's ability to learn and nurse's methods of instruction. |
| 5. Assess client's knowledge and understanding of diabetes, purpose and action of insulin, and reason insulin is required. | Essential for client to know before being able to learn how to give an injection. May need separate teaching plan. |
| 6. If in home, assess likely location where client will prepare injection. | Setting chosen for instruction should be same or similar to one client will use to minimize need to adapt equipment preparation to new setting. |
| 7. Assess family member's interest in and ability to provide injections. | Family member may be principal administrator of medications. If client can self-administer injection, family member should be available as resource person in case client becomes ill. |
| 8. Assess drug dosage and schedule client ordered to receive at home. | Influences nurse's explanations for dosage preparation. |
| 9. If previously instructed on self-injection, assess client's techniques in giving injections. | Nurse's instruction may require only simple reinforcement, depending on client's level of skill. |
| **Nursing Diagnosis** | |
| 1. Cluster data to reveal actual or potential nursing diagnoses: | |
| a. Knowledge deficit regarding disease process or treatment: related to new diagnosis. | Nurse includes discussion and instructions when teaching client. |
| b. Altered health maintenance: related to physical or cognitive limitations. | Perceptual and cognitive impairment or lack of family resources prohibits client's ability to maintain health. |

| Steps | Rationale |
|---|---|
| c. Sensory perceptual alteration, tactile or visual: related to diabetic changes. | Alternate aids may be needed for client to prepare and use syringe. |
| d. Impaired physical mobility: related to upper extremity weakness. | May require family member to learn technique. |

## Planning

| Steps | Rationale |
|---|---|
| 1. Develop individualized objectives for teaching plan. Client will be able to:<br>a. Describe parts of syringe.<br>b. Correctly manipulate parts of syringe and needle without contaminating them.<br>c. Discuss techniques for maintaining asepsis.<br>d. Identify correct insulin dosage and type of insulin.<br>e. Correctly prepare ordered dosage in insulin syringe.<br>f. Discuss sites used for insulin injections.<br>g. Describe purpose for rotating sites.<br>h. Correctly self-administer insulin at a proper site. | Provides organization for teaching plan and guidelines to evaluate client's success. |
| 2. Have client prepare following equipment and supplies: | |
| a. Vial of insulin in correct concentration (U-100) | Symbol of U-100 indicates number of units per milliliter of insulin. |
| b. Two or three insulin syringes (0.5 to 1 ml, calibrated in units) | Syringe comes with preattached needle and is designed for accurate insulin dose preparation. Use extra syringe for client to manipulate parts. |
| c. Antiseptic swabs | |
| d. Bottle of normal saline or sterile water | Used to practice syringe preparation. |
| 3. Instruct client in comfortable environment, e.g., sitting in chair in hospital room or sitting at kitchen table in home. | Client will more likely remain receptive to nurse's explanations. |
| 4. Provide adequate time for teaching session. | Prevents interruptions. Teaching should occur when client is receptive. |

## Implementation

| Steps | Rationale |
|---|---|
| 1. Have client wash hands. Explain importance of handwashing. | Client must understand that aseptic or clean technique is required to perform injections safely. |
| 2. Allow client opportunity to manipulate syringe parts. Explain which parts must remain sterile and which can be touched. | Client must be familiar with how to use equipment. Familiarity with aseptic technique in handling syringe ensures safe drug administration. |
| 3. Have client compare syringe scale with insulin label of concentration on insulin vial. | Concentration of insulin in units and number of units marked on syringe should match; e.g., 100 unit syringe is used only with U-100 insulin. |
| 4. Discuss client's ordered dosage. (Dosage may change depending on course of disease.) | Dosage in units is number of units prepared in syringe. |
| 5. Demonstrate technique for mixing insulin vial by gently rolling bottle between your hands. Then allow client to mix the vial. *Never* shake vial. | After sitting, insulin forms crystals on bottom of vial. Mixing produces uniform solution. Shaking creates air bubbles. |
| 6. Demonstrate and explain steps used to prepare syringe:<br>a. Wipe off top of vial with alcohol and remove needle cover.<br>b. Pull plunger out to same number of units to be removed from vial. This pulls air into syringe.<br>c. Push needle slowly into rubber on top of vial while holding syringe barrel carefully. Do not bend needle.<br>d. Push in plunger to push air into bottle; this prevents vacuum.<br>e. Hold vial and syringe together, turn both upside down. Try to hold vial between thumb and forefinger, and let syringe rest against palm.<br>f. Slowly pull back on plunger to number of units of insulin to be given. Be sure needle stays under fluid in vial.<br>g. Do not touch inside of plunger.<br>h. Check for clear air bubbles inside syringe. Small bubbles are not harmful but take up space in syringe. With bubbles present, you may not prepare right amount of insulin. | Demonstration is most effective technique for teaching motor skill. Use simple step-by-step explanations so client may ask questions at any point during procedure. Explanation should include basic principles for syringe preparation: prevent vacuum in vial; prevent air bubble aspiration; keep syringe and needle sterile; remove air without ejecting fluid. |

| Steps | Rationale |
|---|---|
| i. Remove syringe from vial by pulling it straight out. If bubbles can be seen, tap side of syringe barrel sharply with middle finger while holding syringe upright. When bubbles rise to top of syringe, pull back slightly on plunger and then push it back to correct number of units. This pushes air out through needle. | |
| j. Check to be sure correct amount of insulin is in syringe and no air bubbles exist. | |
| k. Draw up 0.2 ml of air for dead space. | |
| l. Put cover back without touching needle. | |
| 7. Show chart of injection sites and find each accessible site on client's body. | Client must learn correct sites for injecting insulin into subcutaneous tissue. Comparing body parts allows nurse to point out areas that should be avoided, e.g., scars and bruises. |
| 8. Discuss importance of rotating sites systematically and provide client with injection record. | Clients must be responsible for administering injections to prevent irritation of tissues. Changes in fatty tissue interfere with drug absorption. |
| 9. Have client choose injection site in abdomen or thigh where nurse can easily demonstrate injection. | Practice at locating sites increases client's learning. Client should be able to view nurse's demonstration easily. |
| 10. Administer injection while explaining each step slowly, using simple terms: | Nurse's instructions during demonstration should include principles for minimizing pain, injecting needle correctly, checking for blood return, maintaining asepsis. |
| a. Wipe off site with alcohol swab to clean area. | |
| b. Take cover off needle and lay cover on table. | |
| c. Hold syringe as you would a pencil. | |
| d. Grasp injection site between thumb and fingers of free hand. To inject arm, press back of upper arm against wall or back of chair. "Roll" arm down to push up skin. | This technique is simple to perform and increases client's access to more body parts. |
| e. With quick jab, insert needle into cleaned area at an angle. | If client inserts needle at angle of approximately 45°-90° needle should enter subcutaneous tissue. |
| f. Do not push needle in; this may hurt. Gently insert needle to end and always hold onto syringe. | Client should learn methods to minimize discomfort. Partial insertion of needle may result in insulin being injected into dermis or fatty tissue. |
| g. Let go of skin. Use that hand to pull back on plunger about two units' distance. Look for blood inside syringe. If you see blood, pull needle out of skin. | Checking for blood return must become integrated step of procedure. |
| h. If you do not see blood, push plunger in to administer insulin. Be sure to inject all the insulin. | Client must learn to administer all the drug to receive correct dose. |
| i. Put alcohol swab over needle gently and pull needle out quickly. | |
| j. Briefly hold alcohol swab over site. | |
| k. Discard unsheathed needle and attached syringe in a plastic receptacle. | Prevents needle stick. (CDC no longer recommends capping needle.) |
| l. Write on chart where you gave injection. | Ensures rotation of injection sites. |
| 11. Have client ask questions about procedure. | Allows clarification of any misunderstanding. |
| 12. Wash hands. | Reduces transmission of infection. |

## Evaluation

| | |
|---|---|
| 1. Have client prepare syringe using saline or sterile water instead of insulin. | Return demonstration provides feedback for evaluating client's learning. |
| 2. Have client explain usual insulin dosage and type. | Determines understanding of proper dosage. |
| 3. Ask client to select injection site and explain importance of rotating sites. | Ability to select site confirms client's understanding. |
| 4. Have client self-administer injection. | Return demonstration is best way to confirm learning of motor skill. |

### *Expected outcomes*

| | |
|---|---|
| 1. Client is able to successfully meet each learning objective previously identified. | Objectives provide guidelines for evaluation of client's knowledge and skills. |

### *Unexpected outcomes*

| | |
|---|---|
| 1. Client is unable to meet one or more established learning objectives. | Further instruction or practice is necessary. |

| Steps | Rationale |
|---|---|
| **Recording and Reporting** | |
| 1. Describe in nurses' notes content or skills taught to client and client's ability to perform skill. | Information provides continuity for teaching plan so that other staff members will not continue to teach same material. |
| **Follow-up Activities** | |
| 1. Client may need to practice several different steps of procedure with assistance before performing each skill independently. | Practicing skill several times increases client's learning. |

### Special Considerations

- If a family member learns how to administer injection, caution them against capping a used needle. Needle should instead be disposed of uncapped in a box or plastic container.
- Client with glasses should wear them whenever insulin is prepared. Some clients often use magnifying glasses; nurse should assess accuracy of this method. If lens is swollen, glasses may not improve vision.
- Client may select syringe of preference. Be sure client knows 0.5-ml syringe is marked off in 1-unit increments and 1-ml syringe is marked in 2-unit increments.
- Elderly clients often require extra time to learn new motor skills.
- Many clients cannot see air bubbles. Helpful tip: have client gently push plunger back and forth three times. This usually purges syringe of air bubbles.
- U-40 insulin is available but less commonly ordered.

### Teaching Considerations

- Teaching booklets are available for clients of all reading levels.
- Include family, as appropriate, so they might reinforce information or learn skill themselves.
- Nurses may choose to teach only part of a plan during one teaching session. Be sure other staff nurses know progress of teaching plan.
- Instruct client and primary care giver to maintain sterile technique. Observe injection sites for complications and observe for medication side effects.
- Allow several return demonstrations on drawing up medications from vial and ampule and injection technique.
- Instruct proper methods of disposal of needles and equipment.
- Instruct precautions in caring for a client with a potential or positive diagnosis of AIDS.

### Home Care Considerations

- See Skill 21-1.

## *SKILL 21-5 Administering Intramuscular Injections*

An injection given by the intramuscular route deposits medication into deep muscle tissue. The vascularity of muscle tissue results in fast drug absorption. An aqueous solution absorbs in 10 to 30 minutes as opposed to at least 30 minutes when given subcutaneously (McConnell, 1982). However, an increased risk of injecting drugs directly into blood vessels exists. As in the case with subcutaneous injections, any factor that interferes with local tissue blood flow will affect the rate and extent of drug absorption.

A nurse uses a longer and heavier-gauge needle to pass through subcutaneous tissue and penetrate deep muscle tissue. However, weight influences needle size selection. Generally, for the average adult, a 19- to 23-gauge; 1¼ to 1½-inch needle with a medium bevel inserted at a 90° angle will pass through subcutaneous tissue and enter deep muscle (see Fig. 21-5, p. 488). Children usually require a 25- to 27-gauge, ½- to 1-inch needle, since their muscles are smaller and less developed. An elderly or cachectic client may require shorter, smaller-gauged needles because of muscle atrophy. Emaciated muscles, however, absorb medication poorly and should be avoided when possible.

Muscle is less sensitive to irritating and viscous drugs. A normal, well-developed adult client can safely tolerate as much as 3 ml of medication in larger muscles such as the vastus lateralis. Smaller muscles can tolerate only smaller amounts of medication without severe discomfort. Children, the elderly, and thin clients tolerate less than 2 ml of medication. Whaley and Wong (1987) recommend giving no more than 1 ml to small children and older infants.

Intramuscular injection sites for adults include the vastus lateralis, ventrogluteal, dorsogluteal, and deltoid muscles. In children and infants, the gluteus medius, ventrogluteal, and vastus lateralis muscles are preferred.

## VASTUS LATERALIS

The vastus lateralis muscle is a preferred injection site for adults, children, and infants because of the absence of major nerves and blood vessels in the area. The muscle is thick and well developed, is located on the anterior lateral aspect of the thigh, and extends in an adult from a handbreadth above the knee to a handbreadth below the greater trochanter of the femur (Fig. 21-25). The middle third of the muscle is the suggested site for injection. In width the site extends from the midline of the thigh's top to the midline of the thigh's outer side. Fig. 21-26 shows the site of the vastus lateralis in children.

## VENTROGLUTEAL

The ventrogluteal muscle involves the gluteus medius and minimus, is situated deep and away from major nerves and blood vessels, and is a safe site for all clients. Because it is located away from the rectal area, less chance of contamination exists in incontinent clients (a problem when the dorsogluteal site is used).

The nurse locates the muscle by placing the heel of the hand over the greater trochanter of the client's hip. The right hand is used for the left hip, and the left hand is used for the right hip. The nurse points the thumb toward the client's groin and fingers toward the client's head, places the index finger over the anterior superior iliac spine, and extends the middle finger back along the iliac crest toward the buttock. The index finger, the middle finger, and the iliac crest form a V-shaped triangle and the injection site is the center of the triangle (Fig. 21-27).

## DORSOGLUTEAL

The dorsogluteal muscle has been a traditional site for intramuscular injections; however, a risk exists of striking the underlying sciatic nerve, greater trochanter, or major

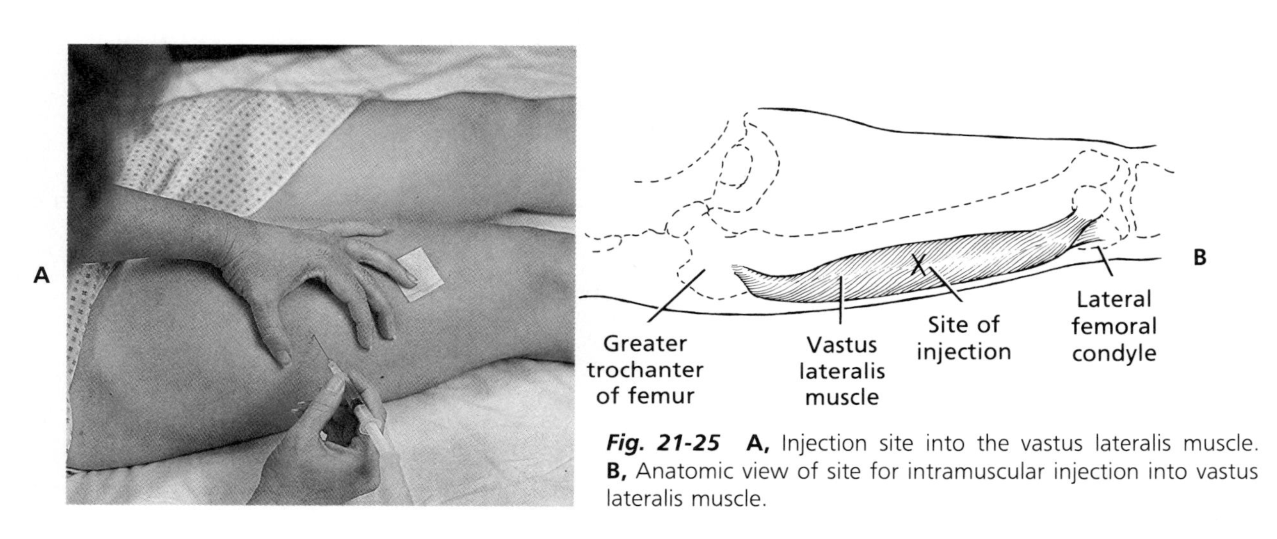


***Fig. 21-25*** **A,** Injection site into the vastus lateralis muscle. **B,** Anatomic view of site for intramuscular injection into vastus lateralis muscle.

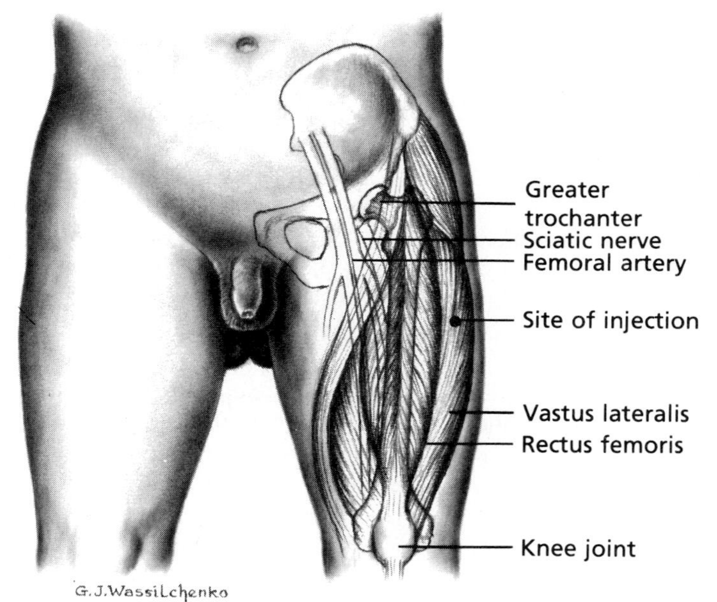


***Fig. 21-26*** Acceptable intramuscular site for children, the vastus lateralis.

From Whaley LF, Wong DL: Nursing care of infants and children, ed 3, St Louis, 1987, The CV Mosby Co.

blood vessels. Insertion of a needle into the sciatic nerve can cause permanent or partial paralysis of the involved leg. In clients with flabby, sagging tissues the site is difficult to locate. In children the muscle is usually too small until they reach 3 years of age. The muscle is developed by walking.

The dorsogluteal site is located in the upper outer quadrant of the buttock, approximately 5 to 8 cm (2 to 3 inches) below the iliac crest (Fig. 21-28, *A*). Clients may lie prone with toes turned medially or in a side-lying position with the upper leg flexed at the hip and knee. Two methods can be used to locate the dorsogluteal site:

1. Locate the posterior superior iliac spine and the greater trochanter of the femur. Draw an imaginary line between the two anatomic landmarks. The sciatic nerve runs parallel and below the line. The injection site is above and lateral to the line (Fig. 21-28, *B*).
2. A less accurate method of locating the dorsogluteal muscle is dividing the buttock into quadrants. The vertical dividing line extends from the gluteal fold up to the iliac crest. The intersecting horizontal line extends from the medial fold to the lateral aspect of the buttock. The injection site is in the upper outer quadrant (Fig. 21-28, *B*). This method for site selection increases the risk of injury to the sciatic nerve.

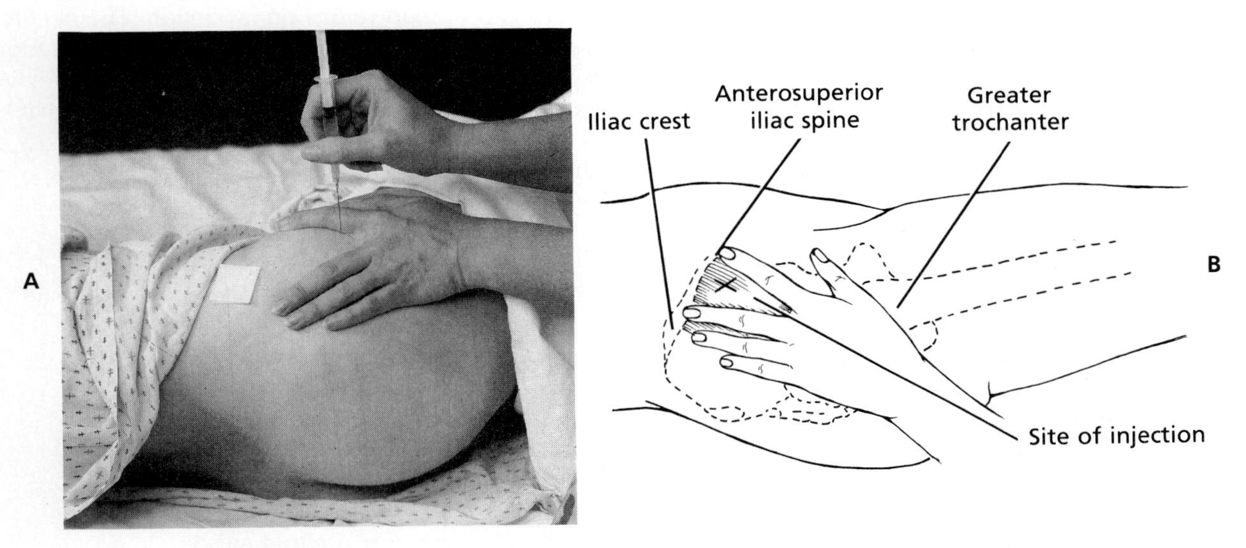


***Fig. 21-27*** **A,** Injection site into ventrogluteal muscle avoids major nerves and blood vessels. **B,** Anatomic view of ventrogluteal muscle injection site.

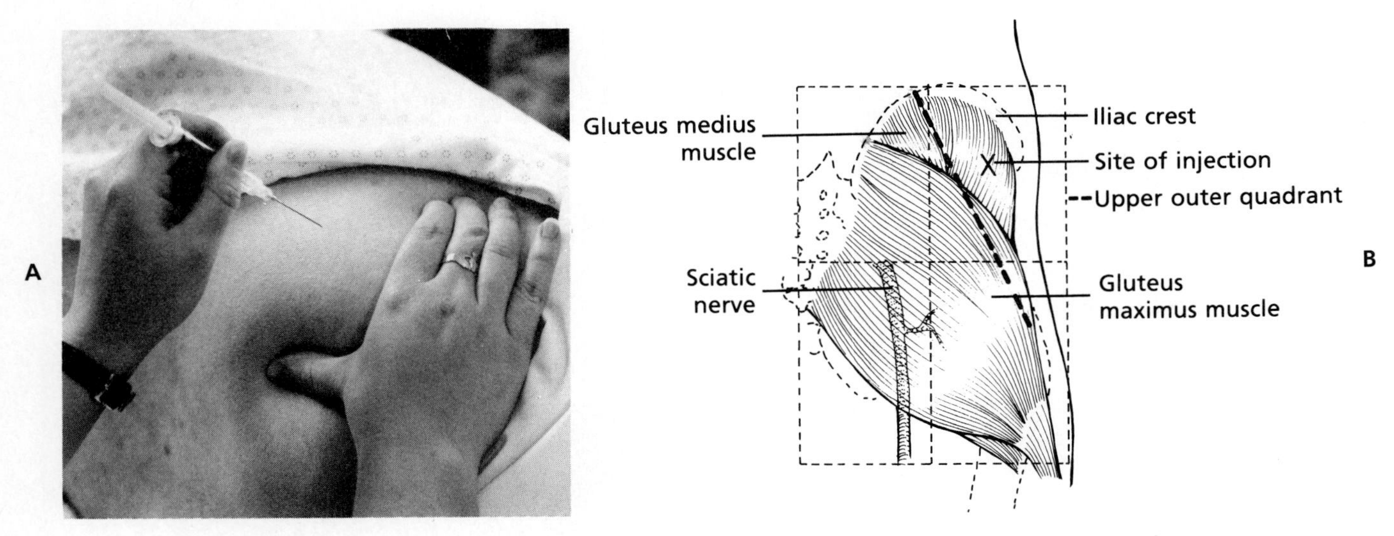


***Fig. 21-28*** **A,** Site of injection into dorsogluteal muscle. **B,** Imaginary diagonal line extending from posterior superior iliac spine to greater trochanter is landmark for selecting dorsogluteal injection site. Alternatively, buttocks may be divided into quadrants for selecting dorsogluteal injection site.

## DELTOID

Although the deltoid site is easily accessible, the muscle is not well developed in many adults. The deltoid should not be used in children or infants. The radial and ulnar nerves and brachial artery lie within the upper arm along the humerus. The nurse should use this site only for small medication volumes or when other sites are inaccessible due to dressings or casts.

To locate the deltoid muscle, the nurse fully exposes the client's upper arm and shoulder. A tight-fitting sleeve should not be rolled up. The nurse has the client relax the arm at the side and flex the elbow. The client may sit, stand, or lie down (Fig. 21-29, *A*). The nurse palpates the lower edge of the acromion process, which forms the base of a triangle in line with the midpoint of the lateral aspect of the upper arm. The injection site is in the center of the triangle, about 2.5 to 5 cm (1 to 2 inches) below the acromion process (Fig. 21-29, *B*). The nurse may also locate the site by placing four fingers across the deltoid muscle, with the top finger along the acromion process. The injection site is then three finger-widths below the acromion process.

## Z-TRACK METHOD

When irritating preparations such as iron or Vistaril are given intramuscularly, the Z-track method of injection minimizes tissue irritation by sealing the drug within muscle tissues.

The nurse selects an intramuscular site, preferably in larger, deeper muscles such as the ventrogluteal. It is important to apply a new needle to the syringe after preparing the drug so no solution remains on the outside needle shaft. The nurse draws up 0.2 ml of air to create an air lock. After preparing the site with an antiseptic swab, the nurse pulls the overlying skin and subcutaneous tissues approximately 2.5 to 3.5 cm (1 to 1½ inches) laterally to the side. Holding the skin taut with the nondominant hand, the nurse injects the needle deep into muscle. With practice the nurse learns to hold the syringe and aspirate with one hand. The nurse injects the drug and air slowly if there is no blood return on aspiration. The needle remains inserted for 10 seconds to allow the medication to disperse evenly. The nurse releases the skin after withdrawing the needle, which leaves a zigzag path that seals the needle track wherever tissue planes slide across each other (Fig. 21-30). The drug is less likely to escape from the muscle tissue.

### Purposes

1. Safely deposit medications in deep muscle tissue.
2. Avoid injury to the client.
3. Ensure proper drug absorption after injection.

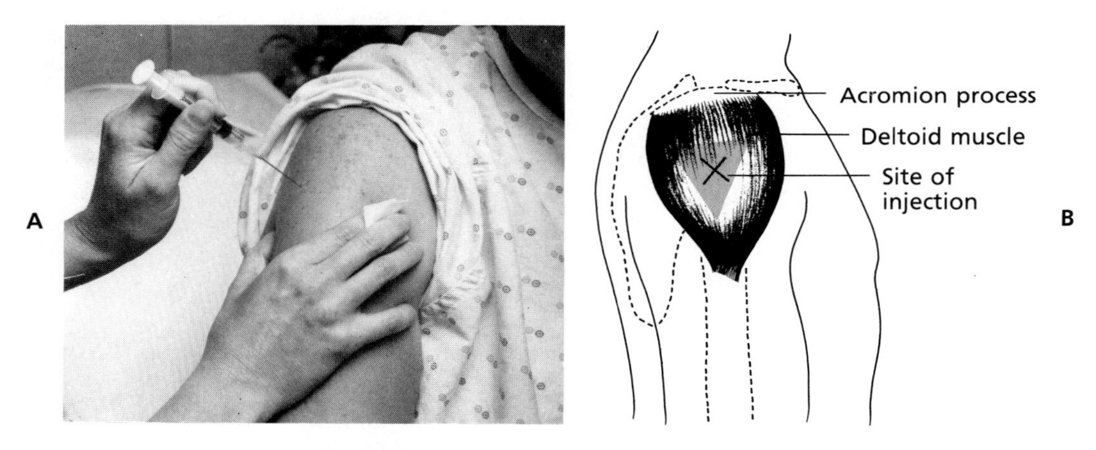


***Fig. 21-29*** **A,** Site of intramuscular injection into deltoid muscle. **B,** Site of deltoid muscle injection below acromion process.

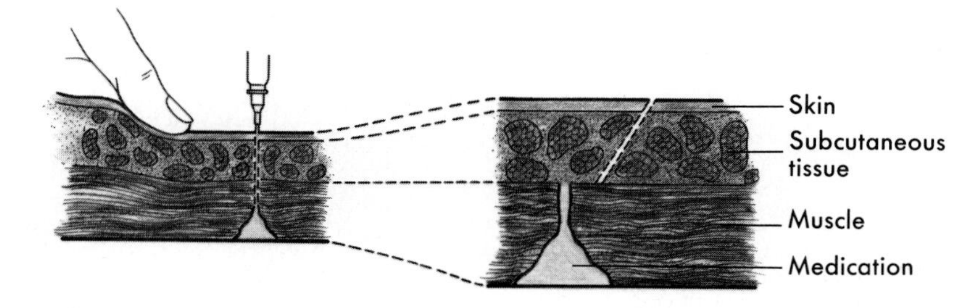


***Fig. 21-30*** Z-track method of injection prevents the deposition of medication through sensitive tissues.

## *Procedure 21-5*

| Steps | Rationale |
|---|---|
| **Assessment** | |
| 1. Review physician's medication order for client's name, drug name, dosage, time, and route of administration. | Ensures safe and correct administration of medication. |
| 2. Gather information pertinent to drug(s) ordered: action, purpose, time of onset and peak action, normal dosage, common side effects, nursing implications. | Nurse must be able to anticipate drug's effects and observe client's response. Allows nurse to judge appropriateness of therapy as client's condition changes. |
| 3. Consider factors that may contraindicate intramuscular injection, e.g., muscle atrophy, reduced blood flow, or circulatory shock. | Atrophied muscle absorbs medication poorly. Factors interfering with blood flow to muscles impairs drug absorption. |
| 4. Assess indications for intramuscular injection: | |
| a. Large volume of medication to inject. | Muscle less sensitive to large volumes of solution. |
| b. Client unable to tolerate oral drugs (Chapter 19). | Results in parenteral route as most suitable. |
| c. Fast action of drug desired. | Intramuscular route chosen in emergencies or when rapid effects are desirable. |
| 5. Assess client's medical history, history of allergies, and medication history. | May influence how certain drug acts. Information also indicates client's need for medication. |
| 6. Consider client's age. | In infants and children many muscle groups are underdeveloped. With aging, muscle fibers are reduced unless person exercises regularly. |
| 7. Assess client's knowledge regarding medication. | Information may pose implications for client education. Assessment may also reveal drug use problems at home. |
| 8. Observe client's verbal and nonverbal responses toward receiving injection. | Injections can be painful. Clients may experience considerable anxiety, which can increase pain. |
| **Nursing Diagnosis** | |
| 1. Cluster data to reveal actual or potential nursing diagnoses: | |
| a. Anxiety: related to receiving injection. | Nurse must use techniques during administration that minimize client's anxiety. |
| b. Altered tissue perfusion: related to hypovolemia. | May indicate need for different drug route. |
| c. Knowledge deficit regarding medication schedule: related to misunderstanding. | Indicates need for education to be incorporated into procedure. |
| **Planning** | |
| 1. Develop individualized goals for client based on nursing diagnoses: | |
| a. Promote optimal relaxation of muscle. | Positioning techniques relax muscle, reducing discomfort of injections. |
| b. Client feels minimal discomfort from injection. | Basic guidelines for administering injections reduce discomfort. |
| c. Client will feel less anxious. | Nurse's technique can control anxiety. Stress from procedure can easily frighten child. |
| d. Promote optimal drug absorption and distribution. | Nurse locates muscles accurately to ensure drug is deposited correctly for optimal therapeutic effect. |
| e. Client attains knowledge of drug therapy. | Giving medications is excellent time to discuss drug implications. |
| 2. Wash hands. | Reduces transmission of infection. |
| 3. Prepare following equipment and supplies: | |
| a. Syringe: 2-3 ml for adult, 1-2 ml for infant or child | Size chosen according to volume of drug to be administered. |
| b. Needle: 19-23 gauge, 1-1½ in for adults; 25-27 gauge, ½ -1 in for children | Needle must be long enough to penetrate muscle. Gauge is determined by viscosity of fluid. |
| c. Antiseptic swab, e.g., alcohol | |
| d. Medication ampule or vial | |
| e. Medication card, form, or printout | Identifies dose ordered and client's name. |
| 4. Prepare correct dosage from ampule or vial (Skill 21-1). Check dosage carefully. | Ensures that medication is sterile. Dosage is accurate. |
| 5. Optional: for irritating medications, e.g., iron, prepare an air lock. Draw 0.1-0.2 ml of air into syringe, being careful not to expel drug dosage. Air moves to end of plunger. (Check agency policy for use of airlock.) | Volume of air will be injected behind bolus of medication to clear needle of medication, preventing tracking of drug through sensitive tissue after needle is withdrawn. However, there is risk that an air lock could deliver excess medication that normally would be left in the needle (Chaplin, et al., 1985) |

| Steps | Rationale |
|---|---|
| 6. Change needle on syringe. | Prevents tracking of irritating substances as needle passes into muscle. |
| 7. Identify client by checking identification armband and asking client's name. Compare with medication ticket. | Ensures correct client is receiving medication. |
| 8. Explain procedure to client and proceed in calm, confident manner. | Helps client anticipate nurse's action. Calm approach minimizes client's anxiety. |

## Implementation

| Steps | Rationale |
|---|---|
| 1. Close room curtains or door. | Provides client privacy. |
| 2. Keep sheet or gown draped over body parts not requiring exposure. | Proper selection of injection site may require exposure of body parts. |
| 3. Select appropriate injection site by assessing size and integrity of muscle. Palpate for areas of tenderness or hardness. Note presence of bruising or area of infection. | Muscle should be soft when relaxed and firm when tense; indicates healthy tissue. |
| 4. Assist client to comfortable position, depending on site chosen: vastus lateralis-client lies flat, supine, with knee slightly flexed; ventrogluteal-client lies on side, back, or abdomen; flexes knee and hip on side to be injected; dorsogluteal-client lies prone with feet turned inward or lies on side with upper knee and hip flexed and placed in front of lower leg; deltoid-client may sit or lie flat with lower arm flexed but relaxed across abdomen or lap. | Position that reduces strain on muscle minimizes discomfort of injection. |

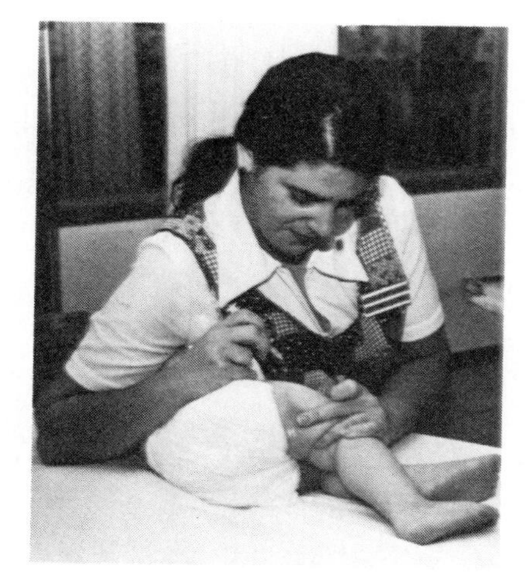

***Fig. 21-31***

From Whaley LW, Wong DL: Nursing care of infants and children, ed 3, 1987, St Louis, The CV Mosby Co.

| Steps | Rationale |
|---|---|
| 5. Relocate site using anatomic landmarks. | Injection into correct anatomic site prevents injury to nerves, bones, and blood vessels. |
| 6. Restrain child (Fig. 21-31). | Children often jerk or pull away unexpectedly, causing injury to themselves. |
| 7. Cleanse site with an antiseptic swab. Apply swab at center of the site and rotate outward in a circular direction for about 5 cm (2 in). | Mechanical action of swab removes secretions containing microorganisms. |
| 8. Hold swab between third and fourth fingers of nondominant hand. | Swab remains readily accessible when needle is withdrawn. |
| 9. Remove needle cap from needle by pulling it straight off. | Preventing needle from touching sides of cap prevents contamination. |
| 10. Hold syringe between thumb and forefinger of dominant hand as you would a dart. Hold it with palm down at 90°. | Quick, smooth injection requires proper manipulation of syringe. Needle must be injected at 90° angle to enter muscle and so air lock rises to top of medication toward plunger. |
| 11. Administer injection: | |
| a. Position nondominant hand at proper anatomical landmarks and spread skin tightly. Inject needle quickly at 90° angle into muscle. | Speeds insertion and reduces discomfort. |
| b. If client's muscle mass is small, grasp body of muscle between thumb and fingers. | Ensures that medication reaches muscle mass. |
| c. If giving irritating preparation, use Z-track method (see Fig. 20-30). (See section on Z-track method.) | Creates zigzag path through tissues that seals needle tract to avoid tracking of medication. |

| Steps | Rationale |
|---|---|
| 12. After needle enters site, grasp lower end of syringe barrel with nondominant hand. Move dominant hand to end of plunger. Avoid moving syringe. | Smooth manipulation of syringe parts reduces discomfort from needle movement. |
| a. If using Z-track method, hold skin tightly with nondominant hand. Use dominant hand to move carefully toward end of plunger. | Skin must remain pulled until after drug is injected. |
| 13. Slowly pull back on plunger to aspirate medication. If blood appears in syringe, remove needle and dispose of medication and syringe properly. Repeat preparation procedure. If no blood appears, inject medication slowly. | Aspiration of blood into syringe indicates intravenous placement of needle. Intramuscular medications are not for intravenous use. Slow injection reduces pain and tissue trauma. |
| 14. Withdraw needle quickly while placing antiseptic swab gently above or over injection. | Support of tissues around injection site minimizes discomfort during needle withdrawal. |
| a. When using Z-track method, keep needle inserted for 10 sec after injecting medication. Then release client's skin after withdrawing needle. | Allows medication to disperse evenly. Tissue planes slide across one another to create zigzag path that seals medication into muscle tissue. |
| 15. Massage skin lightly. In children, place small Band-Aid over puncture site. | Massage can stimulate circulation and improve drug distribution. Band-Aid may provide child with sense of comfort. |
| 16. Assist client to comfortable position. | Gives client sense of well-being. |
| 17. Discard uncapped needle and attached syringe into appropriately labeled receptacles. | Prevents injury to clients and health care personnel. CDC no longer recommends capping needles before disposal. |
| 18. Wash hands. | Reduces transmission of microorganisms. |
| **Evaluation** | |
| 1. Return to room and ask if client feels any acute pain, burning, numbness, or tingling at injection site. | Continued discomfort may indicate injury to underlying bones or nerves. |
| 2. Return to evaluate client's response to medication in 10-30 min. | Intramuscular medications absorb quickly; undesired effects may also develop rapidly. Nurse's observations determine efficacy of drug action. |
| 3. Ask client to explain purpose and effects of medication. | Evaluates client's understanding of information taught. |
| ***Expected outcomes*** | |
| 1. Client experiences temporary mild burning at injection site. | Displacement of tissues during injection causes discomfort. |
| 2. No allergies or undesired effects occur. | Drug action is normal. |
| 3. Client explains purpose and effects of medication. | Demonstrates learning. |
| ***Unexpected outcomes*** | |
| 1. Client continues to complain of localized pain, numbness, or tingling. | Indicates injury to nerves or tissues. |
| 2. Client develops signs and symptoms of allergy or side effects. | Extent of symptoms depends on client's sensitivity to drug and dose of drug. |
| 3. Client unable to explain purpose or effects of medication. | Requires reinstruction or client is unable to learn at this time. |
| **Recording and Reporting** | |
| 1. Immediately after administration, chart medication dosage, route, site, time, and date given in medication record. Correctly sign according to institutional policy (see Fig. 21-24). | Timely documentation prevents future drug administration errors. |
| 2. Report any undesirable effects from medication to nurse in charge or physician. | Client's response may indicate additional medical therapy. |
| 3. Record client's response to pain medications or similar drugs in nurses' notes. | Documents client's response to care. |

## Special Considerations

- Clients who have had cerebrovascular accident (stroke) or spinal cord injuries often have muscle atrophy.
- Be sure client wears allergy bracelet indicating medications and substances to which client is allergic.
- Tuberculin syringe is very useful for infants, especially for calculating small dosages of potent drugs.
- Use good illumination when assessing injection site.
- Never surprise children; always be sure they know they are to receive an injection.
- Infant or child needs to be held or comforted after injection. Parents can provide this support best.

## Teaching Considerations

- Clients requiring regular injections, e.g., vitamin $B_{12}$ should learn importance of rotating sites. Injections may be given by family members, client, or home health nurse.
- Instruct client and primary care giver to maintain sterile technique.

- Instruct client and primary care giver to observe injection sites for complications.
- Instruct client and primary care giver to observe for medication side effects.
- Allow for several return demonstrations on drawing up medications from the vial or ampule and injection technique.
- Instruct proper methods of disposal of needles and equipment.
- Instruct on precautions in caring for a client with a potential or positive diagnosis of AIDS.

### Home Care Considerations

- See Skill 21-1.

## *SKILL 21-6 Administering Intradermal Injections*

The nurse typically gives intradermal injections for skin testing, for example, in tuberculin screening and allergy tests. Because these medications are potent, they are injected into the dermis, where blood supply is reduced and drug absorption occurs slowly. A client may have an anaphylactic reaction if the medications enter the client's circulation too rapidly. For clients with a history of numerous allergies the physician often performs skin testing.

Skin testing requires the nurse to clearly see injection sites for changes in color and tissue integrity. Intradermal sites should be lightly pigmented, free of lesions, and relatively hairless. The inner forearm and upper back are ideal locations.

The nurse uses a tuberculin or small hypodermic syringe with a short (¼ to ½ in), fine-gauge (26 or 27) needle for skin testing. The angle of insertions for an intradermal injection is 5° to 15° (see Fig. 21-5). Only small amounts of medication (0.01 to 0.1 ml) are injected intradermally. If a bleb does not appear or if the site bleeds after needle withdrawal, the medication may enter subcutaneous tissues. In this case skin test results will not be valid.

### Purposes

1. Deposit medication into the dermal skin layer safely.
2. Test a client's sensitivity to specific allergens.
3. Minimize chances of allergic reactions.

## *Procedure 21-6*

| Steps | Rationale |
|---|---|
| **Assessment** | |
| 1. Review physician's medication order for client's name, drug name, dosage, time and route of administration. | Ensures safe and correct administration of medication. |
| 2. Know information regarding expected reaction when testing skin with specific allergen or medication. | Body releases antibodies in response to allergen. Type of reaction depends on client's sensitivity. |
| 3. Assess client's history of allergies and know substance client is allergic to and normal allergic reaction. | Certain substances have similar compositions; nurse should not administer any substance to which client is known to be allergic. |
| 4. Check date of expiration for medication, vial, or ampule. | Drug loses its potency when outdated. |
| 5. Assess client's knowledge of purpose and reactions of skin testing. | Reveals need for client instruction. |
| **Nursing Diagnosis** | |
| 1. Cluster data to reveal actual or potential nursing diagnoses: | |
| a. Potential for injury: related to exposure to potential allergen. | Nurse must carefully observe client's reaction to medication. |
| b. Knowledge deficit regarding skin testing: related to inexperience. | Nurse provides client with information needed to observe results of skin testing. |
| **Planning** | |
| 1. Develop individualized goals for client based on nursing diagnoses: | |
| a. Promote optimal drug absorption and distribution. | Nurse can visually determine if medication is deposited into dermis. |

| **Steps** | **Rationale** |
|---|---|
| b. Determine client's level of sensitivity to allergens. | Extent of skin reaction determines degree of sensitivity. |
| c. Client attains knowledge about expected skin test results. | Client can participate in observing for expected skin changes. |
| 2. Wash hands. | Reduces transmission of microorganisms. |
| 3. Prepare following equipment and supplies: | |
| a. 1 ml tuberculin syringe with preattached 26- or 27-gauge needle | |
| b. Alcohol swabs | |
| c. Vial or ampule of skin test solution | Substance being tested comes in various dilutions or concentrations. |
| d. Medication card, form, or printout | Identifies medication dose ordered and client's name. |
| 4. Prepare correct dosage from vial or ampule (Skill 21-1). Check dosage carefully. | Ensures medication is sterile, dosage is accurate. |
| 5. Identify client by checking identification armband and asking client's name. Compare with medication ticket. | Ensures correct client receives ordered drug. |
| 6. Explain steps of procedure and tell client injection feels like slight burning or sting. | Helps minimize client's anxiety. |

## Implementation

| **Steps** | **Rationale** |
|---|---|
| 1. Close room curtain or door. | Provides privacy. |
| 2. Keep sheet or gown draped over body parts not requiring exposure. | Injection site may require exposure of body parts. |
| 3. Select appropriate injection site. Inspect skin surface over sites for bruises, inflammation, or edema. Note lesions or discolorations of forearm. Select site three to four finger-widths below antecubital space and handwidth above wrist. | Injection sites should be free of abnormalities that may interfere with drug absorption. An intradermal site should be clear so results of skin test can be seen and interpreted correctly. |
| 4. Assist client to comfortable position with elbow and forearm extended and supported on flat surface. | Stabilizes injection site for easiest accessibility. |
| 5. Cleanse site with an antiseptic swab. Apply swab at center of the site and rotate outward in a circular direction for about 5 cm (2 in). | Mechanical action of swab removes secretions containing microorganisms. |
| 6. Hold swab between third and fourth fingers of nondominant hand. | Swab remains readily accessible when needle is withdrawn. |
| 7. Remove needle cap from needle by pulling it straight off. | Preventing needle from touching sides of cap prevents contamination. |
| 8. Hold syringe between thumb and forefinger of dominant hand with bevel of needle pointing up. | Smooth injection requires proper manipulation of syringe parts. With bevel up, medication will less likely be deposited into tissues below dermis. |
| 9. With nondominant hand, stretch skin over site with forefinger or thumb. | Needle pierces tight skin more easily. |
| 10. With needle almost against client's skin, insert it slowly at 5°-15° angle until resistance is felt. Then advance needle through epidermis to approximately 3 mm (⅛ in) below skin surface. Needle tip can be seen through skin (Fig. 21-32). | Ensures needle tip is in dermis. |

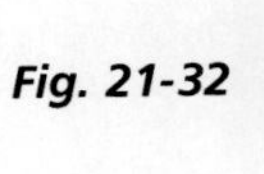

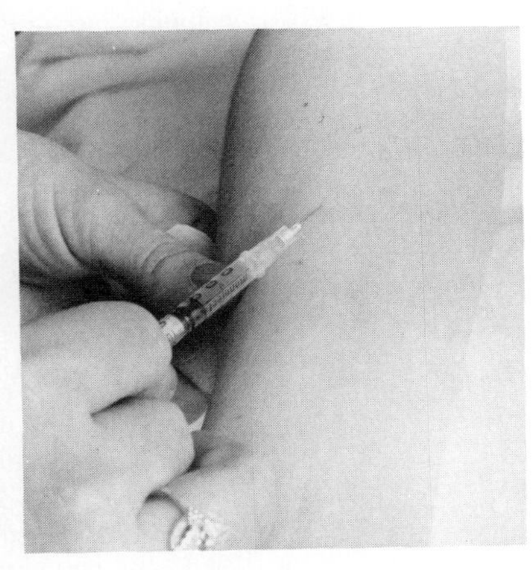

**Fig. 21-32**

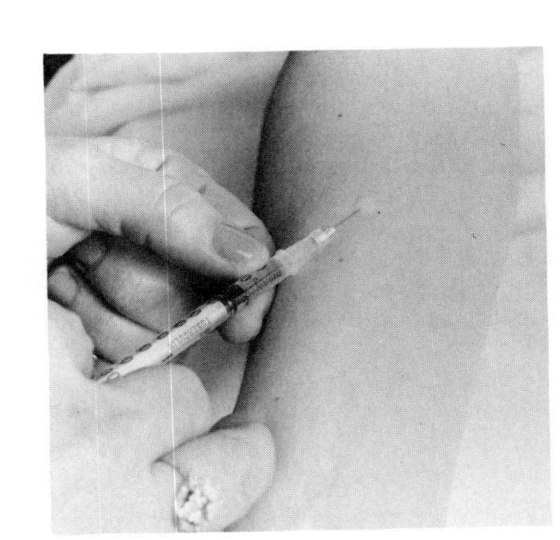

**Fig. 21-33**

| Steps | Rationale |
|---|---|
| 11. Inject medication slowly. Normally, resistance is felt. If not, needle is too deep; remove and begin again. | Slow injection minimizes discomfort at site. Dermal layer is tight and does not expand easily when solution is injected. |
| 12. While injecting medication, notice that small bleb resembling mosquito bite appears on skin's surface (Fig. 21-33). | Wheal indicates medication is deposited in dermis. |
| 13. Withdraw needle while applying alcohol swab gently over site. | Support of tissue around injection site minimizes discomfort during needle withdrawal. |
| 14. Do not massage site. | Massage may disperse medication into underlying tissue layers and alter test results. |
| 15. Assist client to comfortable position. | Gives client sense of well-being. |
| 16. Discard uncapped needle and attached syringe in appropriately labeled receptacles. | Prevents injury to clients and health care personnel. CDC no longer recommends capping of needles. |
| 17. Wash hands. | Reduces transmission of microorganisms. |

## Evaluation

| | |
|---|---|
| 1. Stay with client and observe for any allergic reactions. | Severe anaphylactic reaction is characterized by dypsnea, wheezing, and circulatory collapse. |
| 2. Use skin pencil and draw circle around perimeter of injection site. Read site within 48-72 hr of injection. | Site must be read at various intervals to determine test results. Pencil mark makes site easy to find. |
| 3. Ask client to discuss implications of skin testing and signs of hypersensitivity. | Client's ability to recognize signs of skin testing helps to ensure timely reporting of results. |

### *Expected outcomes*

| | |
|---|---|
| 1. Client experiences very mild burning sensation during injection but no discomfort after injection. | Normal reaction to medication deposited in dermis. |
| 2. Small light-colored wheal approximately 6 mm (¼ in) in diameter forms at site and gradually disappears. Minimal bruising may be present. | Medication is in dermis and is eventually absorbed. Bruising is result of minor bleeding from capillaries. |
| 3. Client is able to identify signs of a skin reaction and their significance. | Demonstrates learning. |

### *Unexpected outcomes*

| | |
|---|---|
| 1. Raised, reddened, or hard zone forms around test site. | Indicates sensitivity to the injected allergen. (Positive test for tuberculin skin testing.) |
| 2. Onset of allergic reaction develops within minutes. | Allergen absorbed into blood stream, causing allergic reaction. |
| 3. Client unable to explain purpose or signs of skin testing. | Client requires reinstruction or unable to learn at this time. |

## Recording and Reporting

| | |
|---|---|
| 1. Record area of injection, amount and type of testing substance, and date and time on medication record and nurses' notes (see Fig. 21-24). | Timely documentation prevents future adiministration errors. |
| 2. Report any undesirable effects from medication to nurse in charge or physician. | Client's response may indicate additional medical therapy. |

## Special Considerations

- Nurse must use caution when testing clients with low concentration of medication. Negative skin test does not mean client is not allergic to larger therapeutic dose.
- Client should wear allergy identification band listing all substances to which client is allergic.
- Not necessary to aspirate, since dermis is relatively avascular.
- If no wheal appears, medication probably entered subcutaneous tissues. Skin test results will not be valid.
- Caution client not to wash off markings around injection site.
- If client has had close contact with a tuberculin carrier, intradermal skin reactions, including induration measuring 5 mm and larger, are significant.
- If tuberculin testing reactions are less than 5 mm, close contacts are retested in 2 mo.

## Teaching Considerations

- When clients are tested in a clinic or other outpatient setting, have them call in results of skin tests if a follow-up appointment is not made.

# SKILL 21-7 *Adding Medications to Intravenous Fluid Containers*

Of all the methods for drug administration, the intravenous (IV) route poses the greatest risks for a client. Medications enter the venous circulation directly and thus can cause rapid effects. The nurse must observe clients closely for symptoms of adverse reactions. Special attention is given to dosage calculation and drug preparation. The nurse carefully checks the "five rights" of safe drug administration and is aware of the desired action and potential side effects of each medication. This is especially important when administering IV drugs to children. A child requires only minute dosages of certain medications. Care must also be taken when infusing medications through a child's veins because they are so small and fragile.

Many parenteral medications are highly alkaline and irritating to muscle and subcutaneous tissue. Thus the IV route is best to minimize client discomfort. The nurse administers drugs intravenously by three methods:

1. As mixtures within large volumes of IV fluids.
2. By "piggyback" infusion of a solution containing the prescribed medication and a small volume of fluid through an adjoining container or existing IV line.
3. By injection of a bolus or small volume of medication through an existing IV infusion line or heparin intravenous lock.

In all three methods the client has either an existing IV infusion line or an IV access site in the form of a heparin lock. In most institutions and settings only physicians are allowed to inject medications directly into a client's veins through venipuncture.

## GUIDELINES

1. Be sure IV line for injecting medications is patent and running.
2. Always observe for clarity of IV solutions after adding a medication. Incompatible drugs in solution cause clouding or crystallization of fluids.
3. Observe condition of an IV site while medications are infusing. Infiltration (Chapter 23) can occur at any time.
4. Always observe the client closely while IV medications are infusing.

## CONTAINERS

Mixing drugs in large volumes of fluids is relatively safe and easy. The nurse or pharmacist dilutes IV medications in large volumes (500 to 1000 ml) of compatible IV fluids such as normal saline, dextrose and water, or lactated Ringer's solution. In many hospital settings the pharmacy adds drugs to primary containers of IV solutions to ensure asepsis. Because a drug is not in a concentrated form, the risk of side effects or fatal reactions is minimal. Vitamins and potassium chloride are two types of drugs commonly added to IV fluids.

### Purposes

1. Minimize likelihood of adverse drug reactions.
2. Provide continuous infusion of a prescribed medication to maintain therapeutic blood levels.
3. Provide electrolyte, mineral, and vitamin replacement for clients unable to eat.
4. Avoid discomforts of giving medications by other parenteral routes.

## *Procedure 21-7*

| Steps | Rationale |
|---|---|
| **Assessment** | |
| 1. Check physician's order to determine type of IV solution to use and type of medication and dosage. | Client's overall physical condition dictates type of IV solution used. Ensures safe and accurate drug administration. |
| 2. Collect information necessary to administer drug safely, including: action, purpose, side effects, normal dosage, time of peak onset, nursing implications. | Allows nurse to give drug safely and to monitor client's response to therapy. |
| 3. When more than one medication is to be added to IV solution, assess for compatibility of medications. | Drugs often are incompatible when mixed together. Chemical reaction that occurs results in clouding or crystallization of IV fluids. |
| 4. Assess client's systemic fluid balance, as reflected by skin hydration and turgor, body weight, pulse and blood pressure. | Danger of continuous IV infusions is that fluids may infuse too rapidly, causing circulatory overload. |
| 5. Assess client's history of drug allergies. | IV administration of drugs causes rapid effects. Allergic response can be immediate. |
| 6. Assess IV insertion site for signs of infiltration or phlebitis. | An intact, properly funcitoning site ensures medication is given safely. |

| Steps | Rationale |
|---|---|
| **Nursing Diagnosis** | |
| 1. Cluster data to reveal actual or potential nursing diagnoses: | |
| a. Potential fluid volume excess: related to rapid IV fluid infusion. | Client at risk unless nurse monitors IV infusion on routine basis. |
| **Planning** | |
| 1. Develop individualized goals for adding medications to IV fluid containers: | |
| a. Ensure accurate dosage and infusion of fluid. | Prevents adverse drug reaction and fluid overload. |
| b. Prevent transfer of infection to container. | Strict aseptic technique keeps container's contents sterile. |
| 2. Prepare the following equipment and supplies: | |
| a. Vial or ampule of prescribed medication | |
| b. Syringe of appropriate size (5-20 ml) | |
| c. Sterile needle (1-1½ in, 19-21-gauge) with special filters (optional) | Larger needle gauge ensures easy aspiration of drugs from vial or ampule. Filter prevents solid material from entering syringe and avoids transfer to fluid container. |
| d. Correct diluent (e.g., sterile water or normal saline) | Certain IV medications are prepared in dry powder form. Diluent must be added for mixing. |
| e. Sterile IV fluid container (bag or bottle, 500-1000 ml in volume) | IV solution bags are kept sterile by being stored in separate intact plastic bag. IV bottles have plastic or metal seal over bottle cap. |
| f. Alcohol or antiseptic swab | |
| g. Label to attach to IV bag or bottle | Continuously infusing medication must be labeled properly for all nurses to observe. |
| h. Medication ticket, form, or printout | Verifies order. |
| 3. Wash hands thoroughly. | Reduces transfer of microorganisms when handling sterile equipment. |
| 4. Assemble supplies in medication room. | Ensures procedure will be orderly with less likelihood of contaminating supplies. |
| 5. Prepare prescribed medication from vial or ampule (if a filter needle is used, replace it with a regular needle before injecting medication into the IV fluid container.) | Different techniques used for each type of container. |
| 6. Identify client by reading identification band and asking name. Compare with medication ticket. | Ensures correct client receives ordered medication. |
| 7. Prepare client by explaining that medication is to be given through existing IV line or one to be started. Explain that no discomfort should be felt during drug infusion. Encourage client to report symptoms of discomfort. | Allows client to understand procedure and minimizes anxiety. Most IV medications will not cause discomfort when diluted. However, potassium chloride can be irritating. Pain at insertion site may be early indication of infiltration. |

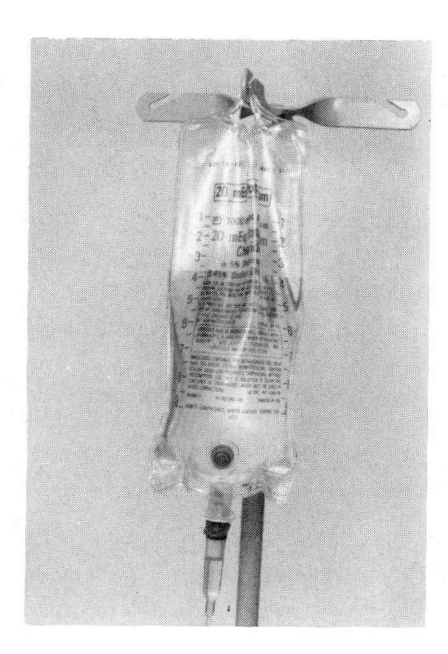

*Fig. 21-34*

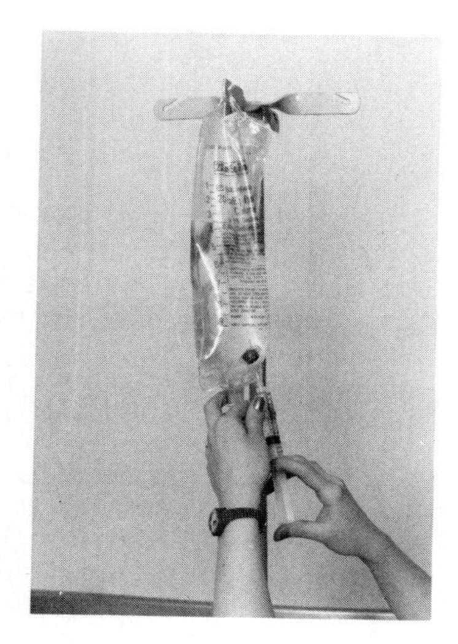

*Fig. 21-35*

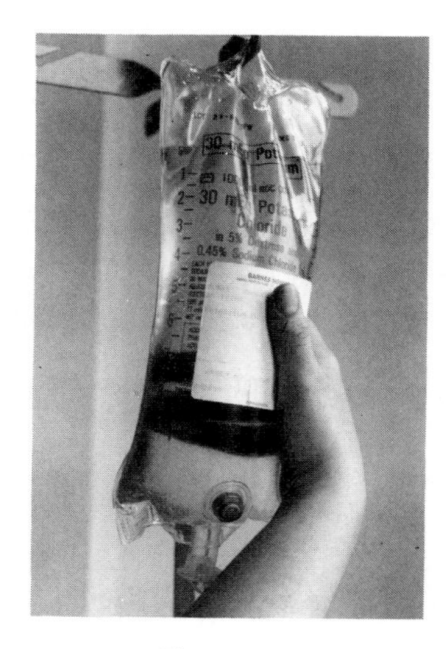

*Fig. 21-36*

| Steps | Rationale |
|---|---|
| **Implementation** | |
| 1. Add medication to new container: | |
| a. Locate medication injection port on plastic IV solution bag. | |
| ▪ Remove plastic cover over port. Port has small rubber stopper at end. Do not select port for the IV tubing insertion or air vent (Fig. 21-34). | Medication injection port is self-sealing to prevent introduction of microorganisms after repeated use. |
| b. Locate injection site on intravenous solution bottle. | |
| ▪ Remove metal or plastic cap and rubber disk. Place cap right side up on countertop. | Cap seals bottle to maintain its sterility. Inside of cap may remain sterile for reuse. |
| ▪ Locate medication injection site on bottle's rubber stopper. Site is usually marked by an **X**, circle, or triangle. | Accidental injection of medication through main tubing port or air vent can alter pressure within bottle and cause fluid leaks through air vent. |
| c. Wipe off port or injection site with alcohol or antiseptic swab. | Reduces risk of introducing microorganisms into bag during needle insertion. |
| d. Remove needle cap from syringe and carefully insert needle of syringe through center of injection port or site, and inject medication. | Injection of needle into sides of port may produce leak and lead to fluid contamination. |
| e. Withdraw syringe from bag or bottle. Cover glass bottle top with antiseptic swab and sterile bottle cap. | Open tubing port in bottle provides direct route for microorganisms to enter solution. Bags have self-sealing port. |
| f. Mix medication and IV solution by holding bag or bottle and turning it gently end to end. | Allows even distribution of medication. |
| g. Complete medication label with name and dose of medication, date, time, and nurse's initials. Stick it upside down on bottle or bag. | Label can be easily read during infusion of solution. Informs nurses and physicians of contents of bag or bottle. |
| h. Spike bag or bottle with IV tubing and hang (see Chapter 23). Regulate infusion at ordered rate. | Prevents rapid infusion of fluid. |
| 1. Add medication to existing container: | |
| a. Prepare vented IV bottle or plastic bag: | |
| ▪ Check volume of solution remaining in bottle or bag. | Proper volume is needed to dilute medication adequately. |
| ▪ Close off IV infusion clamp. | Prevents medication from directly entering circulation as it is injected into bag or bottle. |
| ▪ Wipe off medication port with an alcohol or antiseptic swab. | Mechanically removes microorganisms that could enter container during needle insertion. |
| ▪ Insert syringe needle through injection port and inject medication (Fig. 21-35). | Injection port is self-sealing and prevents fluid leaks. |
| ▪ Lower bag or bottle from IV pole and gently mix. | Ensures medication is evenly distributed. |
| ▪ Rehang bag and regulate infusion to desired rate. | Prevents rapid infusion of fluid. |
| b. Complete medication label and stick it to bag or bottle (Fig. 21-36). | Informs nurses and physicians of contents of bag or bottle. |
| 2. Properly dispose of equipment and supplies. Do not cap needle of syringe. | Proper disposal of needle prevents injury to nurse and client. Capping of needles increases risk of finger stick. |
| 3. Wash hands. | Reduces transmission of microorganisms. |
| **Evaluation** | |
| 1. Observe client for signs or symptoms of drug reaction. | IV medications can cause rapid effects. |
| 2. Observe for signs and symptoms of fluid volume excess. | Rapid uncontrolled infusion can cause circulatory overload. |
| 3. Periodically return to client's room to assess IV insertion site and rate of infusion. | Over time IV site may become infiltrated or needle malpositioned. Flow rate may change according to client's position or volume left in container. |
| ***Expected outcomes*** | |
| 1. Client experiences no medication side effects. | Drugs were given safely. |
| 2. No signs or symptoms of fluid volume excess develop. | IV rate monitored correctly. |
| 3. IV site remains free of swelling or inflammation. | Fluid was delivered intravenously. |
| ***Unexpected outcomes*** | |
| 1. Client has undesired reaction to medication. | Response depends on client's sensitivity and drug's action. |
| 2. Client develops signs of fluid volume excess, e.g., abnormal breath sounds (crackles), blood pressure changes, jugular venous distention, edema, shortness of breath, intake greater than output. | Excess fluid intake can compromise circulatory regulation. |
| 3. IV site becomes swollen, warm, reddened, and tender to touch (Chapter 23). | Indicates signs of phlebitis. |
| 4. IV site becomes cool, pale, and swollen (Chapter 23). | Indicates signs of infiltration. |

**Steps** **Rationale**

**PARENTERAL FLUID**

| AMT. | TYPE OF FLUID | MEDICATION ADDED | DATE/ HR START | RN INIT | DATE/ HR COMP | RN INIT | AMT. REC'D | SITE | IV SITE CARE DATE/HR | TUBING CHANGE DATE / HR | RN INIT |
|---|---|---|---|---|---|---|---|---|---|---|---|
| 1L | $D_5W$ | 20 meq. KCl | 1/8 0900 | P.L. | 1/8 1800 | T.M. | 1000ml | V | 1/8 1000 | | |
| 1L | LR | 20 meq. KCl | 1/8 1800 | T.M. | | | | | | | |
| | | | | | | | | | | | |
| | | | | | | | | | | | |
| | | | | | | | | | | | |
| | | | | | | | | | | | |
| | | | | | | | | | | | |
| | | | | | | | | | | | |
| | | | | | | | | | | | |
| | | | | | | | | | | | |
| | | | | | | | | | | | |
| | | | | | | | | | | | |
| | | | | | | | | | | | |
| | | | | | | | | | | | |
| | | | | | | | | | | | |

*Fig. 21-37*

### Recording and Reporting

1. Record solution and medication added to parenteral fluid on appropriate form (Fig. 21-37).

Information used to monitor type of solutions client receives and fluid intake over 24 hr.

2. Report any side effects to nurse in charge or physician.

Reaction may require therapeutic intervention.

### Special Considerations

- Check with pharmacist or drug literature for drug compatibility.
- When monitoring IV fluid infusion, vitamins, minerals, and most electrolytes are relatively safe. Potassium chloride, if allowed to infuse too quickly, can cause heart dysrhythmias.
- Pharmacies use special plastic caps to seal bottles previously mixed.
- When adding medication to a vented administration set be sure there is sufficient fluid in the bottle or bag. After closing the IV flow clamp, detach the air vent cap while keeping the end sterile. Remove needle from the medication syringe and insert the tip of the syringe into the air vent port. Instill medication and reattach the air vent.

### Home Care Considerations

- See Skill 21-1.

## *SKILL 21-8* Administering Intravenous Medications by Intermittent Infusion Sets

Another way to reduce the risk of rapid drug dose infusion is to dilute IV medications in small volumes of solution and administer over a short period.

The fluid is contained within a secondary fluid container separate from the primary IV fluid bag. The container connects directly to the primary IV line or to a separate tubing that inserts into the primary IV line. Two types of containers are (1) volume-control administration sets (for example, Volutrol or Pediatrol) and (2) piggyback or tandem intravenous sets.

Volume-control administration sets are small (100 to 150 ml) containers that attach just below the primary infusion bag or bottle. The set is attached and filled in a manner similar to a regular IV infusion. However, the priming or filling of the set is different, depending on the type of filter (floating valve or membrane) within the set. Follow package directions for priming sets.

Piggyback sets are small (50 to 100 ml) IV bags or bottles connected to short tubing lines that connect to the upper **Y**-port of a primary infusion line or to an intermittent venous access (Fig. 21-38, *A*). The piggyback tubing is a microdrip or macrodrip system (Chapter 23). The sets are called piggyback because the small bag or bottle is set higher than the primary infusion bottle.

The port of the primary IV line contains a back check valve that automatically stops flow of the primary infusion once the piggyback infusion flows. After the piggyback solution infuses and the solution within the tubing falls below the level of the primary infusion drip chamber, the back check valve opens and the primary infusion again flows.

A tandem set is similar to the piggyback except that both the primary and secondary solutions are at the same height (Fig. 21-38, *B*). The secondary infusion line is inserted into a primary line port without a back check valve and more proximal to the client. The secondary tandem set requires a longer tubing to reach the primary line port. It is necessary to clamp the primary line as the secondary solution infuses if the two solutions are incompatible or if rapid infusion of the solution is required.

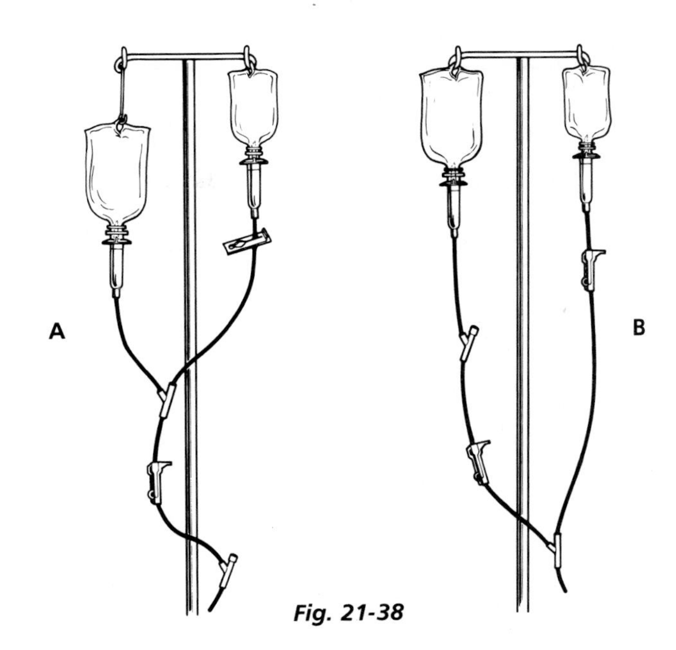

*Fig. 21-38*

**Purposes**

1. Administer IV medications over a limited period to maintain concentrated blood levels of drugs and prevent drug instability.
2. Limit fluid intake during drug administration.
3. Avoid mixing medications that are incompatible with drugs in the primary intravenous solution.
4. Dilute potentially irritating IV medication.
5. Reduce risk of rapid dose infusion by IV push.

## *Procedure 21-8*

| Steps | Rationale |
|---|---|
| **Assessment** | |
| 1. Check physician's order to determine type of IV solution to be used, type of medication, dosage, and route and time of administration. | Client's overall physical condition dictates type of IV solution used. Ensures safe and accurate drug administration. |
| 2. Collect information necessary to administer drug safely, including: action, purpose, side effects, normal dosage, time of peak onset, nursing implications. | Allows nurse to give drug safely and to monitor client's response to therapy. |
| 3. Assess patency of client's existing IV infusion line (Chapter 23) by noting infusion rate of main IV line. | IV line must be patent and fluids must infuse easily for medication to reach venous circulation effectively. |
| 4. Assess IV insertion site for signs of infiltration or phlebitis: redness, pallor, swelling, tenderness, on palpation. | Confirmation of placement of IV needle or catheter and integrity of surrounding tissues ensures medication is administered safely. |
| 5. Assess client's history of drug allergies. | Effects of medications can develop rapidly after IV infusion. Nurse should be aware of clients at risk. |
| 6. Assess client's understanding of purpose of drug therapy. | May reveal need for education. |
| **Nursing Diagnosis** | |
| 1. Cluster data to reveal actual or potential nursing diagnoses: | |
| a. Pain: related to phlebitis or infiltration. | Indicates need to discontinue current IV line and start another. |
| b. Knowledge deficit regarding drug therapy: related to inexperience. | Nurse will instruct client during drug administration. |

| Steps | Rationale |
|---|---|
| **Planning** | |
| 1. Develop individualized goals for client based on nursing diagnoses: | |
| a. Infuse medication at proper rate. | Rapid infusion may present risk of undesired drug action. |
| b. Client's discomfort is minimal. | Slow, controlled infusion prevents irritation of vein at IV insertion site. |
| c. Maintain sterility of IV line. | IV line provides excellent route for infection unless aseptic technique is followed. |
| d. Promote optimal drug absorption and distribution. | IV route provides rapid therapeutic effect. |
| 2. Prepare following equipment and supplies: | |
| a. Piggyback or tandem: | |
| ▪ Medication prepared in a 50-100 ml labeled infusion bag | Used for piggyback administration. Most piggybacks are prepared by pharmacies. |
| ▪ Short microdrip or macrodrip tubing set for piggyback | Long tubing set for tandem. |
| ▪ Needle (21- or 23-gauge) | Medication is "piggybacked" or connected to client main infusion line by needle inserted through IV line injection port. Larger needle would cause leakage at Y-port connector. |
| ▪ Adhesive tape (optional) | |
| ▪ Antiseptic swab | |
| ▪ Metal hook (piggyback only) | To lower primary infusion bag below smaller infusion bag (used only if tubing is shorter than primary infusion tubing). |
| ▪ Medication ticket, form, or printout. | |
| b. Volume-control administration set: | |
| ▪ Volutrol or Burette | Graduated container connects to main IV solution. |
| ▪ Infusion tubing | Connected to administration set used to inject medication into set. |
| ▪ Syringe (5-20 ml) | |
| ▪ Needle (1-1½ in, 21-23-gauge) | |
| ▪ Vial or ampule of ordered medication | |
| ▪ Medication label | |
| ▪ Medication ticket, form, or printout | |
| 3. Wash hands. | Reduces transmission of infection. |
| 4. Assemble supplies at bedside. | Drug preparation usually not required. May assemble infusion tubing and bag of medication in medication or client's room. |
| **Implementation** | |
| 1. Piggyback or tandem: | |
| a. Connect infusion tubing to medication bag (see Chapter 23). Allow solution to fill tubing by opening regulator flow clamp. | Infusion tube should be filled with solution and free of air bubbles to prevent air embolus. |
| b. Hang piggyback medication bag above level of primary fluid bag. (Hook may be used to lower main bag.) Hang tandem infusion at same level as primary fluid bag. | Height of fluid bag affects rate of flow to client. |
| c. Connect covered sterile needle to end of infusion tubing. | Cover keeps needle sterile before connecting it to main IV line. |
| d. Check client's identification by looking at armband and asking name. | Ensures drug is administered to correct client. |
| e. Explain purpose of medication to client and explain that medication is to be given through existing IV line. Encourage client to report symptoms of discomfort at site. | Keeps client informed of planned therapies. |
| f. Piggyback: clean upper injection Y-port of primary IV line with antiseptic swab. Tandem: clean injection Y-port proximal to client on primary line with antiseptic swab. | Prevents introduction of microorganisms during needle insertion. |
| g. Remove cover and insert needle of secondary line through proper injection port of main IV line. Secure with strip of adhesive tape if necessary. | Establishes route for IV medication to enter main IV line. Tape prevents needle from slipping out of port. |
| h. Regulate flow rate of medication solution. (Usually medication should infuse within 30-60 min) | Provides slow, intermittent infusion of medication infusion in 30-60 min, maintains therapeutic blood levels. |
| i. After medication has infused, check flow regulator on primary infusion. Backcheck valve on piggyback stops flow of the primary infusion until medication infuses. The tandem and primary infusions will flow together until the tandem set empties. The primary infusion should automatically begin to flow after the piggyback or tandem solution is empty. | Valve prevents backup of medication into main infusion line. Checking flow rate ensures proper administration of IV fluids. |

| Steps | Rationale |
|---|---|

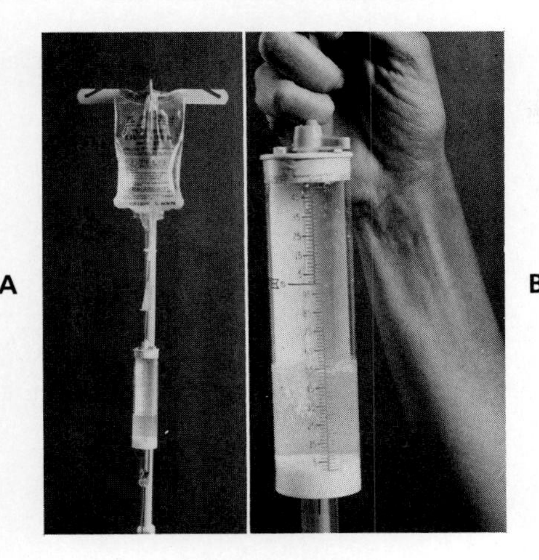


*Fig. 21-39*

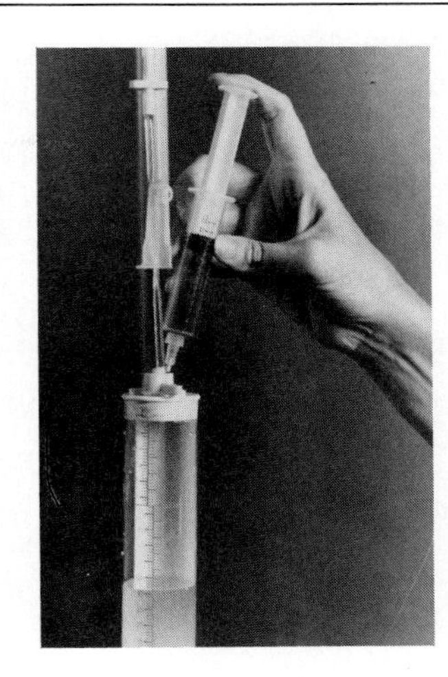

*Fig. 21-40*

| Steps | Rationale |
|---|---|
| j. Regulate main infusion line to desired rate, if necessary. | Infusion of piggyback may interfere with the main line infusion rate. |
| k. Leave secondary bag, tubing, and inserted needle in place for future drug administration or discard in appropriate containers. | Establishment of secondary line produces route for microorganisms to enter main line. Repeated changes in tubing or needles increase risk of infection transmission (check agency policy). |
| 2. Volume-control administration set (e.g., Volutrol): | |
| a. Assemble supplies in medication room. | Controls risk of contaminating IV solution. |
| b. Prepare medication from vial or ampule (Procedure 21-1). | Ensures medication is sterile. |
| c. Check client's identification by looking at armband and asking name. Compare with medication ticket. | Ensures drug administered to correct client. |
| d. Explain procedure to client. Encourage client to report symptoms of discomfort at site. | Keeps client informed of planned therapies. |
| e. Fill Volutrol with desired amount of fluid (50-100 ml) by opening clamp between Volutrol and main IV bag (Fig. 21-39). | Small volume of fluid dilutes IV medication and reduces risk of too rapid infusion. |
| f. Close clamp and check to be sure clamp in air vent of Volutrol chamber is open. | Prevents additional leakage of fluid into Volutrol. Air vent allows fluid in Volutrol to exit at regulated rate. |
| g. Clean injection port on top of Volutrol with antiseptic swab. | Prevents introduction of microorganisms during needle insertion. |
| h. Remove needle cap and insert syringe needle through port, then inject medication (Fig. 21-40). Gently rotate Volutrol between hands. | Rotating mixes medication with solution in Volutrol to ensure equal distribution. |
| i. Regulate IV infusion rate to allow medication to infuse in 30-60 min. | For optimal therapeutic effect, drug should infuse in prescribed time interval. |
| j. Label Volutrol with name of drug, dosage, total volume including diluent, and time of administration. | Alerts nurses to drug being infused. Prevents other medications from being added to Volutrol. |
| k. Dispose of uncapped needle and syringe in proper container. | Prevents accidental needle sticks |
| 3. Wash hands. | Reduces transmission of infection. |

## Evaluation

| | |
|---|---|
| 1. Observe client for signs of adverse reactions. | IV medications act rapidly. |
| 2. During 30-60 min of infusion, periodically check infusion rate and condition of IV site. | IV must remain patent for proper drug administration. Development of infiltration necessitates discontinuing infusion. |

### *Expected outcomes*

| | |
|---|---|
| 1. Drug infuses without adverse reactions. | Drug was given safely with desired therapeutic effect. |
| 2. Medication infuses within desired period. | Intravenous line remains patent. |
| 3. IV site remains intact without signs of swelling or inflammation, or symptom of tenderness at site. | Fluid infuses into vein rather than tissues. |

| Steps | Rationale |
|---|---|
| ***Unexpected outcomes*** | |
| 1. Client develops adverse drug reaction. | Nature of reaction depends on drug, dosage, and client's sensitivity. |
| 2. Medication does not infuse over desired period. | Can result from improper calculation of flow rate, malpositioning of IV needle at insertion site, or infiltration. |
| 3. Client develops signs and symptoms of phlebitis or infiltration. | Fluid infuses into tissues. Vein is inflamed. |
| **Recording and Reporting** | |
| 1. Record drug, dosage, route, and time administered on medication form (see Fig. 21-24). | Timely documentation prevents medication errors, e.g., repeated doses. |
| 2. Record volume of fluid in medication bag or Volutrol on intake and output I & O form. | Fluid balance regulated and monitored on basis of total fluid intake. |
| 3. Report any adverse reactions to nurse in charge or physician. | Reaction may require therapeutic intervention. |
| **Follow-up Activities** | |
| 1. After drug infuses, be sure to add IV solution to Volutrol. | IV can run dry unless solution is added to Volutrol for continuous infusion. |

### Special Considerations

- Never give IV medications via blood products.
- IV medication should never be given when site is swollen and tender to palpation or when infusion flows slowly when regulating clamp is wide open.
- When piggybacking an IV line, a 21- or 23-gauge needle ensures drug will infuse easily into main IV line.
- Secondary line tubing can be used again by adding a new piggyback or tandem container. Check agency policy to determine how long lines are considered sterile.

### Home Care Considerations

- See Skill 21-1.

## *SKILL 21-9* Administering Medications by Intravenous Bolus

An IV bolus involves introducing a concentrated dose of a drug directly into the systemic circulation. The IV bolus is used during emergencies, with critically unstable clients, and as a route of administration when rapid and predictable responses are required (Burman and Berkowitz, 1986). An IV bolus may be given directly into a vein, into an existing IV line through an injection port, or through a heparin lock (Fig. 21-41). A heparin lock consists of an indwelling needle or catheter attached to a plastic tube with a sealed injection port on the end. Institutional policy dictates which medications the nurse may give by IV push.

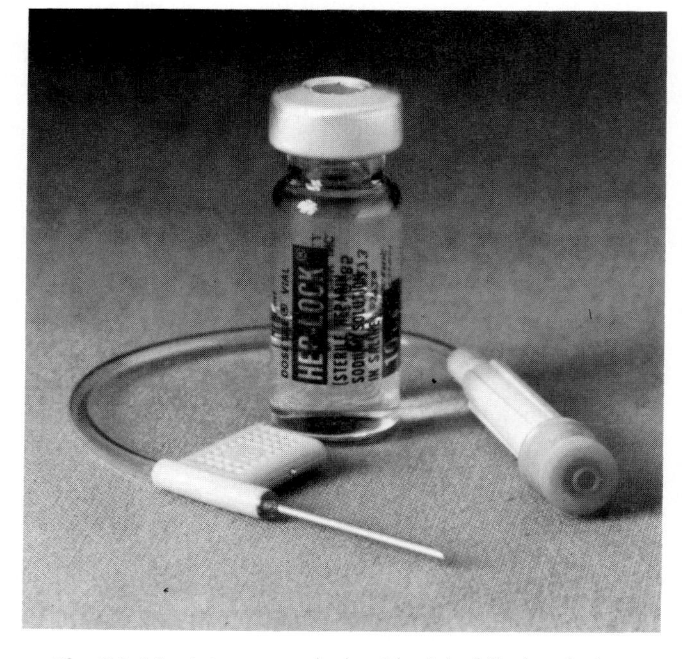

***Fig. 21-41*** Intravenous lock with vial of flush solution.

The IV bolus is the most dangerous method for drug administration because there is no time to correct errors. In addition, a bolus may cause direct irritation to the lining of blood vessels.

Thus the nurse must be sure the IV catheter or needle is correctly positioned in the client's vein. An IV bolus should never be given if the insertion site appears puffy or edematous or if the fluid from a connecting IV line cannot flow at the proper rate. Accidental injection of a medication into tissues surrounding a vein can cause pain, necrotic sloughing of tissues, and abscesses.

### Purposes

1. Deliver a fast-acting drug quickly in emergency situations.
2. Dilute a drug that cannot be diluted in another way.
3. Limit fluid intake during drug administration.
4. Achieve maximal drug effects.

## *Procedure 21-9*

| Steps | Rationale |
|---|---|
| **Assessment** | |
| 1. Check physician's order for type of medication, dosage, time, and route of administration. | Ensures safe and accurate drug administration. |
| 2. Collect information necessary to administer drug safely, including: action, purpose, side effects, normal dosage, time of peak onset, nursing implications. | Allows nurse to give drug safely and to monitor client's response to therapy. |
| 3. If drug is to be given through existing IV line, determine type of additives within IV solution. | IV medication may not be compatible with additives. |
| 4. Assess condition of needle insertion site (IV line or heparin lock) for signs of infiltration or phlebitis. | Drug should not be administered if site is edematous or inflamed. |
| 5. Check client's history of drug allergies. | IV bolus delivers drug rapidly. Allergic reaction could prove fatal. |
| **Nursing Diagnosis** | |
| 1. Cluster data to reveal actual or potential nursing diagnoses: | |
| a. Pain: related to infiltration or needle displacement. | Indicates need to change IV site before drug administration. |
| **Planning** | |
| 1. Develop individualized goals for client based on nursing diagnoses: | |
| a. Ensure drug is properly distributed. | Nurse takes precautions to be sure IV needle is positioned in vein. |
| b. Minimize client's risks. | Careful monitoring may allow nurse to take action to limit any adverse effects of drug. |
| c. Maintain sterility of IV line. | IV line provides direct route for infection unless aseptic technique is followed. |
| 2. Prepare the following equipment and supplies: | |
| a. IV push (existing line): | |
| ▪ Medication in vial or ampule | |
| ▪ Syringe (3-5 ml) | |
| ▪ Sterile needles (21- and 25-gauge) | Large gauge needles used to draw up medication. Small gauge needle used to insert through Y-port of IV tubing. |
| ▪ Antiseptic swab | |
| ▪ Watch with second hand or digital readout | |
| ▪ Medication ticket, form, or printout | |
| ▪ Medication ticket, form or printout | |
| b. IV push (intravenous lock) | |
| ▪ Medication in vial or ampule | |
| ▪ Syringe (3-5 ml) | Used for medication preparation. |
| ▪ Syringes (1-3 ml) | Used for heparin flush or saline solution. |
| ▪ Vial of heparin flush solution (1 ml = 100 units or 1 ml = 10 units, depending on agency policy) (optional) or vial of normal saline | Keeps heparin lock patent and free of clots. Studies have not shown clear advantage of using heparin instead of saline (Dunn and Lenihan, 1987; Harrigan, 1985). |
| ▪ Sterile needles (21- and 25-gauge) | Large-gauge needles used to draw up medication. Small-gauge needle used to insert through heparin lock. |
| ▪ Antiseptic swab | |
| ▪ Watch with second hand or digital readout | |
| ▪ Medication ticket, form, or printout | Verifies order. |
| 3. Wash hands. | Reduces transmission of infection. |
| 4. Prepare ordered medication from vial or ampule (see Procedure 21-1). Read package directions carefully for proper IV dilution of medication. | Ensures medication is sterile. |
| 5. After preparing medication, apply small-gauge needle to syringe. | Used to insert through IV line or heparin lock. |

| Steps | Rationale |
|---|---|
| **Implementation** | |
| 1. IV push (existing line): | |
| a. Check client's identification by looking at armband and asking name. Compare with medication ticket. | Ensures drug is administered to correct client. |
| b. Explain procedure to client and encourage client to report symptoms of discomfort at IV site. | Informs client of planned therapies. |
| c. Select injection port of IV tubing closest to client. A circle on port may indicate site for needle insertion (Fig. 21-42). | Allows for easier fluid aspiration to obtain blood return. Injection ports are self-sealing and will not leak. |
| d. Clean off injection port with antiseptic swab. | Prevents introduction of microorganisms during needle insertion. |
| e. Insert small-gauge needle of syringe containing prepared drug through center of port. | Prevents damage to port's diaphragm and subsequent leakage. |
| f. Occlude the intravenous line by pinching tubing just above the injection port. Pull back gently on the syringe's plunger to aspirate for a blood return (Fig. 21-43). | Final check ensures that medication is being delivered into the bloodstream. |
| g. After noting blood return, inject medication slowly over several min. (Read directions on drug package.) Use a watch to time administrations (Fig. 21-44). | Ensures safe drug infusion. Rapid injection of an IV drug can prove fatal. |
| h. After injecting medication, release tubing, withdraw syringe, and recheck the fluid infusion rate. | Injection of a bolus may alter the rate of fluid infusion. Rapid fluid infusion can cause circulatory fluid overload. |
| 2. IV push (intravenous lock): | |
| a. Check client's identification by looking at armband and asking full name. Compare with medication ticket. | Ensures drug is administered to correct client. |
| b. Heparin flush method: | |
| ▪ Prepare a syringe with 1 ml of heparin flush solution. | Flush solution keeps heparin lock patent after drug is administered. |
| ▪ Prepare a syringe with 1 ml of normal saline. Attach 25-gauge needle to syringe. | Used to assess for blood return in heparin lock. |
| c. Saline flush method: | |
| ▪ Prepare 2 syringes with 2 ml of normal saline each. Attach 25-gauge needle to each syringe. | Normal saline has been found to be effective in keeping intravenous locks patent. |
| d. Administer drug: | |
| ▪ Clean the lock's rubber diaphragm with the antiseptic swab. | Cleaning prevents introduction of microorganisms during needle insertion. |

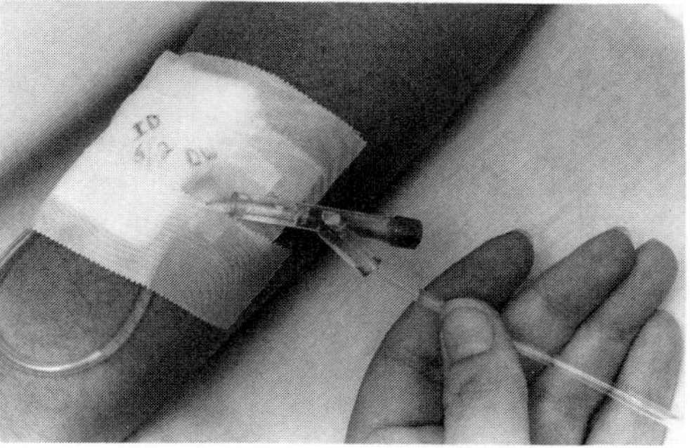
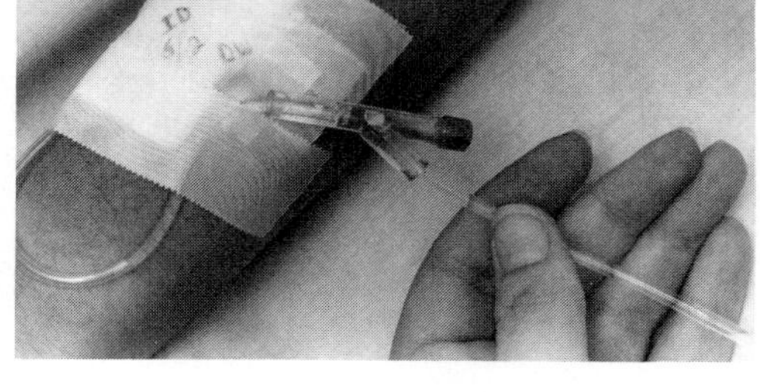

**Fig. 21-42**

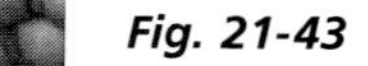

**Fig. 21-43**

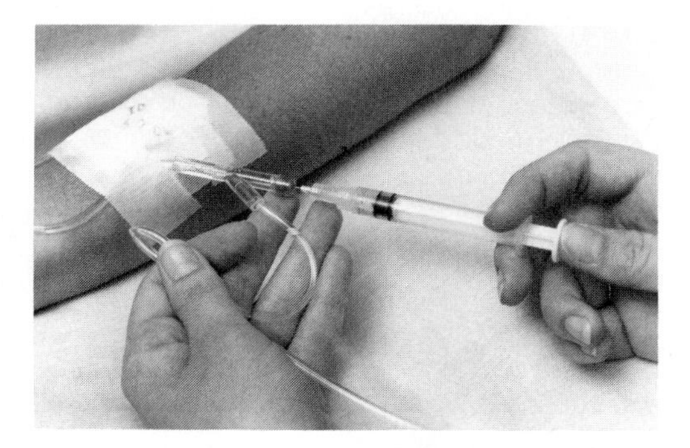

**Fig. 21-44**

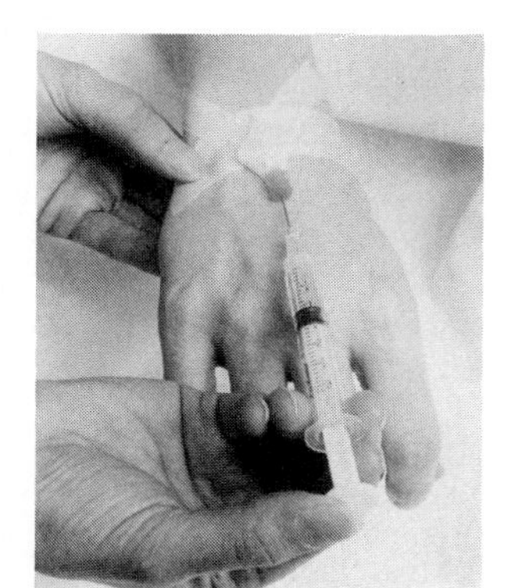

**Fig. 21-45**

| Steps | Rationale |
|---|---|
| ▪ Insert needle of syringe containing normal saline through center of diaphragm. Pull back gently on syringe plunger and look for blood return. | Determines if IV needle or catheter is positioned in vein. (At times a heparin lock will not yield a blood return even though lock is patent.) |
| ▪ Flush reservoir with 1 cc saline by pushing slowly on the plunger. | Cleans needle and reservoir of blood. |
| ▪ Remove needle and saline-filled syringe. | |
| ▪ Clean the lock's diaphragm with the antiseptic swab. | Prevents transmission of infection. |
| ▪ Insert the needle of syringe containing prepared medication through center of diaphragm. | Using center of diaphragm prevents leakage. |
| ▪ Inject medication bolus slowly over several min. (Each medication has a recommended rate for bolus administration. Check package directions.) Use a watch to time the administration Fig. 21-45. | Rapid injection of an intravenous drug can kill a client. |
| ▪ After administering the bolus, withdraw the syringe. | |
| ▪ Clean the lock's diaphragm with an antiseptic swab. | Prevents transmission of infection. |
| e. Heparin flush: | |
| ▪ Insert needle of syringe containing the heparin through the diaphragm. Inject 1 ml heparin slowly, then remove syringe. | Maintains patency of needle by inhibiting clot formation. Diluted heparin avoids anticoagulation. |
| f. Saline flush: | |
| ▪ If using only saline to flush the reservoir, inject 2 cc of saline after each use of the intravenous lock. | |
| 3. Wash hands. | Reduces transmission of microorganisms. |
| 4. Dispose of uncapped needles and syringes in proper container (Fig. 21-46). | Prevents accidental needle sticks. |

## Evaluation

| | |
|---|---|
| 1. Observe client closely for adverse reactions during administration and for several min thereafter. | IV medications act rapidly. |
| 2. Observe IV site during injection for sudden swelling. | Determines development of infiltration into tissues surrounding vein. |

### *Expected outcomes*

| | |
|---|---|
| 1. Drug infuses without adverse reactions occurring. | Drug given safely. |
| 2. IV site remains clear, without swelling. | Fluid infuses into vein. |

### *Unexpected outcomes*

| | |
|---|---|
| 1. Client develops adverse reaction to medication. | Drug's potency may cause maximal responses or side effects. |
| 2. IV site becomes puffy. | Infiltration indicates immediate discontinuation of injection. |

## Recording and Reporting

| | |
|---|---|
| 1. Record drug, dosage, route, and time on medication form. | Timely documentation prevents medication errors. |
| 2. Report any adverse reactions to nurse in charge or physician. | Adverse response to IV bolus drug may necessitate emergency measures. |

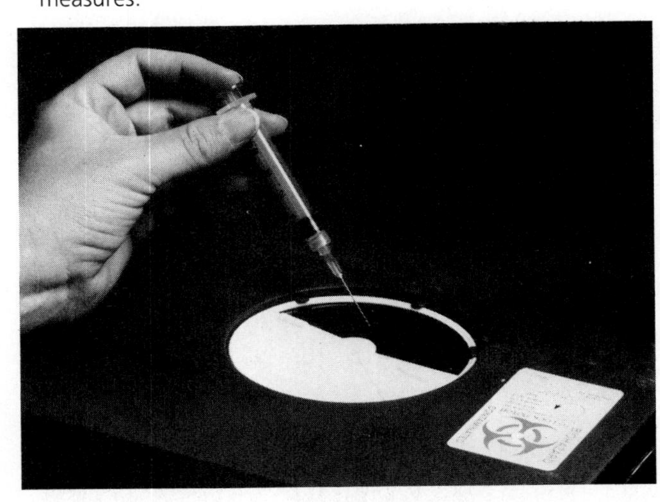

***Fig. 21-46*** Special containers are available in nursing units for the disposal of contaminated syringes.

## Special Considerations

- When administering drug through existing IV line, nurse may inject medication retrograde, back toward infusion set and bag, as tubing is pinched below port. When tube is released, medication enters more slowly.
- Be sure to loosen tape or dressing over IV site in order to see it clearly before administering drug.

---

**BIBLIOGRAPHY**

Bontempo ST, Eggland ET: Nursing implications for home parenteral therapy, Home Health Care Nurse 6(4):14, 1988.
Burman R, Berkowitz H: IV bolus: effective but potentially hazardous Crit Care Nurs 6(1):22, 1986.
Centers for Disease Control: Guidelines for isolation procedures, Atlanta, 1983.
Chaplin G, Shull H, Welk PC: How safe is the air-bubble technique for I.M. injections? Nursing '85 15:59, Sept. 1985.
Clark JB, et al.: Pharmacological basis of nursing practice, ed 3, St. Louis, 1986, The CV Mosby Co.
Cyganski JM, et al.: The case for the heparin flush, Am J Nurs 87:796, 1987.
Dunn DL, Lenihan SF: The case for the saline flush, Am J Nurs 87:798, 1987.
Farley HF, et al.: Will that IM needle reach the muscle? Am J Nurs 86(12):1327, 1331, 1986.
Feldman HR: Practice may make perfect but research makes a difference—IM injection in the ventrogluteal site, Nursing '87 17(3):46, 1987.
Giving Medications, Nursing Photobook, Springhouse, Pa, 1983, Intermed Communications, Inc.
Golden S: Nursing a loved one at home, Philadelphia, 1988, Running Press Book Publishers.
Govoni L, Hayes J: Drugs and nursing implications, New York, 1980, Appleton-Century Crofts.
Harrigan CA: Intermittent IV therapy without heparin: a study, NITA 8:519, 1985.
Hellnick PE: How to teach do-it-yourself IV therapy, RN 50(10):135, 1987.
Hughes CB: Giving cancer drugs I.V.: some guidelines, Am J Nurs 86(1):34, 1986.
Jackson JL, Johnson E: Patient education in home care: a practical guide to effective teaching and documentation, Rockville, Md, 1988, Aspen Publishers, Inc.
Keen MF: Comparison of intramuscular injection techniques to reduce site discomfort and lesions, Nurs Res 35:207, 1986.
Koivisto VA, Felig P: Ann Intern Med 92:59, 1980.
Knott SP, et al.: Teaching self-injection to diabetics; an easier and more effective way, Nursing '84 14(1):57, 1984.
Mascaro J: Managing IV therapy in the home, Nursing '86, 16(5):50, 1986.
McConnell EA: The subtle art of really good injections, RN 45:24, 1982.
Perez S: Reducing injection pain, Am J Nurs 84:7, 1984.
Potter PA, Perry AG: Basic nursing, St. Louis, 1987, The CV Mosby Co.
Potter PA, Perry AG: Fundamentals of nursing concepts, process, and practice, ed 2, St. Louis, 1989, The CV Mosby Co.
Rettig FM, Southby JR: Using different body positions to reduce discomfort from dorsogluteal injection, Nurs Res 31:219, 1982.
Scipien G, et al.: Comprehensive pediatric nursing, New York, 1986, McGraw-Hill Book Co.
Shepherd MJ, Swearingen P: Z-track injections, Am J Nurs 84:746, 1984.
Shlafer M, Marieb E: The nurse, pharmacology, drug therapy, Menlo Park, Calif, 1989, Addison-Wesley Publishing Co.
Smith HA: Teaching family members intrathecal morphine administration, J Neurosci Nurs 18(2):95, 1986.
Smith S, Duell D: Clinical Nursing skills Los Altos, Calif, 1985, Nat Nurs Rev.
Tanner S: IV bolus leaves no room for error, RN 44:54, 1981.
Thatcher G: Insulin injections: the case against random rotation, Am J Nurs 85:690, 1985.
The fine points of insulin injection, Emerg Med, p. 173, June 15, 1980.
Walsh J, Persons C, Wieck L: Manual of home health care nursing, Philadelphia, 1987, JB Lippincott Co.
Whaley LF, Wong DL: Nursing care of infants and children, ed 3, St. Louis, 1987, The CV Mosby Co.
Vanbree NS, et al.: Clinical evaluation of three techniques for administering low-dose heparin, Nurs Res 33(1):15, 1984.

# 22
# CHEMOTHERAPY

## OBJECTIVES

*Mastery of content in this chapter will enable the nurse to:*

- Define key terms.
- Discuss teaching that should occur for the client receiving chemotherapeutic agents.
- State four factors to be considered when selecting a vein for intravenous (IV) chemotherapy administration.
- Identify the type of needle best suited for administration of chemotherapeutic agents.
- List protective clothing the nurse should wear when preparing and administering chemotherapeutic agents.
- Describe the procedure for administration of IV push chemotherapeutic agents.
- Document correctly the procedure for administration of IV chemotherapy agents.
- Describe steps to be taken if a vesicant agent extravasates.
- List signs and symptoms of an allergic reaction to a chemotherapeutic agent.
- List actions to be taken if an allergic reaction to a chemotherapeutic agent occurs.

## KEY TERMS

*Alopecia*
*Anorexia*
*Chemotherapeutic agent*
*Chemotherapy*
*Class II biological safety cabinet*
*Extravasation*
*Intracavitary*
*Intrathecal*
*Leukopenia*
*Metastasis*
*Myelosuppression*
*Neutropenic*
*Remission*
*Stomatitis*
*Thrombocytopenia*
*Vesicant*

## SKILLS

**21-1** Administering Chemotherapeutic Agents by the Intravenous Push Method

Chemotherapy is the use of drugs to prevent cancer cells from multiplying, invading adjacent tissue, and metastasizing. It is recognized as effective in the treatment of cancer. The use of chemotherapy can provide cure, control, long-term remission, and palliation of cancer. The drugs may be used in conjunction with other therapy (surgery, radiotherapy) if there is a possibility that undetected cancerous cells have spread to more than one site in the body. This is termed *adjuvant chemotherapy*.

Chemotherapeutic agents are most frequently given in combinations. Combinations of drugs are used to increase the chances of attaining complete remission, to prolong the length of remission, to prevent the onset of drug resistance, and to enhance the effectiveness of the drugs used. While combination chemotherapy is effective, the use of more than one drug may increase the likelihood of toxic side effects. Attempts are made to use drugs with different toxicities.

Chemotherapy treatments are given according to time sequences or cycles. Cycles are planned to provide maximal exposure of cancer cells to drugs while allowing clients to recover from any drug-induced side effects. Cycle lengths vary according to the type of cancer and the particular client's tolerance of side effects.

Chemotherapeutic agents can be administered by various routes (oral, subcutaneous, intracavitary). The best route allows drugs to reach high concentrations in the tumor mass, and thus intravenous (IV) push administration, which allows drugs to enter the venous system rapidly, is a common method used in administering chemotherapy.

Because chemotherapeutic agents are most active against frequently dividing cells, normal cells that rapidly multiply may be harmed by antineoplastic drugs. Normal cells most commonly affected are:

1. Cellular components of bone marrow (red blood cells, white blood cells, and platelets).
2. Hair follicles.
3. Mucosal lining of the gastrointestinal tract.
4. Skin.
5. Germinal cells (sperm and ova).

The effect of chemotherapeutic agents on these cells may result in myelosuppression, alopecia, stomatitis, or sterility. In addition to these effects, many chemotherapeutic agents cause mild to severe nausea and vomiting. Some drugs have side effects that are unique to the particular medication. It is the responsibility of the nurse giving chemotherapy to be able to anticipate side effects that may occur as the result of a particular treatment regimen. Information obtained from client assessment regarding tolerance of previous therapies together with a thorough familiarity with the effects of the medications administered will allow the nurse to form the most appropriate care plan.

Chemotherapeutic agents should be administered only by registered nurses who have been educated specifically to perform the procedure. Nurses who administer these drugs must be skillful in IV techniques (Chapter 23). They are responsible for knowing drug actions, expected side effects, and complications that may occur during administration. Expert administration of antineoplastic drugs is only the first event in care of clients receiving chemotherapy. Nurses must also be prepared to assist clients in the experiences of nausea, vomiting, and anorexia; stomatitis; alopecia; leukopenia; thrombocytopenia; and anemia.

Many psychosocial issues revolve around chemotherapy treatment. Clients express concern about side effects, the nurse's ability to perform the procedure correctly (including initiating the IV needle), and the effectiveness of the therapy. A competent, supportive nurse can begin to assist clients in exploring these issues. Clients require and have a right to expect accurate information about chemotherapy treatment and resources available to assist with difficulties.

Chemotherapeutic agents should be prepared in a Class II biological safety cabinet to protect both the preparer and the environment from unnecessary exposure to potentially hazardous material. In most institutions this cabinet is located in the pharmacy, where the pharmacist reconstitutes the medication. Because this is the safest environment for preparation, reconstitution of chemotherapeutic agents is not discussed in this chapter.

## PREREQUISITE KNOWLEDGE

1. Principles of teaching and learning.
2. Principles of chemotherapeutic drug pharmacology.
3. Principles of medical asepsis.
4. Principles of IV fluid therapy.
5. Principles of nursing care for the client experiencing anxiety and body image changes.

## PREREQUISITE SKILLS

1. Initiation and maintenance of an IV site (Chapter 23).
2. Proper handwashing techniques (Chapter 37).
3. Measurement of vital signs (Chapter 12).

***TABLE 22-1*** Vesicant/Irritant and Nonvesicant Cancer Chemotherapeutic Drugs

| Generic Name | Other Name | Generic Name | Other Name |
|---|---|---|---|
| **Vesicant Drugs (Commercial Agents)** | | **Nonvesicant Agents** | |
| Dactinomycin | (Actinomycin D) | Bleomycin* | (Blenoxane) |
| Dacarbazine | (DTIC) | Cyclophosphamide | (Cytoxan) |
| Daunomycin | (Cerubidine) | Cytarabine | (ARA-C) |
| Doxorubicin | (Adriamycin) | Floxuridine | (FUDR) |
| Mithramycin | (Mithracin) | Fluorouracil* | (5-FU) |
| Mitomycin C | (Mutamycin) | Methotrexate | |
| Estramustine phosphate | (Estracyte) | Cisplatin† | (Platinol) |
| Mechlorethamine | (Nitrogen mustard) | Thiotepa | |
| Vinblastine | (Velban) | Asparaginase | (Elspar) |
| Vincristine | (Oncovin) | Mitozantrone | (Novantrone) |
| | | **Definitions** | |
| **Irritant Agents** | | Vesicant: Cancer chemotherapeutic agent capable of causing or forming a blister and/or causing tissue destruction. | |
| Carmustine | (BCNU) | Irritant: Cancer chemotherapeutic agent capable of producing venous pain at the site or along the vein, with or without inflammatory reaction. | |
| Etoposide | (VP-16-213 VePesid) | Extravasation: Leakage of a vesicant or irritant drug into subcutaneous tissue that is capable of causing pain, necrosis, and/or sloughing of the tissue. | |
| Streptozocin | (Zanosar) | | |

Modified from Cancer chemotherapy: guidelines and recommendations for nursing education and practice, Oncology Nursing Society, 1984.
*Occasionally causes mild phlebitis.
†Single case report each of cellulitis and fibrosis. (Ca Treat Rep 64(10):1162, 1980).

# SKILL 22-1 Administering Chemotherapeutic Agents by the Intravenous Push Method

### Purposes

1. Ensure safe administration of chemotherapeutic drugs.
2. Educate clients about side effects to expect and how to manage them.
3. Maintain client's comfort.
4. Promote a positive client body image.

## Procedure 22-1

| Steps | Rationale |
|---|---|
| **Assessment** | |
| 1. Review medical order. | Allows nurse to determine special equipment needs, time constraints, pretreatment conditioning, and to validate information regarding drug dosages, route, and expected side effects. |
| 2. Review medical and nursing history. | Allows nurse to educate client regarding plan of therapy and to plan care around client's medical status. |
| 3. Review allergic history. | Several chemotherapeutic agents can cause severe allergic reactions. |
| 4. Determine if ordered laboratory data have been obtained. | Various chemotherapeutic agents cause bone marrow suppression. Adequate hepatic and renal function are necessary for proper metabolism and excretion of chemotherapeutic agents. |
| 5. Assess client's previous experience with chemotherapy treatments. | Previous experience influences client's reaction to present situation. Eliciting information may help nurse in anticipating client needs. |
| 6. Assess condition of veins. For inspection instruct client to remove clothing and jewelry from arms. Solicit client's desires about insertion site. | Some chemotherapeutic agents cause necrosis if infiltrated subcutaneously (vesicants, Table 22-1). Thus, particular caution must be exercised when choosing vein for administration of IV chemotherapy. Thorough assessment of veins allows time to employ methods of distending veins if necessary. Clients become knowledgeable regarding condition of veins and appropriate injection sites. This information should be considered. |
| 7. Obtain current vital sign values and document mental status. | Provides baseline information for future comparisons. Vital signs and mental status may change with anaphylactic reaction. |
| 8. Identify clients at risk for complications during or after chemotherapy treatment: | |
| a. Elderly. | Elderly cilents may have decreased hepatic blood flow, decreased ability to activate carcinogens and drugs, decreased glomerular filtration rate, decreased renal blood flow, and decreased hematopoietic cell reserve. |
| b. Persons with poor venous acess. | Increases risk of extravasation. |
| c. Persons with an allergy history. | Increases risk of an anaphylactic reaction. |
| d. Persons with a history of complications from previous chemotherapy treatments. | Nurse can prepare to prevent or minimize the complication. |
| e. Persons receiving high doses of chemotherapy. | Increases probability of severe side effects. |
| f. Persons who are highly anxious. | May alter client's compliance with therapy. |
| **Nursing Diagnosis** | |
| 1. Cluster data to reveal actual or potential nursing diagnoses: | |
| a. Knowledge deficit regarding chemotherapy treatment and side effects: related to unfamiliarity. | Throughout procedure nurse discusses implications of therapy. |
| b. Potential for injury: related to alteration in immune response. | Results of drug side effects. |
| c. Potential body image disturbance: related to hair loss. | Results of drug side effects. |

| Steps | Rationale |
|---|---|
| d. Potential impaired skin integrity: related to poor venous integrity. | Careful monitoring of IV site is essential. |
| e. Potential altered nutrition: related to nausea and vomiting. | Result of drug side effects. |
| f. Potential altered oral mucous membrane: related to cellular injury. | Result of drug side effects. |
| g. Anxiety: related to chemotherapy procedure. | Understanding of all implications of therapy enhances client coping. |

## Planning

| Steps | Rationale |
|---|---|
| 1. Develop individualized goals for client based on nursing diagnoses: | |
| a. Minimize client's discomfort. | Nurse uses techniques to prevent injury during administration and to minimize side effects. |
| b. Provide psychologic support. | Client will experience considerable anxiety and fear over procedure and disease process. |
| c. Client understands chemotherapy side effects. | Client receives therapy over many days and often in home setting. |
| d. Client manages drug side effects. | Client can learn measures to manage complications. |
| e. Client maintains positive body image. | Good hygiene and grooming can assist in minimizing effects of hair loss. |
| 2. Prepare teaching plan including the following objectives:<br>a. Describe how particular regimen is given.<br>b. State common side effects of treatment.<br>c. State ways to cope with nausea, vomiting, alopecia, stomatitis, and bone marrow suppression.<br>d. State signs and symptoms to report after discharge: temperature over 38° C, rash of any kind, severe constipation or diarrhea, sudden weight gain or loss, persistent bleeding from any site, any pain of unusual intensity or distribution, shortness of breath, severe and persistent vomiting more than 24 hr after treatment.<br>e. State medications that should receive physician approval before taking: aspirin and aspirin-containing compounds, antibiotics, anticoagulants, anticonvulsants, barbiturates, antihypertensives, cough medications, Darvon, hypoglycemics, diuretics, hormones, tranquilizers, nasal sprays, vitamins.<br>f. Discuss effects of chemotherapy on fertility and childbearing. | Informed client can participate in management of side effects. Information about expected events may alleviate fear, anxiety, and other stresses. |
| 3. Assemble required equipment: | |
| a. IV needle (21- or 23-gauge butterfly recommended) | Steel butterfly needles of 21- or 23-gauge size cause least amount of trauma to veins and are associated with lower incidence of phlebitis and infection. Gauge of needle should be smaller than diameter of vein. |
| b. Tourniquet | Aids in venous distention. |
| c. Alcohol swabs | Skin must be cleansed. |
| d. Povidone iodine (Betadine) | Used as cleansing agent in neutropenic persons in addition to alcohol preparation. |
| e. Appropriate IV solution<br>f. IV tubing | IV push or piggyback chemotherapeutic agents should be given through running IV line of compatible solution. Dilution of drug will lessen venous irritation. Patent main IV line should be in place in event of adverse reaction. |
| g. Stopcock | Eliminates use of needles in **Y** sites of IV tubing, which may cause accidental punctures. |
| h. Tape | Secures needle. |
| i. Band-Aid | |
| j. Syringes of ordered chemotherapeutic agents | |
| k. Long-sleeved isolation gown or disposable gown | Provides protection to nurse from medication contact with clothing and skin. |
| l. Polyvinyl chloride gloves | Protect hands from contact with medication. |
| m. Mask (depending on institution's policy) | Prevents possible aerosol inhalation. |
| n. Goggles | Protect eyes from contact with medication. |
| o. Container in which to dispose all equipment used in chemotherapy administration | Prevents personnel exposure to medication or equipment contaminated with medication or aerosols. |

| Steps | Rationale |
|---|---|
| p. Emergency medications: epinephrine (Adrenalin), diphenhydramine (Benadryl), dopamine HCl (Intropin), levarterenol bitartrate (Levophed), sodium bicarbonate, aminophylline, hydrocortisone sodium succinate | For use in treatment of anaphylaxis or extravasation. |
| q. Any special equipment such as scalp hypothermia cap | Scalp hypothermia may be ordered in attempt to decrease or prevent expected alopecia. Hypothermia causes vasoconstriction of scalp vasculature, which decreases medication delivery to hair follicles. Effectiveness is influenced by medications, time period over which they are used, infusion rate, and client's hepatic and renal function. It may not be successful in preventing hair loss. If scalp hypothermia is ordered, variety of hypothermia caps are commercially available. Follow manufacturer's recommendations for optimal use of scalp hypothermia. |
| 4. Explain steps of procedure to client. | Minimizes client anxiety. |
| 5. Administer a test dose when using drug with increased incidence of hypersensitivity. | Determines whether client is hypersensitive to medication and reduces risk of anaphylactic reaction. |

## Implementation

| Steps | Rationale |
|---|---|
| 1. Wash hands. | Reduces transmission of microorganisms. |
| 2. Apply gown, gloves, goggles, and mask (optional) (Fig. 22-1). | Protects nurse from contacting irritating chemotherapeutic agent. |
| 3. Prepare premedication from vial or ampule (Skill 21-1). | |
| 4. Verify prepared medications with physician's orders. | Prevents error in administration of medication. |
| 5. Identify client by checking identification arm band and asking client's name. | Ensures that correct client receives prescribed medication. |
| 6. Examine syringes of medication for clarity. | Medication that is cloudy or has precipitated should not be administered. Various chemotherapeutic agents are stable for only short periods of time. |
| 7. Premedicate with medication as ordered by physician. | Many chemotherapeutic agents alone or in combination cause nausea and vomiting, which may range from mild to severe. Medication with antiemetic regimen before chemotherapy is administered may prevent or minimize nausea and vomiting. |
| 8. Position client comfortably with call bell in reach. Position hand and arm for comfort and stability. | Client movement is restricted after IV push administration has begun. Client is made as comfortable as possible before therapy begins to avoid position changes. Proceed distally (hand) to proximally (forearm). Site should be alternated from arm to arm for daily treatments. |
| 9. Initiate infusion site (Chapter 23). Secure needle with tape so that insertion site is not obstructed from view. | Allows nurse to observe onset of infiltration. |
| 10. Test venous integrity and flow with appropriate IV solution. Observe for infiltration. Solicit client's sensation of comfort at site. | IV site should always be easily viewed by nurse to detect infiltration. IV should flow freely, indicating venous patency. |
| 11. Encourage client to observe for and report adverse reactions. | Assists in early detection of extravasation or anaphylactic reaction. |
| 12. Administer chemotherapeutic agents through the stopcock (Fig. 22-2). | Prevents accidental needle puncture of administrator or intravenous tubing. |

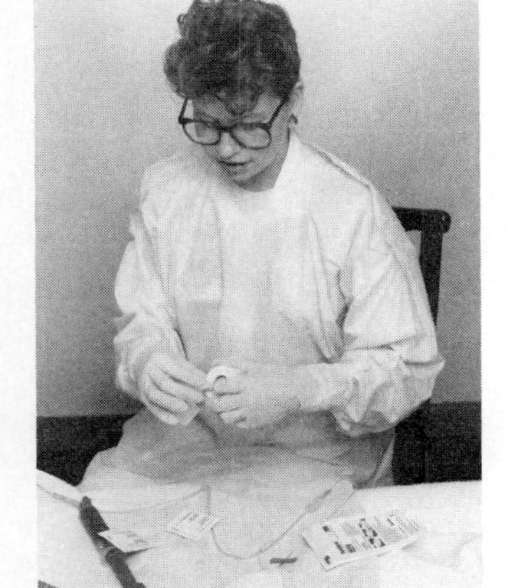

*Fig. 22-1*

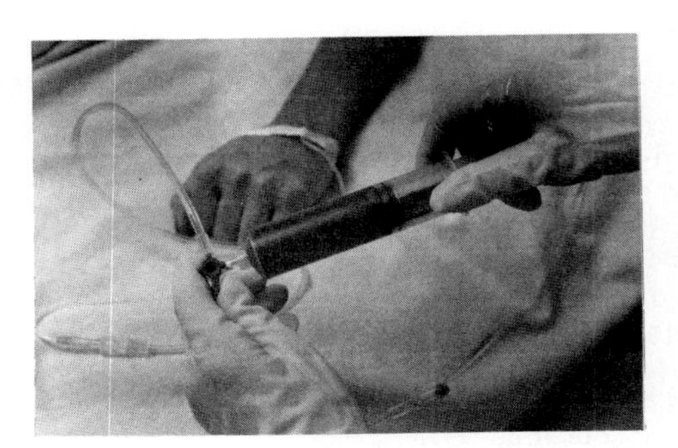

*Fig. 22-2*

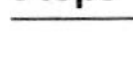

| Steps | Rationale |
|---|---|

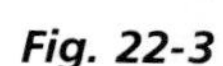

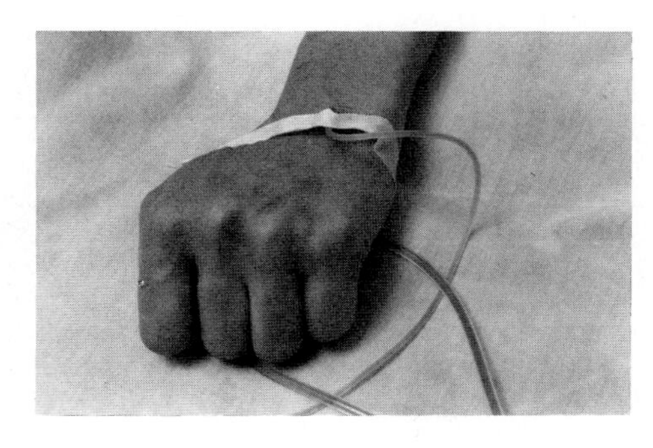

*Fig. 22-3*

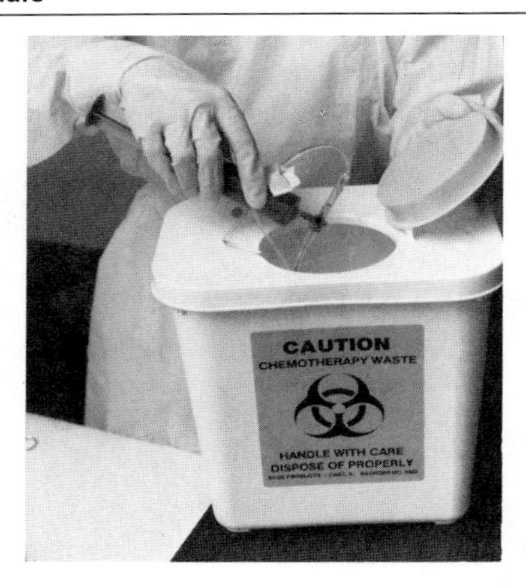


*Fig. 22-4*

| Steps | Rationale |
|---|---|
| a. Follow institutional policy regarding sequencing of drugs (if combination contains vesicant). | Sequencing of vesicant and nonvesicant drugs is controversial. Factors favoring administration of vesicants first: vascular integrity decreases over time; vein is most stable and least irritated at beginning of treatment. Factors favoring administration of vesicants last: vesicants are irritating and may increase vein fragility, necessitating new venipuncture; venous spasm, which may occur at beginning of therapy, may be painful to client. Nurse must decide whether pain is result of spasm or infiltration. |
| b. Administer drug slowly, aspirating blood or lowering IV bag after every 3-4 ml of medication administered. | Venous integrity should not be jeopardized by rapid infusion, which may cause increased intraluminal pressure and venous rupture. Testing for blood return is one way to verify that needle is placed correctly in vein. Slow administration prevents untoward sensations. Site should be observed for redness of swelling, which may indicate infiltration. |
| c. Observe insertion site for swelling, redness, hives, or blebs (Fig. 22-3). | Indicates possible infiltration or hypersensitivity reaction. |
| d. Ask client about sensations during therapy. | Indicates possible venous spasm or infiltration. |
| e. Flush IV line with appropriate fluid between drugs (10-15 ml). | Prevents mixture of medications in IV line. |
| f. At end of all drug administration, flush IV line with appropriate fluid (20-30 ml). | Assists in reducing venous irritation. |
| g. According to physician's orders, IV needle may be left in place or removed. | |
| ▪ If needle is left in place, cover with antimicrobial ointment and sterile dressing and tape securely. | Allows further hydration or administration of IV antiemetics. Care reduces risk of infection. |
| ▪ If needle is removed, apply sterile dressing and bandage. Elevate arm and apply pressure. | Prevents hematoma formation. |
| 13. Dispose of equipment (IV bags, tubing, syringes, alcohol swabs, absorbent pads) according to institutional policy (Fig. 22-4). Remove and dispose of gloves. | Prevents personnel exposure to medication or equipment contaminated with medication or aerosols. |
| 14. Wash hands. | Reduces transmission of microorganisms. |

## Evaluation

| Steps | Rationale |
|---|---|
| 1. Reassess client to determine response to IV push administration of chemotherapeutic drug. | Provides continual monitoring of client for allergic and untoward effects of drugs. |
| 2. Have client describe side effects of medication and management, and steps to take if problems develop. | Evaluates client's understanding of therapy and its implications. |

### *Expected outcomes*

| Steps | Rationale |
|---|---|
| 1. Client accurately states expected side effects of therapy. | Feedback measures client's level of learning. |
| 2. Client states ways to manage expected side effects. | |
| 3. There is no redness, swelling, or pain at injection site. | Nurse's techniques prevented infiltration at IV site. |
| 4. Client has name and number of professional to contact with questions or concerns. | Ensures access to needed resources. |
| 5. 48 hr after procedure client has no severe vomiting or diarrhea, is able to tolerate a bland diet, performs oral hygiene qid, is drinking 2 L of fluids a day. | Gastrointestinal symptoms lessen 48 hr following procedure. |

| Steps | Rationale |
|---|---|
| ***Unexpected outcomes*** | |
| 1. Extravasation of vesicant chemotherapeutic agent is suspected or confirmed. In this situation: | Result of needle displacement or vein rupture. |
| a. Stop administration of chemotherapeutic agent. | If extravasation is suspected, no more drug should be injected. Amount of damage is frequently related to amount of drug extravasated. |
| b. Confirm extravasation. | Extravasation is confirmed by swelling at insertion site. Swelling may or may not be accompanied by redness, blood return, and client report of pain or burning at site. |
| c. Leave needle in place. | Allows administration of antidotes. |
| d. Aspirate any residual drug and blood in IV tubing, needle, and infiltration site. | Decreases amount of drug exposure to tissue. |
| e. Instill IV antidote (Table 22-2). | Reverses effects of chemotherapeutic agent. |
| f. Remove IV needle. | Needle may contain residual amounts of chemotherapeutic drug. |
| g. Inject antidote subcutaneously around site of extravasation, moving clockwise and using new 25-gauge needle with each injection. | Decreases tissue damage. |
| h. Apply topical ointment if ordered. | Decreases tissue damage. |
| i. Cover with occlusive sterile dressing that is changed b.i.d. for 7 days. | Provides protection to damaged area. |
| j. Apply warm or cold compresses according to institutional policy. | Decreases tissue damage by altering blood flow to area. |
| k. Notify physician of incident. | Client may require further therapy. |
| 2. Signs and symptoms of anaphylaxis are present. Guidelines for prevention of and intervention for anaphylaxis include: | |
| a. When administering drug with increased incidence of hypersensitivity, administer test dose before ordered dose. | Determines whether client is hypersensitive to medication. |
| b. Monitor client for at least 15 min after test dose. | Observe for local or systemic reaction to test dose. |
| c. Administer ordered dosage of drug slowly. | Introduces medication into client's system slowly. |
| d. Observe client for 15-30 min after medication administration. | Detects delayed reaction. |
| e. Stop administration if any of the following occur: complaints of uneasiness or agitation, dizziness, nausea, or crampy abdominal pain; desire to urinate or defecate; generalized itching; chills; tightness in chest; inability to speak; local or generalized urticaria; respiratory distress with or without wheezing; flushed appearance; hypotension; cyanosis. | Signs and symptoms of impending anaphylactic reaction. |
| f. Notify physician. | |
| g. Leave needle in place and maintain IV line with normal saline or ordered fluid. | Promotes expansion of vascular space and provides easy access for emergency drugs. |
| h. Place client in supine position. | Promotes perfusion to vital organs. |
| i. Monitor vital signs every 2 min until stable, then every 5 min for 30 min, then every 15 min. | Monitors client's response to medication. |
| j. Maintain airway (Chapter 16). | Airway obstruction can occur with anaphylaxis. |
| 3. Client unable to describe side effects of medication and treatment implications | Reinstruction is necessary |
| **Recording and Reporting** | |
| 1. Record in nurses' notes: procedure, date, time, medications administered, type of needle used, placement of needle, condition of injection site, type of IV fluid used for flushing tubing, client tolerance of procedure, teaching provided. | Timely documentation prevents drug administration errors. |
| 2. Record unexpected outcomes in nurses' notes according to institutional policy. | Provides data to evaluate response of client to therapy. |
| 3. Report extrasavation or anaphylactic reaction immediately to physician or nurse in charge. | Provides prompt initiation of medical follow-up. |
| **Follow-up Activities** | |
| 1. Observe client (at least every hr) after conclusion of therapy. Monitor as follows: intake and output, food intake, episodes of emesis, IV insertion site, bowel function, emotional status. | Allows quick identification of side effects or unexpected reactions. |

***TABLE 22-2*** Antidotes for Vesicant/Irritant Drugs

| Drug Classification | Specific Agent | Local Antidote | Positive Effect: Animal Studies | Positive Effect: Clinical Case Reports | Antidote Preparation |
|---|---|---|---|---|---|
| **Alkylating agent** | Mechlorethiamine (Nitrogen mustard) | Isotonic sodium thiosulfate 1g/10 ml (manufacturer's recommendations) | None | Yes[1] | Mix 4 ml of 10% Na thiosulfate with 6 ml sterile water for injection (1/6 molar solution results) |
| | Mitomycin C (Mutamycin) | Topical DMSO (RIMSO) | Yes[2] | None | 1-2 ml of 1 mmol DMSO 50% - 100% |
| **Plant alkyloids** | Vinblastine (Velban) Vincristine (Oncovin) | Hyaluronidase (Wydase) 150 U/ml (manufacturer's recommendations) | Yes[4] | None | Add 1 ml USP sodium chloride (150 U/ml results) |
| | Vindesine (Eldisine) Teniposide (VM-26) Etoposide (VP-16-213 VePesid) | Hyaluronidase (Wydase) 150 U/ml | Yes[4] | None | |
| **Anthracycline Antibiotics** | Doxorubicin (Adriamycin) Daunomycin (Cerubidine) | Topical cooling | Yes[5,6] | Yes[7,8] | Topical cooling may be achieved using: - ice packs - cooling pad with ice water circulating - cryogel packs changed frequently |
| | Bisantrene | Sodium bicarbonate 1 mEq/1 ml (premixed) | Yes[12] | Yes[12] | Mix equal parts of 1 mEq/ml sodium bicarbonate with sterile normal saline (1:1 solution). Resulting solution is 0.5 mEq/ml |

From Cancer chemotherapy: guidelines and recommendations for the management of extravasation and anaphylaxis, Oncology Nursing Society, 1988.


1. Owen O, Dellatorre DL, Scott EJ, Cohen MR: Accidental intramuscular injection of mechlorethamine, Cancer 45:8, 2225-2226, 1980.
2. Dorr, R.; Soble, M.J.; Liddil, J.D.; Keller, J.H. Mitomycin C skin toxicity studies in mice: reduced ulceration and altered pharmokinetics with topical dimethyl sulfoxide. *Journal of Clinical Oncology* 4:1339-1404, 1986.
3. Dorr, R.T.; Alberts, D.S.; Woods, M.W. Vinca alkaloid ulceration: experimental mouse model and effects of local antidotes, *Proc Am Assoc Ca Res* 23:109, 1982.
4. Dorr, R.T.; Alberts, D.S. Skin ulceration potential without therapeutic anticancer activity for Epipodophyllotoxin commercial diluents. *IND* 1:151-159, 1983.
5. Dorr, R.T.; Alberts D.S.; Stone, A. Cold protection and heat enhancement of doxorubicin skin toxicity in the mouse. *Cancer Treatment Reports* 69(4):431-437, April 1985.
6. Harwood, K.V.; Bachur, N. Evaluation of dimethyl sulfoxide and local cooling as antidotes for doxorubicin extravasation in a pig model. *Oncology Nursing Forum* 14(1):39-44, 1987.
7. Rudolph, R.; Larson, D.L. Etiology and treatment of chemotherapeutic agent and extravasation injuries: a review. *Journal of Clinical Oncology* 5(7):1116-1126, 1987.
8. Larson, D. Treatment of tissue extravasation by antitumor agents. *Cancer* 49:1796-1799, 1982.
9. Banerfee, A.; Brotherston, T.M.; Lamberty, B.G.H.; Campbell, R.C. Cancer chemotherapy agent-induced perivenous extravasation injuries. *Postgraduate Medical Journal* 63(735)5-9, 1987.
10. Preuss, P.; Partoft, S. Cytotoxic extravasations. *Annals of Plastic Surgery* 19(4):323-329, 1987.
11. Loth, T. Minimal surgical debridement for the treatment of chemotherapeutic agent-induced skin extravasations. *Cancer Treatment Reports* 70(3):401-404, 1986.
12. Loth, T.; Eversmann, W.W. Treatment methods for extravasations of chemotherapeutic agents: a comparative study. *The Journal of Hand Surgery* 11A(3):388-396, 1986.

| **Method of Administration** | **Comments** |
|---|---|
| 1. Inject 5-6 ml (0.2-0.24 gm) IV through existing line and SQ into extravasated site with multiple injections<br>2. Repeat dosing SQ over next several hours<br>3. Apply cold compresses<br>4. No total dose established | 1. *Action:* chemical neutralization<br>2. Initiate treatment immediately and liberally |
| 1. Apply topically one time to the site | 1. Probably not effective for distal or delayed ulcers<br>2. Initiate treatment immediately<br>3. *Action:* carrier solvent or oxygen radical scavenger |
| 1. Inject 1-6 ml (150-900 U) SQ into extravasated site with multiple injections<br>2. Repeat dosing SQ over next several hours<br>3. Apply *warm* compresses<br>4. No total dose established | 1. *Action:* enhances adsorption and dispersion of extravasated drug<br>2. Corticosteroids and topical cooling appear to worsen toxicity<br>3. Warm compresses increase systemic absorption of the drug |
| 1. Inject ½ ml (50-100 mg) IV through existing line and SQ into extravasated site with multiple injections<br>2. Apply cold compresses<br>3. Total dose not to exceed 100 mg | |
| 1. Cooling of site to patient tolerance for 24 hours<br>2. Elevate and rest extremity 24-48 hours then resume normal activity as tolerated<br>3. If pain, erythema and or swelling persist beyond 48 hours, refer patient immediately to plastic surgeon for consultation. Surgical debridement may be necessary; however, only one-third of vesicant extravasations lead to ulceration[7, 9-12] | 1. Application of cold compresses inhibit cytotoxicity of drug[13]<br>2. Some studies suggest a role for topical dimethyl sulfoxide (DMSO) and others show no benefit or delayed healing[6, 14-21]<br>3. Local singular injection of low doses (less than 50 mg) soluble hydrocortisone may still be beneficial. Avoid multiple injections into site |
| 1. Inject 2-6 ml (1.0-3.0 mEq) IV through existing line and SQ into extravasated site with multiple injections<br>2. Apply cold compresses<br>3. Total dose not to exceed 10 ml of 0.5 mEq/ml solution (5.0 mEq) | 1. *Action:* chemical activation<br>2. Dilute bicarbonate chemically degrades the drug |


13. Herman, T.; Baustian, A.; Kundrat, M. Enhancement of hyperthermia-induced lethality and modulation of Adriamycin (ADR) cytotoxicity by cooling. *Proceedings of the American Association of Cancer Research and the American Society of Clinical Oncology,* 21:221, 1981.
14. Olver, I.N.; Aisner, J.; Hament, A.; Buchanan, L.; Bishop, J.F.; Kaplan, R.S. A prospective study of topical dimethyl sulfoxide for treating anthracycline extravasation. *Journal of Clinical Oncology.* 6(11):1732-1735, 1988.
15. Desai, M.H.; Teres, D. Prevention of doxorubicin-induced ulcers in the rat and pig with dimethyl sulfoxide (DMSO). *Cancer Treatment Reports* 66:1371-1374, 1982.
16. Svingen, B.A.; Powis, G.; Appel, P.L.; Scott, M. Protection against Adriamycin-induced skin necrosis in the rat with dimethyl sulfoxide and alpha tocopherol. *Cancer Research* 41:3395-3399, 1981.
17. Dorr, R.T.; Alberts, D.S. Failure of DMSO and Vitamin E to prevent doxorubicin skin ulceration in the mouse. *Cancer Treatment Reports* 67:499-501, 1983.
18. Nobbs, P.; Barr, R.D. Soft tissue injury caused by antineoplastic drugs is inhibited by topical dimethyl sulphoxide and alpha tocopherol. *British Journal of Cancer* 48:873-876, 1983.
19. Soble, M.; Dorr, R.; Plezia, P.; Breckenridge, S. Dose dependent skin ulcers in mice treated with DNA binding antitumor antibiotics. *Cancer Chemotherapy and Pharmacy,* 1987.
20. Olver, I.N. Use of dimethyl sulfoxide in limiting tissue damage caused by extravasation of doxorubicin. *Cancer Treatment Reports* 67:407-408, 1983.
21. Lawrence, H.J.; Goodnight, S.H. Dimethyl sulfoxide and extravasation of anthracycline agents. (Letter). *Annals of Internal Medicine* 98:1025, 1983.
22. Dorr, R.T.; Peng, Y.M.; Alberts, D.S. Bisantrene solubility and skin toxicity studies: efficacy of sodium bicarbonate as a local antidote. *Invest New Drug* 2:351-357, 1984.

## Special Considerations

- Use of heat vs. cold for compresses after extravasation is not supported by scientific research
  - The following factors support use of heat treatment: heat increases blood flow to injured area, possibly increasing transport of drug from area; when used with hyaluronidase in treating vinca alkaloid extravasation, heat increases effectiveness of antidote; heat accelerates cellular metabolism.
  - The following support use of cold treatment: cold causes constriction of peripheral veins and decreases blood flow, resulting in localization of extravasated drug; cold slows cell metabolism, improving survival of minimally injured tissues; cold minimizes local pain.
- When determining IV site examine both arms with clothing and jewelry removed. Proceed distally to proximally. Avoid using extremity with restricted circulation: side of mastectomy, lymphadenopathy, superior vena cava syndrome; lower extremities; immobilized fracture; veins that are phlebitic or sclerosed; veins of antecubital fossa or wrist; an extremity from which blood has been recently obtained; a pre-existing IV site. Site should be alternated from arm to arm for daily treatments.
- Possibility of an anapylactic reaction occurring when chemotherapeutic agents are used increases with previous sensitivity to anticancer drugs, drugs given intravenously, crude preparations of investigational drugs. Drugs that commonly cause anaphylactic events include: asparaginase, cisplastin, bleomycin, and etoposide (see Evaluation, Unexpected Outcomes for further information).
- Hospital policies may vary; generally pregnant or lactating women are advised not to administer chemotherapeutic agents.

## Teaching Considerations

- Teaching is not appropriate for clients who do not wish information.
- Information may be given to significant other. The client who is anxious generally will not retain important information.
- Instruct client and family on how particular regimen is given, common side effects, and signs and symptoms of extravasation and anaphylaxis..
- State common side effects of treatment.
- State ways to cope with nausea, vomiting, alopecia, stomatitis, and bone marrow suppression.
- State signs and symptoms to report after discharge: temperature over 38° C, rash of any kind, severe constipation or diarrhea, sudden weight gain or loss, persistent bleeding from any site, any pain of unusual intensity or distribution, shortness of breath, severe and persistent vomiting more than 24 hr after treatment.
- State medications that should receive physician approval: aspirin and aspirin-containing compounds, antibiotics, anticoagulants, anticonvulsants, barbiturates, antihypertensives, cough medications, Darvon, hypoglycemics, diuretics, hormones, tranquilizers, nasal sprays, vitamins.
- Discuss effects of chemotherapy on fertility and childbearing.

## Home Care Considerations

- Chemotherapy may be administered in home setting by bolus, intermittent, or continuous infusion.
- Chemotherapy should be administered with established policies and procedures by qualified RNs who have the ability to assist in management of side effects and adverse reactions.
- After administration of an IV push chemotherapeutic agent the nurse should monitor the client for 30-60 min. A follow-up visit should be made the next day.
- Emergency drugs and equipment must be available at all times (see Table 22-3).
- Clients receiving chemotherapy at home should have electricity, plumbing, and access to telephone and emergency medical services.
- Before administering chemotherapy the nurse should have access to the results of ordered laboratory tests.
- Items used in home chemotherapy administration should be placed in a puncture resistant container and disposed of according to agency and state regulations.

***TABLE 22-3*** Emergency Home Care Kits

| Anaphylaxis Kit | Extravasation Kit |
|---|---|
| Epinephrine (1:1000 IV) | Cold bags |
| Benadryl (50 mg IV) | Solumedrol (80 mg ampule) |
| Benadryl (50 mg PO) | Specific antidote, such as hyaluronidase for Vinca alkaloids |
| Tylenol tablets | Hydrocortisone cream (1%) |
| Airway | Needles and syringes (22 G, 3 ml, and 5 ml) |
| IV fluid solution and tubing | Alcohol swabs |
| | Sterile 4 × 4 gauze bandages |
| | Tape |

(Adapted from Garvey E: Current and future issues in home administration of chemotherapy, Semin Oncol Nurs 3(2):147, 1987.

#### BIBLIOGRAPHY


Bleschik S: The normal physiological changes of aging and their impact on the response to cancer treatment, Semin Oncol Nurs 4(3):178, 1988.

Brands B: A nursing protocol for the client with neutropenia, Oncol Nurs Forum 11(2):24, 1984.

Cancer chemotherapy: guidelines and recommendations for nursing education and practice, Oncol Nurs Soc, 1984.

Garvey EC: Current and future nursing issues in the home administration of chemotherapy, Semin Oncol Nurs 3(2):142, 1987.

Hunt J, Anderson J, Smith I: Scalp hypothermia to prevent adriamycin induced hair loss, Cancer Nurs 5:25, 1982.

Ignoffo R, Friedman M: Therapy of local toxicities caused by extravasation of cancer chemotherapeutic drugs, Cancer Treat Rev 7:17, 1980.

Kaempfer SH: The effects of cancer chemotherapy on reproduction: a review of the literature, Oncol Nurs Forum 8(1):11, 1981.

Kraemer K: Anaphylaxis resulting from chemotherapy, Oncol Nurs Forum 8(4):13, 1981.

Longman A, Rogers B: Altered cell growth in cancer and the nursing implications, Cancer Nurs 7(5):405, 1984.

Maxwell MB: When the cancer patient becomes anemic, Cancer Nurs 7(4):321, 1984.

Miller SA: Nursing actions in cancer chemotherapy administration, Oncol Nurs Forum 7(4):8, 1980.

Miller SA: Issues in cytotoxic drug handling safety, Semin Oncol Nurs 3(2):133, 1987.

# UNIT VII

# FLUID BALANCE

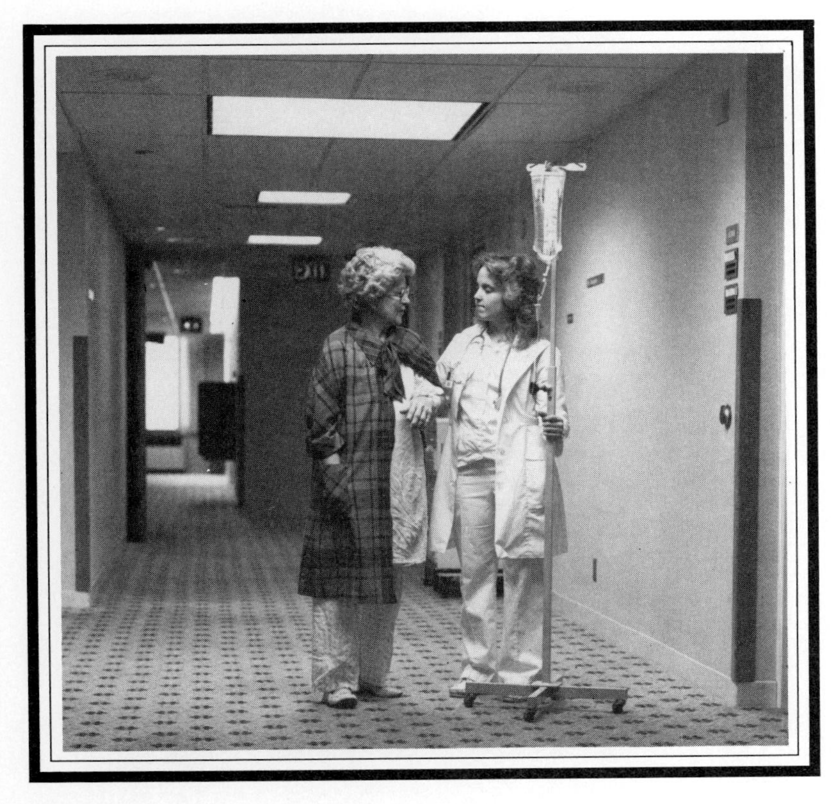

*Fluid and electrolyte balance within the body is necessary to maintain health and function in all body systems. The balance is maintained by the intake and output of water and electrolytes and their distribution in the body. When a client is unable to meet fluid needs or maintain fluid and electrolyte balance, severe, life-threatening situations and death occur.*

*Many variables can change the distribution of body fluid and electrolytes. In the case of pregnancy or exercise, fluid and electrolyte imbalance is a normal and expected response. However, certain disease conditions, such as nausea and vomiting, have more severe consequences. The nurse is responsible for assessing the client's ability to meet fluid needs and determining when and which type of intervention is appropriate.*

*This unit explores nursing measures designed to monitor and restore fluid balance and restore circulating blood volume. In addition, the unit describes interventions necessary to maintain the patency of vascular access devices.*

# 23
# INTRAVENOUS FLUID THERAPY

### OBJECTIVES

*Mastery of content in this chapter will enable the nurse to:*

- Define key terms.
- Discuss conditions requiring intravenous (IV) therapy.
- Identify potential nursing diagnoses for clients requiring IV therapy.
- Explain how to prepare the client and family for IV therapy.
- Identify individualized nursing goals for clients requiring IV therapy.
- Demonstrate in a laboratory or clinical situation initiation of IV therapy, regulation of IV flow rate, changing of IV solutions, changing of IV tubing, and changing of IV dressings.

### KEY TERMS

*Anions*
*Cations*
*Electrolyte*
*Hyperkalemia*
*Hypernatremia*
*Hypokalemia*
*Hyponatremia*
*Infiltration*
*Infusion pump*
*Isotonic*
*Milliequivalent per liter (mEq/L)*
*Patency*
*Phlebitis*
*Solvent*
*Venipuncture*

### SKILLS

***23-1*** Initiating Intravenous (IV) Therapy
***23-2*** Regulating IV Flow Rate
***23-3*** Changing IV Solutions
***23-4*** Changing Infusion Tubing
***23-5*** Changing an IV Dressing

The fluids that circulate throughout the body in extracellular and intracellular fluid spaces are composed of electrolytes, minerals, and cells.

An electrolyte is an element or compound that, when melted or dissolved in water or another solvent, dissociates into ions and is able to carry an electric current. Positively charged electrolytes are cations. (Students may find it helpful to associate the "t" in cation, which has a positive charge with a plus [+] sign.) Negatively charged electrolytes are called anions. Anions have a minus (−) sign after the chemical symbol. Concentrations of electrolytes differ in extracellular and intracellular fluids.

Electrolytes are commonly measured in milliequivalents per liter (mEq/L). This value represents the number of grams of the specific electrolyte (solute) dissolved in 1 liter of plasma (solution). The only electrolyte concentrations not recorded in milliequivalents per liter are calcium and phosphate.

## CATIONS

Major cations within body fluids include sodium, potassium, calcium, and magnesium. Cations may be interchanged when one cation leaves the cell and is replaced by another entering the cell. This replacement occurs because cells tend to maintain electrical neutrality.

### Sodium

Sodium ($Na^+$) is the most abundant cation in extracellular fluid. Sodium ions are involved in the process of maintaining water balance, transmission of nerve impulses, and contraction of muscles. The normal extracellular concentration of sodium is 136 to 144 mEq/L.

An important physiological principle in fluid and electrolyte balance is that water goes where sodium goes. If the kidneys retain sodium, water is retained. Conversely, if the kidneys excrete sodium, water is also excreted. The action of many drugs, such as diuretics, is based on this principle.

### Potassium

Potassium ($K^+$) is the predominant intracellular cation regulating neuromuscular excitability and muscle contraction. The sources of potassium are primarily dietary and include whole grains, meat, legumes, fruits, and vegetables. Potassium is needed for glycogen formation, protein synthesis, and correction of acid-base imbalances. The normal range for serum potassium is 3.5 to 5.5 mEq/L.

### Calcium

Calcium ($Ca^{++}$) is the fifth most abundant element in the body. The body requires calcium for cellular membrane integrity and structure, adequate cardiac conduction, blood coagulation, and bone growth and formation. Calcium is present in three forms in body fluids: (1) ionized (4.5 mg/100 ml), (2) nondiffusible, which is calcium complexed to protein anions (5 mg/100 ml), and (3) calcium salts such as calcium citrate and calcium phosphate (1 mg/100 ml). Calcium in body fluid is a small percentage of the total body calcium. The major portion of calcium is in bones and teeth.

The normal range of calcium in the body fluids is 8.5 to 12 mg/100 ml. These values reflect an ionized calcium range of 4.0 to 5.0 mg/100 ml.

### Magnesium

Magnesium ($Mg^{++}$) is the second most important cation of intracellular fluids and is essential for enzyme activities, neurochemical activities, and muscular excitability. Plasma concentrations of magnesium range from 1.5 to 2.5 mEq/L.

## ANIONS

There are three major anions of body fluids. These negatively charged electrolytes are chloride, bicarbonate, and phosphate ions.

### Chloride

Chloride ($Cl^-$) is the major anion in extracellular and intracellular fluid. It balances cations within extracellular fluid. If a negatively charged ion leaves the extracellular fluid and enters the intracellular fluid, a chloride ion will be exchanged and enter the extracellular fluid. The ion exchange maintains the electrical neutrality of the cell. Normal serum chloride levels range from 95 to 105 mEq/L.

### Bicarbonate

Bicarbonate ($HCO_3^-$) is the major chemical base buffer within the body. The bicarbonate ion is found in extracellular and intracellular fluid. It is regulated primarily through the kidneys. When the body needs to retain more base, the kidneys reabsorb greater quantities of bicarbonate and return it to the extracellular fluid. Normal bicarbonate levels range between 22 and 26 mEq/L.

### Phosphate

Phosphate ($PO_4^-$) is a buffer anion present intracellularly and extracellularly. Phosphate, with calcium, contributes to the development and maintenance of bones and teeth. In addition, phosphate promotes normal neuromuscular action, participates in carbohydrate metabolism, and assists in acid-base regulation. Phosphate is normally absorbed through the gastrointestinal tract in a range of 3 to 12 mg/100 ml.

## PARENTERAL REPLACEMENT OF FLUIDS

Fluids may be replaced through infusion directly into the circulating blood volume in addition to or in place of fluids ingested through the digestive system. Parenteral replacement includes IV fluid and electrolyte therapy, blood therapy (Chapter 25), and total parenteral nutrition (Chapter 28).

The goal of IV fluid administration is correction or prevention of fluid and electrolyte disturbances in clients. When IV therapy is necessary, the nurse must know the correct solution and equipment needed and how to initiate an infusion, regulate the fluid infusion rate, maintain the system, identify and correct problems, and discontinue the infusion.

### Intravenous Solutions

Prepared IV solutions fall into three general categories: isotonic, hypotonic, and hypertonic. An isotonic solution has a total electrolyte content approximating 310 mEq/L. A hypotonic solution has a total electrolyte content less than 250 mEq/L. A hypertonic solution has a total electrolyte content of 375 mEq/L or greater (Metheny and Snively, 1983). The type and amount of IV solution ordered by the physician is determined by serum electrolyte values and fluid volume loss.

In addition to the specific IV fluid ordered, the physician often includes additives such as vitamins or potassium. Clients with properly functioning kidneys who are NPO should have potassium added to the IV solution. If the physician's order does not include potassium, the nurse should double-check the order. Kidneys routinely excrete potassium, and if there is no potassium intake orally or parenterally, hypokalemia can quickly develop.

### Intravenous Needles and Catheters

As nurses prepare equipment for the initiation of an IV infusion (Skill 23-1), they must decide whether to use IV needles or angiocatheters, which are often referred to as IV catheters. Generally, small-bore, 21- or 22-gauge butterfly needles are used when the anticipated duration of therapy is short and it is a nonemergency situation. Small-bore, 21- to 23-gauge butterfly needles may be used for the pediatric client needing IV fluid therapy.

Angiocatheters comprise a metal stylet, which is used to pierce the skin, and a plastic catheter, which is threaded into a vein and remains there for the instillation of fluid. Angiocatheters do not dislodge from the vein as easily as butterfly needles. In addition, large volumes of fluids and medications can be quickly administered through the catheter without a high risk of infiltration. Therefore during emergency situations an angiocatheter is the method of choice for initiating IV fluid therapy. If the duration of therapy is expected to last longer than 24 hours, however, an angiocatheter is used, and if the administration of blood or blood products is anticipated, a size 18 or 19 angiocatheter is necessary to allow infusion of the viscous blood product solutions (Chapter 25).

### PREREQUISITE KNOWLEDGE

1. Factors affecting fluid and electrolyte balance.
2. Anatomy of the circulatory system.
3. Principles of surgical asepsis.
4. Principles of medication administration.

### PREREQUISITE SKILLS

1. Assessment of body systems affected by IV therapy (Chapter 13).
2. Recording of intake and output (Chapter 13).
3. Maintenance of a sterile field (Chapter 38).
4. Proper handwashing techniques (Chapter 37).

### GUIDELINES

1. Know the client's normal range of vital signs. Altered fluid or electrolyte imbalances can affect vital signs. Dehydration can produce hypotension and tachycardia. Fluid overload can result in hypertension and a bounding pulse. Disturbances in serum potassium can result in an irregular pulse.
2. Know the client's developmental stage. The proportion of total body water to body mass changes from infancy to the older adult years.
3. Know the client's weight. Body size affects total body water. Fat contains no water; the obese client thus has proportionately less body water.
4. Know the client's medical history and present medications or therapies. Certain drugs such as diuretics or steroids affect fluid and electrolyte balance. Likewise, a client may be on a specific diet, such as a low-sodium diet for water retention.
5. Beware of prolonged environmental conditions that can affect the client's fluid status. Prolonged exposure to hot, humid weather can lead to fluid and electrolyte imbalances, particularly in the infant, the older adult, or the chronically ill client.
6. Know the client's exercise pattern. Exercise results in the increase of sensible water loss through sweat.
7. Know if the client is right or left handed. When possible place an IV into the nondominant hand.
8. Determine that the present IV system is closed and intact. A system that has remained closed and in which none of the connections have separated ensures that the sterility of the system has been maintained. If the nurse suspects that the infusion tubing has separated from the IV catheter or needle, sterility is no longer assumed, and new, sterile tubing should be attached to the solution and catheter or needle.
9. Note when the last IV tubing and dressing change occurred.

To maintain sterility of a patent IV system, the Centers for Disease Control (CDC, 1987) recommend the following:

1. Change keep-vein-open (KVO) solutions every 24 hours.
2. Change IV tubing every 48 hours.
3. Change IV dressings as follows:
   a. Gauze dressing every 24 hours.
   b. Transparent dressings every 3 to 5 days as per manufacturers directions. NOTE: transparent dressing must remain occlusive for long-term application.

## SKILL 23-1
## INITIATING INTRAVENOUS THERAPY

The goal of IV fluid administration is correction or prevention of fluid and electrolyte disturbances in clients who are or may become acutely ill. For example, a client with third-degree burns over 40% of the body is critically ill and has severe fluid and electrolyte imbalances. Fluid therapy must be continuously regulated in a burn client because of continual changes in fluid and electrolyte balance. A client who is NPO for 2 days after surgery receives IV fluid replacement to prevent fluid and electrolyte imbalances; the infusion is usually discontinued when client resumes oral intake.

### Purposes

1. Restore and maintain fluid and electrolyte balance.
2. Establish a route for intravenous (IV) medication.
3. Establish a route for emergency IV medication.

## Procedure 23-1

| Steps | Rationale |
|---|---|
| **Assessment** | |
| 1. Identify client whose potential for fluid and electrolyte imbalance may require IV fluid therapy. | Identify potential or actual risk factors increasing client's chances of fluid and electrolyte imbalances. All types of chronic diseases can cause fluid or electrolyte imbalances. Because progression of these diseases is usually slow, imbalances can be controlled. However, in clients with exacerbations of chronic illnesses, disease process is often no longer stabilized, and fluid and electrolyte imbalances are present. |
| 2. Observe for signs and symptoms indicating fluid or electrolyte imbalances:<br>a. Sunken eyes.<br>b. Periorbital edema. | Because fluid and electrolyte disturbances can affect every system, nurse must systematically assess client to identify abnormalities related to fluid or electrolyte imbalance. |
| c. Greater than 2% increase or decrease in body weight. | Daily weights document fluid retention or loss. Change in body weight of 1 kg corresponds to 1 L of fluid retention or loss. |
| d. Dry mucous membranes.<br>e. Flattened or distended neck veins.<br>f. Change from baseline vital signs.<br>g. Irregular pulse rhythm.<br>h. Auscultation of rales or rhonchi in lungs.<br>i. Poor skin turgor.<br>j. Increased or decreased bowel sounds. | |
| k. Decreased urine output. | Monitoring urinary output is one method of assessing fluid balance. During dehydration, kidney attempts to restore fluid balance by reducing urine production. |
| l. Behavioral changes.<br>m. Confusion. | |
| 3. Review client's medical record for physician's order, stating type and amount of IV fluid and rate of fluid administration. | IV fluids must be ordered by physician. Verification of orders is ensured when nurse reviews medical record. In addition, nurse follows "five rights" for administration of medications (Unit VI). |
| **Nursing Diagnosis** | |
| 1. Cluster data to reveal actual or potential nursing diagnoses:<br>a. Fluid volume deficit:<br>▪ Related to prolonged vomiting or diarrhea.<br>▪ Related to trauma.<br>b. Potential fluid volume deficit:<br>▪ Related to vomiting or diarrhea.<br>▪ Related to trauma. | Fluid volume deficits usually result from isotonic, hypernatremic, or hyponatremic dehydration. |
| c. Fluid volume excess: related to impaired renal function. | Fluid volume excess frequently results from overhydration and edema or water intoxication. |
| **Planning** | |
| 1. Develop individualized goals for client based on nursing diagnoses:<br>a. Restore client's fluid and electrolyte balance. | Client suffering temporary fluid losses such as that due to specific volume losses in surgery will have fluid and electrolyte balance restored to normal. |
| b. Maintain client's fluid and electrolyte balance. | Client suffering prolonged fluid losses such as with fresh third-degree burns or continual wound drainage requires measures to maintain fluid balance until fluid and electrolytes are no longer lost. |
| c. Client maintains patent IV catheter. | Patency of IV catheter allows for IV fluid administration. |
| 2. Assemble necessary equipment for initiating IV line:<br>a. Correct solution<br>b. Proper needle for venipuncture (Fig. 23-1)<br>c. Infusion set (infants and children require a 60 gtt/ml drip and often a volume control device) | Correct selection and preparation of equipment assist in safe and quick placement of IV line. |

**Steps** | **Rationale**

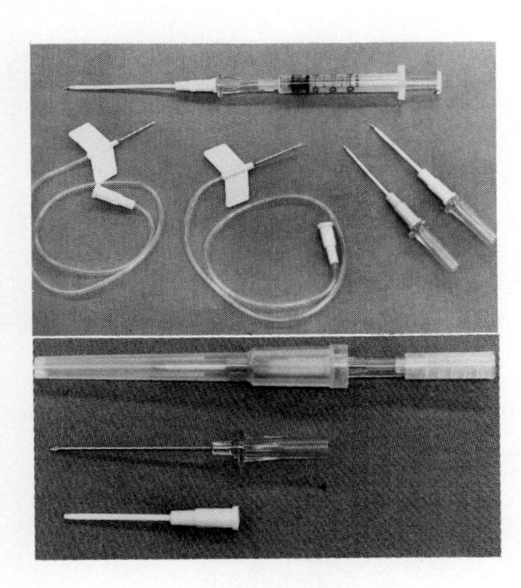

*Fig. 23-1*

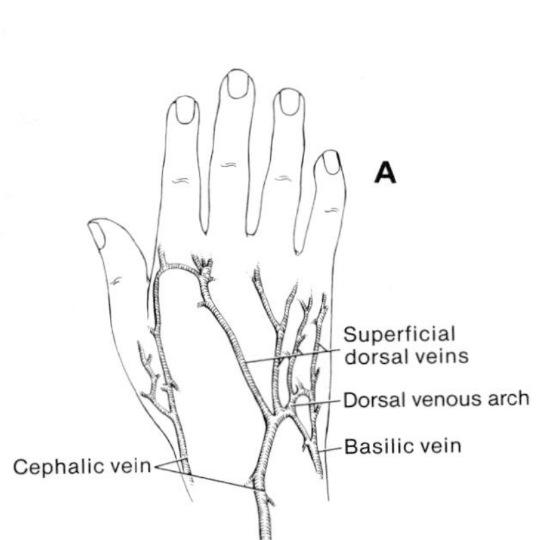


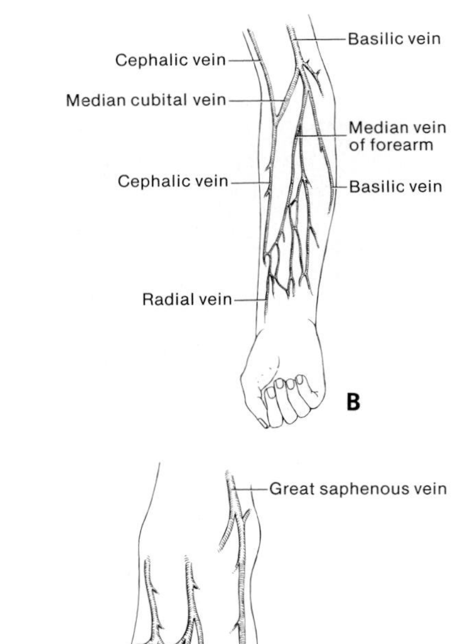


*Fig. 23-2*

d. IV tubing
e. Alcohol and povidone-iodine cleansing swabs
f. Disposable gloves
g. Tourniquet
h. Arm board
i. Gauze and povidone-iodine ointment or transparent dressing and povidone-iodine solution — Dressings provide barrier against bacteria. When transparent dressing is selected, povidone-iodine solution rather than ointment is recommended because ointment interferes with adherence of dressing to skin.
j. Tape, cut and ready to use
k. Towel to place under client's hand
l. IV pole

3. Identify accessible vein for placement of IV needle or catheter (Fig. 23-2, *A-C*). — Selection of appropriate vein promotes ease and placement of IV catheter and needle.
   a. Avoid bony prominences.
   b. Use most distal portion of vein first.
   c. Avoid placing IV over client's wrist.
   d. Avoid placing IV in client's dominant hand.
4. Prepare client and family by explaining procedure, its purpose, and what is expected of client. — Decreases anxiety and promotes cooperation.

## Implementation

1. Wash hands. — Reduces transmission of microorganisms.
2. Organize equipment on clutter-free bedside stand or overbed table (Fig. 23-3). — Reduces risk of contamination and accidents.
3. Open sterile packages using aseptic technique (Chapter 38). — Maintains sterility of equipment and reduces spread of microorganisms.
4. Check solution, using "five rights" of drug administration. Make sure prescribed additives, such as potassium and vitamins, have been added. Check solution for color, clarity, and expiration date. — IV solutions are medications and should be double-checked to reduce risk of error. Solutions that are discolored, contain particles, or are expired are not to be used.

   NOTE: When using bottled IV solution, remove metal cap and metal and rubber disks beneath cap (Fig. 23-4). For plastic IV solution bags, remove plastic sheath over IV tubing port. — Permits entry of infusion tubing into solution.

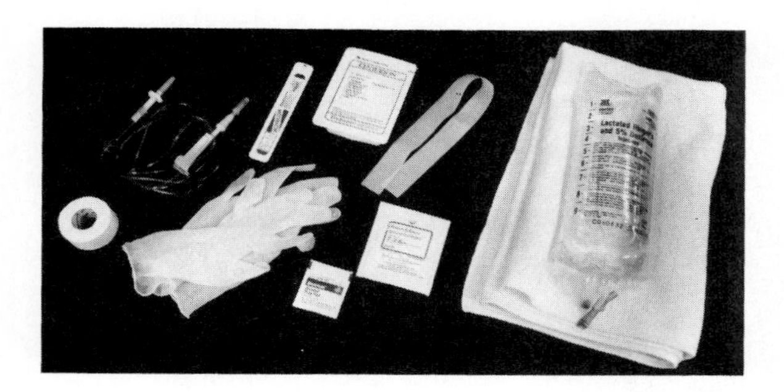

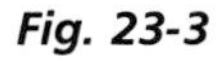

*Fig. 23-3*

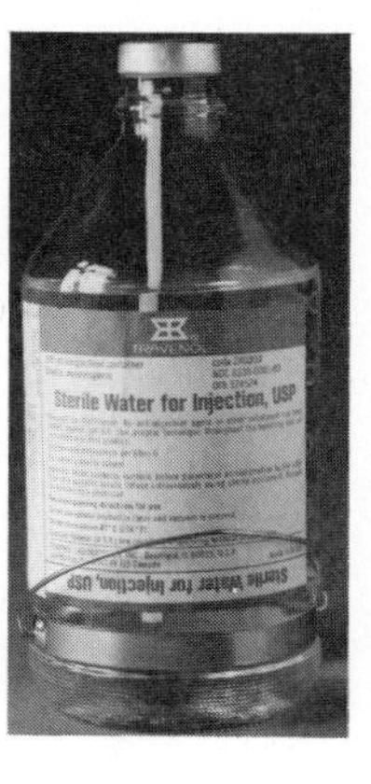


*Fig. 23-4*

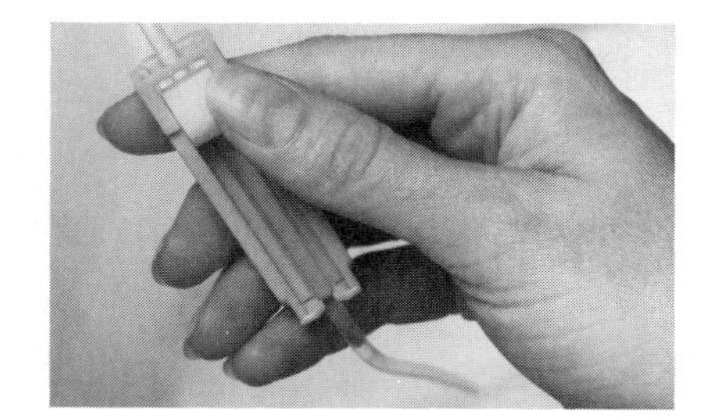

*Fig. 23-5*

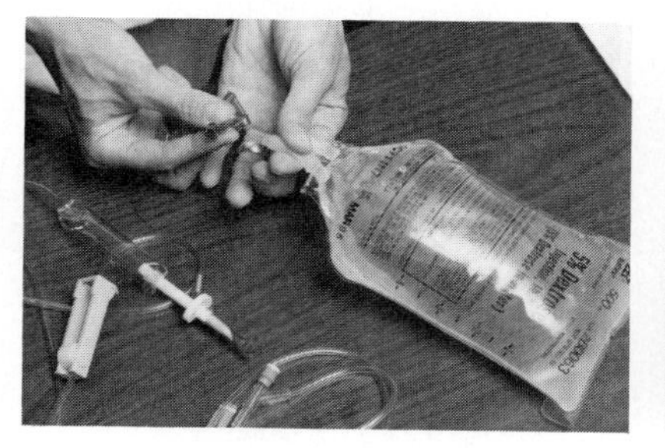

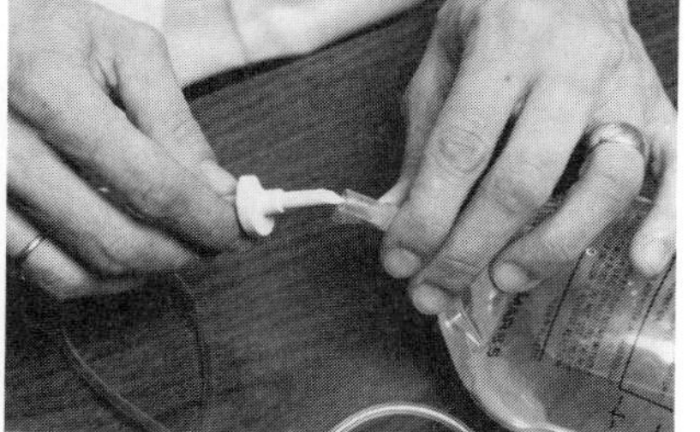

*Fig. 23-6* A, B

| Steps | Rationale |
|---|---|
| 5. Open infusion set, maintaining sterility of both ends. | Prevents bacteria from entering infusion equipment and bloodstream. |
| 6. Place roller clamp (Fig. 23-5) about 2 to 4 cm (1 to 2 in) below drip chamber. | Close proximity of roller clamp to drip chamber allows more accurate regulation of flow rate. |
| 7. Move roller clamp to "off" position. | Prevents accidental spillage of fluid on client, nurse, bed, or floor. |
| 8. Insert infusion set into fluid bag or bottle. | |
| a. Remove protective cover from IV bag without touching opening (Fig. 23-6, *A*). | Maintains sterility of solution. |
| b. Remove protector cap from tubing insertion spike, not touching spike, and insert spike into opening of IV bag (Fig. 23-6, *B*). Or insert spike into black rubber stopper of IV bottle. Cleanse rubber stopper with antiseptic. | Prevents contamination of solution from contaminated insertion spike. |
| 9. Fill infusion tubing. | |
| a. Compress drip chamber and release. | Creates suction effect; fluid enters drip chamber. |
| b. Remove needle protector and release roller clamp to allow fluid to travel from drip chamber through tubing to needle adapter. Return roller clamp to off position after tube is filled. | Removes air from tubing and permits tubing to fill with solution. |
| c. Be certain tubing is clear of air and air bubbles. | Large air bubbles can act as emboli. Remove air by allowing fluid to flow through tubing until tubing is free of air. Collect excess solution in basin and discard. |
| d. Replace needle protector. | Maintains system sterility. |
| 10. Select appropriate IV needle or angiocatheter. | Needle or angiopuncture is necessary to puncture vein and instill IV fluid. |
| 11. Select distal site of vein to be used. | If sclerosing or damage to vein occurs, proximal site of same vein is still usable. |
| 12. If large amount of body hair is present at needle insertion site, shave it off. | Reduces risk of contamination from bacteria on hair. Also assists in maintaining intactness of dressing and makes removal of tape less painful. |
| 13. If possible, place extremity in dependent position. | Permits venous dilation and visibility. |
| 14. Place tourniquet 10 to 12 cm (5 to 6 in) above insertion site. Tourniquet should obstruct venous, not arterial, flow (Fig. 23-7). Check presence of distal pulse. | Diminished arterial flow prevents venous filling. |

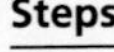

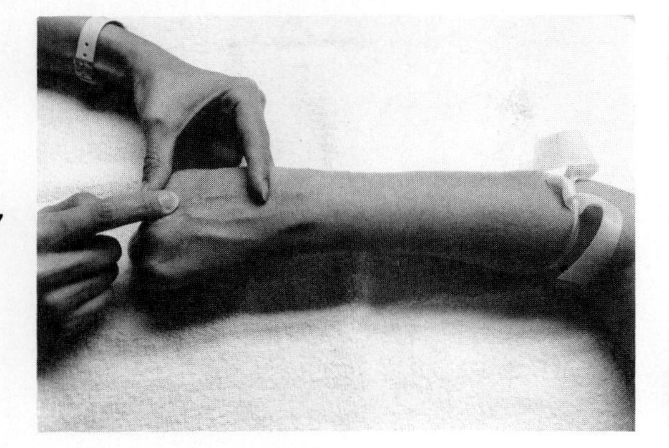

***Fig. 23-7***

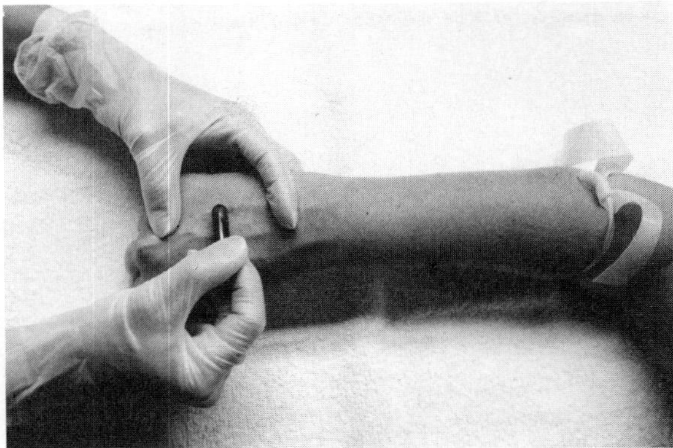

***Fig. 23-8***

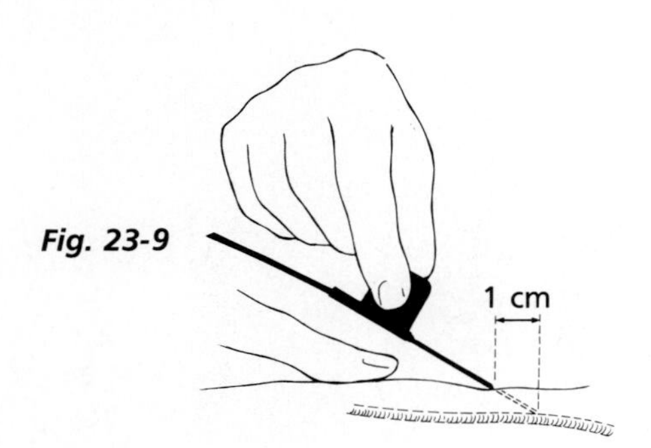


***Fig. 23-9***

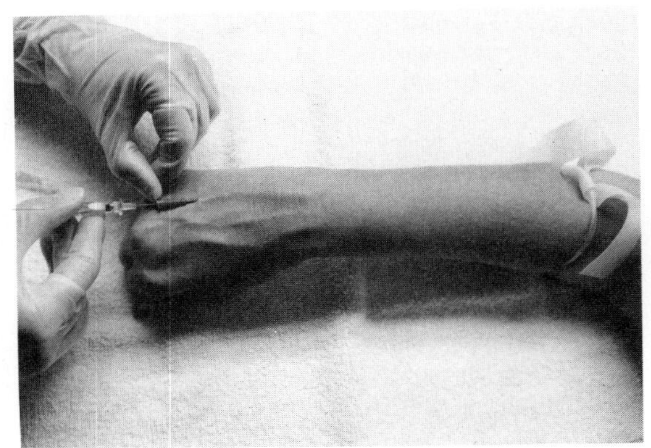

***Fig. 23-10***

| **Steps** | **Rationale** |
|---|---|
| 15. Apply disposable gloves. | Decreases exposure to HIV, hepatitis, and other blood-borne organisms (CDC, 1987). |
| 16. Select well-dilated vein. Client may have to make fist if vein in hand or arm is selected. | Muscle contraction increases venous distention. |
| NOTE: Be sure needle adapter end of infusion set is nearby and on sterile gauze or towel. | Permits smooth, quick connection of infusion to IV needle once vein is punctured. |
| 17. Cleanse insertion site with povidone-iodine solution, followed by alcohol (Fig. 23-8). | Providone-iodine is topical antiinfective; alcohol is topical antiseptic. Together, they reduce skin surface bacteria. |
| 18. Perform venipuncture. *Butterfly needle:* needle at 30-degree angle with bevel up about 1 cm (½ in) distal to actual site of venipuncture (Fig. 23-9). *Angiocatheter:* inserted bevel-up at 30-degree angle distal to actual site of venipuncture. | Allows nurse to place needle parallel with vein. Thus, when vein is punctured, risk of puncturing both sides is reduced. |
| 19. Look for blood return through tubing of butterfly needle or angiocatheter, indicating that needle has entered vein. Advance catheter into vein until hub rests at venipuncture site. Remove stylet from angiocatheter, leaving catheter in place (Fig. 23-10). Small, flexible catheter remains to permit entry of IV fluids. | Increased venous pressure from tourniquet increases backflow of blood into catheter or tubing. |
| 20. Connect needle adapter of infusion set to hub of angiocatheter or needle. To maintain sterility, do not touch point of entry of needle adapter or hub of angiocatheter (Fig. 23-11). | Prompt connection of infusion set maintains patency of vein. |
| 21. Stabilizing catheter with one hand, release tourniquet. Release roller clamp to begin infusion at a rate to maintain patency of IV line. | Permits venous flow and prevents clotting of vein and obstruction of flow of IV solution. |
| 22. If gauze dressing is used, place povidone-iodine ointment at venipuncture site (Fig. 23-12). If transparent dressing is used, place povidone-iodine solution at site. | Topical antiseptic germicide reduces bacteria on skin and decreases risk of local or systemic infection. Use of solution increases adherence of transparent dressing. |
| 23. Secure IV catheter or needle. | Prevents accidental removal of catheter from vein. |
| a. Place narrow piece (½ in) of tape under catheter and cross tape over catheter. | |

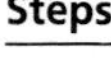

**Steps** | **Rationale**

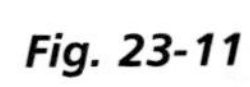
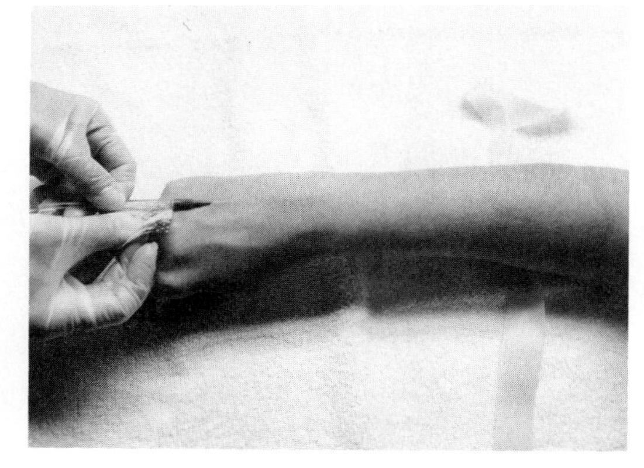

*Fig. 23-11*

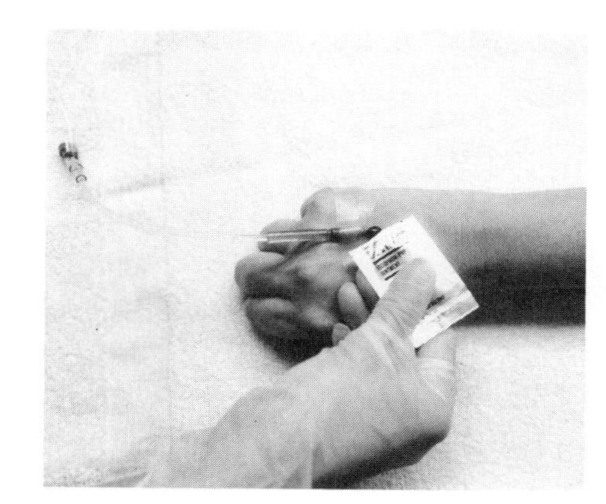

*Fig. 23-12*

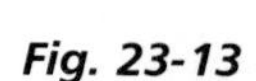
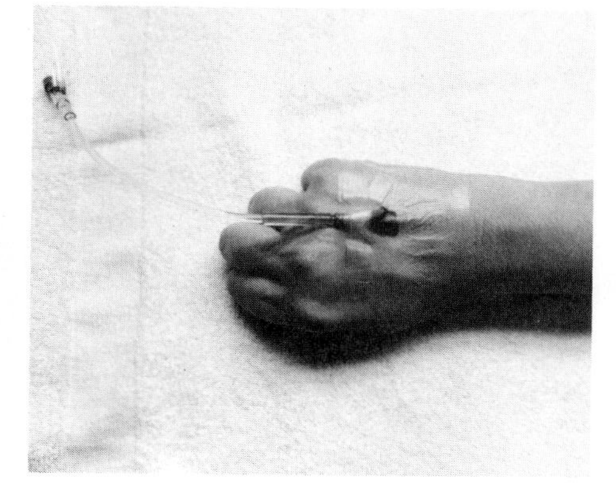

*Fig. 23-13*

b. Place second piece of narrow tape directly across catheter.

c. Place third piece of narrow tape under IV insertion needle adapter and cross tape over infusion tubing. Place 2 × 2 gauze pad over catheter and secure with 1 in piece of tape or place transparent dressing over IV site in direction of hair growth (Fig. 23-13).

Prevents accidental disconnection of IV infusion.
Placing dressing in direction of hair growth decreases discomfort to client when dressing is removed.

d. Secure infusion tubing to dressing with piece of 1 in tape.

Stabilizes connection of infusion to catheter.

24. Write date and time of placement of IV line on dressing.

Provides immediate data as to when IV was inserted and subsequent dressing changes.

25. Adjust flow rate to correct drops per minute (Skill 23-2).

Maintains correct rate of flow for IV solution.

26. Remove gloves. Discard supplies and wash hands.

Reduces transmission of microorganisms.

## Evaluation

1. Observe client every hour to determine response to therapy.
   a. Correct amount of solution infused as prescribed.
   b. Proper flow rate gtt/minutes.
   c. Patency of IV catheter or needle.
   d. Absence of infiltration, phlebitis, or inflammation.

Provides continuous evaluation of type and amount of fluid delivered to client. Hourly inspection prevents accidental fluid overload or inadequate infusion rate and identifies early incidence of vein inflammation.

### *Expected outcomes*

1. Fluid and electrolytes return to normal.

Indicates correction of fluid and electrolyte imbalances.

2. Vital signs and other abnormal assessment parameters stabilize and return to normal.

Indicates circulatory system's response to correction of fluid and electrolyte balance.

3. Patent IV line is indicated by:

Maintains IV infusion.

   a. Adequate blood return to IV line when IV solution is placed below level of venipuncture site.

Blood returns because pressure of venous blood is greater than pressure in IV infusion tubing.

   b. Palpation of cannulated vein distal to site. Observe for slowing or momentary cessation of IV rate.

Palpation results in mechanical compression of vein. When IV line is patent, compression results in slowing or cessation of

| Steps | Rationale |
|---|---|
| | flow rate. If flow does not change, infiltration may be present, vein is palpated too lightly, or vein is palpated too distal to angiocatheter or IV needle. |
| c. Absence of infiltration as indicated by swelling and pallor at venipuncture site. | Infiltration results from dislodging of needle into subcutaneous space. |
| d. Absence of inflammation. | Inflammation results from irritation to vein by catheter or IV solution. |
| ***Unexpected outcomes*** | |
| 1. Uncorrected fluid and electrolyte imbalances can result in: | |
| a. Fluid volume deficit such as isotonic dehydration, related to loss of plasma, associated with burns; hypernatremic dehydration, related to CNS lesion; hyponatremic dehydration, related to chronic malnutrition. | Prolonged fluid volume deficits increase risk for severe dehydration, shock, coma, death. |
| b. Fluid volume excess such as overhydration and edema, related to sodium retention; overhydration and water intoxication, related to excessive water ingestion. | Results when cardiovascular or renal systems cannot adapt to excess fluids and overload occurs. |
| c. Electrolyte imbalances such as hyponatremia, related to use of diuretics; hypernatremia, related to excessive insensible water loss; hypokalemia, related to gastrointestinal losses with diarrhea; hyperkalemia, related to renal failure; hypocalcemia: related to rapid blood transfusion containing citrate; hypercalcemia, related to osteoporosis; hypomagnesemia: related to malnutrition associated with alcoholism; hypermagnesemia, related to hyperparathyroidism; hypochloremia; related to prolonged vomiting; hyperchloremia, related to acid-base disturbances. | Can result from disease, trauma, prescribed therapies. Severity of symptoms relate directly to degree of electrolyte imbalance. |
| 2. Infiltration is indicated by swelling and possible pitting edema, pallor, pain at insertion site, possible decrease in flow rate. | Swelling results from increased tissue fluid. If enough fluid accumulates, pitting edema forms. Pallor is caused by decreased circulation to region. In addition, fluid may be flowing through IV line at decreased rate or may have stopped. Pain may also occur with infiltration. Pain usually results from edema and increases as infiltration worsens. |
| 3. Phlebitis is indicated by pain, increased skin temperature, erythema along path of vein. | Phlebitis is inflammation of vein caused by IV catheter or by chemical irritation of additives and medications given intravenously. |
| 4. Bleeding occurs at venipuncture site. | Bleeding is common in clients who have received heparin or who have bleeding disorder. If bleeding occurs around venipuncture site and catheter is within vein, dressing may be applied over site. Bleeding from vein is usually slow, continuous seepage. Clients do not bleed to death from slight continuous bleeding around venipuncture site. |
| **Recording and Reporting** | |
| 1. Record in nurses' notes type of fluid, insertion site, flow rate, size and type catheter or needle, and when infusion was begun. | Documents initiation of therapy as ordered by physician. |
| 2. Record client's response to IV fluid, amount infused, and integrity and patency of system at least every 8 hr. | Documents ongoing IV therapy and client's tolerance and response to therapy. |
| 3. Report to oncoming nursing staff: type of fluid, flow rate, status of venipuncture site, amount of fluid remaining in present solution, any side effects. | Provides new nursing personnel with status of IV fluid. Allows new nursing staff to plan when new solution should be hung. |
| 4. Report to physician adverse reactions such as congestive heart failure, shock, thrombophlebitis. | Prompt reporting of adverse reactions permits initiation of appropriate medical therapies to treat adverse reactions. |
| **Follow-up Activities** | |
| 1. Monitor resolution of unexpected outcomes every 4 hr, infiltration, phlebitis. | Allows nurse to evaluate response of unexpected outcomes. |
| 2. Observe therapy system and correct flow rate (Skill 23-2), change solution (Skill 23-3), change infusion tubing (Skill 23-4), change dressing (Skill 23-5). | Ongoing observations of IV system ensure that physician's fluid orders are maintained and that interventions are instituted for complications or untoward events. |

### Special Considerations

- Women of child-bearing age may note fluctuations in weight of 2 to 5 lb between ovulation cycle and onset of menstruation. This does not indicate fluid imbalance but rather normal physiological response to fluctuating hormone levels.
- Most IV infusions in pediatric client require a 21- or 23-gauge butterfly needle (Whaley and Wong, 1987). When child is critically ill or long-term IV access is anticipated, surgical cut down may be used to access larger vein.
- Assessment for potential venipuncture sites should consider conditions, cautions, and contraindications that exclude certain sites. Because very young and elderly clients have fragile veins, nurse should avoid sites that are easily moved or bumped. It is often difficult to insert IV line in clients who have had numerous venipunctures because their veins may be sclerosed with scar tissue. Obese clients present problems for venipuncture because of difficulty in locating superficial veins. IVs should not be introduced into lower extremities unless specifically ordered by physician. Lower extremities are more likely to develop thrombophlebitis.
- Avoid using circulatory or neurologically impaired extremities.
- Venipuncture is contraindicated in site with signs of infection, infiltration, or thrombosis. Infected site is red, tender, swollen, and possibly warm to touch. Exudate may be present. Infected site is not used because of danger of introducing bacteria from skin surface into bloodstream.
- When it is anticipated that blood or blood components are going to be administered, large-gauge (19 or 18) needle should be used for infusion of more viscous solution.
- Critically ill clients at all stages of life require more frequent assessment to monitor status of therapy.
- When infiltration occurs, infusion must be discontinued and, if necessary, reinserted into another extremity. Nursing measures to reduce discomfort caused by infiltration are elevation of extremity, which promotes venous drainage and helps decrease edema, and wrapping extremity in warm towel for 20 min every 4 hr, which increases circulation and reduces pain and edema.
- When phlebitis is present, IV line must be discontinued and new line inserted in another vein. Warm, moist heat on site of phlebitis can offer some relief (Chapter 44).
- Phlebitis is potentially dangerous because blood clots (thrombophlebitis) can occur and in some cases result in emboli.
- When solution has less than 100 ml remaining, present nursing shift should have new solution at client's bedside and slow flow rate. This reduces risk of solution emptying during change of shift report.

### Teaching Considerations

- If clients are older children allowing them to select IV site may increase cooperation because they have some control over their treatment.
- If IV is positional, instruct client how to properly position arm to maintain flow.
- Instruct client about signs and symptoms of infiltration, phlebitis, inflammation.
- Instruct client to inform nurse if flow slows or stops.
- Instruct client how to ambulate with IV pole or stand.
- Instruct client and primary care giver about procedures of IV therapy, including sterile technique while manipulating syringes and other supplies.
- Instruct client and primary care giver about administration of IV solutions.
- Teach client and primary care giver to recognize potential problems with infusion and appropriate reaction to problems.
- Instruct primary care giver to keep dressings dry, clean, in place.
- Teach primary care giver to apply pressure with sterile gauge if needle falls out and, if client is on anticoagulant therapy, to tape several pieces of sterile gauze in place for at least 20 min or until bleeding stops.
- Teach client that, when bathing, it is best to take tub bath but not to let IV tubing touch water and to unplug pump first if one is used.
- Instruct client and primary care giver to keep IV solution above waist level when ambulating.
- Instruct client to wear clothes with large sleeves.
- Teach client and family to monitor intake and output using household measuring devices.

### Home Care Considerations

- Assess client and family/primary care giver's willingness to participate in client's care, including procurement of supplies and ability to handle emergency situations.
- Assess home environment for possible safety hazards, cleanliness, adequate storage for supplies, electrical wiring, and availability of running water.
- Coordinate client teaching and develop plan of care to be followed by IV team, client and primary care giver.
- Prepare client and primary care provider to be independent in IV therapy at home.

## *SKILL 23-2*
## *REGULATING IV FLOW RATE*

After the infusion is secured and the line is patent, the nurse is responsible for regulating the rate of infusion according to the physician's orders. An infusion rate that is too slow can lead to further cardiovascular and circulatory collapse in a client who is dehydrated, in shock, or critically ill. If an infusion runs too slowly the chances of the vein clotting off are greater. An infusion rate that is too rapid can result in fluid overload, which is particularly dangerous in certain cardiovascular, kidney, and neurologic disorders. The nurse calculates the infusion rate to prevent too slow or too rapid administration.

Two devices can assist the nurse in maintaining correct

flow rates. An infusion pump is designed to deliver a measured amount of fluid over a period of time. IV infusion pumps monitor IV fluids based on the flow rate or drops per minute. In addition, a volume control device is placed between the IV bag and the insertion spike of the infusion set.

Children, the elderly, clients with severe head trauma, and clients susceptible to volume overload must be protected from sudden increases in infusion volumes. Sudden increases can occur accidentally. For example, a restless client may loosen the roller clamp with a sudden movement and thus increase the flow rate, or the flow rate may be accidentally increased if the client ambulates. A sudden increase in volume can make the client critically ill or cause death.

### Purposes

1. Maintain fluid and electrolyte balance.
2. Infuse IV fluids as ordered.

## Procedure 23-2

| Steps | Rationale |
|---|---|
| **Assessment** | |
| 1. Observe patency of IV line and needle. | For fluid to infuse at proper rate, IV line and needle must be free of kinks, knots, clots. |
| a. Open drip regulator and observe for rapid flow of fluid from solution into drip chamber, then close drip chamber to prescribed rate (see implementation section). | Rapid flow of fluid into drip chamber indicates patency of IV line. Closing drip chamber to prescribed rate prevents fluid overload. |
| b. Lower bottle, bag below level of infusion site and observe for blood return. | Indicates needle is patent and in vein. Venous pressure is greater than pressure in IV tubing. |
| c. Palpate cannulated vein near venipuncture site until rate of flow is occluded. | Cessation of drops from drip chamber indicates catheter or needle is in vein. If fluid continues to drip, infiltration is present. |
| 2. Check client's medical record for correct solution and additives. Usual order includes: solution for 24 hr usually divided into 2 or 3 L. Occasionally, IV order contains only 1 L to keep vein open (KVO). Record also shows time over which each liter is to infuse. | IV fluids are medications. "Five rights" decrease chance of medication error. |
| **Nursing Diagnosis** | |
| 1. Cluster data to reveal actual or potential nursing diagnoses requiring accurate regulation of IV flow rates, including:<br>a. Fluid volume deficit:<br>▪ Related to fluid loss.<br>▪ Related to dehydration.<br>b. Fluid volume excess:<br>▪ Related to fluid retention.<br>▪ Related to sodium retention. | Clients with actual or potential alterations in fluid and electrolyte status who are receiving IV therapy require accurate administration of fluid volumes each hour to meet fluid and electrolyte requirements. |
| **Planning** | |
| 1. Develop individualized goals for client based on nursing diagnoses:<br>a. Restore client's fluid and electrolyte balance.<br>b. Maintain client's fluid and electrolyte balance.<br>c. Maintain accurate IV flow rate. | Proper flow rates restore and maintain fluid and electrolyte balance. Excessive or diminished flow rates have potential to worsen fluid and electrolyte status. |
| 2. Have paper and pencil to calculate flow rate. | Beginning student is unfamiliar with IV fluid rates and should use mathematical calculations to get correct rate. |
| 3. Know calibration in drops per milliliter (gtt/ml) of infusion set:<br>*Microdrip:* 60 gtt/ml<br>*Macrodrip* (Metheny and Snively, 1983):<br>Abbott Lab 15 gtt/ml<br>Travenol Lab 10 gtt/ml<br>McGaw Lab 15 gtt/ml<br>IVAC 20 gtt/ml | Microdroppers, also called minidrip, universally deliver 60 gtt/ml. However, there are different commercial parenteral administration sets for macrodrip. Nurse should know which company's infusion set hospital uses. |
| 4. Select one of following formulas to calculate flow:<br>a. $\text{ml/hr} = \dfrac{\text{total volume}}{\text{hours of infusion}}$ | Once hourly rate has been determined, these formulas will give correct flow rate. |

| Steps | Rationale |
|---|---|

*or*

b. Drop factor × ml/min = drops/minute

*or*

c. $\frac{\text{Total volume} \times \text{drop factor}}{\text{Infusion time in minutes}} = \text{drops/minute}$

5. Place infusion pump or volume control device at bedside if ordered or available. — Reduces risk of infusion of incorrect fluid.

## Implementation

1. Read physician's orders and follow "five rights" for correct solution and proper additives. — IV fluids are medications; following "five rights" decreases chance of medication error.
   a. IV fluids are usually ordered for 24 hr period, indicating how long each liter of fluid should run; e.g., IV order for client is: — Determines volume of fluid that should infuse hourly. Fluid needs vary; rate must be given over time ordered.
      Bottle 1: 1000 ml D5W with 20 mEq KCl 8 AM-4PM
      Bottle 2: 1000 ml D5W with 20 mEq KCl 4PM-12 midnight
      Bottle 3: 1000 ml D5W with 20 mEq KCl 12 midnight-8AM
      Total 24 hr IV intake: 3000 ml
2. Determine hourly rate by dividing volume by hours, e.g., — Provides even infusion of fluid over prescribed hourly rate.

   $\frac{1000 \text{ ml}}{8} = 125 \text{ ml/hr}$

   *or* if 4 liters are ordered for 24 hr:

   $\frac{4000}{24} = 166.7 \text{ ml} = 167 \text{ ml/hr}$

3. Place adhesive or fluid indicator tape on IV bottle or bag next to volume markings. Fig. 23-14 is based on 125 ml in 8 hr period. — Time taping IV bag gives nurse visual cue as to whether fluids are being administered over correct period of time.
4. After hourly rate has been determined, calculate minute rate based on drop factor of infusion set. Minidrip or microdrip infusion set has drop factor of 60 gtt/ml. Regular drip or *macrodrip infusion set used here* has drop factor of 15 gtt/ml. Using formula, calculate minute flow rates: — Allows nurse to calculate minute flow rate based on this formula:

   $\frac{\text{total volume} \times \text{drop factor}}{\text{infusion time in minutes}}$

   Bottle 1: 1000 ml with 20 KCl — Volume is divided by time.

   *Microdrip:*

   $\frac{125 \text{ ml} \times 60 \text{ gtt/ml}}{60 \text{ min}} = \frac{7500 \text{ gtt}}{60 \text{ min}} = 125 \text{ gtt/min}$

   *Macrodrip:*

   $\frac{125 \text{ ml} \times 15 \text{ gtt/ml}}{60 \text{ min}} = 31\text{-}32 \text{ gtt/min}$

5. Time flow rate by counting drops in drip chamber for 1 min by watch, then adjust roller clamp to increase or decrease rate of infusion (Fig. 23-15). — Determines if fluids are administered too slowly or too fast. Rate of infusion should also be checked by watch even if infusion pump is used.

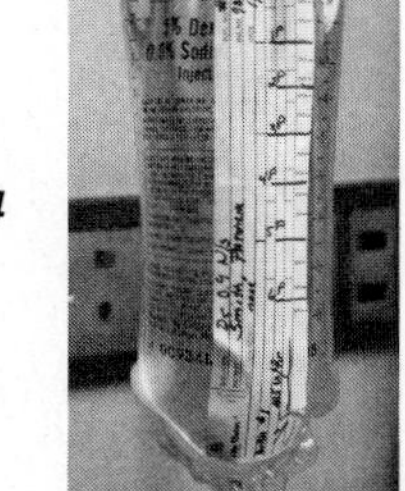

***Fig. 23-14***

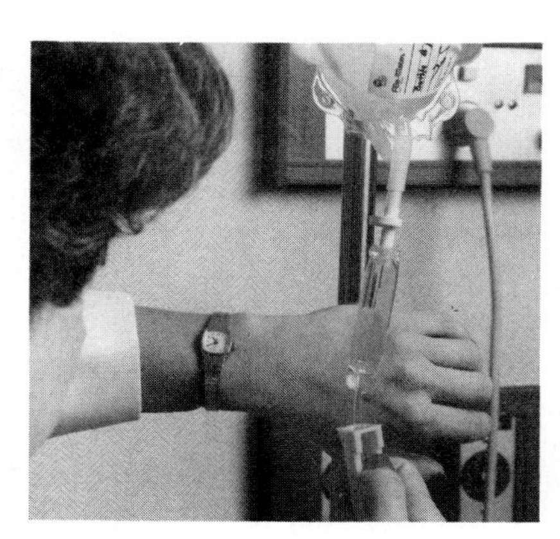

***Fig. 23-15***

| Steps | Rationale |
|---|---|
| 6. Follow this procedure for infusion pump. | |
| a. Place electronic eye on drip chamber below origin of drop and above fluid level in chamber (Fig. 23-16). | IV infusion pumps monitor fluids based on flow rate or drops per minute and have electronic eyes that count number of drops flowing from administration set. |
| b. IV infusion tubing is placed within ridges of control box in direction of flow (i.e., portion of tubing nearest IV bag at top and portion of tubing nearest client at bottom). Required drops per minute are selected, door to control tubing is shut, power button is turned on, and start button is pressed (Fig. 23-17). | Infusion pumps move fluid by compressing and milking IV tubing, thus propelling fluid through tubing. |
| c. Drip regulator must be open while infusion pump is in use. | |
| d. Monitor infusion rates at least hourly. | Infusion pumps are not infallible and do not replace frequent, accurate nursing assessments. |
| e. Assess patency of system when alarm sounds. | Alarm indicates that electronic eye has not noted precise number of drops from drip chamber. Factors triggering alarm on infusion pump can result from empty solution bag or bottle, kink in tubing, closed drip regulator, infiltrated or clotted needle. |
| 7. Follow this procedure for volume control device. | |
| a. Place volume control device between IV bag and insertion spike of infusion set (Fig. 23-18). | Reduces risk of sudden increases in fluid volume. |
| b. Place 2 hours of fluid into device. | Prevents IV line from running dry if nurse does not return in exactly 60 min. In addition, if there is accidental increase in flow rate, client receives at most only 2 hours' allotment of fluid. |
| c. Assess system at least hourly; add fluid to volume control device. Regulate flow rate. | Maintains patency of system. |

## Evaluation

| Steps | Rationale |
|---|---|
| 1. Observe client to determine response to therapy and restoration of fluid and electrolyte balance. | Signs and symptoms of dehydration or overhydration warrant changing rate of fluid infused. |
| 2. Evaluate for signs of infiltration: inflammation at site, clot in catheter, kink or knot in infusion tubing (Skill 23-1). | Prevents decrease or cessation of flow rate. |

### *Expected outcome*

| Steps | Rationale |
|---|---|
| 1. Infusion rate remains within prescribed flow. | Client receives prescribed volume of fluid. |

### *Unexpected outcomes*

| Steps | Rationale |
|---|---|
| 1. Sudden infusion of large volume of solution occurs, causing fluid overload. | Result of rapid administration of large amount of fluid into circulating blood volume. Signs and symptoms indicate client's cardiovascular and/or renal status cannot adapt to large volume. |
| 2. There is empty IV solution container with subsequent loss of IV line patency. | Absence of IV fluid allows clot to form at tip of catheter and occludes line. |

## Recording and Reporting

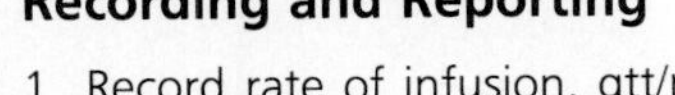

| Steps | Rationale |
|---|---|
| 1. Record rate of infusion, gtt/min and ml/hr, in nurses' notes every 4 hr. | Documents that the prescribed flow is delivered to client. |

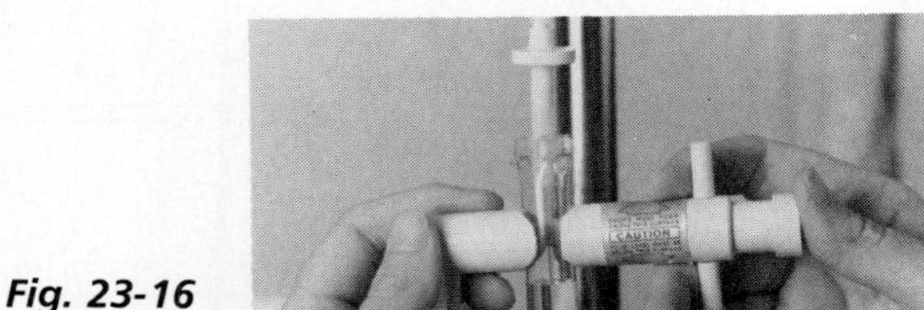

***Fig. 23-16***

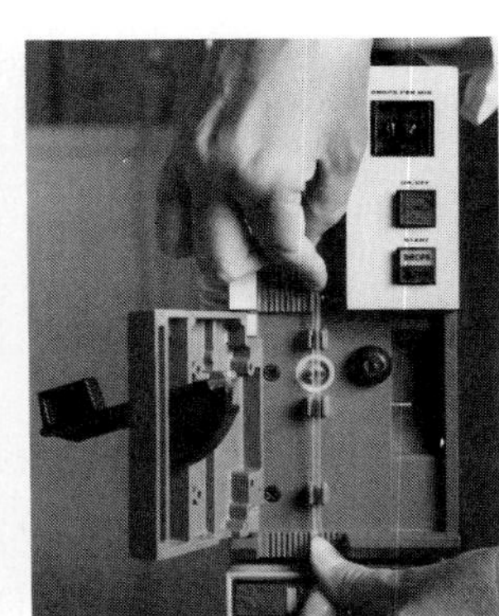

***Fig. 23-17***

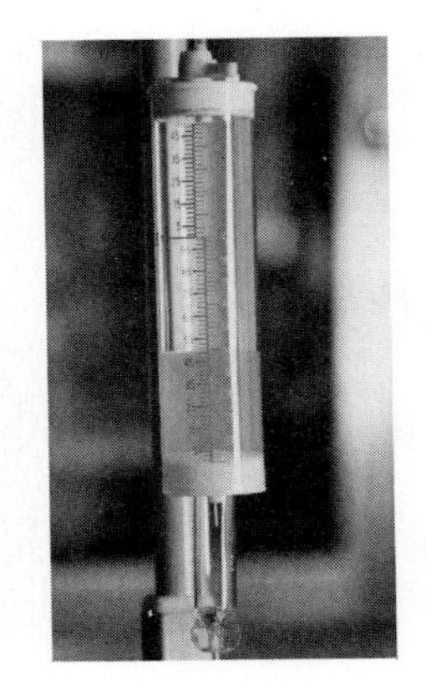

***Fig. 23-18***

| Steps | Rationale |
|---|---|
| 2. Immediately record in nurses' notes any new IV fluid rates. | Specifically documents at what point fluid rate was changed. |
| 3. At change of shift or when leaving on break, report rate of infusion to nurse in charge or next nurse assigned to care for client. | Assists in maintaining continuity of therapy. |
| **Follow-up Activities** | |
| 1. Recalculate flow rate based on volume of fluid remaining, time of infusion, and client's status. | IV fluid orders are calculated for 24 hr period; thus sudden increase or decrease in flow rate requires recalculation of remaining fluid over remaining time of infusion. |

### Special Considerations

- If rapid flow of fluid is not observed and no kinks are visible, nurse may need to remove dressing to allow full observation of needle or catheter (Skill 23-5).
- Some agencies have conversion chart posted in medication area that specifies desired flow for rate in gtt/min for variety of IV fluid prescriptions.
- Many institutions use infusion pump on all clients with fluid and electrolyte disturbances. Pediatric clients or clients with fluctuating fluid and electrolyte status should have volume control devices or infusion pumps to regulate IV fluid solution.
- Nurses should not depend entirely on visual cue provided by time taping. Nurse routinely monitors IV infusion rate and regulates flow accordingly.
- Rate of infusion should be checked by watch, even when infusion pump is used.

### Teaching Considerations

- Client should know the prescribed hourly flow of IV fluids.
- If an infusion pump is used, the client should know its preset rate and the significance of alarms.
- Teach client, primary care giver to time drops per minute using watch with second hand.
- Teach primary care giver why flow rate may decrease and how to correct rate.
- Instruct client, primary care giver not to increase flow rate without checking with nurse.

### Home Care Considerations

- Make sure nurse is in the home when IV pump is delivered. This enables nurse to determine that equipment properly works.
- Ensure that client's electrical outlets are properly grounded.

# *SKILL 23-3*
# *CHANGING IV SOLUTIONS*

Because clients receiving IV therapy may require frequent changing of IV solutions, the nurse should allow adequate time for this procedure.

Occasionally clients have an infusion only to deliver IV medication every 4, 6, or 8 hr (Chapter 20). In this case an hourly infusion flow of about 10-15 ml/hr is used to keep the vein open (KVO) and usually a microdrip infusion set is used. Generally these clients do not use an entire IV solution bag. However, they need to have a new solution bag or bottle at least once every 24 hr because the sterility of the solution cannot be guaranteed for longer than a day.

### Purposes

1. Maintain fluid balance.
2. Follow physician's orders.
3. Ensure sterility of solution.

## *Procedure 23-3*

| Steps | Rationale |
|---|---|
| **Assessment** | |
| 1. Check physician's orders. | Ensures that correct solution will be used. |
| 2. If order is written for KVO, note date and time when solution was last changed. | Sterility of solutions in bag or bottle cannot be guaranteed for longer than 24 hr (CDC, 1982). |

| Steps | Rationale |
|---|---|
| **Planning** | |
| 1. Develop individualized goals for client: | |
| a. Maintain client's fluid and electrolyte balance. | IV solutions promote and maintain adequate fluid and electrolyte balance. |
| b. Promote infusion of client's IV solutions as ordered by physician. | Instillation of correct solution, as ordered by physician, assists in restoring or maintaining fluid and electrolyte balance. |
| 2. Have next solution prepared at least 1 hr before needed. If prepared in pharmacy, be sure it has been delivered to floor. Check that solution is correct and properly labeled. | Adequate planning reduces risk of clot formation in vein caused by empty IV bag. Checking prevents medication error. |
| 3. Prepare to change solution when fluid remains only in neck of bottle or bag. | Prevents air from entering tubing and vein from clotting from lack of flow. |
| 4. Be sure drip chamber is half full. | Provides fluid to vein while bag is changed. |
| **Implementation** | |
| 1. Wash hands. | Reduces transmission of microorganisms. |
| 2. Prepare new solution for changing. If using plastic bag, remove protective cover from entry site. If using glass bottle: remove metal cap and metal rubber disks. | Permits quick, smooth, and organized change from old to new solution. |
| 3. Move roller clamp to reduce flow rate. | Prevents solution remaining in drip chamber from emptying while changing solutions. |
| 4. Remove old solution from IV pole (Fig. 23-19). | Brings work to nurse's eye level. |
| 5. Quickly remove spike from old solution and, without touching tip, spike new bottle. | Reduces risk of solution in drip chamber running dry and maintains sterility. |
| 6. Hang new bag or bottle of solution. | Allows gravity to assist with delivery of fluid into drip chamber. |
| 7. Check for air in tubing. | Reduces risk of air embolus. |
| 8. Make sure drip chamber contains solution. | Reduces risk of air entering tubing. |
| 9. Regulate flow to prescribed rate. | Maintains measures to restore fluid balance and deliver IV fluid as ordered. |
| **Evaluation** | |
| 1. Observe client to determine response to IV fluid therapy. | Provides ongoing evaluation of client's fluid and electrolyte status. |
| ***Expected outcomes*** | |
| 1. Fluid infusion is correct. | Documents that physician's fluid order is being carried out. |
| 2. IV line remains patent. | |
| 3. Fluid and electrolyte balance is maintained. | Documents that prescribed rate of flow is followed. |
| ***Unexpected outcome*** | |
| 1. Infusion hanging or flow rate is incorrect. | Incorrect infusion of solution or infusion of incorrect volume is medication error. |
| **Recording and Reporting** | |
| 1. Record amount and type of fluid infused and amount and type of new fluid. | Documents that solution has infused and new solution has been started. |

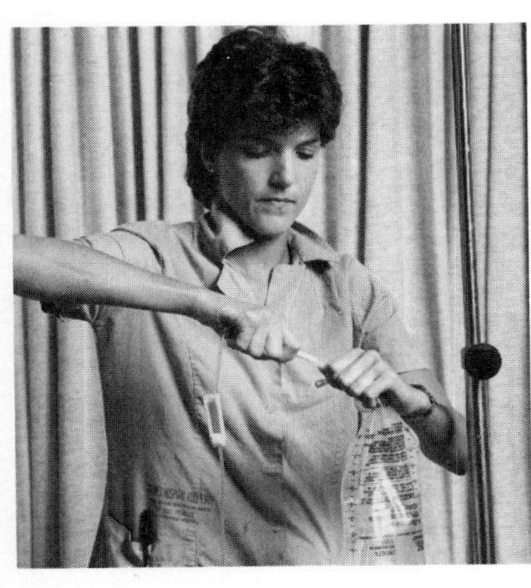

***Fig. 23-19***

| Steps | Rationale |
|---|---|
| **Follow-up Activities** | |
| 1. Complete incident report when incorrect infusion is delivered to client. | Provides institution with specific documentation of error. |

### Special Considerations

- IV fluid orders are written at least daily by physician.
- Contamination of infusion set increases risk of infection.
- If client is critically ill, nurse should plan to review client's medical orders at least every 2 hr.
- Following "five rights" reduces risk of hanging wrong solution. If this happens, stop infusion, replace with correct solution or $D_5W$, notify physician.
- Some agencies require that notations on changes of IV solution be noted in nurses' notes and IV infusion flow sheet.

### Teaching Considerations

- Inform client of new solution and additives.
- Inform client of changes in prescribed flow rate.
- Tell client how long the solution should run (e.g., 4 hours, 8 hours).

### Home Care Considerations

- If client or family must pick up antibiotics or other parenteral fluids from hospital pharmacy, be sure physician's orders have been completed to avoid needless waiting by client or family at hospital.

## *SKILL 23-4*
## *CHANGING INFUSION TUBING*

Technically, IV tubing can remain sterile for 48 hr; however, most institutions recommend that new sterile tubing be used every 24 hr. The hospital or agency policy manual contains specific guidelines as to when tubing is to be changed. The procedure is much simpler and more efficient if the nurse changes the infusion tubing when preparing to hang a new bag or bottle.

However, situations arise when the nurse needs to change tubing without hanging a new bag. Such situations include accidental puncture of the tubing from a "piggyback" IV medication (Chapter 20) or after infusion of packed red cells or whole blood (Chapter 25). To prevent the entry of bacteria into the client's bloodstream when infusion tubing is changed, sterility must be maintained.

### Purposes

1. Maintain infusion therapy.
2. Maintain sterility of IV therapy system.
3. Maintain patency of infusion tubing.

## *Procedure 23-4*

| Steps | Rationale |
|---|---|
| **Assessment** | |
| 1. Determine when new infusion set is warranted: | |
| a. Hanging first solution of day. | IV tubing should be changed daily, and procedure is simplified when changing tubing with new solution. |
| b. Puncture of infusion tubing. | Punctured tubing results in fluid leakage. |
| c. Contamination of tubing. | Contamination of tubing allows entry of bacteria into client's bloodstream. |
| 2. Observe for occlusions in tubing. Such occlusions can occur after infusion of packed red blood cells, whole blood, or albumin. | Whole blood or blood component products can occlude or partially occlude tubing. |
| **Nursing Diagnosis** | |
| 1. Cluster data to reveal actual or potential nursing diagnoses: | |
| a. Potential for infection: | |

| Steps | Rationale |
|---|---|
| ▪ Related to contamination of IV tubing. | Puncture of tubing results in port of entry for bacteria, thus contaminating tubing. |
| ▪ Related to accidental separation of tubing from IV needle or catheter. | Separation of tubing permits port of entry for bacteria. |
| b. Potential fluid volume deficit: related to occlusion of tubing administration of viscous solutions such as blood or blood components. | Viscous solutions adhere to walls of tubing and decrease size of lumen, in some cases totally occluding tubing. |

## Planning

| Steps | Rationale |
|---|---|
| 1. Develop individualized goals for client based on nursing diagnoses: | |
| a. Maintain sterility of infusion tubing. | Break in sterility permits entrance of bacteria, increasing risk of bacteremia. |
| b. Maintain patency of client's IV tubing. | Decreasing patency of infusion tubing can ultimately decrease rate of flow. |
| 2. Assemble the following:<br>a. Infusion tubing<br>b. Sterile 2 × 2 or 4 × 4 gauze pads<br>c. If a new IV dressing must be applied:<br>▪ Sterile 2 × 2 gauze pads<br>▪ Sterile 4 × 4 gauze pads<br>▪ Povidone-iodine ointment<br>▪ Adhesive remover<br>▪ Povidone-iodine solution<br>▪ Alcohol swabs<br>▪ Strips of tape or polyurethane film dressing<br>▪ Disposable gloves | Placement of all equipment at bedside enables nurse to efficiently and safely complete procedure. |
| 3. Explain procedure to client. | Promotes cooperation and prevents sudden movement of extremity, which could dislodge IV needle or catheter. |

## Implementation

| Steps | Rationale |
|---|---|
| 1. Wash hands. | Reduces transmission of microorganisms. |
| 2. Open new infusion set, keeping protective coverings over infusion spike and insertion site for butterfly needle or IV catheter. | Provides nurse with ready access to new infusion set and maintains sterility of infusion set. |
| 3. Apply nonsterile, disposable gloves. | Reduces risk of exposure to HIV, hepatitis, and other blood-borne bacteria (CDC, 1987). |
| 4. Place sterile 2 × 2 or 4 × 4 gauze pads on bed near IV puncture site. | Provides sterile field for new sterile needle adapter before connection to IV needle or catheter. |
| 5. If needle or catheter hub is not visible, remove IV dressing as directed in Skill 23-5. Do not remove tape securing needle or catheter to skin. | Needle hub must be accessible to provide smooth transition when removing old and inserting new tubing. |
| 6. Take new IV tubing and move roller clamp to "off" position. | Prevents spillage of solution after bag or bottle is spiked. |
| 7. Slow rate of infusion by regulating drip rate on old tubing. | Prevents complete infusion of solution remaining in tubing. Complete infusion of solution remaining in tubing increases risk of occlusion of IV catheter or needle. |
| 8. With old tubing in place, compress drip chamber and fill chamber. | Provides surplus of fluid in drip chamber so there is enough fluid to maintain IV patency while changing tubing. |
| 9. Discontinue old tubing from solution and hang drip chamber over IV pole. | Allows fluid to continue to flow through IV catheter while nurse is preparing new tubing. |
| 10. Place insertion spike of new tubing into old solution opening and hang or tape solution on IV pole. | Permits flow of fluid from solution into new infusion tubing. |
| 11. Compress and release drip chamber on new tubing. | Allows drip chamber to fill and promote rapid, smooth flow of solution through new tubing. |
| 12. Open roller clamp, remove protective cap from needle adapter, and flush tubing with solution. | Removes air from tubing and replaces it with fluid. |
| 13. Place needle adapter of new tubing, with protective cap off, between sterile 2 × 2 or 4 × 4 gauze pads near client's site (Fig. 23-20). | Provides smooth, quick insertion of new tubing into needle hub while maintaining sterility of infusion tubing. |
| 14. Turn roller clamp on old tubing to "off" position. | Prevents spillage of fluid as tubing is removed from needle hub. |
| 15. Stabilize hub of catheter or needle and gently pull out old tubing. Maintain stability of hub and insert needle adapter of new tubing into hub (Figs. 23-21 and 23-22). | Prevents accidental displacement of catheter or needle. |

| Steps | Rationale |
|---|---|

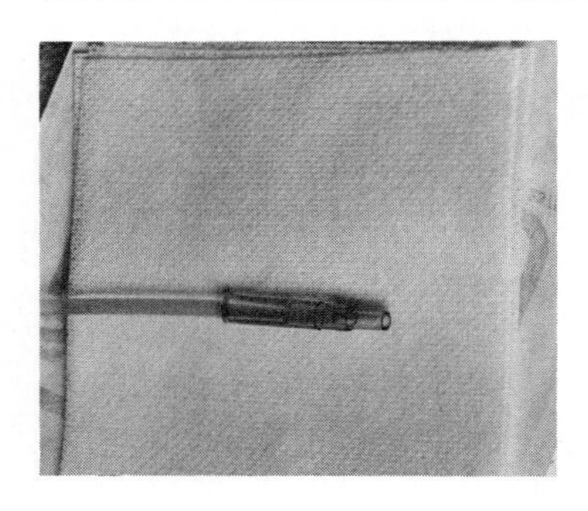

*Fig. 23-20*

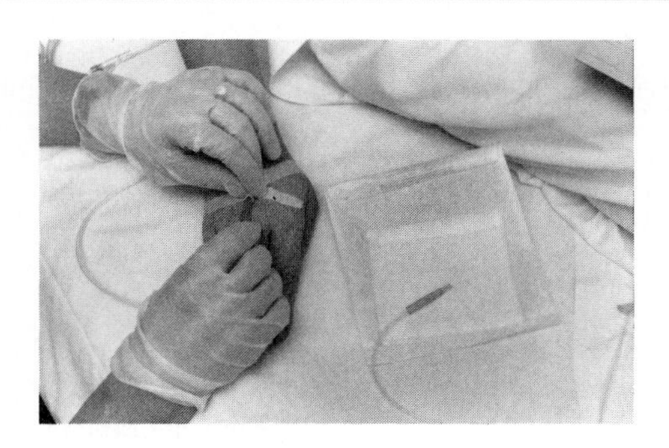

*Fig. 23-21*

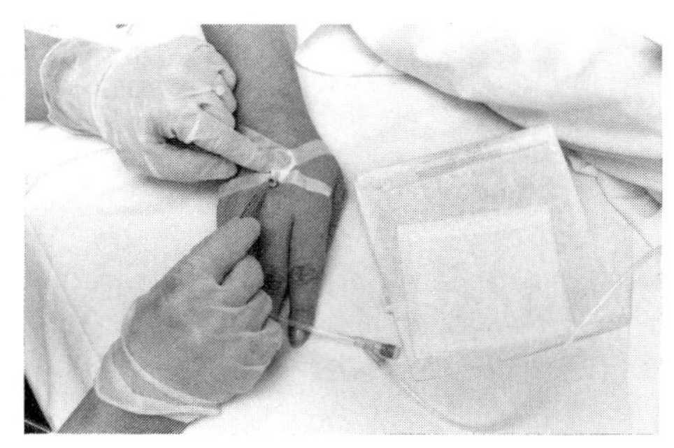

*Fig. 23-22*

| Steps | Rationale |
|---|---|
| 16. Open roller clamp on new tubing. Allow solution to run rapidly for 30 to 60 sec. | Permits IV solution to enter catheter or tubing. |
| 17. Regulate IV drip according to physician's orders and monitor rate hourly. | Maintains infusion flow at prescribed rate. |
| 18. If necessary, apply new dressing (Skill 23-5). | Reduces risk of bacterial infection from skin. |
| 19. Discard old tubing in container for contaminated materials. | Reduces accidental transmission of microorganisms. |
| 20. Remove and disopose of gloves. Wash hands. | Reduces transmission of microorganisms. |

## Evaluation

| | |
|---|---|
| 1. Evaluate flow rate and observe connection site for leakage. | Maintains prescribed rate of flow of IV therapy and determines if fit is secure. |

### *Expected outcomes*

| | |
|---|---|
| 1. Absence of infection. | Maintains sterility. |
| 2. Absence of leakage of solution from tubing. | Prevents contamination of solution through disconnection of connection tubing. |
| 3. Patent IV tubing. | Maintains closed, sterile system and regulation of IV flow. |

### *Unexpected outcome*

| | |
|---|---|
| 1. Decreased or absent flow of IV fluid indicated by decreased rate. | Can occur if nurse fails to open drip regulator and recalibrate drip rate on new tubing. Infiltration or occlusion of catheter can also be the cause. |

## Recording and Reporting

| | |
|---|---|
| 1. Record changing of tubing and solution on client' record. | Documents procedure and records that measures to maintain sterility were carried out. |
| 2. Place piece of tape with date and time below level of drip chamber. | Provides visual cue to all care providers of when IV tubing was changed. |

## Follow-up Activities

| | |
|---|---|
| 1. Determine presence of blood return. | Maintains patency and correct flow of fluids. When tubing is kinked, an infiltration is present or rate of flow is decreased. |
| 2. If solution slowed or increased, recalibrate IV flow in gtt/min to prescribed rate. | Amount of fluid infused is altered. |
| 3. Inspect tubing for kinks and venipuncture site for infiltrations. | |

## Special Considerations

- Flushing tubing with 0.9 normal saline after administration of whole blood or blood components can reduce risk of occlusion of IV tubing.
- If separation of tubing from needle is required to irrigate needle, IV should be turned off and distal end of IV tubing should be placed on sterile 4 × 4 gauze pads, or sterile needle cover placed over distal end.
- If infusion pump is used, remove tubing from pump.

## Teaching Considerations

- Instruct client to notify nurse if fluid leaks around IV site or from the tubing itself.
- Instruct client to notify nurse if tubing separates from catheter, infusion device, or IV container.

# SKILL 23-5
# CHANGING AN IV DRESSING

After an intravenous line is in place, the nurse must have visual access to the insertion site to inspect it for possible signs of infection or early signs of infiltration. When a gauze dressing is selected, the dressing is changed every 24 hours. The newer, clear polyurethane dressings are changed every 3 to 5 days (Lawson, 1986). Sterile dressing changes reduce the risk of infection at the venipuncture site.

## Purposes

1. Decrease bacterial contamination of the venipuncture site.
2. Maintain patency of the IV therapy system.
3. Inspect the venipuncture site for infiltration or infection.

## Procedure 23-5

| Steps | Rationale |
|---|---|
| **Assessment** | |
| 1. Determine when dressing was last changed. Many institutions require nurse to write date and time on dressing. | Provides information regarding length of time that present dressing has been in place. In addition, nurse is able to plan for dressing change. |
| 2. Observe present dressing for moisture. | Moisture is medium for bacterial growth. Moisture on sterile dressing renders dressing contaminated. |
| 3. Observe present dressing for intactness. | Nonadhering dressing increases risk of bacterial contamination to venipuncture site or displacement of IV catheter. |
| 4. Observe IV system for proper functioning or complications: kinks in infusion tubing or IV catheter, infiltration, inflammation. | Unexplained decrease in flow rate or pain and swelling at venipuncture site require nurse to investigate placement and patency of IV catheter. |
| **Nursing Diagnosis** | |
| 1. Cluster data to reveal actual or potential nursing diagnoses, including: | |
| a. Potential for infection: related to old or contaminated IV dressing. | Old or contaminated IV dressings increase risk for developing infection at IV site or for bacterial invasion into blood stream. |
| **Planning** | |
| 1. Develop individualized goals for client based on nursing diagnoses, including: | |
| a. Maintain sterility of venipuncture site. | Break in sterility permits entrance of bacteria and increases risk of bacteremia. |
| b. Maintain patency of IV system. | Break in integrity of IV system increases risk of bacteremia, clot formation within needle or catheter, or infiltration. |
| 2. Assemble necessary equipment<br>a. Sterile 2 × 2 gauze pad<br>b. Sterile 4 × 4 gauze pad<br>c. Povidone-iodine ointment<br>d. Adhesive remover<br>e. Povidone-iodine solution<br>f. Alcohol swabs<br>g. Strips of tape or polyurethane film dressing<br>h. Disposable gloves | Placement of all equipment at bedside enables nurse to efficiently and safely complete procedure.<br><br>Many institutions are adopting clear, thin, adhesive-backed polyurethane dressings (Fig. 23-23) that provide barrier against bacteria, allow continuous observation of venipuncture site, and eliminate necessity of daily dressing changes (Runquist, 1984). |

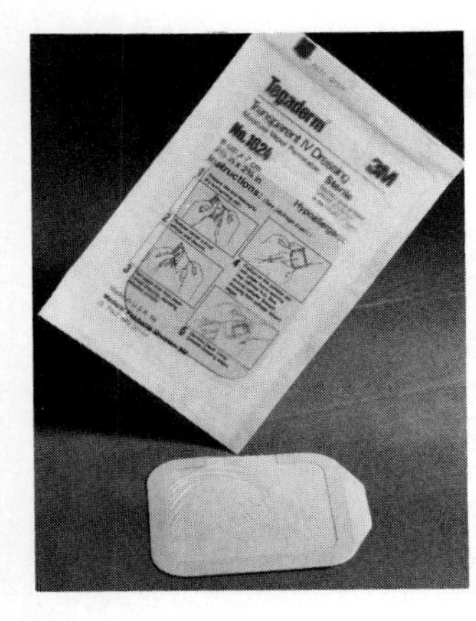


*Fig. 23-23*

| Steps | Rationale |
|---|---|
| 3. Explain procedure to client. Explain that affected extremity must be held still and how long procedure will take. | Assists in obtaining client cooperation; gives client time frame around which personal activities can be planned. |

## Implementation

| Steps | Rationale |
|---|---|
| 1. Wash hands. | Reduces transmission of microorganisms. |
| 2. Apply disposable gloves. | Reduces risk to HIV, hepatitis, and other blood-borne bacteria. |
| 3. Remove tape and gauze from old dressing one layer at a time, leaving tape that secures IV needle or catheter in place. | Prevents accidental displacement of catheter or needle, which can occur if catheter tubing becomes tangled between two layers of dressing. |
| 4. If infiltration, phlebitis or clot occur or if ordered by physician, discontinue infusion. | |
| a. Turn roller clamp to "off" position. | Prevents spillage of IV fluid on bed, client, nurse, or floor. |
| b. Place gauze or alcohol pad over venipuncture site and remove catheter or needle by pulling straight away from site. | Prevents damage to client's vein. |
| c. Apply pressure to site for 1 to 2 min. | Controls bleeding or hematoma formation. |
| 5. If IV is infusing properly, gently remove tape securing needle or catheter. Stabilize needle or catheter with one hand. | Exposes venipuncture site. Stabilization prevents accidental displacement of catheter or needle. |
| 6. Use adhesive remover to cleanse skin and remove adhesive residue. | Adhesive residue decreases ability of new tape to adhere tightly to skin. |
| 7. Using circular motion, cleanse insertion site with povidone-iodine solution followed by alcohol (Fig. 23-24). | Circular motion prevents cross-contamination from skin bacteria near venipuncture site. Povidone-iodine is topical anti-infective; alcohol is topical antiseptic. Together, they reduce skin surface bacteria. |
| 8. Replace single strip of adhesive tape to anchor IV catheter or needle. | Prevents accidental displacement of catheter or needle. |
| 9. Place povidone-iodine ointment or solution on venipuncture site. | Povidone-iodine is topical antiseptic germicide that reduces skin bacteria and therefore reduces risk of local or systemic infection.<br>Manufacturers of polyurethane dressings do not recommend use of antiseptic ointment over puncture site because ointment interferes with adherence of dressing to skin. Instead they recommend use of antiseptic such as povidone-iodine solution on puncture site. Once antiseptic has dried, clear dressing is applied (Runquist, 1984). |
| 10. Place 2 × 2, 4 × 4 or a clear dressing over venipuncture site. If a clear dressing is selected, apply it in the direction of hair growth (Fig. 23-25). | Provides barrier against bacteria. |
| 11. Remove and discard gloves. | |

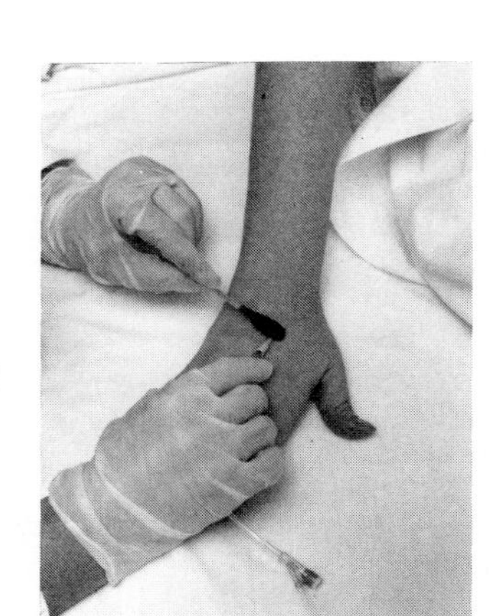

***Fig. 23-24***

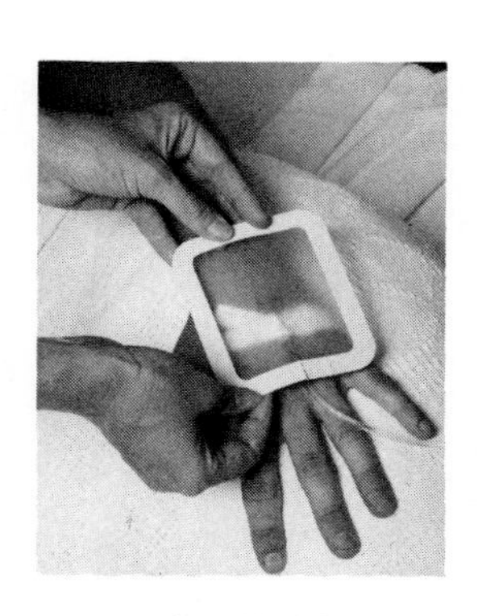

***Fig. 23-25***

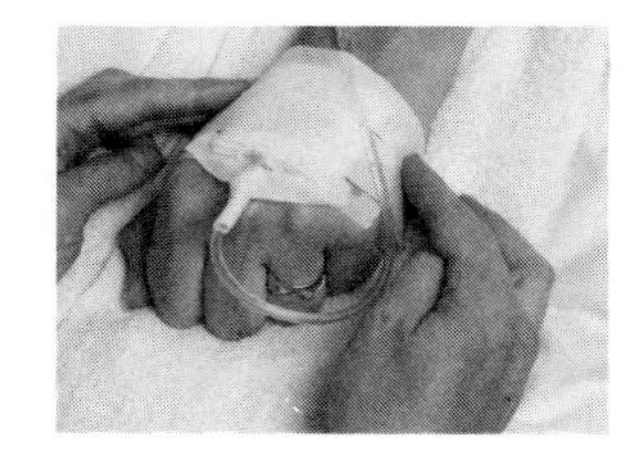

***Fig. 23-26***

| Steps | Rationale |
|---|---|
| 12. Anchor IV tubing with additional pieces of tape (Fig. 23-26). When using polyurethane dressing avoid placing tape directly over dressing. | Prevents accidental displacement of IV needle or catheter or separation of IV tubing from needle adapter. |
| 13. Place date and time of dressing change directly on dressing. | Documents dressing change. |
| 14. Discard equipment and wash hands. | Reduces transmission of microorganisms. |
| **Evaluation** | |
| 1. Observe functioning and patency of IV system in response to changing dressing. | Validates that IV is patent and functioning correctly. |
| ***Expected outcomes*** | |
| 1. IV is patent as evidenced by absence of infiltration, phlebitis, or clot. | Maintains flow rate as prescribed by physician. |
| 2. Absence of infection. | Maintains sterility of system. |
| ***Unexpected outcomes*** | |
| 1. IV catheter or needle is infiltrated, as evidenced by decreased flow rate or edema, pallor, or decreased temperature around insertion site. | Indicates fluid in interstitial space. |
| 2. Phlebitis is present as evidenced by erythema and tenderness along vein pathway. | Results from inflammation of vein. |
| 3. IV catheter or needle, is accidently removed. | Can occur after incorrect removal of dressing. |
| **Reporting and Recording** | |
| 1. Record in nurses' notes time IV dressing was changed. Include patency of system and observation of venipuncture site. | Documents that dressing was changed, functioning of IV system, and that venipuncture site is free of infection. |
| 2. Report to nurse in charge or oncoming nursing shift that dressing was changed and any significant information about integrity of system. | Assists in verification of care delivered and planning of future nursing care. |
| **Follow-up Activities** | |
| 1. When infiltration or phlebitis is present: | |
| a. Remove IV catheter or needle and place warm, moist heat to affected area. | Warm, moist heat improves circulation and decreases edema in interstitial space. |
| b. Initiate another IV using another extremity. | Use of another extremity avoids further injury to already inflamed vein. |
| 2. If IV is accidentally removed, initiate new line. | Maintains therapy as prescribed by physician. |

## Special Considerations

- If there is no date or time on gauze IV dressing, assume that present dressing is at least 24 hours old and plan to change it.
- Pediatric clients may not be able to fully understand nurse's explanation. Presence of parent or security toy during procedure can help to decrease fear and increase cooperation.
- When using polyurethane film dressing, observe venipuncture site. If there is no sign of infection and IV is patent, dressing does not need to be removed.
- Clients who have received heparin require longer pressure (5-10 min or more) on site because of action of heparin on blood-clotting mechanisms.

## Teaching Considerations

- When a transparent dressing is used, instruct client that it may remain in place for approximately 5 days.
- Client should be instructed to notify nurse if skin under dressing or tape becomes reddened, itches, or burns or if dressing becomes dislodged.

## BIBLIOGRAPHY

Barfoot KR, Ross KL: Intravenous therapy at home: an overview, Home Healthc Nurse 6(4):11, 1988.

Bogkoff SC, Boxnell AD, Boxnell JJ: Six ways to clear air from an IV line, Nursing 18(2):46, 1988.

Bulau JM: Clinical policies and procedures for home health care, Rockville, Md, 1986, Aspen Publishers, Inc.

Byers PH: Comparison of application factors among three brands of transparent semipermeable film for peripheral IVs, NITA, 8:315, 1985.

Centers for Disease Control: Guidelines for intravascular infections. Infection control 3:61, 1982.

Centers for Disease Control: Recommendations for prevention of HIV transmission in health care settings. MMWR 36 (suppl 25) 35, 1987.

Golden S: Nursing a loved one at home, Philadelphia, 1988, Running Press Book Publishers.

Gorski L: Effective teaching of home IV therapy, 5(5):10, 12, 16, 1987.

Groer MW: Physiology and pathophysiology of body fluids, ed 2, St Louis, 1989, The CV Mosby Co.

Josephson A, Gombert ME, Sierra MF, et al.: The relationship between intravenous fluid contamination and the frequently of tubing replacement, Infect Control 6(9):367, 1985.

Lawson M, Kavanagh T, McCredie K, et al.: Comparison of transparent dressings to paper tape dressing over central venous catheter sites, NITA 9(1):40, 1986.

Mascaro J: Managing IV therapy in the home, Nursing 86, 16(5):50, 1986.

Mellema SJ, Ponintoveski BC: Geriatric IV therapy, J Intravenous Therapy 11(1):56, 1988.

Metheny NM: Overview of fluid and electrolyte balance, NITA 4:38, 1981.

Metheny NM, Snively WD: Nurse's handbook of fluid balance, ed 4, Philadelphia, 1983, JB Lippincott Co.

Millam DA: Managing complications of IV therapy, Nursing '88 18(3):34, 1988.

Nelms R: Keeping air out of IV lines, Nursing '86 16(3):57, 1986.

Potter PA, Perry AG: Fundamentals of nursing: concepts, process, and practice, ed 2, St Louis, 1989, The CV Mosby Co.

Runquist B, Aspinall J, Hibbard L: A new approach for problem IV dressings, RN 47(6):49, 1984.

Sager D, Bomar S: Intravenous medications, Philadelphia, 1980, JB Lippincott Co.

Walsh J: Persons C, Wieck L: Manual of home health care nursing, Philadelphia, 1987, JB Lippincott Co.

Wetmore N: Extravasation: the dreaded complication, NITA 8:47, 1985.

Whaley LF, Wong DL: Nursing care of infants and children, ed 3, St Louis, 1987, The CV Mosby Co.

Wiseman M: Setting standards for home IV therapy, Am J Nurs 85:421, 1985.

# 24

# VASCULAR ACCESS DEVICES

## OBJECTIVES

*Mastery of content in this chapter will enable the nurse to:*

- Define the key terms.
- Identify types of vascular access devices (VADs) in use today.
- Describe the rationale for selecting a particular type of VAD.
- Assess the educational needs of clients with VADs, including care, maintenance, safety, discharge preparation, and home use.
- Implement appropriate interventions using VADs according to specific plans of therapy.
- Evaluate the effectiveness of interventions to determine ways to prevent or minimize complications in the management of VADs.

## KEY TERMS

*Aspirate*
*Cannula*
*Catheter hub*
*Central venous catheter*
*Cephalic vein*
*Dacron cuff*
*Embolus*
*Exit site*
*External jugular vein*
*Hemodialysis*
*Huber needle*
*Implanted infusion port*
*Injection cap*
*Insertion site*
*Intraclavicular fossa*
*Irrigate*
*Lumen*
*Oncology*
*Percutaneous*
*Plasmapheresis*
*Right atrial catheter*
*Sclerosis*
*Sepsis*
*Silicone septum*
*Subcutaneous tunnel*
*Vascular access device (VAD)*

## SKILLS

**24-1** Caring for Vascular Access Devices

Clients with chronic disease often need long-term IV therapy, which requires safe, repeated access to the venous system for administration of drugs, fluids, nutrition, and blood products. Frequent venipuncture (Chapter 23) and multiple IV lines pose problems and risks, including infection, pain, and bruising. Clients with chronic disease are generally more susceptible to infection and bleeding. Clients receiving multiple doses of chemotherapeutic drugs (Chapter 22) experience vein sclerosis or hardening. Eventually, no suitable peripheral veins remain for drug administration.

The need for safe and convenient long-term IV therapy has led to the development of VADs, which are catheters, cannulas, or infusion ports designed for long-term, repeated access to the venous or arterial systems. The nurse must be able to maintain the integrity of central venous catheters and implanted infusion ports and educate clients about the care of catheters for home use.

Home health nurses frequently administer parenteral nutrition (Chapter 28) and chemotherapy (Chapter 22) in the home using VADs. The trend in the care of oncology clients is expanded home health services. VADs allow clients to go home earlier and receive continued care rather than remain in acute-care settings for several weeks.

Nurses play a role in identifying clients who may benefit from VADs. For example, a client with severe nutritional deficiencies may need long-term parenteral nutrition. The nurse may be the first to recognize the client's intolerance to oral or enteral feedings.

The types of VADs and their therapeutic uses vary according to the the diagnosis. Nurses must have the necessary knowledge, skill, and judgment to maintain and trouble shoot VADs. Client education is also important. Clients and families learn to change dressings around catheters and to recognize signs of complications such as infection, bleeding, or leakage at insertion sites.

## GUIDELINES

1. Know the types of VADs in use today (implanted and indwelling), including indications for the use, complications, and maintenance.
2. Know the manufacturer's recommendations and have reference literature available to give to clients, family, and health care professionals.
3. Know hospital policy and procedure for using each device for repeated safe vascular access.

4. Know the surgical technique for placement of each VAD and the anatomic sites involved in catheter insertion. For example, care for an arterial catheter is different than care for a venous catheter.
5. Know the client's medical diagnosis, past history, stage of disease, and the primary purpose for using the VAD.
6. Know the schedule for administration of fluids, drugs, nutrition, and blood products, as well as for blood sampling, dressing changes, and heparin irrigations of the VAD. This knowledge minimizes the number of times the device must be entered.
7. Flush the catheter after each use and as directed by manufacturer's recommendations and institutional policy and procedure to assure continued patency.
8. Identify whether catheters have single or double lumens. Simultaneous infusion of incompatible fluids should be cautiously performed, especially for drugs with a low solubility factor like phenytoin or doxorubicin.
9. Involve the client and family in care plan so they can obtain skills needed to maintain the VAD.
10. Anticipate discharge needs. Be sure the necessary supplies for dressing changes and irrigations are available for the client. A home care referral may be needed so a nurse can monitor care and ensure that the client is capable of managing the VAD.

### PREREQUISITE KNOWLEDGE

1. Principles of medical asepsis.
2. Principles of IV therapy.
3. Principles of teaching and learning.
4. Anatomy of cardiovascular system.
5. Health care problems of the chronically ill.

### PREREQUISITE SKILLS

1. Initiation, maintenance, and regulation of IV fluids (Chapter 23).
2. Administration of IV medications (Chapter 21). and blood products (Chapter 25).
3. Obtaining blood samples (Chapter 45).
4. Proper handwashing techniques (Chapter 38).
5. Changing a dry, sterile dressing (Chapter 41).
6. Application of sterile gloves, gown, and mask (Chapter 38).
7. Application of a sterile drape (Chapter 38).

## *SKILL 24-1 Caring for Vascular Access Devices*

To manage long-term IV therapy effectively the nurse must know the types of VADs, including central venous catheters, external catheters, and implanted infusion ports.

Central venous catheters are inserted by the physician into a large vein, typically the superior vena cava that leads to the right atrium of the heart (Fig. 24-1). The large vessel lumen minimizes the risks of vessel irritation, inflammation, or sclerosis that commonly occur when smaller peripheral veins are used.

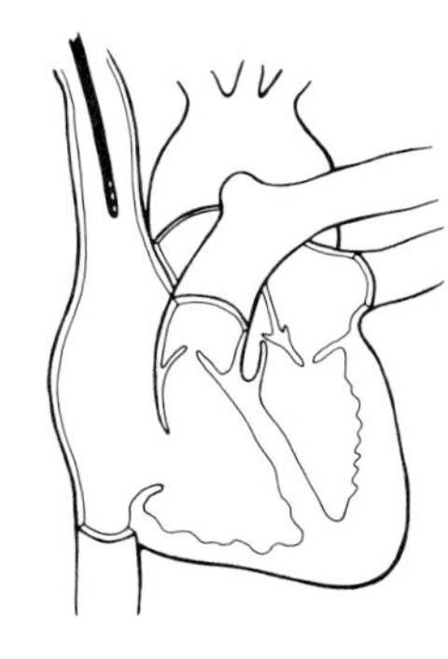

*Fig. 24-1* Catheter tip lies in right atrium.

Atrial catheters are surgically inserted with the client in the operating room under general or local anesthesia. First a tunnel is made through subcutaneous tissue, usually between the clavicle and nipple. The tunnel allows the catheter to remain in place longer because it creates space between the end of the catheter and the actual vein. The risk of infection is less. Then the catheter tip is inserted through the cephalic, internal, or external jugular vein, or a similar large vein, and is threaded into the right atrium (Fig. 24-2). These catheters have single or double lumens; i.e., one or two hollow tubes extend within the inside of the catheter and allow for administration of more than one type of infusion simultaneously.

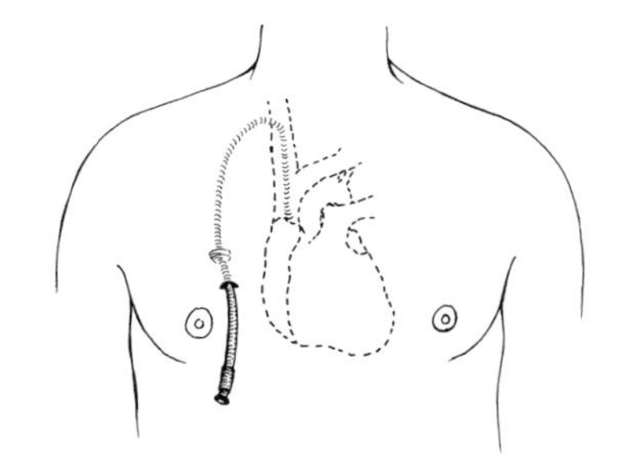

*Fig. 24-2* Small-gauge catheter in place, threaded into right atrium.

A second type of external catheter is the small-gauge central venous catheter, which is inserted directly through the skin and into the subclavian vein of the neck

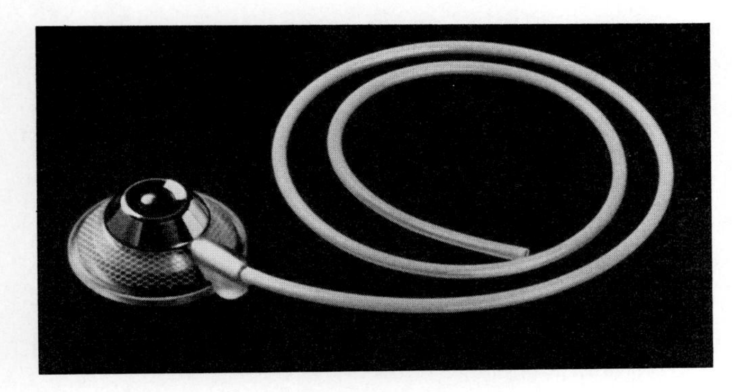

*Fig. 24-3*

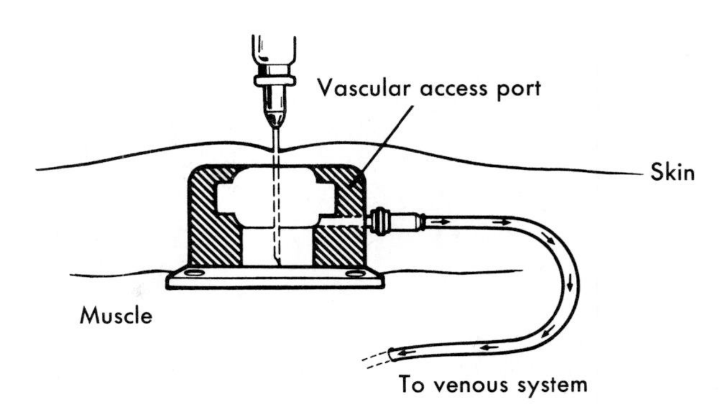


***Fig. 24-4*** Example of a double lumen port.

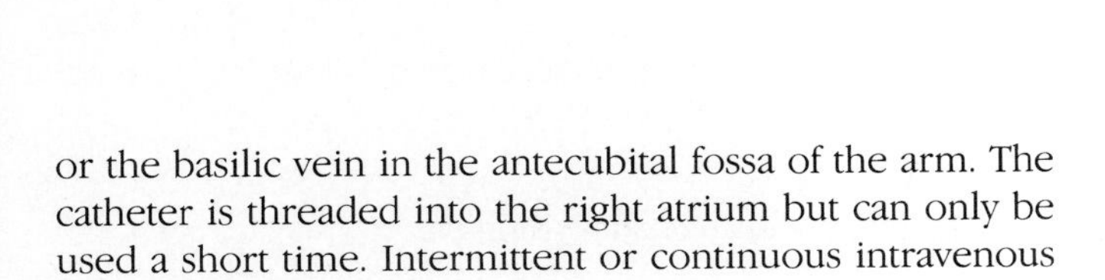

or the basilic vein in the antecubital fossa of the arm. The catheter is threaded into the right atrium but can only be used a short time. Intermittent or continuous intravenous infusions can be given.

The third type of VAD is the implanted infusion port, which consists of a self-sealing injection port housed in a plastic or metal case (Fig. 24-3) and connected to a silicone venous catheter. The port is also now available with a double lumen catheter. The physician implants the infusion port under sterile conditions in an operating room with the client under local anesthesia. The infusion port usually rests in a subcutaneous pocket in the infraclavicular fossa, and the catheter is inserted into a large vein and threaded into the right atrium (Fig. 24-4). The port can be easily palpated to determine placement. Specially designed Huber needles (straight or with 90-degree angles) are inserted through the skin to enter the port (Fig. 24-5). Implanted infusion ports are used for administration of injections and for continuous infusions of all types: medications, chemotherapy, parenteral nutrition, and blood products. The nurse or client heparinizes the port every 4 weeks when not in use to maintain its patency.

Care of VADs is simple as long as nurses and clients are aware of the purpose and function of the devices and the two most common complications, infection and clotting. In the home, most clients learn to use clean technique for dressing changes and catheter care. Within 2 to 3 weeks

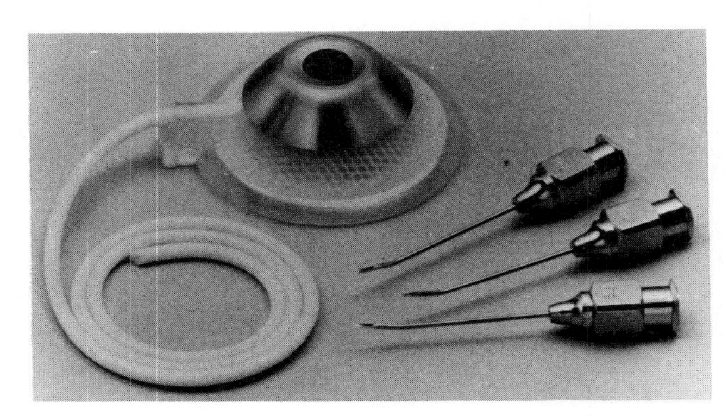

*Fig. 24-5*

an adhesive bandage is sufficient to cover catheter insertion sites. Clients can learn to initiate infusions, heparinize devices, and discontinue infusions.

### Purposes

1. Provide a dependable, safe route for long-term IV therapy.
2. Provide a means of delivering more than one IV infusion simultaneously through a single access.
3. Prevent injury to a client from introduction of infectious organisms or air into the vascular system.
4. Maintain patency of catheters or infusion ports.
5. Prevent damage to VADs.
6. Provide clients with skills needed to care for VADs and to monitor infusions.

## *Procedure 24-1*

| Steps | Rationale |
|---|---|
| **Assessment** | |
| 1. Assess diagnosis of client's stage of disease and plan of therapy by review of medical record. | Allows nurse to understand need for vascular access in treatment of disease and in evaluation of response to therapy and to determine need to educate client about disease process and plan of therapy using VAD. |
| 2. Assess treatment schedule: times for administration of fluids, drugs, blood products, nutrition. | Allows nurse to schedule use of VAD for simultaneous administration of products, to educate client about schedule of administration, and to provide for comfort and reduction of anxiety about therapy. |

| Steps | Rationale |
|---|---|
| 3. Assess type of VAD in place. | Care and management depends on type and size of catheter, number of lumens, type of infusion port. |
| 4. Assess need to use VAD for blood sampling. | Scheduling sampling needs allows nurse to minimize entering VAD system and allows for timely collection of specimens to evaluate therapy. Risk of infection increases with multiple entry into vascular system, especially in immunocompromised clients. |
| 5. Assess VAD placement site for skin integrity and signs of infection: redness, swelling, tenderness, exudate, bleeding. | Clients requiring long-term IV therapy often have conditions placing them at risk for alterations in skin integrity and immune function. |
| 6. Assess for proper function of VAD before therapy: integrity or port or catheter, ability to irrigate or infuse fluid, ability to aspirate blood. | Allows nurse to assure proper function of VAD with minimal complications. |
| 7. Assess need for irrigation and dressing change by referring to medical record, nurses' notes, manufacturer's recommended guidelines for use. | Provides guidelines for catheter patency and prevention of infection. |
| 8. Assess client's reaction to VAD and knowledge of purpose, care, maintenance: ask client to discuss steps in care and to perform procedure (e.g., catheter site cleansing or dressing change). | Determines client's level of understanding. Allows nurse to educate client for home care of VAD. |
| 9. Assess physician's order for medication, fluids, blood products, blood sampling. | Ensures safe, therapeutic administration. |

## Nursing Diagnosis

| Steps | Rationale |
|---|---|
| 1. Cluster data to reveal actual or potential nursing diagnoses: | |
| a. Actual or potential impaired skin integrity: ▪ Related to localized inflammation. | Requires aseptic technique for dressing and site care. |
| b. Knowledge deficit regarding care of VAD: ▪ Related to inexperience. | Indicates need for client education before discharge. |
| c. Potential body image disturbance: ▪ Related to VAD placement. | Client will require emotional and psychosocial support. |
| d. Potential for infection: ▪ Related to frequent venous access. | Nurse must take preventive measures and monitor changes in condition. Daily catheter care is essential. |

## Planning

| Steps | Rationale |
|---|---|
| 1. Develop individualized goals for client based on nursing diagnoses: | |
| a. Skin at catheter exit or placement site remains clear, without inflammation or infection. | Skin care and dressing changes reduce risk or infection or breakdown. |
| b. Client remains free of systemic infection. | Techniques used in care of VAD are important in reducing transfer of microorganisms. |
| c. Client able to independently participate in care. | Maintains client's control in treatment plan. Clients too ill to care for catheters should participate in care through decision making. |
| d. Patency of catheter or cannula ensured. | Routine irrigation and proper monitoring of continuous infusions keep VADs patent. |
| e. Client, family understand knowledge and skills needed to care for VAD: dressing change and heparinization techniques, hygiene and skin care at catheter exit or placement sites, knowledge of emergency situations with ability to contact appropriate professional help, ability to secure supplies necessary for home care. | VAD provides for long-term IV therapy in home. Client, family should be given opportunities to discuss therapies and practice skills before discharge. |
| 2. Assemble equipment: | |
| a. Blood drawing: | |
| ▪ Povidone-iodine and alcohol preparation swabs | Rigorous skin cleansing reduces introducing organisms into system. |
| ▪ 4 to 5 syringes (10 and 20 ml) | Used to collect blood and flush catheter. |
| ▪ Sterile drape | Used to drape area around infusion port. |
| ▪ Vial of saline solution | Used to flush catheter. |
| ▪ Heparin solution (heparin flush or heparin 100 units/ml in saline) or saline solution as recommended by manufacturer or hospital policies and procedures | Used as irrigant for catheter patency. |
| ▪ Plastic clamp | Used to clamp silicone catheters when removing cap from end of catheter to prevent air embolus into system. |

| Steps | Rationale |
|---|---|
| ▪ Sterile Huber needle (20- to 22-gauge) | Used to enter infusion port septum. |
| ▪ Sterile needle (20- to 22-gauge) | Used to enter injection cap on catheter. |
| ▪ Blood tubes, labels, requisitions | Specimen must be labeled properly in correct container. |
| ▪ Sterile gloves, gown, masks | Sterile procedure used with infusion port. |
| b. Administration of drugs, fluids, blood products: | |
| ▪ Povidone-iodine and alcohol swabs | Used for skin preparation and cleansing catheter tip. |
| ▪ Drug, fluid, blood product to be infused | |
| ▪ Sterile IV and extension tubing with stopcock | Protect against entrance of microorganisms into system. |
| ▪ IV pole, infusion pump, blood pump | |
| ▪ Sterile drape | Used to drape area around infusion port. |
| ▪ Saline solution | Used to flush catheter. |
| ▪ Sterile Huber needle (20- to 22-gauge) | Used to enter port septum. |
| ▪ Sterile needle (20- to 22-gauge) | Needle to enter injection cap on catheter. |
| ▪ Dressing supplies as indicated: 4 × 4 gauze pads, tape | Sterile dressing should be applied to insertion or exit site to secure needle or catheter. |
| ▪ Sterile gloves, gown, masks | Sterile procedures used with infusion port. |
| ▪ Label with date, time, size | Ensures dressing and tubing changes are made on schedule. |
| c. Dressing change: | |
| ▪ Povidone-iodine and alcohol swabs | Skin and catheter preparation reduce introducing organisms into system. |
| ▪ Povidone-iodine ointment (used for gauze dressings only) | Recommended at exit or needle insertion site to minimize growth of bacteria. |
| ▪ Dressing supplies (e.g., tape, sterile gauze 4 × 4, 2 × 2, moisture vapor permeable transparent dressings [optional]) | Occlude needle insertion site. Transparent dressing may be used to permit visualization of needle insertion site or catheter exit site. |
| ▪ Sterile gown, gloves, mask | Sterile procedures used with infusion port. |
| ▪ Label with date, time, needle size | Dressing and tubings should be labeled so changes will be made on schedule and needle of same size is used. |
| d. Heparinization: | |
| ▪ Povidone-iodine and alcohol preparation swabs | Used for skin and catheter preparation. |
| ▪ Syringe (5 ml) | |
| ▪ Saline solution | Used to flush or irrigate catheter or port to maintain patency. |
| ▪ Heparin solution (heparin flush or 100 units/ml in saline) | |
| ▪ Cap for catheter | Protects end of catheter and prevents contamination by frequent changing. |
| ▪ Clamp for catheter | Clamp catheter when opening to prevent entrance of air and embolus formation. |
| ▪ Sterile needle (22-gauge) | Used to enter port or injection cap. |
| ▪ Sterile gown, gloves, mask | |
| 1. Position client, in supine position with head slightly elevated. | Stabilizes client and prevents accidental pulling or tugging at catheter. Location of infusion port requires palpation and examination in supine position. |
| 2. Explain procedure to client. Instruct to lie still. | Allows nurse to alleviate client's anxiety by explaining ahead of time. |
| 3. Arrange sterile equipment at bedside. | Provides easy access to equipment. |

## Implementation

***Administration of infusions or sampling of blood from implanted infusion port***

| Steps | Rationale |
|---|---|
| 1. Wash hands thoroughly. | Reduces transfer of microorganisms. |
| 2. Mask self and client. | Prevents spread of airborne microorganisms while needle insertion site is exposed. |
| 3. Prepare sterile field, opening sterile supplies. | Provides work space for use of sterile items. |
| 4. Using povidone-iodine swabs, prepare client's skin overlying port septum, moving in concentric circles from inside out. | Rigorous skin preparation is necessary to prevent introducing bacteria into system. |
| 5. Prepare skin with alcohol in same fashion. | Alcohol has additional antiseptic properties. |
| 6. Apply sterile gloves. | Prevents transmission of microorganisms by nurse's hands. |
| 7. As another nurse holds vial of saline, fill sterile syringe with saline solution. | Second nurse holds vial, which is contaminated on outside, so nurse filling syringe does not contaminate supplies. |
| 8. Attach one end of sterile extension tubing to syringe and special Huber needle to other end. Fill tubing with saline solution. | Removes all air from tubing, reducing risk of air embolus. |
| 9. Apply sterile drape to port site. | Provides sterile work area. |

*Fig. 24-6*

A

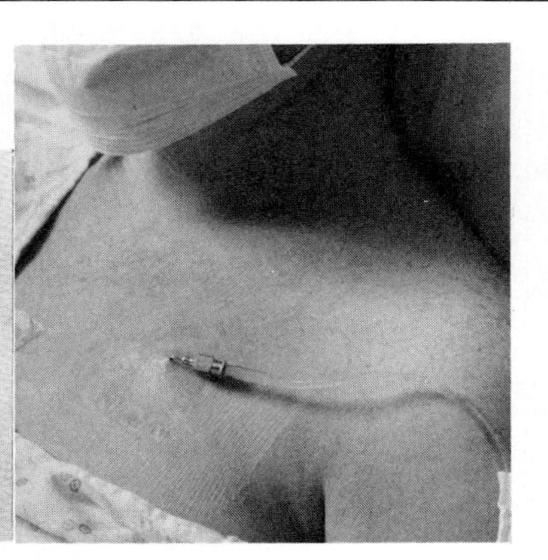

B

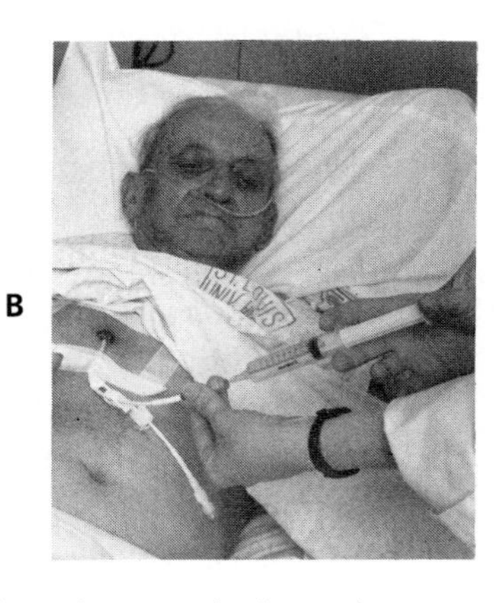

*Fig. 24-7*

| Steps | Rationale |
| --- | --- |
| 10. Palpate port septum, observing strict aseptic technique. | Entry site for needle insertion must be located to ensure proper needle entry. |
| 11. Insert Huber needle through skin and push firmly down until needle penetrates silicone septum and rests firmly against needle stop (Fig 24-6, *A* and *B*). | Ensures proper placement of needle into infusion port. |
| 12. Fill another syringe, as in step 7 and flush port with 20 ml normal saline. Do not irrigate forcefully if resistance is felt. | Forceful irrigation against resistance may propel clotted blood into the client's muscular system. |
| 13. To draw blood samples, first aspirate and discard 7 ml of fluid. | Avoids dilution of sample. |
| 14. Withdraw necessary blood for each sample, using syringe size equal to total volume withdrawn. | Eliminates repeated need to puncture infusion port for sampling. |
| 15. Refill saline syringe and flush port with 20 ml normal saline after sample is obtained. | Any fluid other than normal saline has potential for clotting blood or precipitating in catheter. |
| 16. If continuous infusion is not indicated, heparinize port by flushing with 10 ml heparin flush solution. | Prevents clot formation. |
| 17. If IV fluid will be continuously administered, secure Huber needle with sterile gauze or transparent dressing. | Prevents accidental dislodging of needle and infection at insertion site. |
| 18. Connect IV infusion tubing with sterile tubing connected to Huber needle. | IV infusion system should be closed to maintain sterility. |
| 19. Regulate IV infusion as ordered. | Maintains desired fluid intake and patency of catheter. |
| 20. Dispose of all soiled supplies and used equipment. Send specimens to lab. Wash hands. | Reduces spread of microorganisms. |

***Administration of infusions or sampling of blood from central venous catheter***

| Steps | Rationale |
| --- | --- |
| 1. Wash hands thoroughly. | Reduces transmission of microorganisms. |
| 2. Use povidone-iodine and alcohol preparation swabs to cleanse injection cap or catheter hub. | Prevents introduction of microorganisms into catheter. |
| 3. Prepare two syringes: one with 10 ml normal saline other with 20 ml saline. | Used to flush catheter. |
| 4. If cap will be removed, place strip of tape over catheter before applying clamp. Clamp catheter using plastic clamp only. | Catheter must be clamped if cap is removed to prevent entrance of air. Metal clamps damage silicone catheter. Tape prevents catheter tears. |
| 5. To remove cap, hold outside of catheter firmly, without touching inside of catheter lumen. | Prevents contamination of catheter. |
| 6. If cap is in place, insert needle of syringe containing 10 ml normal saline and flush. If cap is removed, connect syringe tip to catheter hub, release clamp, flush, and reclamp (Fig. 24-7). | Flushing ensures patency of catheter. Catheter must always be clamped between change of syringe or tubing to prevent exposure to air. |
| 7. Connect syringe for blood sampling, release clamp. Aspirate 7 ml fluid, reclamp, and expel aspirate. | Avoids diluting sample. |
| 8. Attach or insert syringe of size equal to volume of blood sample to withdraw to catheter. Release clamp. Withdraw necessary blood for samples and reclamp. | Samples should be collected at one time to minimize time needed to open catheter system. |
| 9. Attach or insert syringe filled with 20 ml normal saline to catheter. If clamp is present, release, flush vigorously, and reclamp. | Catheter should be cleared of all blood or medications that may clog catheter lumen, or precipitate with additives in IV fluids. |
| 10. If no continuous infusion is indicated, heparinize catheter. Connect syringe containing 3 ml heparin flush solution. If clamp is present, release, flush, and reclamp. | A catheter not in use must be heparinized to prevent clot formation. |

| Steps | Rationale |
|---|---|
| 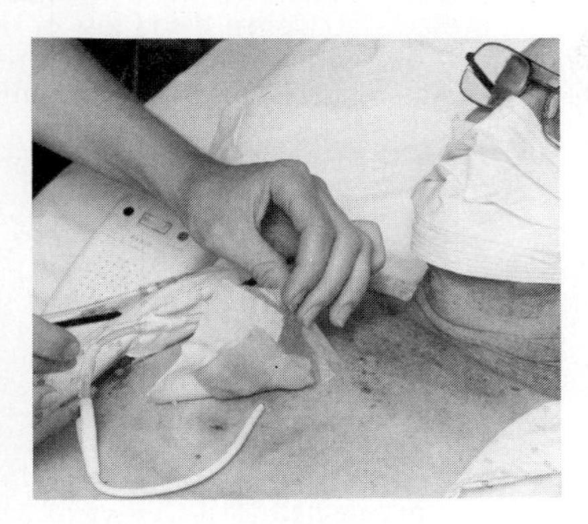 *Fig. 24-8* | 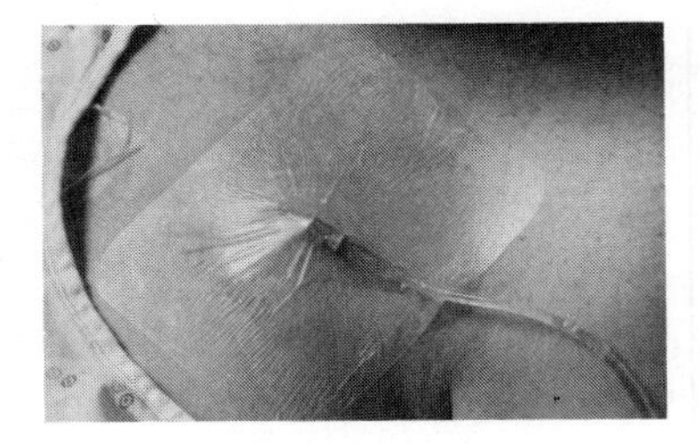 *Fig. 24-9* |
| 11. Replace new cap to end of catheter and remove clamp. | Maintains sterile seal to catheter. |
| 12. If IV fluids will be administered, connect IV tubing to end of catheter, being sure both ends are sterile. | IV system should be closed to maintain sterility. |
| 13. Regulate IV infusion as ordered. | Maintains ordered fluid intake and keeps catheter patent. |
| 14. Tape all tubing connections and pin tubing to client's gown. | Prevents accidental tubing disconnection and catheter displacement. |
| 15. Dispose of soiled equipment and used supplies. Wash hands. | Reduces transmission of microorganisms. |
| ***Dressing change*** | |
| 1. Wash hands. | Reduces transmission of microorganisms. |
| 2. Mask self and client, if indicated. | Prevents exposure of airborne microorganisms to catheter exit or placement site. |
| 3. Carefully remove old dressing, noting drainage and appearance of catheter or needle insertion site (Fig. 24-8). | Remove tape carefully because clients frequently have alterations in skin integrity. |
| 4. Inspect placement or exit site for signs of redness, swelling, inflammation, tenderness, exudate. | Potential site of infection. |
| 5. If catheter is tunneled, palpate dacron cuff in subcutaneous tunnel. | Documenting position of cuff verifies proper placement. |
| 6. Inspect catheter and hub for intactness. | Catheter may become torn, cut, displaced, cracked, split. |
| 7. Apply sterile gloves. | Prevents direct transmission of microorganisms to skin exit site. |
| 8. Clean placement or exit site with povidone-iodine and alcohol swabs by starting from inside moving out in circular fashion, maintaining strict asepsis. Clean about a 3 cm area. | It is impossible to sterilize skin. Organisms that accumulate must be eliminated by mechanical and chemical means. |
| 9. Apply povidone-iodine ointment over exit site if using gauze dressing. Use povidone-iodine solution for transparent dressing. | Further reduces growth of bacteria at site. |
| 10. Redress site using sterile gauze and tape or transparent dressing as indicated (Fig. 24-9). | Prevents entrance of bacteria into exit or placement site. |
| 11. Secure tubing or needle to client's gown. | Prevents accidental pulling and displacement. |
| 12. Label date, time of dressing change, size of needle in place. | Documents dressing change. Provides guideline for time of next change. |
| 13. Dispose of soiled supplies; wash hands. | Reduces transmission of microorganisms. |
| **Evaluation** | |
| 1. When continuous infusions are administered, observe and calculate drip rate hourly. Note ease at which fluid rate can be increased. | To maintain proper fluid infusion, desired drip rate should be regulated continuously. A gradual slowing in rate or inability to increase rate may indicate catheter occlusion. |
| 2. Routinely assess vital signs of client, noting changes symptomatic of fever. | Catheter-related sepsis can cause fever, chills, flushed skin, tachycardia. |
| 3. Observe catheter or port exit or placement site when sites are exposed. | Continual monitoring for signs of inflammation or infection is essential. |

| Steps | Rationale |
|---|---|
| 4. Observe all catheter connection points periodically. | An intact system prevents accidental blood loss or entrance of air. |
| 5. Inspect condition of catheter and connecting tubing daily for leaks, holes, tears, splits, or cracked hubs. | Break in integrity of system predisposes client to hemorrhage or air embolus. |
| 6. Consult x-ray reports for catheter placement. | A routine chest x-ray examination can locate position of catheter tip. |
| 7. Evaluate ability of client, family to provide care and maintain catheter or infusion port through discussion and return demonstrations of dressing changes and skin care. Determine need for restrictions on daily activities. | Measures client's ability to care for self, and any additional learning needs. |
| ***Expected outcomes*** | |
| 1. Site is intact, has normal color, has no swelling. | Local signs of infection are absent. |
| 2. Systemic signs of infection are absent. | Catheter system remains sterile. |
| 3. Fluids, medications, blood products infuse without difficulty. | Patency of catheter is maintained. |
| 4. Blood can be aspirated from catheter. | Indicates patency and good catheter tip positioning in right atrium. |
| 5. Catheter and connecting tube are intact. | Integrity of system is maintained. |
| 6. Catheter tip is correctly placed in right atrium, as confirmed by x-ray examination. | Correct placement minimizes chances of displacement or occlusion. |
| 7. Client, family able to explain purpose of VAD therapy and perform dressing changes and skin care. | Demonstrates that client, family are learning. |
| ***Unexpected outcomes*** | |
| 1. Redness, swelling, inflammation, tenderness are present at exit or placement sites. | Indicate localized skin infection. |
| 2. Client has fever, chills, positive blood cultures. | Signs and symptoms of systemic infection due to catheter related sepsis. |
| 3. There is damage to catheter: displacement, cut or tear, hole; loss of cap, crack in hub or cap. | Requires immediate catheter repair or discontinuation to prevent hemorrhage or air embolus. |
| 4. Catheter is occluded by blood, fibrin, precipitated drugs. | Prevents delivery of IV infusion. |
| 5. Air embolus forms. Symptoms depend on area of body affected. | Air bubbles enter and travel through circulatory system, blocking blood flow after lodged in vessel lumen. |
| 6. Client or family member is unable to explain or perform VAD care. | May indicate need for home health care referral or additional instruction. |

## Recording and Reporting

| | |
|---|---|
| 1. Chart date and time of medications, blood products, parenteral nutrition given, samples obtained in nurses' notes or medication form. | Timely documentation prevents administration errors and repetition of blood sampling. |
| 2. Chart condition of exit site or port implantation site, including skin integrity, signs of infection, placement and integrity of catheter. | Documents ongoing condition and response to catheter site care. |
| 3. Chart dressing change procedure, label date, time, type of needle in port. | Documents nursing care. |
| 4. Chart patency of catheter, ability to draw blood, difficulty with infusions. | If complications arise, it is important to have documentation that preventive measures were performed. |
| 5. Chart measures taken to educate client in self-care, response to education. | Provides continuity of care so other staff members may contribute to education. |
| 6. In emergency situations (damage to catheter, loss of patency, blood loss, air embolus, septic episode, local signs of infection), notify nursing or medical personnel immediately. Instruct client and family when to contact medical personnel. | Allows immediate attention by appropriate personnel. |

## Follow-up Activities

| | |
|---|---|
| 1. In case of occluded catheter, consult institution's policy. Flushing vigorously with normal saline under pressure of infusion pump can restore patency. Instillation of urokinase can effectively dissolve clots. | VADs are designed for long-term use. Clients undergo discomfort and expense if catheters or ports clot and new ones must be inserted. |
| 2. In case of catheter damage, clamp catheter immediately proximal to damaged site. Notify physician. | Prevents blood loss and entrance of air into vascular system. |
| 3. If catheter leak is identified, position client head down and slightly on left side. | Prevents air from entering circulatory system. |

## Special Considerations

- Most common complications are infection, bleeding, leakage at insertion site, occlusion, displacement of catheter or needle in port.
- Special central venous catheter (Groshong) that eliminates need for heparin as irrigant is available. Special three-way valve presents blood from backing into catheter tip and clotting.
- Clients who have undergone radiation therapy or chemotherapy have compromised immune functions that increase risk of infection.
- Ready access to manufacturers' recommendations and familiarity with institutional policies and procedures is essential.
- Have a catheter repair kit available or know where to obtain one immediately.

## Teaching Considerations

- Discuss and provide written emergency measures and telephone numbers of health care personnel to be used in case of catheter damage or needle displacement; swelling, redness, or leakage at insertion site; occlusion of port or catheter; temperature above 100° F; shaking chills.
- Provide written instruction for dressing changes, inspection of insertion site, irrigations, tubing changes.
- Arrange for instruction and return demonstration of skills by client or care giver.
- Have client or care giver maintain list of care givers and telephone numbers (e.g., physician, nurse, social worker, pharmacist, dietician).

## Home Care Considerations

- Initiate referral for discharge planning to social service, counselor, home care coordinator early for assessment of resources.
- Determine client and care giver's acceptance of client's altered body image.
- Provide client with written list of providers for supplies and equipment.
- Assess willingness and ability of primary care giver to assist in home management of device. Acceptance of altered body image influences primary care giver's readiness to assist with care.
- Instruct in adaptations in hospital procedures that can be made at home (e.g., good handwashing instead of sterile gloves).
- Discuss troubleshooting and emergency care routines with care giver in home.
- Assess home environment, determining suitable area for dressing changes and avoiding areas where contaminants are potential hazards.
- Determine ability of client to meet expenses of equipment involved in caring for VAD; attempts by client to try to cut costs may create situation in which sterile technique is compromised.

---

### BIBLIOGRAPHY


Bothe A, et al.: Implantable central venous access systems, Am J Surg 147:565, 1984.

Bothe A, Piccione W, Ambrosino JJ, et al.: Implantable central venous access system, Am J Surg 147:565, 1984.

Brady AM, Schuman E, Winters V: Successful chronic intravenous access via right atrial catheters, Proceedings of the American Society Clinical Oncology 3:95, 1984.

Brincker H, Axelsen F: New techniques for intravenous access and prolonged infusions relevant to new doxorubicin dosage schedules, Anthracyclines Cancer Ther 186-191, Oct 1982.

Champault G: Totally implanted catheters for cancer chemotherapy: French experience on 325 cases, Cancer Drug Deliv 3:131, 1986.

Cruz J, Paschold E, Sterchi M, et al.: Evaluation of a totally implantable system for venous access, Proc Am Soc Clin Oncol 1984.

Dennis EMP: An ambulatory infusion pump for pain control: a nursing approach for home care, Cancer Nurs 7:309, 1984.

Ellerhorst-Ryan JM: Troubleshooting the venous access system, AM J NURS 85(7):795, 1985.

Goodman MS, Wickham R: Venous access devices: an overview, Oncol Nurs Forum 11(S):16-23, 1984.

Goodman MS, Wickham R: Venous access devices: an oncology nurse overview, Hosp Pharm News 20(7):495-511, 1985.

Hughes CB: A totally implantable central venous system for chemotherapy administration: nursing considerations, NITA 8(6):523, 1985.

Keating S, Kelman G: Home health care nursing: concepts and practice, Philadelphia, 1988, JB Lippincott Co.

Lawson M, et al.: The use of urokinase to restore the patency of occluded central venous catheters, Am J IV Ther Clin Nutr Oct 1982, p. 29.

Lokich JJ, et al.: Complications and management of implanted venous access catheters, J Clin Oncol 3(5):710-717, 1985.

Lokich JJ, Bothe A, Benotti P, et al.: Complications and management of implanted venous access catheters, J Clin Oncol 3:710, 1985.

Newton R, De Young JL, Levin H: Volumes of implantable vascular access devices and heparin flush requirements, NITA 8:137, 1986.

Parsa MH, Tabora F: Establishment of intravenous lines for long-term intravenous therapy and monitoring, Surg Clin North Am 65:835, 1985.

Ready AR, Downing R, Fielding JWL, et al.: Venous access using the Hickman catheter, Eur J Surg Oncol 11:155, 1985.

Reilly JJ, Steed DL, Ritter PS: Indwelling venous access catheters in patients with acute leukemia, Cancer 53:219, 1984.

Riser SA: Patient care manual for implanted vascular access devices, NITA 11(2):166, 1988.

Rutherford C: A study of single lumen peripherally inserted central line catheter dwelling time and complications, NITA 11(2):169, 1988.

Strum S, McDermed J, Korn A, et al.: Improved methods for venous access: the Port-A-Cath, a totally implanted catheter system, J Clin Oncol 4:596, 1986.

Wainstock JM: Making a choice: the vein access method you prefer, Oncol Nurs Forum 14(1):79, 1987.

Walsh J, Persons C, Wieck L: Manual of home care nursing, Philadelphia, 1987, JB Lippincott Co.

Welling RE, Hall JM, Meyer RL, et al.: Implantable venous access devices: an alternative method of extended cancer care, J Surg Oncol 33:73, 1986.

Wilkes G, et al.: Long term venous access, Am J Nurs 85(7):793, 1985.

Wilkes G, Vannicola P, Starck P: Long term venous access. Am J Nurs 85:793, 1985.

# 25
# BLOOD THERAPY

### OBJECTIVES

*Mastery of content in this chapter will enable the nurse to:*

- Define key terms.
- Discuss indications for blood therapy.
- Describe various transfusion reactions.
- Demonstrate the following skills on selected clients: initiation of blood therapy, assisting with autotransfusion, monitoring for transfusion reactions.

### KEY TERMS

*Autologous transfusion*
*Autotransfusion*
*Blood group*
*Blood plasma*
*Blood pump*
*Blood transfusion*
*Blood typing*
*Blood-warming coil*
*Erythroblastosis fetalis*
*Hemolysis*
*Serology*
*Transfusion reaction*

### SKILLS

**25-1** Initiating Blood Therapy
**25-2** Assisting with Autotransfusion
**25-3** Monitoring for Transfusion Reactions

Blood replacement or transfusion is the intravenous (IV) administration of whole blood or a component such as plasma, packed red blood cells, or platelets. The objectives for blood transfusions are:

1. To increase circulating blood volume following surgery, trauma, or hemorrhage.
2. To increase the number of red blood cells and to maintain hemoglobin levels in clients with severe chronic anemia.
3. To provide plasma clotting factors to help control bleeding in clients with hemophilia.

When blood or its component is transfused into a client it is important that the appropriate blood group be administered. For this purpose the ABO system of blood grouping is used to type red blood cells. It includes four main groups: A, B, O, and AB.

Individuals with type A blood cells produce anti-B antibodies in their plasma naturally. Similarly, type B individuals produce anti-A antibodies in their plasma naturally. A type O individual produces antibodies to both A and B, but his cells can be transferred into clients with types A, B, or AB blood. A type AB individual produces neither antibody, which is why type AB individuals can be universal recipients. If blood that is mismatched with the client's blood is transfused, a transfusion reaction occurs. The transfusion reaction is an antigen-antibody reaction and can range from a mild response, such as itching, rash, or chilling, to severe anaphylactic shock. The blood group designates the antigen present in blood cells.

Another consideration when matching for blood transfusions is the Rh factor. This is an antigenic substance present in the erythrocytes of most people. A person having the factor is Rh positive, and a person lacking the factor is Rh negative. If the blood administered to an Rh-positive person is Rh negative, hemolysis, or red blood cell destruction, and anemia will occur. Rh-negative blood contains antibodies that will hemolyze the person's own blood cells. An Rh-negative mother, previously exposed to Rh-positive factor (antigen), can transfer anti-Rh-positive antibodies to the fetus, resulting in red blood cell lysis and, in severe cases, erythroblastosis fetalis.

Because of the possibility of transfusion reactions when blood products are administered the technique of autotransfusion has been developed. Autotransfusion is the collection, anticoagulation, filtration, and reinfusion of blood from an active bleeding site.

The decision to administer blood therapy is made by the physician. However, the nurse must perform an individualized pretransfusion assessment to determine the client's probable response to the therapy. In addition, accurate assessment skills enable the nurse to immediately identify any adverse effects of the blood therapy (Table 25-1).

***TABLE 25-1*** Blood Transfusion Products

| Blood Product | Description | Indications | Common Complications |
|---|---|---|---|
| Whole blood | 500 ml unit contains about 200 ml of red blood cells (RBCs) and 300 ml of plasma. | Massive blood loss; exchange transfusion in neonates. | Hemolytic reaction; allergic reaction; hypothermia; electrolyte disturbances; citrate intoxication; hepatitis. |
| Red blood cells (packed) | 250 ml unit contains about 200 ml of RBCs (with same amount of hemoglobin as whole blood) and 50 ml of plasma. | Inadequate oxygen-carrying capacity. | Hemolytic reaction; allergic reaction; hypothermia; electrolyte disturbances; citrate intoxication; hepatitis. |
| Red blood cells (deglycerolized or washed) | 200 ml unit contains RBCs suspended in 50 ml of normal saline, with virtually all leukocytes and plasma proteins removed; deglycerolized RBCs, taken from donors with rare blood types, are first frozen (with glycerol added to preserve RBCs), then thawed and "deglycerolized" before transfusion; washed RBCs are not frozen. | Rare blood types (deglycerolized only); history of repeated febrile nonhemolytic reactions (washed only); immunoglobulin A (IgA) deficiency with sensitivity to IgA (washed preferred, but deglycerolized may be administered). | |
| Plasma (fresh-frozen, single-donor frozen) | 200-300 ml unit of fresh frozen plasma contains all coagulation factors, plus 400 mg of fibrinogen; single-donor frozen plasma contains less of coagulation factors V and VIII. | Coagulation deficiencies for which specific factor concentrates are unavailable. | Allergic reaction; circulatory overload; hepatitis; febrile reaction. |
| Platelet concentrates | 30-60 ml unit contains about half of original platelets in unit of whole blood. | Thrombocytopenia. | Allergic reactions; febrile reactions; hepatitis. |
| Cryoprecipitated antihemophilic factor | Frozen 20 ml unit contains mostly coagulation factor VIII, plus 250 mg of fibrinogen. | Hemophilia A; von Willebrand's disease; hypofibrinogenemia. | Allergic reactions; hepatitis; AIDS. |
| Granulocytes | Units vary in volume but contain mostly granulocytes (exact number depends on method of salvage) plus RBCs, plasma, and platelets. | Severe gram-negative infection, unresponsive to routine forms of therapy, in immunosuppressed patient. | Rash; febrile reaction; hepatitis. |
| Serum albumin (5% and 25%) and plasma protein fraction (PPF) | 25% albumin, which contains higher concentration of albumin than 5%, comes in 50 ml and 100 ml units; 5% albumin and PPF (essentially same product) come in 250 ml units. | Blood volume depletion (used most often for patients in hypovolemic shock and for burn patients); adult respiratory distress syndrome; dehydration; hypoalbuminemia. | Circulatory overload; febrile reaction. |

Data modified from Querin JJ, Stahl LD: Nursing '83 13:34, 1983; Masoorli ST, Piercy S: RN p. 32, Sept. 1984.

## GUIDELINES

1. Know the client's normal range of vital signs. Administration of blood products frequently elevates the client's blood pressure. This elevation may be a desired effect when the client has lost extracellular fluid. However, some clients, particularly the elderly, may become volume overloaded and experience a sudden abrupt elevation in their blood pressure. Furthermore, when a client is having a transfusion reaction, an elevated temperature and pulse may provide the only initial symptoms. When a severe transfusion reaction occurs the client frequently becomes hypotensive and is at risk for developing shock.
2. Know the client's transfusion history. Clients who have had multiple blood transfusions are at risk for transfusion reactions and untoward effects such as hepatitis or acquired immune deficiency syndrome (AIDS).
3. Monitor the client's intake and output measurements. Any client receiving parenteral therapy should have intake and output measurements taken.
4. Be aware of the presence of surgical wound or drainage equipment and the expected "normal amount" of drainage. Knowledge of the amount of normal expected drainage can quickly alert the nurse to abnormal excessive blood loss and the need for medical assistance.
5. Know the client's most recent serum electrolyte measurements. Potassium levels increase in banked or stored blood because potassium is released into the plasma with red cell lysis. Hypocalcemia may occur secondary to citrate binding in clients who have received massive transfusions.
6. Place blood pressure cuff and thermometer at client's bedside. The client's vital signs must be taken before administering blood products, every 5 min for the first 15 min, and hourly thereafter. This enables the nurse to have baseline vital signs to compare with the client's vital signs during the initiation of blood therapy, to detect any early signs of a transfusion reaction.

## PREREQUISITE KNOWLEDGE

1. Fluid and electrolyte therapy.
2. Normal anatomy and physiology of circulatory and respiratory systems.
3. Normal respiration.
4. Factors that influence vital signs.

## PREREQUISITE SKILLS

1. Administration of intravenous therapy (Chapter 23).
2. Physical assessment (Chapter 13).
3. Assessment of vital signs (Chapter 12).

# *SKILL 25-1 Initiating Blood Therapy*

When a client receives blood or blood components, the nurse should understand why the client is to receive the blood, what specific product the client is to receive, and the procedures and hospital policy involved. The nurse's major role in the transfusion of blood or blood components is to monitor the client during and after any transfusion. Developing nursing skills to interpret any adverse effect of a blood transfusion can be life saving. Accurate and quick assessment of clinical signs and symptoms is essential (Pauley, 1985).

Numerous types of blood components are available for clients requiring blood therapy. The indications for use can differ from one product to another, and the physician determines which blood component should be administered to the client.

### Purposes

1. Replace blood volume or blood components lost in surgery, through trauma, or from a disease process.
2. Maintain circulating fluid balance.

## *Procedure 25-1*

| Steps | Rationale |
|---|---|
| **Assessment** | |
| 1. Inspect integrity and intactness of present intravenous line. | Presence of infiltration or signs of infection contraindicates use of the intravenous line for blood therapy. |
| 2. Review hospital/agency procedure and policy regarding administration of blood or blood products. | Hospital/agency policy and procedure is designed to ensure safe and correct blood administration. |
| 3. Observe that venipuncture was performed with 18- or 19-gauge angiocatheter. | Larger catheters promote optimum flow because molecules of blood and its components are larger than molecules of intravenous fluids. In addition, large catheter prevents hemolysis. |

| Steps | Rationale |
|---|---|
| 4. Obtain client's transfusion history. | Identifies client's prior response to transfusion of blood components. If prior reaction occurred, health care team can take measures to reduce present and future risks of reaction. |
| 5. Review baseline vital signs in client's medical record before initiating transfusion. | Changes in vital signs can indicate possible transfusion reaction. |
| 6. Review physician's order. | Blood must be ordered by physician. |

## Nursing Diagnosis

| Steps | Rationale |
|---|---|
| 1. Cluster data to reveal actual or potential nursing diagnoses: | |
| a. Potential or actual fluid volume excess: related to infusion of blood components. | Rapid infusion of whole blood or some of its components such as 25% albumin can result in signs and symptoms of fluid volume overload. |
| b. Decreased cardiac output: related to decreased fluid volume. | Clients requiring transfusion of blood or blood components may have severe blood or fluid losses because of surgery, trauma, or hemorrhage. |

## Planning

| Steps | Rationale |
|---|---|
| 1. Develop individualized goals for client based on nursing diagnoses: | |
| a. Maintain normal fluid status. | Maintain prescribed rate of flow and assessing client's fluid status decrease risk of fluid volume excess. |
| b. Maintain infusion rate at prescribed flow. | |
| c. Reduce client's risk of transfusion reaction. | Use of proper procedures and client assessment before initiation of blood therapy reduces risk of transfusion reaction. |
| 2. Prepare following equipment in addition to primary intravenous infusion: | |
| a. Blood filter (Fig. 25-1) and tubing. | Filters remove large aggregates that form in any blood product containing plasma. They are also used to remove smaller particles called microaggregates that form in all stored units of whole blood and packed red cells (Bahu, 1983). |
| 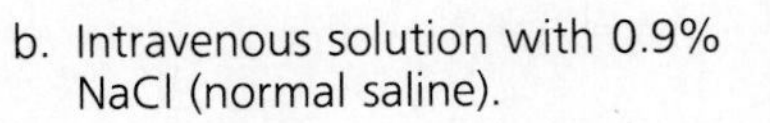 b. Intravenous solution with 0.9% NaCl (normal saline). | Saline is isotonic and reduces hemolysis; 5% dextrose in water ($D_5W$) results in hemolysis of red blood cells. Lactated Ringer's solution results in blood clotting (Bahu, 1983). |
| c. Blood warmer if needed. | Rapid administration of cold blood has hypothermic effect on myocardium, resulting in decreases in cardiac output; metabolic acidosis; conduction defects; possible death (Bahu, 1983). |
| d. Pressure bag. | Increases rate of infusion or maintains flow rate. Frequently used with blood components with greater viscosity such as packed red cells. |
| e. Disposable gloves. | Reduces transmission of blood-borne microorganisms. |

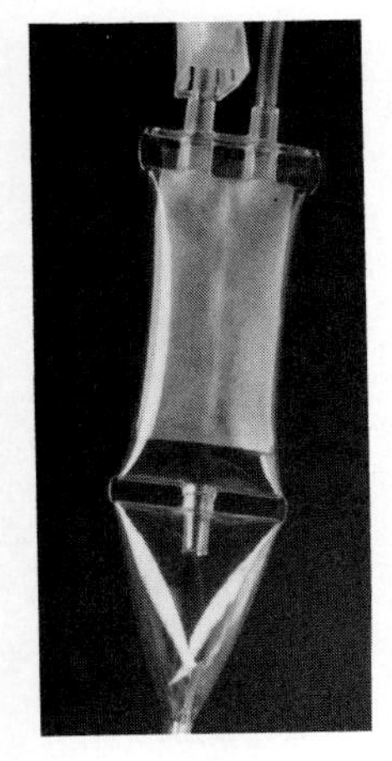

***Fig. 25-1***

| Steps | Rationale |
|---|---|
| 3. Obtain blood from blood bank following agency protocol. Blood banks only send one unit at a time. No more than 20 min should elapse between time blood arrives and time it is administered. | Prevents bacterial growth and destruction of red blood cells. Whole blood or packed red cells should remain in a cold (1° to 6° C) environment. |
| 4. Explain procedure to client and its purpose. | Increases client cooperation and decreases anxiety. |
| 5. Ask the client to report shortness of breath, chills, headache, itching, or rash immediately. | These are signs of a transfusion reaction. Prompt reporting and discontinuation of transfusion can help to minimize a reaction. |
| 6. Have client sign any necessary consent forms. | Some agencies require clients to sign consent forms before receiving any blood component transfusions. |
| 7. With another registered nurse, correctly verify blood product and identify client: | Strict adherence to verification procedures before administration of blood or blood products reduces risk of administering wrong blood to client. When an error is noted during verification procedure, notify blood bank and appropriate personnel as indicated by agency policy. *Do not administer the product.* |
| a. Client's name and identification number (verbally and against his arm band). | |
| b. Client's blood group and Rh type. | |
| c. Crossmatch compatability. | |
| d. Donor blood group and Rh type. | |
| e. Unit and hospital number. | |

| Steps | Rationale |
|---|---|
| f. Expiration date on blood.<br>g. Type of blood component.<br>h. Clots in blood—if clots are present, return blood to blood bank. | An anticoagulant, citrate-phosphate-dextrose (CPD), is added to blood and permits preserved blood to be stored for 21 days. A newer anticoagulant, citrate-phosphate-dextrose-adenine (CPD-A), allows storage for 35 days (Metheny and Snively, 1983). |
| 8. If venipuncture is necessary follow Skill 23-1, Planning, Steps 2-3. | |

## Implementation

| Steps | Rationale |
|---|---|
| 1. Obtain baseline vital signs before administering transfusion. | Verifies client's pretransfusion temperature, pulse, blood pressure, and respirations. |
| 2. Wash hands and apply disposable gloves. | Reduces risk for transmission of HIV, hepatitis, and other blood-borne bacteria. |
| 3. Open blood administration set. | Prepares blood administration tubing. |
| a. For Y-tubing administration, set both roller clamps to "off" position.<br>b. For single tubing administration, set roller clamp to "off" position. | Moving roller clamp(s) to "off" position prevents accidental spilling, and wasting of blood. |
| 4. For Y-tubing only:<br>a. Spike 0.9 normal saline intravenous bag.<br>b. Spike blood or blood component unit and fill drip chamber with blood.<br>c. Prime tubing with 0.9 normal saline.<br>▪ Squeeze sides of drip chamber.<br>▪ Allow chamber to fill and filter to be half covered with normal saline.<br>▪ Open roller clamp and permit infusion tubing to fill with normal saline. | Use of Y-tubing permits nurse to quickly switch from infusion of 0.9 normal saline to blood unit. When unit is finished nurse is able to maintain patency of vein by infusing normal saline. Y-tubing administration sets should be used when multiple blood transfusions are anticipated. |
| 5. For single tubing administration:<br>a. Spike blood unit.<br>b. Squeeze drip chamber; allow filter to be filled with blood.<br>c. Open roller clamp and allow infusion tubing to fill with blood. | Prepares administration filter and tubing with blood. Promotes quick connection of prepared infusion tubing to intravenous catheter. |
| 6. Remain with client during first 15-20 min of transfusion. Initial flow rate during this time should be 2-5 ml/min. | Most reactions occur during the first 15-20 min of a transfusion. Infusing small amount initially prevents client from receiving too much blood if there is reaction (Bahu, 1983). |
| 7. Monitor client's vital signs appropriately: every 5 min for first 15 min; every 15 min for next hour; hourly until unit of blood is infused. | Documents any change in vital signs that could be early warning of transfusion reaction. |
| 8. Regulate infusion according to physician's orders. | Client's condition dictates rate at which blood should infuse. |
| 9. After blood has infused clear intravenous line with 0.9% NaCl. | Infuses remainder of blood in intravenous line and 0.9% NaCl prevents hemolysis of red cells. |

## Evaluation

| Steps | Rationale |
|---|---|
| 1. Observe for any chills, flushing, itching, dyspnea, rash, hives, or other signs of transfusion reaction. | Indicates early sign of transfusion reaction. |
| 2. Observe client and assess lab values to determine response to administration of blood components. | Assessment notes presence or absence of any physiological changes that occur with transfusion reaction. |
| 3. Periodically inspect IV site. | Evaluates presence of infiltration or phlebitis. |

### *Expected outcomes*

| Steps | Rationale |
|---|---|
| 1. Client remains free of signs and symptoms indicating transfusion reaction. | Documents that client was able to tolerate infusion of blood components without any adverse reactions. |
| 2. Client's hemoglobin and hematocrit levels of fluid balance improve. | Indicates that transfusion has had beneficial physiological effect on client's hematological system. |
| 3. Signs and symptoms associated with infiltration or phlebitis at venipuncture site are absent (Chapter 23). | Ensures patency and adequate functioning of IV system for administration of blood, blood components, or fluid therapy. |

### *Unexpected outcomes*

| Steps | Rationale |
|---|---|
| 1. Client displays signs and symptoms of a transfusion reaction: chills; fever; urticaria (Skill 25-3). | Occurs when donor's blood antibodies are incompatible with those of recipient. |

| Steps | Rationale |
|---|---|
| 2. Client has signs and symptoms of anaphylactic shock: hypotension; tachycardia; flushing; mental confusion; cardiac arrest (Skill 25-3). | Although rare, anaphylactic shock occurs when donor blood has been improperly matched in blood bank or wrong blood has been given to wrong client. |
| 3. Infiltration or phlebitis is present at venipuncture site. | Necessitates removal of intravenous line and insertion of new angiocatheter. |

## Recording and Reporting

| | |
|---|---|
| 1. Record type and amount of blood component administered and client's response to blood therapy. | Documents administration of blood component and client's reaction. |

## Follow-up Activities

| | |
|---|---|
| 1. Transfusion reaction: | |
| a. Stop transfusion immediately and follow agency procedure. | Prevents further entry of incompatible blood into recipient. |
| b. Maintain patent intravenous line using normal saline. | Provides route to administer emergency drugs and fluids if necessary. |
| c. Return remaining blood and tubing to blood bank. | Provides prompt testing of administered blood for incompatibilities. |
| 2. Anaphylactic shock: | |
| a. Discontinue transfusion. | Prevents further entry of incompatible blood into recipient. |
| b. Call for emergency assistance. | Anayphalactic shock is medical emergency, life support measures must be initiated. |
| c. Begin CPR as necessary. | Maintains basic life support. |
| d. Maintain patent IV. | Needed to administer emergency medications and fluids. |
| 3. Infiltration or infection at venipuncture site: | |
| a. Stop transfusion. | Prevents worsening of infiltration. |
| b. Restart IV at new venipuncture site. | Reestablishes patent IV to transfuse blood components. |
| c. Institute nursing measures to reduce infiltration or inflammation. | Promotes comfort. |

## Special Considerations

- Saline solution should remain until transfusion is completed to flush line of blood or to keep intravenous line patent for supportive measures in case of transfusion reaction.
- When clients require rapid infusions of multiple units of cold blood, the unit of blood *should not* be warmed, but rather infusion tubing itself should be warmed.
- When a pressure bag is used, pressure should not exceed 300 mm Hg because of potential destruction of red blood cells and hemoglobinuria if blood is infusing under pressure through small bore needle (Bahu, 1983).
- Assess vital signs as each unit of blood is initiated.
- In adult, whole blood and packed cells usually infuse over 1½ to 2 hr. Elderly client may have decreased cardiac function or suffer from chronic anemia, thus may require slower infusion time. If client is bleeding severely, infusion time may be increased with use of blood pump.
- In child, first 50 ml of blood should be infused over 30 min. If no reaction occurs, flow rate is increased accordingly to infuse remainder of 275 ml over 2-hr period (Whaley and Wong, 1987).

## Teaching Considerations

- Client is instructed to notify nurse of signs of itching, swelling, dizziness, dyspnea, or chest pain.
- Client instructed on the anticipated length of transfusion time.
- Client instructed on signs of infiltration, inflammation, or phlebitis.
- Client instructed on the rationale for frequent vital sign monitoring when transfusion is initiated.

## Home Care Considerations

- If blood is given in the home setting, the nurse must follow meticulous cross-check procedures to assure correct administration of blood.
- Blood must be administered as quickly as possible after obtaining it from the blood bank.
- The nurse must plan carefully so the client has nursing personnel available during the entire transfusion period.
- Clients who have had prior transfusion reactions are poor risks for home transfusion.
- Policies and procedures established by the home health agency must be followed. Standards should address such issues as: legal implications, educational preparation of the nurse, client selection process, blood storage, blood transport, location of client's residence, emergency procedures, and specific state's nurse practice act.

# *SKILL 25-2 Assisting with Autotransfusion*

Autotransfusion is the collection, anticoagulation, filtration, and reinfusion of blood from an active bleeding site (Duff, 1983). It is frequently used in the emergency or operating rooms to salvage the client's own blood for reinfusion.

Autotransfusion is not new; it was first attempted in the early 1800s. Recent medical advances in cardiovascular surgery and treatment of trauma victims have resulted in the development of technology to refine the autotransfusion technique.

The advantages of autotransfusion are numerous. First, the risk of technical errors in blood typing and crossmatching are eliminated (Popovsky, 1986). Second, possible adverse effects associated with homologous blood transfusions are eliminated. Third, dependence on homologous blood banks is eliminated. Last, blood obtained by intraoperative autotransfusion has more viable red blood cells because it has not undergone the biochemical changes that occur during storage (Duff, 1983). In addition, possible exposure to serum hepatitis, syphilis, malaria, brucellosis, AIDS, and viral diseases is avoided (Popovsky, 1986).

To administer an autotransfusion a device for processing the client's blood must be available. The generic term for these devices is *cell saver.* A cell saver is composed of a double lumen suction tubing, a collection reservoir, a delivery pump, and a centrifuge. Collected blood is mixed with an anticoagulant filtered to remove fat, surgical debris, white blood cells, and platelets and is concentrated to a hematocrit of 50%-60%. The end product, red blood cells, is washed with one liter of saline (Duff, 1983).

### Purposes

1. Replace blood volume lost in surgery or trauma
2. Maintain circulating fluid balance
3. Reduce the chance of allergic reactions

## *Procedure 25-2*

| Steps | Rationale |
|---|---|
| **Assessment** | |
| 1. Determine integrity of existing intravenous line. | Presence of infiltration or signs and symptoms of infections contraindicate use of the intravenous line for blood supply. |
| 2. If an IV line is present observe that venipuncture was performed with 18- or 19-gauge angiocatheter. | Autotransfusion is replacement of red blood cells; larger catheter is necessary to permit administration of thicker, more viscous red blood cells. |
| 3. Obtain baseline vital signs before initiating autotransfusion. | Clients requiring autotransfusion are experiencing excessive blood loss either from traumatic wound or surgical procedure and have fluctuating vital signs. When severe hemorrhage is present, autotransfusion can be life-saving modality when donated blood is not available quickly. |
| 4. Identify factors that preclude autotransfusion: fecal and urine contamination; preexisting coagulation problems; autotransfusion of blood collected during surgery for malignancies. | Studies have shown that use of autologous blood in patients with bowel contamination does not increase risk of infection. Apparently phagocytic activity found in fresh autologous blood prevents sepsis when blood is reinfused. This, however, is not recommended except in cases of exsanguinating hemorrhage when immediate volume replacement is necessary (Emminizer, 1981). |
| **Nursing Diagnosis** | |
| 1. Cluster data to reveal actual or potential nursing diagnoses:<br>a. Pain: related to infusion equipment.<br>b. Decreased cardiac output: related to trauma or surgical procedure blood loss. | Actual nursing diagnoses identified are related to client's need for autotransfusion. |
| **Planning** | |
| 1. Develop individualized goals for client based on nursing diagnoses:<br>a. Promoting comfort.<br>b. Maintaining adequate tissue perfusion.<br>c. Improving cardiac output. | Improved cardiac output and reduced pain and anxiety lead to decreased oxygen demands by body. |

| Steps | Rationale |
|---|---|
| 2. If autotransfusion procedure is elective phlebotomy, schedule appointments with client at blood bank. | Clients may be requested to donate blood up to 8 weeks before surgery to assure that sufficient amount of autologous blood is available. |
| 3. Collect necessary supplies:<br>a. Large bore venous line<br>b. Cell saver<br>c. Anticoagulant-saline mixture<br>d. Transfer bag<br>e. Label<br>f. Disposable gloves | Immediate access to necessary supplies provides efficient implementation of autotransfusion procedure. |
| 4. To administer autotransfusion, see Skill 25-1, Planning, Steps 1-7. | |

## Implementation

| Steps | Rationale |
|---|---|
| 1. Initiate intravenous line using large bore angiocatheter (size 18 or 19 gauge). | Large bore intravenous catheter is required to remove whole blood from client. Use of small intravenous catheter causes vein to collapse because of pressure required to extract whole blood. |
| 2. Place collected blood into cell saver and follow agency and manufacturer's procedure. | Basic functions of present cell savers are to anticoagulate, separate, filter, and store collected red blood cells. |
| 3. Follow procedure outlined in Skill 25-1, Implementation, for administration of autotransfusion. | Clients receiving autotransfusion are not at risk for transfusion reactions or anaphylactic shock because threat of blood incompatibility does not exist. However, risk of labeling error or giving blood to wrong client with similar name does exist. |

## Evaluation

| Steps | Rationale |
|---|---|
| 1. Observe client and lab values to determine response to administration of autotransfusion. | Reassessment should note improvement in client's vital signs because of restoration of circulating blood volume. |

### *Expected outcomes*

| Steps | Rationale |
|---|---|
| 1. There is improvement in client's vital signs and hemoglobin and hematocrit levels. | Indicates that transfusion has physiologically benefited client's circulatory and hematological system. |
| 2. Signs and symptoms associated with infiltration or infection at venipuncture site are absent (Chapter 23). | Ensures patency and adequate functioning of IV system for administration of blood, blood components, or fluid therapy. |

### *Unexpected outcomes*

| Steps | Rationale |
|---|---|
| 1. Client displays signs and symptoms associated with fluid overload: elevated BP; tachycardia; rales; shortness of breath. | Occurs when client's cardiovascular status is unable to handle additional blood volume. |
| 2. Infiltration or phlebitis at venipuncture site is present. | Necessitates removal of intravenous line and insertion of new angiocatheter. |

## Recording and Reporting

| Steps | Rationale |
|---|---|
| 1. Record amount of blood received by autotransfusion and client's response to blood therapy. | Documents administration of blood and client's response. |
| 2. Report number of units infused at change-of-shift report. | Provides oncoming nursing personnel with an exact number of units transfused. |

## Follow-up Activities

| Steps | Rationale |
|---|---|
| 1. Fluid overload:<br>a. Reduce transfusion rate but maintain patent IV. | Reducing transfusion rate reduces volume of blood entering client's circulatory system. |
| b. Contact client's physician. | Physician may order infusion discontinued or administered more slowly. |
| 2. Infiltration or infection at venipuncture site:<br>a. Stop transfusion. | Prevents worsening of infiltration. |
| b. Restart IV at new venipuncture site. | Reestablishes patent IV to resume transfusion. |
| c. Institute nursing measures to reduce infiltration or inflammation. | Promotes comfort. |

## Special Considerations

- Although threat of transfusion reaction is absent during autotransfusion, client's baseline and serial vital signs should be recorded in nurses' notes.
- Hemolytic reactions occur because blood sample, blood unit, or client was improperly identified. Proper identification is mandatory and agency procedure should be properly followed.
- Febrile nonhemolytic reactions occur in 1% to 2% of transfusions. Clients with prior multiple transfusions frequently develop such antibodies, as can clients with history of multiple pregnancies (Pauley, 1985).

***TABLE 25-2*** Adverse Reactions to Blood Transfusions

| Type | Cause | Onset | Signs or Symptoms | Nursing Actions |
|---|---|---|---|---|
| Febrile nonhemolytic (most common reaction; usually occurs in previous transfusion recipients or multiparous clients). | Antigen-antibody reaction to white blood cells or platelets contained in blood product. | Immediately or within 6 hours after transfusion. | Fever (with or without chills), headache, nausea and vomiting, nonproductive cough, hypotension, chest pain, dyspnea. | 1. Stop transfusion.<br>2. Keep vein open.<br>3. Notify physician and blood bank.<br>4. Take vital signs every 15 min. |
| Allergic urticaria. | Allergic reaction to plasma-soluble antigen contained in blood product. | Anytime during transfusion or within 1 hour after transfusion. | Skin rash. | 1. Slow transfusion to keep-vein-open rate.<br>2. Notify physician and blood bank.<br>3. Take vital signs every 15 min. |
| Delayed hemolytic (more common than acute hemolytic; frequently missed; occurs in previous transfusion recipients or multiparous clients). | Incompatibility of RBC antigens other than ABO group. | Days to weeks after transfusion. | Decreasing hemoglobin level, possible persistent low-grade fever. | 1. Notify physician and blood bank. |
| Acute hemolytic (potentially life threatening). | ABO group incompatibility. | Usually during first 5 to 15 minutes, but may occur any time during transfusion. | *Mild form:* fever, chills, back pain, hypotension, nausea, vomiting, flushing, hematuria, oliguria. *Severe form (in addition to above):* dyspnea, chest pain, anuria, shock, disseminated intravascular coagulation. | 1. Stop transfusion.<br>2. Keep vein open.<br>3. Notify physician and blood bank.<br>4. Take vital signs every 15 min. Assess for signs and symptoms of shock.<br>5. Monitor intake and output; check for decreased urinary output.<br>6. Start resuscitative measures if necessary. |
| Anaphylactic (extremely rare; potentially life threatening). | Idiosyncratic reaction in patients with immunoglobulin A (IgA) deficiency, sensitized to IgA through previous transfusion or pregnancy. | Immediately (after transfusion of only few milliliters of blood). | Severe respiratory and cardiovascular collapse (with dyspnea and tachypnea, tachycardia, hypotension, and cyanosis), severe gastrointestinal disturbances (with nausea, vomiting, diarrhea, and cramping). | 1. Stop tranfusion.<br>2. Keep vein open.<br>3. Notify physician and blood bank.<br>4. Take vital signs every 15 min.<br>5. Start resuscitative measures if necessary. |

Modified from Querin JJ, Stahl LD: Nursing '83 13:34, 1983.

# SKILL 25-3
# MONITORING FOR TRANSFUSION REACTIONS

During the infusion of blood the client is at risk for a reaction, particularly during the first 15 min. Therefore the nurse should remain with the client and assess color, vital signs, and physiological responses. The various kinds of transfusion reactions are described in Table 25-2.

A transfusion reaction is a systemic response by the body to the administration of blood incompatible with that of the recipient. The causes include red cell incompatibility or allergic sensitivity to the leukocytes, the platelets, or the plasma protein components of the transfused blood, or to the potassium or citrate preservative in the blood. Blood transfusions can also transmit disease.

Several types of reactions can result from blood transfusions. General adverse reactions (Table 25-2) range from immediate onset of fever, chills, and skin rash to hypotension, shock, and a delayed reaction that may not occur until several days or weeks later.

A second category of reactions includes diseases transmitted by asymptomatic blood donors. Common diseases that can be transmitted through transfusion are malaria, hepatitis, and AIDS. Since all units of blood collected must undergo serological testing, the risk of acquiring blood-borne bacterial and viral infections is minimized.

## Purposes

1. Identify early signs of a transfusion reaction.
2. Promptly discontinue the transfusion.
3. Provide immediate emergency measures if needed.

## *Procedure 25-3*

| Steps | Rationale |
|---|---|
| **Assessment** | |
| 1. Observe for fever with or without chills; lumbar pain; hypotension; dyspnea; oliguria; shock; abnormal bleeding; anuria. Review laboratory results for hemoglobinemia or hemoglobinuria. | Signs and symptoms indicate acute hemolytic reaction, which occurs when donor red cells are incompatible with recipient's plasma. During mismatch of donor and recipient blood there is intravascular hemolysis and osmotic lysis of red blood cells with release of hemoglobin. In addition, coagulation system stimulates activation of intrinsic clotting cascade, causing small clots in circulation, thus initiating disseminated intravascular coagulation (DIC). Cumulative effect of hemolytic reaction is disastrous for kidneys. Frequently, ultimate cause of death is renal failure (Pauley, 1985). |
| 2. Observe for chills and fever several hours after transfusion. | Indicates delayed hemolytic reaction caused by antibody reacting with its corresponding antigen. |
| 3. Observe for fever; chills; hypotension; lumbar pain; palpitations; headache; malaise. | These symptoms are associated with febrile nonhemolytic reactions. Frequent cause of fever is recipient antibodies reacting with transfused lymphocytes or platelet cell membrane. |
| 4. Observe for local erythema; hives; itching; possible fever. | Urticaria reactions occur with infusion of plasma and are not serious. |
| 5. Observe for life-threatening signs and symptoms: respiratory distress; hypotension; abdominal cramps; vomiting and diarrhea; shock; loss of consciousness. | These signs and symptoms occur with anaphylactic reaction and are rare. Anaphylactic reactions have two distinct features: development of untoward effects following infusion of only a few milliliters of blood or plasma and absence of fever. |
| 6. Observe for dyspnea; cyanosis; severe headache; elevated systolic blood pressure; increased central venous pressure. | Circulatory overload increases client's cardiac burden, producing left ventricular failure with pulmonary edema. |
| 7. Observe for hypothermia and cardiac dysrhythmias. | Occurs when clients require massive transfusions. Cold blood reaches right ventricle by way of central veins, causing an immediate cooling effect. Cardiac conduction system is affected. |
| 8. Observe for signs and symptoms indicating citrate toxicity: circumoral tingling; hypotension; nausea and vomiting; alkalosis; hypokalemia; cardiac dysrhythmias. | Occurs when citrate anticoagulant accumulates in clients with hypothermia or if blood is administered rapidly at rates of 100 ml/min when infused excess citrate combines with calcium and may be excreted in urine. |
| 9. Observe for weakness; fatigue; nausea; jaundice; 1-6 mo following transfusion. | Indicates presence of hepatitis. Hepatitis has long incubation period; it is unlikely that this reaction will occur during hospital stay. |

| Steps | Rationale |
|---|---|
| 10. Observe for signs and symptoms associated with AIDS: fever, night sweats; weight loss; skin lesions; 18-24 mo following transfusion. | AIDS has been transmitted by blood transfusions. |

## Nursing Diagnosis

| Steps | Rationale |
|---|---|
| 1. Cluster data to reveal actual or potential nursing diagnoses:<br>a. Pain: related to urticaria from transfusion reaction.<br>b. Altered cardiopulmonary tissue perfusion: related to administration of improperly matched blood.<br>c. Decreased cardiac output: related to shock secondary to transfusion reaction. | Actual nursing diagnoses identified are related to type or severity of reaction.<br>Some reactions may result in urticaria; other more severe reactions may result in cardiopulmonary arrest. |

## Planning

| Steps | Rationale |
|---|---|
| 1. Develop individualized goals for client based on nursing diagnoses:<br>a. Promote comfort.<br>b. Maintain adequate tissue perfusion.<br>c. Improve cardiac output. | Improved cardiac output and reduction in pain and anxiety result in decreased oxygen demands. |

## Implementation

| Steps | Rationale |
|---|---|
| 1. Stop transfusion. | Reduces further risk. Severity of reaction is related to amount infused. |
| 2. Maintain patent intravenous line, using 0.9% NaCl. | In event of life-threatening anaphylactic shock, essential fluids and medications can be administered to improve cardiac output and to promote adequate tissue perfusion. |
| 3. Obtain two blood samples from arm opposite transfusion. | One blood sample and pretransfusion sample are crossmatched to be sure correct blood was given and check for antibodies was done to determine whether reaction had occurred. Second blood sample is centrifuged and serum is examined for free hemoglobin, which would indicate hemolysis (Cullins, 1979). |
| 4. Return remaining blood to blood bank. | Sample of blood from transfusion will be crossmatched with client's pretransfusion and posttransfusion sample to determine if error in crossmatching occurred. |
| 5. Notify physician of client's transfusion reaction and present physical assessment findings. | Transfusion reactions require prompt and immediate medical intervention. |
| 6. Monitor client's vital signs every 15 min or more frequently if needed. | Maintains ongoing assessment of client's cardiopulmonary status. |
| 7. Administer prescribed medications depending on type and severity of transfusion reaction. | |
| a. Diphenhydramine. | Antihistamine administered parenterally counteracts some allergic response. Sometimes this drug is also ordered pretransfusion. |
| b. Broad-spectrum antibiotics. | Administered when bacterial reaction is suspected. |
| c. Intravenous fluids. | Rapid administration of intravenous fluid helps to counteract symptoms of systemic shock. |
| 8. Obtain first voided urine to test for hemoglobinuria. | Hemoglobinuria occurs with hemolytic transfusion reactions when hemolysis has occurred. Urine specimen may be red or black, indicating potential renal involvement. Renal involvement requires prompt treatment with mannitol to promote diuresis and prevent renal tubular damage. |

## Evaluation

| Steps | Rationale |
|---|---|
| 1. Observe client to determine changes in status as result of discontinuing transfusion or instituting measures to reduce transfusion reaction. | Provides continued monitoring of client's cardiopulmonary status. |

### *Expected outcomes*

| Steps | Rationale |
|---|---|
| 1. Client's vital signs, cardiac output, and physiologic status improve. | Indicates transfusion reaction is under control and client's cardiopulmonary functioning is stabilized. |

| Steps | Rationale |
|---|---|
| ***Unexpected outcomes*** | |
| 1. Client's physiological status worsens. | Progressive decline in client's physiological status occurs with severe transfusion reactions and can progress to cardiac arrest. |

## Recording and Reporting

| | |
|---|---|
| 1. Record exact time of transfusion reaction, client's assessment findings, and nursing and medical actions taken. | Documents presence of transfusion reaction and any follow-up treatment. |
| 2. Immediately report to nurse in charge and physician presence of transfusion reaction and client's physical assessment findings. | Promotes prompt action to reduce adverse effects of transfusion reaction. |

## Follow-up Activities

| | |
|---|---|
| 1. Maintain patent intravenous line. | Provides access for parenteral medications. |
| 2. Initiate CPR. | Restores cardiopulmonary function. |

## Special Considerations

- Some physicians may order antihistamines to be given before transfusion is administered.
- Clients requiring multiple rapid transfusions are at greater risk for citrate toxicity.
- Risk of hepatitis B has been decreased because of hepatitis testing required on all donor blood.
- Hemophiliacs are at risk because of frequent need for antihemophiliac factor, which is prepared from large pools of human plasma (Pauley, 1985).
- In presence of severe reactions, nurse should be prepared to administer cardiopulmonary resuscitation (CPR) (Chapter 18).

### BIBLIOGRAPHY


Bahu GAB: Administering blood safely, AORN 37:1073, 1983.
Birdsall C, Carpender K, Considine R: How is autotransfusion done? Am J Nurs 88:108, 110, 1988.
Cullins LC: Preventing and treating transfusion reactions, Am J Nurs 79:935, 1979.
Duff L: Intraoperative autotransfusion, AORN 37:1102, 1983.
Emminizer S, Klopp EH, Hauer MM: Autotransfusion current status, Heart Lung 10:83, 1981.
Girard NJ, Morgan RC, Orr MD: Autologous salvage of blood: Perioperative nursing considerations, AORN 47(2):492, 498, 502, 1988.
Kemp B, Pillitteri A: Fundamentals of nursing, Boston, 1984; Little, Brown & Co.
Landier WC, Barrell ML, Styfie EJ: How to administer blood components to children, Maternal-Child Nursing 12(3):178, 1987.
Masoorli ST, Piercy S: A lifesaving guide to blood products, RN p. 32, Sept. 1984.
Metheny NM, Snively WD Jr: Nurse's handbook of fluid balance, ed 4, Philadelphia, 1983, JB Lippincott Co.
Pauley SY: Transfusion therapy for nurses, part 2, NITA 8:51, 1985.
Pauley SY: Transfusion therapy for nurses, part 5, NITA 8:51, 1985.
Peck NL: Action stat: blood transfusion reaction, Nursing 17(1):33, 1987.
Phillips A: Are blood transfusions really safe? Nursing '87 17(6):63, 1987.
Pluth NM: A home care transfusion program, Oncol Nurs For 14(5):43, 1987.
Popovsky MA, Taswell HF: Role of IV and transfusion nurses in autologous transfusion, NITA 7:385, 1984.
Popovsky MA: Autologous transfusion: present practice and future trends, NITA 9:292, 1986.
Potter PA, Perry AG: Fundamentals of nursing: concepts, process, and practice, ed 2, St. Louis, 1989, The CV Mosby Co.
Querin JJ, Stahl LD: Twelve simple sensible steps for successful blood transfusion, Nursing '83 13:34, 1983.
Querin JJ, Mesnard JE: Hepatitis and blood transfusions, Nursing 17(11):143, 1987.
Rutman RC, Miller TV: Transfusion therapy: principles and procedures, Rockville, Md, 1982, Aspen Publishing Co.
Scipien G, et al.: Comprehensive pediatric nursing, New York, 1986, McGraw-Hill Book Co.
Smith S, Duell D: Clinical nursing skills, Los Altos, Calif, 1985, National Nursing Review.
Whaley LF, Wong DL: Nursing care of infants and children, ed. 3, St. Louis, 1987, The CV Mosby Co.
Williams WJ, Beutler E, Erslev AJ, Rundles RW: Hematology, New York, 1972, McGraw-Hill Book Co.

# UNIT VIII

# NUTRITION

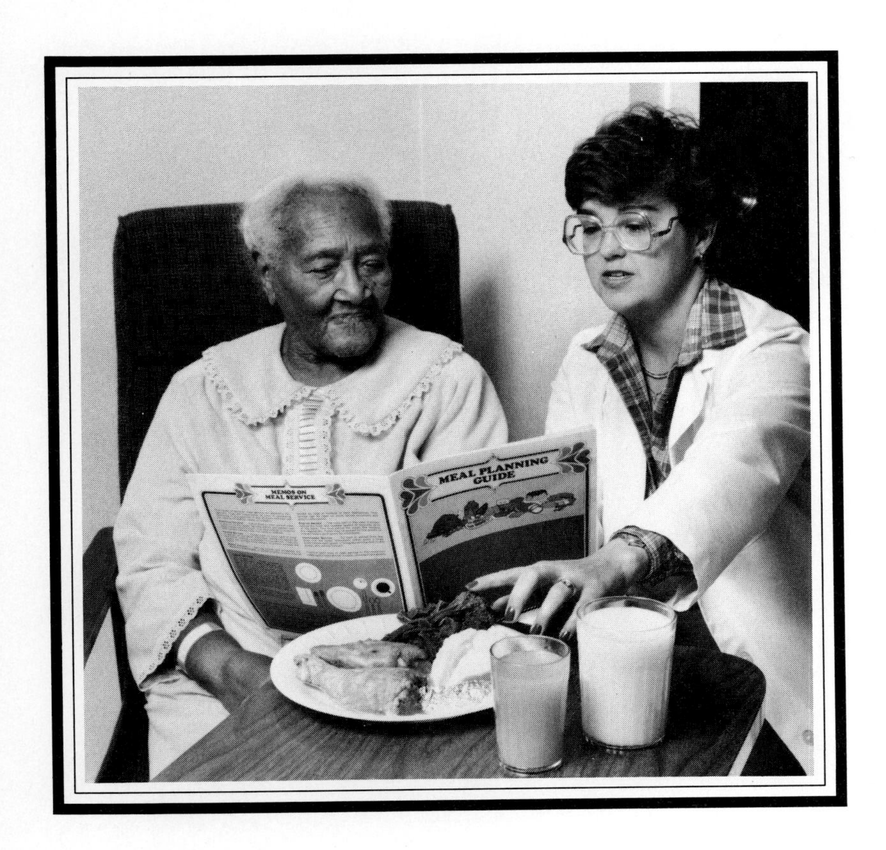


*A client's nutritional status is closely aligned with that client's overall level of health. Clients who enter the health care setting undergo nutritional assessment, often in conjunction with physical assessment, to be screened for existing or potential nutritional deficiencies. Once in the health care system, numerous factors and conditions have the potential to impair clients' nutritional status. Nurses must be responsive to this basic need and plan care accordingly. The chapters in this unit outline the skills and tools necessary to complete nutritional assessment, describe the skills dealing with oral nutrition, duscuss gastric and jejeunal tube feedings, and feature skills to maintain an adequate nutritional status for clients who need additional supplementation in the form of total parenteral nutrition.*

# 26

# ORAL NUTRITION

## OBJECTIVES

*Mastery of the content in this chapter will enable the nurse to:*

- Define key terms.
- Assess client's nutritional status and need for feeding assistance.
- Identify type of diet the client is receiving.
- Determine client's food allergies.
- Assess an infant's level of growth and development.
- Provide a pleasant eating environment for the client.
- Prepare the client to receive appropriate meals.
- Assemble necessary equipment to feed the client.
- Demonstrate appropriate nursing care in assembling the client's tray.
- Demonstrate how to properly assist a client with oral nutrition.
- Evaluate the client's tolerance to oral nutrition.
- Assess the client's extent of visual impairment and how it affects eating.
- Demonstrate how to properly bottle-feed an infant.
- Demonstrate how to assist a mother in breast-feeding an infant.
- Provide a safe environment for the infant.
- Evaluate the infant's tolerance to bottle- or breast-feeding.
- Demonstrate how to properly feed an infant solid food.

## KEY TERMS

*Anergy*
*Anorexia*
*Anthropometry*
*Antibody*
*Antigens*
*ASPEN*
*Cachexia*
*Calipers*
*Emaciation*
*Kilogram*
*MAC*
*Malnutrition*
*MAMC*
*TSF*

## SKILLS



The nutritional needs of hospitalized clients have gained importance in the health care profession. Hospital-wide surveys have demonstrated that malnutrition is unexpectedly high (50%) (Bistrian, 1974; Bistrian, 1976; Milano, 1978; Stetzer, 1979). Malnutrition is a very complex, widespread condition affecting a variety of individuals. Detection and prevention are imperative to the care of the malnourished client.

Nutritional assessment parameters, as related to clinical outcome, have not been established. A complete nutritional assessment requires the nurse to use many evaluation tools. Nutritional assessment, as a clinical tool, is still developing and has not been standardized. However, prevention, identification, and treatment of the malnourished client could be enhanced through the use of a standardized nutritional assessment. Today, nurses are becoming more involved in the nutritional assessment of the client. Although the dietitian frequently performs the nutritional assessment, the nurse should understand the components of this assessment and their interpretation to incorporate this information into the nursing care plan.

Adults are usually able to eat independently, but many clients need help. The amount and type of help is determined by the client's physical and cognitive limitations.

Infants depend entirely on others for their nutritional needs. The newborn's nutritional intake consists of breast milk or formula. This feeding continues until the child is from 3 to 6 months of age. Then, depending on the child's rate of growth, the mother's preference, and the pediatrician's advice, the feeding of solid food is begun.

Some elderly clients may also require feeding assistance because of the numerous physical alterations associated with aging. Other individuals who require feeding assistance are neurologically or orthopedically impaired clients who may be unable to manipulate feeding utensils.

Being fed by another person may cause psychologic problems. The increased need for feeding assistance may lead to depression, because clients feel that they are a burden to either the staff or their family. Therefore it is important for the nurse to be patient and understanding.

### PREREQUISITE KNOWLEDGE

1. Principles of medical asepsis.
2. Principles of enteral nutrition.
3. Principles of fluid and electrolytes.
4. Basic nutrition.
5. Anatomy and physiology of the gastrointestinal system.
6. Principles of growth and development.

### PREREQUISITE SKILLS

1. Proper handwashing techniques (Chapter 37).
2. Physical assessment (Chapter 13).
3. Intradermal injection (Chapter 21).

### GUIDELINES

1. Be aware of clients who are at risk for malnutrition. Certain individuals are known to be at risk and the nurse will be able to provide preventive care and seek appropriate resources for intervention.
2. Be aware of signs and symptoms of malnutrition. Severely underweight individuals are not the only ones who are malnourished. To provide care to all, the nurse needs to be able to detect the client with subtle nutritional changes as well as the obviously malnourished client.
3. Know client's medical history. Certain disease processes alter the digestive process. In addition, some medical problems cannot be treated with enteral nutrition, and alternative therapies need to be chosen.
4. Know client's social, economic, and environmental limitations as related to nutrition. Clients may be very interested in learning about nutrition, but if they do not have the facilities at home, they are unable to apply their information. The nurse needs to be aware of limitations and work with the client to improve nutrition.
5. Be sure equipment is functional before assessment. To properly perform the assessment, the nurse relies on equipment that is accurate and easy to use.
6. Use a systematic and organized approach to nutritional assessment. This allows the nurse to obtain essential information without being either redundant or incomplete.
7. Verify, communicate, and document findings. If others on the health team are unaware of the nurse's findings, the implementation process is halted and incomplete.
8. Be familiar with the different types of oral diets. This knowledge will help the nurse to properly plan for the client's needs.
9. Be aware of the psychologic impact that feeding assistance has on the client.
10. An organized approach when feeding the client will help the client feel more at ease, and appetite may increase in an unhurried atmosphere.
11. Know client's level of physical and cognitive functioning and encourage participation in feeding whenever possible.
12. Promote factors that improve client's appetite such as pleasant and comfortable surroundings and a neat meal tray.

## *SKILL 26-1*
## *PERFORMING NUTRITIONAL ASSESSMENT*

Nutritional assessment has four components: client history (medical, psychologic, social, and dietary), physical examination, anthropometrics, and biochemical parameters.

The client's history is a detailed written description that provides the nurse with data concerning the client's nutritional status. Along with the medical history, it is imperative that the nurse observe and examine the client for signs of malnutrition. Potential problems may be detected during the physical examination that were not discerned from the history. For example, the individual who has given you a detailed description of nutritional intake is assessed as adequately nourished. On physical examination, the client has dry, scaly skin. Upon further investigation, it is found that the client has had very few fat calories in the diet and therefore has an essential fatty acid deficiency.

Evaluation of body size and muscle wasting is accomplished through the use of anthropometrics. Anthropometrics will be discussed later in greater detail. Biochemical deviations that occur in the malnourished client must also be evaluated.

Nutritional assessment goals as outlined by the American Society of Parenteral and Enteral Nutrition (ASPEN) are:

1. Identify nutritional deficiencies that adversely affect health.
2. Obtain specific information to assist in planning and delivering nutritional care.
3. Evaluate the efficacy of nutritional care, modifying the nutritional care plan as needed to obtain the desired result (Forlaw, 1988).

The nutritional assessment must be individualized to adequately assess each client. The nurse must be aware of who is at risk for malnutrition and who is malnourished.

### Purposes

1. Identify nutritional deficiencies of clients.
2. Obtain information to assist in providing nutritional needs of clients.

## *Procedure 26-1*

### Assessment

| Steps | Rationale |
|---|---|
| 1. Determine need to perform nutritional assessment. | Certain conditions place client at risk for malnutrition, i.e., gross underweight (>80% below standard), gross overweight (>120% above standard), recent weight loss of >10%, alcoholism, no oral intake for 10 days on simple IV fluids, malabsorption syndromes, increased metabolic demands, and catabolic states. |
| 2. Assess client for factors that influence nutritional intake. | Social, economic, physical, and psychologic factors play parts in malnutrition. |
| 3. Perform thorough dietary history, e.g., typical meals, food preferences, snacks. | Dietary history reviews food consumption and eating habits that aid in detection of deficiencies. |
| 4. Review results of relevant laboratory tests: albumin and transferrin, total lymphocyte count (TLC), skin test antigens for cellular hypersensitivity (Table 26-1). | These biochemical parameters (ordered by physician) measure visceral and circulating protein status. Albumin and transferrin indicate visceral protein status. TLC and skin antigens assess immunocompetence. |

### Nursing Diagnosis

| Steps | Rationale |
|---|---|
| 1. Cluster data to reveal actual or potential nursing diagnoses: | |
| a. Altered nutrition—less than or more than body requirements: related to poor nutritional intake. | Clients may exhibit physical signs and symptoms of nutritional impairment. Complete nursing assessment helps identify cause of nutritional alteration. |
| b. Altered nutrition—less than or more than body requirements: related to malabsorption or catabolic states. | |
| c. Altered nutrition—less than or more than body requirements: related to social, economic, and psychologic factors. | |

### Planning

| Steps | Rationale |
|---|---|
| 1. Develop individualized goals for assessing a client's nutrition: | |
| a. Identify baseline knowledge (diet history). | Provides nurse with comparison for future follow-up, as well as information to identify if client is at risk for malnutrition. |
| b. Identify client's usual weight. Goals may include weight maintenance, weight gain, weight loss. | |
| c. Identify signs and symptoms associated with nutritional alterations. | |
| 2. Prepare needed equipment: | |
| a. Assessment sheet and pen | Organized, systematic assessment tools will facilitate speed and accuracy of assessment. Sheet will also be used for documentation (Fig. 26-1). |
| b. Tongue blade, stethoscope, penlight | Stethoscope will be needed to auscultate lung sounds (Chapter 13). Tongue blade and light will help nurse see oral mucosa. |
| c. Scale and tape measure (will also be used in anthropometric measurements) | To achieve accurate height and weight. (See Table 13-4, p. 239). |
| d. Set of calipers | Skinfold calipers measure subcutaneous tissue size. |

| Steps | Rationale |
|---|---|
| 3. Explain to client nutritional assessment and its effect on health care. | Clients need to be well informed so that they may actively participate in their health care. |
| 4. Perform assessment in quiet undistracted environment. | Quiet undistracted environment will help nurse to better obtain needed information. |

## Implementation

| | |
|---|---|
| 1. Obtain complete and thorough nursing history to include social, economic, and psychologic information. | Nursing history allows nurse to determine client's nutritional baseline, potential problem areas, and current problems. |
| 2. Either initiate diet diary or perform 24-hr recall interview. | Diet diary and 24-hr recall evaluate food consumption and eating habits. |
| 3. Document findings on nutritional assessment sheet. | Prompt documentation prevents nurse from omitting essential information from late entry. |
| 4. Assist client into bed. | Having client in bed facilitates physical assessment. |
| 5. Perform physical assessment as described in Chapter 13. | Through use of physical assessment, nurse will be able to detect signs and symptoms of malnutrition (Table 26-2). |
| 6. Assist client to standing position, free of restrictive clothing. | Clients must be standing for anthropometric measurements. |
| 7. Have client stand on scale or if client is unable to stand use chair, litter, or sling-type scales. Record weight; convert to kilograms (weight × 2.2 = kg). | Weight is gross but very useful index of client's state of nutrition.<br>Client should be weighed with same scale at same time every day with same amount of clothing. |
| 8. Measure client's height. If client is unable to stand, measure from heel to top of head while lying flat on bed and record. | Correct height will assist in calculating ideal body weight. |
| 9. Using tape, measure smallest portion of wrist distal to styloid process (Fig. 26-2). | Wrist circumference is used to estimate body frame size. |
| 10. With client's nondominant arm relaxed, measure circumference at midpoint of arm in cm (between tip of acromial process of scapula and olecranon process of ulna) and | Mid-upper arm circumference (MAC) determines muscle wasting. |

***TABLE 26-1*** Common Laboratory Tests to Evaluate Nutritional Status

| Test/Normal Range | Purpose | Abnormal Findings/Implications |
|---|---|---|
| Serum albumin normal: 4-5.5 mg/dl | Maintain serum protein levels<br>Maintain fluid and electrolyte balance<br>Useful in determining prolonged protein wasting | Abnormal values may take up to 2 weeks before they are reflected in blood studies<br>Abnormalities in liver and kidney diseases, stress, dehydration, infection<br><2.5 mg/dl indicates severe protein depletion |
| Transferrin normal: 170-250 mg/dl | More specific indicator of protein/calorie malnutrition than albumin<br>Blood protein binds with iron | Abnormal values respond quickly to changes in protein intake<br>Decreased in liver disease and chronic renal failure |
| Total lymphocyte count (TLC) normal: >1800 | Impaired nutritional intake depresses immune system, which is reflected in TLC | Depleted in all immunosuppressed clients |
| Hemoglobin normal: 12-15 g/dl | Measures oxygen and iron carrying capacity of the blood | Decrease may indicate some form of anemia or can be lowered with blood loss |
| Blood urea nitrogen (BUN) normal: 10-20 mg/dl | Measures breakdown of dietary protein<br>Measures urea production in the liver and excretion in the kidneys | Elevated with excessive protein intake<br>Depressed with low protein intake<br>Elevated in liver and renal disease<br>Falsely elevated in hypovolemic dehydration |
| Creatinine excretion in 24-hour urine | Creatinine formation and excretion reflects total muscle mass<br>Indirect measure of skeletal muscle mass depletion | Abnormally low in renal disease<br>Abnormally low in severe malnutrition and starvation |

ST. LOUIS UNIVERSITY MEDICAL CENTER
NUTRITION SUPPORT SERVICES
Nutritional Assessment

ate ________ adm. Date________ Age_____ Sex_____

DIAGNOSIS: ________________________________

ASSOCIATED DISEASES: ________________________________

OPERATION: ________________________________

Stress of Illness: __ Fever __ Infection __ Diarrhea/Emesis __ Respirator
__ Chomotherapy or Radiation __ Surgery

Drug Therapy: __ Insulin __ Steroids __ Narcotics __ Other__________________

Lab Data: $Na/K^{+}$_____ $Cl/CO_2$ _____ Glucose _____ BUN _____ Serum Creatinine_______

$Ca^{+}/Phosphate_4$ _____ Total Protein/Albumin _____ Chol/Triglyceride _______

Hgb/Hct _____ Transferrin _____ WBC _____ LDH _____ Total Bilirubin ______

SGOT _____ Mg _____ $B_{12}$ _____ Folate _____ Pro Time _____ PTT _______

Other ____________________

ht.________ cm Wt. _______ Kg. adm. Wt. _______ Kg Usual Wt. _______ Kg.

Ideal Body Weight _______ Kg. % Wt. change _______ % change in BMR _______

est. metabolic rate ________ est. cal. needs for Wt. maintenance ________

Wt. gain/anabolism_______ est. Nitrogen needs for Nitrogen balance _____ Protein needs _____

ANTHROPOMETRICS: WRIST circumference ______ MAC ____ SEC ____
TSF _____ ____ ____ SUM ____

SKIN ANTIGEN TEST: TETANUS GLYCERIN CONTROL
DIPHTHERIA CANDIDA
STREPTOCOCCUS TRICHOPHYTON
TUBERCULIN PROTEUS

RESULTS: ________________________________

________________________________

RECOMMENDATIONS: ________________________________

________________________________
Signature

D1.05 Rev. 2/83

***Fig. 26-1***
Courtesy St. Louis University Hospital, St. Louis.

***TABLE 26-2*** Clinical Signs of Nutritional Status

| Body Area | Signs of Good Nutrition | Signs of Poor Nutrition |
|---|---|---|
| General appearance | Alert, responsive | Listless, apathetic, cachectic |
| Weight | Normal for height, age, body build | Overweight or underweight (special concern for underweight) |
| Posture | Erect, arms and legs straight | Sagging shoulders, sunken chest, humped back |
| Muscles | Well-developed, firm, good tone, some fat under skin | Flaccid, poor tone, underdeveloped, tender, edema, wasted appearance, cannot walk properly |
| Nervous control | Good attention span, not irritable or restless, normal reflexes, psychologic stability | Inattentive, irritable, confused, burning and tingling of hands and feet (paresthesia), loss of position and vibratory sense, weakness and tenderness of muscles (may result in inability to walk), decrease or loss of ankle and knee reflexes, absent vibratory sense |
| Gastrointestinal function | Good appetite and digestion, normal regular elimination, no palpable organs or masses | Anorexia, indigestion, constipation or diarrhea, liver or spleen enlargement |
| Cardiovascular function | Normal heart rate and rhythm, no murmurs, normal blood pressure for age | Rapid heart rate (above 100 beats per min), enlarged heart, abnormal rhythm, elevated blood pressure |
| General vitality | Endurance, energetic, sleeps well, vigorous | Easily fatigued, no energy, falls asleep easily, looks tired, apathetic |
| Hair | Shiny, lustrous, firm, not easily plucked, healthy scalp | Stringy, dull, brittle, dry, thin, and sparse, depigmented, can be easily plucked |
| Skin (general) | Smooth, slightly moist, good color | Rough, dry, scaly, pale, pigmented, irritated, bruises, petechiae, subcutaneous fat loss |
| Face and neck | Skin color uniform, smooth, pink, healthy appearance, not swollen | Greasy, discolored, scaly, swollen, skin dark over cheeks and under eyes, lumpiness or flakiness of skin around nose and mouth |
| Lips | Smooth, good color, moist, not chapped or swollen | Dry, scaly, swollen, redness and swelling (cheilosis), or angular lesions at corners of the mouth, fissures or scars (stomatitis) |
| Mouth, oral membranes | Reddish pink mucous membranes in oral cavity | Swollen, boggy oral mucous membranes |
| Gums | Good pink color, healthy, red, no swelling or bleeding | Spongy, bleed easily, marginal redness, inflamed, gums receding |
| Tongue | Good pink color or deep reddish in appearance, not swollen or smooth, surface papillae present, no lesions | Swelling, scarlet and raw, magenta color, beefy (glossitis), hyperemic and hypertrophic papillae, atrophic papillae |
| Teeth | No cavities, no pain, bright, straight, no crowding, well-shaped jaw, clean, no discoloration | Unfilled caries, absent teeth, worn surfaces, mottled (fluorosis), malpositioned |
| Eyes | Bright, clear, shiny, no sores at corner of eyelids, membranes moist and healthy pink color, no prominent blood vessels or mound of tissue or sclera, no fatigue circles beneath | Eye membranes pale (pale conjunctivae), redness of membrane (conjunctival injection), dryness, signs of infection, Bitot's spots, redness and fissuring of eyelid corners (angular palpebritis), dryness of eye membrane (conjunctival xerosis), dull appearance of cornea (corneal xerosis), soft cornea (keratomalacia) |
| Neck (glands) | No enlargement | Thyroid enlargement |
| Nails | Firm, pink | Spoon shape (koilonychia), brittle, ridged |
| Legs, feet | No tenderness, weakness, or swelling; good color | Edema, tender calf, tingling, weakness |
| Skeleton | No malformations | Bowlegs, knock-knees, chest deformity at diaphragm, beaded ribs, prominent scapulas |

From Williams SR: Nutritional guidance in prenatal care. In Worthington-Roberts BS, Vermeersch JA, Williams SR: Nutrition in pregnancy and lactation, ed 3, St. Louis, 1985, The CV Mosby Co; Grant JA, Kennedy-Caldwell C: Nutritional support in nursing, Philadelphia, 1988, Grune-Stratton.

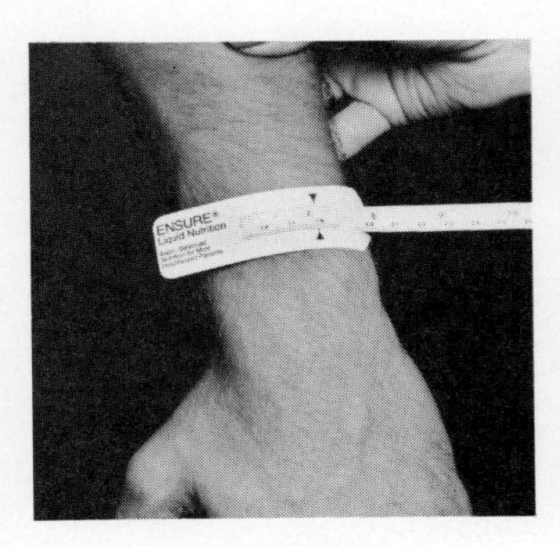


*Fig. 26-2*

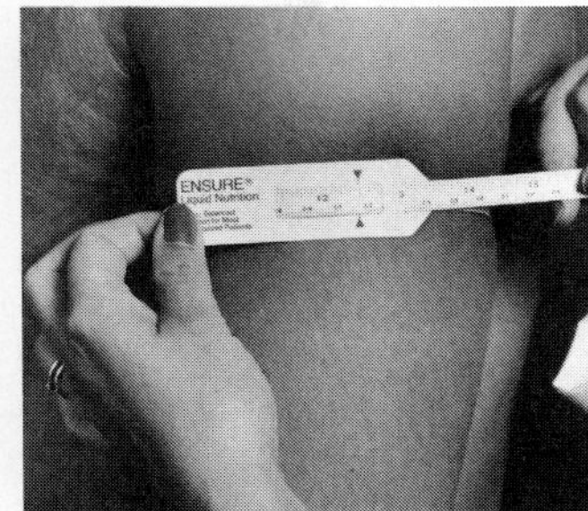
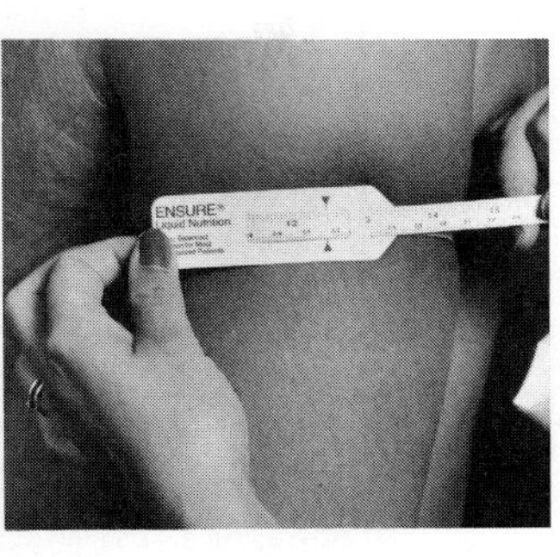


*Fig. 26-3*

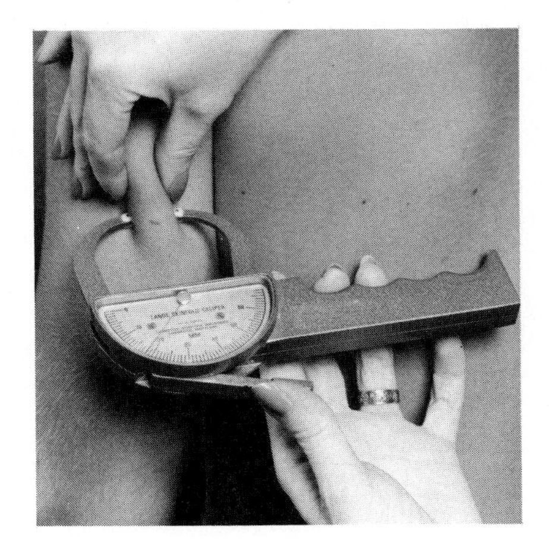

*Fig. 26-4*

| Steps | Rationale |
|---|---|
| record (Fig. 26-3). If client is bedridden, measurements may be taken with arm bent and placed across chest. | |
| 11. With thumb and forefinger, pinch a double fold of fat lengthwise about 1 cm above midpoint of MAC. With other hand, place teeth of calipers on either side of fat fold. Calipers are placed below fingers so pressure is exerted from calipers and not fingers. Record 3 separate readings in mm and document (Fig. 26-4). | Skin fold measurements are used to estimate fat content of subcutaneous tissue (i.e., biceps, scapula, abdominal muscles). Triceps skin fold (TSF) is most common and easiest to measure. Average 3 readings of TSF. |
| 12. Assist client to comfortable position. | Remainder of assessment is comprised of calculations and review of lab work. |
| 13. Calculate mid-arm muscle circumference (MAMC), i.e., MAMC = MAC − (TSF × 3.14) and record. | MAMC is estimation of skeletal muscle mass. |
| 14. Choose site to administer skin antigen test. Select only sites that have enough surface area and subcutaneous tissue (i.e., volar surface of arm or back) (see Chapter 28). | Skin testing evaluates sensitivity to bacteria. Anergy is common in malnutrition and is absence of any response to testing. |
| 15. Cleanse site with alcohol and allow to dry completely. | Alcohol will disinfect skin. |
| 16. Holding premixed antigen kit in right hand, support client's site with other hand. | |
| 17. With skin taut, press antigen skin testing unit onto skin with enough pressure to penetrate skin. Maintain firm contact for 5 sec. | Allows antigen to enter interdermis. |
| 18. Draw line around test area and read results in 24 and 48 hr. | Marking area will allow easy visibility of site injection. |
| 19. Discard supplies appropriately and wash hands. | Reduces transmission of microorganisms. |
| 20. Explain to client that nutritional assessment is complete. | Allows time for client to ask questions about assessment. |

## Evaluation

| Steps | Rationale |
|---|---|
| 1. Review history and physical findings. Note abnormalities or areas of concern. | Completeness of data obtained from history and physical findings permits prompt interventions for nutritional alterations. |
| 2. Review diet diary and 24-hr recall with client. | Determine status of dietary habits and client's knowledge. |
| 3. Compare client's height and weight with normal height and weight for that age group. | Weight may fluctuate with age, size, and height. |
| 4. Review anthropometric data. | Normal MAC: Male 29.5 cm, Female 28.5 cm<br>Normal TSF: Male 12.5 cm, Female 16.5 cm<br>Normal MAMC: Male 25.3 cm, Female 23.2 cm |
| 5. Compare normal albumin, transferrin, and total lymphocyte count with client's values; albumin less than 3.5 gm/dl warrants further evaluation; less than 3.0 gm/dl denotes moderate protein depletion; less than 2.4 gm/dl denotes severe protein depletion. | Normal albumin level is 3.5-5.5 gm/dl, transferrin: >200 mg/dl, total lymphocyte count: white blood count (WBC) × percent lymphocyte (TLC = WBC × % lymphs), greater than 2000 not depleted, 1200-2000 mild, 800-1199 moderate, <800 severe. |

ST. LOUIS UNIVERSITY MEDICAL CENTER
NUTRITION SUPPORT SERVICES
Nutritional Assessment

ate 12-11 adm. Date 12-8 Age 48 Sex M

DIAGNOSIS: Small bowel obstruction

ASSOCIATED DISEASES: radiation enteritis

OPERATION: 12/9 exploratory laparotomy

Stress of Illness: ✓ Fever (T=101°) ✓ Infection __ Diarrhea/Emesis __ Respirator
__ Chomotherapy or Radiation ✓ Surgery

Drug Therapy: __ Insulin __ Steroids __ Narcotics __ Other ______

Lab Data: $Na/K^+$ 131/3.9 $Cl/CO_2$ 109/24 Glucose 98 BUN 10 Serum Creatinine 10
$Ca^+$/$Phosphate_4$ 8.9/3.2 Total Protein/Albumin 4.8/2.3 Chol/Triglyceride 113/100
Hgb/Hct 10/31 Transferrin 121 WBC 12.1 LDH 90 Total Bilirubin 1.0
SGOT 30 Mg 2.0 $B_{12}$ ____ Folate ____ Pro Time 43% PTT 41.0
Other ______

ht. 182.9 cm Wt. 72 Kg. adm. Wt. 70 Kg Usual Wt. 84 Kg.

Ideal Body Weight 83 Kg. % Wt. change 14 % change in BMR 50

est. metabolic rate ____ est. cal. needs for Wt. maintenance ____

Wt. gain/anabolism ____ est. Nitrogen needs for Nitrogen balance ____ Protein needs ____

ANTHROPOMETRICS: WRIST CIRCUMFERENCE 6½" MAC 30 SEC ____
TSF 12.4, 12.4, 12.6 SUM 12.5

SKIN ANTIGEN TEST: TETANUS O GLYCERIN CONTROL O
DIPHTHERIA O CANDIDA O
STREPTOCOCCUS O TRICHOPHYTON O
TUBERCULIN + PROTEUS O

RESULTS: 1 12CM. # OF POSITIVE ANTIGENS/SUM TOTAL OF INDURATION

RECOMMENDATIONS:

______
Signature

D1.05 Rev. 2/83

***Fig. 26-5***
Courtesy St. Louis University Hospital, St. Louis.

| Steps | Rationale |
|---|---|
| 6. Review antigen skin testing at 24 and 48 hr (candida, mumps, trichomonas, coccidiodin, streptokinase, streptodornase, and control). Positive reaction is reported with induration of 2 mm or more. | Virulence to bacterial and viral infection is greater in malnourished clients; basal metabolism is energy needed to maintain body's basic processes with the exclusion of digestion. |
| 7. Determine client's caloric needs. | Most commonly used formula is Harris-Benedict equation: Basal Energy Expenditure (BEE) = 66.47 + 13.75 W (weight) + 5.0 H (height) − 6.76 (age) (males). Basal Energy Expenditure (BEE) = 655.10 = 9.56 W (weight) + H (height) − 4.68 (age) (females). |
| 8. Determine amount of protein client requires. | |
| 9. Determine route of nutrition (enteral or parenteral). | If gastrointestinal tract functions, it should be used. |
| 10. If parenteral nutrition: choose either peripheral or central TPN, and determine whether fat is needed. | Total parenteral nutrition and fat emulsion are necessary to promote and maintain nutritional balance during illness. |
| ***Expected outcomes*** | |
| 1. Physical assessment and laboratory data are consistent with proper nutritional balance. | Indicates that client's nutritional intake and use of nutritional substances are within normal values. |
| ***Unexpected outcomes*** | |
| 1. Nutritional alterations are less than body requirements. | |
| 2. Nutritional alterations are more than body requirements. | Indicates actual or potential malnourished status. |

### Recording and Reporting

1. Make recommendations and document (Fig. 26-5).

### Special Considerations

- Client or significant other should be reliable source of information for a dietary history. Determine what medications client is on, nutritional status (Table 26-2), and possible drug interaction.
- Both diet diary and 24-hr recall are effective methods for taking diet history. Diet diary is obtained over longer period of time and helps to determine food likes and dislikes, as well as allergies. The 24-hr recall is an account of everything the client has consumed over that period of time; it is less time-consuming but not as accurate.
- Ideally, the same person should measure client. Room temperature should be comfortable for client during procedure.
- To determine:

$$\_\% \text{ IBW} = \frac{\text{actual weight} \times 100}{\text{IBW}}$$

or

$$\frac{\text{Percent weight change} = \text{actual weight} \times 100}{\text{usual}}$$

- If patient has lost more than 10% of body weight, weight gain program is begun. 500 Kcals increase in calories provide 1-lb weight gain.
- Albumin is major protein produced by liver. It is useful indicator for chronically malnourished clients; in acute client, greater number of factors influence albumin (e.g., stress, hydration, surgery); transferrin is more specific indicator of protein and calorie malnutrition than albumin.

## *SKILL 26-2*
## *ASSISTING THE ADULT CLIENT WITH ORAL NUTRITION*

Assisting the adult with oral nutrition requires time, patience, knowledge, and understanding. Most people eat without assistance. However, with illness or trauma, the client may be physically unable to eat without assistance. Physical impairments that limit self-feeding include hemiplegia, fractured arm, quadriplegia, debilitating illness, or generalized weakness. The presence of intravenous catheters or tubings, dressings, and bandages can also limit self-feeding. While adult feeding needs and techniques differ from those for infants, the adult who needs help to eat still needs compassion and understanding. Merely feeding the adult can be accomplished with common sense, but providing a socially meaningful mealtime requires education and experience on the part of the nurse.

### Purposes

1. Maintain nutritional status.
2. Promote socialization.

## *Procedure 26-2*

| Step | Rationale |
|---|---|
| **Assessment** | |
| 1. Determine to what extent client is able to self-feed. Assess physical motor skills, level of consciousness, visual acuity and peripheral vision, mood. | Thorough understanding of client's physical and cognitive limitations will alert nurse to client's needs. |
| 2. Identify type of diet that client can tolerate. | Nurse awareness of specific diet order provides appropriate nutrition. |
| 3. Assess client's appetite, tolerance to food, likes and dislikes. | Awareness of client's needs before meals will prevent misunderstanding and frustration for both nurse and client. |
| 4. Assess whether client has food allergies. | Prevents allergic reaction to food groups. |
| **Nursing Diagnosis** | |
| 1. Cluster data to reveal actual or potential nursing diagnoses related to clients nutritional and feeding needs: | |
| a. Altered nutrition: related to inappropriate diet, food intolerances. | Incorrect diet, i.e., regular diet when client needs pureed diet, or food intolerances can decrease client food intake and affect nutritional status. |
| b. Feeding self-care deficit: related to weak hand grasp and reduced vision. | Directs nurse to use techniques that will optimize client's ability to eat. |
| **Planning** | |
| 1. Develop individualized goals for client based on nursing diagnoses: | |
| a. Promote dietary intake. | Adequate dietary intake decreases client's risk for nutritional imbalances. |
| b. Promote independence in feeding. | Allowing participation in feeding activities can increase clients dietary intake. |
| c. Promote socialization during mealtime. | Isolated clients are at risk for decreased nutritional intake, which can result from depression or social isolation. |
| 2. Prepare client's room for mealtime: | Unsightly, odor-filled room can decrease client's appetite. |
| a. Remove any unpleasant sights (i.e. bedpans, dressings, and trash). | |
| b. Remove any unpleasant odors. | |
| c. Clear overhead table. | |
| d. Set up chair for client and for nurse. | |
| 3. Prepare client for meal: | |
| a. Assist client to urinate or defecate. | Oral hygiene will improve taste and increase appetite. |
| b. Assist client with mouth care. | |
| c. Assist client with eyeglasses or contact lenses if used/needed. | Reduces spread of microorganisms. |
| d. Assist client to wash hands. | Upright position is normal position for meals and also helps prevent aspiration. |
| e. Assist client to an upright position. | Facilitates self-feeding. |
| f. Apply/obtain any special devices (i.e., hand splints, pedestal cup, built-up silverware, Tommy-tippy cup). | |
| 4. Wash hands before preparing client's tray. | Reduces spread of microorganisms. |
| 5. Assemble needed supplies to facilitate feeding (Fig. 26-6): utensils, napkins, towels, tray. | Preparing needed equipment before entering room provides organized, unhurried impression. |
| **Implementation** | |
| 1. Assess tray for completeness and correct diet. | Prevents ingestion of incorrect or incomplete meal. |
| 2. Prepare tray to meet client's needs: open cartons, remove lids, cut food, season food by asking client's preferences. | Clients with cognitive or physical impairments may not have fine motor coordination needed to prepare tray for eating. |
| 3. Place small towel or napkin under client's chin. | Protects client's clothes and bed linens. |
| 4. If client is able to eat independently, stop here. Return after 10-20 min. | Determines how well client is tolerating diet. |
| 5. If convenient sit in chair next to client. | It is psychologically more comforting to client if nurse is sitting. |
| 6. Ask in what order client would like to eat. | Allows client to choose which foods to eat first. |
| 7. Cut food into bite-sized pieces. | Small pieces, easier to chew, decrease possibility of aspiration. |

| Step | Rationale |
| --- | --- |

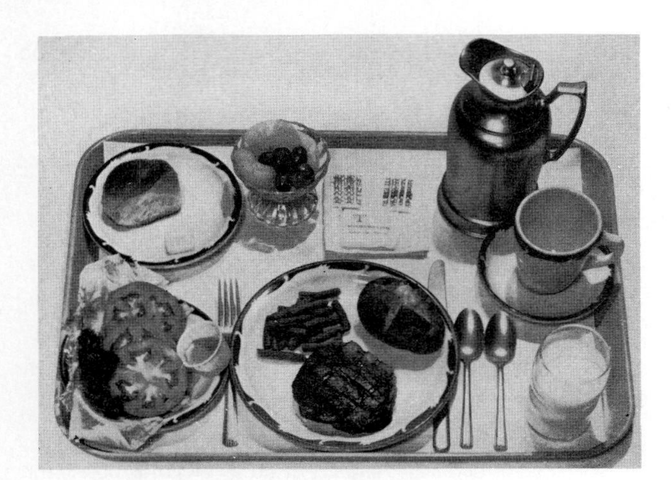

***Fig. 26-6***

From Williams SR: Mowry's basic nutrition and diet therapy, ed 8, St Louis, 1988, The CV Mosby Co.

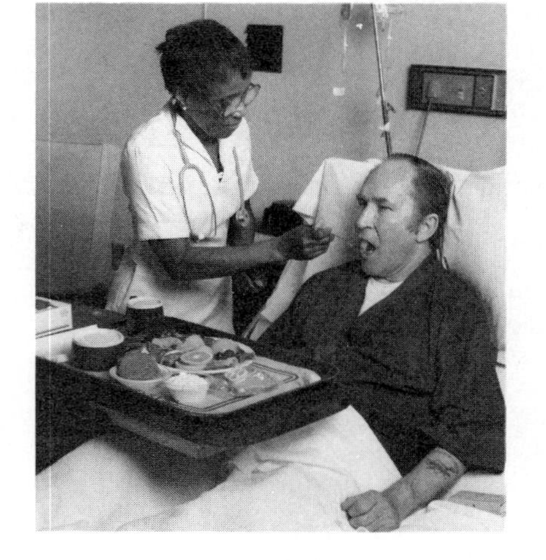

***Fig. 26-7***

| Step | Rationale |
| --- | --- |
| 8. Feed client, placing one type of food on utensil at a time (Fig. 26-7). | Avoids rushing client through the meal. Allows client enough time to chew and swallow food. |
| 9. Provide fluids as requested. Do not allow client to drink all liquids at beginning of meal. | Assists swallowing. Prevents client from filling up on liquids. |
| 10. Talk to client during meal. | Meal should be a pleasant event. Conversation promotes socialization. Too much talk prevents client from eating. |
| 11. Use meal as an opportunity to educate client (i.e., topics related to nutrition, postoperative exercises, discharge plans). | Education can occur whenever nurse and client are together. |
| 12. Assist client to wash hands and perform mouth care. | Mouth care after meals helps prevent dental caries. If client has dentures, wash them as directed by client. |
| 13. Assist client to resting position. | Client may feel tired after full meal. If client is prone to aspiration leave head elevated 45° for 30 min after meal. |
| 14. Return client's tray to appropriate place. | Returning tray promptly will facilitate prompt pick-up by dietary department. |
| 15. Wash hands. | Reduces spread of microorganisms. |

## Evaluation

| Step | Rationale |
| --- | --- |
| 1. Assess client's tolerance to diet. | Overfeeding may cause nausea and vomiting. Underfeeding may leave client feeling hungry. |
| 2. Assess client's fluid and food intake. | Helps to determine whether client's nutritional and fluid needs are being met. |
| 3. Assess client's ability to assist with feeding. | Helps determine if client is gaining independence in feeding. |

### *Expected outcomes*

| Step | Rationale |
| --- | --- |
| 1. Client completes meal. | Prescribed dietary intake has been eaten; decreases risk of nutritional imbalances. |
| 2. Client does not complain of any gastric problems or food intolerances. | Indicates absence of gastric disturbance or food intolerance. |

### *Unexpected outcomes*

| Step | Rationale |
| --- | --- |
| 1. Client is unable to complete meal. | Client may feel that an improper meal was delivered, or there were insufficient personnel to assist with feeding. |
| 2. Client complains of nausea, vomiting, diarrhea, or food intolerances. | Gastrointestinal symptoms may indicate food intolerances, allergies, or presence of bacteria. Presence of such symptoms impairs absorption of nutrients. |

## Recording and Reporting

| Step | Rationale |
| --- | --- |
| 1. Document in client's chart: client tolerance of diet, amount eaten, intake and output. | Documentation facilitates communication among health care professionals. |

| Step | Rationale |
|---|---|
| **Follow-up Activities** | |
| 1. Determine why client is unable to finish meal (i.e., inadequate personnel for feeding assistance, ingestion of large volume of liquids immediately before meal, improper diet). | Identification of cause of unexpected outcome allows nursing personnel to avoid similar situation in future. |
| 2. Notify physician of any unexpected outcomes. | Prompt notification promotes fast interventions. |

### Special Considerations

- Clients require proper-fitting dentures to eat properly.
- Elderly clients may have diminished appetite because of loss of taste, smell, and decreased number of taste buds.
- If client is unable to sit up to eat, elevate head of bed to approximately 90°; if unable to sit up in bed to eat turn client on a side.
- If client is on calorie counts, record caloric intake on appropriate form; if intake and output are being evaluated, record fluid intake on appropriate form.

### Teaching Considerations

- Instruct client and primary care giver in required diet, including elimination of certain foods. Provide written instructions.
- Instruct client and primary care giver to maintain a nutritional balance of foods.
- Instruct client and primary care giver to monitor intake of fluids, calories, fats, salt.
- Instruct client and primary care giver on importance of providing frequent mouth care.

### Home Care Considerations

- Assess familiarity of client and primary care giver with proper nutritional standards.
- Assess financial resources of client and family to determine if they are able to purchase proper foods for the client.
- Assess priority given by client and family to provision of a balanced nutritional plan.
- Verify physician's diet order for the client.
- Verify accuracy of food with physician's diet order.
- Assist client to feed self. Help client do as much as possible in feeding self.
- Assist client, family, and primary care giver to make eating an enjoyable experience.

## *SKILL 26-3*
## *TEACHING BREAST-FEEDING*

Breast-feeding requires special instructions for the hospitalized infant and their mothers. For example, a mother who is breast-feeding should avoid using any soap on her breasts because soap tends to dry and crack nipples. Breast milk is more nutritious than formula feedings. Mother's milk is formed in the acinar or alveolar cells of the mammary glands. These cells secrete colostrum, which is a thin, watery, high-protein fluid that is fairly low in sugar and fat.

Infants who are breast-fed are less likely to have gastrointestinal (GI) disorders. Other advantages include: providing temporary immunity to certain diseases, lessening the risk of allergic reactions, and providing emotional support for the baby.

### Purposes

1. Maintain proper nutritional status.
2. Promote growth and development.
3. Maintain fluid and electrolyte balance.
4. Provide cuddling and bonding between infant and mother.

## *Procedure 26-3*

| Step | Rationale |
|---|---|
| **Assessment** | |
| 1. Assess whether infant has well-developed suck reflex. | Sufficient reflex determines whether infant will be able to suck milk from the breast. |
| 2. Stimulate rooting reflex; brush infant's cheek with nipple. | Rooting reflex causes child to turn toward nipple (food source). |
| 3. Evaluate infant's weight. | Weight gain indicates how well infant is doing nutritionally. |

| Step | Rationale |
|---|---|
| **Nursing Diagnosis** | |
| 1. Cluster data to reveal actual or potential nursing diagnoses: | |
| a. Altered nutrition—less than body requirements: related to improper technique for breast feeding. | Improper technique for breast-feeding results in nutritional deficit. |
| **Planning** | |
| 1. Develop individualized goals for client based on nursing diagnoses: | |
| a. Maintain fluid and electrolyte balance. | Maintain infant's nutrient, fluid, and electrolyte needs. |
| b. Promote bonding and cuddling. | Breast-feeding provides opportunity for play and cuddling between infant and mother. |
| 2. Infant should be awake, hungry, and dry before feeding is initiated. | Awake and comfortable infant will feed better. |
| 3. Dress infant appropriately. | If too warm, infant may fall asleep. If too cool, infant may be fussy and restless. |
| 4. Assemble supplies: a. Clear water b. Cotton balls | |
| 5. Assist breast-feeding mother to prepare self: wash hands, wash nipples with clear water and use cotton to dry. | Washing nipples removes old milk that provides media for bacterial growth. Bacteria may cause GI disturbances. |
| 6. Assist the mother in finding a comfortable position, either sitting (i.e., armchair with pillow to support baby correctly, with a footstool to support the mother's feet during feeding) or lying on her side with a pillow under her head and the baby on the bed beside her. | Proper and comfortable position of the mother will provide comfort and security for her and the baby during breast-feeding. |
| 7. For breast-feeding, check both mother's and infant's identification bands to be sure baby is delivered to correct mother. | Proper identification of mother and baby prevents chance of error (breast-feeding wrong baby). |
| **Implementation** | |
| 1. Position infant at breast in semisitting position with face close to breast. One arm and hand or pillow to support infant. | Proper position will provide comfort and security. |
| 2. Allow baby to root for nipple and touch cheek with breast. | Rooting reflex stimulates baby to open mouth and seek nipple. |
| 3. Lips of the infant should cover areola. | Establishes suction and makes sucking effective. |
| 4. Burp baby at least once during feeding and at end. Place baby in sitting position on mother's or nurse's lap, tilt forward, and gently pat back. Place baby prone on mother's or nurse's shoulder and gently pat back. Place baby in prone position on lap and gently pat back; newborn babies should be burped after each ounce. | Releases swallowed air and promotes completion of breast-feeding. |
| 5. Continue feeding until infant is satisfied. | Complete feeding allows baby to feel satisfied. If infant falls asleep while eating stroke cheek to arouse. |
| 6. When infant has stopped sucking, instruct mother to put her finger to the corner of the baby's mouth and gently pull. | Breaks suction of baby clinging to breast after feeding is completed. |
| 7. Have mother check diaper. | If diaper is wet or soiled, change it before returning infant to crib. |
| 8. Place infant in bed on stomach or right side. | Aids in emptying stomach and prevents regurgitation. |
| **Evaluation** | |
| 1. Assess if infant has spit up in crib or is restless. Burp restless infant. | Indicates presence of air in stomach. |
| 2. Observe mother and infant interaction. | Assesses bonding. |
| 3. Observe infant's response toward sucking and feeding. | Determines infant's tolerance to feeding. |
| ***Expected outcomes*** | |
| 1. Infant does not vomit, spit up excessively, or have diarrhea. | Indicates that allergy or intolerance to feeding is not present. |
| 2. Infant completes feeding. | Ensures complete nutritional, fluid, and electrolyte balance. |
| 3. Mother and infant appear comfortable with nursing. | Indicates positive breast-feeding for both mother and infant. |
| ***Unexpected outcomes*** | |
| 1. Infant refuses breast repeatedly. | May indicate pain, GI upset, or illness. |

### Recording and Reporting

| Step | Rationale |
| --- | --- |
| 1. Record baby's tolerance, amount, regurgitation, length of feeding, and how baby sucked. | Documents intake and infant's ability to tolerate feeding. |

### Follow-up Activities

| Step | Rationale |
| --- | --- |
| 1. Contact pediatrician about any unexpected outcomes. | Provides opportunity to have infant examined to identify illness. |

### Special Considerations

- Infants are born with ability to suck and swallow; small, premature infants may have difficulty sucking.
- Length of time for breast-feeding depends on age of baby and how vigorously baby sucks. Length of time for breast-feeding is usually 5-30 min.
- If mother had a Caesarean section, place a pillow over her lap to protect tender area while she is breast-feeding.

# *SKILL 26-4*
# *BOTTLE-FEEDING AN INFANT*

Feeding time for the infant should be happy, warm, and affectionate. Tenderness shown during feeding affects how well the infant eats, the infant's future personality, and how the infant learns to love.

A variety of formulas are available. The most convenient are the ready-to-use formulas supplied in either bottles or cans. Other types include powdered, concentrated liquid, evaporated milk, iron fortified, and hypoallergenic. Each contains the appropriate nutritional requirements; the choice of a formula is usually made after considering the infant's nutritional needs, cost, preparation, and time involved.

Bottle-feeding the infant is discussed in this skill, but not all mothers bottle-feed. Hospitalized breast-feeding infants and their mothers have special needs as well. Mother's milk surpasses formula feeding nutritionally. It has other advantages as well, such as providing temporary immunity to a number of diseases, decreasing the risk of allergic reactions, and providing emotional support for the baby.

Whether an infant is bottle- or breast-fed does not normally have a major effect on nutritional status. In addition to nutrition the feeding should provide warmth, love, and security.

### Purposes

1. Maintain proper nutritional status.
2. Promote growth and development.
3. Maintain fluid and electrolyte balance.
4. Provide cuddling and bonding for infant.

## *Procedure 26-4*

### Assessment

| Step | Rationale |
| --- | --- |
| 1. Assess whether infant has well-developed suck reflex. | Sufficient reflex determines whether infant will be able to suck formula from bottle. |
| 2. Stimulate rooting reflex; brush infant's cheek with nipple. | Rooting reflex causes child to turn toward nipple (food source). |
| 3. Evaluate infant's weight. | Weight gain indicates how well infant is doing nutritionally; normal gain in early newborn is 1 oz/day. |
| 4. Assess infant for allergic reactions (i.e., skin eruptions, digestive alteration, running nose, increased crying). | Some infants are sensitive or allergic to cow milk or prepared formulas. |
| 5. Assess infant's tolerance to formula. | If infant does not tolerate formula, severe dehydration and electrolyte imbalance may occur. |
| 6. Assess whether proper formula is used. | Physician will recommend type of formula (i.e., premixed commercially prepared, evaporated milk, or self-mix). |

| Step | Rationale |
|---|---|
| **Nursing Diagnosis** | |
| 1. Cluster data to reveal actual or potential nursing diagnoses: | |
| a. Potential nutritional deficit: related to incorrect use of formula. | Incorrect formula or formula intolerance results in nutrition deficit. |
| **Planning** | |
| 1. Develop individualized goals for client based on nursing diagnoses: | |
| a. Promote proper nutritional intake. | Prepared formula is complete meal and should maintain infant's nutrient and fluid and electrolyte needs. |
| b. Maintain fluid and electrolyte balance. | |
| c. Promote bonding and cuddling. | Bottle-feeding provides opportunity for play and cuddling between infant and mother or care giver. |
| 2. Wash hands. | Reduces spread of microorganisms. |
| 3. Assemble supplies: | |
| a. Sterile nipple and bottle | |
| b. Sterile formula | |
| 4. Prepare bottle and nipple (nipple should be firm). | Prevents infant from indigestion or swallowing large quantities of air. |
| 5. Prepare formula: commercially prepared, aseptic method, or terminal-heating method. | Preparation of formula in advance ensures smooth, organized feeding period for infant. |
| 6. Warm bottle to room temperature in deep pan of hot water. | Warm milk soothes infant. *Never* take bottle from refrigerator and let it sit on counter; bacteria may grow. Formula should feel warm when sprinkled on inside of wrist. |
| 7. Identify infant by checking wristband. | Identifying infant will prevent giving wrong formula to infant. |
| 8. Prepare infant: change diaper, dress infant in comfortable clothes, infant should be awake and hungry. | Feeding time should be opportunity to bond with infant. Sleepy baby does not feed well. Dry diaper will help comfortable infant eat better. |
| 9. Arrange for quiet room and comfortable chair. | Quiet room and comfortable chair facilitate increased appetite in infant by producing comfort and security to improve suck and swallow. |
| **Implementation** | |
| 1. Position infant: cradle baby with one hand and arm (football hold) while supporting baby against your body or lap. | Proper position will provide comfort and security. |
| 2. Place bib or small towel under infant's chin. | Protects infant's clothing. |
| 3. Allow baby to root for nipple and touch corner of mouth with nipple. | Rooting reflex will stimulate baby to open mouth and seek nipple. |
| 4. Insert filled nipple. Hold bottle upside down. | Prevents baby from sucking air. Never prop bottle. If baby vomits, aspiration may occur. |
| 5. Burp baby at least once during feeding and at end. Place baby in sitting position on mother's or nurse's lap, tilt forward, and gently pat back. Place baby prone on mother's or nurse's shoulder and gently pat back. Place baby in prone position on lap and gently pat back. Newborn babies should be burped after each ounce. | Releases swallowed air and promotes completion of bottle-feeding. |
| 6. Take nipple out of mouth periodically. | Allows baby to rest and to let air into the bottle, preventing nipple collapse. |
| 7. Continue feeding until infant is satisfied. | Complete feeding allows baby to feel satisfied. If infant falls asleep while eating, stroke cheek to arouse. |
| 8. Check diaper. | If diaper is wet or soiled, change it before returning infant to crib. |
| 9. Place in bed on stomach or right side. | Aids in emptying stomach and prevents regurgitation. |
| 10. Dispose of bottles appropriately and wash hands. | Reduces transmission of microorganisms. |
| **Evaluation** | |
| 1. Assess if infant has spit up in crib or is restless. Burp restless infant. | Indicates presence of air in stomach. |
| 2. Observe mother and infant interaction. | Assesses bonding. |
| 3. Observe infant's response toward sucking and feeding. | Determines infant's tolerance to feeding. |

| Steps | Rationale |
|---|---|
| ***Expected outcomes*** | |
| 1. Infant completes feeding. | Ensures complete nutritional, fluid, and electrolyte balance. |
| 2. Infant does not vomit, spit up excessively, or have diarrhea. | Indicates that allergy or intolerance to formula is not present. |
| 3. Mother and infant cuddle and appear content. | Indicates initial bonding. |
| ***Unexpected outcomes*** | |
| 1. Infant refuses formula repeatedly. | May indicate pain, GI upset, or illness. |
| 2. Infant vomits or has diarrhea or rash. | May indicate intolerance to formula or GI upset. |
| **Recording and Reporting** | |
| 1. Record baby's tolerance, amount, regurgitation, length of feeding, and how baby sucked. | Documents intake and infant's ability to tolerate formula. |
| **Follow-up Activities** | |
| 1. Contact pediatrician about any unexpected outcomes. | Provides opportunity to obtain new formula or to have infant examined to identify illness. |

### Special Considerations

- Infants are born with ability to suck and swallow; small, premature infants may have difficulty sucking and may require premie nipple.
- Two types of bottles are used: commercially prepared (bottle and nipple are one unit and presterilized); glass bottle that must be sterilized. Holes in nipple are correct if warm milk comes out in large single drops when bottle is shaken.
- There are three methods to prepare formula: commercially prepared formula is premixed, requires very little assistance; aseptic method—formula and bottle are sterilized separately; terminal heating—formula is prepared and placed in clean bottles; formula and bottles are sterilized together. Refrigerate formula when cooled. Always check that appropriate formula is given to infant.
- Length of time for bottle-feeding depends on age of baby and how vigorously baby sucks. Length of time for bottle-feeding is usually 10-25 min.
- If mother had a Caesarean section, place a pillow over her lap to protect tender area while she is bottle-feeding.

# *SKILL 26-5*
# *FEEDING AN INFANT SOLID FOODS*

The age at which an infant is started on solid foods varies. Many physicians introduce solids at about 4 to 6 months but each child is different. There is no specific age at which infants must be started on solid foods.

There are two choices of solid food available for infants; commercially available baby food or food prepared in the home (blenderized). Allergies may become evident with the introduction of solids. The box provides a list of "safe" foods, and foods that cause common food allergies.

Begin solid foods by giving the infant a taste of the new food; then gradually work up to several tablespoons at feeding. Introduce one new food at a time. Allow the infant time to get used to the taste before initiating another food. If the infant appears to dislike a particular food, do not force but instead wait a few weeks and retest the food.

Cereal is usually the first food to be introduced. If the infant dislikes it, fruit may be substituted, and cereal tried again at a later time. After the infant is tolerating fruit and cereal, vegetables are begun. Loose bowels or mucus in stool are strong indications that the infant is not tolerating vegetables. Meat is usually added last. The order in which food is introduced varies; follow the program that the infant's pediatrician recommends.

When feeding the infant for the first time, patience is a virtue. The infant will be confused and startled over this new taste and unsure as to what to do. The food will ooze out of the infant's mouth. Be patient and try again. With time, usually a few days, the infant adapts to solid food.

### Purposes

1. Maintain proper nutritional status.
2. Promote growth and development.
3. Maintain fluid and electrolyte balance.
4. Provide cuddling and bonding for the infant.
5. Promote independent feeding.

### COMMON FOOD ALLERGIES

**Foods that cause allergies**

Milk and milk-containing foods: cheese, creamed vegetables, creamed soups, cottage cheese, gravy, ice cream, margarine, sherbet
Orange juice
Egg
Wheat

**Safe foods**

| | | | |
|---|---|---|---|
| Apples | Cranberries | Pears | Squash |
| Apricots | Ginger ale | Pineapple | Sugar |
| Bacon | Grapes | Poi | Sweet potatoes |
| Barley | Honey | Raisins | Tapioca |
| Beets | Lamb | Rice | Tea |
| Carrots | Lettuce | Rye | Vanilla extract |
| Capon | Oats | Salt | Vinegar (cider) |
| Coffee | Peaches | Soybeans | |

From Good eating for the person sensitive to cow milk or other foods, Columbus, Ohio, 1977, Ross Laboratories.

## *Procedure 26-5*

| Step | Rationale |
|---|---|
| **Assessment** | |
| 1. Assess infant's developmental abilities in relation to feeding, e.g., ability to sit in high chair; need to be held by nurse. | Knowledge of infant's level of development helps nurse to plan appropriate meal and provide proper level of assistance. |
| 2. Assess infant for allergic reactions. | Infants may be sensitive to milk or other foods. Symptoms associated with allergy to cow milk protein or sugar include: skin eruptions (eczema, rashes, or hives), digestive problems (colic, diarrhea, constipation), respiratory problems (runny nose, ear problems, postnasal drip), irritable disposition, failure to gain weight. |
| 3. Assess infant's likes or dislikes of foods. | When infant is ill maintain adequate nutrition, fluid, and electrolyte balances by increasing food that child likes. |
| 4. Assess infant's record for information pertaining to feeding schedule. | Adherence to home feeding schedule may help ill infant adapt to hospital environment. |
| **Nursing Diagnosis** | |
| 1. Cluster data to reveal actual or potential nursing diagnoses related to infant nutrition and feeding needs: | |
| a. Potential altered nutrition: related to inability to tolerate diet. | Incorrect diet or food intolerance results in nutritional deficiency. |
| **Planning** | |
| 1. Develop individualized goals for infant based on nursing diagnoses: | |
| a. Promote proper nutritional intake. | Solid foods supplement and replace some of quantity of formula needed. Proper introduction of solid foods provides nutritionally balanced diet. |
| b. Provide socialization. | Feeding increases contact with care givers and parents. |
| 2. Wash hands. | Reduces transfer of microorganisms. |
| 3. Assemble supplies: | |
| a. Small feeding spoon and dish | Small spoon facilitates introduction of solids into child's mouth. |
| b. Food at room temperature | |
| c. Bib | |
| d. Infant seat or high chair | |
| 4. Prepare food and dish. | |
| 5. Identify infant. | Identification of infant prevents giving infant improper diet. |
| 6. Prepare infant. Change diaper, dress infant in comfortable clothes. | Dry, comfortable baby usually eats better. |
| 7. Arrange for quiet uninterrupted environment. | At this age, infant is very interested in the environment and therefore is easily distracted from the meal. |
| **Implementation** | |
| 1. Position infant. Infants can be fed while in high chair, sitting on your lap, or in infant seat. | Proper position provides comfort and security. |
| 2. Place bib on infant. | Protects clothes from being soiled. |

| Step | Rationale |
|---|---|
| 3. Sit comfortably next to infant. | Unhurried infant acquires good eating habits. |
| 4. Hold infant's hands. | Prevents infant from hitting spoon and smearing food. |
| 5. Initiate feeding. Offer taste of new food and gradually work up to several tablespoons. | Allows infant to adapt to solid foods. |
| 6. Communicate with infant during meal. | Provides socialization. |
| 7. Wash infant and change diaper. | Promotes hygiene. |
| 8. Give formula. | Allows infant to increase solid intake gradually. Formula first causes satisfied infant to refuse solid food. |
| 9. Dispose of utensils and wash hands. | Reduces transfer of microorganisms. |

## Evaluation

| | |
|---|---|
| 1. Evaluate infant after feeding. Observe for vomiting or diarrhea. | Indicates food intolerances. |
| 2. Observe infant and care giver interaction. | Evaluates bonding and socialization. |

### *Expected outcomes*

| | |
|---|---|
| 1. Infant completes feeding. | Ensures complete nutritional intake. |
| 2. Infant does not vomit, spit up excessively, or have diarrhea. | Indicates that allergies or food intolerances are not present. |

### *Unexpected outcomes*

| | |
|---|---|
| 1. Infant refuses solid foods. | May indicate dislike of food introduced. |
| 2. Infant has rash or runny nose, or crying increases. | May indicate likelihood of food allergy. |
| 3. Infant vomits or has diarrhea. | May indicate GI upset or intolerance to new solid food. |

## Recording and Reporting

| | |
|---|---|
| 1. Document infant's tolerance to diet. | Facilitates communication among health care professionals. |

## Follow-up Activities

| | |
|---|---|
| 1. Do not force infant to eat; reintroduce the solid food later. | Some infants accept a solid food on the second attempt. |

## Special Considerations

- Infant's mother can provide nurse with information about child's likes and dislikes and usual feeding schedule.
- When initiating solid food, do not place food on highchair. Infant will attempt to play with food.

### BIBLIOGRAPHY


Baby care basics, New Jersey, 1983, Johnson and Johnson.

Bistrian BR, et al.: Protein status of general surgical patients, JAMA 230:858, 1974.

Bistrian BR, et al.: Prevalence of malnutrition in general medical patients, JAMA 235:1567, 1976.

Bobak IM, Jensen MD, Zalar MK: Maternity and gynecologic care: the nurse and the family, ed 4, St Louis, 1989, The CV Mosby Co.

Brunner L, Suddarth D: The Lippincott Manual of Nursing Practice, ed 4, Philadelphia, 1986, JB Lippincott Co.

Bulau J, Clinical policies and procedures for home health care, Rockville, Md, 1986, Aspen Publishers, Inc.

Curtas S: Nutritional assessment. In: Kennedy-Caldwell C, Guenter P: Nutrition support nursing, Core Curriculum, Silver Springs, 1988, Aspen Publishers, Inc.

Feeding Baby, Gerber Products Co.

Forlaw B, Grant P: Introduction to nutritional and physical assessment of the adult patient for the nurse, Aspen, Colo., 1983, ASPEN.

Forlaw L.: Nutritional assessment. In: Grant J, Kennedy-Caldwell C, eds: Nutritional support in nursing, Philadelphia, 1988, Grune and Stratton.

Golden S: Nursing a loved one at home, Philadelphia, 1988, Running Press Book Publishers.

Good eating for the person sensitive to cow milk or other foods, Columbus, Ohio, 1977, Ross Laboratories, Inc.

Grant JA, Kennedy-Caldwell C: Nutritional support in nursing, Philadelphia, 1988, Grune and Stratton.

Hamilton P: Basic pediatric nursing, ed 6, St. Louis, 1987, The CV Mosby Co.

Marlow D, Redding B: Textbook of pediatric nursing, ed 6, Philadelphia, 1988, WB Saunders Co.

Metheny N: Fluid and electrolyte balance: nursing considerations, ed. 1, Philadelphia, 1987, JB Lippincott Co.

Milano J, et al.: Serum prealbumin, retinol binding, protein, transferrin, and albumin levels in patients with large bowel cancer, J Nat Cancer Inst 61:687, 1978.

Nolte J.: The first year of life, American Baby, New York, 1982.

Potter PA, Perry AG: Fundamentals of nursing: concepts, process, and practice, ed 2, St Louis, 1989, The CV Mosby Co.

The primer on infant nutrition, Columbus, Ohio, 1977, Mead Johnson Nutritional Division.

Stetzer MH, et al.: Instant nutritional assessment, J Parenter Enteral Nutr 3:157, 1979.

Williams SR: Nutrition and diet therapy, ed 6, St. Louis, 1989, The CV Mosby Co.

Your baby's iron nutrition, Columbus Ohio, 1980, Ross Laboratories, Inc.

# 27

# ENTERAL FEEDINGS

### OBJECTIVES

*Mastery of content in this chapter will enable the nurse to:*

- Define key terms.
- Assess client to receive enteral tube feedings.
- Determine the appropriate route of intubation for the client.
- Demonstrate ability to intubate the client.
- Demonstrate the appropriate technique for administering bolus tube feedings.
- Demonstrate the appropriate technique for administering continuous tube feedings.
- Evaluate the client's tolerance to feeding.
- Demonstrate the appropriate technique for administering jejunal feedings.
- Demonstrate appropriate gastrostomy and jejunostomy tube exit site care.

### KEY TERMS

*Enteral nutrition*
*Gastrostomy feeding tube*
*Jejunal feeding tube*
*Nasogastric feeding tube*
*Nasointestinal feeding tube*

### SKILLS

**27-1** Intubating the Client with a Large-Bore Nasogastric Feeding Tube
**27-2** Intubating the Client with a Small-Bore Nasogastric Feeding Tube
**27-3** Verifying Tube Placement for a Large-Bore Feeding Tube
**27-4** Verifying Tube Placement for a Small-Bore Feeding Tube
**27-5** Administering Enteral Feedings via Nasogastric Tube (Large- or Small-Bore)
**27-6** Administering Enteral Feedings via Gastrostomy Tube
**27-7** Administering Enteral Feedings via Nasointestinal Tube
**27-8** Administering Enteral Feedings via Jejunostomy Tube

Enteral nutrition is the administration of nutrients directly through the gastrointestinal (GI) tract. The most desirable and appropriate method of providing nutrition is the oral independent route; unfortunately, this is not always possible. For clients with a functional GI tract, enteral tube feedings are the logical choice.

Several different formulas that are presterilized to prevent bacterial contamination are available commercially (Table 27-1).

This chapter discusses the methods for providing enteral support. Before initiating enteral support, the nurse must be able to provide a route of administration (i.e., nasogastric or nasointestinal intubation) and be prepared to care for surgically implanted feeding devices (gastrostomy or jejunostomy).

The skills presented in this chapter focus on the administration of nutritional feedings directly into the gastrointestinal tract and the goal to restore the client's nutritional status. The nurse bases care on specific assessment findings.

### GUIDELINES

1. Be aware of the purpose for the feeding and who are appropriate candidates. A feeding tube may not be appropriate for the client and harm could occur at the time of insertion (i.e., upper GI bleeding or inadvertent placement of nasoenteral tube in the respiratory tract).
2. Be aware of the psychological implications associated with the insertion of a feeding tube. The client may become frightened and will need reassurance and encouragement throughout the insertion procedure.
3. Be aware of safety measures to prevent dislodgment of the feeding tube and aspiration of gastric contents by the client. Clients who are disoriented or comatose are at greater risk for aspiration than those who are alert and oriented.

**TABLE 27-1** Enteral Nutrition Products in the Tube Feedings Categories

| Products in Each Category | Calories (kilocalories/ml) | Osmolality (mOsm/kg) | Protein (g/liter) | Protein Source |
|---|---|---|---|---|
| **Isotonic tube feedings*** | | | | |
| Ensure | 1.06 | 450 | 37.2 | Casein, soy |
| Precision Isotonic Diet | 0.96 | 300 | 29 | Egg albumin |
| Osmolite | 1.06 | 300 | 37.2 | Casein, soy |
| Isocal | 1.06 | 300 | 34 | Casein, soy |
| **High calorie/high nitrogen tube feedings†** | | | | |
| Travasorb MCT‡ | 2.00 | 475 | 98 | Casein, lactalbumin |
| Magnacal | 2.00 | 590 | 70 | Casein |
| Isocal HCN | 2.00 | 690 | 75 | Casein |
| **High nitrogen tube feedings§** | | | | |
| Vivonex High Nitrogen Diet | 1.00 | 810 | 46 | Amino acids |
| Travasorb HN | 1.00 | 560 | 45 | Lactalbumin |
| Precision High Nitrogen Diet | 1.05 | 525 | 44 | Egg albumin |
| Vital HN | 1.00 | 460 | 42 | Soy, whey, meat, amino acids |
| Criticare HN | 1.06 | 650 | 38 | Casein, amino acids |
| Osmolite HN | 1.06 | 310 | 44.8 | Casein, soy |
| **Blenderized tube feedings** | | | | |
| Compleat-B | 1.00 | 490 | 40 | Milk, beef |
| Compleat-Modified Formula | 1.07 | 300 | 42.7 | Beef, cereal |
| Formula 2 | 1.00 | 435-510 | 38 | Milk, meat, wheat |
| Vitaneed | 1.00 | 310 | 35 | Beef, casein |

Modified from: Sandoz: Sandoz Nutrition your source for nutrition, Clinical Products Division, 1985, Sandoz Nutrition Corporation.
From Hopefel AW, Herrmann VM: Am J Hosp Pharm 39:5114, 1982. Used with permission.
*Specifications: lactose free, osmolality <350 mOsm/kg, caloric density approximately 1 kcal/ml, and nutritionally balanced.
†Specifications: lactose free, osmolality <600 mOsm/kg, caloric density 2 kcal/ml, protein content >70 g/L, and nutritionally balanced.
‡*MCT,* Medium-chain triglyceride.
§Specifications: lactose free, protein content >40 g/L, high biological value protein, low tar, and low residue.
¶*RTU,* Ready to use.

4. Consider the client's medication. It is recommended that mixing medications with tube feeding formula should be avoided when possible. Some medications, particularly antibiotics and syrups, may lose their therapeutic effectiveness, as well as cause disruption of emulsion of the feeding formula, resulting in a formula that resembles undigested milk.
5. Know the client's exercise pattern. Clients requiring physical or occupational therapy should have their tube feedings completed at least 1 hr before activity.

## PREREQUISITE KNOWLEDGE

1. Principles of fluid and electrolytes.
2. Anatomy and physiology of the gastrointestinal system.
3. Anatomy and physiology of the respiratory system.
4. Basic nutrition.
5. Principles of medical asepsis.

## PREREQUISITE SKILLS

1. Proper handwashing technique (Chapter 37)
2. Physical assessment (Chapter 13)

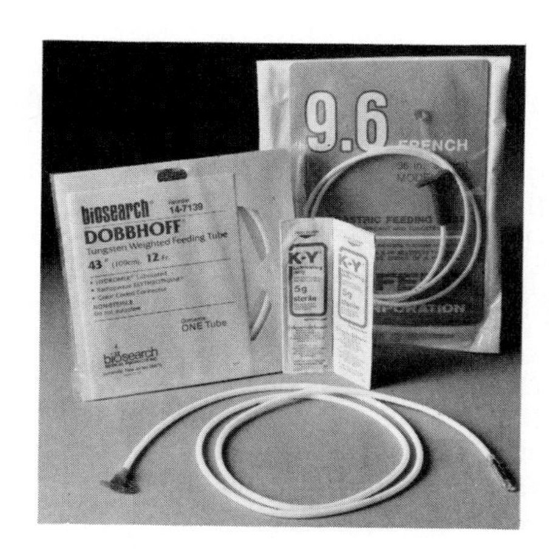


*Fig. 27-1*

| Fat (g/liter) | Fat Source | Sodium (meq/liter) | Form | Manufacturer |
|---|---|---|---|---|
| 37.2 | Corn | 36.8 | Liquid | Ross |
| 30 | Hydrogenated soy | 19.7 | Powder | Sandoz |
| 38.5 | Soy, MCT, corn | 27.6 | Liquid | Ross |
| 44 | Soy, MCT | 23.1 | Liquid | Mead Johnson |
| 66 | MCT, sunflower | 15.2 | Powder | Travenol |
| 80 | Hydrogenated soy | 43.5 | Liquid | Chesebrough-Ponds |
| 91 | MCT, soy | 3.5 | Liquid | Mead Johnson |
| 0.87 | Safflower | 23 | Powder | Norwich-Eaton |
| 13 | MCT, sunflower | 40.0 | Powder | Travenol |
| 0.5 | Hydrogenated soy | 42.7 | Powder | Sandoz |
| 10 | Safflower, MCT | 20.3 | Powder | Ross |
| 3.0 | Safflower | 27.2 | Liquid | Mead Johnson |
| 36.8 | Soy, MCT, corn | 40.5 | Liquid | Ross |
| 40 | Corn, beef fat | 55.1 | RTU¶ | Sandoz |
| 36.7 | Corn, beef fat | 29.1 | RTU | Sandoz |
| 40 | Corn, egg yolk, beef fat | 26.1 | RTU | Cutter |
| 40 | Soy, beef | 21.7 | RTU | Chesebrough-Ponds |

## *SKILL 27-1*
## *INTUBATING THE CLIENT WITH A LARGE-BORE NASOGASTRIC FEEDING TUBE*

There are many types of nasogastric tubes that are passed via the nares into the stomach (Fig. 27-1). Some are firm, polyvinyl large-bore tubes. Others are soft, flexible small-bore tubes (usually made of polyurethane or silicone) (Skill 27-2). Nasogastric tubes may have lubricants adhering to the surface; when wet, they pass more easily than a nonlubricated tube. The nurse needs to know the types of tubes used in a particular setting.

Placing a nasogastric (NG) or nasointestinal (NI) tube requires a physician's order. Placement needs to be verified by x-ray film to determine that it is in the stomach or in the intestine and not in the airways. Complications of prolonged intubation may include nasal erosion, sinusitis, esophagitis, gastric ulceration, and pulmonary aspiration.

### Purposes

1. Administer medications and feedings.
2. Maintain nutritional intake.

## Procedure 27-1

| Steps | Rationale |
|---|---|
| **Assessment** | |
| 1. Assess client for enteral tube feedings and intubation: impaired swallowing, head or neck surgery, decreased level of consciousness, surgeries involving upper alimentary tract, or facial trauma. | Identifying clients who need tube feedings before they become nutritionally depleted facilitates preparation of nursing care plan and promotes client education. |
| 2. Assess client for appropriate route of intubation. Have client close each nostril alternately and breathe. Examine each naris for patency. | NG tubes are usually passed nasally. They may be passed orally if nares are irritated or septal defect or facial fractures are present. Nares may be obstructed; assessment determines which naris to use for intubation. |
| 3. Assess client's medical history: nosebleeds; nasal surgery; deviated septum. | If client has history of any of the problems listed, nurse may need to seek physician's order to change route of nutritional support. |
| 4. Assess client for gag reflex. Place tongue blade in client's mouth, touching uvula. | Checking gag reflex assists nurse in identifying client's ability to swallow and reduces risk of aspiration. |
| 5. Assess client's mental status. | Alert client will be better able to cooperate with procedure. If vomiting should occur, an alert client can usually expectorate vomitus with reduced risk of aspiration. |
| **Nursing Diagnosis** | |
| 1. Cluster data to reveal actual or potential nursing diagnoses: | |
| a. Altered nutrition less than body requirements: related to reduced caloric intake. | Previous or concurrent illness may reduce client's ability to orally ingest nutrients. |
| b. Impaired skin integrity: related to placement of NG tube at naris. | Prolonged pressure on external naris from NG tube can result in skin breakdown. |
| c. Body image disturbance: related to invasive feeding tube. | Presence of NG tube may cause embarrassment to some clients. |
| d. Pain: related to NG tube placement. | NG tube can cause gagging and places pressure on external nares. |
| **Planning** | |
| 1. Develop individualized goals for client based on nursing diagnoses: | |
| a. Maintain nutritional and fluid and electrolyte balance. | Schedule of tube feedings is planned to meet these needs. |
| b. Skin remains intact. | Proper placement of tube at naris prevents skin irritation. |
| c. Improve body image. | |
| d. Promote comfort. | Increases client's cooperation with intubation procedure. |
| 2. Explain procedure to client. | Well-informed client is more cooperative at time of insertion. |
| 3. Assemble and examine equipment: | Examination of equipment before use prevents difficulty during the procedure. |
| a. NG tube (14-18 Fr) | |
| b. Water-soluble lubricant | Lubricant facilitates insertion of tube. |
| c. 60 ml catheter tip syringe | Syringe is necessary to inject air into tube to check placement. |
| d. Stethoscope | Stethoscope is used to auscultate air in stomach. |
| e. Hypoallergenic tape and tincture of benzoin | Tube is taped in place to prevent dislodgment. Tincture of benzoin protects skin and helps tape adhere. |
| f. Glass of water and straw | Facilitates client's ability to swallow while tube is being placed. |
| g. Emesis basin | Nasogastric intubation may stimulate gag reflex and cause nausea and vomiting. |
| h. Tongue blade | Tongue blade is essential for testing gag reflex. |
| i. Towel | Towel is placed under client's chin to protect bedclothes. |
| j. Clean gloves | Protects nurse from transmission of infection from gastric contents. |
| k. Facial tissue | Remove excess lubricant from naris. |
| l. Normal saline solution | Used to flush feeding tubing. |
| 4. Instruct client to raise index finger during intubation to indicate gagging or discomfort. | It is important for client to have way of communicating to alleviate stress. |
| 5. Remove dentures (if client is being intubated orally). | Dentures may obstruct oral intubation. |
| 6. Position client in sitting or high Fowler's position with neck hyperextended. If client is comatose, place in semi-Fowler's position. | Reduces risk of pulmonary aspiration if client should vomit. |
| 7. Examine feeding tube for flaws, e.g., rough or sharp edges on distal end and closed or clogged outlet holes. | Flaws in feeding tube hamper tube intubation. |

| Steps | Rationale |
|---|---|
| 8. Determine length of tube to be inserted and mark with tape. | |
| a. Traditional method (Fig. 27-2): measure distance from tip of nose to earlobe to xyphoid process of sternum. | Being aware of proper length to intubate determines approximate depth of insertion. |
| b. Hanson method: first mark 50 cm point on tube; then do traditional measurement. Tube insertion should be to midway point between 50 cm (25 in) and traditional mark. | |
| 9. Prepare nasogastric tube for intubation: | |
| a. Plastic tubes should not be iced. | Tubes will become stiff and inflexible, causing trauma to mucous membranes. |

*Fig. 27-2*

## Implementation

| Steps | Rationale |
|---|---|
| 1. Wash hands. | Reduces spread of microorganisms. |
| 2. Put on clean gloves. | Protects nurse from transmission of microorganisms from gastric contents. |
| 3. Lubricate nasogastric tube 10-20 cm. | Lubrication decreases friction between nasal mucous membrane and tube. |
| 4. Alert client that insertion is to begin. Insert tube gently through nostril to back of throat (posterior nasopharynx). May cause client to gag. Aim back and down toward ear. | Natural contours facilitate passage of tube into gastrointestinal tract. |
| 5. Flex client's head toward chest after tube has passed through nasopharynx. Allow client to relax a moment. | Closes off glottis and reduces risk of tube entering trachea. Allows client to "catch breath" and remain calm. |
| 6. Encourage client to swallow by giving small sips of water or ice chips when possible. Advance tube as client swallows. Rotate tube 180 degrees while inserting. | Swallowing facilitates passage of tube past oropharynx. Rotating tube decreases friction. |
| 7. Emphasize need to mouth breath and swallow during procedure. | Helps facilitate passage of tube and alleviates client's fears during procedure. |
| 8. Advance tube each time client swallows until desired length has been passed. | Reduces discomfort and trauma to client. |
| 9. Do not force tube. When resistance is met or client starts to gag, choke, or become cyanotic, stop advancing tube and pull tube back. Check for position of tube in back of throat with tongue blade. | Tube may be coiled, kinked, in oropharynx or entering trachea. |
| 10. Check placement of tube. (See Skill 27-3.) | Proper position is essential before initiating feedings. |
| 11. Apply tincture of benzoin on tip of client's nose and tube. Allow to dry. | Helps tape adhere better. |
| 12. Remove gloves. Secure tube with tape and avoid pressure on naris. | Prevents trauma to nasal mucosa and permits client mobility. |
| a. Cut 10 cm (4 in) long piece of tape. Split one end lengthwise 5 cm (2 in). Place other end of tape over bridge of client's nose. Wrap 1.3 cm (½ in) strips around tube as it exits nose (Fig. 27-3). | Prevents tissue necrosis to naris. Secures tape to nares. |

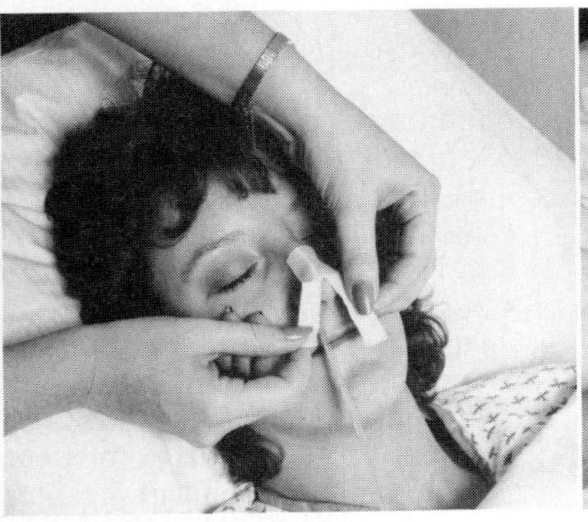
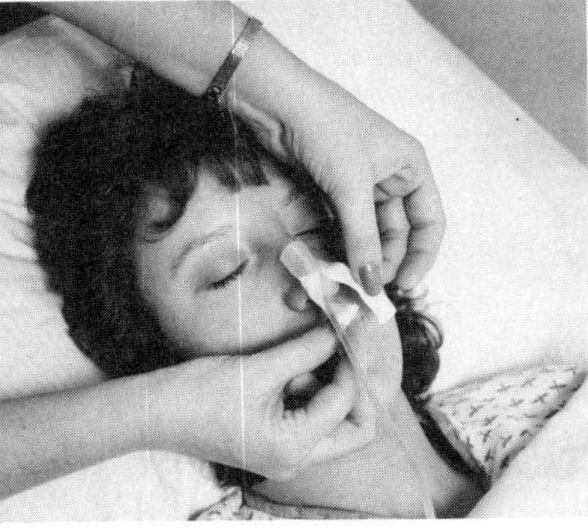

*Fig. 27-3*

| Steps | Rationale |
|---|---|
| b. Fasten end of nasogastric tube to client's gown by looping rubber band around tube in slip knot. Pin rubber band to gown. | Reduces traction on the naris if tube moves. Provides slack to take if client moves. |
| 13. Obtain x-ray of abdomen (tube must be radiopaque). | Determines placement of tube. |
| 14. Administer oral hygiene frequently (Chapter 8). Cleanse tubing at nostril. | Promotes client comfort and integrity of oral mucous membranes. |
| 15. Remain and talk with client. | Decreases anxiety after tube insertion. |

## Evaluation

| | |
|---|---|
| 1. Reassess client to determine response to nasogastric tube intubation: | |
| a. Persistent gagging. | Indicates prolonged irritation and stimulation of client's gag reflex. Can result in vomiting and increased risk of aspiration. |
| b. Paroxysms of coughing. | May indicate presence of nasogastric tube in client's airway. |
| 2. Confirm x-ray results. | Verifies tube position. |

### *Expected outcomes*

| | |
|---|---|
| 1. Tube is positioned in stomach. | Correct placement. |
| 2. Feeding tube will remain patent. Flushing with 30 ml of warm water every 4 hr will ensure patency and continued smooth infusion of feeding formula into client's GI tract. | Feeding tubes can become occluded with formula or medications; occlusion of feeding tube can result in need to reinsert new feeding tube. |
| 3. No complaints or observations of discomfort or nasal trauma. | Intubation can cause trauma to nares. |

### *Unexpected outcomes*

| | |
|---|---|
| 1. Inability to introduce air because of kinking or occlusion of tube. | Kinked or occluded tube will prevent feeding from entering GI tract and subsequent absorption of nutrients. |
| 2. Displacement of feeding tube to another site (i.e., from stomach to esophagus or duodenum to stomach). | May occur when client coughs or vomits, or if frequent nasotracheal suctioning is done. |

## Recording and Reporting

| | |
|---|---|
| 1. Report to oncoming nursing staff: type of tube placed and client's tolerance to procedure. | Provides new nursing personnel with status of GI feeding. Allows new nursing staff to plan for next feeding. |

## Follow-up Activities

| | |
|---|---|
| 1. Pulmonary aspiration of vomitus: notify physician; suction client; obtain chest x-ray. | X-ray film verifies presence of pulmonary infiltrate. Notifying physician can result in prompt treatment of infiltrate. |
| 2. Displaced or occluded feeding tube: remove old tube and reinsert new tube. | Provides for correct tube placement and continuation of tube feedings. |

## Special Considerations

- Risk of pulmonary aspiration is increased when nasally placed feeding tube is present.
- Do not intubate client who is lying supine or lying on side unless head is elevated.
- For unconscious client, stroke throat to stimulate reflex swallowing during intubation.
- Using traditional method to determine length of feeding tube to be inserted provides estimated distance from nose to stomach in 98% of clients.
- Large-bore NG feeding tubes may also be used to decompress stomach (Chapter 39).

## Teaching Considerations

- Instruct client and primary care giver as to possible side effects: diarrhea, nausea, or vomiting associated with tube feedings.
- Instruct primary care giver to offer oral hygiene frequently and to keep client's lips moistened.
- Teach primary care giver correct method for taping indwelling tube to nose to eliminate pressure on nose and face and to allow enough tubing for movement.

## Home Care Considerations

- Although contraindicated for feeding purposes in home environment because of irritation to GI tract and pressure necrosis, these tubes may still be used.
- Assess client and primary care giver's ability and commitment to insert NG feeding tube before feeding session.
- Assess primary care giver's desire to assist client in maintaining tube and feeding program.
- Assess environmental sanitation of the client to determine potential for infection.
- Assess home environment for appropriate storage space for equipment and supplies.

# *SKILL 27-2 Intubating the Client With a Small-Bore NG or NI Feeding Tube*

The typical small-bore feeding tubes are tungsten weighted to facilitate natural peristalic movement to carry the end of the tube through the pyloric sphincter and into the duodenum or jejunum (Fig. 27-1). Because the tubes are flexible, a small nylon guidewire or stylet is used to provide rigidity to facilitate intended position. These tubes can be left for an extended period without causing irritation to the gastric mucossa.

### Purposes

1. Administer medications and feedings.
2. Maintain nuritional intake.

## *Procedure 27-2*

| Steps | Rationale |
|---|---|
| **Assessment** | |
| 1. Assess client for enteral tube feedings and intubation: impaired swallowing, head or neck surgery, decreased level of consciousness, surgeries involving upper alimentary tract, or facial trauma. | Identifying clients who need tube feedings before they become nutritionally depleted will facilitate preparation of nursing care plan and will promote client education. |
| 2. Assess client for appropriate route of intubation. Have client close each nostril alternately and breathe. Examine each naris for patency. | Nares may be obstructed or irritated or septal defect or facial fractures may be present. Assessment determines which naris to use for intubation. |
| 3. Assess client's medical history: nosebleeds; nasal surgery; deviated septum. | If client has history of any of the problems listed, nurse may need to seek physician's order to change route of nutritional support. |
| 4. Assess client for gag reflex. Place tongue blade in client's mouth, touching uvula. | Checking gag reflex assists nurse in identifying client's ability to swallow and reduces risk of aspiration. |
| 5. Assess client's mental status. | Alert client will be better able to cooperate with procedure. If vomiting should occur, an alert client can usually expectorate vomitus with reduced risk of aspiration. |
| **Nursing Diagnosis** | |
| 1. Cluster data to reveal actual or potential nursing diagnoses: | |
| a. Altered nutrition: less than body requirements: related to reduced caloric intake. | Disease process or trauma may reduce clients ability to orally ingest nutrients. |
| b. Impaired skin integrity: related to placement of NG or NI tube at naris. | Prolonged pressure on external naris from NG or NI tube can result in skin breakdown. |
| c. Body image disturbance: related to invasive feeding tube. | Presence of NG or NI tube may cause embarrassment to some clients. |
| d. Pain: related to NG or NI tube. | NG or NI tube can cause gagging and places pressure on external nares. |
| **Planning** | |
| 1. Develop individualized goals for client based on nursing diagnoses: | |
| a. Maintain nutritional and fluid and electrolyte balance. | Tube feeding schedule is planned to meet these needs. |
| b. Skin around nares remains intact. | Proper positioning and taping reduces irritation. |
| c. Improve body image. | |
| d. Promote comfort. | Increases client's cooperation with intubation procedure. |
| 2. Explain procedure to client. | Well-informed client is more cooperative at time of insertion. |
| 3. Assemble and examine equipment: | Examination of equipment before use prevents difficulty during the procedure. |
| a. Nasogastric or nasojejunal tube (8-12 Fr) | |
| b. 30 ml or larger luer-lok or tip syringe | Using a syringe less than 30 ml for injecting air to check placement or clear blockage may cause rupture of the tube. |
| c. Stethoscope | Stethoscope is used to auscultate air in stomach. |
| d. Hypoallergenic tape and tincture of benzoin | Tube is taped in place to prevent dislodgment. Tincture of benzoin protects skin and helps tape adhere. |

| Steps | Rationale |
|---|---|
| e. Glass of water and straw | Purposes: a. Activates lubricant (at distal tip and inner lumen) to facilitate insertion of tube b. Aids in guidewire or stylet insertion c. Facilitates client's ability to swallow while tube is being placed |
| f. Emesis basin | Nasal intubation may stimulate gag reflex and cause nausea and vomiting. |
| g. Tongue blade | Tongue blade is essential for testing gag reflex. |
| h. Towel | Towel is placed under client's chin to protect bedclothes. |
| i. Guidewire or stylet | Guidewire is needed to help place soft, flexible feeding tube (such as Dobhoff, Keofeed, etc.). |
| j. Facial tissue | Remove excess lubricant from naris. |
| k. Clean gloves | Protects nurse from transmission of infection from GI contents. |
| 4. Explain to client how to communicate during intubation by raising his index finger to indicate gagging or discomfort. | It is important for client to have way of communicating to alleviate stress. |
| 5. Position client in sitting or high Fowler's position with neck hyperextended. If client is comatose place in semi-Fowler's position. | Reduces risk of pulmonary aspiration in event client should vomit. |
| 6. Examine feeding tube for flaws: rough or sharp edges on distal end and closed or clogged outlet holes. | Flaws in feeding tube hamper tube intubation. |
| 7. Determine length of tube to be inserted and mark with tape. | Being aware of proper length to intubate determines approximate depth of insertion. |
| a. Traditional method (Fig. 27-2): measure distance from tip of nose to earlobe to xyphoid process of sternum. Add additional 20 to 30 cm (8-12 in) for nasointestinal tube. | |
| b. Hanson method: first mark 50 cm point on tube; then do traditional measurement. Tube insertion should be to midway point between 50 cm (25 in) and traditional mark. Add additional 20 to 30 cm (8-12 in) to nasogastric mark for NI tube. | |
| 8. Prepare NG or NI tube for intubation: | |
| a. Plastic tubes should not be iced. | Tubes will become stiff and inflexible, causing trauma to mucous membranes. |
| b. Wash hands. | Reduces spread of microorganisms. |
| c. Inject 10 ml of water from 30 ml or larger luer-lok tip syringe into the tube. | Aids in guidewire or stylet insertion. |
| d. Insert guidewire or stylet into tube, making certain it's securely positioned against weighted tip and that both luer-lok connections are snugly fitted together. | Promotes smooth passage of tube into GI tract. Improperly positioned stylet can induce serious trauma. |
| e. Dip weighted tip of tube into glass of water. | Activates lubricant to facilitate passage of tube into naris to GI tract. |

## Implementation

| Steps | Rationale |
|---|---|
| 1. Put on clean gloves. | Protects nurse from transmission of infection from GI contents. |
| 2. Insert tube through nostril to back of throat (posterior nasopharynx). May cause client to gag. Aim back and down toward ear. | Natural contours facilitate passage of tube into GI tract. |
| 3. Flex client's head toward chest after tube has passed through nasopharynx. | Closes off glottis and reduces risk of tube entering trachea. |
| 4. Encourage client to swallow by giving small sips of water or ice chips when possible. Advance tube as client swallows. Rotate tube 180 degrees while inserting. | Swallowing facilitates passage of tube past oropharynx. Rotating tube decreases friction. |
| 5. Emphasize need to mouth breath and swallow during the procedure. | Helps facilitate passage of tube and alleviates client's fears during the procedure. |
| 6. Advance tube each time client swallows until desired length has been passed. | Reduces discomfort and trauma to client. |
| 7. Do not force tube. When resistance is met or client starts to cough, choke, or become cyanotic, stop advancing the tube and pull tube back. Check for position of tube in back of throat with tongue blade. | Tube may be coiled, kinked, or entering trachea. |
| 8. Check placement of tube. (See Skill 27-4.) | Proper position is essential before initiating feedings. |
| 9. Apply tincture of benzoin on tip of client's nose and tube. Allow to dry. | Helps tape adhere better. |
| 10. Secure tube with tape (Skill 27-1) and avoid pressure on naris. Anchor tubing to client's gown when possible. | Prevents trauma to nasal mucosa and permits client mobility. |

| Steps | Rationale |
|---|---|
| 11. Position client on right side when possible until radiological confirmation of correct placement has been verified. | Allow tube to pass small intestine (duodenum or jejunum). |
| 12. Obtain x-ray of abdomen (tube must be radiopaque.) | Placement of tube is verified by x-ray examination. |
| 13. Leave stylet in place until correct position is assured by x-ray. Never attempt to reinsert partially or fully removed stylet while feeding tube is in place. | Guidewire or stylet may perforate GI tract, especially esophagus or nearby tissue and seriously injure the client. |
| 14. Remain and talk with client. | Decreases anxiety after tube insertion. |
| 15. Administer oral hygiene frequently (Chapter 8). Cleanse tubing at nostril. | Promotes client comfort and integrity of oral mucous membranes. |
| 16. Remove gloves, dispose of equipment, wash hands. | Reduces transmission of microorganisms. |

## Evaluation

| | |
|---|---|
| 1. Reassess client to determine his response to NG or NI tube intubation: | |
| a. Persistent gagging. | Indicates prolonged irritation and stimulation of client's gag reflex. Can result in vomiting and increased risk of aspiration. |
| b. Paroxysms of coughing. | May indicate presence of NG or NI tube in client's airway. |
| 2. Confirm x-ray results. | Verifies tube position. |

### *Expected outcomes*

| | |
|---|---|
| 1. Feeding tube will remain patent. Flushing with 30 ml of warm water every 4 hr will ensure patency and continued smooth infusion of feeding formula into client's GI tract. | Feeding tubes can become occluded with formula or medications; occlusion of feeding tube can result in need to reinsert new feeding tube. |
| 2. No complaints or signs of discomfort. | Intubation can cause irritation to nares. |
| 3. Tube is in stomach or intestine. | Correct placement. |

### *Unexpected outcomes*

| | |
|---|---|
| 1. Inability to introduce air or formula because of kinking or occlusion of tube. | Displaced or occluded tube will prevent feeding from entering GI tract and subsequent absorption of nutrients. |
| 2. Displacement of feeding tube to another site (i.e., from stomach to esophagus, or duodenum to stomach). | May occur when client coughs or vomits, or if frequent nasotracheal suctioning is done. |

## Recording and Reporting

| | |
|---|---|
| 1. Report to oncoming nursing staff: type of tube placed and client's tolerance to procedure. | Provides new nursing personnel with status of GI feeding. Allows new nursing staff to plan for next feeding. |

## Follow-up Activities

| | |
|---|---|
| 1. Pulmonary aspiration of vomitus: notify physician; suction client; obtain chest x-ray. | X-ray film verifies presence of pulmonary infiltrate. Notifying physician can result in prompt treatment of infiltrate. |
| 2. Displaced or occluded feeding tube: remove old tube and reinsert new tube. | Provides for correct tube placement and continuation of tube feedings. |

## Special Considerations

- NG or NI feeding tubes are inserted in clients with decreased level of consciousness, but risk of pulmonary aspiration is increased.
- Do not intubate client who is lying supine or lying on side unless head is elevated.
- The equipment needed for infant includes:
  a. Feeding tube (5-10 Fr)
  b. Feeding bag
  c. Syringe (size 0.5-1 cc)
  d. Stethoscope
  e. Water for lubrication
  f. Tape
  g. Formula
- Premature infant and neonate: measure from bridge of nose to just beyond tip of sternum. Older child: measure from tip of nose past ear, to tip of sternum.
- In infant, observe for vagal stimulations during intubation of feeding tube.

## Teaching Considerations

- Instruct client and primary care giver on possible side effects: diarrhea, nausea, or vomiting associated with tube feedings.
- Instruct primary care giver to offer oral hygiene frequently and to keep client's lips moistened.
- Teach primary care giver correct method for taping indwelling tube to nose to eliminate pressure on nose and face and to allow enough tubing for movement.

## Home Care Considerations

- Assess client and primary care giver's ability and commitment to insert NG feeding tube before feeding session.
- Assess primary care giver's desire to assist client in maintaining tube and feeding program.
- Assess environmental sanitation of client to determine potential for infection.
- Assess home environment for appropriate storage space for equipment and supplies.

# SKILL 27-3 Verifying Tube Placement for a Large-Bore Feeding Tube

Testing placement for a large-bore or a small-bore (Skill 27-4) feeding tube is a major problem for nurses, since nurses are responsible for verifying proper tube position before each intermittent feeding and at least once a shift when continuous feedings are given. In addition, nurses are confronted with the difficult task of testing for gastric versus respiratory placement when tubes are initially inserted.

Inadvertent respiratory placement or dislocation of feeding tubes must be detected to maintain client safety. Displacement of soft small-bore tubes is less easily detected than is firm large-bore tubes. However, failure to detect pulmonary placement in large- or small-bore tubes can lead to complications, especially if feedings are instilled. Therefore, the most accurate method for verifying tube placement is x-ray confirmation.

### Purposes

1. Rule out inadvertent respiratory placement.
2. Rule out dislocation of feeding tubes (i.e., from stomach to esophagus).

## Procedure 27-3

| Steps | Rationale |
|---|---|
| **Assessment** | |
| 1. Identify signs, symptoms and interventions of inadvertent respiratory placement. Observe for coughing, choking, or cyanosis, especially in alert, conscious clients. | These signs and symptoms may indicate inadvertent respiratory placement. |
| 2. Identify signs and symptoms that increase risk of tube dislocation. a. Coughing. b. Retching. c. Nasotracheal suctioning. | Feeding tubes may become dislocated (i.e., stomach to esophagus or stomach to lungs). |
| 3. Review client's record for history of prior tube displacement. | Recurring tube displacements may increase clients risk for passing large-bore tube into clients respiratory tract. |
| **Nursing Diagnosis** | |
| 1. Cluster data to reveal actual or potential nursing diagnoses: | |
| a. Impaired gas exchange: related to aspiration of gastric contents into respiratory tract. | Aspiration pneumonia results when GI feedings enter respiratory tract. |
| b. Altered nutrition—less than body requirements: related to clogging of tube (i.e., formula residue adhering to the lumen or inadequately crushed medications administered through the tube). | Measures to prevent tube clogging are selecting proper drug forms for tube administration (i.e., thoroughly crushing solid forms of medications) and flushing tubes routinely (i.e., 30 ml of warm water after each intermittent feeding, 30 ml of warm water every 6 to 8 hours if client is receiving continuous feeding, and 30 ml of warm water before and after medication administration). |
| c. Pain: related to pressure against nares from nasogastric tube. | Irritation increases if tube is improperly placed. |
| **Planning** | |
| 1. Develop individualized goals for client based on nursing diagnoses: | |
| a. Maintain nutritional and fluid and electrolyte balance. | Schedule of tube feedings is planned to meet client's nutritional and fluid and electrolyte needs. |
| b. Prevent aspiration of gastric feeding. | Correct verification of tube placement reduces risk of aspiration. |
| c. Promote comfort. | Increases client's cooperation. |
| 2. Explain procedure to client. | Well-informed client is more cooperative and relaxed. |
| 3. Assemble equipment: | |
| a. 60 ml catheter tip syringe. | Syringe is necessary to inject air into tube to check placement. |
| b. Stethoscope. | Stethoscope is used to auscultate air entering the stomach. |
| c. Clean gloves. | Protects nurse from transmission of infection from GI contents. |

| Steps | Rationale |
|---|---|
| **Implementation** | |
| 1. Wash hands and put on gloves | Reduces transmission of microorganisms. |
| 2. Perform measures to verify placement of tube: | |
| a. Aspirate GI contents with a syringe. | Obtain recognizable GI contents to determine proper placement |
| b. Auscultate with stethoscope over left upper quadrant of abdomen and quickly inject 10 to 20 ml of air without resistance via syringe into tube. | Air (i.e., whooshing or gurgling sound) can be heard entering stomach. This method is not consistently reliable since a tube inadvertently placed in the lungs, pharynx, or esophagus can transmit a sound similar to that of air entering the stomach. |
| 3. Remove and dispose of gloves. Wash hands. | Reduces transmission of microorganisms. |
| **Evaluation** | |
| 1. Reassess client to determine his response to nasogastric tube: | |
| a. Persistent gagging. | May indicate prolonged irritation and stimulation of client's gag reflex can result in vomiting and increased risk of aspiration. |
| b. Paroxysms of coughing. | May indicate presence of nasogastric tube in client's airway. |
| ***Expected outcomes*** | |
| 1. Tube feeding infuses smoothly into client's GI tract. | Feeding tube is patent. |
| ***Unexpected outcomes*** | |
| 1. Feeding tube is displaced (i.e., stomach to airways) because of severe coughing, nasotracheal suctioning, or vomiting. | Severe respiratory distress may indicate displacement of feeding tube. |
| **Recording and Reporting** | |
| 1. Report to oncoming nursing staff: type of tube and client's tolerance to verifying tube placement. | Provides new nursing personnel with status of GI feeding. Allows new nursing staff to plan for next feeding. |
| **Follow-up Activities** | |
| 1. Displaced or occluded feeding tube: remove old tube and reinsert new tube. | Provides for correct tube placement and continuation of tube feeding. |

## Special Considerations

- If muffled or faint sound is present after injected air, tube may be in lungs.
- For obese clients, sound produced by injected air may be very faint, requiring air injection two or three times.
- In clients with gastric resections, do not withdraw or advance tube, since suture line could be interrupted, causing hemorrhage.

## Teaching Considerations

- Instruct primary care giver to check that tube is in correct position before instilling formula or medications.
- Instruct primary care giver not to proceed with feedings if there is any doubt as to proper placement of tube.

# SKILL 27-4 Verifying Tube Placement for a Small-Bore Feeding Tube

## Purposes

1. Rule out inadvertent respiratory placement.
2. Rule out dislocation of feeding tubes (i.e., from stomach to esophagus).

## Procedure 27-4

| Steps | Rationale |
|---|---|
| **Assessment** | |
| 1. See Assessment, Skill 27-3 on p. 610. | |
| **Nursing Diagnosis** | |
| 1. Cluster data to reveal actual or potential nursing diagnoses: | |
| a. Impaired gas exchange: related to aspiration of gastric contents into respiratory tract. | Aspiration pneumonia results when GI feedings enter respiratory tract. |
| b. Altered nutrition—less than body requirements: related to kinking or clogging of tube (i.e., formula residue adhering to lumen or inadequately crushed medications administered through tube). | If feeding tube remains kinked, new tube may be inserted. Prevention of tube clogging includes selecting proper drug forms for tube administration (i.e., crushing solid forms of medications thoroughly or using liquid forms of medications) and flushing tubes routinely (i.e., 30 ml of warm water after each intermittent feeding, 30 ml of warm water every 6-8 hours if client is receiving continuous feeding, and 30 ml of warm water before and after medication administration). |
| c. Pain related to pressure from nasogastric feeding tube. | While pressure with small-bore feeding tubes are not as great, some clients may experience pain or discomfort with these tubes. |
| **Planning** | |
| 1. Develop individualized goals for client based on nursing diagnoses: | |
| a. Prevent aspiration of GI feeding. | Correct verification of tube placement reduces risk of aspiration. |
| b. Maintain nutritional and fluid and electrolyte balance. | Schedule of tube feedings is planned to meet client's nutritional and fluid and electrolyte needs. |
| c. Promote comfort. | Increase client's cooperation. |
| 2. Explain procedure to client. | Well-informed client is more cooperative and feels more at ease. |
| 3. Assemble equipment: | |
| a. 30 ml or larger luer-lok or tip syringe | Syringe is necessary to inject air into tube to check placement. |
| b. Stethoscope | Stethoscope is used to auscultate air entering the stomach. |
| c. Clean gloves | Protects nurse from transmission of infection from GI contents. |
| **Implementation** | |
| 1. Wash hands and put on gloves. | Reduces transmission of microorganisms. |
| 2. Perform measures to verify placement of tube: | |
| a. Aspirate GI contents with syringe. | Obtain recognizable GI contents to determine proper placement |
| b. Auscultate with stethoscope over left upper quadrant of abdomen and quickly inject 10 to 20 ml of air without resistance via syringe into tube. | Air (i.e., whooshing or gurgling sound) can be heard entering stomach. This method is not consistently reliable since tube inadvertently placed in lungs, pharynx, or esophagus can transmit sound similar to that of air entering stomach. |
| c. Ensure that x-ray of tube placement needs to be done. | Determines that small-bore feeding tube is not in airway. |
| 3. Remove and dispose of gloves. Wash hands. | Reduces transmission of microorganisms. |

| Steps | Rationale |
|---|---|
| **Evaluation** | |
| 1. Reassess client to determine response to NG or NI tube: | |
| a. Persistent gagging. | May indicate prolonged irritation and stimulation of client's gag reflex can result in vomiting and increased risk of aspiration. |
| b. Paroxysms of coughing. | May indicate presence of nasogastric or nasointestinal tube in client's airway. |
| ***Expected Outcomes*** | |
| 1. Feeding tube is patent as indicated by smooth infusion of tube feeding into client's GI tract. | Patent tube allows smooth infusion of feeding into GI tract. |
| ***Unexpected outcomes*** | |
| 1. Feeding tube is displaced (i.e., stomach to airways) because of severe coughing, nasotracheal suctioning, or vomiting. | Severe respiratory distress may indicate displacement of feeding tube. |
| **Recording and Reporting** | |
| 1. Report to oncoming nursing staff: type of tube and client's tolerance to verifying tube placement. | Provides new nursing personnel with status of GI feeding. Allows new nursing staff to plan for next feeding. |
| **Follow-up Activities** | |
| 1. Displaced or occluded feeding tube: remove old tube and reinsert new tube. | Provides for correct tube placement and continuation of tube feeding. |

### Special Considerations

- If muffled or faint sound is present after injected air, tube may be in lungs.
- For obese clients, sound produced by injected air may be very faint, requiring air injection two or three times.
- After injection of air, client may belch if tube is in esophagus.
- In infant only, inject 0.5 cc-1 cc air.

### Teaching Considerations

- Instruct primary care giver to check that tube is in correct position before instilling formula or medications.
- Instruct primary care giver not to proceed with feedings if there is any doubt as to proper placement of tube.

## *SKILL 27-5* *Administering Enteral Feedings via Nasogastric Tube (Large- or Small-Bore)*

Enteral feeding is preferred over parenteral nutrition because it improves utilization of nutrients, is safer for clients, and is less expensive. Not all clients are able to be fed enterally, but if the bowel can handle nutrients, it should be used. The indications for enteral feeding include:

1. Clients who cannot eat (comatose clients with a functional gastrointestinal system or clients receiving mechanical ventilation).
2. Clients who will not eat (elderly or confused clients).
3. Clients who cannot maintain adequate oral nutrition (clients with cancer, sepsis, infection, trauma, or head injury).

### Purposes

1. Promote and improve nutritional status.
2. Administer medications.

## *Procedure 27-5*

| Steps | Rationale |
|---|---|
| **Assessment** | |
| 1. Identify signs and symptoms of malnutrition (Chapter 26). | Certain conditions place client at risk for malnutrition. |
| 2. Assess client for food allergies. | Prevents client from developing localized or systemic allergic responses. |
| 3. Assess client's need for enteral tube feedings (Skill 27-1): impaired swallowing; decreased level of consciousness; head or neck surgery; facial trauma; surgeries of upper alimentary canal. | Identifies clients who need tube feedings before they become nutritionally depleted. |
| 4. Auscultate for bowel sounds before feeding. | Bowel sounds indicate presence of peristalsis and ability of GI tract to digest nutrients. |
| 5. Verify physician's order for formula, rate, route, and frequency. | Tube feedings must be ordered by physician. |
| **Nursing Diagnosis** | |
| 1. Cluster data to reveal actual or potential nursing diagnoses: | |
| a. Pain: related to placement of nasogastric tube. | Placement of tubes can cause localized discomfort at insertion site. |
| b. Diarrhea: related to initiation of tube feedings. | Clients receiving tube feedings are at risk for developing diarrhea. |
| c. Altered nutrition—less than body requirements: related to intolerance of tube feedings | Prolonged vomiting or diarrhea decreases absorption and use of nutrients. |
| d. Impaired gas exchange: related to aspiration of gastric contents into respiratory tract. | Aspiration pneumonia results when gastric feedings enter respiratory tract. |
| **Planning** | |
| 1. Develop individualized goals for client based on nursing diagnoses: | |
| a. Maintain nutritional and fluid and electrolyte balance. | Schedule of tube feedings is planned to meet client's nutritional and fluid and electrolyte needs. |
| b. Prevent aspiration of gastric feeding. | Correct verification of tube placement reduces risk of aspiration. |
| c. Prevent nausea and diarrhea. | Symptoms result from rapid infusion of feeding. |
| 2. Wash hands. | Reduces transmission of microorganisms. |
| 3. Assemble equipment: | |
| a. Disposable gavage bag and tubing | Serves as container for formula. |
| b. 60 ml catheter tip syringe (large-bore) or 30 ml or larger luer-lok or tip syringe (small-bore) | Formula can be administered via syringe for bolus feedings. Syringe is also used to check tube placement. |
| c. Stethoscope | Stethoscope is used to auscultate air entering stomach. |
| d. Formula | |
| e. Infusion pump: use pump designed for tube feedings | Helps regulate flow of continuous feeding. |
| 4. Prepare bag and tubing to administer formula: | |
| a. Connect tubing and bag. | Tubing must be free of contamination to prevent bacterial growth. |
| b. Fill bag and tubing with formula. | Placement of formula through tubing prevents excess air from entering gastrointestinal tract. |
| 5. Explain procedure to client. | Well-informed client is more cooperative and at ease. |
| 6. Place client in high Fowler's position or elevate head of bed 30 degrees. | Elevated head helps prevent chance of aspiration. |
| **Implementation** | |
| 1. Check placement of gastric tube (Skills 27-3 and 27-7). | |
| a. Aspirate gastric secretions and check gastric residual. | Presence of gastric secretions indicates that the distal end of the tube is in the stomach. Residual volume indicates if gastric emptying is delayed. Delayed gastric emptying means that 150 ml or more remains in the client's stomach. |
| b. Auscultate over left upper quadrant with stethoscope and inject 10 to 20 ml of air into tube. | Air (i.e., whooshing or gurgling sound) can be heard entering stomach. This method is not consistently reliable since tube inadvertently placed in lungs, pharynx, or esophagus can transmit sound similar to that of air entering stomach. |

| Steps | Rationale |
|---|---|
| 2. Initiate feeding. | |
| a. **Bolus or intermittent feeding** | |
| ▪ Pinch proximal end of the feeding tube. | Prevents air from entering client's stomach. |
| ▪ Attach syringe to end of tube and elevate to 18 inches above the client's head. | |
| ▪ Fill syringe with formula. Allow syringe to empty gradually, refilling until prescribed amount has been delivered to the client. | |
| ▪ If gavage bag is used, attach bag to the end of the feeding tube and raise bag 18 inches above client's head. Fill bag with prescribed amount of formula, allow bag to empty gradually over 30 min. | Gradual emptying of tube feeding by gravity from syringe or gavage bag reduces risk of diarrhea induced by bolus tube feedings. |
| b. **Continuous drip method** (Fig 27-4) | |
| ▪ Hang gavage bag to IV pole.<br>▪ Connect end of bag to the proximal end of the feeding tube.<br>▪ Connect infusion pump and set rate. | Continuous feeding method is designed to deliver prescribed hourly rate of feeding. This method reduces risk of diarrhea. Clients who receive continuous drip feedings should have residuals checked every 4 hours. |
| 3. When tube feedings are not being administered, clamp the proximal end of the feeding tube. | Prevents air from entering stomach between feedings. |
| 4. Administer water via feeding tube as ordered with or between feedings. | Provides client with source of water to help maintain fluid and electrolyte balance. |
| 5. Rinse bag and tubing with warm water after all bolus feedings. | Rinsing bag and tube with warm water clears old tube feedings and prevents bacterial growth. |
| 6. Advance tube feeding (box on p. 616). | Tube feedings should be advanced gradually to prevent diarrhea and gastric intolerance of formula. |

## Evaluation

| | |
|---|---|
| 1. Evaluate amount of aspirate (residual) every 4 hr. | Evaluates tolerance of tube feeding. |
| 2. Monitor urine for sugar and acetone (S and A) every 6 hr. | Urine for S and A alert nurse to client's tolerance of glucose. |
| 3. Monitor intake and output every shift. | Intake and output are indications of fluid balance. |
| 4. Weigh client daily. | Weight gain is indicator of improved nutritional status. |
| 5. Observe return of normal laboratory values. | Improving laboratory values, i.e., WBC or electrolytes, indicate return to normal nutritional status. |
| 6. Observe client's level of comfort. | |

### *Expected outcome*

| | |
|---|---|
| 1. Nutritional status is improved as evidenced by increasing weight and improving laboratory values. | Indicates that client's nutritional needs are being met. |

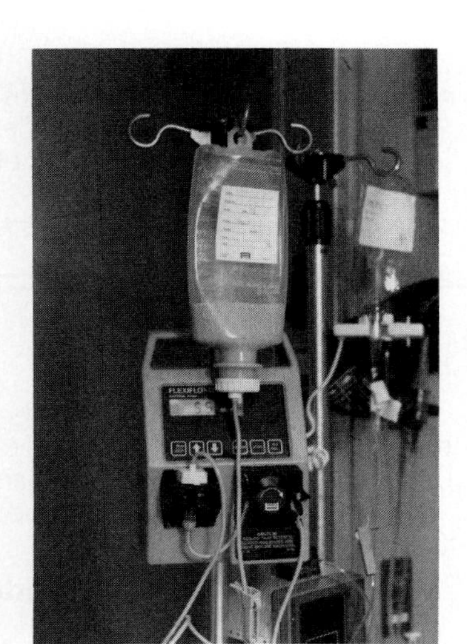

***Fig. 27-4***

### ADVANCE TUBE FEEDING

**Bolus**

1. Advance concentration before increasing volume.
2. After client has tolerated desired concentration of feeding, advance volume over 24 to 48 hour period until maximum nutrient requirements are reached.
3. Aspirate before each feeding.
   a. Volume: 150 ml or more. Notify physician and withhold feeding. Check residual in 2 hours (if volume 150 ml or more again notify the physician so that client can be evaluated for delayed gastric emptying.
   b. Volume: less than 150 ml. Give tube feeding as ordered.

**Continuous feeding**

1. Advance concentration, then volume.
2. Initial infusion rate is usually 50 ml/hr.
3. After determining tolerance, advance in increments of 25 ml/hr daily until the necessary volume is reached or an infusion rate of 125 ml/hr.

| Steps | Rationale |
|---|---|
| ***Unexpected outcomes*** | |
| 1. Client aspirates formula. | Aspiration can occur when tube is inappropriately placed or client coughs and misplaces tube. |
| 2. Client develops diarrhea. | Clients receiving tube feedings may have loose stools but diarrhea or liquid stools (3 times or more in 24 hrs) indicates intolerance. |
| 3. Client develops nausea and vomiting. | Vomiting is usually not caused by feeding but may indicate gastric ileus. |
| **Recording and Reporting** | |
| 1. Record amount and type of feeding. | Documents amount and type of feeding administered to client. |
| 2. Record client's response to tube feeding, patency of tube, and any untoward effects. | Documents client's reaction to therapy and identifies presence of any adverse reactions (i.e., aspiration). |
| 3. Report to oncoming nursing staff: type of feeding; status of feeding tube; client's tolerance; adverse effects. | Provides new nursing personnel with status of gastric feeding. Allows new nursing staff to plan for next feeding. |
| **Follow-up Activities** | |
| 1. Aspiration: suction client; notify physician; obtain chest x-ray. | Suctioning removes gastric contents from respiratory tract. Chest x-ray verifies presence of pulmonary infiltrate. |
| 2. Diarrhea: decrease feeding. | Decrease amount of liquid delivered to lower gastrointestinal tract. |
| 3. Nausea and vomiting: hold tube feeding for 12 hrs. | Reduces gastric distention. |

## Special Considerations

- Some tube feedings are ordered as continuous drip over 24 hrs while others are ordered for specified amount given at intermittent intervals (i.e., 250 ml Ensure every 4 hrs).
- Formula can be hung 8 to 12 hrs at room temperature.
- If bowel sounds are absent, notify physician before initiating feeding.
- Intermittent feeding is preferred in infants because of possible perforation of stomach, nasal airway obstruction, ulceration, and irritation to mucous membrane.
- Can also use disposable gavage bag. With gavage bag, adjust drip rate to infuse over 30 min. Hold tubing approximately 18 in above client, 6-8 in above syringe, allow 10 min to infuse. Gavage bag: infuse over 15 min.
- Aspiration may be lessened if head of bed is elevated 30-45 degrees during feeding and 1 hr after feeding.
- May need antidiarrheal agents (codeine, Kaopectate, Lomotil) when diarrhea occurs.

## Teaching Considerations

- Instruct primary care giver to administer feedings at room temperature, keeping feedings refrigerated between feedings.
- Teach client and primary care giver to keep tubing clamped between feedings and to give feedings with client in sitting position. If tolerated, client should remain upright for 1 hr after feedings.

- Instruct primary care giver to keep air from entering tubing via irrigating syringe and to irrigate with small amount of water before and after feedings.
- Instruct primary care giver that client may complain of feelings of fullness, increased gas, belching, or diarrhea.
- Instruct primary care giver to crush all pills and mix with some water or feeding formula before administration through tube.
- Instruct primary care giver to rinse tube with water to clear tube after giving medications.
- Instruct primary care giver and client to monitor intake and output using household measuring devices.

# *SKILL 27-6* *Administering Enteral Feedings via Gastrostomy Tube*

Gastric feeding is the ideal method for enteral feeding, since the stomach serves as a natural reservoir, permitting delivery of partially digested nutrients to the bowel at a slow rate. Gastric feedings may be given through a nasogastric or a gastrostomy tube. The nasogastric tube can be inserted by the nurse (Skill 27-1).

A gastrostomy tube is an alternative route for gastric feedings. The tube is inserted in the operating room by a surgeon. A large tube, usually a Foley catheter, is placed in the stomach and exits through an incision in the upper left quadrant of the abdomen. It is used for clients unable to tolerate nasogastric tubes.

See p. 613 for purposes.

## *Procedure 27-6*

| Steps | Rationale |
|---|---|
| **Assessment** | |
| 1. Identify signs and symptoms of malnutrition (Chapter 26). | Certain conditions place client at risk for malnutrition. |
| 2. Assess client for food allergies. | Prevents client from developing localized or systemic allergic responses. |
| 3. Assess client's need for enteral tube feedings (Skill 27-1): impaired swallowing; decreased level of consciousness; head or neck surgery; facial trauma; surgeries of upper alimentary canal. | Identifies clients who need tube feedings before they become nutritionally depleted. |
| 4. Auscultate for bowel sounds before feeding. | Bowel sounds indicate presence of peristalsis and ability of gastrointestinal tract to digest nutrients. |
| 5. Verify physician's order for formula, rate, route and frequency. | Tube feedings must be ordered by physician. |
| 6. Assess gastrostomy site for breakdown, irritation, or drainage. | Infection, pressure from gastrostomy tube, or drainage of gastric secretions can cause skin breakdown. |
| **Nursing Diagnosis** | |
| 1. Cluster data to reveal actual or potential nursing diagnoses: | |
| a. Pain: related to placement of gastrostomy tube. | Tube placement can cause localized discomfort at insertion site. |
| b. Diarrhea: related to initiation of tube feedings. | Clients receiving tube feedings are at risk for developing diarrhea. |
| c. Altered nutrition—less than body requirements: related to intolerance of tube feedings. | Prolonged vomiting or diarrhea decreases absorption and use of nutrients. |
| d. Impaired skin integrity: related to leakage at gastrostomy site. | Presence of infection or secretions at gastrostomy site can increase client's risk for skin breakdown around stoma. |
| e. Potential impaired gas exchange: related to aspiration of gastric contents. | Aspiration results if abdominal distention causes vomiting. |
| **Planning** | |
| 1. Develop individualized goals for client based on nursing diagnoses: | |
| a. Maintain nutritional and fluid and electrolyte balance. | Schedule of tube feedings is planned to meet client's nutritional and fluid and electrolyte needs. |

| Steps | Rationale |
|---|---|
| b. Promote comfort. | Increases client's cooperation and, in some cases, participation with tube feeding. |
| c. Prevent aspiration of gastric feeding. | Correct verification of tube placement reduces risk of aspiration. |
| d. Maintain skin integrity. | |
| 2. Wash hands. | Reduces transmission of microorganisms. |
| 3. Assemble equipment: | |
| a. Disposable gavage bag and tubing | Serves as container to place formula in. |
| b. 60 ml catheter tip syringe | Formula can be administered via syringe for bolus feedings. Syringe is also used to check tube placement. |
| c. Stethoscope | Stethoscope is used to auscultate air entering the stomach. |
| d. Formula | |
| e. Infusion pump: use pump designed for tube feedings | Helps regulate flow of continuous feeding. |
| 4. Prepare bag and tubing to administer formula: | |
| a. Connect tubing and bag. | Tubing must be free of contamination to prevent bacterial growth. |
| b. Fill bag and tubing with formula. | Placement of formula through tubing prevents excess air from entering gastrointestinal tract. |
| 5. Explain procedure to client. | Well-informed client is more cooperative and feels more at ease. |
| 6. Place client in high Fowler's position or elevate head of bed 30 degrees. | Elevating client's head helps prevent chance of aspiration. |

## Implementation

| Steps | Rationale |
|---|---|
| 1. Check placement of gastric tube. | |
| a. Aspirate gastric secretions and check gastric residual. | Presence of gastric contents indicates that end of tube is in stomach. Gastric residual determines if gastric emptying is delayed. Delayed gastric emptying means that 150 ml or more remains in client's stomach from previous feeding. |
| b. Auscultate over left upper quadrant with stethoscope and inject 10 to 20 ml of air into tube. | Air (i.e., whooshing or gurgling sound) can be heard entering stomach. |
| 2. Initiate feeding. | |
| a. **Bolus or intermittent feeding** | |
| ▪ Pinch proximal end of the gastrostomy tube. | Prevents air from entering the client's stomach. |
| ▪ Attach syringe to end of tube and elevate to 18 inches above the client's abdomen. | |
| ▪ Fill syringe with formula. Allow syringe to empty gradually, refilling until prescribed amount has been delivered to the client. | Gradual emptying of tube feeding by gravity from a syringe or gavage bag reduces the risk of diarrhea induced by bolus tube feedings. |
| ▪ If gavage bag is used, attach bag to the end of the feeding tube and raise bag 18 inches above client's abdomen. Fill bag with prescribed amount of formula, allow bag to empty gradually over 30 minutes. | |
| b. **Continuous drip method** | |
| ▪ Hang gavage bag to IV pole.<br>▪ Connect end of bag to the proximal end of the gastrostomy tube.<br>▪ Connect infusion pump and set rate. | Continuous feeding method is designed to deliver a prescribed hourly rate of feeding. This method reduces the risk of diarrhea. Clients who receive continuous drip feedings should have their residuals checked every 4 hours. |
| 3. When tube feedings are not being administered, clamp the proximal end of the gastrostomy tube. | Prevents air from entering the stomach between feedings. |
| 4. Administer water via feeding tube as ordered with or between feedings. | Provides client with source of water to help maintain fluid and electrolyte balance. |
| 5. Rinse bag and tubing with warm water after all bolus feedings. | Rinsing bag and tube with warm water clears old tube feedings and prevents bacteria growth. |
| 6. Advance tube feeding (box on p. 616). | Tube feedings should be advanced gradually to prevent diarrhea and gastric intolerance of formula. |
| 7. Change gastrostomy exit site dressing as needed; inspect exit site every shift. | Leakage of gastric drainage may cause irritation and excoriation. Skin around feeding tube should be cleansed daily with warm water and mild soap; small gauze dressing may be applied to exit site. |
| 8. Dispose of supplies and wash hands. | Reduces transmission of microorganisms. |

| Steps | Rationale |
|---|---|
| **Evaluation** | |
| 1. Evaluate client's tolerance of tube feeding. | Tolerance of tube feeding is evaluated by checking amount of aspirate (residual) every 4 hrs. |
| 2. Monitor urine for sugar and acetone (S and A) every 6 hrs. | Urine for S and A alert nurse to client's tolerance of glucose. |
| 3. Monitor intake and output every shift. | Intake and output are indications of fluid balance. |
| 4. Weigh client daily. | Weight gain is indicator of improved nutritional status. |
| 5. Observe return of normal laboratory values. | Improving laboratory values, i.e., WBC or electrolytes, indicate return to normal nutritional status. |
| 6. Observe stoma site for skin integrity. | Gastric secretion can cause injury and necrosis at stoma site. |
| ***Expected outcome*** | |
| 1. Nutritional status is improved as evidenced by increasing weight and improving laboratory values. | Indicates that client's nutritional needs are being met. |
| ***Unexpected outcomes*** | |
| 1. Client aspirates formula. | Aspiration can occur when tube is inappropriately placed. |
| 2. Client develops diarrhea. | Clients receiving tube feedings may have loose stools, but diarrhea or liquid stools (3 times or more in 24 hrs) indicates intolerance. |
| 3. Client develops nausea and vomiting. | Vomiting is usually not caused by feeding but may indicate gastric ileus. |
| **Recording and Reporting** | |
| 1. Record amount and type of feeding. | Documents amount and type of feeding administered to client. |
| 2. Record client's response to tube feeding, patency of tube, and any untoward effects. | Documents client's reaction to therapy and identifies presence of any adverse reactions (i.e., aspiration). |
| 3. Report to oncoming nursing staff: type of feeding; status of gastrostomy tube; client's tolerance; adverse effects. | Provides new nursing personnel with status of gastric feeding. Allows new nursing staff to plan for next feeding. |
| **Follow-up Activities** | |
| 1. Aspiration: suction client; notify physician; obtain chest x-ray. | Suctioning removes gastric contents from respiratory tract. Chest x-ray verifies presence of pulmonary infiltrate. |
| 2. Diarrhea: decrease feeding. | Decrease amount of liquid delivered to lower gastrointestinal tract. |
| 3. Nausea and vomiting: hold tube feeding for 12 hrs. | Reduces gastric distention. |

## Special Considerations

- If bowel sounds are absent, notify physician before initiating feeding.
- Formula can be hung 8 to 12 hrs at room temperature.
- Gastrostomy tube is much easier for client because of location and is more appropriate for long-term use.
- Intermittent feeding is preferred in infants because of possible perforation of stomach and irritation to mucous membrane. Can also use disposable gavage bag. With gavage bag, adjust drip rate to infuse over 30 min. Hold tubing approximately 18 in above client. 6-8 in above syringe, allow 10 min to infuse. Gavage bag: infuse over 15 min.
- Aspiration may be lessened if head of bed is elevated 30-45 degrees during feeding and for 1 hr after feeding.
- May need antidiarrheal agents (codeine, Kaopectate, Lomotil) when diarrhea occurs.
- Some tube feedings are ordered as continuous drip over 24 hrs while others are ordered for specified amount given at intermittent intervals (i.e. 250 ml Ensure every 4 hrs).

## Teaching Considerations

- Teach primary care giver to clean around tube with warm water or hydrogen peroxide and to protect skin with gauze squares.
- Instruct primary care giver to clean skin often to protect against damage of skin by gastric juices.

# SKILL 27-7 Administering Enteral Feedings via Nasointestinal Tube

Nasointestinal (NI) i.e., duodenal or jejunal, and jejunostomy feedings are given to clients who have had gastric resections precluding delivery of nutrients into the stomach and to neurologically impaired clients who are unable to handle their own vomitus. Therefore clients with gastric cancer, chronic nausea and vomiting, surgical intervention, or extensive peptic ulcer disease are candidates for these types of feedings.

As with the gastric feeding tube, the jejunostomy tube is surgically inserted. Clients who do not require long-term support can also benefit through use of the NI route. The advantage of these feedings is decreased gastric reflux, thereby reducing the risk of aspiration.

The duodenal and jejunal feedings bypass the stomach, a natural reservoir, thereby necessitating continuous feedings. The small intestines adapt better to volume changes versus concentration, and many authorities recommend that the volume be increased before increasing caloric concentration.

NI and jejunostomy have advantages and disadvantages, as with all forms of enteral nutrition. The advantages include decreased incidence of aspiration and allowance of feeding immediately postoperatively. Nutrients must be delivered by continuous infusion and not by bolus, which may cause diarrhea.

### Purposes

1. Deliver nutritional supplements to the lower intestinal tract.
2. Administer medication.

## Procedure 27-7

| Steps | Rationale |
| --- | --- |
| **Assessment** | |
| 1. Identify signs and symptoms of malnutrition (Chapter 26) | Certain conditions place client at risk for malnutrition. |
| 2. Assess client for food allergies. | Prevents client from developing localized or systemic allergic responses. |
| 3. Assess client's need for enteral tube feedings (Skill 27-1): impaired swallowing; decreased level of consciousness; head or neck surgery; facial trauma; surgeries of upper alimentary canal. | Identifies clients who need tube feedings before they become nutritionally depleted. |
| 4. Auscultate for bowel sounds before feeding. | Bowel sounds indicate presence of peristalsis and ability of gastrointestinal tract to digest nutrients. |
| 5. Verify physician's order for formula, rate, route, and frequency. | Tube feedings must be ordered by physician. |
| **Nursing Diagnosis** | |
| 1. Cluster data to reveal actual or potential nursing diagnoses: | |
| a. Pain: related to placement of feeding tube. | Placement of tubes can cause localized discomfort at insertion site. |
| b. Diarrhea: related to initiation of tube feedings. | Clients receiving tube feedings are at risk for developing diarrhea. |
| c. Altered nutrition—less than body requirements: related to intolerance of tube feedings | Prolonged vomiting or diarrhea decreases absorption and use of nutrients. |
| **Planning** | |
| 1. Develop individualized goals for client based on nursing diagnoses: | |
| a. Maintain nutritional and fluid and electrolyte balance. | Schedule of tube feedings is planned to meet client's nutritional and fluid and electrolyte needs. |
| b. Promote comfort. | Increases client's cooperation. |
| c. Prevent aspiration of GI feeding. | Correct verification of tube placement reduces risk of aspiration. |
| 2. Assemble equipment: | |
| a. Disposable gavage bag | Serves as container for formula. |

| Steps | Rationale |
|---|---|
| b. 30 ml or larger luer-lok or tip syringe | Syringe is used to check for residual. |
| c. Formula | |
| d. Infusion pump: use pump designed for tube feedings | Helps regulate flow of continuous feeding. |
| 3. Prepare bag and tubing to administer formula: | |
| a. Connect tubing and bag. | Tubing must be free of contamination to prevent bacterial growth. |
| b. Fill bag and tubing with formula. | Placement of formula through tubing prevents excess air from entering gastrointestinal tract. |
| 4. Explain procedure to client. | Well-informed client is more cooperative and feels more at ease. |
| 5. Place client in high Fowler's position or elevate head of bed 30 degrees. | Elevating client's head helps prevent chance of aspiration. |

## Implementation

| Steps | Rationale |
|---|---|
| 1. Wash hands. | Reduces transmission of microorganisms. |
| 2. Aspirate intestinal secretions and check for residual. | Presence of intestinal fluid indicates that end of tube is in small intestine (i.e., duodenum or jejunum). Large residual indicates slow small intestinal emptying. |
| 3. Initiate continuous tube feeding (Skill 27-5, Implementation, Step 2b, p. 615). | NI feedings are given continuously to ensure proper absorption. |
| 4. Advance tube feeding (p. 616). | To provide maximum nutrition, formula needs to be increased to meet client's nutritional requirements. |

## Evaluation

| Steps | Rationale |
|---|---|
| 1. Evaluate amount of aspirate (residual) every 4 hr. | Evaluates tolerance of tube feeding. |
| 2. Monitor urine for sugar and acetone (S and A) every 6 hr. | Urine for S and A alert nurse to client's tolerance of glucose. |
| 3. Monitor intake and output every shift. | Intake and output are indications of fluid balance. |
| 4. Weigh client daily. | Weight gain is indicator of improved nutritional status. |
| 5. Observe return of normal laboratory values. | Improving laboratory values, (i.e., WBC or electrolytes,) indicate return to normal nutritional status. |
| 6. Inspect nares for signs of pressure. | Nasointestinal tubes can cause uncomfortable pressure areas on client's nares. |

### *Expected outcome*

| Steps | Rationale |
|---|---|
| 1. Nutritional status is improved as evidenced by increasing weight and improving laboratory values. | Indicates that client's nutritional needs are being met. |

### *Unexpected outcomes*

| Steps | Rationale |
|---|---|
| 1. Client develops diarrhea. | Clients receiving tube feedings may have loose stools, but diarrhea or liquid stools (3 times or more in 24 hrs) indicates intolerance. |
| 2. Client develops nausea and vomiting. | Vomiting is usually not caused by feeding but may indicate intestinal ileus. |

## Recording and Reporting

| Steps | Rationale |
|---|---|
| 1. Record amount and type of feeding. | Documents amount and type of feeding administered to client. |
| 2. Record client's response to tube feeding, patency of tube, and any untoward effects. | Documents client's reaction to therapy and identifies presence of any adverse reactions (i.e., aspiration). |
| 3. Report to oncoming nursing staff: type of feeding; status of feeding tube; client's tolerance; adverse effects. | Provides new nursing personnel with status of intestinal feeding. Allows new nursing staff to plan for next feeding. |

## Follow-up Activities

| Steps | Rationale |
|---|---|
| 1. Diarrhea: decrease feeding. | Decrease amount of liquid delivered to lower gastrointestinal tract. |
| 2. Nausea and vomiting: hold tube feeding for 12 hr. | Reduces intestinal filling and allows for peristalsis to return. |

### Special Considerations

- Formula can be hung 8 to 12 hrs at room temperature.
- Aspiration may be lessened if head of bed is elevated 30-45 degrees during feeding.
- If bowel sounds are absent, notify physician before initiating feeding.
- Advance as follows: begin at half strength at 50 ml/hr (give isotonic feedings at full strength); proceed to half strength at 75 ml/hr; then to half strength at 100 ml/hr; then to half strength at 125 ml/hr; then advance to full strength. Add food coloring to formula to facilitate identification of aspirated tube feeding and to prevent inadvertent introduction of formula into IV line. Formula without color could be mistaken for IV intralipids.
- May need antidiarrheal agents (codeine, Kaopectate, Lomotil) when diarrhea occurs.

### Teaching Considerations

- Instruct primary care giver to clean skin often to protect against damage by gastric juices.

# *SKILL 27-8* *Administering Enteral Feedings via Jejunostomy Tube*

### Purposes

1. Deliver nutritional supplements to the lower intestinal tract.
2. Administer medication.

## *Procedure 27-8*

| Steps | Rationale |
|---|---|
| **Assessment** | |
| 1. See Assessment, Skill 27-7 on p. 620. | |
| 2. Assess skin integrity around jejunostomy. | Pressure, local infection, or gastric secretion can cause localized skin breakdown. |
| **Nursing Diagnosis** | |
| 1. Cluster data to reveal actual or potential nursing diagnoses: | |
| a. Pain: related to placement of feeding tube. | Placement of tubes can cause localized discomfort at insertion site. |
| b. Diarrhea: related to initiation of tube feedings. | Clients receiving tube feedings are at risk for developing diarrhea. |
| c. Altered nutrition—less than body requirements: related to intolerance of tube feedings. | Prolonged vomiting or diarrhea decreases absorption and use of nutrients. |
| d. Impaired skin integrity: related to leakage at jejunostomy site. | Presence of infection or secretions at jejunostomy site can increase client's risk for skin breakdown around stoma. |
| **Planning** | |
| 1. Develop individualized goals for client based on nursing diagnoses: | |
| a. Maintain nutritional and fluid and electrolyte balance. | Schedule of tube feedings is planned to meet client's nutritional and fluid and electrolyte needs. |
| b. Promote comfort. | Increases client's cooperation and, in some cases, participation with tube feeding. |
| c. Maintain skin integrity. | Regular cleansing of jejunostomy site will reduce irritation. |
| 2. Assemble equipment: | |
| a. Disposable gavage bag | Serves as container to place formula in. |
| b. 60 ml catheter tip syringe | Syringe is used to check for residual. |
| c. Formula | |
| d. Infusion pump: use pump designed for tube feedings | Helps regulate flow of continuous feeding. |
| 3. Prepare bag and tubing to administer formula: | |
| a. Connect tubing and bag. | Tubing must be free of contamination to prevent bacterial growth. |
| b. Fill bag and tubing with formula. | Placement of formula through tubing prevents excess air from entering gastrointestinal tract. |

| Steps | Rationale |
|---|---|
| 4. Explain procedure to client. | Well-informed client is more cooperative and feels more at ease. |

## Implementation

| Steps | Rationale |
|---|---|
| 1. Wash hands. | Reduces transmission of microorganisms. |
| 2. Aspirate intestinal secretions and check for residual. | Presence of intestinal fluid indicates that end of tube is in jejunum. A large residual indicates slow small intestinal emptying. |
| 3. Initiate continuous tube feeding (Skill 27-5, Implementation, Step 2b, p. 615). | Jejunal feedings are given continuously to ensure proper absorption. |
| 4. Advance tube feeding (p. 616). | To provide maximum nutrition, formula needs to be increased to meet client's nutritional requirements. |
| 5. Change jejunostomy exit site dressing as needed; inspect exit site every shift. | Leakage of intestinal drainage may cause irritation and excoriation. Skin around feeding tube should be cleansed daily with warm water and mild soap; small gauze dressing may be applied to exit site. |

## Evaluation

| Steps | Rationale |
|---|---|
| 1. Evaluate client's tolerance of tube feeding. | Tolerance of tube feeding is evaluated by checking amount of aspirate (residual) every 4 hr. |
| 2. Monitor urine for sugar and acetone (S and A) every 6 hr. | Urine for S and A alert nurse to client's tolerance of glucose. |
| 3. Monitor intake and output every shift. | Intake and output are indications of fluid balance. |
| 4. Weigh client daily. | Weight gain is indicator of improved nutritional status. |
| 5. Observe return of normal laboratory values. | Improving laboratory values, i.e., WBC or electrolytes, indicate return to normal nutritional status. |
| 6. Observe skin around jejunostomy tube. | |

### *Expected outcome*

| Steps | Rationale |
|---|---|
| 1. Nutritional status is improved as evidenced by increasing weight and improving laboratory values. | Indicates that client's nutritional needs are being met. |

### *Unexpected outcomes*

| Steps | Rationale |
|---|---|
| 1. Client develops diarrhea. | Clients receiving tube feedings may have loose stools, but diarrhea or liquid stools (3 times or more in 24 hrs) indicates intolerance. |
| 2. Client develops nausea and vomiting. | Vomiting is usually not caused by feeding but may indicate intestinal ileus. |

## Recording and Reporting

| Steps | Rationale |
|---|---|
| 1. Record amount and type of feeding. | Documents amount and type of feeding administered to client. |
| 2. Record client's response to tube feeding, patency of tube, and any untoward effects. | Documents client's reaction to therapy and identifies presence of any adverse reactions (i.e., aspiration). |
| 3. Report to oncoming nursing staff: type of feeding; status of feeding tube; client's tolerance; adverse effects. | Provides new nursing personnel with status of intestinal feeding. Allows new nursing staff to plan for next feeding. |

## Follow-up Activities

| Steps | Rationale |
|---|---|
| 1. Diarrhea: decrease feeding. | Decrease amount of liquid delivered to lower gastrointestinal tract. |
| 2. Nausea and vomiting: hold tube feeding for 12 hr. | Reduces intestinal filling and provides time for peristalsis to return. |

## Special Considerations

- Formula can be hung 8 to 12 hrs at room temperature.
- Add food coloring to formula to facilitate identification of aspirated tube feeding and to prevent inadvertent introduction of formula into IV line. Formula without color could be mistaken for IV intralipids.
- Pump is only necessary for clients receiving continuous feedings.
- If bowel sounds are absent, notify physician before initiating feeding.
- May need antidiarrheal agents (codeine, Kaopectate, Lomotil) when diarrhea occurs.

## Teaching Considerations

- Teach primary care giver to clean skin around tube with warm water or hydrogen peroxide and to protect skin with gauze squares.
- Instruct primary care giver to clean skin often to protect against damage of skin by gastric juices.

---

### BIBLIOGRAPHY

Bernard M, Forlaw L: Complications and their prevention. In Rombeau J, Caldwell M (eds): Enteral and tube feeding: Clinical nutrition, vol. I, Philadelphia, 1984, WB Saunders Co.

Bernstein L, Grieco A, Dete M. Primary care in the home, Philadelphia, 1987, JB Lippincott Company.

Biosearch: Entriflex feeding tube, 1984, Biosearch Medical Products.

Cataldo C: Tube feedings: clinical applications, Columbus, Ohio, 1982, Ross Laboratories.

Chernoft R: Nutritional support formulas and delivery of enteral feeding, J Am Diet Assoc 29:430, 1981.

Covell M. The home alternative to hospitals and nursing homes, New York, 1983, Rawson Associates.

Crocker K: Metabolic monitoring during nutritional support therapy. In Grant J, Kennedy-Caldwell C: Nutritional support in nursing, Philadelphia, 1984, Grune and Stratton.

Dobb G: Diarrhea in the critically ill, Intens Care Med 12:113, 1986.

Enteral P&P, St. Louis, St. Louis University Hospital.

Gebbie K: Summary of the national conference—Classification of nursing diagnosis, St. Louis, 1975, St. Louis University School of Nursing.

Golden S. Nursing a loved one at home, Philadelphia, 1988, Running Press.

Griggs and Hoppe: Nasogastric tube feedings, ASN, p. 481, 1979.

Guinness R: How to use the new small-bore feeding tubes, Nursing 86 16(4):51, 1986.

Hansen B: Feeding methods and gastrointestinal function. In Rombeau J, Caldwell M (eds): Enteral and tube feeding: clinical nutrition, vol I, Philadelphia, 1984, WB Saunders Co.

Hanson RL: Predictive criteria for length of nasogastric tube insertion for tube feeding, JPEN 3:160, 1979.

Hoover H, et al.: Nutritional benefits of immediate postoperative jejunal feeding of an elemental diet, Am J Surg 139:153, 1980.

Hopefl AW, Herrmann VM: Developing a formulary for enteral nutrition products, Am J Hosp Pharm 39:1514, 1982.

Johnson VH: Tube feeding complications: causes, prevention, and therapy, Nutritional Support Services 6(3):17, 24, 1986.

Kennedy-Caldwell C: Pediatric nutritional support. In Grant J, Kennedy-Caldwell C: Nutritional support in nursing, Philadelphia, 1988, Grune and Stratton.

Melnik G, Wright K: Pharmacologic aspects of enteral nutrition. In Rombeau J, Caldwell M (eds): Enteral and tube feeding: clinical nutrition, vol I, Philadelphia, 1984, WB Saunders Co.

Metheny N: Measures to test placement of nasogastric and nasointestinal feeding tubes: a review, Nurs Res November/December, 1988.

Metheny N: 20 ways to prevent tube-feeding complications, Nursing 85 15(1):47, 1985.

Moore EE, Dunn EL, Jones TN: Immediate jejunostomy feeding, Arch Surg 116:681, 1981.

Patterson R: Enteral nutrition delivery systems. In Grant J, Kennedy-Caldwell C: Nutritional support in nursing, Philadelphia, 1988, Grune and Stratton.

Rombeau J, Jacobs D: Nasoenteric tube feeding. In Rombeau J, Caldwell M (eds): Enteral and tube feeding: clinical nutrition, Vol I, Philadelphia, 1984 WB Saunders Co.

Ross G: Geriatric enteral hyperalimentation. II. Nutritional support services, 1:7, 1981.

Sandoz Nutrition Corporation: Sandoz nutrition, your source for nutrition, Ridgewood, New Jersey, 1985, Clinical Products Division.

Walsh J, Persons C, Wieck L: Manual of home health care nursing, Philadelphia, 1987, JB Lippincott Co.

Williams P: How do you keep medicines from clogging feeding tubes? Am J Nurs February 1989.

Woldrum K, et al.: Patient education. Rockville Md, 1985, Aspen Publishers, Inc.

# 28

# TOTAL PARENTERAL NUTRITION

## OBJECTIVES

*Mastery of content in this chapter will enable the nurse to:*

- Define key terms.
- Identify clients who are candidates for peripheral vein parenteral nutrition.
- Identify appropriate site to administer vein parenteral nutrition.
- Evaluate and implement a peripheral vein IV to administer solution.
- Demonstrate appropriate nursing care of the client receiving peripheral nutritional support.
- Demonstrate appropriate nursing care of the client receiving fat emulsions.
- Demonstrate appropriate nursing care of the client receiving home nutritional support.
- Identify clients who are candidates for central vein solution.
- Assist the physician with placement of a central vein catheter.
- Demonstrate a central line dressing change.
- Evaluate and inspect catheter exit sites for signs and symptoms of infection.

## KEY TERMS

| | |
|---|---|
| *Amino acid* | *Infusate* |
| *Bacteriostatic* | *Iso-osmotic solution* |
| *Basal metabolism* | *Malabsorption* |
| *Calorie (Kcal)* | *Osmolality* |
| *Dextrose* | *Parenteral nutrition* |
| *Enteral nutrition* | *Thrombophlebitis* |
| *Fenestrated drape* | *Trendelenburg's position* |
| *Hydrothorax* | *Visceral protein status* |

## SKILLS

**28-1** Caring for the Client Receiving Peripheral Vein Parenteral Nutrition
**28-2** Caring for the Client Receiving Fat Emulsions
**28-3** Caring for the Client Receiving Central Venous Placement for Central Parenteral Nutrition

Total parenteral nutrition (TPN) (hyperalimentation) is the intravenous (IV) infusion of amino acids (protein/nitrogen), glucose (hypertonic, isotonic solutions), and additives (vitamins, electrolytes, minerals, trace elements). Nutrition through the gastrointestinal tract is best and should be used before initiating parenteral nutrition. However, certain disease states limit enteral nutrition and TPN is indicated (see box on p. 626).

To provide comprehensive care, the nurse must be able to detect clients at risk for malnutrition and assess malnourished hospitalized clients. Detection and assessment of these clients is discussed in Skill 26-1. Through the use of complete nutritional assessment, the nurse is able to determine the regimen that best meets the client's nutritional needs as well as the appropriate route of administration. Parenteral nutrition can be administered peripherally or centrally. This chapter covers peripheral vein parenteral nutrition (PPN), fat emulsions, and central vein parenteral nutrition (CPN) and concludes with the home application of TPN.

TPN has physiologic and psychologic implications. When no longer able to maintain an adequate nutritional status enterally a client becomes socially isolated. A majority of social events focus around food, thereby excluding the client from complete participation. The nurse plays an important part in the client's psychological well-being by becoming well-informed about the condition, prognosis, length of therapy, and personal views on nutrition. Client and family education help to alleviate many of the client's fears and concerns.

The nursing committee of the American Society of Parenteral and Enteral Nutrition (ASPEN) has defined nutritional support nursing practice, the scope of nutritional support nursing, and the goals of nutritional support.

*Nutritional support nursing practice* is the care of individuals with potential and/or known nutrition alterations that are inherent in all disease states. Nutritional support nursing involves use of interventions that enhance the maintenance and/or restore the individual's nutritional health within the context of a person's life goals. Physiologic, metabolic, behavioral, and technologic principles and skills are applied when planning support. Nurses generally function as equal members of multidisciplinary nutritional support services (Forlaw, 1983). Nursing activities are holistic and based on scientific principles. Activities are revised when changes occur in the individual's situation and/or when current research data can be translated into new or different clinical measures (Forlaw, 1983).

The following outcomes are specific to individuals requiring nutritional support nursing care. Identification of measurable outcomes requires assessment of the health of the individual.

1. The individual or significant other demonstrates a knowledge of nutritional requirements and of measures necessary to meet them.
2. The client uses measures of nutritional support that maintains or improves nutritional status.
3. The client demonstrates appropriate responses to nutritional support intervention.
4. The client suffers no preventable adverse effects from nutritional support modalities or nursing interventions (Forlaw, 1984).

### ***INDICATIONS FOR TPN***

1. Client unable to ingest or absorb sufficient nutrients through the GI tract because of:
   - Interstitial obstruction.
   - Mucositis from chemotherapy.
   - Nausea and vomiting.
   - Ileus from therapy and/or surgery.
   - Lack of enzymatic digestion.
   - Absorptive malfunction.
2. Client's oral intake inadequate because of:
   - Anorexia.
   - Elevated metabolic demands related to trauma, tumor, infection, and sepsis.
3. Clients at risk for malnutrition because of:
   - Gross underweight (>80% below standard).
   - Gross overweight (>120% above standard).
   - Recent weight loss of >10%.
   - Alcoholism.
   - NPO for >5 days.

## GUIDELINES

1. Know which clients are candidates for TPN. Clients unable to take nutrition orally or enterally should be considered for TPN. In addition, clients who are severely burned or injured may receive TPN and oral nutrition.
2. Know when peripheral vein access is desired over central vein access. Clients with altered sugar metabolism or liver disease do better with hypocaloric peripheral solutions than with high-calorie central solutions.
3. Know the solutions used for peripheral versus central vein access. Certain solutions, such as hyperosmolar solutions, must be administered into a central vein.
4. Be aware of complications associated with TPN. The nurse must continually assess for and quickly identify complications.
5. Know the client's normal range of vital signs. Clients receiving hyperosmolar solutions may have sudden unexpected changes in vital signs.
6. Know the client's recent temperature. Clients with peripheral or central IV lines are susceptible to septicemia; an elevated temperature can be an early indicator of a bacterial process.

## PREREQUISITE KNOWLEDGE

1. Principles of fluid and electrolyte balance.
2. Principles of blood osmolality.
3. Principles of IV care.
4. Central and peripheral vascular systems anatomy and physiology.
5. Principles of surgical aspesis.

## PREREQUISITE SKILLS

1. Perform proper handwashing technique (Chapter 38).
2. Initiate a peripheral IV (Chapter 23).
3. Care for a client with a peripheral IV (Chapter 23).
4. Complete a nutritional assessment (Chapter 26).
5. Conduct a physical assessment (Chapter 13).
6. Monitor vital signs (Chapter 12).

# *SKILL 28-1 Caring for the Client Receiving Peripheral Vein Parenteral Nutrition*

PPN is a form of nutritional support reserved for maintenance therapy of client's nutritional status or for actual correction of a mild nutritional deficiency. PPN involves the use of isotonic solutions infused through small peripheral veins (i.e., forearm and hand). The indications for PPN include:

1. Delay in central venous catheter placement (i.e., central venous access cannot be obtained or insertion of a central venous catheter is unnecessary).
2. Marginal nutritional status.
3. Short-term expectancy for need of parenteral nutrition (i.e. postoperatively, NPO for greater than 5 days, or not requiring PPN for greater than 7 to 10 days).
4. History of repeated sepsis making central vein cannulation unsafe.
5. At times, clients receive PPN as well as enteral feedings to further increase nutrient intake.

Peripheral access requires the use of lower concentrations of dextrose and amino acids to lower tonicity and lessen the risk of vein damage. For example, PPN consists of 5% to 10% dextrose and amino acids supplemented by IV fat emulsion to provide 2000 Kcal/day. PPN is usually administered in conjunction with fat emulsion. Unfortunately, PPN is usually more difficult to maintain because of frequent episodes of phlebitis of superficial arm veins and infiltrations of solutions into subcutaneous tissue. Therefore, the final dextrose concentration must be no greater than 10% because the peripheral vein will sclerose at higher concentrations. However, solutions of lower concentration make it difficult to supply adequate calories and amino acids through a peripheral vein. This problem, with the scarcity of adequate access sites, is the reason many experts recommend PPN for only short periods of time. Nutrients given through central veins may be very concentrated (i.e., 1800 mOsm). However, concentrations this great are not tolerated in peripheral veins because of their relatively low blood flow.

## Purpose

1. Maintain or improve nutritional status in clients requiring short-term nutritional support.

## *Procedure 28-1*

| Steps | Rationale |
|---|---|
| **Assessment** | |
| 1. Assess client's nutritional status (Skill 26-1). | Nurse needs to be aware of client's nutritional needs to judge response to therapy. |
| 2. Determine if client is candidate to receive PPN: client is NPO more than 5 days, there is no metabolic or renal disease, signs and symptoms of malnutrition are absent. | PPN has advantages and disadvantages and must be evaluated to provide safe care. |
| 3. Assess factors influencing PPN administration. | IV access and fluid status can influence tolerance to PPN. If client has IV, check for patency and rapid blood return. |
| 4. Assess for an appropriate site to begin an IV for PPN (Skill 23-1). | Large vein must be free of phlebitis, infection, or tortuosity. |
| 5. Verify physician's order for nutrients, minerals, electrolytes, as well as flow rate. | PPN must be ordered by physician. |
| **Nursing Diagnosis** | |
| 1. Cluster data to reveal actual or potential nursing diagnoses: | |
| a. Altered nutrition: related to less than body requirements. | Client unable to tolerate enteral nutrition. |
| b. Fluid volume excess: related to increased volume of solution to provide adequate calories and protein. | Peripheral parenteral solutions may cause fluid and electrolyte imbalances. |
| c. Bathing/hygiene self-care deficit: related to peripheral IV. | IV can decrease client's ability to meet hygiene, grooming, or toileting needs. |
| **Planning** | |
| 1. Develop individualized goals for client based on nursing diagnoses: | |
| a. Maintain or improve nutritional status and fluid status. | Directs nurse to pursue supportive treatment. |
| b. Establish patent IV line. | Produces safe route of administration of solution. |

| Steps | Rationale |
|---|---|
| c. Promote client's ability to independently perform ADLS. | Continuous monitoring is necessary due to mixture of additives in IV solution. |
| 2. Prepare needed equipment: | |
| a. Tubing (IV) | Tubing is chosen on basis of nurse's assessment. Microdrip tubing is used when administering less than 100 ml/hr. Macrodrip tubing is used for greater than 100 ml/hr. |
| b. PPN solution (IV) | |
| c. IV filter (optional) | Filter is used to stop in-line microorganisms. |
| d. IV catheter (22 gauge) | |
| e. All other equipment used to start IV (Chapter 23) | |
| f. Infusion pump | Pump will help to regulate flow rate. |
| 3. Explain purposes of PPN. | Promotes understanding and relieves anxiety. |
| 4. Place client in comfortable position in bed. | Facilitates initiation of IV line. |

## Implementation

| Steps | Rationale |
|---|---|
| 1. Wash hands. | Reduces transmission of microorganisms. |
| 2. Follow Skill 23-1, Implementation, for initiating IV care and dressing of IV. | |
| 3. Insert IV tubing into infusion pump and set flow rate (Chapter 23). | Flow rates are based on physician's order. Rate must be maintained to prevent sudden electrolyte imbalances. |

## Evaluation

| Steps | Rationale |
|---|---|
| 1. Reassess client to determine response to administration of PPN: improved weight, laboratory values, caloric intake. | Provides for modification of nursing care plan. |
| 2. Inspect status of IV site every 2-4 hr. | Determines presence of infiltration or phlebitis. |
| 3. Auscultate lung sounds. | Evaluates risk of pulmonary edema. |

### *Expected outcomes*

| Steps | Rationale |
|---|---|
| 1. Venipuncture site is free of redness, swelling, or inflammation. | Infiltrated or phlebotic IV is very painful. |
| a. Change dressing every 48 to 72 hr and tubing and bag every 24 hr. | Prevents cross-contamination. |
| b. Rotate IV site every 72 hr. | Reduces chance for thrombophlebitis and infection. |
| 2. Client's ideal weight gain is usually between ½ and 1 lb/day. | Weight is excellent indication of how well patient is doing nutritionally and determines fluid volume. Weight gain of more than 1 lb/day indicates fluid retention. |
| 3. Breath sounds are clear to auscultation. | Occurrence of rales (crackles) indicates fluid overload. |
| 4. Urine sugar and acetone (S & A) level is negative or 1+. | Urine S & A level is used to determine tolerance to dextrose. |
| 5. Client is able to complete ADLs. | |

### *Unexpected outcomes*

| Steps | Rationale |
|---|---|
| 1. There is phlebitis of the vein. | Indicates irritation to vein, usually the most common of PPN. |
| 2. Weight gain greater than 1 lb/day. | Indicates fluid retention, not restoration of body proteins. |
| 3. Crackles auscultated over lung fields. | When fluid overload is present, excess fluid accumulates in lung fields. |
| 4. Urine S & A level greater than 1+. | May indicate inability to successfully metabolize dextrose in solution, catheter sepsis. |

## Recording and Reporting

| Steps | Rationale |
|---|---|
| 1. Record condition of IV and rate of infusion. | Documents status of IV infusion rate. |
| 2. Record intake and output every shift. | Indicates fluid status. |
| 3. Record temperature every 4 hr. | Gradual elevation of temperature may indicate catheter sepsis. |
| 4. Record urine for S & A every 6 hr. | Documents metabolic response to glucose solution. |

## Follow-up Activities

| Steps | Rationale |
|---|---|
| 1. Phlebitis: | |
| a. Initiate new IV line. | Removes irritation from vein. |
| b. Apply warm, moist packs to extremity. | Promotes circulation and reduces redness and swelling. |
| 2. Weight gain, rales, or increased urinary sugar: | |
| a. Notify physician. | Solution changes require physician's order. |
| b. Change solution. | If fluid overload is present, physician may also wish to treat client with diuretics and fluid restrictions. |

### Special Consideration

- Rate of PPN does not need to be gradually increased to receive maximum therapy. PPN is iso-osmolar and is tolerated well by most clients.

### Teaching Considerations

- Instruct primary care giver about the proper methods for storing patenteral nutrition supplies.
- Teach client, primary care giver to monitor client's weight, calorie count, intake and output, and urine assessment.
- Teach client, primary care giver about actions to take in case of emergency.

### Home Care Considerations

- Observe client, primary care giver perform procedure in hospital before discharge.
- Assess client's home for suitability to provide PPN safely.
- Use aseptic technique when assembling equipment for dressing changes on clean surface in home.

## *SKILL 28-2 Caring for the Client Receiving Fat Emulsions*

Fat comprises 40% to 50% of the calorie content in the American diet. Fats supply essential fatty acids that are used as energy. Maintaining essential fatty acids, especially in clients with increased metabolic demands requiring long-term parenteral nutrition, is very difficult. The essential fatty acid important to parenteral nutrition is linoleic acid. Linoleic acid, which cannot be made from other fats in humans, must be supplied. Thus, the development of fat emulsion (Intralipid, Liposysn, and Travamulsion) is a form of parenteral nutrition providing linoleic acid, which prevents or reverses essential fatty acid deficiency (EFAD). Signs and symptoms of EFAD include dry scaly skin, sparse hair growth, impaired wound healing, decreased resistance to stress, increased susceptibility to respiratory tract infections, anemia, thrombocytopenia, and liver function abnormalities.

Fat emulsion is a soybean or safflower oil base that is isotonic and may be infused with amino acid and dextrose solution through a central or peripheral vein. Fats may be administered through a separate IV, given piggyback through a Y-connector near the port of entry, or admixing the amino acid, dextrose, and fat emulsion solution in one container (i.e., 3-in-1 system) to infuse over 24 hr. Emulsified fats are used to provide a high-calorie intake. For example, 500 ml of a 10% solution supply 550 Kcal, and 500 ml of a 20% solution supply 1000 Kcal.

Not all clients should receive fat emulsion. Individuals for whom fat emulsions are contraindicated include those who have a disturbance of normal fat metabolism, such as pathologic hyperlipemia, lipid nephrosis, acute pancreatitis, or jaundice. In these conditions the client is unable to metabolize fat.

### Purposes

1. Prevent or reverse essential fatty acid deficiency.
2. Maintain nutritional status.
3. Improve nutritional status.

## *Procedure 28-2*

| Steps | Rationale |
|---|---|
| **Assessment** | |
| 1. Assess client for fat deficiency: serum triglyceride level. Serum triglyceride should be drawn before initiation of fat therapy (baseline) and 6 hr after fat has infused. | Determines client's ability to metabolize and use fat. |
| 2. Assess client for EFAD: dry, scaly skin; sparse hair growth; impaired wound healing. | Indicates need for fat emulsions. |
| 3. Find appropriate functional IV site to administer fat emulsion. | Fat emulsions may be given through separate IV, piggybacked through peripheral or central line, admixed in solution bag. |
| 4. Decide on best time to administer fats. | Fat emulsions may cause nausea, strange taste, full feeling and are better tolerated at night. |
| 5. Check physician's order for volume of fat emulsion. | Fat emulsions must be ordered by physician. |
| **Nursing Diagnosis** | |
| 1. Cluster data to reveal actual or potential nursing diagnoses: | |
| a. Altered nutrition—less than body requirements: related to inability to tolerate enteral nutrition. | Absence of essential fatty acids results in nutritional deficit, and impaired wound healing may occur. |

| Steps | Rationale |
|---|---|
| **Planning** | |
| 1. Develop individualized goals for client based on nursing diagnoses: | |
| a. Promote adequate nutritional intake. | Clients receiving TPN through peripheral vein need fat emulsions for balanced parenteral nutrition. Fat emulsions can be given as calorie source, EFA replacement, or to help wean client from ventilator. |
| b. Establish patent IV line. | Successful delivery of fat emulsion requires intact IV system to minimize vascular complications. |
| 2. Prepare needed equipment: | |
| a. Fat emulsion: (Remove fat emulsion from refrigerator 1 hr before administering). | |
| b. IV tubing | |
| c. Small gauge needle (19 gauge) or stop cock. | Needle or stopcock used to insert IV tubing into primary IV line. |
| d. Alcohol swab | |
| e. Infusion pump | |
| 3. Explain why client is receiving fat emulsions. | Reduces anxiety and promotes cooperation. |
| **Implementation** | |
| 1. Wash hands. | Reduces transmission of microorganisms. |
| 2. Connect tubing to solution and run fat emulsion into IV tubing. | To prevent air from entering vascular system, all tubing must be purged. |
| 3. Clean peripheral line tubing injection port with alcohol swab. (Optional: add stopcock to connection point.) | Removes surface organisms at injection site and prevents organisms from entering blood system. |
| 4. Inject needle and tubing of fat emulsion into injection port of primary IV line. Tape injection site. (Optional: connect fat emulsion tubing to stopcock and turn to "on" position.) | Taping prevents needle from dislodging. Tight connection prevents leakage of fluid. |
| 5. Set flow rate on infusion pump. | Up to 2.5 gm fat/kg/day may be infused but should not exceed 60% of total Kcal. |
| 6. Discard supplies and wash hands. | Prevents transmission of infection. |
| **Evaluation** | |
| 1. Evaluate client to determine response to fat emulsion: improved weight and laboratory values. | Provides for modification of care plan and nutritional supplement if needed. |
| 2. Monitor temperature every 4 hr. | Determines onset of fever, a complication of fat intolerance or sepsis. |
| ***Expected outcome*** | |
| 1. Triglyceride level is stable. | Increased level indicates poor tolerance to fat. |
| 2. IV site is free of redness. Line is patent. | Insures proper fat administration. |
| ***Unexpected outcome*** | |
| 1. There is intolerance to fat emulsion as evidenced by increased triglyceride levels, increased temperature (3° to 4° F), chills, headache, nausea and vomiting, muscle ache, backache, chest pain. | Lipoprotein lipase, which is responsible for clearance of fat from circulation, may not be activated; excess fat accumulation occurs. |
| **Recording and Reporting** | |
| 1. Record intake and output every shift. | Indicates fluid status. |
| 2. Record temperature every 4 hrs. | Gradual elevation of temperature may indicate catheter sepsis. |
| 3. Record condition of IV site and status of infusion. | Documents status of IV site. |
| **Follow-up Activity** | |
| 1. If fat emulsion is not tolerated, therapy must be discontinued per physician's order. | Client is unable to properly metabolize parenteral fat solution. |

### Special Considerations

- Children have increased need for essential fatty acids because of growth.
- When fat rather than glucose is used as energy source, carbon dioxide output is decreased, which results in circulating free fatty acids and increased ketone levels.
- If admixing fat and TPN, solution bag is only equipment.
- Do not shake fat emulsion bottle excessively; this disrupts physical stability of microscopic fat globules. Inspect bottle for opacity and consistency in texture and color. Use tubing provided by manufacturer. Do not use filters because fat particles are larger than filters.
- 10% fat emulsions are infused over 4 hrs and 20% fats are infused over 6 hrs. All fats can hang for 12 hrs and admixing fats for 24 hrs. Initial rate 1 ml/min × 15 to 30 min.

### Teaching Considerations

- Instruct primary care giver about proper methods for storing parenteral nutrition supplies.
- Teach client, primary care giver to monitor client's weight, calorie count, intake and output, urine assessment.
- Teach client, primary care giver about actions to take in case of emergency.

### Home Care Considerations

- Observe client, primary care giver perform procedure before discharge.
- Assess client's home for suitability to provide TPN safely.
- Use aseptic technique when assembling equipment for IV dressing changes on clean surface in home.

## *SKILL 28-3 Caring for the Client Receiving Central Venous Placement for Central Parenteral Nutrition*

CPN is a form of nutritional support administered through central vein cannulation (Fig. 28-1). A catheter is usually placed in the subclavian vein through an infraclavicular venipuncture. This is the preferred method of cannulation, primarily because it provides a flat, relatively immobile area on the chest for a clear adhesive dressing. The vessels have a high flow rate, thereby decreasing the risk of phlebitis or thrombus formation.

The standard solution for CPN is hyperosmolar as compared to the osmolality of a PPN solution (Table 28-1). There are four general classifications of clients who require CPN: 1) clients unable to eat for prolonged periods because of trauma or comatose state; 2) clients unable to absorb food because of primary gastrointestinal disease,

**TABLE 28-1** Comparison of CPN and PPN

| | CPN | PPN |
|---|---|---|
| Osmolality | 1800-2000 mOsm | 600-700 mOsm |
| Route of administration | Central venous catheter | Small peripheral vein |
| Usual daily caloric intake | 2000-4000 | 700-2000 |
| Fat emulsion | Minor caloric source; provides essential fatty acid | Major caloric source; provides essential fatty acid |
| Objectives | Weight maintenance; weight gain | Weight maintenance |
| Duration of therapy | 6 days or longer | 3-7 days |

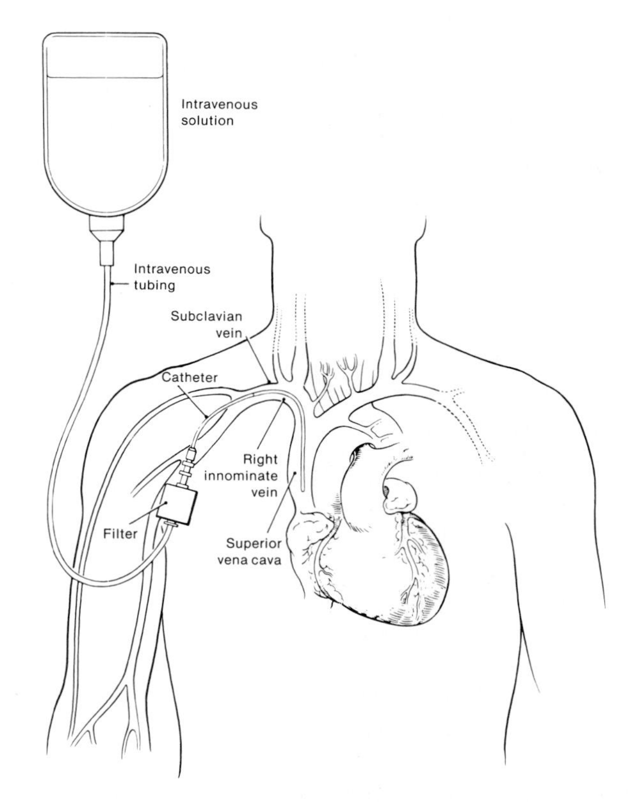


***Fig. 28-1*** Hyperalimentation showing catheter placed directly into subclavian vein and threaded into innominate vein and superior vena cava.

From Phipps WJ, Long BC, Woods NF: Medical-surgical nursing: concepts and clinical practice, ed 3, St Louis, 1987, The CV Mosby Co.

fistulas, or gastrointestinal obstruction; 3) clients in whom malnutrition occurs in a preoperative or postoperative condition such as malignancy; and 4) clients in whom the bowel or other organs need to rest, such as those with pancreatitis or inflammatory bowel disease.

### Purposes

1. Maintain nutritional status.
2. Improve nutrition status in clients requiring long-term nutritional support.

## *Procedure 28-3*

| Steps | Rationale |
|---|---|
| **Assessment** | |
| 1. Assess need for CPN by nutritional assessment (Skill 26-1), physical assessment (Chapter 13), and frequent laboratory data monitoring. | Provides baseline to compare changes after CPN is started. |
| 2. Check physician's order for nutrients, minerals, electrolytes, as well as flow rate. | Parenteral therapy must be ordered by physician. |
| **Nursing Diagnosis** | |
| 1. Cluster data to reveal actual or potential nursing diagnoses: | |
| a. Potential for infection: related to central venous puncture. | Placement of central line has risks. Complications include sepsis and pneumothorax. |
| b. Altered nutrition—less than body requirements: related to inability to tolerate enteral nutrition. | Clients with or who are at risk for serious nutritional deficiency are candidates for CPN. |
| **Planning** | |
| 1. Central IV lines are inserted by physicians. | |
| 2. Develop individualized goals for client based on nursing diagnoses: | |
| a. Maintain surgical asepsis of venipuncture site. | Reduces risk of line asepsis. |
| b. Promote adquate nutritional intake. | CPN required for balanced nutrition and weight gain. |
| 3. Prepare needed equipment: | All equipment must be accessible for nurse to assist with insertion of central venous catheter. Organization of equipment results in smooth and organized insertion of central IV line. |
| a. 2 caps | |
| b. 2 sterile gowns | |
| c. 2 masks | |
| d. Nonsterile gloves | |
| e. 3 pair sterile gloves | |
| f. 4 × 4 gauze pads | |
| g. Bottle of alcohol | |
| h. Towel | |
| i. Pad | |
| j. Povidone-iodine scrub soap | |
| k. Povidone-iodine swabsticks (3) | |
| l. 1% lidocaine (Xylocaine) | Anesthetizes venipuncture site. |
| m. Central line catheter insertion kit | |
| n. Sterile barrier | Provides sterile field for catheter insertion. |
| o. 500 ml bottle D5W | |
| p. Sterile 6" extension tubing | |
| q. 3 alcohol swabs | |
| r. 3 povidone-iodine swabs | |
| s. 1 povidone-iodine ointment | |
| t. 1 clear adhesive dressing | |
| u. 2 pieces of tape (3 × 1) | |
| v. Tincture of benzoin (optional) | |
| w. Infusion pump | |
| 4. Explain to client steps for central line insertion and need for CPN and follow-up care. | Promotes understanding and alleviates anxiety. |

| Steps | Rationale |
|---|---|
| **Implementation** | |
| 1. Nurse and physician wash hands. | Reduces transmission of microorganisms. |
| 2. Physician with the assistance of nurse positions client flat in bed lying supine. Place rolled towel between scapulas and place protective pad under shoulder area. | Opens angle between clavicle and first rib. |
| 3. Nurse puts on cap, mask, and unsterile gloves. Physician should don cap, gown, mask, and sterile gloves. | |
| 4. Nurse saturates 1 4 × 4 gauze pad with alcohol, and physician scrubs area using circular motion from shoulder to ear to chin to nipple for approximately 1 min. | Alcohol cleans and defats skin. |
| 5. Discard 4 × 4 gauze pad. | |
| 6. With povidone-iodine scrub, physician cleans above area 1 min with soap. | Removes surface skin bacteria. |
| 7. Physician wipes away excess soap with sterile 4 × 4 gauze pad. | |
| 8. Physician cleans area with povidone-iodine swab three times in circular motion. Discard gloves. | Prevents transmission of infection to sterile equipment. |
| 9. Physician puts on sterile gloves. | |
| 10. Nurse opens first wrapping of central vein kit and hands to physician. Physician will aseptically pick up wrapped central line kit. | Maintains sterile asepsis. |
| 11. Physician will open second wrapping and prepare sterile field. Physician will find anatomical landmarks and place fenestrated drape appropriately. | Provides sterile work space. |
| 12. Physician will review kit and put needles on syringe. | |
| 13. Nurse sets up IV bag and fills tubing. | IV tubing ready to be connected to IV catheter. |
| 14. Nurse opens 6″ sterile tubing, and physician places on sterile field, following aseptic technique. | Maintains sterile asepsis. |
| 15. Nurse places client in Trendelenburg's position and turns client's head away from site of insertion. | Promotes maximal filling and distention of subclavicular vein. |
| 16. Nurse wipes off top of 1% lidocaine bottle and turns upside down. | Removes surface bacteria; allows physician to withdraw lidocaine while maintaining asepsis. |
| 17. Physician injects needle into bottle and withdraws approximately 3 to 4 ml lidocaine. Physician injects needle into site for subclavian puncture and anesthetizes venipuncture site. | Minimizes discomfort client will feel during venipuncture. |
| 18. Have client perform Valsalva maneuver (holding breath while bearing down). | Increases venous pressure and reduces risk of air entering central line and subsequent air embolism. |
| 19. Physician inserts subclavian IV catheter into subclavian vein. | Large vein is less irritated by CPN solution. |
| 20. Nurse checks on client throughout to assess tolerance of procedure. For example, when physician is threading catheter into the vein, ask how client is tolerating this. | If client complains of pains in neck area, it indicates that line is floating into neck and not subclavian vein. Alert physician. |
| 21. While physician is cannulating central vein, aseptically connect IV tubing to 6 in extension tubing and flush with IV fluid. | |
| 22. When physician has rapid blood return, physician connects IV tubing to client's subclavian catheter. | Prevents air from entering venous system. |
| 23. Nurse opens IV fluids wide open. | Assesses whether fluid is infusing easily. |
| 24. Nurse lowers IV bag below heart level. | Provides blood return to determine presence of IV in venous system. |
| 25. Nurse raises IV bag and slows rate to 30 ml/hr until chest x-ray study is obtained. | Central line cannulations increase risk of pneumothorax. Chest x-ray verifies absence of pneumothorax before fluids are regulated at a rapid flow. |
| 26. Physician sutures central venous catheter in place. | Suturing catheter to chest wall if possible prevents accidental dislodgement and helps occlusive dressing to adhere better. |
| 27. Physician removes sterile clothes and completes procedure. | Occurs only if physician is not applying occlusive dressing to IV site. |
| *Applying occlusive dressing.* | |
| 1. Put on sterile gloves. | Maintains surgical asepsis. |
| 2. With alcohol swab, start at catheter exit site and work in circular motion outward approximately 2 to 3 in. (Do three times.) | Removes blood and defats skin. |
| 3. With povidone-iodine swabs, repeat above step. Allow area to dry. | Disinfects skin. (Do not blow or fan dry). |
| 4. Apply small amount of povidone-iodine ointment at catheter exit site. | Povidone-iodine is bacteriostatic ointment. |

| Steps | Rationale |
|---|---|
| 5. Apply clear, adhesive dressing over site (Chapter 23). | Reduces transmission of microorganisms to venipuncture site and allows observation of site. |
| 6. Connect tubing to infusion pump and set rate (Chapter 23). | Maintains prescribed rate of infusion flow. Check infusion rate every hr. When solution is begun, start at 1 L/24 hr (42 ml/hr) first day. |
| 7. Assist with chest x-ray examination. | Documents line position or presence of hydrothorax. |
| 8. Reposition client. | Maintains comfort. |
| 9. Dispose of supplies and wash hands. | Reduces transmission of microorganisms. |

## Evaluation

| | |
|---|---|
| 1. Inspect site and dressing daily for redness, swelling, exudate, unocclusiveness. | Indicates inflammation or irritation at venipuncture site. |
| 2. Evaluate client for complications associated with parenteral nutrition (Table 28-2). | Complications of TPN can be systemic or localized. |

### *Expected outcomes*

| | |
|---|---|
| 1. Venipuncture site is free of inflammation. | Denotes absence of infection at central venous site. |
| 2. Client's ideal weight gain is usually between ½ and 1 lb/day. | Weight is excellent indication of how well client is doing nutritionally and is used to determine fluid volume. Weight gain of more than 1 lb/day indicates fluid retention. |
| 3. Breath sounds are clear to auscultation. | Occurrence of rales (crackles) indicates fluid overload. |
| 4. Urine S & A level is negative or 1+. | Urine S & A level is used to determine tolerance to dextrose. |

### *Unexpected outcomes*

| | |
|---|---|
| 1. There is sepsis of the central venous site. | Indicates infection at the catheter site. Catheter sepsis is common complication of CPN. |
| 2. Weight gain greater than 1 lb/day. | Indicates fluid retention, not restoration of body proteins. |
| 3. Crackles auscultated over lung fields. | When fluid overload occurs, excess fluid accumulates in lung fields. |
| 4. Urine S & A level is greater than 1+. | May indicate inability to successfully metabolize dextrose in solution and catheter sepsis. |

## Recording and Reporting

| | |
|---|---|
| 1. Record condition of IV and rate of infusion. | Documents status of IV infusion rate. |
| 2. Record intake and output every shift. | Indicates fluid status. |
| 3. Record temperature every 4 hrs. | Gradual elevation of temperature may indicate catheter sepsis. |
| 4. Record urine for S & A levels every 6 hrs. | Documents metabolic response to glucose solution. |

## Follow-up Activities

| | |
|---|---|
| 1. Sepsis: | |
| a. Remove central venous catheter. | Removes source of infection. |
| b. Obtain culture of catheter tip and blood cultures. | Identifies microorganisms causing infection. |
| 2. Weight gain, rales, increased urinary sugar: | |
| a. Notify physician. | Solution changes require physician's order. |
| b. Change solution. | If fluid overload is present, physician may also wish to treat client with diuretics and fluid restrictions. |

## Special Considerations

- Central IV lines are inserted by physicians.
- Tubing and solution are changed every 24 hr. Clean, adhesive dressing is changed every 7 days unless it becomes unocclusive.

## Teaching Considerations

- Instruct primary care giver about proper methods for storing parenteral nutrition supplies.
- Teach client, primary care giver to monitor client's weight calorie count, intake and output, and urine assessment.
- Teach client, primary care giver about actions to take in case of emergency.

## Home Care Considerations

- Observe client, primary care giver perform procedure before discharge.
- Assess client's home for suitability to provide TPN safely.
- Use aseptic technique when assembling equipment for dressing changes on clean surface in home.

***TABLE 28-2*** Complications Associated with CPN

| Problem | Cause | Symptoms | Immediate Action | Prevention |
|---|---|---|---|---|
| Air embolism | IV tubing disconnected.<br>Rubber-tipped injection port, syringe, tubing removed without clamp on.<br>Injection port fell off. | Coughing<br>Shortness of breath<br>Chest pain<br>Cyanosis | Clamp catheter.<br>Lie on left side with head down.<br>Call physician. | Tape junctions.<br>Clamp catheter. |
| Infection | Poor aseptic technique.<br>Contaminated tubing or heparin. | Redness, swelling, drainage at insertion site<br>Temperature above 100° F (37.7° C)<br>Chills<br>Sweating<br>Lethargy<br>Urine spot checks showing glucose levels greater than ½ % | Call physician. | Use proper aseptic technique. |
| Hyperglycemia | Fluids infused too fast.<br>Too little insulin in infusion solution.<br>Infection. | Nausea<br>Weakness<br>Thirst<br>Headache<br>Urine spot checks showing glucose levels greater than ½ % | Call physician.<br>May need to decrease infusion rate or add insulin to solution. | Maintain prescribed drip rate—never try to "catch up" if rate slows.<br>Maintain aseptic technique.<br>Have glucose tolerance tested in hospital before discharge.<br>Monitor blood glucose levels monthly. |
| Hypoglycemia | Fluids stopped abruptly.<br>Too much insulin in infusion solution. | Sweating<br>Pale facial color<br>Heart palpitations<br>Nausea<br>Headache<br>Shaky feeling<br>Blurred vision<br>Hunger pangs | Call physician.<br>May need to adjust infusion rate or decrease insulin in infusion.<br>If hypoglycemia is suspected, have client drink glass of orange juice with 2 teaspoons of sugar.<br>If client is unable to tolerate fluids by mouth, place hard candy or cake decorating gel under tongue. | Have glucose tolerance tested in hospital before discharge.<br>Monitor blood glucose levels monthly. |

Modified from Wilhelm L: Helping your patient "settle in" with TPN, Nursing 85, p 63, April 1985.

## BIBLIOGRAPHY


Anderson AR: Are your IV chemo skills up-to-date? RN 89(1):40, 1989.

Atkins J, Oakley C: A nurse's guide to TPN, RN 49(6):20, 1986.

Blackburn G, Flatt J, Hensle T: Peripheral amino acids infusions. In Fischer J, editor: Total parenteral nutrition, ed 1, Boston, 1976, Little, Brown, & Co, Inc.

Blackburn G, et al.: Peripheral intravenous feeding with isotonic amino acid solution, Am J Surg 125:447, 1973.

Carr P: When the patient needs TPN at home, RN 49(6):25, 1986.

Cerra F: Parenteral nutrition. In Pocket manual of surgical nutrition, St Louis, 1984, The CV Mosby Co.

Colley R: Parenteral nutrition. In Metheny N, editor: Fluid and electrolyte balance: nursing considerations, ed 3, Philadelphia, 1987, JB Lippincott Co.

Colley R, Wilson J: Meeting patients' nutritional needs with hyperalimentation, Nursing 79 9:76, 1979.

Crocker K: Metabolic monitoring during nutritional support therapy. In Grant J and Kennedy-Caldwell C: Nutritional support in nursing, Philadelphia, 1988, Grune & Stratton, Inc.

Dirks I, Shipley L: Intravenous fat emulsion as a component of tpn, Nutrit Support Serv 4(4):41, 1984.

Englert D: Rational use of fat emulsions, Nutrit Support Serv p 35, Sept 1982.

Fleming C, Nelson J: Nutritional options. In Kinney J, Jeejeehoy K, Hill G, Owen O: Nutrition and metabolism in patient care, Philadelphia, 1988, WB Saunders Co.

Fong, Grimley: Peripheral intravenous infusion of amino acids, Am J Hosp Pharm 38:652, 1981.

Forlaw L, Torosian M: Central venous catheter care. In Rombeau J, Caldwell M, editors: Clinical nutrition. Vol. II. Parental nutrition, Philadelphia, 1986, WB Saunders Co.

Forlaw L, Bayer, Grant: Introduction to nutritional and physical assessment of the adult patient for the nurse, Silver Spring, Md, 1983, ASPEN.

Forlaw L, et al.: Nursing care standards for nutritional support of the hospitalized patient, Silver Spring, Md, 1984, ASPEN.

Gahart B: Intravenous medications: a handbook for nurses and other allied health personnel, ed 5, St Louis, 1989, The CV Mosby Company.

Griggs B: Indications for nutritional support in the adult patient. In Grant J, Kennedy-Caldwell C: Nutritional support in nursing, Philadelphia, 1988, Grune & Stratton, Inc.

Gullatte M: Managing an implanted infusion device, RN 89(1):45, 1989.

Haddad A: High touch needs of high-tech patients, Caring 7(9):9, 1988.

Keithley JK: Proper nutritional assessment can prevent hospital malnutrition, Nursing 79 9:68, 1979.

Kruzic P, Grundfast D, Stites L, John E: Home Care IV therapy manual, Rockville, Md, Aspen Publishers, Inc.

Liposysn 11: Intravenous fat emulsion, May 1988, Abbott Laboratories.

Loludice T: Total parenteral nutrition: the do's and dont's, Nutr Support Serv 1(2):30, 1981.

Maker V: Applications of central vs. peripheral T.P.N., NITA 6:357, 1983.

Miller L, Devin G, Yen R, Kaminski M: Enteral and parenteral nutrition in the critically ill patient, Hospital Formul 21:672, 1986.

Phillips G, Odgers C: Indications and contraindications. In Parenteral and enteral nutrition: a practical guide, New York, 1986, Churchill Livingstone, Inc.

Phillips G, Odgers C: Special techniques—protein sparing, cyclic nutrition. In Parenteral and enteral nutrition: a practical guide, New York, 1986, Churchill Livingstone, Inc.

Ryder M: Parenteral nutrition. In Kennedy-Caldwell C, Guenter P: Nutrition support nursing: core curriculum, Silver Spring, Md., 1988, ASPEN.

Scholl D, Rago R: Total parenteral nutrition. In Nutrition and diet therapy, Oradell, NJ, 1986, Medical Economics Books.

# UNIT IX

# ELIMINATION

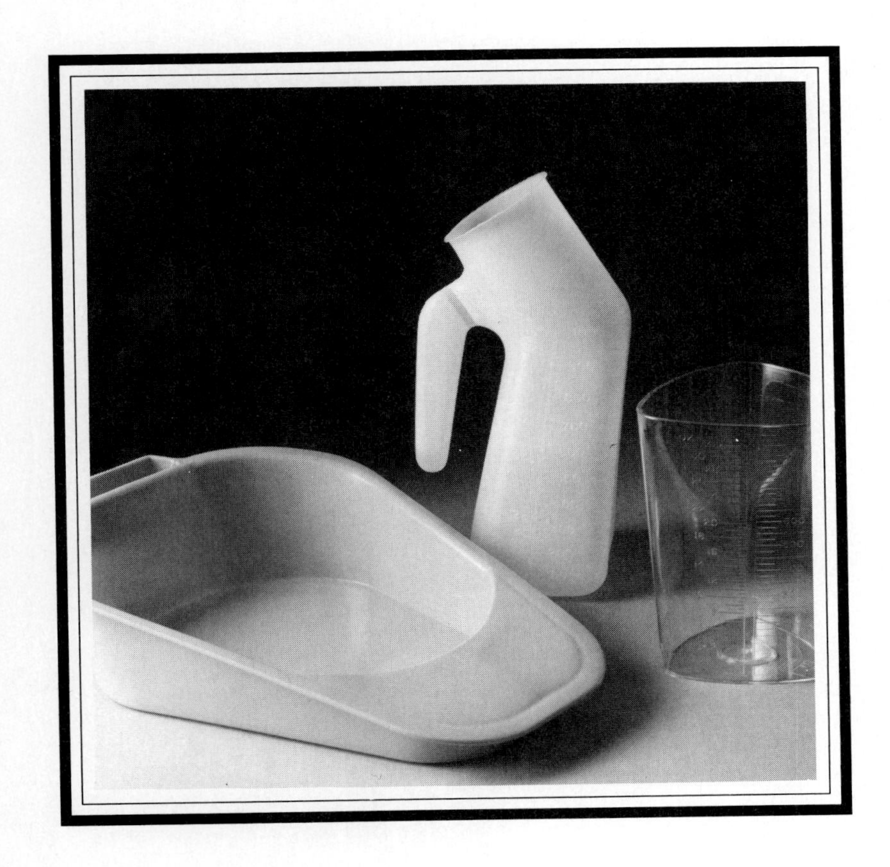

*Depending on mobility status and the kinds of treatment and procedures a client must undergo, urinary and bowel elimination may pose myriad problems. Physically the client may not be able to perform normal patterns of elimination and may need assistance from staff and/or special devices. It is imperative that the nurse display understanding and respect the client's privacy when meeting these basic needs.*

*Chapter 30 contains basic skills such as assisting the client to use a urinal and more advanced skills of catheterization.*

*Chapter 31 presents skills to assist the client with bowel elimination, including bedpan use and enema adminsistration.*

*Chapter 32 features special skills for ostomy care, a rapidly growing specialty in any health care setting. Client teaching is also stressed.*

# 29

# URINARY ELIMINATION

## OBJECTIVES

*Mastery of content in this chapter will enable the nurse to:*

- Define key terms.
- Identify factors that alter normal voiding.
- Describe devices used to promote urinary drainage.
- Identify techniques used to minimize urinary tract infection.
- Teach clients self-catheterization.
- Select appropriate clients for measurement of intake and output.
- Evaluate a client's hydration status.
- Develop a teaching plan for clients to measure and record their intake and output in a community setting.
- Perform the following skills: measure and record intake and output, place and remove urinal, insert urinary catheter, complete routine catheter care, obtain residual urines, irrigate a catheter, remove a retention catheter, apply a condom catheter.

## KEY TERMS

*Aldosterone*
*Catheterization*
*Incontinence*
*Intake*
*Micturition*
*Nosocomial infection*
*Output*
*Residual urine*
*Urethral sphincter*
*Urinary retention*
*Urinary tract infection*
*Urine*
*Urine specific gravity*

## SKILLS

**29-1** Measuring and Recording Intake and Output
**29-2** Assisting a Client to Use a Urinal
**29-3** Inserting a Straight or Indwelling Catheter
**29-4** Performing Routine Catheter Care
**29-5** Obtaining Catheterized Specimens for Residual Urine
**29-6** Teaching Self-Catheterization
**29-7** Performing Catheter Irrigation
**29-8** Removing a Retention Catheter
**29-9** Applying a Condom Catheter
**29-10** Peritoneal Dialysis and Continuous Ambulatory Peritoneal Dialysis

Urinary elimination is a natural process individuals take for granted until it is altered by some uncontrollable physiologic factor. Clients needing assistance with urinary elimination may require physiologic and psychologic assistance from the nurse. Often physiologic support requires use of an invasive procedure, such as the insertion of a catheter into the bladder. Psychologic assistance is needed to assist the client in an adjustment to a visible urine collection drainage bag. Therefore the nurse must be competent in performing technical skills and sensitive to a client's psychologic needs.

The urinary tract is susceptible to infections, particularly when invaded, as is the case when a sterile catheter is inserted. Therefore the nurse must be able to apply the principles of sterile asepsis.

When clients have altered or impaired urinary elimination, they require intake and output measurements to assist in monitoring fluid and electrolyte balance. This balance can include the measurement of intake and output.

Placing a client on intake and output measurements requires cooperation and assistance from the client and family. Intake measurements must include all liquids and semiliquids, such as gelatin and ice cream, and liquid medication taken orally. Fluids administered as enteral feedings through nasogastric, gastrostomy, or jejunostomy tubes are considered oral intake and should be recorded as such (Chapter 27). IV solutions (Chapter 23), blood components (Chapter 25), and TPN (Chapter 28) are recorded as fluid intake.

Output includes the measurement and recording of all liquid excreted or drained from the client. Thus all urine, vomitus, and liquid stools are recorded as output. Drainage from wounds, fistulas, and nasogastric and wound suction equipment is also considered output (Chapter 44). The recording of all types of intake and output is a procedure used to monitor fluid and electrolyte balance.

Certain disease processes, medications, and stages of growth and development influence fluid and electrolyte status. Physical assessment findings can indicate that a fluid or electrolyte imbalance exists. The nurse must know the factors influencing fluid and electrolyte balance and the signs and symptoms of fluid imbalances. When there is a potential or actual fluid and electrolyte imbalance, the nurse should place the client on intake and output measurements.

## GUIDELINES

1. Know the client's usual fluid intake pattern, including the types and amount of fluids and when they are ingested.
2. Know the client's normal range of vital signs. Abnormal fluid and electrolyte balances can affect the amount of circulating blood volume. During dehydration, the blood pressure is decreased and the pulse and body temperature are elevated. Overhydration usually produces a bounding pulse in which the rate may be either increased or decreased. Blood pressure may rise slightly, but body temperature remains unchanged.
3. Know the client's medical history and therapies the client is receiving. Clients with cardiopulmonary or renal disease frequently have fluid imbalances. Diuretics are often used to regulate fluid balance, and they usually have beneficial effects. However, side effects can further potentiate fluid and electrolyte imbalances.
4. Be aware of environmental conditions that can affect fluid balance. Prolonged or extreme environmental temperatures can cause increased loss of body fluids through perspiration.
5. Place the client on intake and output measurements when there is an anticipated or suspicious change in fluid balance. Although the physician orders intake and output measurements for clients, the nurse has a responsibility to determine if more frequent measurements are required. For example, a client who is one day postoperative for abdominal surgery and is NPO (nothing by mouth), is receiving IV therapy, has a nasogastric (NG) tube attached to suction, and has an indwelling Foley catheter may suddenly develop an increase in gastric drainage. One of the nurse's appropriate actions may be to increase the intake and output measurements from every 8 hours to every 2 hours to determine if there is an increased trend for fluid loss necessitating increased fluid replacement. The nurse also should not hesitate to initiate intake and output measurements when a client suddenly develops vomiting, diarrhea, or hemorrhage, and is immediately postoperative.
6. Know the client's most recent serum electrolyte measurements. Abnormal electrolyte values can affect fluid balance and, if uncorrected, can lead to deterioration of the client's health status or even death.
7. Maintain perineal hygiene patterns. Because urinary tract infections are the most prevalent nosocomial infections, it is imperative that the nurse adhere to the principles of medical asepsis. Handwashing after caring for each client is critically important. The nurse should teach clients, particularly girls and women, proper perineal hygiene habits.
8. Know the client's level of comfort. A client uncomfortable physically or psychologically may be unable to relax the external urethral sphincter to void or completely empty the bladder. The nurse can promote comfort measures by providing privacy, offering the client a warm bedpan, assisting the client into a normal voiding position (standing for a man, squatting for a woman), or reducing pain by administering a prescribed analgesic before assisting the client to ambulate to the bathroom. Distraction measures, such as turning on a water tap so that the client can hear water running, will help the person to void.
9. Identify conditions that weaken abdominal or pelvic muscles, such as multiple abdominal or gynecologic surgeries or pregnancies. Clients with weak abdominal or pelvic floor muscles can be taught exercises to strengthen these muscles and increase the ability of the bladder to contract and promote better control of the external urethral sphincter.
10. Know the client's normal patterns of micturition. The client should be taught never to ignore the urge to void. The nurse can assist by responding readily to the client's request to use a bedpan, urinal, or bathroom or commode. The nurse can also offer a client the opportunity to void after meals and before bedtime. Clients should receive diuretic medications early in the morning so they do not need to void during the night.
11. Consider the client's age when assessing how the aging process affects micturition habits.

## PREREQUISITE KNOWLEDGE

1. Principles of fluid and electrolyte balance.
2. Effect of specific electrolyte imbalance on body function.
3. Fluid balance alterations of dehydration and overhydration.
4. Anatomy and physiology of the urinary system.
5. Principles of medical and surgical asepsis.
6. Principles of normal micturition.
7. Principles of teaching and learning.
8. Concepts of osmosis, diffusion, and fluid balances.

## PREREQUISITE SKILLS

1. Perform proper handwashing techniques (Chapter 37).
2. Perform physical assessment (Chapter 13).
3. Perform sterile technique (Chapter 38).
4. Perform perineal hygiene (Chapter 6).
5. Obtain a urine specimen (Chapter 45).

# SKILL 29-1 Measuring and Recording Intake and Output

Measuring and recording all intake and output during a 24 hr period helps to complete the assessment data base for fluid and electrolyte balance. The nurse is responsible for collecting and recording these data. Intake includes all liquids taken orally, by feeding tube, and parenterally. Liquid output includes urine, diarrhea, vomitus, gastric suction, and drainage from postsurgical tubes, such as chest tube or Penrose drains. Frequently, the recording of such data is referred to as the client's I & O.

### Purposes

1. Maintain ongoing assessment data of the client's fluid status.
2. Document the client's ability to tolerate oral fluids.
3. Document significant fluid losses.
4. Document the exact amount of fluids given to the client.

## Procedure 29-1

| Steps | Rationale |
|---|---|
| **Assessment** | |
| 1. Review client's graphic chart for elevations in body temperature (Chapter 12). | Prolonged fever diminishes body fluids by increasing insensible water losses from lungs through increased respiratory rate and from the skin through diaphoresis. |
| 2. Assess for surgical wound drainage. Wound drains are frequently present in clients suffering trauma and in those who have had chest or abdominal surgery. | Wound drainage represents plasma or whole blood loss. If drainage is significant or prolonged, fluid and electrolyte imbalance results. Wound suction removes plasma and whole blood. Excessive fluid loss from wound must be replaced. Accurate recording of output assists in fluid replacement. |
| 3. Identify presence of any wound or gastric suction equipment. Clients with abdominal surgery, gastrointestinal hemorrhage, pancreatitis, cholecystitis have nasogastric suction. | Gastric suction removes hydrochloric acid (HCl), potassium (K), and other fluids from stomach. Gastric suction decompresses stomach and keeps stomach empty. |
| 4. Assess patency and flow rate of IV and TPN solutions (Chapters 23 and 28). | Incorrect IV solutions and inaccurate flow rates can result in fluid and electrolyte imbalances. |
| 5. Identify conditions that can influence fluid balance status: | |
| a. Major burns: second degree, 20% of body surface; third degree, 10% of body surface. | Fluid volume loss is directly proportional to amount and depth of injury. Average adult with burn of 40% of body increases body surface fluid loss from 20 to 100/ml/hr/sq meter of body surface. Major vascular fluid loss occurs during the first 24 to 48 hr. |
| b. Diuretics. | Cause excretion of water and sodium. Some diuretics can be potassium wasters (furosemide) or potassium savers (spironolactone). |
| c. Steroids. | Steroids (e.g., prednisone, cortisone), cause sodium and water retention and excretion of potassium. |
| d. Severe trauma, especially crush injuries. | Hyperkalemia occurs from release of intracellular potassium from injured cells. |
| e. Head injuries with cerebral edema. | Cerebral edema creates pressure on pituitary gland causing alterations of antidiuretic hormone (ADH) secretion: *Diabetes insipidus:* too little ADH is secreted and large amounts of dilute urine are excreted. *Syndrome of inappropriate secretion of antidiuretic hormone* (SIADH): excessive secretion of ADH with water retention (Metheny, 1987). |
| f. Endocrine imbalances: | |
| ▪ Cushing's disease or Cushing's syndrome. | Excessive amount of corticosteroids causes sodium and water retention with potassium excretion. |
| ▪ Addison's disease. | Insufficient amounts of corticosteroids cause sodium and water excretion. |
| ▪ Diabetic ketoacidosis. | Osmotic diuresis due to increased blood sugar causes severe fluid volume deficit. |

| Steps | Rationale |
|---|---|
| g. Gastroenteritis. | Excretion of potassium and chloride ions affects fluid and electrolyte balance. Excretion of hydrogen ion alters acid-base status. |
| 6. Observe for weight changes that occur within 24 to 48 hr.<br>2%-5% loss Mild dehydration<br>6%-9% loss Moderate dehydration<br>10%-14% loss Severe dehydration<br>20% loss Death<br>2%-4% gain Mild volume overload<br>5%-7% gain Moderate overload<br>8% or more gain Severe volume overload | Allows nurse to identify early assessment finding for dehydration or volume overload. |
| 7. Inspect client for signs of fluid overload or dehydration:<br>a. Eyes—*dehydration:* sunken eyes; dry conjunctivae; decreased or absence of tearing; *fluid overload:* periorbital; blurred vision; papilledema.<br>b. Mouth—*dehydration:* sticky, dry mucous membrane; dry, cracked lips; decreased saliva; increased viscosity of saliva; *fluid overload:* longitudinal furrows on tongue, swollen tongue, excessive salivation.<br>c. Cardiovascular—*dehydration:* increased pulse rate, decreased pulse rate, weak pulse, decreased capillary filling; *fluid overload:* bounding pulse rate, blood pressure low with or without orthostatic changes, third heart sound ($S_3$), distended neck veins.<br>d. Gastrointestinal—*dehydration:* sunken abdomen; *dehydration or fluid overload:* vomiting, diarrhea, abdominal cramps.<br>e. Renal—*dehydration:* oliguria or anuria, specific gravity of urine increased; *fluid overload:* decreased specific gravity, diuresis (if kidneys normal).<br>f. Skin—*dehydration:* increased skin temperature; dry, scaly skin; poor turgor; *fluid overload:* edema. | Body compensates for overhydration by maintaining excess volume in extracellular fluid spaces and transferring fluid into tissues, causing edema. Signs of dehydration result from reduction in fluid within tissues and circulatory system. |
| 8. Inspect urine color and specific gravity (normal 1.010 to 1.030) (Chapter 45). | Kidneys attempt to excrete excess fluid during periods of overhydration and conserve body water during periods of dehydration. |

## Nursing Diagnosis

| | |
|---|---|
| 1. Cluster data to reveal actual or potential nursing diagnoses:<br>a. Fluid volume deficit related to:<br>▪ Inadequate intake.<br>▪ Excess fluid loss. | Clients at risk include infants, immobilized clients, disoriented clients, clients with unstable health status, handicapped clients, older adults. |
| b. Fluid volume excess: related to electrolyte imbalance or impaired renal functioning. | Clients at risk include those with chronic or acute cardiopulmonary or renal disease, clients receiving diuretics, IV therapy, TPN, and steroids. |

## Planning

| | |
|---|---|
| 1. Develop individualized goals for client based on nursing diagnoses: | |
| a. Maintain 24 hr fluid intake within 600 ml to 900 ml of 24 hr output measurement. | Insensible fluid losses from lungs, skin, and intestine are approximately 600 to 900 ml. Insensible fluid loss varies with body size and age. |
| b. Maintain a minimum of 1500 ml oral intake per 24 hr. | Adult male weighing 70 kg requires average fluid intake of 2600 ml/day; approximately 1300 ml is from fluid intake (Metheny 1987). |
| c. Physical assessment and laboratory values return to and remain within normal limits. | Dehydration or overhydration can cause decrease or increase in laboratory values. |
| 2. Select appropriate clients whose I & O should be measured. | Any client can be placed on I & O measurements by nurse. Clients whose conditions are unstable or potentially unstable require I & O measurements at least every 4 hr. |
| 3. Assemble necessary equipment in room or near bedside:<br>a. Chart for door or bedside (Fig. 29-1).<br>b. I & O sheet (Fig. 29-2). | Allows for consistent implementation of measurements. |

Barnes Hospital
DAILY INTAKE AND OUTPUT RECORD **B-8**

17-4 Rev. 2/83

**FROM 0700 / / TO 0700 / /** Addressograph Plate

**INTAKE**

Coffee mug - 180cc
Ice tea container to clear line (without ice) - 250cc
Ice cream container (melted) - 30cc
Sherbet container (melted) - 50cc
Juice container - 120cc
Milk carton - 240cc
Paper cup (1/4 from brim) - 240cc
Soup bowl (broth) - 180cc
Gelatin container (melted) - 100cc

RATE GTTS/MIN. CC/HR.

ORDERS: (CIRCLE)
NPO
WATER
CLEAR FLUIDS (circled)
FULL FLUIDS

AMT. DESIRED CC

**OUTPUT**

SOURCE KEY:
V = VOIDED
C = CATHETER
INC = INCONTINENT

SOURCE KEY:
VOM. = VOMITUS
LIQ. S. = LIQUID STOOL
HV. = HEMOVAC
L.T. = LEVIN TUBE
T.T. = T. TUBE
OTHER

| | PARENTERAL | | | ORAL | | URINE | | OTHER | |
|---|---|---|---|---|---|---|---|---|---|
| TIME | SOLUTION IN BOTTLE KIND | AMT. (CC) | AMT. (CC) ABSORBED | KIND | AMT. (CC) | SOURCE | AMT. (CC) | SOURCE | AMT. (CC) |
| 0700 0800 | | | | Juice | 120 | | | | |
| 0800 0900 | | | | Jello | 100 | V | 200 | | |
| 0900 1000 | | | | Maalox | 30 | | | | |
| 1000 1100 | | | | Soup | 180 | | | | |
| 1100 1200 | | | | Juice | 120 | | | | |
| 1200 1300 | | | | Jello | 100 | ✓ | 180 | | |
| 1300 1400 | | | | | | | | | |
| 1400 1500 | | | | | | | | | |
| | 8 HR. TOT. | | | 8 HR. TOT. | 650 | 8 HR. TOT. | 380 | 8 HR. TOT. | |
| 1500 1600 | | | | | | | | | |
| 1600 1700 | | | | | | | | | |
| 1700 1800 | | | | | | | | | |
| 1800 1900 | | | | | | | | | |
| 1900 2000 | | | | | | | | | |
| 2000 2100 | | | | | | | | | |
| 2100 2200 | | | | | | | | | |
| 2200 2300 | | | | | | | | | |
| | 8 HR. TOT. | | | 8 HR. TOT. | | 8 HR. TOT. | | 8 HR. TOT. | |
| 2300 2400 | | | | | | | | | |
| 2400 0100 | | | | | | | | | |
| 0100 0200 | | | | | | | | | |
| 0200 0300 | | | | | | | | | |
| 0300 0400 | | | | | | | | | |
| 0400 0500 | | | | | | | | | |
| 0500 0600 | | | | | | | | | |
| 0600 0700 | | | | | | | | | |
| | 8 HR. TOT. | | | 8 HR. TOT. | | 8 HR. TOT. | | 8 HR. TOT. | |
| | 24 HR. TOT. | | | 24HR. TOT. | | 24 HR. TOT. | | 24 HR. TOT. | |

***Fig. 29-1***
Courtesy Barnes Hospital, St Louis.

B-17

**BARNES HOSPITAL**
**24 HOUR**
**INTAKE AND OUTPUT SUMMARY**
**(Retain in Patient's Record)**

STAMP ADDRESSOGRAPH PLATE HERE

| | | INTAKE | | OUTPUT | | |
|---|---|---|---|---|---|---|
| DATE | SHIFT | ORAL and/or TUBE FEEDING | IV (Incl. Blood and Plasma) | URINE | GASTRIC | OTHER (specify) |
| | 07000 1500 | | | | | |
| | 1500 2300 | | | | | |
| | 2300 0700 | | | | | |
| | TOTAL | | | | | |
| | 07000 1500 | | | | | |
| | 1500 2300 | | | | | |
| | 2300 0700 | | | | | |
| | TOTAL | | | | | |
| | 07000 1500 | | | | | |
| | 1500 2300 | | | | | |
| | 2300 0700 | | | | | |
| | TOTAL | | | | | |
| | 07000 1500 | | | | | |
| | 1500 2300 | | | | | |
| | 2300 0700 | | | | | |
| | TOTAL | | | | | |
| | 07000 1500 | | | | | |
| | 1500 2300 | | | | | |
| | 2300 0700 | | | | | |
| | TOTAL | | | | | |
| | 07000 1500 | | | | | |
| | 1500 2300 | | | | | |
| | 2300 0700 | | | | | |
| | TOTAL | | | | | |
| | 07000 1500 | | | | | |
| | 1500 2300 | | | | | |
| | 2300 0700 | | | | | |
| | TOTAL | | | | | |

***Fig. 29-2*** Twenty-four hour intake and output record.
Courtesy Barnes Hospital, St Louis.

| Steps | Rationale |
|---|---|
| c. Sign with I & O sheet of measurements of containers commonly used (see Fig. 29-1). | |
| d. Graduated metric container for measuring output in or near bathroom. | |

## Implementation

| Steps | Rationale |
|---|---|
| 1. Explain to client and family why I & O measurements are important. | Ambulatory clients need to be active participants so that if they have coffee or juice in hospital cafeteria, they can record intake. |
| 2. Provide client with copy of hospital's metric conversion chart. | Provides easy and accurate conversion method for recording intake. |
| 3. Measure and record all fluids taken by mouth: | |
| a. Liquids with meals, gelatin, custards, ice cream, Popsicles, sherbets, ice chips. | Liquids frozen into solid substances (e.g., ice cream, ice chips) or semisolid foods (e.g., custards, gelatin) are liquid intake. |
| b. Liquid taken with medications. | Clients receiving frequent medicines such as antacids may have additional 160 to 240/ml of daily intake or more. |
| c. Parenteral fluids: IV (Chapter 23), blood components (Chapter 25), total parenteral fluid (Chapter 28). | Parenteral fluids are instilled directly into extracellular fluid and should be recorded as intake. |
| d. Enteral tube feedings (Chapter 27). | High-calorie liquid meals are instilled directly into gastrointestinal system through nasogastric, gastrostomy, or jejunostomy tubes. |
| 4. Instruct client not to empty urinal, Foley drainage bag, bed pan, or commode but to ask nurse to empty and record amount. | Maintains accurate record of output. |
| 5. Measure and record all drainage from Foley catheter, nasogastric suction, and wound suction at least every 8 hr. | Allows nurse to tabulate total output for each nursing shift. |
| 6. If using toilet, ask client to record each urination and whether amount was small, moderate, large. | Toward end of postoperative or postpartum period frequency of voiding is recorded with approximation of amount voided. |
| 7. Wash hands after measuring and recording output fluids. | Reduces transmission of microorganisms. |

## Evaluation

| Steps | Rationale |
|---|---|
| 1. Reassess client's fluid status as per Assessment, pp. 641-642. | Continual monitoring of client's fluid intake and output provides opportunity to identify and correct actual or potential fluid imbalances. |

### *Expected outcomes*

| Steps | Rationale |
|---|---|
| 1. Oral intake is 600 to 900 ml greater than output and at least 1500 ml/24 hours. | Difference allows for insensible water loss from lungs, intestine, skin. |
| 2. Trend is toward return to normal fluid balance as demonstrated by physical assessment and laboratory findings. | Monitors improving fluid status. |

### *Unexpected outcomes*

| Steps | Rationale |
|---|---|
| 1. Fluid volume deficit is present. | Result of prolonged loss without replacement of circulating and interstitial fluid volume. |
| 2. Fluid volume overload is present. | Result of chemical or physiologic imbalance within body that causes abnormal retention of excessive volume. |

## Recording and Reporting

| Steps | Rationale |
|---|---|
| 1. At end of each nursing shift, calculate total intake and output for each client on I & O (Fig. 29-1). | Provides assessment data on fluid balance for next nursing shift. |
| 2. Calculate and record total 24 hr intake and output on 24 hr fluid record sheet located in client's medical record (Fig. 29-2). | Allows entire health care team to review client's 24 hr I & O records over specific period. |

## Special Considerations

- Infant and older adult are more susceptible to fluid and electrolyte imbalances secondary to prolonged fever. Clients with chronic illnesses or acute trauma, such as burns and abdominal injuries, have potential for further fluid and electrolyte imbalances with fever.
- All postoperative clients are at risk for severe plasma or whole blood loss from incision site (Chapter 39).
- Clients who have severe fluid restriction (e.g., congestive heart failure) are at risk for fluid imbalances.

- Symptoms of endocrine imbalances may also be present in clients receiving synthetic steroid preparations such as prednisone.
- Clients under age 10 or over age 60 are at greater risk of fluid electrolyte imbalances secondary to gastroenteritis.
- Postoperative clients are frequently placed on clear liquid diets and advanced to solid foods as tolerance increases.
- Actual time for calculation of 24 hr I & O totals can vary. In some institutions totals are calculated at 12 midnight, in others at 6 AM.

### Teaching Considerations

- Ambulatory client may require frequent reminders of need to measure and record all liquid I & O.
- Severely ill or disoriented client may be unable to understand reason for I & O or to actively participate in any measuring or recording. However, family members may be able to assist in maintaining accurate output.
- Clients with visual impairments may not be able to use standard metric conversion I & O guide.
- Instruct client, primary care giver on use of household measuring devices to measure I & O.
- Instruct client, primary care giver on signs and symptoms of fluid imbalance.

### Home Care Considerations

- Assess client, primary care giver to determine ability and motivation to maintain accurate records of client's I & O.
- Provide client, primary care giver with appropriate measuring containers and an I & O chart. I & O measurements require a conversion chart for household measures to metric measures. Demonstrate proper manner for measuring I & O.
- Provide opportunity for client, primary care giver to demonstrate understanding of procedure for measuring I & O.

# *SKILL 29-2 Assisting a Client to Use a Urinal*

The client's ability to void depends on feeling the urge to urinate and on being able to control the urethral sphincter. One factor that can interfere with micturition is bed rest or immobility, which does not allow the client to assume the normal position for emptying the bladder. The female client is accustomed to squatting, which promotes contraction of the pelvis and intra-abdominal muscles that assist in sphincter control and bladder contraction. The nurse assists the bedridden woman to use a bedpan for voiding (Chapter 31). A man voids more easily in the standing position. If a man cannot reach the toilet facilities, he may stand at the bedside and void into a urinal, a plastic or metal receptacle for urine. If he is unable to stand at the bedside, the nurse needs to assist him to use the urinal in bed.

### Purposes

1. Promote elimination of urine.
2. Prevent skin breakdown resulting from incontinence.

## *Procedure 29-2*

| Steps | Rationale |
|---|---|
| **Assessment** | |
| 1. Assess client's normal urinary elimination habits. | Identifies normal pattern of urination; helps nurse to recognize when client may require use of urinal. |
| 2. Palpate for distended bladder. | Indicates if bladder is full and client needs to void. |
| 3. Assess client's cognitive and physical status. | Provides nurse with information about how much assistance is required to use urinal. |
| **Nursing Diagnosis** | |
| 1. Cluster data to reveal actual or potential nursing diagnoses: | |
| a. Toileting self-care deficit related to: ▪ Impaired ambulation. ▪ Bed rest. | Indicates client is unable to use toilet facilities. |
| b. Impaired skin integrity: related to urinary incontinence. | Urinal provided often enough will minimize incontinence. |
| c. Potential body image disturbance: related to use of urinal. | Men may have difficulty using urinal. |

| Steps | Rationale |
|---|---|
| **Planning** | |
| 1. Develop individualized goals for client based on nursing diagnoses: | |
| a. Promote normal patterns of urinary elimination. | Nurse offers urinal when client feels urge to void. |
| b. Skin remains intact without inflammation. | Perineal hygiene maintained. |
| c. Maintain body image. | Nurse maintains client's privacy. |
| 2. Prepare necessary equipment and supplies: | Ensures an organized procedure. |
| a. Urinal | |
| b. Supplies for diagnostic urine tests or specimen collection | |
| c. Graduated cylinder | Used for measuring output, if needed. |
| d. Disposable gloves | |
| 3. Obtain assistance from other nurses to position client, if necessary. | Men find it easier to void when standing. Unless contraindicated, one or more nurses may help client to stand at bedside. |
| 4. Explain procedure to client. | Promotes maximal cooperation. |
| **Implementation** | |
| 1. Wash hands and don gloves. | Reduces transmission of microorganisms. |
| 2. Provide privacy by closing bedside curtain or room door. | Promotes relaxation. |
| 3. Assist client into appropriate position: position on side, back, or sitting with head of bed elevated, or assist to standing position. | Men find it easiest to void and empty bladder while standing. |
| 4. If possible, client should hold urinal and position penis in urinal. If client needs assistance, position penis completely within urinal and hold urinal in place or assist client to hold urinal. | Penis is placed completely within urinal to avoid spillage of urine on bed linen. |
| 5. Once client has finished voiding, remove urinal, empty it, cleanse it, and return it to client for future use. | Avoids spilling and reduces odors. Prevents growth of microorganisms. |
| 6. Allow client to wash hands after voiding. | Reduces spread of microorganisms. |
| 7. Remove and dispose of gloves; wash hands. | Reduces spread of microorganisms. |
| **Evaluation** | |
| 1. Reassess client to determine ability to use urinal. | Promotes modification of nursing care plan to include more assistance or increased frequency to assist client to use urinal. |
| 2. Note amount and characteristics of urine. | Indicates abnormalities. |
| ***Expected outcome*** | |
| 1. Client is able to assist self with urinal. | Promotes self-care for toileting needs. |
| 2. Client remains continent. | |
| ***Unexpected outcomes*** | |
| 1. Client is incontinent. | Increases risk of skin breakdown. |
| 2. Client is unable to use urinal. | Increases risk of incontinence or urinary retention. |
| **Recording and Reporting** | |
| 1. Record and report client's ability to use urinal and characteristics of urinary output. | Communicates pertinent information to all health care personnel. |
| 2. If client is on I & O, include output data on flow sheet (Skill 29-1). | Monitors fluid balance. |
| **Follow-up Activities** | |
| 1. Incontinence: | |
| a. Offer urinal more frequently. | Reduces risk of incontinence. |
| b. Place urinal near client. | |
| c. Provide frequent skin care. | Maintains skin integrity. |
| 2. Inability to use urinal: | |
| a. Attempt placing client in standing position. | Promotes normal micturition. |
| b. Provide privacy. | |
| c. Provide relaxing environment. | |

### Special Considerations

- Nurse must consider client's social and cultural habits. Men are accustomed to sharing public urinals and privacy may not be major concern.
- Nurse must consider possibility of orthostatic hypotension occurring in clients who are immobilized or who have been recumbent for prolonged period.
- If client is allowed privacy while voiding, ensure that call-bell is within easy access so nurse can be summoned to empty and, if necessary, remove urinal.
- Aging process impairs micturition; elderly man may require urinal more frequently to avoid urinary incontinence.

### Home Care Considerations

- Assess client, primary care giver to determine ability and willingness to use urinal.
- Assess level of assistance required by client to determine if additional medical equipment is necessary (e.g., over-bed trapeze, bedside commode).

## *SKILL 29-3 Inserting a Straight or Indwelling Catheter*

Catheterization of the bladder involves introduction of a rubber or plastic tube through the urethra and into the bladder. The catheter provides for a continuous flow of urine in clients unable to control micturition or in those with obstruction to urine outflow. Because bladder catheterization carries the risk of the development of urinary tract infection, it is preferable to rely on other measures to promote bladder emptying.

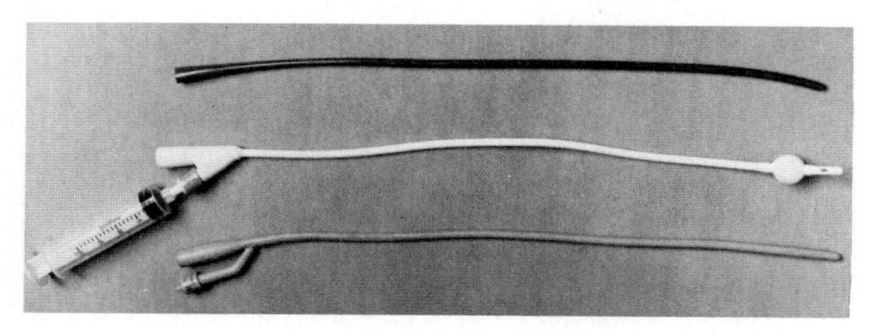

*Fig. 29-3*

Intermittent catheterization, in which a straight catheter is used, can be repeated as necessary. An indwelling or Foley catheter remains in place for an extended period. It may be necessary to change indwelling catheters periodically (Fig. 29-3). The nurse uses sterile asepsis to reduce the risk of bladder infections.

### Purposes

1. Obtain a sterile urine specimen.
2. Maintain patent urinary flow.
3. Relieve bladder distention.
4. Measure residual urine.
5. Maintain urinary continency for client with incompetent bladder.

## *Procedure 29-3*

| Steps | Rationale |
|---|---|
| **Assessment** | |
| 1. Assess status of client: | |
| a. When client last voided. | May indicate likelihood of bladder fullness. |
| b. Level of awareness or developmental stage. | Reveals client's ability to cooperate. |
| c. Mobility and physical limitations of client (nurse can request additional nursing personnel to assist with this procedure if necessary). | Affects way that nurse will position client. |
| d. Client's sex and age. | Determines catheter size to use. No. 8-10 Fr gauge is generally used for children. No. 14-16 Fr gauge for women and no. 12 Fr gauge may be considered for young females. No. 16-18 Fr gauge is used for male client unless larger size is ordered by physician. |
| e. Distended bladder. | Causes pain. Can indicate need to insert catheter if client unable to void independently. |
| f. Any pathologic condition that may impair passage of catheter (i.e., enlarged prostate gland). | Obstruction prevents passage of catheter through urethra into bladder. |
| g. Allergies. | Determines allergy to antiseptic, tape, rubber. |
| 2. Review client's medical record, including physician's order. | Determine purpose of inserting catheter: preparation for surgical procedure, urinary irrigations, collection of sterile urine specimen or measurement of residual urine. |

| Steps | Rationale |
|---|---|
| **Nursing Diagnosis** | |
| 1. Cluster data to reveal actual or potential nursing diagnoses: | |
| a. Urinary retention related to: ▪ Perineal edema. ▪ Enlarged prostrate. | Retention impairs normal removal of urinary wastes and can cause discomfort. |
| b. Potential impaired skin integrity: related to exposure to urine. | Forms of retention may cause stress incontinence. |
| c. Pain related to urinary retention. | Bladder distension is uncomfortable. |
| **Planning** | |
| 1. Develop individualized goals for client based on nursing diagnoses: | Promotes development of individualized care plan based on client needs. |
| a. Promote patent urinary drainage system. | Catheter allows free flow of urine with relief of bladder distention. |
| b. Maintain skin integrity. | Until client can void, catheter provides for urinary elimination. |
| c. Maintain physical comfort. | Patent catheter system keeps bladder empty. |
| 2. Prepare necessary equipment and supplies (Fig. 29-4): | Promotes organization of nurse's activities, thereby increasing efficiency. |
| a. Sterile gloves* (extra pair optional) b. Sterile drapes, one fenestrated c. Lubricant* d. Antiseptic cleansing solution* e. Cotton balls f. Forceps g. Prefilled syringe with normal saline to inflate balloon of indwelling catheter h. Catheter of correct size and type for procedure (i.e., intermittent or indwelling) | Sterile technique required with insertion of catheter into sterile bladder. |

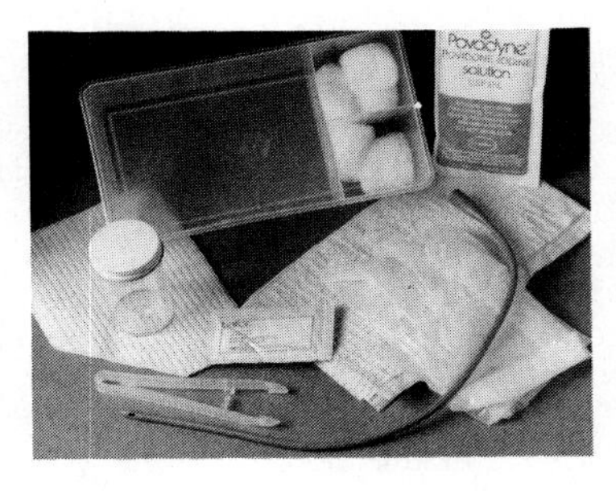


*Fig. 29-4*

| Steps | Rationale |
|---|---|
| i. Flashlight or gooseneck lamp | Helps in visualizing urinary meatus of female client. |
| j. Bath blanket | Promotes privacy by draping client. |
| k. Waterproof absorbent pad | Positioning under client prevents soiling of bed linens. |
| l. Trash receptacle | |
| m. Disposable gloves, basin with warm water, soap, face cloth, towel | Providing perineal care before introducing catheter helps to reduce risk of urinary tract infection. Provides opportunity to examine female's urethral meatus or to retract foreskin of uncircumcised male. |
| n. Sterile drainage tubing and collection bag, tape, safety pin, elastic band | If indwelling catheter will be inserted, tape, elastic band, and pin help secure position of catheter, thus preventing trauma to external urethral sphincter. |
| o. Receptacle or basin (usually bottom of catheterization tray) | Provides area for urine to drain when straight or indwelling catheter is used. |
| p. Specimen container | For sterile urine specimen to determine presence of bacteria. It is wise to obtain sterile urine specimen even if not specified on physician's order. It can document presence or absence of urinary bacteria at time of catheterization. |
| 3. Explain procedure to client. | Reduces anxiety and promotes cooperation throughout procedure. |
| 4. Arrange for extra nursing personnel to assist, if appropriate. | May be necessary to assist with positioning dependent client. Promotes use of correct body mechanics and client's safety. |
| **Implementation** | |
| 1. Wash hands. | Reduces transmission of microorganisms. |
| 2. Raise bed to appropriate working height. | Promotes use of proper body mechanics. |

*These items may be contained on the catheterization tray or may have to be added after the sterile field is established. May depend on whether disposable or nondisposable trays are used by the institution.

| Steps | Rationale |
|---|---|
| 3. Facing client, stand on left side of bed if right-handed (on right side if left-handed). Clear bedside table and arrange equipment. | Successful catheter insertion requires nurse to assume comfortable position with all equipment easily accessible. |
| 4. Raise side rail on opposite side of bed. | Promotes client safety. |
| 5. Close cubicle or room curtains. | Reduces client's embarrassment and aids in relaxation during procedure. |
| 6. Place waterproof pad under client. | Prevents soiling of bed linen. |
| 7. Position client: | Provides good visualization of perineal structures. |
| *Female client:* | |
| a. Assist to dorsal recumbent position (supine with knees flexed). Ask client to relax thighs so as to externally rotate them. | Legs may be supported with pillows to reduce muscle tension and promote comfort. |
| b. Position female client in side-lying (Sims') position with upper leg flexed at knee and hip if unable to be supine. If this position is used, nurse must take extra precautions to cover rectal area with drape during procedure to reduce chance of cross-contamination. | Alternate position if client cannot abduct leg at hip joint (e.g., arthritic joints). Also, this position may be more comfortable for client. Support client with pillows, if necessary, to maintain position. |
| *Male client:* | |
| a. Assist to supine position with thighs slightly abducted. | Prevents tensing of abdominal and pelvic muscles. |
| 8. Drape client. | Avoids unnecessary exposure of body parts and maintains client's comfort. |
| *Female client:* | |
| a. Drape with bath blanket. Place blanket diamond fashion over client, one corner at client's neck, side corners over each arm and side, last corner over perineum. | |
| *Male client:* | |
| a. Drape upper trunk with bath blanket and cover lower extremities with bed sheets, exposing only genitalia. | |
| 9. Using disposable gloves, wash perineal area with soap and water as needed; dry. | Reduces microorganisms near urethral meatus. |
| 10. If inserting indwelling catheter, open package containing drainage system. Place drainage bag over edge of bottom bed frame. Bring drainage tube up between side rail and mattress. | After catheter is inserted, nurse will immediately connect drainage system. Easy access prevents possible contamination. System is positioned to promote gravity drainage. |
| 11. Position lamp to illuminate perineal area. (When using flashlight, assistant holds it.) | Permits accurate identification and good visualization of urethral meatus. |
| 12. Open catheterization kit according to directions, keeping bottom of container sterile. | Prevents transmission of microorganisms from table or work area to sterile supplies. |
| 13. Don sterile gloves (Chapter 38). | Allows nurse to handle sterile supplies without contamination. |
| 14. Organize supplies on sterile field: open sterile package containing catheter; pour sterile package of antiseptic solution in correct compartment containing sterile cotton balls. Lubricate tip of the catheter; remove specimen container (lid should be loosely placed on top) and prefilled syringe from collection compartment of tray and set them aside on sterile field. | Maintains principles of surgical asepsis and organizes work area. |
| 15. Nurse may want to ensure that inflatable balloon of indwelling catheter is intact by inserting syringe tip through valve of intake lumen and injecting sterile fluid until balloon inflates. Then aspirate all fluid out of inflated lumen. | Checks integrity of balloon. Replace balloon that leaks or inflates improperly. |
| 16. Apply sterile drape: | Outer surface of drape covering hands remains sterile. Sterile drape against sterile gloves is sterile. |
| *Female client:* | |
| a. Allow top edge of drape to form cuff over both hands. Place drape down on bed between client's thighs. Slip cuffed edge just under buttocks, taking care not to touch contaminated surface with gloves. | |
| b. Pick up fenestrated sterile drape and allow it to unfold without touching an unsterile object. Apply drape over perineum, exposing labia and being sure not to touch contaminated surface. | Maintains stability of work surface. |
| *Male client:* | Maintains sterility of work surface. |
| a. Apply drape over thighs just below penis. Pick up fenestrated sterile drape, allow it to unfold, and drape it over penis with fenestrated slit resting over penis. | |
| 17. Place sterile tray and contents on sterile drape between thighs. | Provides easy access to supplies during catheter insertion. Maintains aseptic technique during procedure. |

| **Steps** | **Rationale** |
|---|---|
| 18. Determine that catheter tip is properly lubricated:<br>*Females:* 2.5 to 5 cm (1 to 2 in)<br>*Males:* 12.5 to 17.5 cm (5 to 7 in) | Allows easy insertion of catheter tip through urethral meatus. |
| 19. Cleanse urethral meatus:<br>*Female client:*<br>a. With nondominant hand carefully retract labia to fully expose urethral meatus. Maintain position of nondominant hand throughout procedure. | Full visualization of meatus is provided. Full retraction prevents contamination of meatus during cleansing. Closure of labia during cleansing requires that procedure be repeated because area has become contaminated. |
| b. With dominant hand pick up cotton ball with forceps and clean perineal area, wiping front to back from clitoris toward anus. Use new clean cotton ball for each wipe: along near labial fold, directly over meatus, and along far labial fold. | Cleansing reduces number of microorganisms at urethral meatus. Use of single cotton ball for each wipe prevents transfer of microorganisms. Preparation moves from area of least contamination to that of most contamination. Dominant hand remains sterile. |
| *Male client:*<br>a. If client is not circumcised, retract foreskin with nondominant hand. Grasp penis at shaft just below glans. Retract urethral meatus between thumb and forefinger. Maintain nondominant hand in this position throughout procedure. | Minimizes chance of erection occurring (if an erection develops, discontinue procedure). Accidental release of foreskin or dropping of penis during cleansing requires process to be repeated because area has become contaminated. |
| b. With dominant hand pick up cotton ball with forceps and clean penis. Move it in circular motion from meatus down to base of glans. Repeat cleansing two more times using clean cotton ball each time. | Reduces microorganisms at meatus and moves from areas of least to most contamination. Dominant hand remains sterile. |
| 20. Pick up catheter with gloved, dominant hand 7.5 to 10 cm (3 to 4 in) from catheter tip (Fig. 29-5). Hold end of catheter loosely coiled in palm of dominant hand (optional: may grasp catheter with forceps). Place distal end of catheter in urine tray receptacle. | Holding catheter near tip allows easier manipulation during insertion into meatus and prevents distal end from striking contaminated surface.<br>Collection of urine prevents soiling of bed linen and allows accurate measurement of urinary output. |
| 21. Insert catheter:<br>*Female client:*<br>a. Ask client to bear down gently as if to void and slowly insert catheter through meatus. | Relaxation of external sphincter aids in insertion of catheter. |
| b. Advance catheter approximately 5 to 7.5 cm (2 to 3 in) in adult, 2.5 cm (1 in) in child, or until urine flows out catheter's end. When urine appears, advance catheter another 5 cm (2 in). Do not force against resistance. | Female urethra is short. Appearance of urine indicates that catheter tip is in bladder or lower urethra. Advancement of catheter ensures bladder placement. If no urine is obtained in a few min, check if catheter has inadvertently been inserted into vagina. If so, leave catheter in place as landmark indicating where not to insert, and insert another. |
| c. Release labia and hold catheter securely with nondominant hand. | Bladder or sphincter contraction may cause accidental expulsion of catheter. |
| *Male client:*<br>a. Lift penis to position perpendicular to client's body and apply light traction (Fig. 29-6). | Straightens urethral canal to ease catheter insertion. |
| b. Ask client to bear down as if to void and slowly insert catheter through meatus. | Relaxation of external sphincter aids in insertion of catheter. |

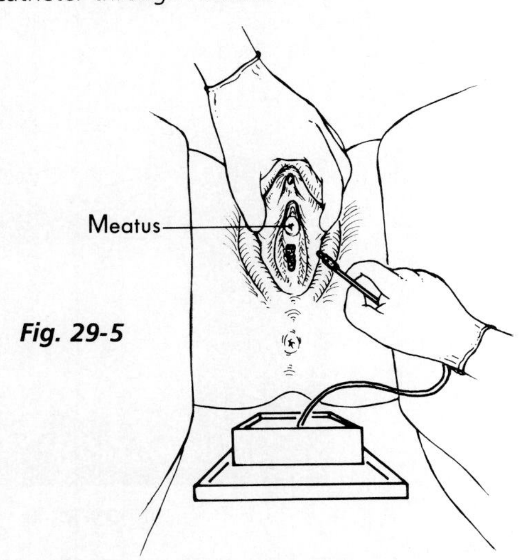

**Fig. 29-5**

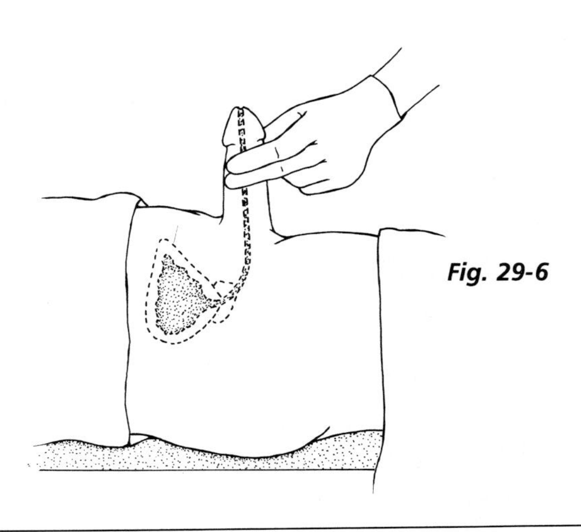
**Fig. 29-6**

| Steps | Rationale |
|---|---|
| c. Advance catheter 17.5 to 22.5 cm (7 to 9 in) in adult and 5 to 7.5 cm (2 to 3 in) in young child, or until urine flows out catheter's end. If resistance is felt, withdraw catheter; do not force it through urethra. When urine appears, advance catheter another 5 cm (2 in). | Adult male urethra is long. It is normal to meet resistance at the prostatic sphincter. When resistance is met, nurse should hold catheter firmly against sphincter without forcing catheter. After few seconds, sphincter relaxes and catheter is advanced. Appearance of urine indicates catheter tip in bladder or urethra. Further advancement of catheter ensures proper placement. |
| d. Lower penis and hold catheter securely in nondominant hand. Place end of catheter in urine tray receptacle. | Catheter may be accidentally expelled by bladder or urethral contraction. Collection of urine prevents soiling and provides output measurement. |
| 22. Collect urine specimen as needed: Fill specimen cup or jar to desired level (20 to 30 ml) by holding end of catheter in dominant hand over cup. With dominant hand, pinch catheter to stop urine flow temporarily. Release catheter to allow remaining urine in bladder to drain into collection tray. Cover specimen cup and set aside for labeling. | Allows sterile specimen to be obtained for culture analysis. |
| 23. Allow bladder to empty fully (about 750 to 1000 ml) unless institution policy restricts maximal volume of urine to drain with each catheterization. | Retained urine may serve as reservoir for growth of microorganisms. |
| 24. Remove straight, single-use catheter:<br>a. Withdraw catheter slowly but smoothly until removed. | Minimizes discomfort to client. |
| 25. Inflate balloon of indwelling catheter:<br>a. While holding catheter with thumb and little finger of nondominant hand at meatus, take end of catheter and place it between first two fingers of nondominant hand. | Catheter should be anchored while syringe is manipulated. |
| b. With free, dominant hand, attach syringe to injection port at end of catheter. | Port connects to lumen leading to inflatable balloon. |
| c. Slowly inject total amount of solution. If client complains of sudden pain, aspirate back solution and advance catheter farther. | Balloon within bladder is inflated. If balloon is malpositioned in urethra, pain will occur during inflation. |
| d. After inflating balloon fully, release catheter with nondominant hand and pull gently to feel resistance (Fig. 29-7). | Inflation of balloon anchors catheter tip in place above bladder outlet to prevent removal of catheter. |
| 26. Attach end of catheter to collecting tube of drainage system (Fig. 29-8). Drainage bag must be below level of bladder. | Establishes closed system for urine drainage. |
| 27. Tape catheter:<br>*Female client:*<br>a. Tape catheter tubing to inner thigh with strip of nonallergenic tape. Allow for slack so movement of thigh does not create tension on catheter. | Anchoring of catheter minimizes trauma to urethra and meatus during movement. Nonallergenic tape prevents skin breakdown. |
| *Male client:*<br>a. Tape catheter tubing to top of thigh or lower abdomen (with penis directed toward chest). Allow slack in catheter so movement does not create tension on catheter. | Anchoring catheter to lower abdomen is thought to reduce pressure on urethra at junction of penis and scrotum, thus reducing possibility of tissue necrosis in this area. |
| 28. Be sure there are no obstructions or kinks in tubing. Place excess coil of tubing on bed and fasten it to bottom sheet with clip from drainage set or with rubber band and safety pin. | Patent tubing allows free drainage of urine by gravity and prevents backflow of urine into bladder. |

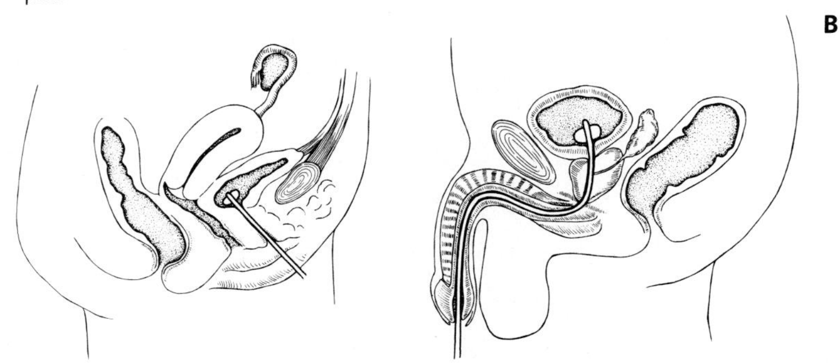


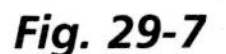

*Fig. 29-7*

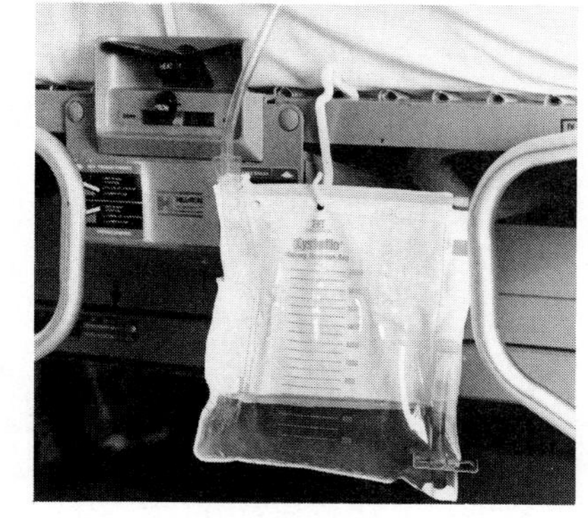

*Fig. 29-8*

| Steps | Rationale |
|---|---|
| 29. Remove gloves and dispose of equipment, drapes, urine in proper receptacles. | Reduces transmission of microorganisms. |
| 30. Assist client to comfortable position. Wash and dry perineal area as needed. | Maintains comfort and security. |
| 31. Instruct client on ways to lie in bed with catheter: side-lying facing drainage system with catheter and tubing draped over thigh; side-lying facing away from system, catheter and tubing extending between legs. | Urine should drain freely without obstruction. Placing catheter under extremities can result in obstruction as from compression of tubing from client's weight. When client is on one side facing away from system, catheter should not be placed over upper thigh; this forces urine to drain uphill. |
| 32. Caution client against pulling on catheter. | Reduces trauma to urethral meatus. |
| 33. Wash hands. | Reduces spread of microorganisms. |

## Evaluation

| | |
|---|---|
| 1. Palpate bladder and ask if client remains uncomfortable. | Determines if distention is relieved. |
| 2. Observe character and amount of urine in drainage system. | Determines if urine is flowing adequately. |
| 3. Determine that there is no urine leaking from catheter or tubing connections. | Prevents injury to client's skin. |

### *Expected outcomes*

| | |
|---|---|
| 1. Bladder distention and related discomfort are relieved. | Removal of urine from bladder relieves sensation of fullness and urge to void. |
| 2. Urine is present in drainage tray or urinary collection bag. | Documents presence of catheter in bladder. |

### *Unexpected outcomes*

| | |
|---|---|
| 1. No urine is present. *Female:* Catheter may be in vaginal opening. *Male:* Catheter may not be advanced far enough. | Absence of urine usually indicates that catheter is not advanced to the bladder or client has oliguria secondary to renal disease, shock, decreased cardiac output. |
| 2. Catheter in male client cannot be advanced. | May indicate prostate hypertrophy. |
| 3. Bladder distention is present. | Catheter is not in place. |
| 4. Leakage of urine from catheter. | May indicate need to inflate balloon or insert a larger catheter. |

## Recording and Reporting

| | |
|---|---|
| 1. Report and record: type and size of catheter inserted, amount of fluid used to inflate balloon, characteristics of urine, amount of urine. | Communicates pertinent information to all members of health care team. |

## Follow-up Activities

| | |
|---|---|
| 1. No urine: reposition or advance catheter. | Advances catheter tip to bladder. |
| 2. Unable to advance catheter in client: seek assistance from physician. | Forcibly advancing catheter in male client can cause urethral tract damage. |

## Special Considerations

- Female client unable to abduct hip joint can be positioned on side with upper leg flexed at hip and knee.
- When client is incontinent, nurse should try alternate measures such as decreasing night-time fluids or offering urinal or bedpan more frequently. Inserting catheter carries risk for urinary tract infections.
- If nondisposable catheter tray is used it may have to be assembled in clean utility room and transported to bedside. Ensure that sterile field is maintained to reduce risk of urinary tract infection.
- When catheterizing male client, erection may develop. Discontinue procedure momentarily.
- Check institution policy before beginning; some agencies restrict maximal amount of urine that can be drained off at one time. This amount may vary from 800 to 1000 ml. This is done to avoid hypotension resulting from sudden release of pressure against pelvic floor blood vessels under bladder.
- Women who are newly postpartum or who have had gynecologic surgery and clients immediately postoperative for bladder surgery are at risk for bladder distention.
- If catheter is definitely in bladder and no urine is produced, absence of urine should immediately be reported to physician.

## Teaching Considerations

- For infant or child, nurse will need to explain procedures to parent.
- Explain to client that burning sensation may be experienced during catheter insertion.
- Caution client against lying on tubing.

# SKILL 29-4 Performing Routine Catheter Care

Clients with indwelling catheters have specific perineal hygiene needs to reduce the risk of urinary tract infection. Any secretions or encrustations at the catheter insertion site must be completely removed. In some institutions, iodophor solutions such as povidone-iodine are used for cleansing and iodophor ointments are applied at the urethral meatus. The use of powders or lotions on the perineum is contraindicated because of the risk of growth of microorganisms, which may ascend the urinary tract.

## Purposes

1. Reduce the risk of infection.
2. Inspect the catheter insertion site for drainage or encrustations.

## Procedure 29-4

| Steps | Rationale |
|---|---|
| **Assessment** | |
| 1. Determine how long catheter has been in place. Check hospital policy to determine how often indwelling catheter must be changed. | Catheters in place for 3 or more days are more likely to cause urethral irritation and build-up of encrustations. |
| 2. Observe any discharge or encrustation around urethral meatus. | Indicates inflammatory process; encrustation could be from diet that is too alkaline. |
| 3. Assess for complaints of pain or discomfort; determine location and type of pain client is experiencing. | Indicates potential urinary tract infection. |
| 4. Monitor client's temperature. | Possible symptom of urinary tract infection. |
| 5. Determine client's fluid intake. | Lack of fluid intake reduces natural flushing of urinary system and increases chance of bacterial growth. |
| **Nursing Diagnosis** | |
| 1. Cluster data to reveal actual or potential nursing diagnoses: | |
| a. Pain: related to presence of indwelling catheter. | Catheter causes local urethral irritation. |
| b. Fluid volume deficit: related to decreased fluid intake. | Predisposes client to risk of urinary infection and dehydration. |
| c. Potential for infection: related to presence of indwelling catheter. | Catheter increases risk of bacteria ascending into urinary tract. |
| **Planning** | |
| 1. Develop individualized goals for client based on nursing diagnoses: | |
| a. Maintain and promote comfort. | Cleansing relieves local discomfort. |
| b. Increase fluid intake. | Helps to lower risk of infection. |
| c. Reduce risk of urinary tract infection. | Cleansing removes microorganisms that can ascend urethra. |
| 2. Prepare necessary equipment and supplies: | |
| a. Soap and wash cloth | To cleanse perineum before catheter care. |
| b. Antiinfective solution | Decreases bacteria at urethral meatus. Type of solution varies with agency policy. |
| c. Antibiotic ointment (e.g., neomycin, povidone-iodine) | Topical antibiotic ointment decreases bacterial encrustations at urethral meatus. |
| d. Sterile swabs | Used to cleanse urethra meatus and apply ointment. |
| e. Forceps | |
| f. Tape | Tape securing catheter to client may have become dislodged or contaminated with fecal material. |
| g. Measurement container | Used if urine collection bag will be emptied. |
| h. Sterile gloves | |
| i. Sterile drape | |
| 3. Explain procedure to client. | Reduces anxiety and promotes cooperation throughout procedure. |

| Steps | Rationale |
|---|---|
| **Implementation** | |
| 1. Wash hands. | Reduces transmission of microorganisms. |
| 2. Close curtains around bed or close door to room. | Reduces embarrassment to client, thus promoting relaxation. |
| 3. Raise bed to appropriate working height. Raise side rails on opposite side of bed. | Promotes use of proper body mechanics and client safety. |
| 4. Organize equipment for perineal care. | Increases efficiency of procedure. |
| 5. Position client correctly and cover with bath blanket, exposing only perineal area. | Reduces client's embarrassment. |
| a. Female in dorsal recumbent position. | |
| b. Male in supine position. | Ensures easy access to perineal tissues. |
| 6. Place waterproof pad under client. | Protects bed linen from soiling. |
| 7. Drape bath blanket on bed clothes so that only perineal area is exposed. | Prevents unnecessary exposure of body parts. |
| 8. Open sterile catheter care kit using sterile aseptic technique. | Maintains organized, sterile work area. |
| 9. Put on sterile gloves (see Chapter 43). | Allows nurse to handle sterile supplies without contamination. |
| 10. Apply sterile drapes over client's perineum. | Outer surface of drape provides a sterile work area. |
| 11. Pour antiseptic solution on cotton balls or swabs. Apply antiseptic ointment to cotton ball (check client for allergies to antiseptic). | Prepares solutions for easy application, minimizing risk of contamination. |
| 12. With nondominant hand: | |
| a. Gently retract labia of female client to fully expose urethral meatus and catheter insertion site; maintain position of hand throughout procedure. | Provides full visualization of urethral meatus. Full retraction of tissues prevents contamination of meatus during cleansing. Accidental closure of labia or dropping of penis during cleansing requires process to be repeated. |
| b. Retract foreskin if client not circumsized, and hold penis at shaft just below glans, maintain position of hand throughout procedure. | |
| 13. Assess urethral meatus and surrounding tissues for inflammation, swelling, discharge. Note amount, color, odor, consistency of discharge. Ask client if burning or discomfort is felt. | Determines local infection and status of hygiene. |
| 14. Cleanse perineal tissues: | Reduces microorganisms at the urethral meatus. Use of single cotton ball for each wipe prevents transfer of microorganisms. Cleansing moves from area of least to most contamination. Dominate hand remains sterile. |
| *Female client:* | |
| a. Use a separate cotton ball and forceps to cleanse each labium majora, moving down toward the anus. Repeat process to cleanse labia minora, then cleanse around the urethral meatus, moving down catheter; be sure to cleanse each side. | |
| *Male client:* | |
| a. While spreading urethral meatus, cleanse around the catheter first, then use clean cotton ball to wipe in circular motion around meatus and glans. | |
| 15. Reassess urethral meatus for discharge. | Determines if cleansing is complete. |
| 16. Take new cotton ball and wipe in circular motion along length of catheter for about 10 cm (4 in). | Reduces presence of secretions or drainage on outside catheter surface. |
| 17. Apply antiseptic ointment at urethral meatus and along 2.5 cm (1 in) of catheter. | Further reduces growth of microorganisms at insertion site. |
| 18. Replace adhesive tape anchoring catheter to client as necessary. Remove adhesive tape residue from skin. | Secures catheter, thus reducing risk of catheter being pulled on and exposing portion that was in urethra. Also prevents drag on catheter and avoids pressure from balloon on bladder floor. |
| 19. Replace urinary tubing and collection bag, if necessary, adhering to principles of surgical asepsis. | Urinary tubing and collection bag should be changed if there are signs of leakage, odor, sediment buildup; usually changed at least once each week. |
| 20. Check drainage tubing to ensure: | |
| a. No tubing loops hang below level of bladder. | Prevents pooling of urine and reflux of urine into bladder. |
| b. Tube is coiled and secured onto bed linen. | Prevents looping of tubing and subsequent pooling of urine. |
| c. Tube is not kinked or clamped. | Prevents stasis of urine in bladder. Also ensures client is not lying on tubing, causing pressure on skin and increasing risk of pressure sore. |
| 21. Collection bag should be emptied as necessary but at least q8h. | Urine in collection bag is excellent medium for growth of microorganisms. |

| Steps | Rationale |
|---|---|
| 22. Assist client to safe, comfortable position. | Promotes safety and comfort. |
| 23. Dispose of contaminated gloves and supplies and wash hands. | Reduces transmission of microorganisms. |
| **Evaluation** | |
| 1. Inspect condition of urethra. | Determines if area is cleansed properly. |
| 2. Note character of urine. | Helps to indicate if infection is present. |
| 3. Assess client's temperature. | Helps to indicate if infection is present. |
| ***Expected outcomes*** | |
| 1. Urethral meatus is free of secretions and encrustations. | Indicates absence of irritation. |
| 2. Urine is clear and volume is sufficient. | Indicates absence of urinary tract infection and adequate output. |
| 3. Client is afebrile. | Indicates absence of infection. |
| ***Unexpected outcomes*** | |
| 1. Odor is present. | Indicates bacterial process. |
| 2. Urethral meatus is reddened and swollen. | Indicates irritation from catheter or tension from drainage bag. |
| 3. Client has fever. | Source of fever can be urinary infection. |
| **Recording and Reporting** | |
| 1. Record in nurses' notes when catheter care was given, assessment of urethral meatus, character of urine. | Documents care delivered and assessment factors to support presence or absence of inflammatory process or external irritation. |
| 2. Report to nursing staff procedure and presence or absence of unexpected outcomes. | May require further therapy. |
| **Follow-up Activities** | |
| 1. Odor: | |
| a. Investigate for infection: obtain sterile urine specimen, observe for fever, increase fluid intake. | Sterile collection of urine specimen and fever assist to document urinary bacteria. Increasing fluid intake assists in flushing kidney of bacteria. |
| 2. Reddened, swollen urethral meatus: | |
| a. Increase frequency of catheter care. | Reduces external irritation from catheter. |
| b. Observe for incorrect taping of catheter. | |
| c. Instruct client not to pull on catheter tubing. | |

## Special Consideration

- Silastic catheters may be less irritating than latex catheters and can be left in place longer.
- Instruct client to hold drainage bag below level of catheter when ambulating.

## Teaching Considerations

- Unless contraindicated, clients with catheter should drink at least 2000 ml of fluid per day to promote continuous flushing of lumen catheter.

## Home Care Consideration

- Assess client, primary care giver for ability and motivation to participate in routine catheter care.

# SKILL 29-5 Obtaining Catheterized Specimens for Residual Urine

Residual urine is the volume of urine in the bladder after a normal voiding. Residual urines are obtained in clients suspected of retaining urine. Urinary retention is the inability of the bladder to fully empty.

Clients at risk for large residual volumes include those receiving bladder training exercises, such as those with spinal cord injuries or who have suffered a cerebral vascular accident, or those who have had bladder surgery.

### Purposes

1. Measure residual urine.
2. Document decrease in quantity of residual urine.

## Procedure 29-5

| Steps | Rationale |
|---|---|
| **Assessment** | |
| 1. Review prior I & O record. | Identifies usual amount of urine voided during each voiding. |
| 2. Determine if client experiences pain or discomfort when voiding. | Pain may be associated with bladder spasms. |
| 3. Review physician's order to determine how often residual urine must be checked. | Order must be obtained from physician before nurse can catheterize client. Physician's order will indicate when this procedure is no longer necessary (e.g., check residual urine bid until amount obtained is 60 ml or less). |
| **Nursing Diagnosis** | |
| 1. Cluster data to reveal actual or potential nursing diagnoses: | |
| a. Urinary retention: related to bladder spasms. | Retained urine indicates client is unable to empty bladder. |
| b. Potential for infection related to: | |
| ▪ Catheterization procedure. | Repeated catheterizations increase risk of infection. |
| ▪ Incomplete bladder emptying. | Stasis of urine provides medium for bacterial growth. |
| **Planning** | |
| 1. Develop individualized goals for client based on nursing diagnoses: | |
| a. Promote bladder emptying. | Reducing residual volume improves ability to contract and empty bladder. |
| b. Reduce risk of infection. | Urinary retention promotes infection. Procedure requires use of asepsis. |
| 2. Consider time factor involved. | Client must be catheterized immediately after voiding to obtain accurate information about amount of urine remaining in bladder. |
| 3. Assemble equipment and supplies (Skill 29-3). | Increases efficiency for performing procedure. |
| 4. Explain procedure to client. | Helps to minimize anxiety. |
| **Implementation** | |
| 1. Ask client to void completely and measure volume of urine. | Determines how much client is able to void compared to how much urine remains in bladder after catheterization. |
| 2. Wash hands. | Reduces transmission of infection. |
| 3. Proceed as for inserting straight intermittent catheter (Skill 29-3, Implementation). | Insertion of straight catheter drains residual urine. |
| 4. Accurately measure urine obtained. | Allows amount retained to be compared to amount voided. |
| **Evaluation** | |
| 1. Compare amount of urine voided and amount obtained on catheterization. | Difference will indicate whether procedure will be repeated. Client who retains more urine than the amount voided has reduced bladder function. |

| Steps | Rationale |
|---|---|
| ***Expected outcomes*** | |
| 1. Successive catheterizations result in decreasing amount of residual urine. | Client gains improved bladder control. |
| 2. Urinary tract remains free of infection. | Removal of retained urine reduces media for bacterial growth. |
| ***Unexpected outcomes*** | |
| 1. Catheterization results in large and increasing volume of urine. | Indicates inadequate bladder emptying. |
| 2. Urinary incontinence of small amount of urine occurs. | Results from overflow incontinence from bladder distention. |
| 3. Client has signs and symptoms associated with bladder infection. | Retained urine contains bacterial growth. |
| **Recording and Reporting** | |
| 1. Report and record amount of urine voided, amount obtained from catheterization, client's response. | Communicates information to all members of health care team, indicating progress of therapy. |
| **Follow-up Activities** | |
| 1. Instruct client on Credé technique for emptying bladder. | Manual compression of bladder can facilitate emptying. |
| 2. Notify physician about signs and symptoms of urinary tract infection. | Physician's order is needed to begin treatment of urinary tract infections. |

### Special Considerations

- Straight catheters are used for residuals; however, physician may order an indwelling Foley catheter insertion if residuals exceed certain volume. If physician's order is written in such manner, nurse may elect to perform residual catheterization with Foley catheter.

### Teaching Considerations

- Teach client to obtain I & O measurements (Skill 29-1).
- Clients need to be informed about symptoms of urinary tract infection: frequency with small amount of voiding, urgency, hesitancy and burning. Infections can increase bladder spasms and lead to worsening of retention.

# *SKILL 29-6 Teaching Self-Catheterization*

Self-catheterization enables the client who no longer has voluntary bladder control to independently maintain urinary continence. Self-catheterization can be taught to clients with paraplegia, hemiplegia, or other illnesses that limit voluntary bladder control. When self-catheterization is included in the care plan, the nurse must also teach a family member or significant other to complete the procedure. It is necessary for another person to know the technique in case the client becomes incapacitated and is unable to empty the bladder.

Self-catheterization is an important component of a client's rehabilitation and return to maximal level of functioning. Therefore instruction is integrated into the rehabilitation program at an early stage and not merely tacked onto the end of the hospital stay.

Some clients maintain bladder continence with self-catheterization using medical asepsis without recurrent urinary tract infections. Other clients must use surgical asepsis because of susceptibility to recurrent urinary tract infections. Deciding to use clean (medical asepsis) versus sterile (surgical asepsis) technique is individualized.

Self-catheterization is taught to clients requiring intermittent straight catheterization and those with indwelling Foley catheters. However, the greater proportion of clients using this technique require intermittent catheterization.

### Purposes

1. Promote urinary continency.
2. Maximize the level of independent functioning.

## Procedure 29-6

| Steps | Rationale |
|---|---|
| **Assessment** | |
| 1. Assess status of client to determine: (1) Learning needs. What does client need to know about self-catheterization? (2) Readiness to learn. Does client want to learn to perform this skill? What does client already know about procedure? (3) Ability to learn. Consider developmental stage, cognitive status, physical attributes. (4) Learning environment. Choose setting where nurse can help client to focus on learning task. | Aids in developing appropriate teaching strategy and selecting proper environment for teaching sessions. It is important to include client and family member in this process. |
| **Nursing Diagnosis** | |
| 1. Cluster data to reveal client's training capabilities and needs and identify appropriate nursing diagnoses: | |
| a. Impaired physical mobility related to: ▪ Pain. ▪ Joint immobility or muscular weakness. | May impair client's ability to manipulate catheter, requiring family member's assistance. |
| b. Knowledge deficit of self-catheterization: related to inexperience. | Client will require careful instruction and opportunity to practice skill. |
| **Planning** | |
| 1. Identify learning objectives for teaching plan (e.g., client will be able to correctly identify urethral meatus, discuss importance of washing hands before beginning procedure and using aseptic technique; correctly identify equipment and supplies used for procedure, position self correctly, cleanse perineal area correctly before insertion of catheter, state how far catheter should be inserted, demonstrate inserting catheter into bladder, demonstrate caring for equipment after it is used). | Based on identified learner needs. Objectives relate to psychomotor, cognitive, affective domain, are stated in behavioral terms, serve as bases to measure learning. Nurse should collaborate with client when developing objectives. |
| 2. Select environment and time suitable to teach procedure. Consider privacy, comfort status, mental alertness, how long or much to include with each session. | Pain and fatigue reduces learner's attention. Analgesics reduce alertness. Consider client's attention span; choose time of day when client is rested. |
| 3. Consider variety of teaching aids: diagrams, slides, articles, models, samples of self-catheterization kits available commercially, individual with similar physical disability. | Sometimes clients learn more quickly with peer (person who has experienced similar problems). Variety of teaching aids ensures using teaching technique beneficial to client. |
| 4. Determine when client will be discharged from health care facility. | Determine time allowed to teach skill. Clients should learn skill early in hospital stay. |
| **Implementation** | |
| 1. Carry out individualized plan, allowing client to return demonstrations each time: | |
| a. Reduction of microorganisms: ▪ Teach theory and importance of hand washing. Demonstrate how to wash hands thoroughly (medical asepsis). ▪ Explain and demonstrate opening catheterization package and manipulation of supplies. (Read directions on label.) ▪ Explain and demonstrate technique for handling catheter. ▪ Explain and demonstrate preparation of urethral meatus. | Starting with simple concepts and working toward more complex ones facilitates learning. Return demonstration actively involves client in performing procedure on self, or client may need to start with model and work up to performing procedure on self with nurse's supervision. |
| b. Insertion of catheter into bladder: ▪ Explain suitable position for client to assume. ▪ Explain and demonstrate insertion of catheter: how to separate labia or hold penis, cleansing urethra, distance to insert catheter. Explain normal sensations client will feel. | Practicing psychomotor skills after cognitive learning allows client to apply and practice principles learned. |

| Steps | Rationale |
|---|---|
| c. Care of equipment:<br>▪ Discuss and demonstrate principles of aseptic technique. | Proper care of equipment ensures maintenance of aseptic technique. |

## Evaluation

| Steps | Rationale |
|---|---|
| 1. Have client independently demonstrate entire procedure. | Feedback on independent demonstration of psychomotor skill is means of evaluating ability. |
| 2. Ask client questions about procedures related to self-catheterization (short quiz could be developed). | Evaluates client's theoretical knowledge. |

### *Expected outcomes*

| Steps | Rationale |
|---|---|
| 1. Client successfully completes self-catheterization. | Indicates appropriate cognitive and psychomotor learning skills. |
| 2. No signs of urinary tract infection are present (clear urine, absence of foul odor, no pain). | Indicates absence of excessive bacteria in urinary tract. |

### *Unexpected outcomes*

| Steps | Rationale |
|---|---|
| 1. Client is unable to complete procedure. | Lack of successful completion of procedure can be due to cognitive or psychomotor learning deficit or personal feelings about self-catheterization. |
| 2. Signs of urinary tract infection are present (fever; cloudy, foul-smelling urine; pain). | Associated with urinary bacteria. Client may be incorrectly cleansing equipment. |

## Recording and Reporting

| Steps | Rationale |
|---|---|
| 1. Document teaching content and learner's progress in client's record. | Documents client's learning for other health care workers. |

## Follow-up Activities

| Steps | Rationale |
|---|---|
| 1. Reinforce teaching. | Encourages client and family to perform catheterization procedure. |
| 2. Teach family members catheterization technique. | |
| 3. Contact physician for antibiotic for urinary tract infection. | |

## Special Considerations

- Be prepared for setbacks. Client may have "bad day" so day's instruction may have to be postponed.
- Positioning may depend on physical ability. Paraplegics frequently assume sitting position.
- Clients with spinal cord injuries may be unable to perceive pain associated with urinary tract infections.

## Teaching Considerations

- Client with hearing problem may respond best to visual material.
- Female client may need mirror to visualize perineal area.
- Video tape demonstrations can be used as long as teacher is available for feedback or discussion. Include family member's participation if appropriate. Implement individualized plan with step-by-step skill progression. Client gradually performs independent self-catheterization.
- Disposable supplies are preferred. If it is necessary to reuse catheters, client should learn boiling technique. (Boil rubber catheter 20 min and wrap in clean cloth.)
- Use learning objectives related to psychomotor skill as bases for evaluating client's performance.
- Use learning objectives related to cognitive ability as criteria for evaluating responses.
- Clients should be instructed to switch from clean to sterile catheter technique when signs of urinary tract infection occur.

# SKILL 29-7 Performing Catheter Irrigation

Catheter irrigations are done on an intermittent basis to maintain catheter patency. There are two types of irrigation systems: closed bladder irrigation systems and disposable irrigation trays. A closed bladder irrigation system provides intermittent or continuous irrigation of the system without disrupting the sterile alignment of the catheter and drainage system (Fig. 29-9). The closed system is used most frequently in clients who have had genitourinary surgery. These clients are at risk for small blood clots and mucous fragments occluding the Foley catheter; they are also at risk for urinary tract infections. The closed bladder irrigation system allows for bladder irrigation to maintain catheter patency without disrupting the system and increasing the risk of entry of bacteria into the urinary tract.

The disposable irrigation system is also used to maintain catheter patency. However, this system is used when bladder irrigations are required less frequently (such as every 8 hr) and there are no blood clots or large mucous shreds in the urinary drainage. This type of irrigation requires the nurse to aseptically break the closed drainage system and maintain surgical asepsis throughout the procedure.

Both systems can be used to irrigate the bladder with a medication to treat an infection or local bladder irritation.

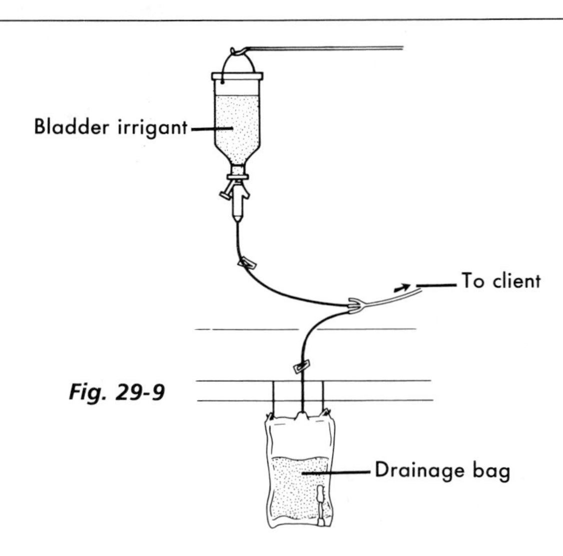

*Fig. 29-9*

If a medication is used, the nurse must verify the order as she would with any other medication (Unit VI).

### Purposes

1. Maintain patency of the urethral catheter.
2. Deliver medication to the bladder to treat an infection or irritation.

## *Procedure 29-7*

| Steps | Rationale |
|---|---|
| **Assessment** | |
| 1. Check client's record to determine: | |
| a. Purpose of closed bladder irrigation. | Allows nurse to anticipate observations to make (e.g., blood or mucus in urine). |
| b. Physician's order. | Order required to initiate therapy. |
| c. Type of irrigating solution to be used. | Ensures that right medication or solution will be administered. |
| d. If client is to receive continuous or intermittent flow into bladder. | Allows nurse to select proper equipment. In continuous irrigation, clamp regulates slow, steady flow into bladder. Because outflow should correspond to regulated irrigation drip, patency of catheter must be checked frequently to prevent distention of bladder. For intermittent irrigation, flow from irrigating solution is clamped for specified time then opened, and designated amount of irrigating solution is allowed to flush into bladder. |
| e. Frequency of irrigation, (such as q8h). | Requires close observation of catheter patency between irrigations. |
| f. Type of catheter used: | |
| ▪ Triple lumen (one lumen to inflate balloon, one to instill irrigation solution, and one to allow outflow of urine) (Fig. 29-9). | Indicates if it is necessary to break system for irrigation. |
| ▪ Double lumen (one lumen to inflate balloon, one to allow outflow of urine). | |
| 2. Assess the following: | |
| a. Color of urine and presence of mucus or sediment. | Determines if client is bleeding or sloughing tissue. |

| Steps | Rationale |
|---|---|
| b. Patency of drainage tubing. | Ensures drainage tubing is not kinked, clamped off incorrectly, or looped below bladder level. |
| c. Closed system: | |
| ▪ Note if fluid entering bladder and fluid draining from bladder are in appropriate proportions. | Determines if system is obstructed by blood clots. One would expect more output than fluid instilled because of urine production. |
| ▪ Note amount of fluid remaining in existing irrigating solution container. | Irrigating solution infuses into bladder by principles of gravity. |
| ▪ Check irrigation solution tubing to ensure it has no kinks and is opened or clamped according to physician's order. | Maintains patency of irrigation system. |
| 3. Review I & O record. | Determines baseline for prior output measures. All clients with continuous bladder irrigations should have I & O measurements (Skill 29-1). |

## Nursing Diagnosis

| Steps | Rationale |
|---|---|
| 1. Cluster data to reveal actual or potential nursing diagnoses: | |
| a. Potential for infection: related to catheter. | Presence of catheter and need to open system increases risk of infection. |
| b. Pain related to: | |
| ▪ Presence of catheter or bladder surgery. | Surgery involving bladder and urethral structures results in discomfort. |
| ▪ Urinary retention. | Clots forming in postoperative phase can obstruct outflow drainage. |

## Planning

| Steps | Rationale |
|---|---|
| 1. Develop individualized goals of care for client based on nursing diagnoses: | |
| a. Maintain patent, free-flowing urinary drainage system. | Prevents urine retention that can cause discomfort. |
| b. Minimize risk of infection. | Aseptic technique is used throughout procedure. |
| c. Minimize discomfort. | Retention and bladder spasms are painful. |
| 2. Collect necessary equipment and supplies: | Promotes organization and efficiency. |
| a. Closed intermittent method: | |
| ▪ Sterile irrigating solution | Sterile irrigating solution is not considered sterile 24 hr after opening. |
| ▪ Sterile graduated cup | |
| ▪ Sterile 30 to 50 ml syringe | Used to instill irrigant into catheter. |
| ▪ Sterile 19- to 22-gauge, 1 in needle | |
| ▪ Antiseptic swab | |
| ▪ Screw clamp | Used to temporarily occlude catheter as irrigant is instilled. |
| ▪ Bath blanket | |
| b. Closed continuous method: | |
| ▪ Sterile irrigating solution, correct bag or solution | |
| ▪ Irrigation tubing with clamp (with or without **Y** connector) | Clamp regulates irrigation flow rate. **Y**-connector allows IV bags to be connected to tubing. |
| ▪ Metric container | Used to measure urine output in drainage bag. |
| ▪ IV pole | |
| ▪ Antiseptic swab | |
| ▪ **Y** connector (optional) | Used to connect irrigation tubing to double-lumen catheter. |
| ▪ Bath blanket | |
| c. Open intermittent method: | |
| ▪ Disposable, sterile irrigation tray and set | |
| ▪ Bulb syringe or 60 ml, piston-type syringe | Provides necessary force to maintain patency. |
| ▪ Sterile collection basin | |
| ▪ Waterproof drape | |
| ▪ Sterile solution container | |
| ▪ Antiseptic swabs | |
| ▪ Sterile gloves | |
| ▪ Ordered irrigating solution at room temperature | Cold solution may cause bladder spasm. |
| ▪ Tape | |
| ▪ Bath blanket | |
| 3. Explain procedure to client. | Helps client to relax and promotes cooperation. |

## Implementation

| Steps | Rationale |
|---|---|
| 1. Wash hands. | Reduces transmission of microorganisms. |

| **Steps** | **Rationale** |
|---|---|
| 2. Provide privacy: pull curtains around bed, fold back covers so catheter is exposed at junction where it connects to drainage tubing. Cover client's chest with bath blanket. | Promotes client's self-esteem; shows respect for client while exposing area nurse must see. |
| 3. Position client in dorsal, recumbent supine position and remove tape anchoring catheter to client. Be careful not to pull on catheter so portion inside urethra is not exposed. | Allows for client comfort; removing tape enables nurse to manipulate catheter. |
| 4. Assess lower abdomen for signs of bladder distention. | Detects if catheter or closed irrigating system is malfunctioning, blocking urinary drainage. |
| 5. **Closed intermittent irrigation:** | |
| a. Prepare prescribed sterile irrigating solution in sterile graduated cup. | |
| b. Draw sterile solution into syringe using aseptic technique. | Ensures sterility of irrigating fluid. |
| c. Clamp indwelling retention catheter below soft injection port. | Occlusion of catheter will provide resistance against which irrigant can be forcefully instilled into catheter. |
| d. Cleanse catheter injection port with antiseptic swab (same port used for specimen collections). | Reduces transmission of infection. |
| e. Insert needle of syringe through port at 30-degree angle. | Ensures needle tip enters lumen of catheter. |
| f. Slowly inject fluid into catheter and bladder. | Slow, continuous pressure will dislodge clots and sediment without traumatizing bladder wall. |
| g. Withdraw syringe and remove clamp; allow solution to drain into urinary drainage bag. (It is optional to keep tubing clamped to allow instilled fluid to remain in bladder.) | Allows drainage to flow via gravity. |
| 6. **Closed continuous irrigation:** | |
| a. Using aseptic technique, insert tip of sterile irrigation tubing into bag containing irrigation solution. | Reduces transmission of microorganisms. |
| b. Close clamp on tubing and hang bag of solution on IV pole. | Prevents loss of irrigating solution. |
| c. Open clamp and allow solution to flow through tubing, keeping end of tubing sterile; close clamp. | Removes air from tubing. |
| d. Wipe off irrigation port of triple-lumen catheter or attach sterile **Y**-connector to double-lumen catheter, then connect to irrigation tubing. | The third catheter lumen or **Y** connector provides means for irrigating solution to enter bladder. System must remain sterile. |
| e. Be sure drainage bag and tubing are securely connected to drainage port of triple-**Y**-connector to double lumen catheter. | Ensures that urine and irrigating solution will drain from bladder. |
| f. For intermittent flow, clamp tubing on drainage system, open clamp on irrigation tubing, and allow prescribed amount of fluid to enter bladder (100 ml is normal for adult); close irrigation tubing clamp, then open drainage tubing clamp. | Fluid instills through catheter into bladder, flushing system. Fluid drains out after irrigation is complete. |
| g. For continuous irrigation, calculate drip rate and adjust clamp on irrigation tubing accordingly; be sure clamp on drainage tubing is open and check volume of drainage in drainage bag. | Ensures continuous, even irrigation of catheter system. Prevents accumulation of solution in bladder, which may cause bladder distention and possible injury. |
| 7. **Open irrigation:** | |
| a. Open sterile irrigation tray; establish sterile field, and pour required amount of sterile solution into sterile solution container. Replace cap on large container of solution. | Adheres to principles of surgical asepsis. |
| b. Don sterile gloves. | Reduces transmission of infection. |
| c. Position waterproof drape under catheter. | Prevents soiling of bed linen. |
| d. Aspirate 30 ml of solution into irrigating syringe. | Prepares irrigant for instillation into catheter. |
| e. Move sterile collection basin close to client's thigh. | Prevents soiling of bed linen and prohibits reaching over sterile area. |
| f. Disconnect catheter from drainage tubing, allowing urine to flow into sterile collection basin; cover open end of drainage tubing with sterile protective cap and position tubing so it stays coiled on top of bed. | Maintains sterility of inner aspect of catheter lumen and drainage tubing; reduces potential of introducing pathogens into bladder. |
| g. Insert tip of syringe into lumen of catheter and gently instill solution. | Reduces incidence of bladder spasm but clears catheter of obstruction. |

| Steps | Rationale |
|---|---|
| h. Withdraw syringe, lower catheter, allow solution to drain into basin; repeat, instilling solution and draining several times until drainage is clear. | Allows drainage to flow by gravity. Provides for adequate flushing of catheter. |
| i. If solution does not return, have client turn onto side facing nurse; if changing position does not help, reinsert syringe and gently aspirate solution. | Change in position may move tip of catheter in bladder, increasing likelihood that fluid instilled will flow out. |
| j. After irrigation is complete, remove protector cap from drainage tubing adaptor, cleanse adaptor with alcohol swab, and reinsert into lumen of catheter to reestablish closed drainage system. | Reduces entrance of microorganisms into system. |
| k. Remove gloves. | |
| 8. Reanchor catheter to client with tape. | Prevents trauma to urethral tissue. |
| 9. Assist client into comfortable position. | Promotes relaxation and rest. |
| 10. Lower bed to lowest position, side rails down if appropriate. | Promotes client safety. |
| 11. Dispose of contaminated supplies and wash hands. | Reduces spread of microorganisms. |

## Evaluation

| | |
|---|---|
| 1. Calculate fluid used to irrigate bladder and catheter and subtract from volume drained. | Determines accurate urinary output. |
| 2. Assess characteristics of output: viscosity, color, presence of clots. | Data serve as baseline to judge response to therapy. |
| 3. Observe catheter patency. | |

### *Expected outcome*

| | |
|---|---|
| 1. Output is greater than volume of irrigating solution used. | Indicates patency of drainage system. |
| 2. Absence of pain or discomfort. | |

### *Unexpected outcome*

| | |
|---|---|
| 1. Irrigating solution is not returned. | Indicates possible occlusion of Foley catheter, which can lead to urinary retention. |
| 2. Client complains of pain. | May indicate retention. |
| 3. Signs of fever or cloudy, foul urine. | May indicate infection. |

## Recording and Reporting

| | |
|---|---|
| 1. Record amount of solution used as irrigant, amount returned as drainage, consistency of drainage in nurses' notes and I & O sheet. | Documents procedure and client's tolerance of it. |
| 2. Report catheter occlusion, sudden bleeding, infection, or increased pain to physician. | May require more aggressive therapy. Reduces risk of urinary retention. |

## Follow-up Activity

| | |
|---|---|
| 1. Notify physician if irrigant is retained and bladder is distended. | Danger of ruptured bladder or pressure on bladder must be avoided. If client is immediately postoperative, physician may be required to change catheter. |

## Special Considerations

- Triple-lumen catheter system does not have to be broken when irrigating bladder.
- Double lumen catheter system requires nurse to break system to irrigate bladder.
- Bleeding is common after transurethral prostatectomy. Nurse should expect bright, red-tinged urine during first 48 hr, followed by pink-tinged to clear urine by fifth postoperative day.
- Supplies for closed system may be kept at bedside. Irrigating solution should be at room temperature. This is similar to adding bag of IV fluid to IV infusion. Check right solution, dose, client, route, time.
- Room-temperature, sterile normal saline is usually used; cold solution can cause bladder spasms.
- If blood is present, flow rate may need to be increased to keep system patent. Rate of infusion may be independent nursing judgment.
- Amount of solution used to flush system may be dictated by physician or institutional policy. Frequency of irrigation is based on need of client (e.g., client who has just had surgery on prostate gland may require irrigations q5-10min in first hr, then tapering off to q4h). When nurse is not in attendance, irrigation is clamped off.

### Teaching Consideration

- Instruct client, primary care giver to observe urine daily for changes in color, presence of mucus or blood, changes in consistency.

### Home Care Considerations

- Assess the client, primary care giver for ability and motivation to perform catheter irrigation.
- Assess client's environment for appropriate storage space for materials needed for procedure.
- Observe client, primary care giver perform procedure.

## *SKILL 29-8 Removing a Retention Catheter*

Removal of a retention catheter is a skill requiring clean technique. When removing a retention catheter, the nurse must prevent trauma to the urethra. If the retention catheter balloon is not fully deflated its removal can result in trauma and subsequent swelling of urethral meatus, and urinary retention can occur.

If the catheter was in place for more than several days, the client may experience dysuria resulting from inflammation of the urethral canal. Because of decreased bladder muscle tone, the client may urinate frequently.

### Purposes

1. Promote normal urinary elimination.
2. Promote normal bladder function.
3. Prevent trauma to the urethra.

## *Procedure 29-8*

| Steps | Rationale |
|---|---|
| **Assessment** | |
| 1. Review client's medical record for physician's order and the reason for removing catheter. | Physician may have ordered catheter removed, enabling client to void after removal. It may be removed to replace with another indwelling catheter. |
| 2. Note period of time catheter was in place. | Assesses risk for loss of bladder tone. |
| **Nursing Diagnosis** | |
| 1. Cluster data to reveal actual or potential nursing diagnoses: | |
| a. Urinary retention: related to recent indwelling catheterization. | After catheter removal, client may not be able to empty bladder, and urinary retention results. |
| b. Pain: related to local urethral irritation. | Catheter that remains in place for prolonged period causes urethral irritation. Client may experience dysuria for several days after catheter removal. |
| **Planning** | |
| 1. Develop individualized goals for client based on nursing diagnoses: | |
| a. Promote return of normal micturition. | Removal of catheter and bladder conditioning restore ability to voluntarily void. |
| b. Reduce risk of urinary tract infection. | Catheter provides direct route for infection. |
| 2. Prepare necessary equipment and supplies: | |
| a. Syringe (same size as volume of solution used to inflate balloon) (Check balloon inflate valve, which has this information printed on it.) | Used to remove normal saline from inflated balloon. |
| b. Waterproof pad | |
| c. Sterile specimen container, labeled correctly | Will need if a specimen for culture and sensitivity is to be obtained before removal (Chapter 46). This may be policy in some institutions. |
| d. 25-gauge ½" needle | |
| e. Alcohol swab | |
| f. Nonsterile, disposable gloves | |
| 3. Explain procedure to client. | Reduces anxiety and promotes cooperation. |

| Steps | Rationale |
|---|---|
| **Implementation** | |
| 1. Wash hands and don gloves. | Reduces transmission of microorganisms. |
| 2. If bladder conditioning is to be performed: | |
| a. 10 hr before removal, clamp indwelling catheter for 3 hr. | Volume of urine stretches bladder's walls to stimulate muscle tone. |
| b. Unclamp and drain urine for 5 min. | Simulates voiding. |
| c. Repeat clamping for 3 hr and draining for 5 min two more times. | Clients who receive bladder conditioning are able to feel urge to void sooner than those who have no conditioning. |
| 3. Provide privacy by closing room door or bedside curtain. | Shows respect for client's self-esteem. |
| 4. Raise bed to appropriate working height. Raise side rail on opposite side of bed. | Promotes use of good body mechanics and client safety. |
| 5. Position client in supine position. | Provides easy access to visualize urethral meatus. |
| 6. Place waterproof pad between female's thighs (if in supine position) or over male's thighs. | Prevents soiling bed linen. Provides wrapper to cover contaminated catheter after removal, thus eliminating possibility of urine contaminating nurse's hand. |
| 7. Obtain sterile urine specimen, if required. | Determines if bacteria is present in urine. |
| 8. Remove adhesive tape anchoring catheter. Cleanse any residue from skin. | Removes source of irritant on skin. |
| 9. Insert hub of syringe into inflate valve. Aspirate entire amount of fluid used to inflate balloon. | Deflates balloon to allow for removal. If portion of solution remains, partially inflated balloon will cause trauma to urethral wall as catheter is removed. |
| 10. Pull catheter out smoothly and slowly. (Stop if resistance is met; balloon is probably still inflated.) | Prevents trauma to urethral mucosa. |
| 11. Wrap contaminated catheter in waterproof pad. Unhook collection bag and drainage tubing from bed. | Prevents contamination of nurse's hands. |
| 12. Reposition client as necessary. Lower level of bed, and position side rails accordingly. | Promotes client comfort and safety. |
| 13. Measure and empty contents of collection bag. | Provides accurate recording of urinary output. |
| 14. Dispose of all contaminated supplies correctly and wash hands. | Reduces spread of microorganisms. |
| 15. If another catheter is to be inserted, proceed according to procedure for insertion of retention catheter. | |
| **Evaluation** | |
| 1. Observe time and amount of first voided specimen. | Indicates return of bladder function and ability of bladder to empty fully. If volume is small, residual urine may be required. |
| 2. Note any discomfort experienced by client when voiding. | It is normal for client to experience dysuria, especially if catheter has been in place for several days or weeks. |
| 3. Note condition of skin from adhesive tape. | Determines presence of skin irritation. |
| ***Expected outcomes*** | |
| 1. Client voids large volume of urine within 8 hr of catheter removal. | Indicates return of voluntary bladder function. |
| 2. Client voids without discomfort. | Indicates absence of urethral trauma. |
| 3. Skin under tape site is clear. | |
| ***Unexpected outcomes*** | |
| 1. Client is unable to void in 8 hr. | Indicates urinary retention. |
| 2. Bladder is distended; client voids small amounts frequently and complains of burning or pain. | Indicates urinary retention with overflow incontinence. Urinary tract infection may be present. |
| 3. Skin under tape site is reddened and weeping fluid. | Indicates tape burn or allergic response. |
| **Recording and Reporting** | |
| 1. Record and report time catheter was removed, time and amount of next voiding. | Communicates pertinent information to all members of health care team. |
| **Follow-up Activity** | |
| 1. Notify physician if bladder distends, client has not voided for 8 hrs, client complains of increasing urge to void. | Can indicate urinary retention and possible need for recatheterization. |

### Special Considerations

- Check to see if physician has ordered bladder conditioning before removal. This may be dependent or independent nursing function; check institutional policy.
- Keep track of I & O for at least 24 hr after removal of catheter.
- If client has not voided within 8 hr after catheter removal, the catheter (intermittent or indwelling, depending on order of physician) may have to be reinserted. Assess for signs of retention.

### Teaching Considerations

- Explain to client that burning sensation may be felt as catheter is withdrawn.

## *SKILL 29-9 Applying a Condom Catheter*

The external application of a urinary drainage device is a convenient, safe method of draining urine in male clients. The condom catheter is suitable for incontinent or comatose clients who still have complete and spontaneous bladder emptying. The condom is a soft, pliable rubber sheath that slips over the penis. A strip of elastic adhesive is placed around the top of the condom to secure it (Fig. 29-10). The catheter may be attached to a leg drainage bag or a standard urinary drainage bag.

A condom catheter may remain in place 1 to 2 days. With each catheter change, the nurse cleans the urethral meatus and penis thoroughly and looks for signs of skin irritation.

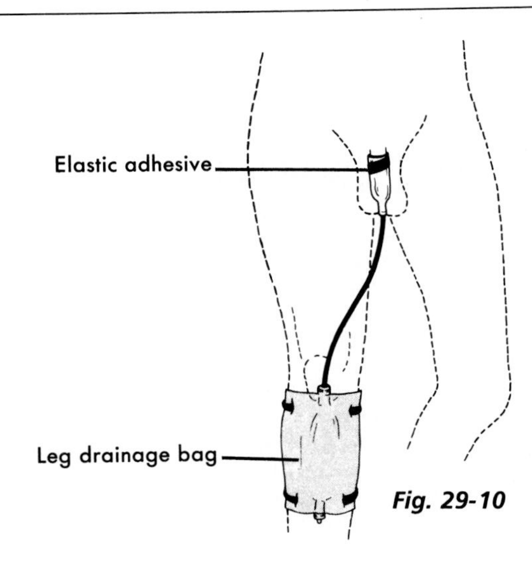

*Fig. 29-10*

### Purposes

1. Provide external urinary drainage.
2. Maintain skin integrity.

## *Procedure 29-9*

| Steps | Rationale |
|---|---|
| **Assessment** | |
| 1. Assess status of client to determine need for condom catheter. | Client continuously incontinent of urine is at risk for skin breakdown. |
| 2. Assess mental status of client so appropriate teaching related to condom can be implemented. | Some male clients may be incontinent only at night. Teaching can be implemented to instruct client on self-application. |
| 3. Assess condition of penis. | Provides baseline to compare changes in condition of skin after condom application. |
| **Nursing Diagnosis** | |
| 1. Cluster data to reveal actual or potential nursing diagnoses: | Allows identification of individualized needs. |
| a. Total incontinence, related to: ▪ Impaired bladder function. ▪ Decreased perception of sensation to void. | Client loses ability to control micturition. |
| b. Potential or actual impaired skin integrity: related to exposure to urine. | Urine causes maceration and irritation of skin. |
| c. Self-esteem disturbance: related to condom catheter. | |

| Steps | Rationale |
|---|---|
| **Planning** | |
| 1. Develop individualized goals for client based on nursing diagnoses: | |
| a. Improve continency. | Control of incontinent drainage prevents continual exposure of skin to urine. |
| b. Prevent skin breakdown. | |
| c. Maintain comfort and self-esteem. | Client gains self-esteem from avoiding embarrassment of incontinence. |
| 2. Prepare necessary equipment and supplies: | |
| a. Rubber condom sheath (proper size) | |
| b. Strip of elastic or Velcro adhesive | |
| c. Urinary collection bag with drainage tubing or leg bag and straps, skin prep | Urinary leg bag allows client to remain mobile. |
| d. Basin with warm water and soap | |
| e. Towels and wash cloths | |
| f. Bath blanket | |
| g. Disposable gloves | Protects nurse's hands; reduces client's risk of infection. |
| 3. Explain procedure to client. | Reduces anxiety and promotes cooperation. |
| 4. Arrange for extra nursing personnel to assist with moving dependent client. | Promotes client safety and proper use of body mechanics by nurse. |
| **Implementation** | |
| 1. Wash hands. | Reduces transmission of microorganisms. |
| 2. Provide privacy by closing room door or bedside curtain. | Maintains client's self-esteem. |
| 3. Assist client into supine position. Place bath blanket over upper torso. Fold sheets so lower extremities are covered; only genitalia should be exposed. | Promotes comfort; draping prevents unnecessary exposure of body parts. |
| 4. Prepare urinary drainage collection bag and tubing. Clamp off drainage exit ports. Secure collection bag to bed frame; bring drainage tubing up through siderails onto bed. Prepare leg bag for connection to condom, if necessary. | Provides easy access to drainage equipment after condom is in place. |
| 5. Put on disposable gloves. Provide perineal care (Chapter 6) and dry thoroughly. | Removes irritating secretions. Rubber sheath rolls onto dry skin more easily. |
| 6. Apply skin preparation to penis and allow to dry. If client is uncircumsized, return foreskin to normal position. | |
| 7. With nondominant hand, grasp penis along shaft. With dominant hand, hold condom sheath at tip of penis and smoothly roll sheath onto penis. | Prepares penis for easy condom placement. |
| 8. Allow 2.5 to 5 cm (1 to 2 in) of space between tip of glans penis and end of condom catheter. | Allows free passage of urine into collecting tubing when client passes urine. |
| 9. Encircle penile shaft with strip of elastic adhesive. Strip should touch only condom sheath. Apply snugly, but not tightly. | Condom must be secured so it is snug and will stay on but not tight enough to cause constriction of blood flow. |
| 10. Connect drainage tubing to end of condom catheter. Be sure condom is not twisted. | Allows urine to be collected and measured. Keeps client dry. Twisted condom obstructs urine flow. |
| 11. Place excess coiling of tubing on bed and secure to bottom sheet. | Prevents looping of tubing and promotes free drainage of urine. |
| 12. Place client in safe, comfortable position. | Promotes comfort. |
| 13. Dispose of contaminated supplies and wash hands. | Reduces spread of microorganisms. |
| **Evaluation** | |
| 1. Observe urinary drainage. | Determines if normal voiding is occurring. |
| 2. Remove condom and inspect skin on penile shaft for signs of breakdown or irritation at least daily during hygiene and when condom is reapplied. | Indicates if condom or urine is causing irritation or if adhesive is too restrictive. Frequent assessment of circulation of glans penis is important to determine if condom has been applied too tightly. |
| ***Expected outcomes*** | |
| 1. Client is continent with condom catheter intact. | Catheter is secure; normal voiding occurs. |
| 2. Penile shaft is free of skin irritation or breakdown. | Indicates absence of irritation. |
| ***Unexpected outcomes*** | |
| 1. Skin around penis is reddened and excoriated. | Results from pressure of adhesive or contact with urine. |
| 2. Urination is reduced or infrequent. | Indicates urinary retention. |
| 3. Urine leaks from tubing. | Catheter is improperly secured to drainage, or catheter has been improperly applied. |

| Steps | Rationale |
|---|---|
| **Reporting and Recording** | |
| 1. Report and record pertinent information: condom application, condition of skin, voiding pattern. | Communicates information to all members of health care team. |
| **Follow-up Activities** | |
| 1. Increase perineal skin care to every 2 to 4 hr. | Removes skin surface bacteria and decreases risk of skin breakdown. |
| 2. Remove condom catheter for 20 min every 2 to 4 hr. | Allows skin on penis to dry. |
| 3. Insert Foley catheter. | Removes urinary distention. |

### Special Considerations

- Condom catheter is suitable for incontinent or comatose male clients with complete and spontaneous bladder emptying.
- Check institutional policy to ascertain if physician's order is required to apply condom.
- Procedure should be explained, even if client is comatose because he may be able to hear.
- Some institutions apply thin layer of plasticized skin spray to skin of penile shaft to protect skin from ulceration and irritation caused by rubber condom and adhesive holding it in place.
- Never use adhesive tape because it is too constrictive.
- It may be necessary to trim some pubic hair to secure condom to penile shaft.

## *SKILL 29-10 Peritoneal Dialysis and Continuous Ambulatory Peritoneal Dialysis*

The kidneys are organs that filter and excrete excess fluid and solute wastes. When the kidneys fail, little to no urine is produced, electrolyte imbalances occur, and toxins accumulate in the blood. If excess fluid and toxins are not removed, death results.

Hemodialysis is one method to remove fluid and solute wastes. Hemodialysis nursing is a specialty practice; although students may observe this procedure, they do not actively participate in it.

There are two additional forms of dialysis that students may encounter. Students may provide direct care to clients receiving these dialysis methods.

The first is peritoneal dialysis (PD), which is used as a therapy to osmotically remove fluid and waste products from the blood. The process takes place in a hospital and involves the surgical insertion of a temporary catheter into the peritoneal cavity (Fig. 29-11). The peritoneal membrane is used to filter excess water, electrolytes, and toxins from the blood. To achieve this, a hypertonic dialysate solution is instilled into the peritoneal cavity. The solution remains for a specific period of time and is then drained through the catheter. Because the dialysate solution is hypertonic, excess water and wastes in the body diffuse through the peritoneal membrane. The peritoneal process has three steps, each lasting approximately 20 minutes: 1) filling the cavity with the dialysate, 2) allowing the fluid to dwell in the cavity, and 3) draining the fluid from the cavity (Strangio, 1988).

A second form of peritoneal dialysis is continuous ambulatory peritoneal dialysis (CAPD). CAPD is a type of therapy that has made home dialysis feasible for the client with end stage renal disease (ESRD). With this type of dialysis, a permanent peritoneal catheter is surgically implanted into the peritoneal cavity, and the processes of osmosis and diffusion remove fluid, excess electrolytes, and toxins from the blood (Perras, 1983). CAPD has the same three phases as routine peritoneal dialysis; however, the time cycle changes. The dwell time ranges from 4 to 8 hr. During this time an empty plastic bag and drainage tubing are folded and concealed under the client's clothes. Afterward, the client drains the abdominal cavity, which is followed by reinstilling fresh dialysate into the peritoneal cavity. The dialysate must be changed three to five times a day. One major advantage of CAPD is that it allows the client to be out of the hospital, maintain the system at home, and continue with daily activities. This method is not appropriate for all clients with ESRD and requires thorough education from nursing and routine follow-up in an outpatient renal clinic (Perras 1983; Lane, 1982).

## Purposes

1. Promote the removal of fluid, electrolytes, and toxins from the blood.
2. Maintain surgical asepsis when providing catheter care or instilling dialysate.
3. Assist in returning normal renal function when ESRD is not present (PD only).
4. Assist the client with ESRD in returning to routine daily activities (CAPD only).

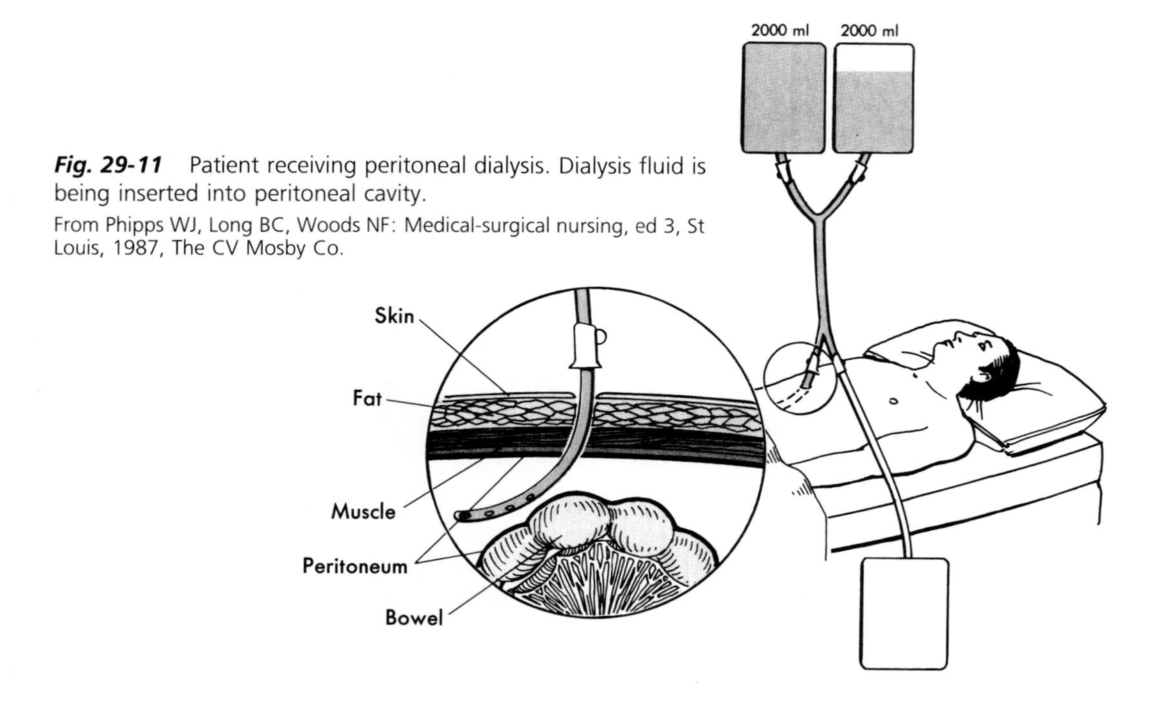


***Fig. 29-11*** Patient receiving peritoneal dialysis. Dialysis fluid is being inserted into peritoneal cavity.

From Phipps WJ, Long BC, Woods NF: Medical-surgical nursing, ed 3, St Louis, 1987, The CV Mosby Co.

## *Procedure 29-10*

| Steps | Rationale |
|---|---|
| **Assessment** | |
| 1. Obtain client's weight. | Provides baseline information about weight attributed to fluid retention. A daily weight gain of 1 kg is equilavant to 1 L of fluid. |
| 2. Obtain vital signs. | Fluid volume changes associated with PD increase risk for hemodynamic blood pressure changes, especially for clients having PD in hospital. |
| 3. Measure abdominal girth.<br>a. Mark midpoint of client's abdomen. Keep mark as reference for future measurements. | Provides baseline data regarding amount of fluid in peritoneal cavity. |
| 4. Inspect catheter site for erythema, tenderness, drainage. | Indicates infection at catheter entry site. Increases risk for peritonitis (Breckenridge, 1982). |
| 5. Measure body temperature. | Provides baseline data about client's febrile status. |
| 6. Review hospital or dialysis unit's procedure for PD or CAPD. | There may be institutional variations regarding ordering of supplies; fill, dwell, and drain times; catheter care; discharge teaching plan. |
| 7. Review physician's orders:<br>a. PD: usually include 24 exchanges with specific dialysate volume and composition, as well as specific dwell time, which is commonly 20 min.<br>b. CAPD: usually include three to five exchanges with specific dialysate volume and composition, as well as specific dwell time, which can range from 4 to 8 hr. | PD and CAPD require specific orders individualized to client's fluid needs and disease process. |
| 8. Obtain laboratory data as ordered:<br>a. PD: every 12 to 24 hours.<br>b. CAPD: can vary depending on individual needs. | Documents fluid and electrolyte status and changes that occur from PD or CAPD. |

| Steps | Rationale |
|---|---|
| **Nursing Diagnosis** | |
| 1. Cluster data to reveal actual or potential nursing diagnoses:<br>a. Fluid volume excess: related to impaired renal function.<br>b. Fluid volume deficit: related to excessive dialysis.<br>c. Potential for infection: related to indwelling peritoneal catheter. | Nursing diagnoses can result from fluid retention from ESRD, fluid depletion from excessive dialysis, or break in aseptic technique during dialysis. |
| **Planning** | |
| 1. Develop individualized goals for client based on nursing diagnoses: | |
| a. Achieve normal fluid and electrolyte balances. | PD and CAPD should result in near-normal fluid and electrolyte balances. |
| b. Prevent infection:<br>▪ No erythema, tenderness, drainage at catheter site.<br>▪ Afebrile. | Presence of temporary or permanent peritoneal catheter and routine manipulation of catheter increases risks for infection. |
| c. Stabilize vital signs. | Changes in fluid volume can increase risk for pulse and blood pressure changes. |
| d. Maintain weight within expected ranges. | Dialysis is designed to restore normal or near-normal weight at end of exchanges. |
| e. Maintain abdominal girth within expected range. | PD client should have no or minimal increase in abdominal girth. Increase indicates fluid retention. |
| 2. Wash hands. | Reduces transmission of microorganisms. |
| 3. If PD is started at bedside, obtain equipment: | Insertion of PD catheter is physician responsibility. Nurse should be familiar with equipment to assist in procedure. |
| a. Ordered dialysate at room temperature (Dialysate is warmed by placing solution bag on warming pad, not into warming solution.) | Dialysate that is too cold results in intolerance, cramps, hypothermia. (Plastic dialysate bags are permeable. Immersing them in warm water when protective wrapper is removed risks introduction of bacteria from nonsterile water; in addition, osmotic concentration of dialysate can change [Strangio, 1988].) |
| b. Deane prosthesis or PD button to leave at bedside. | Aseptically applied to PD site at end of treatment; maintains patency of insertion site for another treatment. |
| c. Sterile gloves | Maintains sterile asepsis. |
| d. Occlusive dressing materials | Prevents entry of bacteria into PD site after treatment. |
| e. Hydrogen peroxide | Used to cleanse around catheter site. |
| f. Povidone-iodine solution<br>g. Povidone-iodine ointment | Anti-infective solutions and ointments reduce risk for bacterial growth. |
| h. Mask | Reduces transmission of microorganisms. |
| i. IV pole | Used to place dialysate solution during instilling cycle. |
| j. Y-connector tubing (CAPD clients may not need) | Allows the nurse to hang two warmed bags. |
| k. Sterile drainage bag | Permits proper collection of fluid from peritoneal cavity during drain cycle. |
| l. Waxed pencil or non-water-soluble marker (PD only) | Allows for proper marking of solution bag. Nurse marks bag with run number and medications added to dialysate. |
| m. Obtain PD set, which should contain:<br>▪ Peritoneal catheter<br>▪ Lidocaine for local anesthesia<br>▪ 3 ml syringe with 25-gauge needle<br>▪ Povidone-iodine solution<br>▪ Alcohol swabs<br>▪ Scalpel<br>▪ Gauze sponges<br>▪ Sterile drape<br>▪ Trocar<br>▪ Connector tubing for instillation of fluid<br>▪ Connector tubing for drainage<br>▪ Y-connector<br>▪ Clamps for connector tubings<br>▪ Drainage bag<br>▪ Sutures and suture needle<br>▪ Nonallergic tape<br>▪ Sterile cap, gown, masks | |
| 4. Explain procedure to client. | Assists in reducing anxiety and promoting cooperation. |

| Steps | Rationale |
|---|---|
| **Implementation** | |
| *Insertion of peritioneal catheter:* | |
| 1. Wash hands. | Reduces transmission of microorganisms. |
| 2. Close client's room door and draw curtains. | Maintains client's right to privacy. |
| 3. Organize equipment at bedside (see #2 under Planning). | Promotes organized and quick insertion of catheter. |
| 4. Administer analgesia or antianxiety medication if required by client and ordered by physician. | Procedure is uncomfortable; although local anesthetic is administered, analgesia or antianxiety medications can result in greater cooperation by client. |
| 5. If client is producing urine and does not have Foley catheter in place, catheterize with straight catheter. | Empty bladder reduces risk of bladder puncture as catheter trocar is inserted into peritoneal cavity. |
| 6. Place client in supine position. | Catheter is inserted in umbilical region. Supine position assists in relaxing abdominal muscles. |
| 7. Clear bedding from umbilical region. | Permits establishment of sterile field without risk of contamination from bedding. |
| 8. Physician and nurse complete sterile scrubs and don sterile masks, caps, gowns, gloves. | Insertion of peritoneal catheter is sterile procedure. Strict surgical asepsis is required to reduce entry of bacteria into peritoneal cavity, which increases risk of peritonitis. |
| 9. Physician follows surgical procedure to insert catheter into peritoneal cavity. | Placement of catheter requires surgical entry into peritoneal cavity. |
| *Initiating dialysis exchanges:* | |
| 1. Wash hands. | Reduces transmission of microorganisms. |
| 2. Place client in semi-Fowler's or high-Fowler's position. | Instilling fluid into peritoneal cavity decreases diaphragmatic excursion and semi or high Fowler's position promotes optimal lung expansion. |
| 3. Make sure all clamps on inflow and outflow tubings are in "off" positions. | Prevents accidental instillation of air or dialysate into peritoneal cavity. Also prevents unscheduled removal of dialysate from cavity before completion of ordered dwell time. |
| 4. Add medications as listed in physician's order: | |
| a. Heparin. | Reduces accumulation of fibrin around catheter tip. |
| b. Local anesthetic. | Aids in reducing back or abdominal pain related only to infusion of dialysate (Birdsall, 1988). |
| c. Prophylactic antibiotics. | Reduces risk of peritonitis. |
| 5. Attach two warmed dialysate bags to inflow tubing (Fig. 29-11) and attach to IV pole. Bags are punctured exactly as IV solution bags (Chapter 23). | Promotes timely, organized follow-up exchanges. Standard PD usually includes 24 exchanges. CAPD clients are instructed to hang only one bag because these clients have three to five exchanges daily. |
| 6. Prime inflow tubing by removing protective cap and maintaining sterility Hold tubing over basin or sink, open inflow clamp, and allow fluid to run through tubing until all air is removed. | Maintaining sterility of cap allows safe, sterile reapplication of cap on inflow tubing. Allowing fluid to run through tubing prevents air from entering peritoneal cavity. |
| 7. Open clamp on dialysate bag #1. Infuse solution over prescribed time (usually 2 L/15 to 20 min). | Permits instillation of dialysate into peritoneal cavity. |
| 8. Clamp inflow tubing for prescribed dwell time: a. PD: usually 15 to 20 min. b. CAPD: 3 to 5 hr. (CAPD client folds tubing and infusion bag on abdomen, which is concealed by clothing, and uses same bag and tubing for drain cycle.) | Prevents air from entering peritoneal cavity. Dwell time permits peritoneal membrane to exchange fluid, electrolytes, toxins from blood. |
| 9. Remove dialysate bag #1 from IV pole. Place warmed bag #3 on pole. | Promotes organized procedure. When multiple exchanges are ordered, nurse should have two dialysate bags on IV pole. |
| 10. Unclamp outflow tubing and drain (usually for 20 min). | Permits drainage of dialysate and wastes from abdominal cavity. During first two to three exchanges, it is common for dialysate to remain in cavity; excess should drain with later exchanges. |
| 11. Clamp outflow tubing. | Prevents untimed drain during subsequent exchange. |
| 12. Empty and measure fluid in drainage bag. | Provides assessment of fluid balance of dialysate solution. If volume of fluid infused, is more than amount drained, balance is negative (e.g., if 2000 ml of dialysate was infused and 1800 ml was drained, balance is negative 200 ml [−200 ml].) |
| 13. Repeat steps 3 thru 10 until all exchanges are complete. | |
| 14. During first exchanges, monitor client's vital signs every 15 min. | Promotes timely documentation of hemodynamic effects of PD. |
| 15. When all exchanges are complete: | |
| a. Cover catheter with sterile cap or remove catheter and | Catheter remains in place if future PD is anticipated. |

| Steps | Rationale |
|---|---|
| insert Deane button into insertion site. This can be a medical procedure or designated to nurses in speciality units. | Maintains patency of catheter insertion site. |
| 16. Inspect catheter dressing. If dressing is reapplied, apply a clear transparent occlusive dressing. | Intact and dry dressing reduces risk of infection. |
| 17. Wash hands and dispose of contaminated supplies according to agency policy. | Reduces transmission of microorganisms and blood-borne pathogens. |
| **Evaluation** | |
| 1. Obtain weight. | Decrease indicates removal of excess fluid; increase indicates retention of fluid. |
| 2. Obtain dialysis fluid balance. | Determines adequacy of fluid removal. |
| 3. Obtain vital signs. | Documents tolerance to PD. |
| 4. Measure abdominal girth. | Provides an indirect measurement of retention of fluid in peritoneal cavity. |
| 5. Inspect catheter site for erythema, tenderness, drainage. | Documents symptoms of infection. |
| 6. Obtain body temperature. | Denotes presence or absence of infection. |
| 7. Inspect returned dialysate solution. | Notes blood, fecal contents, urine. |
| ***Expected outcomes*** | |
| 1. Decreased weight. | Indicates excess fluid removed. |
| 2. Positive fluid balance. | Indicates more dialysate removed than instilled. |
| 3. Stable vital signs. | Indicates no adverse hemodynamic responses. |
| 4. Decreased abdominal girth. | Indicates no fluid retained in peritoneal cavity. |
| 5. No erythema, tenderness, drainage at catheter site. | Indicates absence of local inflammation at catheter site. |
| 6. No fever. | Indicates no systemic bacteria. |
| 7. Dialysate return is clear or slightly light yellow. | Expected color of returned fluid, indicates absence of blood or bacteria. |
| ***Unexpected outcomes*** | |
| 1. Increased weight or no weight change. | Indicates fluid retained in peritoneal cavity. |
| 2. Negative fluid balance. | Indicates excess fluid retained (e.g., total of twelve 2 L (24,000 ml) exchanges instilled; Total output: 20 L. Four L (4000 ml) remains in peritoneal cavity). |
| 3. Decreased blood pressure and tachycardia. | Client unable to tolerate fluid volume, or catheter may have perforated bowel. |
| 4. Increased abdominal girth. | Indicates retained fluid. |
| 5. Erythema, tenderness, drainage at catheter site. | Indicates local inflammatory response. |
| 6. Fever. | Indicates systemic infection. |
| 7. Dialysate drainage abnormal: | |
| a. Cloudy. | Indicates possible infection. |
| b. Bright red blood. | Indicates perforation of organ or major vessel. |
| c. Brown color or presence of stool. | Indicates perforation of bowel. |
| 8. Cramps. | Indicates dialysate too cold, infusion too rapid, volume too much for client to tolerate, or electrolyte imbalances have occurred. |
| 9. Sudden respiratory distress. | Indicates excessive volume for client to tolerate. |
| 10. Poor instillation flow. | Indicates kink in inflow tubing or catheter. |
| 11. Poor drainage. | Indicates kink in outflow tubing or catheter. |
| 12. Scrotal swelling. | Indicates catheter displacement (Birdsall, 1988). |
| 13. Leak at catheter site. | Indicates catheter displacement toward abdominal surface. |
| **Recording and Reporting** | |
| 1. Document client's weight, abdominal girth, dialysis fluid balance before and after PD. | Notes presence or absence of retained fluid in abdominal cavity. |
| 2. Document client's vital signs before, during, after dialysis. | Notes hemodynamic response. |
| 3. Document temperature and status of catheter site. | Notes presence or absence of local or systemic infection. |
| 4. Record color of drainage. | Notes abnormalities in drainage color. |
| 5. Record condition of catheter dressing or if new dressing applied. | Records status of dressing's condition and most recent change. |
| 6. Note any unexpected outcomes and action taken by nurse and physician. | Records continuing care of client and possible future complications. |

| Steps | Rationale |
|---|---|
| **Follow-up Activities** | |
| 1. Remove catheter if following occur: | |
| a. Signs of local infection. | Increases risk of peritonitis. |
| b. Catheter displacement. | Causes danger of organ perforation. |
| 2. Stop dialysis and notify physican for: | |
| a. Change in vital signs. | Indicates intolerace to procedure. |
| b. Respiratory distress. | Causes distention of peritoneal cavity, which limits diaphragmatic excursion. |
| c. Bright red blood. | Indicates perforation of organ or vessel. |
| d. Fecal contents in drainage. | Indicates bowel perforation. |
| e. Scrotal swelling. | Indicates catheter displacement. |
| f. Complaints of cramps. | Warmer dialysate needed, there is too much fluid, or there is electrolyte imbalance. (In latter case, obtain serum electrolyte levels.) |

## Special Considerations

- Fever is early sign of catheter-induced peritonitis (Perras, 1986).
- Changes in blood pressure and increased respiratory rate may signal intolerance to amount of fluid instilled in peritoneal cavity.
- A 1 kg weight gain in 24 to 48 hr can be correlated with 1 L of retained fluid.
- Large volume of dialysate instilled may give client urge to defecate.
- Client receiving PD should be encouraged to move around in bed. However, movements should avoid stressing catheter or tubing.
- Individual hospitals have individual flow sheets to record PD fluids.
- CAPD clients have increased abdominal girth during dwell time of exchange.
- Clients on CAPD may experience fresh weight gain caused by dextrose absorption (Lane, 1982).

## Teaching Considerations

- Teach CAPD clients scrub and exchange procedures according to policy.
- Review teaching plan with client before discharge and during each clinic visit.
- Ask client to correctly demonstrate scrub and exchange procedure.
- Periodically review potential complications and signs and symptoms.
- Review medications and dietary and fluid restrictions.
- Instruct client when and who to contact in emergency.
- Instruct client to correctly take blood pressure.
- Instruct client to correctly weigh self.
- Instruct client about common symptoms associated with peritonitis.

## Home Care Considerations

- CAPD clients must do the following to correctly complete CAPD exchanges:
  a. Achieve goals under Planning.
  b. Demonstrate CAPD scrub and aseptic exchange.
  c. State signs of infection.
  d. Adhere to fluid, dietary, medication therapies.
  e. Perform activities of daily living. CAPD is designed so client can maintain normal daily activities.

### BIBLIOGRAPHY


Barnes SH: The development of a comprehensive instructional package for teaching intermittent self-catheterization, J Entero Therapy 13(6):238, 1986.

Birdsall C: How do you teach female self-catheterization? Am J Nurs (85):1226, 1985.

Birdsall C: How do you manage peritoneal dialysis? Am J Nurs 88:592, 1988.

Birdsall C, Brassil D: How do you use renal irrigations? Am J Nurs 87:909, 1987.

Breckenridge DM, Cupit MC, Raimondo JM: Systematic nursing assessment tool for the CAPD client, Nephrol Nurse 4:24, 1982.

Bulau J: Clinical policies and procedures for home health care, Rockville, Md, 1986, Aspen Publishers, Inc.

Burgener S: Justification of closed intermittent urinary catheter irrigation/instillation: a review of current research and practice, J Adv Nurs 12:229, 1987.

Dudley MN, Barriere SL: Antimicrobial irrigations in prevention and treatment of catheter-related urinary tract infections, Am J Hosp Pharm 38:59, 1981.

Golden S: Nursing a loved one at home, Philadelphia, 1988, Running Press Book Publishers.

Greengold BA, Ouslander JG: Bladder retraining, J Gerontol Nurs 12:31, 1986.

Gurenich I: How to make every culture count, RN 51:49, 1988.

Kane RL, et al.: Essentials of clinical geriatrics, New York, 1984, McGraw-Hill, Inc.

King C: Hydrocele: a complication of CAPD, Nephrol Nurse 3:37, 1981.

Lane T, Stroshal V, Waldorf P: Standards of care for the CAPD patient, Nephrol Nurse 4(5):34, 1982.

McCormick KA: Urinary incontinence in the elderly, Nurs Clin North Am 23:135, 1988.

Metheny NM: Overview of fluid and electrolyte balance: nursing considerations, Philadelphia, 1987, JB Lippincott Co.

Mulhall A, et al.: Emptying urinary drainage bags, Nurs Times 84(4):64, 1988.

Newman DK, et al.: Helping geriatric patients master self-catheterization, RN 51:86, 1988.

Nolph KD: The current status of CAPD and CCPD, Dialysis and Transplantation 17(9):457, 1988.

Orzeck S, Ouslander JG: Urinary incontinence: an overview of causes and treatment, J Entero Therapy 14:20, 1987.

Perras ST, Zappacosta AR: Reduction of peritonitis with patient education and the Travenol CAPD germicidal exchange device, ANNA J 13(4):219, 1986.

Perras ST, Mattern ML, Hughues C, et al.: Primary nursing is the key to success in an outpatient CAPD teaching program, Nephrol Nurse 5(4):8, 1983.

Plymat K, Turner S: In-home management of urinary incontinence, Home Health Nurse 6(4):30, 1988.

Potter PA, Perry AG: Fundamentals of nursing: concepts, process, and practice, ed 2, St Louis, 1989, The CV Mosby Co.

Robb SS: Urinary incontinence verification in elderly men, Nurs Res 34:278, 1985.

Roe B: Aspects of catheter care, Geriatr Nurs Home Care 7(8):21, 1987.

Roe B: Teaching patients about their catheters, Nurs Times 84(12):68, 1988.

Rogers W: Shampoo urethritis (letter), Am J Dis Child 139:748, 1985.

Sandoval M, Parks C: The evolution to CAPD, Nephrol Nurse 3:27, 1981.

Shurr M, Roy C, Atcherson E: CAPD: Dialysis 365 days a year, J Nephrol Nurs 1(1):20, 1984.

Strangio L: Believe it or not . . . Peritoneal dialysis made easy, Nurs 88 18:43, 1988.

Walsh J, Persons C, Wiech L: Manual of home health care nursing, Philadelphia, 1987, JB Lippincott Co.

Whaley LF, Wong DL: Nursing care of infants and children, ed 3, St Louis, 1987, The CV Mosby Co.

Williamson ML: Reducing post-catheterization bladder dysfunction by reconditioning, Nurs Res 31:28, 1982.

Wong ES: Guidelines for the prevention of catheter-associated urinary tract infections. In Guidelines for the prevention and control of nosocomial infections, Atlanta, 1982, U.S. Centers for Disease Control.

# 30

# BOWEL ELIMINATION

### *OBJECTIVES*

*Mastery of content in this chapter will enable the nurse to:*

- Define key terms.
- Describe factors that impede normal bowel elimination.
- Discuss methods to relieve constipation or impaction.
- Implement the following skills: assist client to use a bedpan, insert a rectal tube, digitally remove stool, administer an enema.

### *KEY TERMS*

| | |
|---|---|
| *Cathartic* | *Flatulence* |
| *Cleansing enema* | *Impaction* |
| *Colon* | *Medicated enema* |
| *Constipation* | *Oil retention enema* |
| *Defecation* | *Rectal tube* |
| *Enema* | *Rectum* |

### *SKILLS*

***30-1*** Assisting the Client to Use a Bedpan
***30-2*** Inserting a Rectal Tube
***30-3*** Removing Fecal Impaction Digitally
***30-4*** Administering an Enema

The act of defecating is a normal body process essential to eliminate wastes from the body. People develop their own normal elimination patterns. However, these patterns may be disturbed by physiologic and psychologic factors. When ill at home or in a health care setting, people may not be able to maintain normal elimination habits and therefore may require a nurse's assistance to help with this body process.

To assist clients with bowel elimination, the nurse must have a clear understanding of normal elimination and factors that create alterations. The nurse must be able to assist immobilized clients with the elimination process by helping them on and off bedpans. Often a nurse may be responsible for collecting stool specimens and ensuring that they are properly handled. If clients have constipation, the nurse may be expected to competently administer enemas or to digitally remove impacted stool. While completing any of these skills, the nurse must always show respect for clients' privacy and emotional needs.

## GUIDELINES

1. Determine a client's normal pattern of bowel elimination and try to accommodate that pattern while the client is in a health care setting. Determine the time the client normally has a bowel movement; offer a bedpan or assist the client to the bathroom at that time. Determine habits that normally precede a bowel movement (e.g., does the client normally defecate after breakfast? Does the client routinely take a stool softener?) Last, respond readily to a client's request to use a bedpan or the bathroom.
2. Provide privacy and try to reduce the client's embarrassment. If possible, the client should be encouraged to use the bathroom. However, if the nature of the illness limits physical activity, ensure as much privacy as possible for the bedpan or bedside commode. Pull the curtains around the bed or close the door to the room. Reduce unpleasant odors of defecation by using room deodorizers or ceiling fans.

   Discuss the client's elimination needs in a professional, open manner. Do not use nonverbal body language that indicates disapproval or revulsion.
3. Be aware of foods that promote normal peristaltic movement, including high-fiber foods such as raw fruit, whole grains, and green leafy vegetables. Some foods such as onions, cauliflower, and beans stimulate peristalsis by forming gas, which may cause discomfort. Determine how various foods affect the client's normal elimination pattern and adjust dietary intake accordingly.

   Immobilized clients should receive foods that promote peristalsis but not those that adversely affect bowel routine.
4. Unless contraindicated, encourage adequate hydration.

Normally, a person should drink 6 to 8 glasses of water per day. Hot fluids are especially effective in softening stool and increasing peristalsis. Fluids help to promote passage of food through the intestines by keeping the bowel contents liquid or soft. A reduction of fluid intake slows the passage of food through the intestines. As peristalsis slows, there is increased absorption of fluid and hardening of feces.

5. Encourage clients to be as active as physically possible. Physical activity promotes peristalsis, whereas immobilization decreases it.
6. Promote client comfort. The client must be in a comfortable position to defecate. Consider individual needs and make adjustments as necessary (e.g., raise the level of the toilet seat, position pillows around the bedridden client to support a sitting position, use the correct type of bedpan, warm a bedpan before giving it to the client).

   The client must also be as free of physical discomfort or pain as possible to avoid suppressing the urge to defecate. The nurse may consider administering a prescribed analgesic about a half hour before the normal time of defecation.
7. Be aware of the side effects of medications the client is receiving. Some drugs may impair the normal elimination pattern by causing diarrhea or constipation. Also, general anesthetic agents used during surgery cause temporary cessation of peristalsis, which can affect the normal elimination pattern after surgery.
8. Consider the developmental changes that affect bowel functioning throughout the life span. For example, an elderly person may become less active, his muscle tone is decreased, and eating patterns change. These factors could result in problems with constipation.

### PREREQUISITE KNOWLEDGE

1. Principles of good body mechanics.
2. Principles of medical asepsis.
3. Anatomy and physiology of the colon.
4. Anatomy and physiology of the central nervous system.

### PREREQUISITE SKILLS

1. Proper handwashing techniques (Chapter 37).
2. Skin and perineal care (Chapter 6).
3. Physical assessment of abdomen (Chapter 13).
4. Vital signs (Chapter 12).
5. Principles of medical asepsis (Chapter 37).
6. Proper body mechanics (Chapter 32).

## *SKILL 30-1* *Assisting the Client to Use a Bedpan*

A client restricted to bed must use a bedpan for defecation. Women use bedpans to pass urine and feces, while men use bedpans only for defecation. Sitting on a bedpan can be extremely uncomfortable. The nurse should help the client assume a position similar to the natural squatting position.

Two types of bedpans are available (Fig. 30-1). The regular bedpan, made of metal or hard plastic, has a curved, smooth upper end and a sharp-edged lower end. The pan is approximately 5 cm (2 in) deep. A fracture pan, designed for clients with body or leg casts, has a shallow upper end approximately 1.3 cm (½ in) deep that slips easily under a client. The upper end of either pan fits under the client's buttocks toward the sacrum, with the lower end just under the upper thighs.

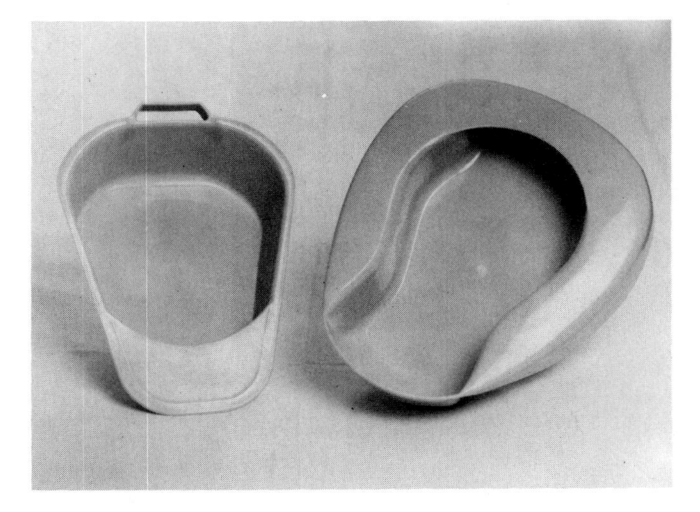

***Fig. 30-1*** Types of bedpans. *Left,* Fracture bedpan; *right,* regular bedpan.

### Purposes

1. Promote independent and normal elimination patterns.
2. Maintain body image.
3. Maintain skin integrity.

## Procedure 30-1

| Steps | Rationale |
|---|---|
| **Assessment** | |
| 1. Assess client's normal bowel elimination habits: routine pattern, effect of certain foods on bowel elimination, effect of stress on normal bowel elimination patterns, current medications, normal fluid intake. | Nurse's competence in managing client's elimination problems depends on thorough understanding of normal elimination and factors that may create alterations. Mass peristalsis is strongest during hour after meal. |
| 2. Assess client to determine level of mobility and amount of assistance required. | Nurse should know how much activity client is allowed. Elderly, obese, debilitated clients may require assistance of two or more nurses to help them on or off bedpans. Assistance from additional personnel promotes safety for client and nurses. |
| 3. Assess if client is allowed to sit up or lie flat when using bedpan. | Determines most appropriate type of bedpan. |
| 4. Assess for rectal or abdominal pain. | Rectal or abdominal pain can reduce client's ability to bear down during defecation. |
| **Nursing Diagnosis** | |
| 1. Cluster data to reveal actual or potential nursing diagnoses: | |
| a. Constipation, related to: ▪ Immobility. ▪ Improper dietary patterns. ▪ Medications. | Prevents client from using toilet facilities. |
| b. Diarrhea, related to: ▪ Fecal impaction. ▪ Nutritional problems. ▪ Medications. | |
| c. Pain, related to: ▪ Abdominal incision. ▪ Rectal irritation. | Pain that impedes client's ability to bear down during defecation can be reduced with timely administration of analgesics. |
| d. Impaired physical mobility, related to: enforced bedrest. | |
| **Planning** | |
| 1. Develop individualized goals for client based on nursing diagnoses: | |
| a. Promote client's comfort. | Proper positioning prevents back strain. |
| b. Promote normal defecation. | Normal squatting position eases defecation. |
| c. Maintain skin integrity. | Correct placement of pan prevents exposing skin to feces. Incontinent stool predisposes client to skin breakdown. |
| 2. Collect appropriate equipment: | Increases efficency. |
| a. Appropriate type of clean bedpan | |
| b. Bedpan cover | |
| c. Toilet tissue | |
| d. Air freshener | |
| e. Specimen container (if necessary) clearly labeled with client's name and identification number | If stool specimen must be obtained, nurse must know what type of specimen is to be collected and appropriate collection container to be used (Chapter 45). Check agency policy. |
| f. Wash basin, face cloths, towels, soap | Used to wash client's hands after wiping the perineal area and to cleanse anal area, thus preventing excoriation and skin breakdown. |
| g. Disposable gloves | Reduces nurse's exposure to blood-borne microorganisms. |
| h. Disposable, padded, plastic pads (incontinence pads) | Protects linen in case of spillage or incontinence. |
| i. Clean draw sheet (optional) | Used to replace linen if client has been incontinent or if bedpan contents are spilled. |
| j. Powder or cornstarch | *Light* application of power or cornstarch on back and buttocks prevents skin from sticking to bedpan. |
| 3. Explain procedure to client, including self-help tips. | Client's knowledge about procedure promotes independence and helps to reduce anxiety. |
| 4. Obtain assistance from additional nursing personnel if client's condition warrants assistance. | Promotes safety for client and nurses by preventing muscle strain. |

| **Steps** | **Rationale** |
|---|---|
| **Implementation** | |
| 1. Wash hands and don gloves. | Reduces transmission of microorganisms. |
| 2. Provide privacy by closing curtains around bed or door of room. | Reduces embarrassment and promotes bowel elimination. |
| 3. Warm bedpan by placing it under warm, running water for few seconds, then dry. Be careful that pan is not too hot. | Metal bedpans are very cold. Warm pan helps client to relax anal sphincter. Although plastic bedpans may not be as cold to touch as metal, it is still wise to warm them before use. |
| 4. Put side rail up on side of bed opposite to working side. | Protects client from falling out of bed when bed is in high position. Client can use side rail to grasp onto and assist self to move about in bed. |
| 5. Position bed in high level according to nurse's height. | Promotes use of good body mechanics and prevents muscle strain for nurse and client. |
| 6. Ensure that client is positioned properly. | Client and bed should bend at corresponding places. |
| *For client who is mobile in bed and can assist with procedure:* | |
| a. Raise client's head 60 degrees. | Prevents hyperextension of back and provides support to upper torso when client raises hips. Sitting position promotes defecation. |
| b. Remove upper bed linens just enough so they are out of the way, but do not unduly expose client. | Prevents embarrassment to client; demonstrates respect for client's sense of dignity. |
| c. Remove bedpan cover and place in accessible location. | |
| d. Instruct client to flex knees and lift hips upward. | Little effort should be required of client, whose body weight is supported by lower legs and feet and upper torso and arms. |
| e. Place hand closest to the client under client's sacrum to assist lifting. At the same time, use other hand to slip bedpan under client. Be sure open rim of bedpan is facing toward foot of bed. (Or have the client use overhead trapeze frame. See Teaching Consideration 1.) | Nurse must ensure that bedpan is placed high enough under buttocks so feces enter pan. Incorrect placement of bedpan can cause discomfort for client and spillage of contents. |
| *For immobile client:* | |
| a. Position bed in flat or level position. | Assists client for whom it is unsafe to exert effort when lifting hips, who must remain flat, who is unable to lift hips to roll onto bedpan. |
| b. Remove top linens as necessary to turn client with minimal exposure. | Prevents embarrassing client; demonstrates respect for client's sense of dignity. |
| c. Ask client to roll into side-lying position or turn client into side-lying position. Simultaneously, place bedpan firmly against client's buttocks and down into mattress. Be sure that open rim of bedpan is facing toward foot of bed. Regular bedpan or fracture pan can be positioned this way. Client then rolls onto back with bedpan securely positioned under buttocks. | Incorrect placement can cause discomfort to client and spillage of contents. |
| d. Client's head can then be raised 30 degrees, unless contraindicated. | Client can assume sitting position unless the condition necessitates maintaining flat position. Sitting position promotes defecation. |
| 7. Ensure that client is comfortable; cover client for warmth. Small pillow or rolled towel placed under lumbar curve of back provides added comfort. | Pain reduces or eliminates urge to defecate, which can result in bowel elimination problems. |
| 8. Ensure that call-bell and toilet tissue are in easy reach for client. | Promotes safety by preventing client from reaching over edge of bed for objects out of reach. |
| 9. Ensure that bed is in lowest position and side rails are up. | Promotes client safety. |
| 10. Allow client to be alone but monitor status. | Reassures client that nurse has not forgotten. Clients may not be able to call nurse; it is nurse's responsibility to assess client's status while on bedpan. |
| 11. Remove gloves and wash hands if tending other clients. | Reduces transmission of microorganisms. |
| 12. Respond to client's call signal immediately. | Promotes client safety. Some clients will try to be independent and remove themselves from bedpan, causing injury or spillage. |
| 13. Position client's bedside chair close to working side of bed. | Can place bedpan and contents on chair after removal from client; adheres to principles of medical asepsis. Also, prevents spillage that could occur if full bedpan was placed on bed. |

| Steps | Rationale |
|---|---|
| 14. Collect basin of warm water. | Allows client to wash hands after wiping perineal area if appropriate; also allows nurse, wearing gloves, to use water to wash client's perineal area if client is unable to wipe thoroughly. |
| 15. Remove upper linens, minimally exposing client. | Prevents undue embarrassment; maintains privacy. |
| 16. Determine if client is able to wipe own perineal area. If not, wearing gloves, using several layers of toilet tissue, wipe from mons pubis toward rectal area (for female client only); dispose of contaminated tissue in bedpan. | Cleansing from area of less contamination to greater contamination reduces spread of microorganisms. |
| 17. Remove bedpan. | |
| *For mobile, independent client:* | |
| a. Ask client to flex knees, placing body weight on lower legs, feet, and upper torso; lift buttocks up from bedpan. At same time, place hand farthest from client on side of bedpan to support it (prevent spillage) and place other hand (closest to client) under sacrum to assist in lifting. After client is completely lifted off bedpan, remove pan and place it on bedside chair. | Nurse should avoid pulling or shoving pan from under hips because this action can pull skin and cause tissue injury. |
| b. Offer client opportunity to wash hands after having wiped perineal area (if appropriate). | Reduces spread of microorganisms. |
| *For immobile client:* | |
| a. Lower head of bed. | Facilitates turning of client. |
| b. Assist client to roll onto side and off bedpan. Hold bedpan steady while client is rolling off it; otherwise spillage will occur. Place bedpan and contents on bedside chair. | Cleansing from area of less contamination to greater contamination reduces spread of microorganisms. Prevents excoriation and skin breakdown. |
| c. Wipe client's anal area with tissue, depositing contaminated tissue in bedpan. If necessary, wash perineal area with warm, soapy water, drying area thoroughly. | Promotes personal hygiene. Excellent time to perform perineal hygiene (Chapter 6). |
| 18. Cover bedpan and contents with bedpan cover as soon as possible. | Reduces spread of offensive odors, thereby reducing embarrassment. |
| 19. Return client to comfortable position, ensuring that bottom linens are clean and as wrinkle-free as possible. If soiled, drawsheet will require changing. | Reduces chance of skin breakdown when bedridden client lies on dry, wrinkle-free linens. |
| 20. Position bed in its lowest position. Ensure that call-bell, drinking water, and desired personal items (e.g., books) are within easy access. | Promotes safety and prevents injury to client. |
| 21. Wearing gloves, empty contents of bedpan into toilet or in special receptacle in appropriate utility room. Spray faucet attached to most institution toilets allows bedpan to be rinsed thoroughly. Client uses same bedpan each time. (If it becomes very soiled, it could be replaced with clean one and soiled one sent for resterilizing). | Should be done as soon as possible to prevent spread of offensive odor. NOTE: Time this is performed depends on situation. However, when done, nurse must not leave client in position that would jeopardize safety (e.g., bed in high position with side rails down). Replacing soiled bedpan reduces growth of microorganisms. Resterilizing prevents spread of microorganisms by cross-contamination. |
| 22. Replace all used equipment in appropriate location. | For easy location when they are subsequently required. |
| 23. Dispose of soiled linens correctly. | Reduces spread of microorganisms. |
| 24. Remove gloves and wash hands. | Reduces spread of microorganisms. |

## Evaluation

| | |
|---|---|
| 1. Assess characteristics of stool. Note color, odor, consistency, frequency, amount, shape, constituents. Also assess characteristics of urine, if client voided in bedpan. | Identifies significant changes or findings, which must be reported to correct member of health care team and recorded on appropriate sheet in client's record. |
| 2. Evaluate client's ability to use bedpan. | Provides continual assessment of ability to use bedpan. |
| 3. Inspect client's skin while removing bedpan. | Liquid stool predisposes client to skin breakdown. |

### *Expected outcomes*

| | |
|---|---|
| 1. Client is able to successfully eliminate body waste products in bedpan. | Indicates normal elimination. |
| 2. Stool is soft and formed. | Normal characteristics. |
| 3. Skin is clear and intact. | There is no irritation. |
| 4. Client eliminates without pain. | There is no rectal inflammation. |

| Steps | Rationale |
|---|---|
| ***Unexpected outcomes*** | |
| 1. Incontinence. | Frequently caused by client's embarrassment in using bedpan or nursing staff delay in offering bedpan. |
| 2. Constipation. | Results from immobility and unnatural position for defecation. |
| 3. Skin breakdown. | Results from irritation of skin caused by urine or fecal materials. |
| 4. Blood in stool. | Important diagnostic finding that requires further testing. |

## Reporting and Recording

| Steps | Rationale |
|---|---|
| 1. Report and record character and amount of stool in nurses' notes. Record urine output if client also voids. | Communicates pertinent information to all members of health care team. |
| 2. Complete laboratory requisition if stool or urine specimen was collected and send to lab. | Proper labelling ensures client receives correct test results. |

## Follow-up Activities

| Steps | Rationale |
|---|---|
| 1. Incontinence: | |
| a. Offer client bedpan every 2 hrs and after meals. | Reduces risk of incontinency. |
| b. Reassess client's elimination pattern. | May reveal cause of incontinence. |
| 2. Constipation: | |
| a. Increase fluids unless contraindicated. | Increases amount of liquid in stool and reduces risk of constipation. |
| b. Provide fruits, vegetables, grains. | Increases bulk in stool and reduces constipation. |
| 3. Skin breakdown: | |
| a. Increase perineal care to every 4 hrs and after each bedpan use (Chapter 6). | Reduces contact between skin and eliminated material. |
| 4. Blood in stool: | |
| a. Test specimen for occult blood in stool (Chapter 45). | Guaiac (hemocult) test verifies substance as blood. |

## Special Considerations

- Barium, used as contrast medium when x-raying bowel, can cause constipation if not evacuated after procedure.
- If client is sharing room, roommates may wish to leave room to provide privacy. Request visitors to leave.
- Extra assistance may be required to turn totally or partially dependent client.
- Nurse must use correct body mechanics while positioning client to prevent muscle strain on client or self.
- Dependent client should be repositioned to ensure proper body alignment (Chapter 33).
- If stool specimen is to be obtained this is appropriate time to collect it.
- If client has urinated in bedpan, amount of urine may need to be measured.

## Teaching Considerations

- Some bedridden clients have overhead trapeze frame connected to bed to help lift themselves on and off bedpan. Teaching this activity can help to maintain strength of client's arms.
- Teach female clients to cleanse from area of less contamination to greater contamination, wiping from front to back. This reduces transmission of anal bacteria to urinary meatus and reduces risk of urinary tract infections.

## Home Care Considerations

- Assess client, primary care giver to determine ability and motivation to carry out care of client.
- Assess client's environment to determine availability of privacy and adequate time to use bedpan.

# SKILL 30-2 *Inserting a Rectal Tube*

A rectal tube is occasionally used for postoperative clients to aid in the relief of abdominal distention secondary to flatus. Such distention frequently occurs after abdominal surgery. The tube may remain in place for several minutes to allow flatus to escape.

### Purpose

1. Relieve abdominal distention secondary to flatus.

## *Procedure 30-2*

| Steps | Rationale |
|---|---|
| **Assessment** | |
| 1. Assess client for abdominal distention, amount of flatus client is passing, existing pathologic condition related to intestinal disorders, bowel sounds. | Indicate extent of distention and/or status of peristalsis. |
| 2. Check physician's order regarding specific instructions for use of rectal tube. | Depending on institutional policy, may or may not be independent nursing function. |
| **Nursing Diagnosis** | |
| 1. Cluster data to reveal actual or potential nursing diagnoses: | |
| a. Pain: related to inability to pass flatus. | Accumulation of gas in intestines can cause abdominal cramping. |
| **Planning** | |
| 1. Develop individualized goal for client based on nursing diagnoses: | |
| a. Relief from abdominal distention. | Passage of flatus relieves distention of intestinal walls. |
| 2. Collect appropriate equipment: | |
| a. Rectal tube of correct size: *Adult:* 22-26 Fr *Infant or child:* 10-12 Fr | Should be large enough to permit passage of flatus but not damaging to external rectal sphincter. |
| b. Water-soluble lubricant | Rectal tube should be well lubricated to prevent injury to rectal mucosa when tube is inserted into rectum. |
| c. Disposable gloves | Prevents transmission of microorganisms from rectal area. |
| d. Waterproof absorbent pad | Protects bed linens if fecal material drains out of rectal tube. |
| e. Tape (Check to see if client has allergies to tape; use appropriate type of tape if allergies are present.) | Prevents tube from being dislodged. Promotes client safety. |
| 3. Explain procedure. | Promotes relaxation and reduces anxiety. Clients should lie quietly in bed while rectal tube is in place to prevent dislodging and irritation of rectal mucosa. |
| **Implementation** | |
| 1. Wash hands. | Reduces transmission of microorganisms. |
| 2. Provide privacy by pulling curtains. | Reduces client's embarrassment; helps client to maintain sense of dignity. |
| 3. Raise bed to appropriate working height. Put side rail up on opposite side of bed. | Promotes good use of body mechanics by nurse and client safety. |
| 4. Ask client to turn onto left side and assume side-lying or Sim's position. Assist client as necessary. Keep client draped except for rectal area. | Allows rectal tube to follow natural curve of rectum and sigmoid colon, thus reducing incidence of irritation or injury to rectal mucosa. |
| 5. Don disposable gloves. | Reduces transmission of microorganisms. |
| 6. Place waterproof pad along buttocks. | Prevents soiling bed linens if fecal material leaks from tube. |
| 7. Lubricate tip of rectal tube generously. | Prevents trauma to rectal mucosa and facilitates easier entry into rectum. |
| 8. Take care to expose client minimally. Gently separate buttocks, locate anus, and ask client to take deep breath and slowly exhale through mouth. | Promotes relaxation and maintains client's sense of self-esteem. Slow exhalation helps to relax external rectal sphincter, thereby decreasing discomfort caused by insertion of rectal tube. |

| Steps | Rationale |
|---|---|
| 9. Insert tip of rectal tube slowly, pointing it in direction of umbilicus. Distance tube can be inserted: *Adult:* 15 cm (6 in) *Child:* 5 to 10 cm (2 to 4 in) | Careful insertion prevents trauma to rectal mucosa. Insertion beyond proper limit or forcing tube can result in bowel perforation. If obstruction or resistance is encountered, *do not continue.* Report problem to appropriate member of health care team. |
| 10. After inserting tube, tape it to lower buttock. | Prevents dislodging. |
| 11. Allow rectal tube to remain in place for no longer than 30 min. Ensure bed is in lowest position. Leave call-bell within easy access. | Can cause irritation to rectal mucosa. Call-bell promotes client's safety. |
| 12. Remove gloves and wash hands after leaving bedside and before removing rectal tube. | Reduces spread of microorganisms. |
| 13. Don gloves and remove rectal tube. Clean client's rectal area. Note characteristics of drainage from rectal tube. | Removes excess lubricant and tape residue. |
| 14. Return client to comfortable position. | Promotes sense of well-being. |
| 15. Dispose of used supplies appropriately. | Reduces transfer of microorganisms. |
| 16. Remove gloves and wash hands. | Reduces transmission of microorganisms. |

## Evaluation

| | |
|---|---|
| 1. Palpate client's abdomen for firmness and distention. Auscultate bowel sounds. | Determines effectiveness in removing flatus and ascertains if procedure must be repeated. |
| 2. Ask client if relief was obtained from rectal tube. | Reveals effect of therapy. |

### *Expected outcomes*

| | |
|---|---|
| 1. Abdomen is flat and soft. | Indicates procedure was effective. |
| 2. Flatus has passed through rectal tube. | |
| 3. Client states that distention and cramping are relieved. | Indicates relief. |

### *Unexpected outcomes*

| | |
|---|---|
| 1. Abdomen remains distended with hyperactive bowel sounds. | Flatus is unrelieved. |
| 2. Client continues to complain of discomfort. | |
| 3. Nurse unable to pass rectal tube. | Possible obstruction due to feces in rectum or unknown pathology. |

## Follow-up Activity

| | |
|---|---|
| 1. Notify physician if rectal tube is unable to be placed due to resistance. | Physician needs to determine cause of resistance. Anal trauma can result from improper insertion of enema tip or rectal tube (Saltzstein, 1988). |

## Recording and Reporting

| | |
|---|---|
| 1. Report and record physical assessment findings before and after procedure and tube insertion. | Communicates data to all members of health care team. |

## Special Considerations

- If this is independent nursing function, nurse should check institution's procedural manual for guidelines.
- Because fluid is not being instilled, rectal tube can be advanced further than when administering enema to reach areas where flatus has accumulated.
- Time between insertions, if flatulence persists, should be determined by physician.

# *SKILL 30-3 Removing Fecal Impaction Digitally*

When an impaction is present, the fecal mass may be too large or hard to be passed voluntarily. Suppositories and enemas may be ordered to promote evacuation of stool. However, if the enema fails to promote defecation, the nurse must use the fingers to break up and remove the fecal mass. This procedure can be very uncomfortable and embarrassing for the client. Excessive rectal manipulation may cause irritation to the mucosa, bleeding, and stimulation of the vagus nerve, which can cause a reflex slowing of the heart rate.

### Purposes

1. Cleanse the rectum of a large or hard fecal mass.
2. Promote the return of normal defecation patterns.

## *Procedure 30-3*

| Steps | Rationale |
|---|---|
| **Assessment** | |
| 1. Assess client to determine: | |
| a. Last bowel movement. | Infrequent defecation increases chances of hard stool forming in rectum. |
| b. Consistency of stool, seepage of liquid stool. This situation may occur particularly in immobilized client. Client seems to continuously or frequently be incontinent of liquid stool. | Symptomatic of an impaction high in colon. Client may be able to pass small pieces of hard stool or there may be episodes of passing small amounts of liquid stool. |
| c. Expression of desire to defecate but inability to do so | Large fecal mass causes rectal distention. |
| d. Complaints of pain when trying to defecate. | Pain often suppresses urge to defecate and compounds problem. |
| e. Abdominal distention, normal bowel patterns, eating habits, exercise pattern or level of mobility, medications, especially narcotic analgesics. | Can contribute to constipation. Nurse must determine if they are contributing factors and attempt to include nursing actions in care plan that may help to prevent situation from recurring. |
| f. Client's normal vital signs. | Vagus nerve stimulation during digital stimulation may result in reflex slowing of heart rate. |
| g. Bowel sounds. | Indicates presence of peristalsis. |
| 2. Check client's record to determine if physician's order exists to remove stool manually. | Because this procedure may involve excessive stimulation of vagus nerve, physician's order must be written in client's record so nurse can perform procedure. |
| **Nursing Diagnosis** | |
| 1. Cluster data to reveal actual or potential nursing diagnoses: | |
| a. Constipation: related to impaction. | Inhibits normal defecation. |
| b. Pain: related to bowel impaction. | Abdominal distention related to fecal mass causes discomfort. Inability to defecate adds to discomfort. |
| **Planning** | |
| 1. Develop individualized goals for client based on nursing diagnoses: | |
| a. Minimize discomfort. | Digital stimulation can be painful, particularly if client is anxious. |
| b. Promote normal defecation. | Clearing of rectum, coupled with proper diet and exercise, aids bowel evacuation. |
| 2. Assemble supplies needed before beginning procedure: | Prevents having to leave client after procedure is started. |
| a. Disposable gloves | Protects nurse's hands and prevents transmission of microorganisms. |
| b. Water-soluble lubricant | Reduces incidence of trauma when gloved finger is inserted into anus. |
| c. Waterproof absorbent pad | Protects bed linens. |
| d. Bedpan | Used to dispose of fecal matter. |
| e. Bedpan cover | Covers bedpan contents during transport to place of disposal. |

| Steps | Rationale |
|---|---|
| f. Bath blanket | Used to drape client during procedure. |
| g. Face cloth, towel, basin | Used to wash client's perineal area when completed. |
| 3. Explain procedure to client. Indicate that manipulation of rectum can cause discomfort. | Promotes client safety. Explanation reduces client's anxiety and helps to acquire cooperation, which is necessary to reduce risk of injury. |

## Implementation

| Steps | Rationale |
|---|---|
| 1. Wash hands. | Prevents transmission of microorganisms. |
| 2. Obtain assistance to help change client's position, if necessary. | Promotes client safety and use of good body mechanics by nurse. |
| a. Assist client to left side-lying position with knees flexed. | Provides access to rectum. |
| 3. Provide for privacy: pull curtains around bed or close door to room, drape bath blanket over client so client is minimally exposed. | Maintains client's dignity. |
| 4. Raise bed to comfortable working height. Put side rail up on opposite side of bed. | Incorporates good body mechanics; promotes client's safety. |
| 5. Drape client's trunk and lower extremities with bath blanket. | Prevents unnecessary exposure of body parts. |
| 6. Place waterproof pad under buttocks. | Prevents soiling of bed linen. |
| 7. Place bedpan next to client. | Bedpan is receptacle for stool. |
| 8. Don disposable gloves. | Reduces transmission of microorganisms. |
| 9. Lubricate glove's index finger with lubricating jelly. | Permits smooth insertion of finger into anus and rectum. |
| 10. Insert index finger into rectum and advance finger slowly along rectal wall toward umbilicus. | Allows nurse to reach impacted stool high in rectum. |
| 11. Gently loosen fecal mass by massaging around it. Work finger into hardened mass. | Loosening and penetrating mass allows nurse to remove it in small pieces, resulting in less discomfort to client. |
| 12. Work stool downward toward end of rectum. Remove small sections of feces. | Prevents need to force finger up into rectum and minimizes trauma to mucosa. |
| 13. Periodically assess heart rate and look for signs of fatigue. Stop procedure if heart rate drops or rhythm changes. | Vagal stimulation slows heart rate and may cause arrhythmias. Procedure may exhaust client. |
| 14. Continue to clear rectum of feces and allow client to rest at intervals. | Rest improves client's tolerance of procedure. |
| 15. After disimpaction, provide washcloth and towel to wash buttocks and anal area. | Promotes client's sense of comfort and cleanliness. |
| 16. Remove bedpan and dispose of feces. Remove gloves by turning inside out and discarding in proper receptacle. | Reduces transmission of microorganisms. |
| 17. Assist client to toilet or clean bedpan. | Disimpaction may stimulate defecation reflex. |
| 18. Wash hands. (Procedure may be followed by enema or cathartic.) | Reduces transmission of microorganisms. |

## Evaluation

| Steps | Rationale |
|---|---|
| 1. Perform rectal examination for stool. | Determines if rectum is clear. |
| 2. Reassess vital signs and compare to baseline values. | Determines extent of vagal stimulation. |
| 3. Assess bowel sounds. | Determines peristaltic activity. |
| 4. Abdomen is soft and nontender. | Discomfort is relieved. |

### *Expected outcomes*

| Steps | Rationale |
|---|---|
| 1. Impacted stool is successfully removed. | Indicates rectum is clear of stool. |
| 2. Client is able to subsequently evacuate stool voluntarily. | Removal of impacted stool should result in normal defecation. |
| 3. Vital signs remain normal. | Absence of vagal stimulation. |

### *Unexpected outcomes*

| Steps | Rationale |
|---|---|
| 1. There is seepage of liquid fecal material. | Indicates continued presence of hard fecal material high in colon. |
| 2. There is bradycardia, decreased blood pressure, decreased level of consciousness. | Vagal stimulation can decrease heart rate, which lowers blood pressure and cardiac output, resulting in decreased level of consciousness. |
| 3. There is presence of blood on gloved finger or in stool. | May result from trauma to rectal mucosa. |

## Recording and Reporting

| Steps | Rationale |
|---|---|
| 1. Report and record client's tolerance to procedure, amount and consistency of stool removed, and adverse effects. | Communicates relevant data to all members of health care team. |

| Steps | Rationale |
|---|---|
| **Follow-up Activities** | |
| 1. Seepage of liquid stool: | |
| a. Contact physician for cleansing enema and cathartics. | Cleansing enemas and cathartics can cause expulsion of fecal mass that cannot be removed digitally. |
| b. Increase intake of fluids orally and parenterally if needed; increase bulk in diet and activity. | May increase peristalsis in colon and reduce constipation. |
| 2. Decreased pulse, blood pressure, level of consciousness: | |
| a. Discontinue procedure. If client experiences shock or cardiac arrest occurs, institute emergency measures. | Relieves vagal stimulation and pulse should elevate. |

### Special Considerations

- Some institutions allow only physician to perform this procedure. Check policy manuals.
- Physician may order oil-retention enema several hours before this procedure to soften stool for easier extraction (Skill 30-4).
- Physician may order analgesic to be administered before procedure.
- Physician may order procedure to be followed by administration of cleansing enema or cathartics.

### Teaching Considerations

- If constipation and subsequent impaction is diet-related, teach client about high-fiber nutritional products to increase bulk.
- If necessary, teach ancillary care givers about the effects of immobility, hydration, nutrition on normal bowel elimination.

## *SKILL 30-4* Administering an Enema

An enema is the instillation of a solution into the rectum and sigmoid colon. Cleansing enemas promote complete evacuation of feces from the colon. They act by stimulating peristalsis through infusion of large volumes of solution. Oil-retention enemas act by lubricating the rectum and colon. Feces absorb oil and become softer and easier to pass. Medicated enemas contain pharmacologic therapeutic agents and are used to reduce dangerously high serum potassium levels, as with a sodium polystyrene sulfonate (Kayexalate) enema, or to reduce bacteria in the colon before bowel surgery, as with a neomycin enema.

The primary reason for an enema is promotion of defecation. The volume and type of fluid instilled breaks up the fecal mass, stretches the rectal wall, and initiates the defecation reflex. Clients should not rely on enemas to maintain bowel regularity because they do not treat the cause of irregularity or constipation. Frequent enemas disrupt normal defecation reflexes, resulting in dependence on enemas for elimination.

Types of enemas:

- *Tap water (hypotonic)*—should not be repeated, because water toxicity or circulatory overload can develop.
- *Physiologic normal saline*—safest. Infants and children can only tolerate this type because of their predisposition to fluid imbalance. If solution is prepared at home, mix 500 ml (1 pint) of tap water with 1 tsp table salt.
- *Hypertonic solution*—useful for clients who cannot tolerate large volumes of fluid because 120 to 180 ml (4 to 6 oz) is usually effective (e.g., commercially prepared Fleets enema).
- *Soapsuds solution*—pure soap may be added to either tap water or normal saline, depending on client's condition and frequency of administration. Use only castile pure soap. Recommended ratio of pure soap to solution is 5 ml (1 tsp) to 1000 ml (1 quart) warm water/saline. Soap should be added to enema bag after water is in place.
- *Oil retention*—an oil-based solution. Permits administration of a small volume, which is absorbed by the stool. The absorption of the oil softens stool for easier evacuation.

### Purposes

1. Relief of constipation.
2. Removal of an impaction.
3. Emptying the bowel in preparation for diagnostic or surgical procedure.
4. Evacuation of feces to institute a program for bowel training for a client with hemiplegia, quadriplegia, or paraplegia.

## Procedure 30-4

| Steps | Rationale |
|---|---|
| **Assessment** | |
| 1. Assess status of client: last bowel movement, level of awareness/developmental stage (so nurse can incorporate appropriate teaching instructions), normal bowel patterns, hemorrhoids, mobility, external sphincter control. | Determines factors indicating need for enema and influencing method of administration. Particular care must be taken when inserting rectal tube to reduce irritation of hemorrhoidal tissues; use generous amount of lubricating jelly to reduce friction when passing rectal tube. |
| 2. Determine client's level of understanding of purpose of enema. | Allows nurse to plan for appropriate teaching measures. |
| 3. Check client's medical record. | Determines purpose of enema administration: preparation for special procedure or reduction of constipation. |
| 4. Review physician's order for enema. | Order by physician is usually required for hospitalized client. Used to determine how many enemas client will require, type of enema to be given (e.g., oil retention, carminative, medicated). Nurse must know this information to organize equipment and prepare client accordingly. |
| **Nursing Diagnosis** | |
| 1. Cluster data to reveal actual or potential nursing diagnoses: | |
| a. Constipation: related to immobility. | Infrequent passage of hard stool impairs normal bowel evacuation. |
| b. Pain: related to bowel distention. | Retained feces distend intestinal walls. |
| **Planning** | |
| 1. Develop individualized goals for client based on nursing diagnoses: | |
| a. Minimize discomfort of procedure. | Anxiety can heighten client's discomfort. Too-rapid infusion of fluid causes cramping. |
| b. Promote normal defecation. | Cleansing of colon, coupled with normal diet and exercise, promotes bowel elimination. |
| 2. Collect appropriate equipment: *Enema bag administration:* | Increases efficiency. |
| a. Enema container (Fig. 30-2) | Contains enema solution. |

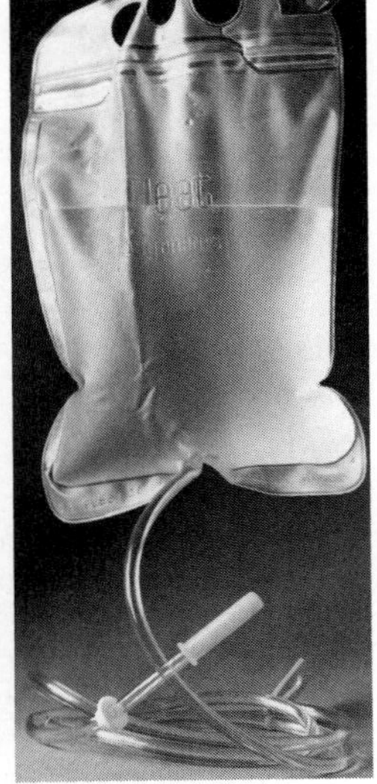

**Fig. 30-2**

| Steps | Rationale |
|---|---|
| b. Tubing and clamp, if not already attached to container, as in disposable set | |
| c. Appropriate size rectal tube:<br>*Adult:* #22-#30 Fr<br>*Child:* #12-#18 Fr | Rectal tubing should be small enough to fit diameter of anus and large enough to prevent leakage of solution from around tube. |
| d. Ordered correct volume of warmed solution:<br>*Adult:* 750 to 1000 ml, 40.5° to 43° C (105° to 109° F)<br>*Child:* 37° C (98.6° F)<br>150 to 250 ml, infant<br>250 to 350 ml, toddler<br>300 to 500 ml, school-age child<br>500 to 700 ml, adolescent | Nurse must be aware of how much fluid a client can safely tolerate; hot water can burn intestinal mucosa; cold water can cause abdominal cramping and is difficult to retain. |
| e. Bath thermometer to measure temperature of solution | If bath thermometer is unavailable, enema solution temperature can be checked by pouring small amount over inner aspect of wrist. |
| f. Lubricating jelly | Reduces friction and irritation to rectal mucosa. |
| g. Waterproof pad | Prevents soiling bed linens. |
| h. Bath blanket | Covers trunk and lower extremities and reduces exposure of body parts. |

| Steps | Rationale |
|---|---|
| i. Toilet tissue | Used to cleanse perineal area after defecation. |
| j. Bedpan, plus commode chair or access to toilet | Depends on client's level of mobility. |
| k. Disposable gloves | Protects nurse's hands and reduces spread of microorganisms. |
| l. Wash cloth, towel, basin | Used to cleanse client after procedure. Depends on client's level of mobility. |
| m. IV pole | Used to hang solution container. |
| *Prepackaged enema* | |
| a. Prepackaged disposable container or prepackaged bottle with rectal tip (Fig. 30-3) | Contains solution and smooth tip for insertion. |
| b. Disposable gloves | |
| c. Lubricating jelly | |
| d. Waterproof pad | |
| e. Bath blanket | |
| f. Toilet paper | |
| g. Bedpan or commode | |
| h. Washcloth, towel, basin | |

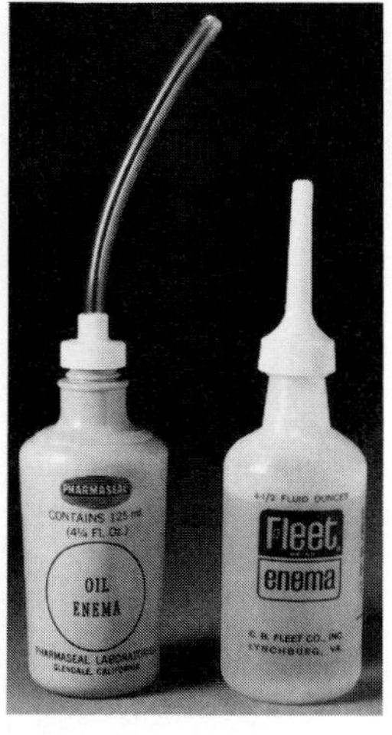


***Fig. 30-3***

| Steps | Rationale |
|---|---|
| 3. Correctly identify client and explain procedure. Check client's identification bracelet to ensure that enema is being given to correct person. | Reduces client's anxiety and promotes cooperation. |
| 4. Assemble enema bag with appropriate solution and rectal tube. | Should be organized before entering client's room. |

## Implementation

| Steps | Rationale |
|---|---|
| 1. Wash hands. | Reduces transmission of microorganisms. |
| 2. Provide privacy by closing curtains around bed or closing door. | Reduces embarrassment for client. |
| 3. Raise bed to appropriate working height for nurse; raise side rail on opposite side. | Promotes good body mechanics and client safety. |
| 4. Assist client into left side-lying (Sims') position with right knee flexed. Children may also be placed in dorsal recumbent position. Position clients with poor sphincter control on bedpan in comfortable dorsal recumbent position. | Allows enema solution to flow downward by gravity along natural curve of sigmoid colon and rectum, thus improving retention of solution. (Clients with poor sphincter control cannot retain all of enema solution.) |
| 5. Place waterproof pad under hips and buttocks. | Prevents soiling of linen. |
| 6. Cover client with bath blanket, exposing only rectal area. | Provides warmth, reduces exposure of body parts, allows client to feel more relaxed and comfortable. |
| 7. Place bedpan or commode in easily accessible position. If client will be expelling contents in toilet, ensure that toilet is free. (If client will be getting up to bathroom to expel enema, place client's slippers and bathrobe in easily accessible position.) | Used in case client is unable to retain enema solution. |
| 8. Don disposable gloves. | Reduces transmission of microorganisms from feces. |
| 9. Administer enema using prepackaged disposable container (Fig. 30-3): | |
| a. Remove plastic cap from rectal tip. Tip is already lubricated, but more jelly can be applied as needed. | Lubrication provides for smooth insertion of rectal tube without causing rectal irritation or trauma (Saltzstein, 1988). |
| b. Gently separate buttocks and locate rectum. Instruct client to relax by breathing out slowly through mouth. | Breathing out promotes relaxation of external rectal sphincter. |
| c. Insert tip of bottle gently into rectum:<br>*Adult:* 7.5 to 10 cm (3 to 4 in)<br>*Child:* 5.0 to 7.5 cm (2 to 3 in)<br>*Infant:* 2.5 to 3.75 cm (1 to 1.5 in) | Gentle insertion prevents trauma to rectal mucosa. |
| d. Squeeze bottle until all of solution has entered rectum and colon. (Most bottles contain approximately 250 ml of solution.) | Hypertonic solutions require only small volumes to stimulate defecation. |
| 10. Administer enema using enema bag: | |
| a. Add warmed solution to enema bag: warm tap water as it flows from faucet, place saline container in basin of | Hot water can burn intestinal mucosa. Cold water can cause abdominal cramping and is difficult to retain. |

| Steps | Rationale |
|---|---|
| hot water before adding saline to enema bag, check temperature of solution with bath thermometer or by pouring small amount of solution over inner wrist. | |
| b. Raise container, release clamp, and allow solution to flow long enough to fill tubing. | Removes air from tubing. |
| c. Reclamp tubing. | Prevents further loss of solution. |
| d. Lubricate 6 to 8 cm (3 to 4 in) of tip of rectal tube with lubricating jelly. | Allows smooth insertion of rectal tube without risk of irritation or trauma to mucosa. |
| e. Gently separate buttocks and locate rectum. Instruct client to relax by breathing out slowly through mouth. | Breathing out promotes relaxation of external anal sphincter. |
| f. Insert tip of rectal tube slowly by pointing tip in direction of client's umbilicus. Length of insertion varies:<br>*Adult* 7.5 to 10 cm (3 to 4 in)<br>*Child* 5 to 7.5 cm (2 to 3 in)<br>*Infant* 2.5 to 3.75 cm (1 to 1½ in) | Careful insertion prevents trauma to rectal mucosa from accidental lodging of tube against rectal wall. Insertion beyond proper limit can cause bowel perforation. |
| g. Hold tubing in rectum constantly until end of fluid instillation. | Bowel contraction can cause expulsion of rectal tube. |
| h. Open regulating clamp and allow solution to enter slowly with container at client's hip level. | Rapid infusion can stimulate evacuation of rectal tube. |
| i. Raise height of enema container slowly to appropriate level above anus: 30 to 45 cm (12 to 18 in) for high enema, 30 cm (12 in) for low enema, 7.5 cm (3 in) for infant. Infusion time varies with volume of solution administered (e.g., 1 L/10 min). | Allows for continuous, slow infusion of solution. Raising container too high causes rapid infusion and possible painful distention of colon. High pressure can cause rupture of bowel in infant. |
| j. Lower container or clamp tubing if client complains of cramping or if fluid escapes around rectal tube. | Temporary cessation of infusion prevents cramping, which may prevent client from retaining all fluid, altering effectiveness of enema. |
| k. Clamp tubing after all solution is infused. | Prevents entrance of air into rectum. |
| 11. Place layers of toilet tissue around tube at anus and gently withdraw rectal tube. | Provides for client's comfort and cleanliness. |
| 12. Explain to client that feeling of distention is normal. Ask client to retain solution as long as possible while lying quietly in bed. (For infant or young child, gently hold buttocks together for few minutes.) | Solution distends bowel. Length of retention varies with type of enema and client's ability to contract rectal sphincter. Longer retention promotes more effective stimulation of peristalsis and defecation. |
| 13. Discard enema container and tubing in proper receptacle or rinse out thoroughly with warm soap and water if container is to be reused. | Reduces transmission and growth of microorganisms. |
| 14. Remove gloves by pulling inside out and discarding in trash can. | Reduces transmission of microorganisms. |
| 15. Assist client to bathroom or help to position client on bedpan. | Normal squatting position promotes defecation. |
| 16. Observe character of feces and solution (caution client against flushing toilet before inspection). | When enemas are ordered "until clear," it is essential to observe contents of solution passed. |
| 17. Assist client as needed to wash anal area with warm soap and water (If nurse administers perineal care, use gloves). | Fecal contents can irritate skin. Hygiene promotes client's comfort. |
| 18. Wash hands. | Reduces transmission of microorganisms. |

## Evaluation

| Steps | Rationale |
|---|---|
| 1. Inspect color, consistency, amount of stool and fluid passed. | Determines if stool is evacuated or fluid is retained. Note abnormalities such as blood or mucus. |
| 2. Assess condition of abdomen. | Determines if distention is relieved. |
| ***Expected outcomes*** | |
| 1. Stool is evacuated. | Solution clears rectum and lower colon of stool. |
| 2. There is clear enema return. | All feces in colon have passed. |
| 3. Abdominal distention is absent. | Gas and feces have been expelled. |
| ***Unexpected outcomes*** | |
| 1. Abdomen is rigid and distended. | Results from perforation of bowel. Enemas should never be given when there is suspicion of appendicitis or bowel obstruction. |
| 2. Abdominal cramping occurs. | Results from volume or inaccurate temperature of instilled solution. |

| Steps | Rationale |
|---|---|
| **Recording and Reporting** | |
| 1. Record pertinent information:<br>a. Type and volume of enema given.<br>b. Characteristics of results. | Communicates pertinent information to all members of health care team. Improves documentation of treatment results. |
| 2. Report failure of client to defecate to physician. | May indicate need for further therapies. |
| **Follow-up Activities** | |
| 1. Stop enema for severe cramping, bleeding, sudden abdominal pain. Physician should be notified for any adverse effect. | Indicates potential trauma to gastrointestinal tract. |

## Special Considerations

- If client cannot control external sphincter, such as a client with paralysis, then client must be placed on bedpan because these clients cannot retain enema solution.
- Administering enema with client sitting on toilet is unsafe because curved rectal tubing can abrade rectal wall.
- For infant or child, nurse may wish to involve parent in procedure.
- "Enema until clear" order means that enemas are repeated until client passes fluid that is clear and contains no fecal matter. Check agency policy, but usually client should only receive three consecutive enemas to avoid disruption of fluid and electrolyte balance.
- Some commercial enema kits come with rectal tube, so ensure that size is appropriate.
- Some disposable kits come with prelubricated tip. Add additional lubricant as needed.
- Children and infants usually do not receive prepackaged hypertonic enemas.

## Teaching Considerations

- Client should be instructed that enemas should not be given to treat cause of constipation.
- If this procedure occurs in client's home, explain procedure to family member.
- For self-administrations, client should be instructed to lie in dorsal recumbent position with knees and hips flexed toward chest.
- Caution client against flushing toilet before nurse has inspected contents.

## Home Care Considerations

- Assess client, primary care giver's ability and motivation to administer enema.
- Assess client's ability to administer enema if enema ordered is self-administrative type.
- Assess client's environment to identify location where enema may be administered with privacy.

## BIBLIOGRAPHY


Alterescu V: Theoretical foundations for an approach to fecal incontinence, J Entero Ther 13:44, 1986.

Aman RA: Treating the patient, not the constipation, Am J Nurs 80:1634, 1980.

Bernstein L, Grieco A, Dete M: Primary care in the home, Philadelphia, 1987, JB Lippincott Co.

Briterman RA: Getting the bowels under control, Emerg Med 19:69, 1987.

Bulau J: Clinical policies and procedures for home health care, Rockville, Md, 1986, Aspen Publishers, Inc.

Burggraf V, Donlin B: Assessing the elderly, Am J Nurse 85:872, 1985.

Davis A, Nagelhout N, Hoban M, Bernard B: Bowel management: a quality assurance approach to upgrading programs, J Gerontol Nurs 12(5):13, 1986.

Erickson EP: Bowel management plan for homebound elderly J Gerontol Nurs 14(1):16, 1988.

Golden S: Nursing a loved one at home, Philadelphia, 1988, Running Press Book Publishers.

Kee JL: Laboratory and diagnostic tests with nursing implications. Norwalk, Conn, 1983, Appleton-Century-Crofts.

Kemp B, Pillitteri A: Fundamentals of nursing, Boston, 1984, Little, Brown & Co, Inc.

Lewis N: Nursing management of altered patterns of elimination, J Home Health Care Pract 1(1):35, 1988.

Lind CD, et al.: Diagnosis: GI complaints in the geriatric patient, Hosp Med 23(10):183, 1987.

Phipps WJ, Long BC, Woods NF: Medical-surgical nursing: concepts and clinical practice, ed 3, St Louis, 1987, The CV Mosby Co.

Potter PA, Perry AG: Fundamentals of nursing: concepts, process, and practice, ed 2, St Louis, 1989, The CV Mosby Co.

Saltzstein R, et al.: Anorectal injuries incident to enema administration: a recurring avoidable problem, Am J Phys Med Rehabil 67:186, 1988.

Tedesco FJ: Laxative use in constipation, Am J Gastroenteral, 80:303, 1985.

Walsh J, Persons C, Wiech L: Manual of home health care nursing, Philadelphia, 1987, JB Lippincott Co.

Whaley LF, Wong DL: Nursing care of infants and children, ed 3, St Louis, 1987, The CV Mosby Co.

# 31
# OSTOMY CARE

## OBJECTIVES

*Mastery of content in this chapter will enable the nurse to:*

- Define key terms.
- Explain differences in color and consistency of drainage based on the location of an ostomy.
- Identify types of bowel and bladder diversions.
- Describe methods used to maintain skin integrity during pouching of ostomies.
- Discuss factors influencing enterostomy drainage.
- Correctly pouch an enterostomy.
- Correctly pouch a urostomy.
- Irrigate a colostomy correctly.
- Catheterize a urostomy correctly.

## KEY TERMS

*Allergen*
*Caput medusa*
*Colostomy*
*Conduit*
*Effluent*
*Enterostomy*
*Fascia*
*Ileostomy*
*Ileal conduit*
*Maceration*
*Peristomal*
*Peritonitis*
*PES*
*Skin barrier*
*Stent*
*Stoma*
*Transilluminate*
*Ureterostomy*
*Urostomy*

## SKILLS

**31-1** Pouching an Enterostomy
**31-2** Irrigating a Colostomy
**31-3** Pouching a Urostomy
**31-4** Catheterizing a Urostomy

Certain diseases or conditions require surgical intervention to create an opening into the abdominal wall for fecal or urinary elimination. A portion of intesti nal mucosa or segment of ureter is brought out to the abdominal wall and a stoma or opening is formed to allow feces or urine to drain.

An *ostomy* is an opening made to allow passage of urine or feces. An enterostomy is any surgical procedure that produces an artificial stoma in a portion of intestine through the abdominal wall. The forms of enterostomy are ileostomy, which involves the ileum of the small intestine, and colostomy, which can involve various segments of the colon (Fig. 31-1). The surgical procedures involved in creating a stoma for urinary drainage are called urostomies and include an ileal conduit and various forms of ureterostomies (Fig. 31-2). A person with an ostomy covers the stoma with a plastic pouch or bag to collect urine or feces.

For diseases or conditions of the bowel, the location of the ostomy determines the consistency of stool passed. An ileostomy bypasses the entire large intestine; thus stools are liquid, frequent, and contain digestive enzymes. The same fecal characteristics hold true for a colostomy of the ascending colon. A colostomy of the transverse colon generally results in a thicker, formed stool. The sigmoid colostomy emits stool almost identical to that normally passed through the rectum.

Ostomies that emit frequent liquid stools create a management challenge. A bag or pouch must be worn at all times. The bag must be emptied throughout the day. Skin care is vital to prevent exposure to fecal irritants.

A colostomy in the transverse colon may be difficult to manage. The client may have to wear a pouch at all times, even though bowel movements occur only two to four times daily. The regularity of bowel movements is unpredictable, so the transverse colostomy cannot usually be

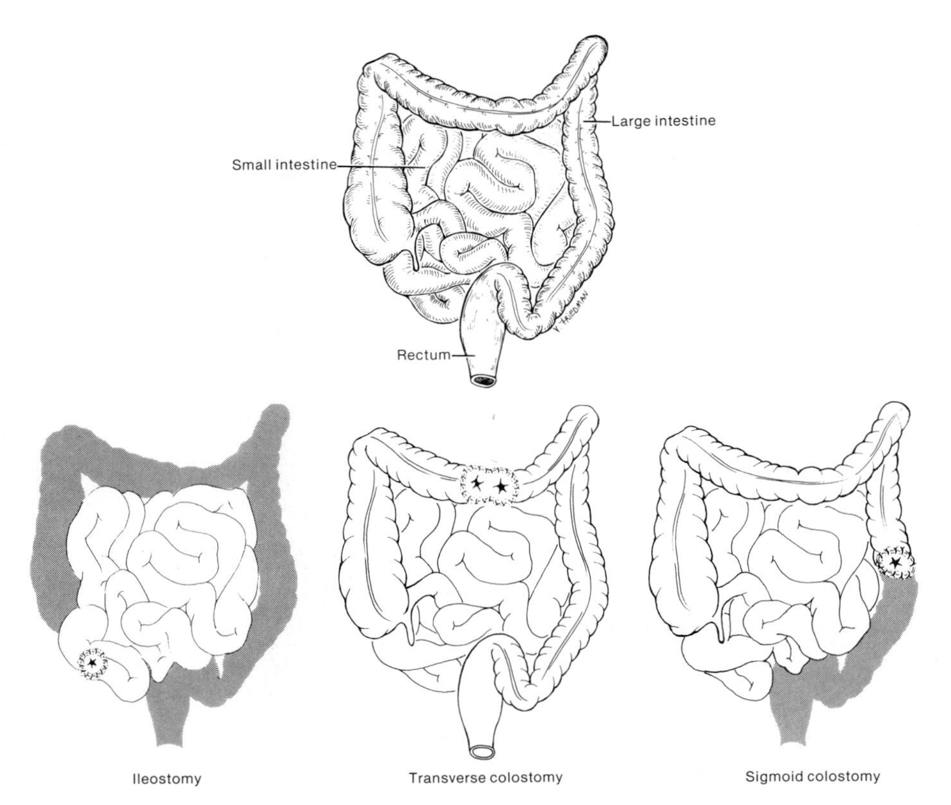


***Fig. 31-1*** Types of enterostomies: ileostomy, transverse colostomy, sigmoid colostomy.

managed by daily irrigation. A sigmoid colostomy can be managed (no fecal output) by daily irrigation because of its anatomical location. Routine irrigations of the descending or sigmoid colostomy, similar to administration of an enema, allow the person to empty the bowel daily and eliminate the need for a pouch. Some clients continue to wear pouches for a feeling of security. Irrigation may be optional.

Fig. 31-2 illustrates an ileal loop and several types of ureterostomies. The ileal loop may be called an ileal conduit, ileal segment, urinary diversion, or urostomy. The surgical procedure may or may not involve cystectomy or removal of the bladder. Usually, 6 to 8 inches of small bowel or ileum is separated from the rest of the bowel. One end is used to create a stoma or opening on the right side; the ureters are implanted into this piece of bowel and a pouch is worn to collect the urine. The rest of the bowel is sutured together so the client has normal bowel movements as before surgery.

A ureterostomy involves bringing the end of one or both ureters directly to the abdominal surface. To avoid the need for two collecting devices, a transureterostomy connects the ureters and brings only one out through the abdominal wall. This procedure is usually performed only in an infant, and a diaper is used. When the child reaches school age, a standard ileal conduit is usually per-

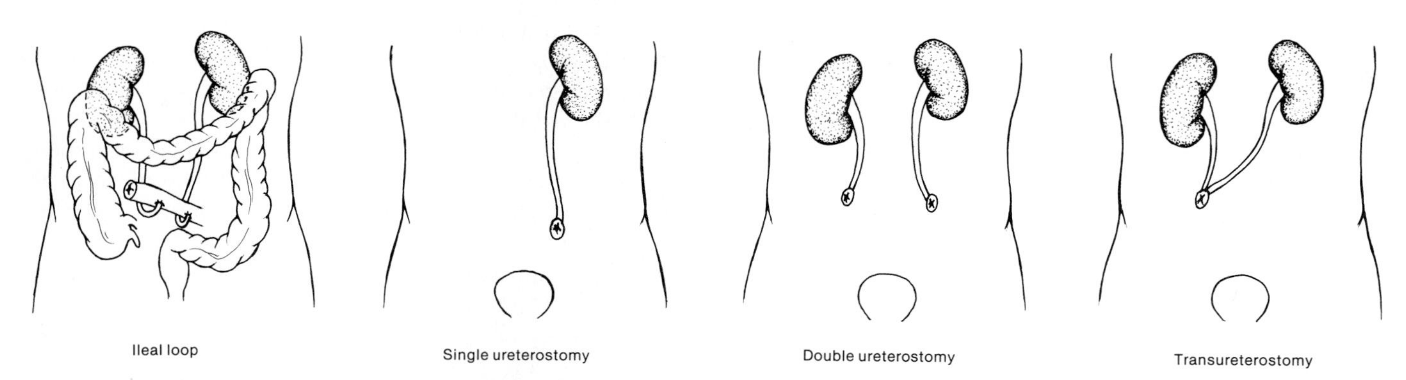


***Fig. 31-2*** Types of ureterostomies: ileal loop, single ureterostomy, double ureterostomy, transureterostomy.

formed because a ureterostomy is difficult to pouch, may become occluded in certain body positions, or may become constricted so there is no urine flow.

A client with a urostomy must wear a pouch because of continuous urinary drainage. There is serious risk of skin breakdown. The client learns to empty the pouch before it becomes heavy with urine because the weight may loosen the seal.

Regardless of the type of ostomy a client may have, a serious threat to body image is created. The client has fears of mutilation, rejection by friends or family, and even a loss of normal sexual function. Foul-smelling odors, spillage, or leakage of liquid stools or urine, and the inability to regulate bowel movements give the client a sense of powerlessness and loss of self-esteem. The nurse must help the client to understand that a normal life-style is possible with an ostomy.

### GUIDELINES

1. Know what type of drainage is expected from the ostomy. Some ostomies, such as an ileostomy, normally have liquid drainage; an ileal conduit, though draining urine, normally has mucus because the bowel still produces mucus.
2. Know the normal elimination pattern so the client can return to or maintain a normal schedule while receiving nursing care.
3. Know the client's routine for self-care of the ostomy. A client who has independently cared for an ostomy should be encouraged to maintain self-care as soon as possible.
4. Know the equipment options available. Many types of equipment are used for different types of stomas, skin irritations, and ostomy drainage.

### PREREQUISITE KNOWLEDGE

1. Principles of medical and surgical asepsis.
2. Anatomy and physiology of the gastrointestinal and urinary tract.
3. The normal process of elimination.

### PREREQUISITE SKILLS

1. Proper handwashing techniques (Chapter 38).
2. Physical assessment (Chapter 13).
3. Preparation of a sterile field (Chapter 38).
4. Donning of sterile gloves (Skill 38-4).
5. Enema administration (Skill 30-4).

## *SKILL 31-1 Pouching an Enterostomy*

Immediately after surgical diversion or removal of a portion of bowel, it is necessary to place a pouchlike appliance over the newly created stoma. The pouch collects all drainage and protects the skin from irritating secretions. A pouch should fit comfortably, cover the skin surface around the stoma, and create a good seal.

The technique of pouching a newly formed stoma differs from those used to pouch a stoma several days or weeks old. The new stoma undergoes varying stages of edema formation during the postoperative healing process. An incision line from the bowel resection may closely approximate the stoma. The stoma itself often has a series of small stitches around its perimeter. A pouch must be applied so it does not constrict the stoma or traumatize healing tissues. Initially, the pouch over a postoperative enterostomy may have to be emptied frequently because of the volume of secretions. It takes several days before a client's normal elimination pattern returns. In the case of an ileostomy, the client will always have frequent drainage. Many types of pouches are available; the urinary pouches have a narrow spout, whereas fecal pouches have a wide opening for easy drainage.

### Purposes

1. Protect the skin from drainage.
2. Contain drainage and odor.
3. Provide visualization of the stoma and sutures.
4. Allow incisional dressing to be changed as needed.

### *Procedure 31-1*

| Steps | Rationale |
|---|---|
| **Assessment** | |
| 1. Check pouch for leakage, length of time in place; ask client about skin tenderness or discomfort. Check stoma for color, healing (Fig. 31-3). Check incision (if present) for relationship to stoma for proper placement of pouch. | To prevent skin irritation, pouch should be changed if leaking, every 4 to 7 days, or when checking skin for irritation. Stoma should be moist, pink to red, well healed. |
| 2. Note drainage from stoma. Keep I & O. | Pouches should be emptied when half to two-thirds full. Ileostomy output is most damaging to skin and appliance. Copious output may result in electrolyte imbalance. |

| Steps | Rationale |
|---|---|

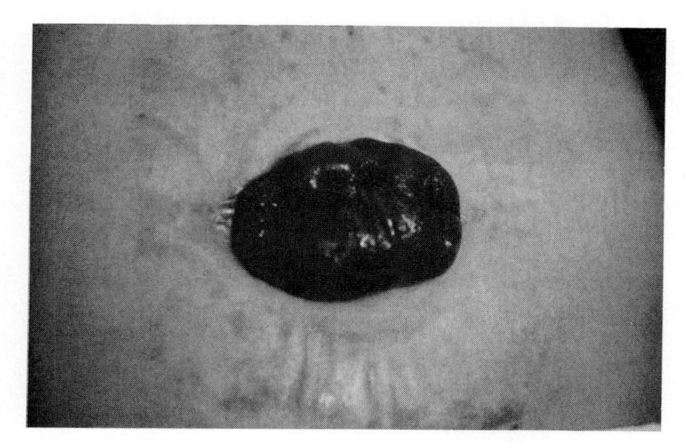

***Fig. 31-3*** Viable, matured transverse loop colostomy and normal peristomal skin.

From Broadwell DC, Jackson BS: Principles of ostomy care, St Louis, 1982, The CV Mosby Co. Reprinted by permission of Hollister Incorporated.

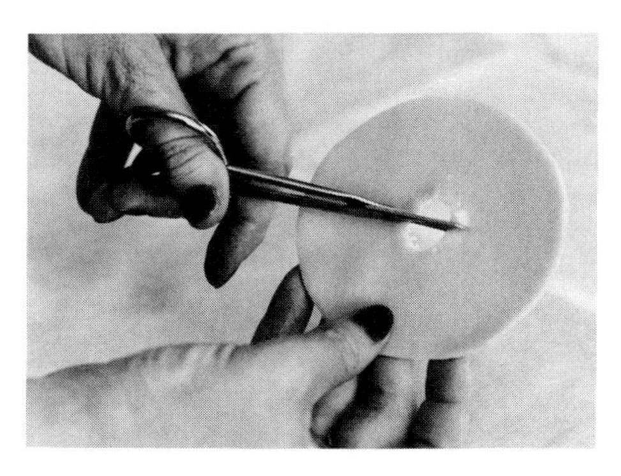

***Fig. 31-4***

| Steps | Rationale |
|---|---|
| 3. Assess site for pouch placement. Allow 1½ to 2 in of skin barrier on all sides of stoma to ensure secure seal. Opening around stoma should be 1/16 to 1/8 in larger than stoma. | Skin barriers ensure secure protective seal. Opening on pouch prevents pressure and trauma to newly formed ostomy. |
| 4. Assess skin around stoma, noting scars, folds, skin breakdown. | Determines need for paste type skin barriers and placement of the pouch. |
| 5. Assess bowel sounds. | Determines presence of peristalsis. |
| 6. Determine client's knowledge and understanding of ostomy. | Assists nurse in determining extent to which client should be encouraged to participate in care. |

## Nursing Diagnosis

| Steps | Rationale |
|---|---|
| 1. Cluster data to reveal actual or potential nursing diagnoses: | |
| a. Potential impaired skin integrity: related to fecal secretions. | Fecal irritants can cause maceration and breakdown of skin. |
| b. Pain: related to abdominal incision. | Incisional discomfort is to be expected after surgery, but incision should be observed for proper healing. |
| c. Knowledge deficit regarding ostomy care: related to inexperience. | Client will require instruction on care and management. |
| d. Alteration in bowel elimination: related to bowel diversion. | Ostomy creates change in passage of stool through intestine. |

## Planning

| Steps | Rationale |
|---|---|
| 1. Develop individualized goals for client based on nursing diagnoses: | |
| a. Skin remains intact without irritation. | Nurse prevents skin breakdown by using correct equipment and applying bag properly. |
| b. Client acquires sense of comfort. | Prompt removal of ostomy drainage prevents skin irritation. |
| c. Client acquires knowledge for self-care. | Client must become independent to perform own ostomy care and show self-acceptance. |
| 2. Prepare equipment and supplies: | |
| a. Skin barrier (unless pouch is manufactured as one piece with barrier) (Cut hole in barrier slightly larger than stoma, 1/16 in larger [Fig. 31-4].) Allow 1½ to 2 in of skin barrier on all sides. | Close fit of barrier around stoma prevents contact of skin with effluent. Barrier cut too tight will loosen from peristalsis of stoma and irritate stoma. Rounded corners adhere better to skin. Maintains skin integrity. |
| b. Prepare ostomy pouch (Cut hole in center of faceplate 1/16 to 1/8 in larger than hole in barrier.) | Avoids risk of cutting stoma. Ensures better seal of barrier. Pouch contains stool; hole allows emptying from bottom without removal of pouch and can be altered to fit changing stoma size. |
| c. Clamp | Pouch should be drainable to avoid frequent changes; therefore requires clamp. |
| d. Gloves (if required by agency policy) | |

| Steps | Rationale |
|---|---|
| d. Hypoallergenic tape (Some one-piece pouches come with tape as part of pouch.) | Used to reinforce appliance to skin barrier. Does not cause skin irritation. |
| e. 4 × 4 gauze sponge or washcloth and towel | |
| f. Washbasin with warm water | |
| g. Skin cleanser (e.g., Sween, Bard) or mild soap (e.g., Ivory, Dial) as long as it contains no oil or lanolin | Used to clean around stoma. |
| 3. Determine optimal time to change ostomy pouch: client is comfortable, client is not eating, before administration of medications that may influence bowel function. When pouch is leaking, change it. | Teaching is ineffective when client is distracted by pain. Signs and smells associated with care are not conducive to appetite. Care goes smoother when done at time when ostomy is least likely to function. Best time for ileostomy is early morning, before meal. |
| 4. Position client supine or standing for pouch application. | When client is lying or standing, there are fewer wrinkles in skin and pouching is easier. When client is sitting, wrinkles are more pronounced. Although care differs, basic principles are same, and review and demonstration aids learning. |
| 5. Explain steps of procedure to client. Ideally client should observe procedure and be involved as much as possible. | Promotes client involvement in care, ultimately preparing self-performance of ostomy management. |

## Implementation

| Steps | Rationale |
|---|---|
| 1. Wash hands, and don gloves, if required. | Reduces transmission of infection. |
| 2. Close room curtains or door. | Provides privacy. |
| 3. Remove old appliance gently as one piece. | Reduces trauma; jerking can cause skin tears. |
| 4. Wash skin gently with skin cleanser or with regular soap and water. Remove all secretions from skin. | Secretions act as irritant to skin. Bacteria in fecal secretions can enter incisional area and cause infection. |
| 5. Rinse soap off thoroughly. Blot dry. | Use of soap could result in film or residue being left behind, causing chemical reactions or burns and premature leakage because of interference with pouch adhesion. Blot dry gently. |
| 6. If blood appears when washing, reassure client that small amount is normal. Continuous bleeding is abnormal after pouch is in place. | Minimizes anxiety because bowel has rich vascular supply. Client must be able to recognize complications. |
| 7. Observe condition of skin, stoma, sutures; encourage client to make these observations at time of pouch change or if skin feels irritated. | Allows for early monitoring of complications. Stoma is at risk for necrosis during first postoperative week; necrosis is evidenced by dark color, dry appearance, failure to bleed, sloughing. Client observation aids in acceptance and adjustment; client develops habit of observing for skin-stomal problems, which are more easily correctable if detected and reported early. |
| 8. If abdominal crease is present or if contour is irregular, use a paste-type barrier. | Provides smooth surface for application of skin barrier and faceplate and better adhesion. |
| 9. Allow paste to dry for 1 to 2 min. | Prevents alcohol burns to skin. |
| 10. Skin must be absolutely dry. May use paper to pat skin or hair dryer set on cool to assist with drying. | Pouch will not stick if skin is damp. |
| 11. Have pouch ready by removing backing from barrier and applying it and pouch as unit to skin after cleaning and drying skin (Fig. 31-5). Smooth out from center. Hold in place firmly for 1 to 3 min. Apply in position that facilitates emptying. | Creates wrinkle-free, secure seal onto skin. |
| 12. Apply hypoallergenic tape as needed to edges of faceplate over skin barrier. Some pouches are manufactured with tape in place. Use of tape may be optional. | Adds extra reinforcement and gives client sense of security. |
| 13. Fold bottom edges of pouch over to fit over clamp. Secure clamp. | Prevents leakage of pouch contents. |
| 14. Dispose of old appliance in plastic bag and in trash chute. (Be sure it is not reusable because it should be washed and reused several times.) | Avoids odors lingering in room, which is unpleasant to client and staff. |
| 15. Wash hands. | Reduces transmission of infection. |

## Evaluation

| Steps | Rationale |
|---|---|
| 1. Note appearance of stoma around skin and existing incision (if present) while pouch is removed and skin is cleansed. | Determines condition of tissues and progress of healing. |
| 2. Reinspect condition of faceplate and skin barrier. | Determines presence of leaks. |
| 3. Ask if client feels discomfort around stoma. | Determines presence of skin irritation. |
| 4. Note client's nonverbal behaviors as pouch is applied. | Indicates level of acceptance of stoma and interest in learning. |
| 5. Ask if client has any questions about pouching. | Determines level of understanding of procedure. |

**Steps** | **Rationale**

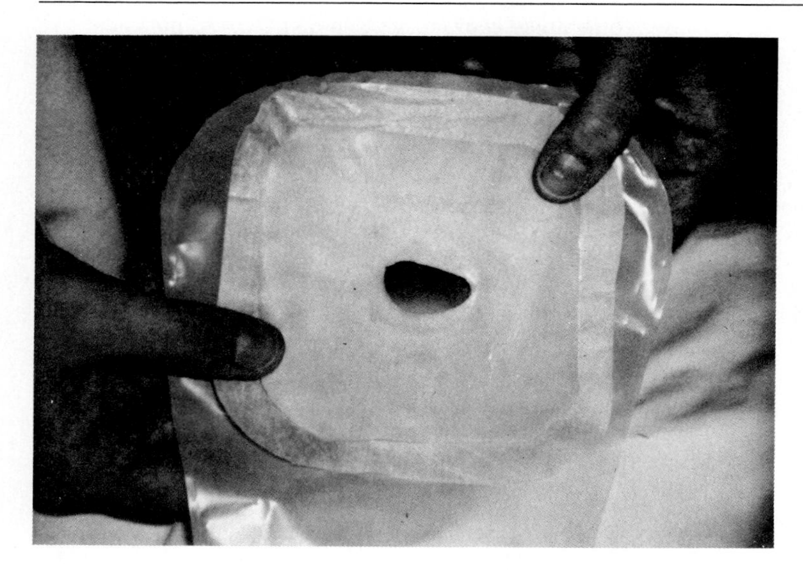

***Fig. 31-5***

Photo from "Managing the ostomy patient" © copyright 1980. Hollister Incorporated. All rights reserved. In Broadwell DC, Jackson BS: Principles of ostomy care, St Louis, 1982, The CV Mosby Co.

### *Expected outcomes*

1. Ostomy is healthy, red, bleeds readily. Skin is healthy, and sutures are intact; stoma is functioning, with moderate amount of liquid or soft stool and flatus in pouch. (Flatus is noted by bulging of pouch in absence of drainage.)

   Normal findings in client with postoperative enterostomy that is healing. Stoma present long-term appears red and moist.
2. Pouch and skin barrier are intact, without leakage.

   Snug seal around stoma has been attained.
3. Client denies discomfort.

   Skin is free of irritation.
4. Client observes stoma and steps of procedure carefully.

   Reveals acceptance of body alteration and interest in self-care.
5. Client asks questions about procedure and may attempt to assist with pouch change.

   Indicates readiness to learn and begin self-care.

## Unexpected outcomes

1. Skin around stoma is irritated.

   May be caused by undermining of pouch seal by fecal contents. An allergic reaction can be manifested by erythema and blistering usually confined to one area immediately under allergen. (Stop use of suspected allergen.) Can result from chemical reaction to cleanser, scrub, soap. Rapid removal of pouch can cause redness or irritation of skin.
2. Mucosal layer of stoma separates from skin.

   May indicate breakdown of sutures or poor healing.
3. Necrotic stoma is manifested by purple or black color, dry instead of moist texture, failure to bleed when washed gently, tissue slough.

   Can reveal inadequate circulation to stoma caused by excessive edema or excessive tension on bowel suture line.
4. Client complains of irritation and burning around stoma.

   Symptoms of skin inflammation, maceration, breakdown.
5. Client refuses to view stoma or participate in care.

   Client denies body change. Each person moves through grieving phase at different rate. Knowledge and acceptance by staff facilitate understanding, acceptance, self-esteem. Acceptance and understanding of significant others should be encouraged by staff because it is integral part of acceptance by client.

## Recording and Reporting

1. Chart type of pouch and skin barrier applied in nurses' notes.

   Documents care provided. Indicates specific pouch and appropriateness for client.
2. Record amount and appearance of effluent in pouch, size of stoma, color, texture, condition of peristomal skin and sutures.

   Determine normal postoperative course. Document ongoing condition of skin.
3. Report abnormal appearance of stoma, suture line, character of effluent to nurse in charge or physician.

   Can indicate need for closer medical and nursing observation.
4. If there is no stool by fifth day, report to physician and nurse in charge. Note abdominal distention and tenderness.

   Can indicate postoperative ileus. May indicate need for irrigation if ordered by physician.

### Special Considerations

- Historically, gloves were not worn when changing pouch to keep the client from feeling they were "dirty" or "messy." Now, with AIDS, many hospital policies require that gloves be worn when personnel change pouch or deal with body fluids.
- Pouch should be used 4 to 7 days if client is not irrigating colostomy.
- If necessary, Stomahesive and other pectin skin barriers may be applied over suture line, if it is not infected, to help to maintain good seal.
- If client is ambulatory, pouch should be directed downward to facilitate emptying; if client is confined to bed or if it is the immediate postoperative period, the pouch should be directed at angle over iliac crest so gravity will take drainage down into pouch. If placed directly to side, pouch will not drain properly.
- Keep in mind that ileostomy drainage is much more corrosive to skin and equipment. Skin barrier should be durable. Ileostomy output is much more liquid and copious. If it exceeds 2400 ml/day, it places client at risk for fluid and electrolyte imbalance; physician should be notified.
- Depending on amount of colon removed or diverted, there may not be effluent drainage for 1 to 5 days or longer; drainage also depends on intake.
- Before disposing of old pouch, save clamp and measure output.
- Client can develop allergy or chemical reaction to substance or piece of ostomy appliance; signs include erythema, blistering, itching. Skin should be observed every time pouch is changed for irritation.
- Notify physician of signs of necrosis or vascular problem with stoma. First 24 to 72 hr presents greatest risk for stoma necrosis, indicated by darkening color. Notify physician of delay in healing or mucosal separation where skin and bowel mucosa do not adhere. Stoma normally bleeds easily. If there is abnormal bleeding (i.e., continuous or more than 100 ml), physician should be informed. Stoma edema is normal part of postoperative healing process.
- Initially, ileostomy output is usually copious, dark green liquid, which then gradually thickens and changes to dark brown. Monitor I & O. Colostomy may not function for first 5 days. Sigmoid colostomy output will initially be diarrhea; it changes to normal, formed stool. Transverse colostomy output is thick liquid, brown, and mushy.

### Teaching Considerations

- Include family members, significant others in teaching because it will increase acceptance of client and in turn client's self-esteem. Client should be encouraged to perform self-care when possible.
- Client's acceptance can be judged by willingness to look at ostomy, questions about bag placement or ostomy function, and requests to participate in care. If apprehensive about touching or looking at ostomy, have client hold 4 × 4 pad over stoma and clean around stoma. This helps to increase client's ability to perform self-care and lessens apprehension.
- Some clients accept stoma very quickly; some never completely accept it. Clients cured of debilitating chronic disease may accept ostomy readily. Clients with diagnosis of cancer may progress more slowly because they also have to work through feelings caused by diagnosis and its threat. Clients who have unexpected ostomy in emergency situation also need more time to adjust. It is important to remember that each client is an individual; Teaching should occur with client's readiness to learn. Eventually, client or family member must be able to change pouch independently.
- Multiple distractions occurring first few days postoperatively may interfere with teaching and learning. Client may benefit from receiving analgesic 30 min before pouch change. Pick an appropriate time for teaching such as several hours after meal or time agreeable to client such as before or after bath.
- Care can be done in one of three positions if physical problems require. Standing position is preferable, but it may also be done lying down or sitting. Sitting position is least desirable because there are usually more wrinkles in skin.
- If client has limitations affecting dexterity, such as arthritis, select clamp and pouch easily managed by client.
- Teach client to avoid soaps containing cold cream, oil, lanolin. Skin must be dry.

## *SKILL 31-2 Irrigating a Colostomy*

Irrigation of a colostomy is a simple procedure that clients can learn. The muscular quality of the colon allows it to be safely irrigated with a relatively large amount of fluid. Clients who perform irrigations at home learn to establish an irrigation procedure so regular emptying of the bowel occurs without stomal discharge between irrigations.

It is rarely necessary to irrigate an ileostomy, except in cases of food blockage. However, a gentle lavage must be performed because of risk of bowel perforation. An ileostomy produces a liquid drainage containing a high concentration of electrolytes such as sodium, chloride, potassium, magnesium, and bicarbonate. Excessive irrigation could lead to a serious fluid and electrolyte imbalance.

When colostomy irrigation is used to manage bowel elimination, the procedure must be performed the same way on a regular basis, either every day or every other day. In addition, it may be several weeks after surgery before any success in effecting bowel regulation can occur. The best candidates for successful irrigation for management seem to be clients who meet five criteria. First, they have a history of regular bowel habits of daily or less than daily frequency. Second, they are able to learn and perform the procedure because they are not hampered by physical or cognitive limitations. Third, they have a good prognosis (i.e., they are not terminally ill). Fourth, they are willing to irrigate the colostomy; some clients have an aversion to inserting anything into their bodies. Last, the best candidates have a bathroom of sufficient size to allow the procedure to be comfortably performed.

### Purposes

1. Manage time of bowel elimination.
2. Stimulate function of the bowel.
3. Cleanse the colon before a procedure or surgery.

## Procedure 31-2

| Steps | Rationale |
|---|---|
| **Assessment** | |
| 1. Assess frequency of defecation and character of stool. | May indicate need to irrigate to stimulate elimination function. |
| 2. Assess time when client normally irrigates ostomy. | Maintains established routine for bowel emptying. |
| 3. In the case of a new ostomy, confer with physician about when irrigations can begin. Obtain written order. | Bowel must be healed totally so irrigating fluid will not cause perforation. Irrigation will initiate attempt to establish regular bowel emptying. This usually occurs 5 to 10 days after surgery. |
| 4. Review orders for diagnostic or surgical procedure involving bowel. | Procedures may indicate need to cleanse bowel of fecal contents. |
| 5. Assess client's understanding of procedure and ability to perform techniques. | Determines level of participation to expect from client and level of explanations nurse should provide and if irrigation is appropriate for client. |
| **Nursing Diagnoses** | |
| 1. Cluster data to reveal actual or potential nursing diagnoses: | |
| a. Colonic constipation, related to: ▪ Bowel diversion. ▪ Dietary changes. | Irrigation will clean bowel; client should follow dietary and exercise guidelines to promote normal defecation. |
| b. Knowledge deficit regarding colostomy care and irrigation: related to inexperience. | Clients with new colostomies must learn to irrigate for home care management. Client will require support and knowledge to attain bowel control and learn irrigation procedure. |
| c. Potential fluid volume deficit: related to excess irrigation. | Can cause extensive loss of liquid fecal material. |
| **Planning** | |
| 1. Develop individualized goals for client based on nursing diagnoses: | |
| a. Promote normal elimination pattern. | Regular irrigation establishes pattern of elimination. |
| b. Improve client's knowledge of irrigation procedure. | Provides client with ability to eventually assume self-care. |
| c. Ensure accurate x-ray studies and safe surgical procedures. | Bowel must be cleansed of all fecal contents for accurate x-ray interpretation and safe exploration of bowel. |
| d. Prevent fluid and electrolyte imbalance. | Excessive fluid instillation or repeated irrigations promotes electrolyte loss. |
| 2. Prepare necessary equipment and supplies: | |
| a. Irrigator with cone (Fig. 31-6) and tube with backflow device 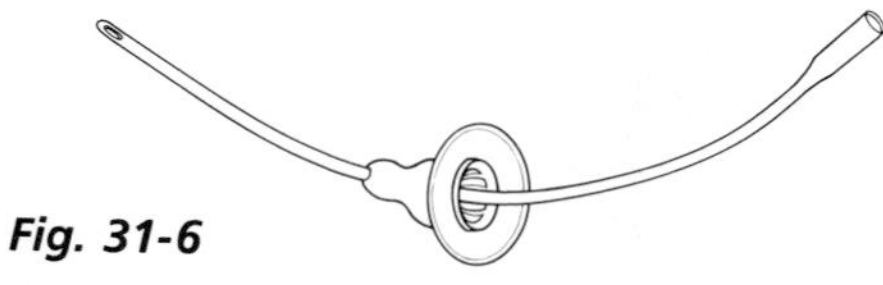 *Fig. 31-6* | Because stoma has no sphincters, there is no way for client to willfully retain solution. Therefore it is given through cone or tube with backflow device, to prevent loss of solution prematurely. |
| b. Irrigation sleeve, with or without belt | Directs flow of irrigating fluid from stoma into toilet. |
| c. Water-soluble lubricant | Makes insertion of cone into stoma easier. Water soluble lubricants will not harm plastic equipment. |
| d. Clamps | May use to close top and bottom of sleeve, allowing ambulation after solution has returned and while awaiting results. |
| e. New appliance or dressing | Will need new pouch or dressing when irrigation completed. |
| f. Bedpan or disposable irrigation sleeve for one-time use | Used if client is confined to bed. Irrigation sleeve can be closed at top and bottom and disposed of after irrigation. |
| g. Washcloth, towel, washbasin, disposable gloves | |
| 3. Prepare client by explaining procedure. Client may feel pressure, fullness, cramping of the bowel but not trauma. | Allays fears by explaining stoma will not be injured and that it has no nerve endings. With care and proper knowledge, irrigation is safe. |

| Steps | Rationale |
|---|---|
| 4. Choose proper times for teaching irrigation (e.g., 1 hr after meal). | Client should be as receptive to teaching as possible. Choosing a time when the irrigation can be done with minimal disturbance will make learning easier. |
| 5. Assist client with positioning: | |
| a. If ambulatory, have client sit on chair in front of toilet. | Allows for directing sleeve into toilet for drainage of fecal contents and irrigant. |
| b. If confined to bed rest, have client lie in comfortable position with head slightly elevated. | Allows client to observe procedure. |

## Implementation

| Steps | Rationale |
|---|---|
| 1. Wash hands. | Reduces transmission of microorganisms. |
| 2. Close bathroom door or room curtains. | Provides privacy. |
| 3. Remove appliance and cleanse skin as in changing enterostomy pouch (Skill 31-1). | Allows access to stoma. |
| 4. Apply irrigation sleeve over stoma. Roll up so bottom just touches water in toilet. (For client confined to bed, clip bottom of drain sleeve.) | Directs flow of stool into toilet. Rolling up sleeve prevents it from stopping up plumbing when toilet is flushed; also keeps end of sleeve clean. |
| 5. Fill irrigator with required solution (usually 500 to 1000 ml tepid water). | 500 to 1000 ml sufficient to distend colon and trigger effective emptying. Cold water results in syncope; hot water could damage stoma or intestine. |
| 6. Attach cone to irrigating tube. Allow fluid to run through entire length of tube. | Flushes air out of tube. Air is expelled from tubing because it causes air lock and will not let solution flow. |
| 7. Apply lubricant to cone. | Prevents trauma to stoma. |
| 8. Insert cone through top of irrigation sleeve. | Ensures containment of irrigation solution and stool within sleeve. |
| 9. Don nonsterile gloves. | |
| 10. Hang irrigation solution so it is between head and shoulder of client. | If solution is too low, it will not flow easily. If too high, it will flow too fast and will not irrigate colon completely. |
| 11. Insert cone gently but firmly into stoma (Fig. 31-7). Stoma should be digitalized before first irrigation with gloved, lubricated finger to determine direction of bowel lumen. | Inserting tube toward direction of bowel facilitates introduction of irrigant. |
| 12. Begin flow of solution and readjust position of cone as necessary. Fig. 31-8 illustrates client performing self-irrigation; gloves are not required. | Nurse may need to redirect cone and slowly increase firmness against stoma until solution flows in easily and leakage around cone ceases. |
| 13. For first irrigation, administer 300 to 500 ml solution; for routine irrigation, administer 500 to 1000 ml solution slowly over 15 min. Pause when client cramps or if there is reflux into irrigation tube. Clamp tube and have client take slow, deep breaths and relax; resume irrigation. Leave cone in place when stopping irrigation. | Usually 500 to 1000 ml is required to empty colon. Pauses prevent premature leakage of solution and keep client comfortable. |

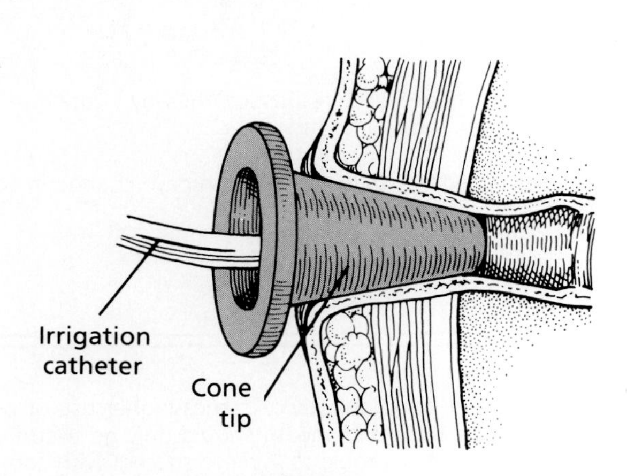

*Fig. 31-7*

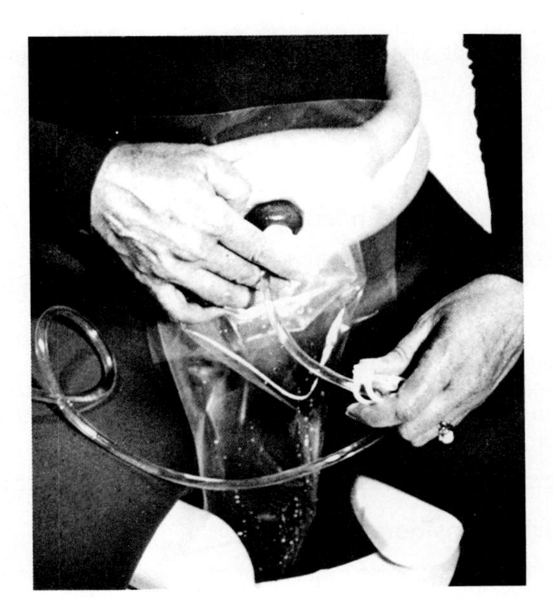
*Fig. 31-8*

| Steps | Rationale |
|---|---|
| 14. When solution flows in, clamp tubing and remove cone. Should obtain small gush of fluid almost immediately. | Clamping tubing prevents return of flow into irrigator. Sleeve should be placed properly to avoid gush over top. |
| 15. Clamp top of sleeve. | Prevents leakage at top. |
| 16. When most of solution has returned, clamp bottom of sleeve. Usually, most active return occurs first 15 to 20 min, although it continues for another 30 to 45 min. | Allows ambulation; prevents leakage. Procedure takes approximately 1 hr, and client may become tired of sitting. |
| 17. When all fecal results have returned, rinse sleeve with water and special liquid cleanser and remove. Then wash sleeve with soap and water rinse and air dry if it is not disposable. | Prevents sleeve from deteriorating, permitting reuse. Controls odor. |
| 18. Apply new pouch according to procedure 31-1. If client experiences no discharge between irrigations, small 4 × 4 dressing may be applied over stoma. | Avoids leakage, skin problems, soiling of clothes. |
| 19. Dispose of equipment no longer needed. | Reduces transmission of microorganisms. |
| 20. Remove gloves and wash hands. | Prevents cross-contamination. |

## Evaluation

| | |
|---|---|
| 1. Inspect volume and character of fecal material and fluid that returns after irrigation. | Determines if irrigant is retained. If client is dehydrated, bowel may absorb irrigation solution. Character and amount of stool reveals success in cleaning bowel or stimulating elimination. |
| 2. Note client's response during irrigant infusion. Ask if cramping or abdominal pain are felt. | Reveals tolerance of irrigation. |
| 3. Ask client to describe steps of procedure. | Evaluates client's learning. |

### *Expected outcomes*

| | |
|---|---|
| 1. Irrigation bag returns volume of fluid equal to amount of irrigant instilled. Large amount of formed stool returns. | Normal defecation with full return of irrigating solution. |
| 2. Client denies abdominal pain or cramping. | Irrigant instilled at proper rate and volume. |
| 3. Client understands and can perform procedure with minimal assistance. | Client is ready to perform self-care. |

### *Unexpected outcomes*

| | |
|---|---|
| 1. Client is unable to retain sufficient solution to result in desired effect. | May be caused by nausea, instillation that is too rapid, or water that is too cold. |
| 2. Client retained all of solution with no returns. | Frequently seen when client is dehydrated or tense. Very common on day of discharge. |
| 3. Client experiences pain during insertion and during or after administration. Abdomen is hard and painful with no bowel sounds. There is no output through ostomy except for small amount of blood. | Symptoms of perforation. |
| 4. Client experiences diarrhea or spillage between irrigation. | May be due to medication or diet. If obstructed, may put out some liquid stool, but irrigation does not return properly. Spillage between irrigation may indicate that problem cannot be managed by irrigation. |
| 5. Client unable to explain or perform procedure. | Indicates additional instruction needed. |

## Recording and Reporting

| | |
|---|---|
| 1. Record procedure, volume, and type of solution administered, amount and type of return, client's tolerance in nurses' notes. | Documents procedure and results of therapy. Data used for comparison for future irrigations. |
| 2. Record reapplication of pouch and condition of stoma and skin in nurse's notes. | Documents procedure. Data used to compare change in condition of skin or stoma. |
| 3. Report symptoms of extreme discomfort, onset of severe diarrhea, poor results, excessive bleeding to nurse in charge or physician. | Indicates need for additional therapy. |

## Special Considerations

- Debilitated, confused, or unconscious clients are at risk for constipation or impaction. Irrigate if obstruction is suspected only with physician's order.
- Use of tube and backflow device carries higher risk of perforation of colon. Tube and sheath should only be used if necessary and if client is unable to achieve success with cone irrigations.

- Some clients feel more secure with small, closed pouch; others use gauze pads or 3-M colostomy dressings or stoma caps with charcoal gas filters. Normally irrigation is done in bathroom.
- Reassure client that slight bleeding is normal because of rich blood supply of colon.
- Clients that develop diarrhea should discontinue irrigation until stool thickens. Diarrhea can be caused by diet, medication, radiation, chemotherapy, bacterial infection.

### Teaching Consideration

- Client should be instructed in community resources such as ostomy groups, enterostomal therapists, home health agencies, suppliers.

### Home Care Considerations

- Assess home environment for bathroom privacy for ostomy care.
- Establish scheduled time for ostomy care during which there will be no interruptions.
- Assess bathroom for towel rack or other device from which irrigation device may be hung; device should hang at shoulder level.
- Drain sleeve may attach with belt, stick on, or attach to flange or skin barrier. For home care, two-piece system is easier to use and more cost effective. Two-piece systems such as Hollister and Squibb-Surfit allow client to remove pouch from flange on barrier wafer and apply snaps of irrigation sleeve. These fit on like Tupperware lids.

## *SKILL 31-3 Pouching a Urostomy*

Because urine flows continuously from a urinary diversion, a urostomy pouch is usually placed over the opening immediately after surgery. Placement of the pouch may be more difficult than the enterostomy because urine flow keeps the skin moist.

The stoma of the urostomy is normally red or pink. It is made from a portion of the gastrointestinal tract. Ideally the stoma should protrude ½ to ¾ inches above the skin. An ileal conduit is usually located in the right lower quadrant; a colon conduit is usually located in the left lower quadrant. Ureterostomies are usually performed in infants, and a conduit is performed when the child approaches school age.

### Purposes

1. Protect the skin from drainage.
2. Contain urine.
3. Accurately measure output for fluid replacement.
4. Provide visualization of the stoma and sutures.
5. Allow the incisional dressing to be changed as needed.
6. Prevent backflow pressure on the ureterobowel anastomosis by use of an antireflux-type pouch.

## *Procedure 31-3*

| Steps | Rationale |
|---|---|
| **Assessment** | |
| 1. Assess existing pouch for leakage, noting condition of underlying skin, stoma, surgical incision. Stoma should be changed if client reports skin is irritated or if pouch has been in place 4 to 7 days. | Determines need to change pouch. Condition of stoma and incision are assessed for complications of healing. Pouch is changed often enough to allow for assessment of peristomal structures and to avoid leakage and contamination of incision. |
| 2. Observe output from stoma, stents, ureteral catheters. Stents are usually left in place 7 to 10 days. | Urinary output should be monitored on all postoperative urostomy clients to monitor renal status. Stents or catheters are used to maintain patency of urinary drainage system and stabilize anastomosis of ureters into segment of bowel while healing. |
| 3. Assess abdomen for most appropriate placement of pouch. Avoid areas with creases or irregular contour if possible. | Ensures secure fit with minimal chance of leakage. Should allow 1½ to 2 in of skin barrier on skin on all sides of stoma for secure seal. Should not overlap sutures of incision, if possible, to avoid unnecessary tension on incision. |
| 4. Assess client's knowledge of purpose of pouching procedure. | Determines need for education on self-care. Response may also reveal level of acceptance of ostomy. |

| Steps | Rationale |
|---|---|

## Nursing Diagnosis

| Steps | Rationale |
|---|---|
| 1. Cluster data to reveal actual or potential nursing diagnoses: | |
| a. Alteration in urinary elimination: related to urostomy. | Creation of ostomy bypasses normal urinary tract. |
| b. Knowledge deficit regarding care of ostomy: related to inexperience. | Clients with newly formed ostomy or poor understanding of ostomy care techniques require instruction. |
| c. Potential alteration in skin integrity: related to urinary drainage. | Continuous flow of urine from stoma may cause maceration and breakdown of skin. |
| d. Body image disturbance: related to stoma. | Change in normal urinary tract with creation of stoma poses threat to body image. |

## Planning

| Steps | Rationale |
|---|---|
| 1. Develop individualized goals for client based on nursing diagnoses: | |
| a. Client attains sense of comfort. | Keeping skin clean and dry prevents irritation. |
| b. Skin remains intact and free of irritation. | Proper pouching technique protects skin from urinary drainage. |
| c. Client acquires knowledge to perform self-care. | Demonstration of good techniques helps client to learn home care. |
| d. Body image improves. | Client is encouraged to participate in self-care to improve self-acceptance. |
| e. Maintain urinary drainage. | Observation of urethral stents until removal at 7 to 9 days and an accurate I & O are vital in maintaining proper functioning of urostomy. |
| 2. Prepare equipment and supplies: | |
| a. Skin barrier | Protects skin and facilitates healing of peristomal breakdown or irritation. Allows more secure seal of pouch. |
| b. Urinary drainage pouch, prepared by cutting hole in center of faceplate $\frac{1}{16}$ to $\frac{1}{8}$ in larger than hole in skin barrier | Contains urine; allows emptying from bottom through valve and hookup to straight drainage; is cut to fit size of and prevent injury to stoma. Skin barrier and pouch should be put together as unit to make application easier. |
| c. Bath basin with water, soap, towel | Used to cleanse skin around stoma. |
| d. Hypoallergenic tape | Used for reinforcement of pouch faceplate as needed. Minimizes skin irritation. |
| e. Gauze (4 × 4 pads) | Used to absorb urine while changing pouch. Also used to wash around stoma. |
| f. Sterile gloves (optional) and sterile forceps | Used to maintain asepsis if stents are present. Stents can be handled comfortably with forceps. |
| g. Karaya powder | Used to treat skin if irritated. |
| h. Trash bag | |
| 3. Plan to change pouch when client is comfortable: early morning, after administration of pain medication; afternoon may be more convenient if family member or significant other is to be included. | Demonstration and teaching are ineffective when client is distracted by pain. Early morning urine output is reduced, thus reducing moisture on peristomal area during pouch change. Moist skin prevents secure skin seal. If pouch leaks, change it as soon as possible. Including family member or significant other helps client's body image. |
| 4. If client is unable to participate with pouch change, place in supine position. If client is able to observe or participate, place in supine or standing position. | In lying and standing positions, there are fewer wrinkles in skin and pouching is easier. If client is too weak to stand, supine position may allow better view. |
| 5. Explain procedure and encourage client to view stoma and ask questions during pouch change. Encourage participation. | Client must view and learn about ostomy to incorporate it as part of self-image and attain adjustment and acceptance. Participation will help to increase self-esteem. |

## Implementation

| Steps | Rationale |
|---|---|
| 1. Wash hands. | Reduces transmission of microorganisms. |
| 2. Close curtains or room door. | Provides privacy. |
| 3. Have all equipment ready. Pouch should be prepared and paper covering removed. | Ensures smooth change with minimal leakage of urine from stoma. |
| 4. Apply gloves. | Prevents transmission of infection. |
| 5. Remove old appliance as one piece, gently pushing skin away from equipment. Stabilize stent with forceps when removing pouch. | Reduces trauma; jerking can cause skin tears. Ureteral catheters or stents are used by surgeons to protect bowel-to-ureter anastomosis. Dislodging can injure anastomosis or interfere with patency. |

**Steps** | **Rationale**

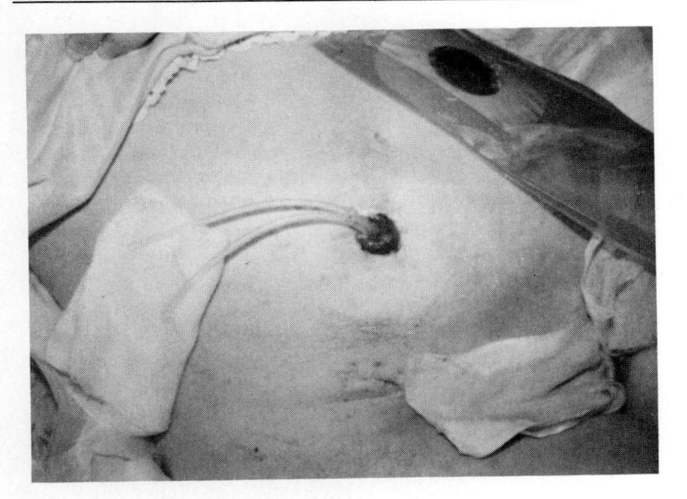

***Fig. 31-9*** Urinary stoma with stents.

From Broadwell DC, Jackson BS: Principles of ostomy care, St Louis, 1982, The CV Mosby Co.

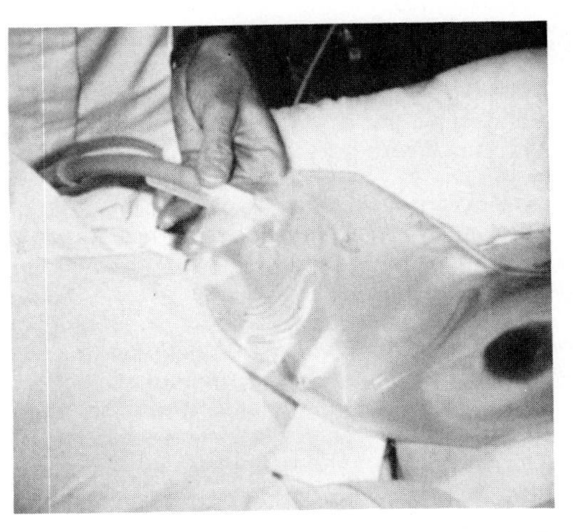

***Fig. 31-10*** Urinary pouch connected to bedside drainage collector.

From Broadwell DC, Jackson BS: Principles of ostomy care, St Louis, 1982, The CV Mosby Co.

6. Apply gauze directly over stoma if stents are out of place. If stents are in place, use gauze under stents as shown in Fig. 31-9.
   Contains urine flow from stent and stoma while pouch is off, keeping skin dry.
7. Cleanse skin with water or use soap without oil and lanolin.
   Soaps with oil and lanolin leave film and prevent adherence of skin barrier.
8. Dry skin thoroughly.
   If skin is moist, pouch will not stick and form good seal.
9. Check skin for irritation while keeping dry gauze near stoma.
   If skin is irritated, use light dusting of Karaya powder and remove excess.
10. Inspect abdominal surface for creases, scars, unusual contours. If irregular surface is present near stoma, fill in with paste to form skin barrier.
    Provides smooth, flat surface for pouch application.
11. Tap stoma twice after checking skin and when ready to apply pouch if stents are out. (NOTE: minimal bleeding of stoma is normal.)
    Causes stoma to contract and gives extra few seconds to apply pouch and keep skin dry.
12. Apply pouch, observing and instructing client on condition of stoma, skin, equipment. Encourage participation and questions.
    Involvement of client in instruction increases likelihood that self-care will be assumed.
13. Apply hypoallergenic tape over edge of pouch faceplate to skin as needed. Apply like picture frame and place small wedge of tape in each corner to reinforce.
    Reinforces seal. Normally pouch adhesive extends over wafer.
14. Attach pouch to straight drainage with valve open when client is in bed or at night after client is home (Fig. 31-10).
    Rapid and constant flow of urine during IV infusion results in frequent emptying of pouch and risk of overfilling. Overfilling can break pouch seal. Continuous drainage to gravity container prevents problems.
15. Dispose of old appliance and soiled gauze in proper receptacle outside room. Remove gloves; wash hands.
    Reduces transmission of infection and avoids unpleasant odors in room.

## Evaluation

1. Note condition of stoma, skin, suture line during pouch change.
   Determines status of integument and progress of wound healing.
2. Evaluate character and volume of urinary drainage.
   Determines if stoma or stents are patent. Character of urine can reveal degree of concentration and alterations in renal function.
3. Note client's or family member's willingness to view stoma and ask questions about procedure.
   Determines level of acceptance and understanding of stoma care and pouch application.
4. Ask if client notes discomfort around stoma.
   Evaluates presence of skin irritation.

| Steps | Rationale |
|---|---|
| ***Expected outcomes*** | |
| 1. Stoma is healthy, red, bleeds minimally. Peristomal skin is clean and intact. Sutures are intact, and incision is well approximated. | These are normal findings in client with postoperative urostomy that is healing. Long-term ostomy stoma is red and moist. |
| 2. Urine draining from stoma and stents is clear and pale yellow with mucous shreds. Volume is approximately equal to fluid intake. | This is normal renal output with patent drainage system. Mucous shreds are normal if bowel is used as conduit; if stents or catheters are present, urine should flow from them without difficulty. |
| 3. Client, family member is willing to view stoma and asks questions about procedural steps. | Shows acceptance of body image change and willingness to learn self-care. |
| 4. Client denies discomfort. | Skin around stoma is free of irritation. |
| ***Unexpected outcomes*** | |
| 1. Skin is irritated (reddened and tender) in peristomal area. Maceration or breakdown may be present. | Can be caused by allergy to pouch and soaps, chemical reaction, mechanical trauma, infection. Opening of pouch may be too large, allowing urine to pool on skin. If opening is too small, may have leakage because of poor seal. |
| 2. Sutures are pulled, and incision is open. | Can be caused by mechanical trauma to wounds, abdominal distention from inability to pass flatus, poor healing due to radiation effect or diabetes. |
| 3. Stoma is necrosed (blackened and dry) and fails to bleed when cleansed. | Results from inadequate blood supply to bowel segment, which can be caused by pouch or barrier being too constrictive, stoma being excessively edematous, or excessive suture line tension on bowel and ureters. |
| 4. There is mucosal separation of stoma from skin. | Can be caused by nutritional deficiency and impairment in wound healing. |
| 5. There is no urine output for several hours or urine output is less than 30 ml/hr. | Findings may reveal obstruction of urinary outflow (with risk of backflow toward kidney) or reduced renal function. There may be leak at anastomosis of ureter to bowel. Client may be dehydrated. |
| 6. Client or family member fails to observe stoma, ask questions, participate in procedure. | Process of grieving has not allowed client to accept body image change and implications of illness. Each person progresses at different rate. |
| 7. Client reports burning discomfort around stoma. | Indicates peristomal skin irritation. |
| **Recording and Reporting** | |
| 1. Record pouch change, condition and appearance of stoma and peristomal structures, character of urine in nurse's notes. | Documents procedure. Provides data on condition of urostomy for future comparisons. |
| 2. Record urinary output on intake and output flow sheet. | Provides ongoing record of fluid balance and functioning of urostomy. |
| 3. Note client's and family's reaction to stoma and procedure in nurses' notes. | Allows staff to provide continuity of care while supporting client and family through grieving and education. |
| 4. Report abnormalities in stoma or peristomal structures and absence of urinary output to nurse in charge or physician. | Even though changes may require immediate surgical intervention or other forms of medical therapy, the sooner proper treatment is initiated, the less chance there will be that the client will have to return to the operating room. |

## Special Considerations

- In immediate postoperative period, stoma should be observed for necrosis or separation.
- Bleeding of stoma over long period is abnormal and may indicate stomal injury or bleeding problem.
- During hospitalization, pouch should be connected to straight drainage when client is in bed.

## Teaching Considerations

- Instruction should be given according to client's ability and readiness.
- Include families and significant others in teaching if possible.
- Those who need assistance in activities of daily living because of physical or mental limitations should be encouraged to do as much for themselves as possible. Nurse must arrange to provide instruction when those who will assist the client at home are available. Self-care and independence are goals.
- Client should be instructed to observe skin for irritation and allergic reactions.
- Choose equipment clients can easily and comfortably handle.

## Home Care Consideration

- Assess home environment to assist client in arranging for privacy, adequacy of lighting, equipment storage, and emergency backup procedures.
- At home, pouch should be unclamped and connected to straight drainage at night.

# SKILL 31-4 Catheterizing a Urostomy

When it is necessary to obtain a specimen from a urostomy, the best way to do it is to insert a catheter into the stoma. Obtaining a specimen from the pouch does not provide a true finding.

The nurse may be apprehensive about causing injury to the client when performing this procedure. However, with the use of strict aseptic technique, catheterization is relatively safe and easy. To prevent trauma of tissues, the nurse should understand how the stoma and ureteral tract are constructed. Because clients with urostomies are at risk for reflux of urine into the stoma, kidney infections are common. Thus catheterization is often performed as a regular means to screen for infection and is the only way to obtain an accurate culture and sensitivity specimen (Chapter 45).

The risk for reflux of urine can be reduced by attaching straight drainage to the urinary pouch during sleep or when high urinary output is expected. Incorrect bag placement, stagnant urine, or large volumes of urine promote backflow into the urostomy stoma. A client must understand the importance of draining urostomy pouches frequently and using clean aseptic technique during stomal and skin care.

### Purposes

1. Determine whether bacteria are present in the urine in sufficient amounts to indicate kidney infection.
2. Assess flow of urine from the urostomy.

## Procedure 31-4

| Steps | Rationale |
|---|---|
| **Assessment** | |
| 1. Determine need to obtain a sterile specimen from urostomy; note signs and symptoms of urinary tract infection such as elevated temperature, chills, foul-smelling urine. | Urostomy may pose risk for reflux of urine back to kidneys and concomitant infection. May be performed as part of routine testing. |
| 2. Obtain physician's order for catheterization. | Invasive procedure requires physician's order. |
| 3. Assess client's understanding of need for procedure and risk of infection. | Determines willingness to cooperate and indicates extent of explanation nurse should provide. |
| **Nursing Diagnosis** | |
| 1. Cluster data to reveal actual or potential nursing diagnoses: | |
| a. Knowledge deficit regarding risk of infection: related to unfamiliarity with procedure. | Client requires instruction to facilitate cooperation and to become prepared to recognize signs and symptoms of infection. |
| b. Potential for infection related to: ▪ Invasive procedure. ▪ Urinary reflux. | Nurse follows preventive steps to avoid introducing microorganisms into urinary system; results of testing after catheterization allows for diagnosis of infection. |
| **Planning** | |
| 1. Develop individualized goals for client based on nursing diagnoses: | |
| a. Urine remains free of infection. | Procedure performed aseptically. |
| b. Client understands risks for urinary infection. | Prepares client to manage urostomy without introducing infection. |
| 2. If possible, provide hydration to client 1 hr before procedure, especially if NPO previous night for diagnostic testing. | Increases volume of urine production. |
| 3. Prepare needed equipment: | |
| a. Plastic bag | For disposal of old appliance and contaminated materials. |
| b. Sterile 4 × 4 gauze pad | Contains urine while pouch is removed and specimen is obtained. |
| c. Supplies that are separate or in sterile catheter kit: | |
| ▪ Sterile, water-soluble lubricant | Facilitates insertion of catheter. |
| ▪ Cleansing solution (povidone-iodine swabs) | Used to rid surface of stoma of contaminants. |
| ▪ Sterile gloves | Used to maintain sterility. |
| ▪ Sterile specimen container | |
| ▪ Sterile rubber catheter | |
| d. Bath towels | Used to help to maintain dryness and cover client. |

| Steps | Rationale |
|---|---|
| e. Properly prepared label and laboratory requisition | Ensures correct identification of specimen |
| f. Equipment for applying new appliance (Skill 31-3) | Client requires appliance to contain urine and protect skin. |
| 4. Explain procedure to client. Also attempt to obtain specimen when client is normally due to change pouch or as close to this time as possible. | Reduces fear and ensures cooperation in obtaining specimen. Changing appliance too frequently can result in skin breakdown. |
| 5. Position client supine. | Facilitates maintaining sterile field and entering stoma without undue difficulty. |

## Implementation

| Steps | Rationale |
|---|---|
| 1. Wash hands. | Reduces transmission of microorganisms. |
| 2. Close room door or bedside curtain. | Provides privacy. |
| 3. Open sterile kit and supplies. Set up equipment within easy reach. | To avoid excessive leakage and client discomfort, have equipment readily available to save time in catheterizing and repouching. |
| 4. Open sterile gloves, use inside of wrapper or inside of kit for sterile field. Prepare 4 × 4 gauze pad and catheter on sterile field. Squeeze small amount of lubricant on section of field. | Avoid contamination; sterile technique is essential. |
| 5. Fold down linen so only area of pouch is revealed. | Maintains client's comfort, avoiding unnecessary exposure of body parts. |
| 6. Place on towel across pubic region and toward side nearest stoma. Place second towel at client's side. | Absorbs urine not contained by gauze; avoids soiling linen and client. Helps to maintain privacy. |
| 7. Remove old appliance gently; cleanse skin. | Protects skin from trauma. |
| 8. Don sterile gloves. | Reduces risk of contamination. |
| 9. Cleanse stoma and surrounding 3 in of skin with gauze moistened with cleanser (povidone-iodine), starting from stoma and working outward *in a circular motion.* Repeat two times. | Removes surface bacteria from skin, moving from area of least bacteria out. |
| 10. Allow some urine to flow out of stoma. | Initial droplets of urine may contain some povidone-iodine. Povidone-iodine will alter results if in specimen. |
| 11. Lubricate catheter with water-soluble lubricant. | Lubricant facilitates passage of catheter through stoma. |
| 12. Remove lid from specimen container. Place distal end of catheter into specimen container. Hold catheter in container with nondominant hand. | Only a few drops of urine will be obtained; care should be used to direct all into container. |
| 13. With dominant hand, insert catheter into stoma gently. Redirect course as needed. Use gentle but firm pressure similar to regular catheterization of urethra. Have client cough or turn slightly to facilitate passage of catheter (most conduits are 15 to 20 cm (6 to 8 in. long). | Care must be taken to avoid perforation. Some resistance is common at muscle level in conduit. Allow catheter to enter slowly. |
| 14. Maintain container below level of stoma. Have client cough as needed. Urine may flow around and through catheter. This is acceptable, but only urine from catheter is desired. Normally, wait 5 min; if no urine is in container, pinch catheter and remove; direct urine "trapped" in catheter into cup. | Facilitates drainage of urine. Only 3 to 15 ml of urine are needed for studies. |
| 15. After withdrawing catheters, place 4 × 4 gauze pad over stoma. | Gauze contains urine, keeping skin dry. |
| 16. Apply lid to specimen container. | Prevents accidental spillage. |
| 17. Remove gloves and label specimen with required information. | Labeling ensures acceptance of specimen by laboratory and processing. |
| 18. Dispose of equipment used for obtaining specimen. Reapply new pouch (Skill 31-3). | Pouch necessary to protect skin; proper technique important to avoid skin and stoma irritation. |
| 19. Remove old pouch and equipment and dispose of properly. | Avoids unpleasant odor in room and eliminates source of infection. |
| 20. Wash hands. | Avoids transmission of infection. |
| 21. Send specimen to laboratory at once. | Allowing urine to sit for long periods at room temperature affects results. |

## Evaluation

| Steps | Rationale |
|---|---|
| 1. Refer to laboratory report and compare results of culture and sensitivity with normal expected findings. | Determines presence of infection. If contamination appears likely, second specimen will need to be sent. |
| 2. Evaluate condition of skin and stoma of client. | Determines condition of skin to detect onset of complications. |

| Steps | Rationale |
|---|---|
| 3. Have client explain need for procedure and possible risks of infection. | Evaluates client's learning. |
| ***Expected outcomes*** | |
| 1. There is no bacteria in urine. | No infection is present. |
| 2. Skin and stoma are clean, intact, without signs of irritation or breakdown. | Urinary drainage system intact and functioning well. |
| 3. Client describes risks of and techniques to prevent infection. | Demonstrates client's learning. |
| ***Unexpected outcomes*** | |
| 1. Culture reveals evidence of bacteria in urine. | Infection is present. |
| 2. Skin or stoma reveal complications. | Indicates infection, allergy, urine leakage, mechanical trauma. |
| 3. Client unable to describe risks of infection. | Indicates need for further instruction. |
| **Recording and Reporting** | |
| 1. Record time specimen collected, client's tolerance of procedure, appearance of urine, skin, stoma. | Documents procedure. Provides data for future comparison. |
| 2. Report results of laboratory test to nurse in charge or physician. | Infection will require supportive therapies. |

## Special Considerations

- Obtain only small amount of urine when inserting catheter if urostomy is functioning properly.
- Client may want to remove and apply appliance by self while nurse does actual catheterization. Client confused or unable to cooperate may require restraint to avoid contamination of specimen.
- Allow a 30 min wait for specimen, especially if client has been NPO for intravenous pyelogram or other test, if possible. If client complains of severe pain or if urine flow is diminished, perforation of conduit or severe infection may be indicated.
- Slight bleeding from newly formed ostomy is normal. Avoid forcing catheter because conduit has no sensory fibers. Bleeding from older urostomy indicates traumatic catheterization.
- Some pouches are reusable and expensive. Always check with client regarding what to do with appliance and assist as needed.
- Be patient and do not expect to obtain specimens within a short period.

## Teaching Considerations

- Explain common symptoms of urinary tract infection: flank pain, dark or bloody urine, foul-smelling urine, fever, nausea.
- Encourage client to maintain fluid intake and notify physician if symptoms of infection develop.
- Instruct primary care giver about aseptic technique.
- Teach proper care of urine specimen.
- Allow primary care giver to return several demonstrations.

## BIBLIOGRAPHY

Airey S, et al.: An innovation in stoma care, Nurs Times 84(6):56, 1988.

Alterescu KB: Colostomy, Nurs Clin North Am 22:281, 1987.

Alterescu V: The ostomy, Am J Nurs 85:1241, 1985.

Alterescu V: The ostomy: what do you teach the patient? Am J Nurs 85:1250, 1985.

Belliveau P, Rolstad BS, Rothenberger DA: Ileal-anal reservoir: an alternative to permanent ileostomy, J Enterostom Ther 9:44, 1982.

Broadwell DC, Jackson BS: Principles of ostomy care, St Louis, 1982, The CV Mosby Co.

Brunner LS, Suddarth DS: Textbook of medical-surgical nursing, ed. 6, Philadelphia, 1989, JB Lippincott Co.

Dudas S: Rehabilitation concepts of nursing, J Enterostom Ther 11(1):6, 1984.

Erickson PJ: Ostomies: the art of pouching, Nurs Clin North Am 22:311, 1987.

Gillies DA: Body image changes following illness and injury, J Enterostom Ther 11(5):186, 1984.

Golden S: Nursing a loved one at home, Philadelphia, 1988, Running Press Book Publishers.

Hampton BG: Colostomy clues for the urological nurse, J Urol Nurs 7(1):357, 1988.

Kelly M: Adjusting to ileostomy, Nurs Times 83(33):29, 1987.

Kobza L: Impact of ostomy on the spouse, J Enterostom Ther 10(2):54, 1983.

Lind CD, et al.: Diagnosis: GI complaints in the geriatric patient, Hosp Med 23(10):183, 1987.

May HJ: Information for ileostomy patients, J Enterostom Ther 9:10, 1982.

Morris EJ, et al.: Urinary findings in 20 asymptomatic patients with ileal conduit, J Enterostom Ther 9(2):24, 1982.

Postier RG, O'Malley V, Pruitt L: Continence preserving operations for ulcerative colitis and multiple polyposis, J Enterostom Ther 11:237, 1984.

Prasad ML: Surgical options for the patient with inflammatory bowel disease, Nurs 88 10(3):141, 1988.

Rodriquez DB: Radiotherapy and the ostomy patient, J Enterostom Ther 8:21, 1981.

Smith DB: The ostomy: how is it managed? Am J Nurs 85:1246, 1985.

Spencer MM, Barnett WO: The continent ileal reservoir (Kock pouch): a new approach, J Enterostom Ther 9:8, 1982.

Spencer MM, Barnett WO: Strategic use of whole-bowel irrigation, Emerg Med 19(18):37, 1987.

Sullivan JW, Grabstold H, Whiteman WF Jr: Complications of ureteroileal conduit with radical cystectomy: review of 336 cases, J Urol 124:797, 1980.

Sullivan JW, Grabstold H, Whiteman WF Jr: Suprapubic cystostomy, Emerg Med 19(15):86, 1987.

Thomas D, et al.: Management of the temporary loop ileostomy following colectomy, mucosal proctectomy, and ileal pouch-anal anastomosis, J Enterostom Ther 14(5):194, 1987.

Thompson J, et al.: Mosby's manual of clinical nursing, ed 2, St Louis, 1989, The CV Mosby Co.

Tosh N: Life following a ileostomy: a personal account, Nurs 87 3(21):790, 1987.

Tranes S: Ileal pull-through surgery, Nurs 87 17(11):92, 1987.

# UNIT X

# POSTURE, MOBILITY, AND AMBULATION

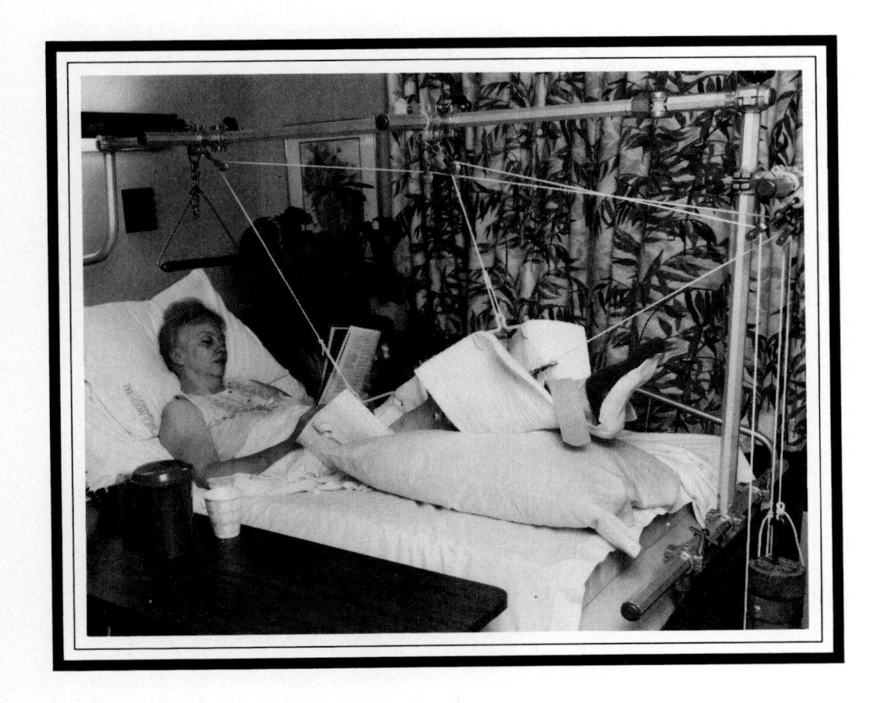

*When a client's health status is impaired, the ability to maintain posture, to move freely, or to ambulate may be restricted. It is the nurse's responsibility to assess the client's mobility status and to design nursing interventions to optimize posture, mobility, and ambulation and thereby reduce hazards from permanent or temporary immobility resulting from illness, trauma, or congenital defects.*

*This unit is divided into five chapters, each of which presents nursing measures designed to improve or maintain posture, mobility, or ambulation. Chapter 32, "Body Alignment and Mechanics," describes nursing skills to improve body alignment and mechanics of the client and the nurse. Chapter 33, "Transfer and Positioning," presents techniques for safely transferring a client from the bed to chair or bed to bed and various therapeutic positions used for clients with restricted mobility. Chapter 34, "Orthopedic Measures," details casting procedures and skills for care of the client in traction. Chapter 35, "Beds, Frames, and Mattresses," describes therapeutic beds used for immobilized, burned, or traumatized clients. Chapter 36, "Exercise and Ambulation," presents nursing therapies to improve mobility and ambulation, including the use of adaptive aids such as crutches.*

# 32

# BODY ALIGNMENT AND MECHANICS

### OBJECTIVES

*Mastery of content in this chapter will enable the nurse to:*

- Define key terms.
- Describe normal body alignment for standing, sitting, and lying down.
- Assess for alterations in body alignment.
- Describe the correct procedures for lifting.

### KEY TERMS

*Base of support*
*Body alignment*
*Body mechanics*
*Center of gravity*
*Gravity*
*Line of gravity*
*Posture*
*Weight*

### SKILLS

**32-1** Maintaining Proper Body Alignment
**32-2** Performing Correct Lifting Techniques

Coordinated body movement involves the integrated function of the skeletal system, skeletal muscles, and nervous system. Because these systems cooperate so closely in the mechanical support of the body, they can almost be considered a single functional unit. The skeleton and skeletal muscles contribute to the body's shape in length and width and to the individual distribution of fat determining the type of body construction.

The skeleton is the supporting framework of the body and consists of 206 bones. The four types of bones in the skeleton are long, short, flat, and irregular. Long bones contribute to height (femur, fibula, and tibia in the leg) and length (phalanges of the fingers and toes). Short bones occur in clusters and, when combined with ligaments and cartilage, usually permit movement of the extremities; two examples of short bones are the carpal bones in the foot and the patella in the knee. Flat bones provide structural contour, such as bones in the skull and the ribs in the thorax. Irregular bones make up the vertebral column and some bones of the skull, such as the mandible.

The muscles concerned primarily with movement are located near the skeletal region, where leverage results in movement. Leverage occurs when specific bones, such as the humerus, ulna, and radius, and the associated joints, such as the elbow joint, act together as a lever. Thus force is applied to one end of the bone to lift a weight as another point tends to rotate the bone in the direction opposite that of the applied force. The muscles that attach to the bones of leverage provide the necessary strength to move the object.

Muscles associated primarily with maintaining posture are short and appear featherlike because they converge obliquely at a common tendon. Muscles of the lower extremities, trunk, neck, and back are concerned primarily with posture. These muscle groups work together to stabilize and support body weight when the person is standing or sitting. The work of these muscles allows the individual to maintain a sitting or standing posture over time.

Movement and posture are regulated by the nervous system. The major voluntary motor area, located in the cerebral cortex, is the precentral gyrus, or motor strip, and crosses at the level of the medulla. Thus the motor fibers from the right motor strip initiate voluntary movement for the left side of the body, and vice versa for the right side.

Body mechanics are the coordinated effort of the musculoskeletal and nervous systems to maintain proper balance, posture, and body alignment during lifting, bending, moving, and performing activities of daily living. Proper body mechanics reduce the risk of injury to the musculoskeletal system. Body mechanics also facilitate body movement so a person can carry out a physical activity without using excessive muscle energy.

The knowledge and application of body mechanics enables the nurse to care safely for clients with varying levels of independent mobility throughout the life span. Correct body mechanics protect the client and nurse from injury to their musculoskeletal systems.

Correct application of body mechanics enables the nurse to use certain muscle groups when completing nursing care. Thus the nurse is able to position, transfer, and ambulate clients safely and efficiently. In addition, knowledge of correct body mechanics provides the nurse with a basis for assessing a client's body alignment and position and further reduce the risks from immobility.

### GUIDELINES

1. Know the physiological influences on body alignment and mobility that affect clients throughout the life span. The greatest impact of the physiologic changes on the musculoskeletal system is observed at the beginning and later years of the life span.
2. Know pathologic conditions that affect a client's alignment and mobility. Postural abnormalities, congenital or acquired, can affect body mechanics. For example, a client with severe kyphosis may not be able to lift an object safely because the center of gravity is out of alignment. Second, diseases that affect bone formation, such as osteoporosis, alter alignment and mobility. Third, degenerative joint diseases, impaired muscle development, and central nervous system damage can alter normal alignment and mobility; as a result, the client's risk of musculoskeletal injury is increased.
3. Know the client's medical history and medication taken that can affect body alignment. Specific medications such as tranquilizers can affect coordination, and steroids can affect bone formation.
4. Control factors that can indirectly affect body mechanics by altering the safety of the environment. Cluttered hallways and bedside areas increase the client's risk of falling (Chapter 4).
5. Use an organized, systematic approach to assess and improve body mechanics. Continued nursing assessment promptly identifies risks to normal alignment and promotes immediate nursing interventions.

### PREREQUISITE KNOWLEDGE

1. Normal growth and development.
2. Hazards of immobility.
3. Anatomy of the musculoskeletal system.
4. Physiology of positioning and movement.

### PREREQUISITE SKILL

1. Physical assessment (Chapter 13).

## *SKILL 32-1 Maintaining Proper Body Alignment*

Body alignment refers to the condition of the joints, tendons, ligaments, and muscles in various body positions. Whether a person is standing, sitting, or lying, there are correct and incorrect body alignments. During correct body alignment, no excessive strain is put on the joints, tendons, ligaments, or muscles, and muscle tone is adequate.

Proper body alignment contributes to body balance. An improperly balanced body displaces the center of gravity and increases the force of gravity, and the person can fall. Body balance is achieved when a wide base of support exists, the center of gravity falls within the base of support, and a vertical line can be drawn from the center of gravity through the base of support.

Body balance also is enhanced by posture. The more correct the posture, the greater is the balance. Clinical nursing activities require the nurse to maintain proper body alignment.

### Purposes

1. Identify altered body alignment.
2. Provide an opportunity for the client to observe posture.
3. Identify the client's learning needs for maintaining correct body alignment.
4. Identify trauma, muscle damage, or nerve dysfunction.

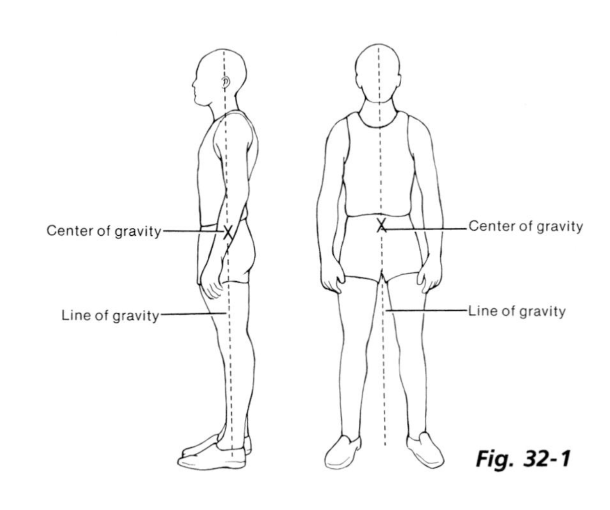

***Fig. 32-1***

## *Procedure 32-1*

| Steps | Rationale |
|---|---|
| **Assessment** | |
| 1. Observe alignment of client in standing, sitting, or lying position. | Determines if client assumes proper body alignment. |
| *Standing* (Fig. 32-1): | |
| a. Head is erect and at midline. | Maintains correct body alignment in relation to normal center of gravity. |
| b. Shoulders and hips are straight and parallel. | Maintains correct body alignment in relation to body's normal center of gravity. |
| c. Vertebral column appears straight when viewed posteriorly. | Maintains correct body alignment in relation to body's normal center of gravity. |
| d. Lateral observation indicates head is erect and spinal curves are aligned in reverse **S** pattern. | In reverse **S** pattern, cervical vertebrae are anteriorly convex, thoracic vertebrae are posteriorly convex, and lumbar vertebrae are anteriorly convex. |
| e. Lateral observation documents that abdomen is comfortably tucked in and knees and ankles are slightly flexed. | Maintains abdomen and trunk directly over body's center of gravity. |
| f. Arms are comfortably positioned at each side. | |
| g. Feet are placed slightly apart, with toes pointed forward. | Produces broad base of support and improves balance. |
| h. Center of gravity is located midline and forms vertical line from middle of forehead to midpoint between feet. Pregnant woman's center of gravity is more anterior to adapt to normal weight gain and growing fetus. Thus she leans slightly backward, and spinal column is slightly swaybacked (Fig. 32-2). | Laterally, line of gravity runs vertically from middle of skull to posterior one third of foot. |
| *Sitting* (Fig. 32-3): | |
| a. Head is erect, and vertebrae are in straight alignment. | |
| b. Body weight is evenly distributed on buttocks and thighs. | Prevents increased pressure over bony prominences and reduces damage to underlying musculoskeletal system. |
| c. Thighs are parallel and in horizontal plane. | Maintains flexion of hips and provides broad base of support. |
| d. Both feet are supported on floor, and ankles are comfortably flexed. | Maintains plantar flexion and reduces risk of foot-drop. |
| e. If client is unable to flex one or both knees, nurse should make sure that elevated legs are supported and ankle is flexed. | |
| f. A 2.5 to 5 cm (1 to 2 in) space is maintained between edge of seat and popliteal space on posterior surface of knee. | Ensures that no excessive pressure is put on popliteal artery or nerve, which could decrease circulation or impair nerve function. |
| g. Client's forearms should be supported on armrest, in lap, or on table in front of chair. | Reduces force of gravity on shoulder joint and chance of accidental shoulder dislocation. |
| *Lying* (Fig. 32-4): | |
| a. Client is in lateral position, with positioning supports removed. | Allows nurse to observe spinal alignment and any pressure points. |
| b. Client's body should be supported by adequate mattress. | Reduces strain on joints and ligaments. |

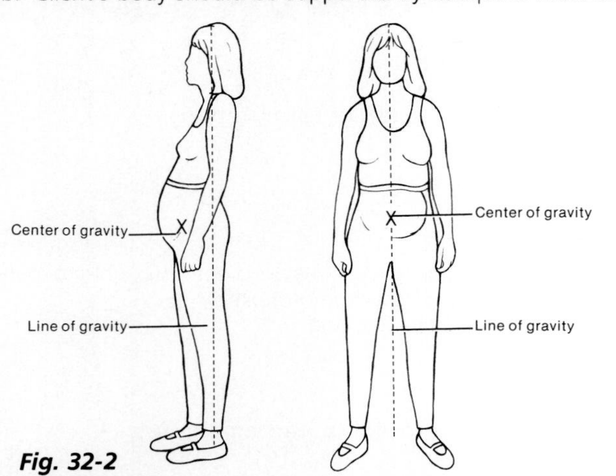

*Fig. 32-2*

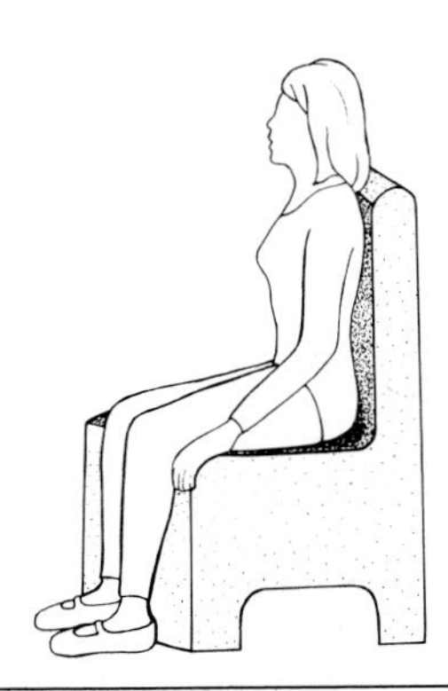
*Fig. 32-3*

| Steps | Rationale |
|---|---|

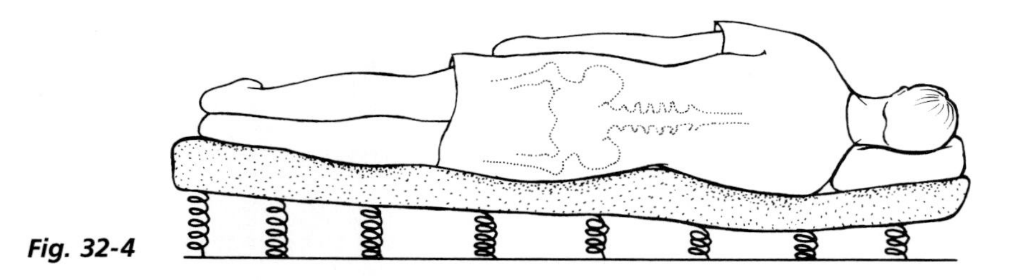

*Fig. 32-4*

| Steps | Rationale |
|---|---|
| c. Vertebral column should be in straight alignment with any observable curves. | Allows for even distribution of body weight. |

## Nursing Diagnosis

| Steps | Rationale |
|---|---|
| 1. Cluster data to reveal actual or potential nursing diagnoses: | |
| a. Impaired skin integrity: related to improper body alignment. | Improper body alignment increases risk of skin breakdown because of increased pressure over joints and bony prominences. |
| b. Potential impaired physical mobility: related to improper body alignment. | Improper body alignment over long period can impede physical mobility. |

## Planning

| Steps | Rationale |
|---|---|
| 1. Develop individualized goals for client based on nursing diagnoses: | |
| a. Reduce injuries to skin and musculoskeletal system secondary to impaired body alignment. | Improves posture and reduces risk of further damage to musculoskeletal system. |
| b. Restore proper body alignment. | Techniques improve alignment, which reduces strain on muscle groups. |
| 2. Explain to client how body alignment is altered and what measures are needed to improve it. | Improves cooperation and enables client and nurse to work together to improve body alignment. |

## Implementation

| Steps | Rationale |
|---|---|
| 1. Instruct client or family on proper body alignment for standing, sitting, or lying. | Provides client or family with necessary knowledge to identify potential altered body alignments. |
| 2. Demonstrate to client or family correct body alignment for standing, sitting, or lying. | Demonstration is reliable technique for teaching psychomotor skill and enables client to ask questions. |
| 3. Have client or family demonstrate correct body alignment for standing, sitting, or lying. | Return demonstration provides nurse with opportunity to identify and correct errors. |
| 4. Discuss with client or family hazards of prolonged immobility on body alignment and mobility (Chapter 36). | Alerts client or family to early assessment factors associated with incorrect body alignment or impaired mobility. |
| 5. Provide client or family with resources (community health agency, physician) to contact when mobility or body alignment is impaired. | Alerts resource persons to assist with minor problems of body alignment before severe, irreversible problems occur. |

## Evaluation

| Steps | Rationale |
|---|---|
| 1. Evaluate client or family to determine ability to monitor and maintain: | Determines effectiveness of teaching plan. |
| a. Correct body position for standing, sitting, or lying. | |
| b. Absence of injury to skin and musculoskeletal system. | |

### *Expected outcomes*

| Steps | Rationale |
|---|---|
| 1. Client independently demonstrates proper body alignment for standing, sitting, or lying. | Provides feedback to nurse and client through independent demonstration of psychomotor skills. |
| 2. Client identifies common assessments of impaired body alignments and injuries to musculoskeletal system. | Documents cognitive learning. |

### *Unexpected outcomes*

| Steps | Rationale |
|---|---|
| 1. Incorrect body alignment is indicated by poor posture or decreased joint mobility. | Indicates need for follow-up learning activities. |
| 2. Damage to skin and musculoskeletal system (e.g., pressure sore, contracture) occurs. | |

| Steps | Rationale |
|---|---|
| **Recording and Reporting** | |
| 1. Record information presented to client and progress toward learning selected knowledge. | Documents client teaching with plan of care. |
| 2. Report information taught to client at change of shift. | Alerts oncoming nursing personnel to information already presented. |
| **Follow-up Activity** | |
| 1. Review teaching plan with client or family and modify as needed. | Reinforces prior learning and identifies cognitive and psychomotor deficiencies. |

### Special Considerations

- Musculoskeletal system in infants is highly flexible. As they continue to grow, musculoskeletal stability increases, and they are able to sit, stand, and walk.
- During aging process, cervical vertebrae may become more flexed, and kyphotic posture may result.
- Toddler balances with feet unusually far apart and slightly everted. Elderly client may take smaller steps with feet closer together and may be at risk for falling.
- Clients with lower extremity weakness, paralysis, or immobilization are at risk for musculoskeletal trauma because of uneven or prolonged distribution of body weight.
- Clients with upper extremity weakness or paralysis are at risk for shoulder dislocation if their forearms are unsupported.
- Clients with impaired mobility, decreased sensation, or lack of voluntary muscle control are at risk for musculoskeletal damage and must have their positions changed frequently.

### Teaching Considerations

- Parents are taught that a toddler walks with abdomen protruding forward and thus is at greater risk for imbalance and falls easily.
- Shorter clients should be taught to use a footstool when sitting.
- Clients at risk for thrombophlebitis, such as postoperative or postpartum clients or clients taking anticoagulants or medication that can increase platelet production, should be taught to maintain space between edge of chair and popliteal space and not cross their legs.
- If client has cognitive or sensory impairment, is younger child, or is severely debilitated, family is primary focus of instruction.
- When client is immobilized or confined to bed, family must be taught proper positioning and transfer techniques (Chapter 33).

# *SKILL 32-2 Performing Correct Lifting Techniques*

The rate of injuries in occupational settings has increased during recent years. More than half of these are back injuries and the direct result of improper lifting and bending techniques. The most common back injury is strain on the lumbar muscle group, which includes the muscles surrounding the lumbar vertebrae. Muscle injury to these areas affects the person's ability to bend forward, backward, and side to side. In addition, the ability to rotate the hips and lower back from left to right and right to left decreases.

### Purposes

1. Prevent injury to the musculoskeletal system.
2. Prevent injury to the client.
3. Promote safe transfer techniques.

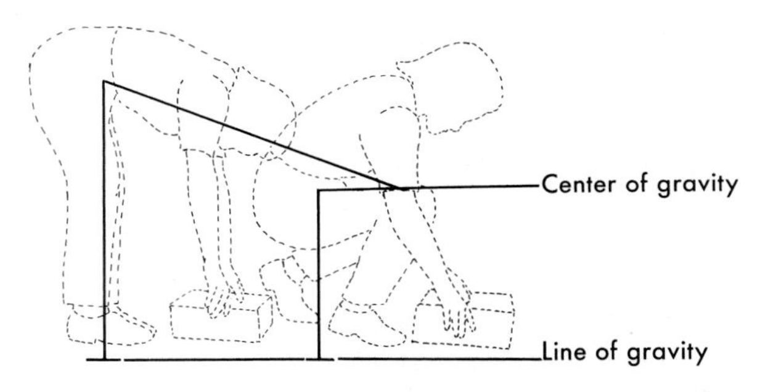


*Fig. 32-5*

## Procedure 32-2

| Steps | Rationale |
|---|---|
| **Assessment** | |
| 1. Assess position of weight to be lifted. Client whose position is restricted because of traction, trauma, body cast requires two or more persons to lift regardless of weight or height. | Position of weight to be lifted should be as close to lifter's center of gravity as possible. |
| 2. Assess height of object to be lifted. | Best height for lifting vertically is slightly above level of middle finger when arm is hanging at person's side (Owens, 1980). |
| 3. Evaluate lifter's body position. | Body should be positioned so multiple muscle groups are able to work together. |
| 4. Know maximal weight that can be safely carried. | Maximal weight that can be safely carried is 35% more than person's body weight. |
| **Nursing Diagnosis** | |
| 1. Cluster data to reveal actual or potential nursing diagnoses: a. Potential for injury: related to improper lifting techniques. b. Impaired mobility: related to improper body alignment while lifting. | Use of improper body alignment and lifting techniques increases risk for musculoskeletal injury, particularly to lumbosacral region. |
| **Planning** | |
| 1. Develop individualized goals for client based on nursing diagnoses: a. Reduce risk of injury to lifter's musculoskeletal system. b. Promote correct body alignment while lifting. | Goals are aimed at reducing risk of injury to nurse and client during lifting technique. |
| 2. When lifting involves transferring client, prepare client by removing excess linen from bed or chair and explaining procedure. | Removal of excess linen or clutter reduces risk of injury from tripping. Explanation increases understanding and cooperation. |
| 3. When lifting object, remove excess clutter from environment. | Provides clear pathway to lift and transfer object. |
| **Implementation** | |
| 1. Lift object correctly from below center of gravity (Fig. 32-5). | |
| a. Come close to object to be moved. | Increases body balance during lifting procedure. |
| b. Enlarge base of support. | Maintains better body balance and reduces risk of falling. |
| c. Lower center of gravity to object. | Increases body balance and enables muscle groups to work together. |
| d. Maintain proper alignment of head and neck with vertebrae. | Reduces risk of injury to lumbar vertebrae and muscle groups. |
| 2. Lift object correctly from shelf above center of gravity. | |
| a. Use safe, stable step stool. | Raises center of gravity closer to object. |
| b. Stand as close to shelf as possible. | Moves center of gravity closer to object. |
| c. Quickly transfer weight of object from shelf to arms and over base of support. | Reduces danger of falling by moving lifted object close to center of gravity over base of support. |
| **Evaluation** | |
| 1. Observe nurse and client to determine ability to use lifting techniques correctly. | Determines effective use of correct lifting techniques. |
| ***Expected outcome*** | |
| 1. Nurse and client safely use lifting techniques. | Provides feedback that safe lifting techniques are used. |
| 2. No injuries result from lifting procedure. | Avoids strain on musculoskeletal system. |
| **Unexpected outcome** | |
| 1. Incorrect lifting techniques are indicated by injury to lifter's musculoskeletal system or injury to client during transfer technique. | Indicates need for follow-up learning activities. |

| Steps | Rationale |
|---|---|
| **Recording and Reporting** | |
| 1. Record type of lifting techniques taught to client or family. | Provides documentation of information given client or family regarding lifting techniques. |
| 2. Immediately report any lifting injury occurring to nurse or client. | Alerts nursing personnel of potential for injury to client or nurse. |

## Special Considerations

- If lifting injury is sustained, some institutions also require incident report to be completed and filed in nursing office.

## Teaching Considerations

- Lifting load that is too heavy can result in muscle tears. Sudden twisting or bending also can tear muscles and ligaments.
- Teach primary care giver to use correct body mechanics in moving, lifting, transferring, positioning client.

### BIBLIOGRAPHY

Alvarez AR, Russell MT: Emergency evacuation: removal of the critically ill patient, Focus Crit Care 14(6):18, 1987.

Bilger AJ, Grun EH: Winger's protective body mechanics: a manual for nurses, New York, 1973, Springer Publishing Co, Inc.

Bulau J: Clinical policies and procedures for home health care, Rockville, Md, 1986, Aspen Publishers, Inc.

Daniels L, Worthington C: Therapeutic exercise for body alignment and function, ed 2, Philadelphia, 1977, WB Saunders Co.

Farrell J: Illustrated guide to orthopedic nursing, Philadelphia, 1982, JB Lippincott Co.

Gates SJ, Starkey RD: Back injury prevention: a holistic approach, AAOHN J 34(2):58, 1986.

Jacobs B, Young M: Transferring patients safely and efficiently, Nurs 81 11(8):64, 1981.

Jensen RC: Disabling back injuries among nursing personnel: research needs and justification, Res Nurs Health 10(1):29, 1987.

Kemp B, Pillitteri A: Fundamentals of nursing, Boston, 1984, Little, Brown & Co, Inc.

Marchette L, Marchette B: Back injury: a preventable occupational hazard, Orthop Nurs 4(6):25, 1985.

Nyhuis AW: Reducing the costs of patient transfers, JONA 17(7/8):11, 1987.

Owens BD: How to avoid that aching back, Am J Nurs 80:984, 1980.

Owens BD: Personal characteristics important to back injury, Rehabil Nurs 11(4):12, 1986.

Owens BD: Procedures Nursing Reference Library Springhouse, Penn, 1985, Springhouse Corp.

Rantz M, Courtial D: Lifting, moving, and transferring patients: a manual, St Louis, 1977, The CV Mosby Co.

Saywell RM, Woods JR, Holmes GL, et al.: Reducing the costs of patient transfers, JONA 17(7/8):11, 1987.

# 33

# TRANSFER AND POSITIONING

### OBJECTIVES

*Mastery of content in this chapter will enable the nurse to:*

- Define key terms.
- Describe normal body alignment for standing, sitting, and lying.
- Describe positioning techniques for the supported Fowler's, supine, prone, side-lying, and Sims' positions.
- Describe the procedures for helping a client to move up in bed, helping a client to a sitting position, and transferring a client from a bed to a chair.
- Describe the procedure for a three-person carry.

### KEY TERMS

*Body mechanics*
*Footboard*
*Foot-drop*
*Friction*
*Gravity*
*Hand roll*
*Hoyer lift*
*Joint*
*Ligament*
*Muscle tone*
*Paralysis*
*Paresis*
*Posture*
*Proprioception*

### SKILLS

***33-1*** Using Proper Transfer Techniques
***33-2*** Moving and Positioning Clients in Bed

Transfer and positioning are some of the most basic nursing skills and are learned early in the student nurse's training. It is easy to forget how vital the correct performance of these skills is to maintaining the client's mobility and independence and the nurse's own health.

No area of knowledge is more important to the nurse in transferring and positioning dependent clients than the principles of proper body mechanics and alignment (Chapter 32). Practical application of these principles reduces the risk of injury to clients and health care personnel. Back injuries are a significant problem for nursing personnel; a sizable number of these injuries are sustained each year as a result of improper lifting and bending techniques.

Too often the client develops complications independent of illness because the principles of alignment and body mechanics are not followed. Improper alignment of the dependent client can result in joint contractures or injuries that may take months to correct or even result in permanent disability.

To maintain correct posture, proper preventive positioning is essential. Improper positioning has many implications. Incorrect positioning, especially of the client with circulatory system impairments, may result in a decubitus ulcer, which can develop in 24 hours and require months of time and thousands of dollars to correct. Contractures and foot-drop occur within a few days when muscles, tendons, and joints become less flexible because of lack of mobility and incorrect alignment. The force of gravity pulls an unsupported, weakened foot into a foot-drop position, and calf muscles and heel cords shorten, complicating future attempts at walking. Pillows under the knees or an elevated bed knee gatch can produce knee and hip contractures. A sagging mattress increases the risk of hip contractures. These knee and hip contractures can cause future gait and posture problems, making mobility more difficult.

Some clients are at especially high risk for complications of improper positioning and have increased risk of injury during transfer. A number of pathologic factors and congenital or acquired postural abnormalities alter alignment, mobility, or both. Pathophysiologic mechanisms altering bone formation or joint mobility present special risks, as does impaired muscle development, which results in muscle wasting and weakness. Central nervous system (CNS) damage may result in motor impairment, proprioceptive loss, or cognitive dysfunction, all of which affect mobility. Direct trauma also affects body mechanics.

The client's goal is to achieve the greatest level of independence possible. This independence can mean the difference between dependence and self-care, living at home or living in a nursing home, isolation and its psychologic effects or mobility and social involvement. The implications of these skills are vitally important to the client's well-being.

### GUIDELINES

1. Know the client's fluid and electrolyte status. Dehydration or edema may require more frequent position changes because clients with fluid or electrolyte disturbances are prone to skin breakdown.
2. Know the client's range of joint motion (ROJM). Contractures or spasticity limit joint and muscle mobility; the nurse must take care not to position the limb in a dysfunctional position.
3. Identify circulatory alterations such as venous ulcers, which may prevent the client from having the extremity in a dependent position. A history of deep vein thrombosis may restrict the length of time a client can remain in a sitting position.
4. Determine the client's level of sensory perception. Loss of sensation increases vulnerability to the hazards of immobility. Clients with decreased sensation must have their positions evaluated and changed frequently to avoid damage to the integumentary and musculoskeletal systems.
5. Know the client's baseline vital signs. The client with low blood pressure may not be able to tolerate sudden position changes and is at risk of fainting while transferring from bed to chair. The febrile client who becomes diaphoretic may require more frequent position changes to avoid skin breakdown.
6. Know underlying chronic conditions such as disease or malnutrition. Clients with underlying chronic conditions are at risk for skin breakdown and other hazards of immobility and as a result require more frequent position changes.
7. Know the client's cognitive status and stage of psychologic adaptation to illness. Both factors affect the ability to learn and participate in transfer and positioning.

### PREREQUISITE KNOWLEDGE

1. Principles of body mechanics.
2. Principles of body alignment.
3. Special transfer needs of clients with neurologic deficits or trauma.
4. Regulation and coordination of body movements by the skeletal, muscular, and nervous systems.
5. Hazards of immobility.

### PREREQUISITE SKILLS

1. Proper handwashing technique (Chapter 37).
2. Assessment of correct body alignment (Chapter 32).
3. Lifting techniques (Chapter 32).
4. Physical assessment (Chapter 13).
5. Assessment of vital signs (Chapter 12).
6. ROJM exercises (Chapter 36).

## *SKILL 33-1 Using Proper Transfer Techniques*

Transfer is an important nursing skill. It helps the dependent client to attain positions to regain optimal independence as quickly as possible. Physical activity maintains and improves joint motion, increases strength, promotes circulation, relieves pressure on skin, and improves urinary and respiratory functions. It also benefits the client psychologically by increasing social activity and mental stimulation and providing a change in environment. Thus mobilization plays a crucial role in the client's rehabilitation.

One of the major concerns during transfer is the safety of client and nurse. The nurse prevents self-injury by use of proper body mechanics, good posture, and correct lifting techniques (Chapter 32).

The nurse must be aware of the client's motor deficits, ability to aid in transfer, and body weight. As a rule of thumb, nurses should never attempt to lift more than 35% of their body weight and must always get assistance if in doubt of the ability to transfer a client.

Many special problems must be considered in transfer. A client immobile for several days or longer may be weak or dizzy or may develop orthostatic hypotension when transferred. A client with neurologic deficits may have paresis (muscle weakness) or paralysis unilaterally or bilaterally, which will complicate safe transfer. A flaccid arm may sustain injury during transfer if unsupported. The nurse may use innovative skills for the transfer of trauma clients. As a general rule, a nurse should use a transfer belt and obtain assistance for mobilization of such clients.

### Purposes

1. Mobilize the client without injury to the client or nurse.
2. Use minimum muscle strength on part of nurse.
3. Offset the systemic hazards of immobility in the client.
4. Increase client independence and aid rehabilitation.

## *Procedure 33-1*

| Steps | Rationale |
|---|---|
| **Assessment** | |
| 1. Assess physiologic capacity to transfer: | Determines neuromuscular integrity for transfer and special adaptive techniques necessary. |
| a. Muscle strength. | Immobile clients have decreased muscle strength, tone, mass. |
| b. Joint mobility and contracture formation. | Large, immobile clients may need to be transferred with Hoyer lift. |
| c. Paralysis or paresis (spastic or flaccid). | Immobility or inflammatory processes (i.e., arthritis) may lead to contracture formation and impaired joint mobility. Client with CNS damage may have bilateral paralysis (requiring transfer by swivel bar, sliding bar, Hoyer lift) or unilateral paralysis, which requires belt transfer to "best" side. Weakness (paresis) requires stabilization of knee while transferring. Flaccid arm must be supported with sling during transfer. |
| d. Bone continuity (trauma, amputation). | |
| e. Upper arm strength. | Clients with trauma to one leg or hip may be non–weight bearing when transferred. Amputees may use sliding board to transfer. |
| 2. Assess presence of weakness, dizziness, postural hypotension. | Determines risk of fainting, falling during transfer. Immobile clients may have decreased ability for autonomic nervous system to equalize blood supply, resulting in drop of 15 mm Hg or more in blood pressure when rising from sitting position. |
| 3. Assess level of bed activity, endurance: | Estimates ability to participate in transfer. |
| a. Assess ability to use arms and legs for moving up and down in bed and repositioning. | |
| b. Assess level of fatigue on activity. | Ability to transfer may be limited by fatigue. Strength may be evaluated by participation in activities of daily living (ADL). Planned rest periods before transfer may enhance function. Vital sign change such as increased pulse and respiration may indicate activity intolerance (Chapter 12). |
| 4. Assess client's proprioceptive function: | Determines stability of balance for transfer. |
| a. Ability to maintain balance while sitting in bed or on side of bed. | Determines risk of fainting or falling during transfer. |
| b. Tendency to sway to or position self to one side. | Clients with brain dysfunction may have proprioceptive losses that cause them to lean to one side or lose balance during transfer. |
| 5. Assess client's sensory status: | Determines influence of sensory loss on ability to make transfer. Visual field loss decreases client's ability to see in direction of transfer. Peripheral sensation loss decreases proprioception. Clients with visual and hearing losses will need transfer techniques adapted to deficits. Clients with cerebrovascular accidents (CVA) may lose area of visual field, which affects vision and perception profoundly. Clients with hemiplegia also may "neglect" one side of body (deny its existence), which distorts perception of the visual field. |
| a. Adequacy of central and peripheral vision. | |
| b. Adequacy of hearing. | |
| c. Loss of peripheral sensation. | |
| 6. Assess client's level of comfort: | Pain may reduce client's motivation and ability to be mobile. Pain relief before transfer enhances client participation. |
| a. Pain. | |
| b. Muscle spasm. | |
| 7. Assess client's cognitive status: | Determines client's ability to follow directions and learn transfer techniques. May indicate clients at risk for injury. Clients with short-term memory deficits may have difficulty in transfer, in initial learning or consistent performance. Clients with head trauma or CVA may have perceptual cognitive deficits that create safety risks. If client has difficulty in comprehension, simplify instructions, maintain consistency. Teach one step at a time, use short commands, repeat often, use gestures, be patient, reinforce performance with praise. |
| a. Ability to follow verbal instructions. | |
| b. Short-term memory. | |
| c. Appropriateness of response. | |
| d. Recognition of physical deficits and limitations to movement. | |
| 8. Assess client's level of motivation: | Determine fears, depressed state, anxiety, grieving. |
| a. Clients eagerness to be mobile. | |
| b. Whether client avoids activity and offers excuses. | Altered psychological states reduce client's desire to engage in activity. |

| Steps | Rationale |
|---|---|
| 9. Previous mode of transfer (if applicable). | Determines mode of transfer and assistance required to provide continuity. Transfer belts should be used with hemiplegic clients being transferred for the first time and all other high-risk clients. |
| 10. Assess client's specific risk of falling when transferred, sustaining injury in fall. | Certain condition increase client's risk of falling or potential for injury. Neuromuscular deficits, motor weakness, calcium loss from long bones, cognitive and visual dysfunction, balance alteration increase risk of injury. |

## Nursing Diagnosis

| Steps | Rationale |
|---|---|
| 1. Cluster data to reveal actual or potential nursing diagnoses: | |
| a. Activity intolerance, related to: ▪ Muscle weakness. ▪ Immobility. | Transfer will increase muscle tone and strength through weight bearing and movement. |
| b. Potential for injury, related to: ▪ Altered cognitive status. ▪ Altered neuromuscular status. ▪ Decreased vision. ▪ Postural hypotension. | Proper use of transfer techniques with adaptation for specific situations reduces risk of injury. |

## Planning

| Steps | Rationale |
|---|---|
| 1. Develop individualized goals for client based on nursing diagnoses: | |
| a. Increase activity tolerance. | Increases in activity tolerance increase the client's ability to participate in transfer techniques. |
| b. Increase ability to bear weight. | Promotes safe transfer. |
| c. Prevent injury during transfer. | Proper technique avoids injury to nurse and client. |
| d. Increase self-care ability. | Participation in transfer techniques increases client's self-care activities. |
| 2. Prepare needed equipment and supplies: | |
| a. Transfer belt (if needed), sling or lapboard (as needed), nonskid shoes, bath blankets, pillows. | Reduces risk of injury. Should be used with all clients who require moderate to maximum assistance or have high risk of falling or injury. |
| b. Wheelchair: if transferring to wheelchair, position chair at 45° angle to bed, lock brakes, remove footrests, lock bed brakes. | Position of wheelchair or stretcher facilitates quick transfer from bed to wheelchair or bed to stretcher. |
| c. Stretcher: if using stretcher, position at right angle (90°) to bed, lock brakes on stretcher, lock brakes on bed. | |
| d. Hoyer lift: if using Hoyer lift, use Hoyer frame, canvas strips or chains, and hammock or canvas strips. | Initially, Hoyer lift may require two or more nurses. Hoyer lifts safely transfer large, immobile clients unable to maintain weight bearing. |
| 3. Explain procedure to client. Repeat instructions simply and with continuity to client with cognitive dysfunction. | Promotes cooperation and reduces anxiety. |

## Implementation

| Steps | Rationale |
|---|---|
| 1. Wash hands. | Reduces transfer of microorganisms. |
| 2. Assist client to sitting position: | |
| a. Place client in supine position. | Enables nurse to continually assess client's body alignment and to administer additional care, such as suctioning or hygiene needs. |
| b. Remove all pillows from bed. | Decreases interference while sitting client up in bed. |
| c. Face head of bed. | Reduces twisting of nurse's body when moving client. |
| d. Place feet apart with foot nearer bed behind other foot. | Improves nurse's balance and allows transfer of body weight as client is moved to sitting position. |
| e. Place hand farther from client under shoulders, supporting client's head and cervical vertebrae. | Maintains alignment of head and cervical vertebrae and allows for even lifting of client's upper trunk. |
| f. Place other hand on bed surface. | Provides support and balance. |
| g. Raise client to sitting position by shifting weight from front to back leg. | Improves nurse's balance, overcomes inertia, and transfers weight in direction in which client is moved. |
| h. Push against bed using arm that is placed on bed surface. | Divides activity between nurse's arms and legs and protects back from strain. By bracing one hand against mattress and pushing against it as client is lifted, part of weight that would be lifted by nurse's back muscles is transferred through her arms onto mattress. |

| Steps | Rationale |
|---|---|

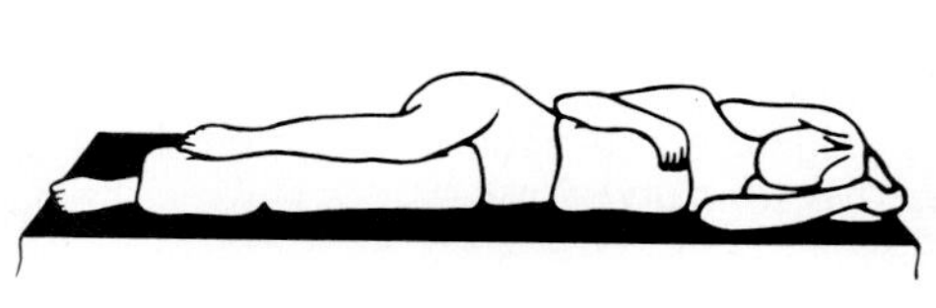

*Fig. 33-1*

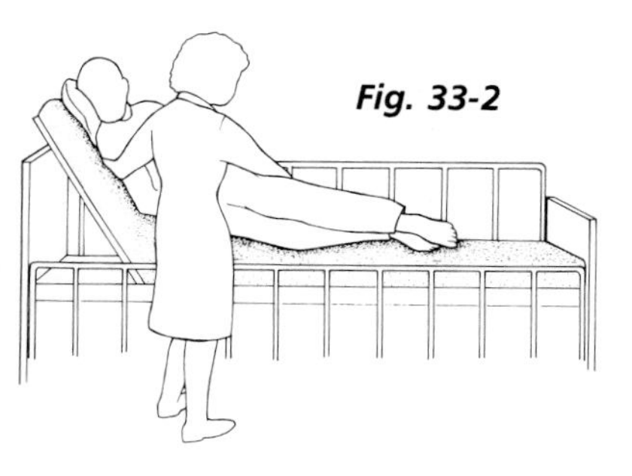

*Fig. 33-2*

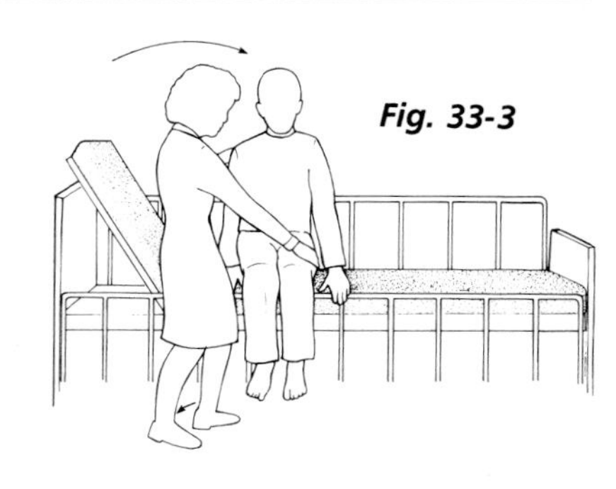

*Fig. 33-3*

| Steps | Rationale |
|---|---|
| 3. Assist client to sitting position on side of bed: | |
| a. Place client in side-lying position, facing nurse on side of bed on which client will be sitting (Fig. 33-1). | Prepares client to move to side of bed and protects from falling. |
| b. Raise head of bed to highest level client is able to tolerate. | Decreases amount of work needed by client and nurse to raise client to sitting position. |
| c. Stand opposite client's hips. | Places nurse's center of gravity nearer client. |
| d. Turn diagonally so nurse faces client and far corner of foot of bed. | Reduces twisting body because nurse is facing direction of movement. |
| e. Place feet apart with foot closer to head of bed in front of other foot. | Increases balance and allows nurse to transfer weight as client is brought to sitting position at side of bed. |
| f. Place arm nearer head of bed under client's shoulders, supporting head and neck. | Maintains alignment of head and neck as nurse brings client to sitting position. |
| g. Place other arm over client's thighs (Fig. 33-2). | Supports hip and prevents client from falling backward during procedure. |
| h. Move client's lower legs and feet over side of bed. | Decreases friction and resistance. |
| i. Pivot toward rear leg, allowing client's upper legs to swing downward. | Allows gravity to lower client's legs. |
| j. At same time, shift weight to rear leg and elevate client (Fig. 33-3). | Allows nurse to transfer weight in direction of motion. |
| k. Remain in front until client regains balance. | Reduces risk of falling. |
| l. Continue to provide physical support to weak or cognitively impaired client. | These clients are at high risk of falling. |
| m. Lower level of bed until client's feet touch floor. | Supports client's feet in dorsal flexion and allows client to easily stand at side of bed. |
| 4. Transferring client from bed to chair: | |
| a. Assist client to sitting position on side of bed. Have chair in position at 45-degree angle to bed. | Positions chair within easy access for transfer. |
| b. Apply transfer belt transfer aids, if needed. | Transfer belt allows nurse to maintain stability of client during transfer, reduces risk of falling. Client's arm should be in sling if flaccid paralysis is present. |
| c. Ensure client has stable nonskid shoes. Weight-bearing, or strong leg forward, weak foot back. | Nonskid soles decrease risk of slipping during transfer. Always have clients wear shoes during transfer; bare feet increase risk of falls. Client will stand on stronger or weight-bearing leg. |
| d. Spread feet apart. | Ensures balance with wide base of support. |
| e. Flex hips and knees, aligning knees with client's (Fig. 33-4). | Flexion of knees and hips lowers nurse's center of gravity to object to be raised; aligning knees with client's allows for stabilization of knees when client stands. |
| f. Grasp transfer belt from underneath, if used, or reach through client's axilla and place hands on client's scapulae. | Lifting client with hands on scapulae reduces pressure on axilla and maintains client stability. Clients with upper extremity paralysis or paresis should never be lifted by or under arms. Transfer belt is grasped at each side to provide movement of client at center of gravity. |
| g. Rock client up to standing on count of 3 while straightening hips and legs, keeping knees slightly flexed (Fig. 33-5). Client may be instructed to use hands to push up if applicable. | Rocking motion gives client's body momentum and requires less muscular effort to lift client. Uses correct body mechanics to raise client to standing position. |
| h. Maintain stability of client's weak or paralyzed leg with knee. | Ability to stand can often be maintained in paralyzed or weak limb with support of knee to stabilize. |
| i. Pivot on foot farther from chair. | Maintains support of client while allowing adequate space for client to move. |
| j. Instruct client to use arm rests on chair for support and ease into chair (Fig. 33-6). | Increases client stability. |

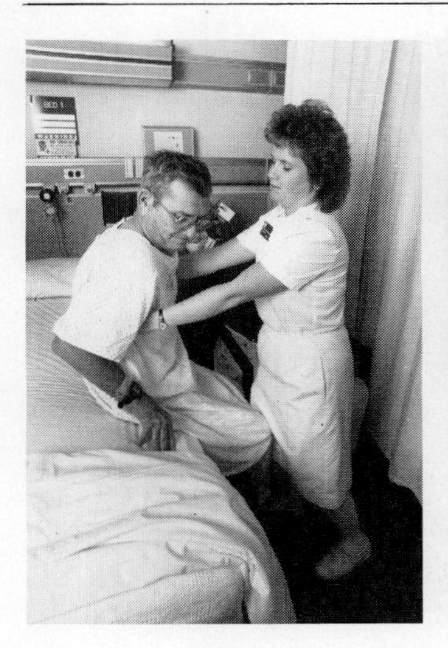

*Fig. 33-4*

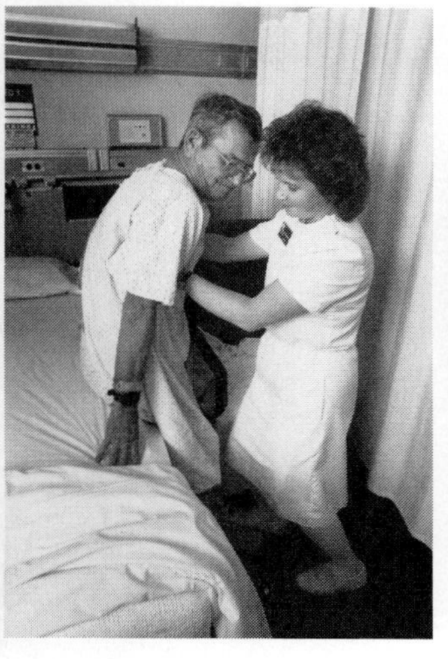

*Fig. 33-5*

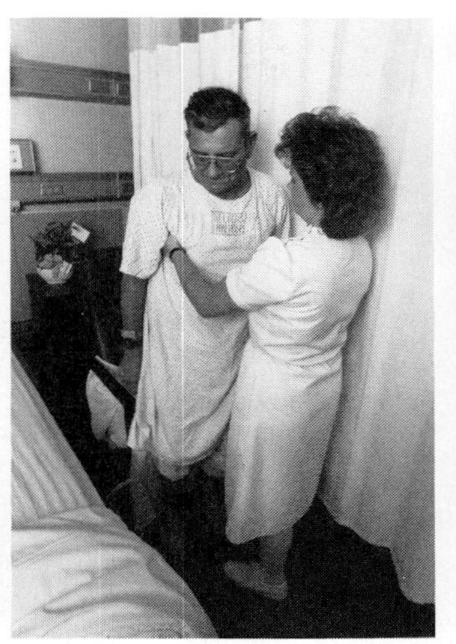

*Fig. 33-6*

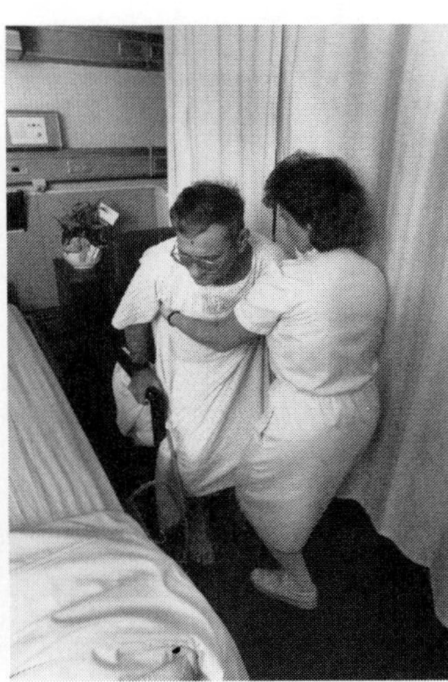

*Fig. 33-7*

| Steps | Rationale |
|---|---|
| k. Flex hips and knees while lowering client into chair (Fig. 33-7). | Prevents injury to nurse from poor body mechanics. |
| l. Assess client for proper alignment for sitting position. Provide support for paralyzed extremities. Lap board or sling will support flaccid arm. Stabilize leg with bath blanket or pillow. | Prevents injury to client from poor body alignment. |
| m. Praise client progress, effort, performance. | Continued support and encouragement provide incentive for client perserverance. |
| 5. Perform three-person carry from bed to stretcher: | |
| a. Three nurses stand side by side facing side of client's bed. The people performing the procedure should be of equal height. | Prevents twisting of nurses' bodies. Client's alignment is maintained. |
| b. Each person assumes responsibility for one of three areas: head and shoulders, hips, thighs and ankles. | Distributes client's body weight. |
| c. Each assumes wide base of support with foot closer to stretcher in front, knees slightly flexed. | Increases balance and lowers lifters' centers of gravity. |
| d. Lifters' arms are placed under client's head and shoulders, hips, and thighs and ankles, with fingers securely around other side of client's body (Fig. 33-8). | Distributes client's weight over lifters' forearms. NOTE: **Spinal cord injuries must be stabilized before transfer.** |
| e. Lifters roll client toward their chests. | Moves workload over lifters' base of support. |
| f. On count of 3, client is lifted and held against nurses' chests. | Enables lifters to work together and safely lift client. |
| g. On second count of 3, nurses step back and pivot toward stretcher, moving forward if needed. | Transfers weight toward stretcher. |
| h. Nurses gently lower client onto center of stretcher by flexing knees and hips until elbows are level with edge of stretcher. | Maintains nurses' alignment during transfer. |
| i. Nurses assess client's body alignment, place safety straps across body, and raise side rails. | Reduces risk of injury from poor alignment or falling. |
| 6. Use Hoyer lift (Fig. 33-9) to transfer client from bed to chair: | |
| a. Bring Hoyer frame to bedside. | Ensures safe elevation of client off bed. (Before using Hoyer lift, be thoroughly familiar with its operation.) |
| b. Position chair near bed and allow adequate space to maneuver lift. | Prepares environment for safe use of lift and subsequent transfer. |
| c. Raise bed to high position, mattress flat. Lower side rail. | Allows nurse to use proper body mechanics. |
| d. Keep bed side rail up on opposite side to nurse. | Maintains client safety. |
| e. Roll client away from nurse. | Positions client for use of Hoyer lift sling. |
| f. Place hammock or canvas strips under client to form seat; with two canvas pieces, lower edge fits under client's knees (wide piece), upper edge fits under client's shoulders (narrow piece). | Two types of seat are supplied with Hoyer lift: hammock style is better for clients who are flaccid, weak, and need support; canvas strips can be used with those with normal muscle tone. Hooks should face away from client's skin. Places Hoyer sling under client's center of gravity and greatest portion of body weight. |

| Steps | Rationale |
|---|---|
| 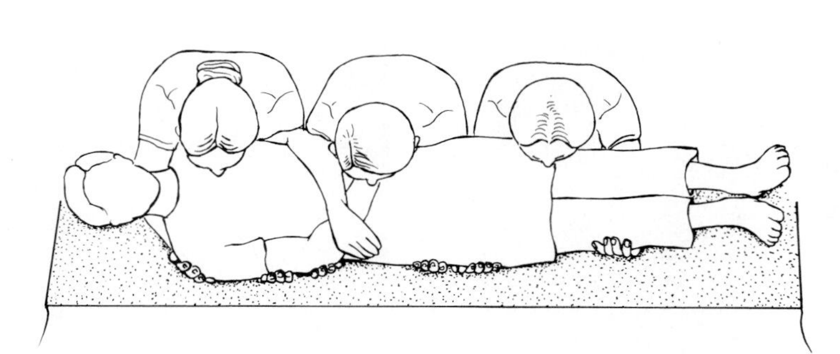 *Fig. 33-8* | 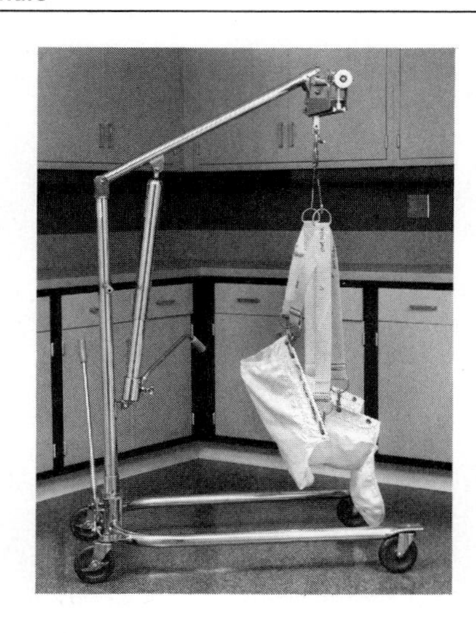 *Fig. 33-9* |
| g. Raise bed rail. | Maintains client safety. |
| h. Go to opposite side of bed and lower siderail. | |
| i. Roll client to opposite side and pull hammock (strips) through. | Completes positioning of client on Hoyer sling. |
| j. Roll client supine onto canvas seat. | Sling should extend from shoulders to knees (hammock) to support client's body weight equally. |
| k. Remove client's glasses, if appropriate. | Swivel bar is close to client's head and could cause breakage of eye glasses. |
| l. Place lift's horseshoe bar under side of bed (on side with chair). | Positions Hoyer lift efficiently and promotes smooth transfer. |
| m. Lower horizontal bar to sling level by releasing hydraulic valve. Lock valve. | Positions hydraulic lift close to client. Locking valve prevents injury to client. |
| n. Attach hooks on strap (chain) to holes in sling. Short chains or straps hook to top holes of sling; longer chains hook to bottom of sling. | Secures hydraulic lift to Hoyer sling. |
| o. Elevate head of bed. | Positions client in sitting position. |
| p. Fold client's arms over chest. | Prevents injury to paralyzed arms. |
| q. Pump hydraulic handle using long, slow, even strokes until client is raised off bed. | Ensures safe support of client during elevation. |
| r. Use steering handle to pull lift from bed and maneuver to chair. | Moves client from bed to chair. |
| s. Roll base around chair. | Positions lift in front of chair in which client is to be transferred. |
| t. Release check valve slowly (turn to left) and lower client into chair. | Safely guides client into back of chair as seat descends. |
| u. Close check valve as soon as client is down and straps can be released. | If valve is left open, boom may continue to lower and injure client. |
| v. Remove straps and Hoyer lift. | Prevents damage to skin and underlying tissues from canvas or hooks. |
| w. Check client for proper sitting alignment. | Prevents injury from poor posture. |
| 7. Wash hands. | Reduces transmission of microorganisms. |

## Evaluation

| | |
|---|---|
| 1. Observe for correct body alignment and presence of pressure points on skin. | Minimizes risk of immobility complications. |
| 2. Monitor vital signs. | Evaluates client's response to postural changes. |
| 3. Observe for increased activity tolerance. | |
| 4. Note client's behavioral response to transfer. | Reveals level of motivation and self-care potential. |

### *Expected outcomes*

| | |
|---|---|
| 1. Client dangles legs or sits without dizziness, weakness, orthostatic hypotension. | Transfer ability is influenced by cause of dependence, length of immobility, ability to follow directions, psychosocial factors. |
| 2. Client tolerates increased activity. | Repeated transfers usually result in greater independence of client. |
| 3. Client can bear more weight. | |

| Steps | Rationale |
|---|---|
| 4. Client transfers without injury. | |
| 5. Client is more motivated to be mobile. | |
| 6. Client transfers with minimal or no assistance. | |
| 7. Client increases independence in ADL. | |
| 8. Skin is clear of pressure areas. | Absence of pressure ulcer formation. |
| ***Unexpected outcomes*** | |
| 1. Client is unable to comprehend and follow directions for transfer. | Cognitive impairments affect learning and retention. Reassess continuity and simplicity of instruction. |
| 2. Client sustains injury on transfer. | Indicates improper transfer technique was used. Evaluate incident that caused injury (e.g., assessment inadequate, change in client status, or improper use of equipment). |
| 3. Client's level of weakness does not permit active transfer. | Physical impairments require increased assistance from nursing personnel. Increase bed activity, exercise to increase tolerance. |
| 4. Client continues to bear weight on non–weight-bearing limb. | Certain conditions (e.g., hip fractures) need to be non–weight bearing through healing process. Reassess client's understanding of weight-bearing status. |
| 5. Client transfers well on some occasions, poorly on others. | Transfers may be difficult when client is fatigued; periodic confusion may alter performance. |
| 6. Client is unable to stand for time required in transfer. | Results from increased fatigue, orthostatic hypotention, pain. |
| 7. Localized areas of erythema that do not disappear quickly. | Early signs of pressure sore. |

## Recording and Reporting

| | |
|---|---|
| 1. Record procedure, including pertinent observations: (weakness, ability to follow directions, weight-bearing ability, balance, ability to pivot, number of personnel needed to assist, amount of assistance (muscle strength) required. | Documents transfer procedure and client's response to transfer. |
| 2. Report any unusual occurrence to nurse in charge. Report transfer ability and assistance needed to next shift or other care givers. Report progress or remission to rehabilitation staff (physical therapist, occupational therapist). | Transfer techniques and adaptive aids used for client, as well as client's response, must be conveyed to other health care personnel to provide continuity of care. |

## Follow-up Activities

| | |
|---|---|
| 1. Schedule transfer after periods of rest. | Client will transfer with greater ease if rested. |
| 2. Increase number of transfers and period of time up gradually. | Increase activity tolerance with graded exercise. |
| 3. Assess special transfer equipment needed for home setting. | Adaptive devices used in hospital should be anticipated for use in home. |
| 4. Assess home environment for hazards. | Doorways or bathrooms may not be adequate for easy transfer, toilet access. |

## Special Considerations

- Infant or toddler, elderly client with short-term memory loss, or client with cognitive dysfunction secondary to disease or trauma may be unable to follow directions regarding positioning and transfer.
- Cognitive immaturity or memory loss creates potential safety hazards because client may attempt to climb out of bed or get up from chair.
- Alterations in neuromuscular function, alterations in physiology of bone formation secondary to disease or aging process, loss of joint mobility, CNS damage, and hazards of immobility increase risk of injury during transfer.
- Profound weakness, cardiac dysfunction, hypotension are also risk factors. Many facilities have developed "risk of falls" assessments to aid in identifying such high-risk persons.
- Psychologic support and encouragement are very important considerations for immobile clients.

## Teaching Considerations

- For many clients, return to home is coupled with enhanced psychologic well-being and increased levels of motivation and ability for self-care function. Appropriate teaching of self-care skills and use of aids to maximize ability enhance outcome.
- Teach family, client transfer skills. Information should include principles of body mechanics and hazards of immobility. Incorporate return demonstration into discharge planning.

## Home Care Considerations

- Transfer ability at home is greatly enhanced by prior teaching of family and support persons, assessment of home for safety risks and functionality, provision of applicable aids.
- Family, support person should practice transfer in hospital to achieve success before taking client home. Alternately, client (if living alone) should practice transfer skills in bed that will be used at home, commode, bath. Clients should be taught to transfer to chairs with arms for ease of rising and sitting.

- Home should be free of risks (i.e., throw rugs, electric cords, slippery floors). If wheel-chair is used, access must be possible through all doors, and space for transfer must be available in bedroom and bathroom.
- Aids that enhance transfer ability are shower stools, commode elevators, hand rails on tub, nonskid shower surface. Many self-care devices are available for wheel-chair-bound client or client with weak or poor muscle function. These are best prescribed by occupational or physical therapist; however, many medical supply stores can provide excellent information and catalogs of such supplies. Another helpful source is the *Red Cross Home Nursing Handbook,* which supplies helpful home-made ideas to enhance self-care.

# *SKILL 33-2 Moving and Positioning Clients in Bed*

Correct positioning of clients is crucial for maintaining proper body alignment and preventing injury to the musculoskeletal system. A client with impaired mobility, decreased sensation, impaired circulation, or lack of voluntary muscle control can develop damage to the musculoskeletal system while lying down. The nurse must minimize this risk by maintaining proper body alignment while moving, turning, or positioning the client.

The following procedures are written for positioning clients who are immobilized or have limited voluntary motor control. Clients who have complete mobility, motor control, and sensory perceptions and who are conscious and oriented usually change positions frequently and assume a position of comfort.

### Purposes

1. Maintain proper client body alignment.
2. Prevent deformities or complications to the skin and musculoskeletal system.
3. Maintain client's comfort.
4. Maintain unrestricted circulation.
5. Provide client with sensory, motor, and cognitive stimulation.

## *Procedure 33-2*

| Steps | Rationale |
|---|---|
| **Assessment** | |
| 1. Assess client's body alignment and comfort level while lying down. | Provides baseline data concerning client's body alignment and comfort level. Determines ways to improve position and alignment. |
| 2. Assess for risk factors that may contribute to complications of immobility: | Increased risk factors require client to be repositioned more frequently. |
| a. Paralysis: hemiparesis resulting from CVA, decreased sensation. | Paralysis impairs movement; muscle tone changes; sensation is affected. Because of difficulty in moving and poor awareness of involved body part, client is unable to protect and position body part for self. |
| b. Impaired mobility: traction or arthritis or other contributing disease processes. | Traction or arthritic changes of affected extremity result in decreased range of joint motion. |
| c. Impaired circulation. | Decreased circulation predisposes client to pressure sores. |
| d. Age: very young, aged. | Premature and young infants require frequent turning because their skin is fragile. Normal physiologic changes associated with aging predispose older adults to greater risks for developing complications of immobility. |
| 3. Assess client's level of consciousness. | Determines need for special aids or devices. Clients with altered levels of consciousness may not understand instructions and be unable to help. |
| 4. Assess client's physical ability to help with moving and positioning: a. Age. b. Level of consciousness. c. Disease process. d. Strength. e. ROJM f. Coordination. | Enables nurse to use client's mobility and strength. Determines need for additional help. Ensures client and nurse safety. |
| 5. Assess for tubes, incisions, equipment (e.g., traction). | Will alter positioning procedure. |

| Steps | Rationale |
|---|---|
| **Nursing Diagnosis** | |
| 1. Cluster data to reveal actual or potential nursing diagnoses: | |
| a. Pain, related to:<br>▪ Restricted movement.<br>▪ Recent surgery.<br>▪ Pressure on bony prominences. | Repositioning aids in alleviating discomfort. |
| b. Impaired skin integrity, related to:<br>▪ Altered circulation from immobility.<br>▪ Infrequent or improper positioning.<br>▪ Physiologic changes resulting from aging. | Requires client's position to be changed at least every 2 hr. |
| c. Impaired physical mobility, related to:<br>▪ Trauma to musculoskeletal system secondary to decreased joint movement.<br>▪ Improper positioning of extremity.<br>▪ Immobility. | Decreases client's ability to independently maintain body alignment and joint mobility. |
| **Planning** | |
| 1. Develop individualized goals for client based on nursing diagnoses: | |
| a. Maintain client's proper body alignment.<br>b. Prevent or reduce injury to client's musculoskeletal system.<br>c. Skin remains intact. | Maintaining client's proper body alignment is crucial to reducing risk of poor alignment and potential injury to skin and musculoskeletal system. |
| d. Promote client's comfort. | Improved comfort level increases participation in positioning procedures. |
| 2. Prepare following equipment and supplies: | |
| a. Pillows | Used to support body parts, extremities or joints; elevates body part. |
| b. Footboard (Fig. 33-10) | Prevents foot-drop by maintaining foot in dorsiflexion. Stimulation to ball of foot by hard surface increases muscle tone. |
| c. Trochanter roll | Used to prevent external rotation of hip when client is supine. |
| d. Sandbag | May be used in place of or in addition to trochanter rolls. Used to immobilize extremity or maintain proper body alignment. |
| e. Hand rolls | Maintains hand, thumb, and fingers in functional position. |
| f. Restraints (as appropriate) | Used to immobilize clients and provide for safety. |
| g. Side rails | Aids weak client to roll from side to side in bed. Ensures client's safety. |
| 3. Raise level of bed to comfortable working height. | Raises level of work toward nurse's center of gravity. |
| 4. Remove all pillows and devices used in previous position. | Reduces interference from bedding during positioning procedure. |
| 5. Get extra help as needed. | Provides for client and nurse safety. |
| 6. Explain procedure to client. | Helps to decrease anxiety and increase cooperation. |
| **Implementation** | |
| 1. Wash hands. | Reduces transmission of infection. |
| 2. Provide for client privacy. Close door to room or close bedside curtains. | Ensuring client's mental comfort is as important as ensuring physical comfort. |
| 3. Put bed in flat position. | Provides easy access to client and allows nurses to reposition client without working against gravity. |
| 4. Move helpless client up in bed (one nurse): | |
| a. Place client on back with head of bed flat. Stand on one side of bed. | Enables nurse to assess body alignment. Reduces gravity's pull on client's upper body. |
| b. Place pillow at head of bed. | Prevents striking client's head against head of bed. |
| c. Begin at client's feet. Face foot of bed at 45-degree angle. Place feet apart with foot nearest head of bed behind other foot (forward-backward stance). Flex knees and hips as needed to bring arms level with client's legs. Shift weight from front to back leg and slide client's legs diagonally toward head of bed. | Positioning is begun at client's legs because they are lighter and easier to move. Facing direction of movement ensures proper balance. Shifting nurse's weight reduces force needed to move load. Diagonal motion permits pull in direction of force. Flexing knees lowers nurse's center of gravity and uses thigh muscles rather than back muscles. |
| d. Move parallel to client's hips. Flex knees and hips as needed to bring arms level with client's hips. | Maintains nurse's proper body alignment. Brings nurse closest to object to be moved and lowers center of gravity. Uses thigh muscles rather than back muscles. |
| e. Slide client's hips diagonally toward head of bed. | Aligns client's hips and feet. |

*Fig. 33-10*

| Steps | Rationale |
|---|---|
| f. Move parallel to client's head and shoulders. Flex knees and hips as needed to bring arms level with client's body. | Maintains nurse's proper body alignment. Brings nurse closer to object to be moved. Lowers nurse's center of gravity. Uses thigh muscles rather than back muscles. |
| g. Slide arm closest to head of bed under client's neck, with hand reaching under and supporting client's shoulder. | Supports client's head and neck, maintaining proper alignment and preventing injury during movement. |
| h. Place other arm under client's chest. | Supports client's body weight and reduces friction during movement. |
| i. Slide client's trunk, shoulders, head, and neck diagonally toward head of bed. | Realigns client's body on one side of bed. |
| j. Elevate side rail. Move to other side of bed and lower side rail. | Protects client from falling out of bed. |
| k. Repeat procedure, switching sides until client reaches desired height in bed. | |
| l. Center client in middle of bed, moving body in same three sections. | Maintains proper body alignment. Provides ample room for turning, positioning, other nursing activities. |
| 5. Assist client to move up in bed (one or two nurses): | |
| a. Place client on back with head of bed flat. | Enables nurse to assess body alignment. Reduces gravity's pull on client's upper body. |
| b. Place pillow at head of bed. | Prevents striking client's head against head of bed. |
| c. Face head of bed: | Facing direction of movement prevents twisting nurse's body while moving client. |
| ▪ Each nurse should have one arm under client's shoulders and one arm under client's thighs. | |
| ▪ Alternate position: position one nurse at client's upper body. Nurse's arm nearest head of bed should be under client's head and opposite shoulder; other arm should be under client's closest arm and shoulder. Position other nurse at client's lower torso. This nurse's arms should be under client's lower back and torso. | Prevents trauma to client's musculoskeletal system by supporting shoulder and hip joints and evenly distributing weight. |
| d. Place feet apart with foot nearest head of bed behind other foot (forward-backward stance). | Wide base of support increases nurse's balance. Stance enables nurse to shift body weight as client is moved up in bed, thereby reducing force needed to move load. |
| e. Ask client to flex knees with feet flat on bed. | Enables client to use femoral muscles during movement. |
| f. Instruct client to flex neck, tilting chin toward chest. | Prevents hyperextension of neck when moving client up in bed. |
| g. Instruct client to assist moving by pushing with feet on bed surface. | Reduces friction. Increases client mobility. Decreases nurse's workload. |
| h. Flex knees and hips, bringing forearms closer to level of bed. | Increases balance and strength by bringing nurse's center of gravity closer to client. Uses thigh instead of back muscles. |
| i. Instruct client to push with heels and elevate trunk while breathing out, thus moving toward head of bed on count of 3. | Prepares client for move. Reinforces assistance in moving up in bed. Increases client cooperation. Breathing out avoids Valsalva maneuver. |
| j. On count of 3, rock and shift weight from front to back leg. At the same time, client pushes with heels and elevates trunk. | Rocking enables nurse to improve balance and overcome inertia. Shifting nurse's weight counteracts client's weight and reduces force needed to move load. Client's assistance reduces friction and nurse's workload. |
| 6. Move helpless client up in bed using drawsheet (two nurses): | |
| a. Place drawsheet under client extending from shoulders to thigh. | Supports client's body weight and reduces friction during movement. |
| b. Place client on back with head of bed flat. | |
| c. Position one nurse at each side of client. | Distributes weight equally between nurses. |
| d. Grasp drawsheet firmly near the client. | |
| e. Place feet apart with forward-backward stance. Flex knees and hips. Shift weight from front to back leg and move client and drawsheet to desired position in bed. | Facing direction of movement ensures proper balance. Shifting weight reduces force needed to move load. Flexing knees lowers nurses' center of gravity and uses thigh instead of back muscles. |
| 7. Realign client in proper body alignment. | Prevents injury to musculoskeletal system. Nurses may assist client to one of the positions listed here (a-h). |
| a. Position client in supported Fowler's position: | |
| ▪ Elevate head of bed 45 to 60 degrees. | Increases comfort, improves ventilation, and increases client's opportunity to socialize or relax. |
| ▪ Rest head against mattress or on small pillow. | Prevents flexion contractures of cervical vertebrae. |
| ▪ Use pillows to support arms and hand if client does not have voluntary control or use of hands and arms. | Prevents shoulder dislocation from effect of downward pull of unsupported arms, promotes circulation by preventing venous pooling, prevents flexion contractures of arms and wrists. |

| Steps | Rationale |
|---|---|
| ▪ Position pillow at lower back. | Supports lumbar vertebrae and decreases flexion of vertebrae. |
| ▪ Place small pillow or roll under thigh. | Prevents hyperextension of knee and occlusion of popliteal artery from pressure from body weight. |
| ▪ Place small pillow or roll under ankles. | Prevents prolonged pressure on heels from mattress. |
| ▪ Place footboard at bottom of client's feet (Fig. 33-11). | Maintains dorsal flexion and prevents foot-drop. |
| b. Position hemiplegic client in supported Fowler's position: | |
| ▪ Elevate head of bed 45 to 60 degrees. | Increases comfort, improves ventilation, increases client's opportunity to relax. |
| ▪ Sit client up as straight as possible. | Counteracts tendency to slump toward affected side. Improves ventilation, cardiac output; decreases intracranial pressure. Improves client's ability to swallow and helps to prevent aspiration of food, liquids, gastric secretions. |
| ▪ Position head with chin slightly forward. | Support reduces risk of joint dislocation. Although muscle tone is decreased and muscles do not actively respond, limbs can be injured. |
| ▪ Provide support for involved arm and hand on overbed table in front of client; place arm away from client's side and support elbow with pillow. | Paralyzed muscles do not automatically resist pull of gravity as they do normally. As result, shoulder subluxation, pain, edema may occur. |
| ▪ Position *flaccid* hand in normal resting position with wrist slightly extended, arches of hand maintained, and fingers partially flexed; may use section of rubber ball cut in half; clasp client's hands together. | Maintains hand in functional position. Prevents contractures. |
| ▪ Position *spastic* hand with wrist in neutral position or slightly extended; fingers should be extended with palm down or may be left in relaxed position with palm up. | Maintains hand in functional position. Inhibits flexor spasticity. |
| ▪ Flex knees and hips by using pillow or folded blanket under knees. | Ensures proper alignment. Flexion prevents prolonged hyperextension, which could impair joint mobility. |
| ▪ Support feet in dorsiflexion with soft pillow or footboard. | Prevents foot-drop. Stimulation of ball of foot by hard surface has tendency to increase muscle tone in client with extensor spasticity of lower extremity. |
| c. Position client in supine position: | |
| ▪ Place client on back with head of bed flat. | Necessary for positioning in supine position. |
| ▪ Place small rolled towel under lumbar area of back. | Provides support for lumbar spine. |
| ▪ Place pillow under upper shoulders, neck, head. | Maintains correct alignment and prevents flexion contractures of cervical vertebrae. |
| ▪ Place trochanter rolls or sandbags parallel to lateral surface of client's thighs. | Reduces external rotation of hip. |
| ▪ Place small pillow or roll under ankle to elevate heels. | Reduces pressure on heels, helping to prevent pressure sores. |
| ▪ Place footboard or soft pillows against bottom of client's feet. | Maintains feet in dorsiflexion. Prevents foot-drop. |
| ▪ Place pillows under pronated forearms, keeping upper arms parallel to client's body (Fig. 33-12). | Reduces internal rotation of shoulder and prevents extension of elbows. Maintains correct body alignment. |
| ▪ Place hand rolls in client's hands. | Reduces extension of fingers and abduction of thumb. Maintains thumb slightly adducted and in opposition to fingers. |
| d. Position hemiplegic client in supine position: | |
| ▪ Place head of bed flat. | Necessary for positioning in supine position. |
| ▪ Place folded towel or small pillow under shoulder or affected side. | Decreases possibility of pain, joint contracture, subluxation. Maintains mobility in muscles around shoulder to permit normal movement patterns. |
| ▪ Keep affected arm away from body with elbow extended and palm up. (Alternative is to place arm out to side with elbow bent and hand toward head of bed.) | Maintains mobility in arm, joints, muscles around shoulder to permit normal movement patterns. (Alternative position counteracts limitation of ability of arm to rotate outward at shoulder [external rotation]. External rotation must be present to raise arm overhead without pain.) |
| ▪ Position affected hand in one of recommended positions for flaccid or spastic hand. | Maintains hand in functional position. |
| ▪ Place folded towel under hip of involved side. | Diminishes effect of spasticity in entire leg by controlling hip position. |
| ▪ Flex affected knee 30 degrees by supporting it on pillow or folded blanket. | Slight flexion breaks up abnormal extension pattern of leg. Extensor spasticity is most severe when client is supine. |
| ▪ Support feet with soft pillows at right angle to leg. | Maintains foot in dorsiflexion and prevents foot-drop. Pillows prevent stimulation to ball of foot by hard surface, which has tendency to increase muscle tone in client with extensor spasticity of lower extremity. |

*Fig. 33-11*

| Steps | Rationale |
|---|---|

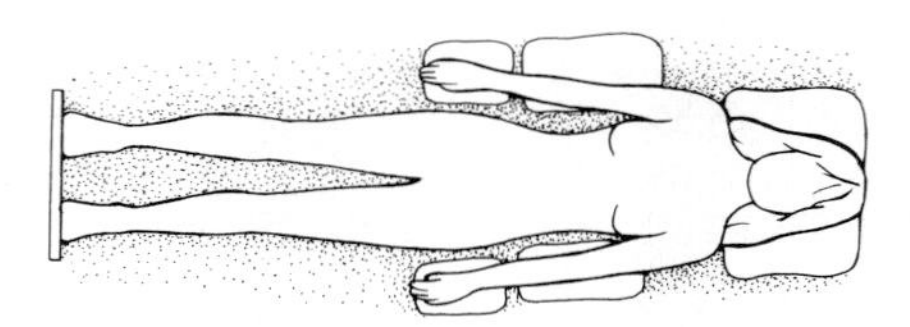

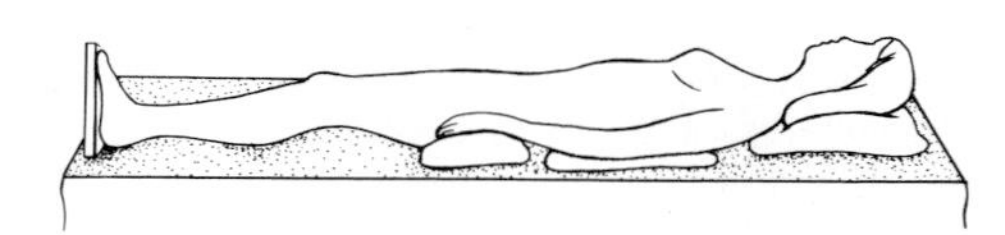

**Fig. 33-12**

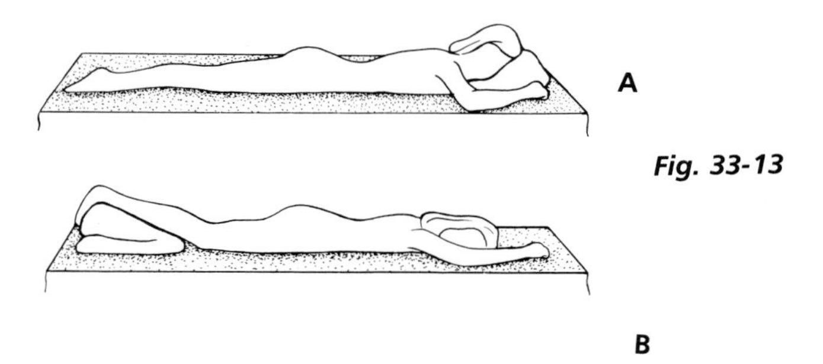


**Fig. 33-13**

e. Position client in prone position:
   - Roll client over arm positioned close to body with elbow straight and hand under hip. Position on abdomen in center of bed.
     Positions client correctly so alignment can be maintained.
   - Turn client's head to one side and support with small pillow (Fig. 13-13, *A*).
     Reduces flexion or hyperextension of cervical vertebrae.
   - Place small pillow under client's abdomen below level of diaphragm.
     Reduces pressure on breasts of some female clients, decreases hyperextension of lumbar vertebrae and strain on lower back. Improves breathing by reducing mattress pressure on diaphragm.
   - Support arms in flexed position level at shoulders.
     Maintains proper body alignment. Support reduces risk of joint dislocation.
   - Support lower legs with pillow to elevate toes (Fig. 33-13, *B*).
     Prevents foot-drop. Reduces external rotation of legs. Reduces mattress pressure on toes.

f. Position hemiplegic client in prone position:
   - Move client toward unaffected side.
     Ensures proper client alignment in center of bed when client is rolled onto abdomen.
   - Roll client onto side.
   - Place pillow on client's abdomen.
     Prevents sagging of abdomen when client is rolled over; decreases hyperextension of lumbar vertebrae and strain on lower back.
   - Roll client onto abdomen by positioning involved arm close to client's body with elbow straight and hand under hip. Roll client carefully over arm.
     Prevents injury to affected side.
   - Turn head toward involved side.
     Promotes development of neck and trunk extension, which is necessary for standing and walking.
   - Position involved arm out to side with elbow bent and hand toward head of bed, fingers extended if possible.
     Counteracts limitation of arm's ability to rotate outward at shoulder (external rotation). External rotation must be present to raise arm over head without pain.
   - Flex knees slightly by placing pillow under legs from knees to ankles.
     Flexion prevents prolonged hyperextension, which could impair joint mobility.
   - Keep feet at right angles to legs by using pillow high enough to keep toes off mattress.
     Maintains feet in dorsiflexion.

g. Position client in lateral (side-lying) position:
   - Lower head of bed completely or as low as client can tolerate.
     Provides position of comfort for client, removes pressure from bony prominences on back.
   - Position client to side of bed.
     Provides room for client to turn to side.
   - Turn client onto side:
     Prevents injury to joints as client is rolled to side.
     - To turn helpless client onto side, flex knee that will not be next to mattress. Place one hand on client's hip and one hand on shoulder.
       Client positioned so leverage on hip makes turning easy.
     - Roll client onto side.
       Rolling client toward nurse causes less trauma to tissues.
   - Place pillow under client's head and neck.
     Maintains alignment. Reduces lateral neck flexion. Decreases strain on sternocleidomastoid muscle.
   - Bring shoulder blade forward.
     Prevents client's weight from resting directly on shoulder joint.
   - Position both arms in slightly flexed position. Upper arm is supported by pillow level with shoulder, other arm by mattress.
     Decreases internal rotation and adduction of shoulder. Supporting both arms in slightly flexed position protects joint. Ventilation is improved because chest is able to expand more easily.
   - Place tuck-back pillow behind client's back. (Make by folding pillow lengthwise. Smooth area is slightly tucked under client's back.)
     Provides support to maintain client on side.

| Steps | Rationale |
|---|---|

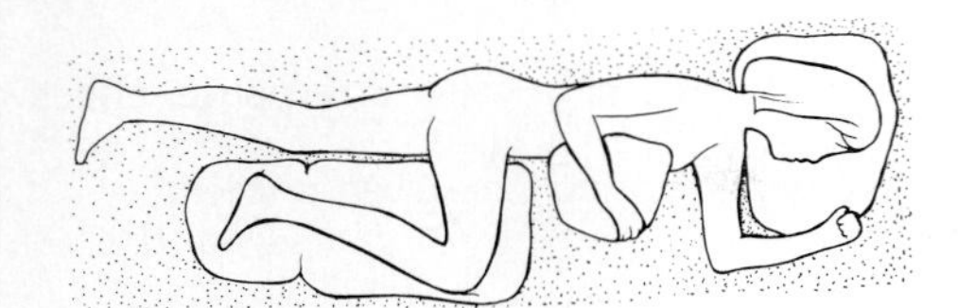
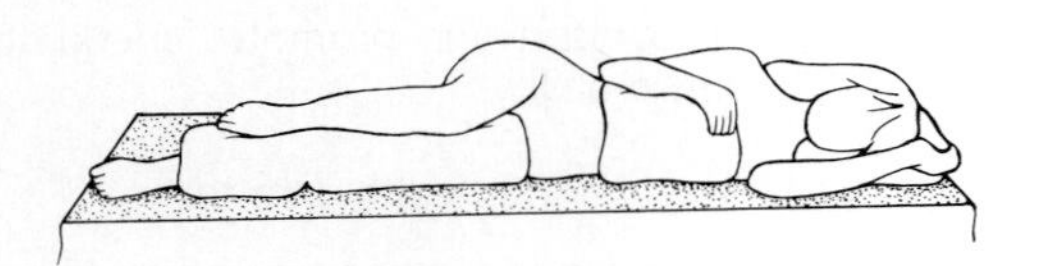
Fig. 33-14

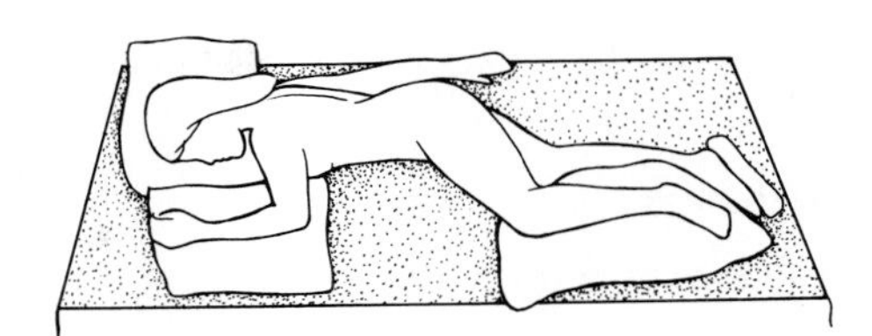
Fig. 33-15

- Place pillow under semiflexed upper leg level at hip from groin to foot (Fig. 33-14). — Flexion prevents hyperextension of leg. Maintains leg in proper alignment. Prevents pressure on bony prominence.
- Place sandbag parallel to plantar surface of dependent foot. — Maintains dorsiflexion of foot. Prevents foot-drop.

h. Position client in Sims' (semiprone) position: — Provides for proper body alignment while client is lying down.
- Lower head of bed completely. — Prepares client for position.
- Place client in supine position. — Client is rolled only partially on abdomen.
- Position client in lateral position, lying partially on abdomen.
- Place small pillow under client's head. — Maintains proper alignment and prevents lateral neck flexion.
- Place pillow under flexed upper arm, supporting arm level with shoulder. — Prevents internal rotation of shoulder. Maintains proper alignment.
- Place pillow under flexed upper legs, supporting leg level with hip. — Prevents internal rotation of hip and adduction of leg. Flexion prevents hyperextension of leg. Reduces mattress pressure on knees and ankles.
- Place sandbags parallel to plantar surface to foot (Fig. 33-15). — Maintains foot in dorsiflexion. Prevents foot-drop.

8. Wash hands. — Reduces transmission of infection.

## Evaluation

1. Assess client's body alignment, position, level of comfort. — Determines effectiveness of positioning. Additional supports (pillows, bath blankets), may be added or removed to promote comfort and correct body alignment.
2. Assess for existence of joint contractures, areas of erythema, or breakdown involving skin. — Provides ongoing observation regarding client's skin and musculoskeletal systems. Indicates complications of immobility or improper positioning of body part.

### *Expected outcomes*

1. Body alignment and joint mobility are improved. — Effectiveness of nursing care is based on client achievement of optimal joint mobility and alignment.
2. Skin remains intact, without evidence of breakdown. — Frequent position changes decrease risk of skin breakdown.
3. Client's comfort is increased. — Proper positioning reduces stress on joints.
4. Level of independence in completing ADL is increased. — Maintaining good body alignment and joint mobility increases client's level of independence and overall mobility. Client with inadequate joint mobility must receive assistance to carry out ADL.

### *Unexpected outcomes*

1. Joint contractures develop or worsen. — Joint contractures may develop or worsen because of improper or ineffective positioning.
2. Client is unable to maintain proper position without assistance. — Client may lean toward affected side (e.g., hemiplegia) and further injure the skin or musculoskeletal system.
3. Skin becomes reddened or breaks down. — Pressure points not properly identified. Frequency of turning is inadequate. Circulation may be impeded.
4. Client is unwilling to move. — Indicates fear of pain or discomfort.

| Step | Rationale |
|---|---|
| **Recording and Reporting** | |
| 1. Record procedure and observations (e.g., condition of skin, joint movement, client's ability to assist with positioning). | Documents procedure, client's response, effectiveness of nursing care. |
| 2. Report observations at change of shift and document in nurses' notes. | Individualizes nursing care given to client. |
| **Follow-up Activities** | |
| 1. Increase frequency of positioning if pressure sores begin to appear, joint mobility becomes impaired or worsened, or client complains of discomfort. | Provides for client comfort and promotes adequate circulation and optimal joint mobility. |
| 2. Consult with physical and occupational therapists as needed. | Provides consistency among health care team. |

## Special Considerations

- Client experiencing severe pain may require analgesia before moving or positioning.
- Some positions may be contraindicated in certain situations (e.g., respiratory difficulties, certain neurologic conditions, presence of incisions, drains, or tubings).
- Use aids such as pillows to relieve concentrated areas of pressure under client's body.
- Reposition clients, especially debilitated, unconscious, or paralyzed clients, at least every 2 hours.

## Teaching Considerations

- Include family in explanations, especially when caring for infant, young child, confused or unconscious client.
- Teach client ways to assist with positioning.
- Provide opportunity for return demonstration.
- Teach client, family signs and symptoms of pressure sores and contractures.

## Home Care Considerations

- Assess ability and motivation of client, family members, primary care giver to participate in moving and positioning client in bed.
- Assess home to determine the compatibility of environment with assistive devices (e.g., over-bed trapeze, Hoyer lift, hospital bed).
- Assess skin for pressure areas and friction burns.

### BIBLIOGRAPHY

Bulau J: Clinical policies and procedures for home health care, Rockville, Md, 1986, Aspen Publishers, Inc.

Gordon M: Assessing activity intolerance, Am J Nurs 76:72, 1976.

Kemp B, Pillitteri A: Fundamentals of nursing, Boston, 1984, Little, Brown & Co, Inc.

Milde EK: Impaired physical mobility, J Geron Nurs 14(3):20, 1988.

Nursing Reference Library: Procedures, Springhouse, Penn, 1985, Springhouse Corp.

Potter PA, Perry AG: Basic nursing, St Louis, 1987, The CV Mosby Co.

Potter PA, Perry AG: Fundamentals of nursing: concepts, process, and practice, ed 2, St Louis, 1989, The CV Mosby Co.

Root L, Kiernan T: Oh, my aching back, New York, 1973, Signet Books.

Saywell RM, Woods JR, Holmes GL, et al.: Reducing the costs of patient transfers, JONA 17(1-8):11, 1987.

Stryker R: Rehabilitative aspects of acute and chronic nursing care, Philadelphia, 1977, WB Saunders Co.

Tolbot D: Principles of therapeutic positioning: a guide for nursing action, Minneapolis, 1978, Sr Kenny Institute.

Walsh J, Persons C, Wieck L: Manual of home health care nursing, Philadelphia, 1987, JB Lippincott Co.

Yates J: Moving and lifting patients: principles and techniques, Minneapolis, 1970, Sr Kenny Institute.

# 34
# ORTHOPEDIC MEASURES

## OBJECTIVES

*Mastery of content in this chapter will enable the nurse to:*

- Define key terms.
- List benefits of the use of casts for clients with musculoskeletal injuries.
- Assemble materials necessary for application of casts.
- Describe how to assist with the application of casts.
- Describe neurovascular checks of a client in specific casts.
- List nutritional factors necessary for clients in casts.
- Describe techniques for drying casts.
- Describe toileting techniques for clients in casts.
- Describe turning and positioning techniques for clients in casts.
- Describe factors for client education for after removal of casts.
- List the purposes of placing clients in skin or skeletal traction.
- Differentiate among rationale for the use of skin or skeletal traction.
- Describe client conditions requiring the use of each form of skin or skeletal traction.
- Describe steps for applying each form of skin or skeletal traction.

## KEY TERMS

*Cast*
*Cast brace*
*Cast saw*
*Cast shoe*
*Cast stabilization*
*Cast syndrome*
*Casting tape*
*Countertraction*
*Four-poster cast*
*Gypsum*
*Harris splint*
*Head halter*
*Knee exercise*
*Knee sling*
*Minerva jacket*
*Neurovascular checks*
*Pearson's attachment*
*Pelvic belt*
*Pelvic sling*
*Petaling*
*Postcast care*
*Pulley*
*Sheet wadding*
*Spica cast*
*Spreader bar*
*Stockinette*
*Thomas splint*
*Traction*
*Traction boot*
*Walking heel*
*Webril*
*Weight holder*
*Windowing*

## SKILLS

**34-1** Assisting with Cast Application
**34-2** Assisting with Cast Removal
**34-3** Assisting with Application of Skin Traction
**34-4** Assisting with Insertion of Pins or Nails for Skeletal Traction

Clients in a cast or traction are susceptible to problems that can affect all body systems. Depending on the extent of a client's injury or illness, an orthopedic device may affect a single body part or the entire body. The resultant immobility requires extensive nursing care.

The adequacy of central and peripheral circulation must be carefully assessed because delivery of oxygenation and removal of wastes are vital for bone healing, muscle growth and strength, and regaining mobility. Color, temperature, and capillary refill assessments provide data about the adequacy of circulation to the casted extremity. Inflammation, cellulitis, or edema may indicate venous stasis or infection.

Integumentary tissues inside and outside the cast must remain healthy and well nourished. Careful assessment of the tissues is vital to detect pressure, inflammation, or lesions that could lead to infections of pressure sores. Gentle and thorough cleansing of skin, careful drying, lubrication with lotions, and gentle, frequent massage provide moisture and stimulation to the integumentary tissues to maintain a healthy state.

Proper turning and positioning help to maintain the health of integumentary and musculoskeletal tissues of individuals in casts. After application of a cast, especially a spica or body cast (Fig. 34-1) or minerva jacket, the client must be turned from side to side and prone to facilitate thorough drying of the cast. Turning the client every 2 to 3 hr while keeping the damp cast uncovered facilitates drying. Turning also aids circulation throughout the body and helps to maintain muscle strength and tone. Placement of pillows, rolls, or blankets helps the client to maintain the side-lying or prone position. In addition, musculoskeletal tissues maintain strength through regularly performed active range-of-motion (ROM) exercises with or without resistance or weight. Quadriceps-, gluteus-, and triceps-, biceps-, and hamstring-setting exercises, performed routinely and steadily, help to maintain muscle mass and tone (Chapter 36).

A major challenge for nurses caring for clients in body, spica, or minerva jacket casts is to maintain the functions of respiratory tissues. Turning facilitates moving air and fluids in the respiratory tissues, but it is vital for full functioning that clients be encouraged to breathe deeply and cough and to practice these exercises. Bed rest over time affects the respiratory tissues, resulting in decreased functioning. Clients who develop respiratory complications may require respiratory therapy and at times administration of antibiotics. Preventive measures should be sufficient to avoid such necessities.

Additional challenges center around intake and maintenance of functions of the gastrointestinal and renal/urinary systems. Clients in casts who are confined to bed frequently develop anorexia, constipation, and at times fecal impaction. Maintaining a high (3000 ml or more) fluid intake plus a high-bulk or high-residue diet fosters proper bowel elimination. Fluid intake also facilitates renal circulation and urinary output to lessen the possibility of a urinary tract infection or renal calculi.

Clients immobilized in casts or traction may lose much weight. Diets should be high in protein, carbohydrates, vitamins, bulk, and fluids and should contain moderate fat, unless contraindicated. Because of individual metabolic and endocrine stress responses, the client will experience catabolism with muscle mass loss for a period of 10 to 20 or more days. With proper diet this trend is followed, it is hoped, by anabolism, muscle mass regain, and weight gain, and blood chemistry changes (levels of sodium and calcium being higher in the plasma, whereas those of potassium and magnesium are lower).

Motor and sensory functions associated with the neurological tissues are greatly affected when a client is placed in a cast. Motor changes may lead to muscle and joint weakness from disuse or pressure, and sensory changes, also from pressure or trauma, may lead to complaints of pain, numbness, and tingling. When such sensory signs are present, they may be relieved by changing the client's position. In addition, bivalving, or cutting the cast removes the pressure or tightness and increases circulation. Permanent damage may result if the circulation is not restored or pressure is not removed. Motor weakness may be restored to normal ranges through ROM exercises and physical therapy. Full muscle function returns slowly, and consistent performance of exercises is required.

Psychologically, clients in casts may experience alterations in self-concept and body image. They may lose some independence, mobility, and work income during their "cast days;" however, if they perceive these changes as temporary, they usually regain full independence and mobility and return to work sooner than those in casts who do not experience regression periods.

Clients in traction or those with casts who are confined to bed may become easily tired during the day and may take short, frequent naps. Thus they may be less sleepy at bedtime and may lie awake past their usual bedtime. To

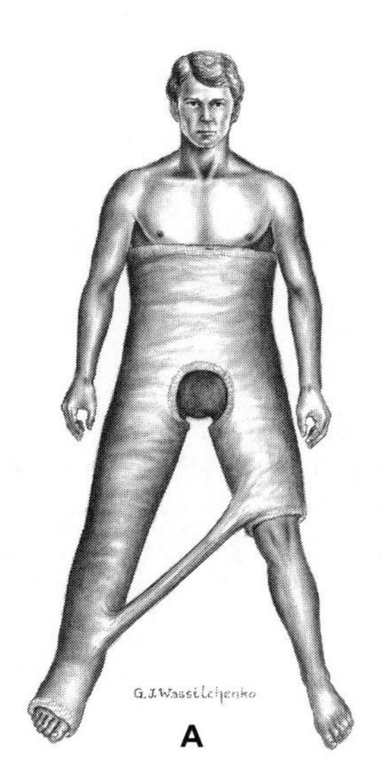


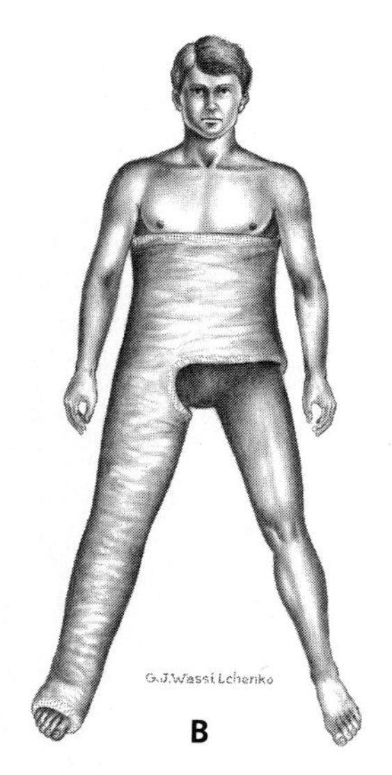


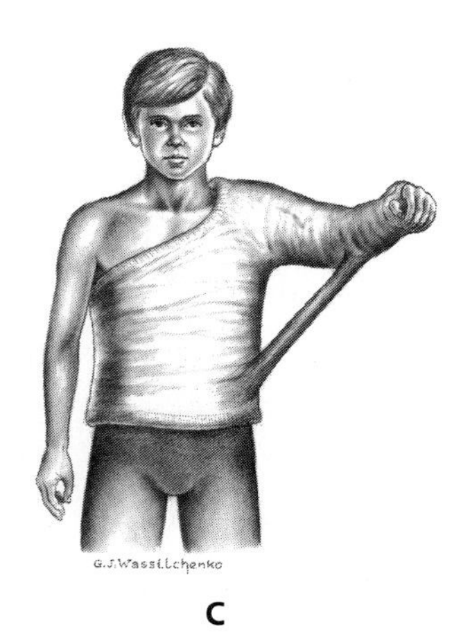


***Fig. 34-1*** Spica casts. **A,** Unilateral hip spica. **B,** One-and-a-half hip spica. **C,** Shoulder spica.
From Thompson JM, et al: Mosby's manual of clinical nursing, ed 2, St Louis, 1989, The CV Mosby Co.

offset this syndrome, clients should maintain active, stimulating activities to become tired at bedtime rather than during the day.

Traction is a force or pull applied to the bones directly or indirectly to overcome deformity and to help to restore alignment. When bones are fractured, muscle spasms pull the distal fragments out of their normal positions (Table 34-1). Sufficient pull must be applied to the injured tissues to overcome muscle spasms and thus permit the bones to realign themselves in the usual anatomical positions. In situations of severe muscle spasms, marked deformity, or displacement, traction must be applied directly to the distal fragments by means of a strong nail or pin to which traction is applied through a bar, ropes, pulleys, and weights. Such skeletal traction may be applied to one or more bones, including the bones of the skull, upper and lower extremities, and pelvic bones.

Traction to the skin, and thus indirectly to the bones (so-called skin traction), can also be applied to these bones. Skeletal traction is commonly used for minor trauma. Because of the lower tolerance of skin tissues, traction should be applied for shorter periods with less weight, and at times can be interrupted.

Skeletal traction, if used for severe trauma, is applied for longer periods, requires much heavier weights, and is never interrupted but always continuous.

The nurse uses her knowledge of normal mobility and the findings from the nursing assessment to provide care to the client with a cast or traction. The following guidelines can assist the nurse in individualizing her nursing care plan.

## GUIDELINES

1. Know the client's dietary preferences. Wound healing and repair of bone and tissues require additional calorie intake. Providing foods the client can enjoy meets these additional calorie needs.
2. Know the limits of ROJM to the casted extremity or extremity in traction. Although it is important to maintain joint mobility, the nurse must not move the affected extremity beyond the limits imposed by the cast or traction. Excessive movement can impair wound healing, extremity alignment, and new bone growth.
3. Determine the client's level of independent functioning. Knowing what the client is capable of doing enables the nurse to properly plan for assisting the client with ADL such as bathing, eating, dressing, and grooming.
4. Know the client's normal elimination patterns. Restrictions on mobility imposed by the cast or traction can result in altered elimination patterns. Knowledge of normal patterns can help the nurse to design a nursing care plan to meet the client's normal patterns.
5. Determine the client's understanding of the normal

***TABLE 34-1*** Description of Types of Fractures

| Type of Fracture | Persons Affected | Description of Fracture | Force or Power Causing Fracture |
|---|---|---|---|
| Avulsed | Children and young adults | Bone and other tissues are pulled away from usual attachments; frequently occurs in ankle, knee (patella), and elbow. | Direct or indirect force pulls tissues away. |
| Closed | All ages | Bone is fractured, but skin over site remains intact. | Force is minor, but bone is broken. |
| Comminuted | Young or older adults | Fracture results in more than two pieces and much soft tissue trauma. | Crushing force is applied directly to tissue. |
| Compression | All ages | Bone is squeezed or wedged together at one side or at cortex. | Axial compressive force is applied directly to superior skeleton. |
| Greenstick | Children and older (geriatric) adults | Break is in one outer covering (cortex) of bone. | Force is minor, and direct or indirect. |
| Oblique | All ages | Fracture is obliquely across both cortices of bone. | Force is twisting or angulating with axial compression. |
| Open | All ages | Skin is open; bones are fractured. | Moderate or severe force exceeds tissue tolerance. |
| Pathologic | Older ages | Fracture may be transverse, oblique, or spiral. | Minor direct or indirect force is applied to bone weakened by tumor or other condition. |
| Spiral | Young and older adults | Fracture curves around both cortices, which may twist to become displaced. | Force is direct or indirect and twisting. |
| Stress | Young and older adults | One cortex is cracked. | Applications of force are repetitive, such as from striking a level. May also occur in bones weakened from medication. |
| Transverse | All ages | Horizontal break occurs across both bone cortices. | Force is direct or indirect and moderate. |

bone-healing process. This knowledge assists the nurse in developing a teaching plan for the client to care for the casted extremity at home.
6. Know the results of recent laboratory tests. Serum calcium levels may rise, particularly in children.
7. Know the frequency and type of analgesics ordered for the client by the physician. The client may experience acute, continuous pain during the first 4 to 7 days (the acute inflammatory stage), and thus require 24-hour administration of analgesics during this time.
8. Know the materials used in cast application and traction setup. Various materials affect drying time, resistance to pressure, weight bearing.

**PREREQUISITE KNOWLEDGE**

1. Functions of the muscles, bones, other supporting tissues.
2. Principles of body mechanics.
3. Factors of wound and bone healing.
4. Hazards of immobility.

**PREREQUISITE SKILLS**

1. Techniques for lifting, moving, carrying clients (Chapters 32 and 33).
2. Physical assessment (Chapter 13).
3. Hygiene assistance (Unit III).

## *SKILL 34-1 Assisting with Cast Application*

A cast is an externally applied structure used to hold musculoskeletal tissues in a specific position to permit healing of injuries or fractures or to align malpositioned tissues, such as in clubfoot or congenital hip dislocation. The rigidity of the cast overcomes the tension, tone, or rotational forces of the muscles or bones for the time required to heal or align the diseased or injured tissues. Because a cast holds tissue in the position in which it is applied, it must be applied carefully and properly to achieve the goals for its use. Assisting with the application of a cast is a standard nursing skill.

Casts are made from plaster of paris or synthetic materials. A plaster of paris cast has multiple rolls of open-weave cotton saturated with calcium sulfate crystals. These casts are heavier than synthetic casts and take 48 hours with no weight bearing or application of pressure to dry. Synthetic casts are composed of polyester and cotton, which is impregnated with a water-activated polyurethane resin. In addition, synthetic casts are also made of fiberglass or plastic. The newer synthetic casts are lightweight, set in 15 minutes, and can sustain weight-bearing or pressure in 15 to 30 minutes.

### Purposes

1. Facilitate the application of the cast for the safety of the client and health care personnel.
2. Provide optimal care to the client before, during, and after the application of the cast.

## *Procedure 34-1*

| Steps | Rationale |
|---|---|
| **Assessment** | |
| 1. Assess client's previous health status, including conditions affecting wound healing (e.g., diabetes, malnutrition). | Client's health status is pertinent to potential healing of tissues enclosed by cast. Nurse may need to provide special hygiene, mobility, or psycho support interventions. |
| 2. Assess client's understanding of upcoming cast application. | Relieves client's anxiety and helps nurse to determine whether additional information is needed. |
| 3. Assess condition of tissues to be in the cast. Note presence of skin breakdown, bruising, rash, irritation. Skin of babies, children, older persons may contain less subcutaneous fat. | Determines need for additional skin care before cast application. |
| 4. Determine client's pain status. | Fractures are painful; client responses vary as does need for analgesic. |
| **Nursing Diagnosis** | |
| 1. Cluster data to reveal actual or potential nursing diagnoses:<br>a. Impaired physical mobility, related to:<br>▪ Fractured bone (Table 35-1).<br>▪ Congenital deformities. | Use of cast provides rest to affected tissues to promote healing. Fractured bones must be held in contact with one another and immobile for union to transpire. Congenital deformities must be realigned and immobilized for correction to occur. |

| Steps | Rationale |
|---|---|
| b. Potential impaired skin integrity, related to: ▪ Presence of cast. ▪ Impaired circulation. | Underlying skin is at risk for breakdown resulting from pressure from cast or moisture trapped under cast. |
| c. Pain: related to fracture. | As fracture becomes realigned, pain should decrease. |
| **Planning** | |
| 1. Develop individualized goals for client based on nursing diagnoses: | |
| a. Maintain comfort and avoid additional trauma. | Additional trauma impedes healing and can cause malunion of fractured bone. |
| b. Maintain integrity of cast for time required for healing. | Proper cast care in acute and long-term settings promotes proper alignment during healing process. |
| c. Maintain muscle and joint functions within limitations of cast. | Unless instructed by physician, client should never keep casted extremity totally immobile (e.g., if forearm is casted, client should move shoulder joint). |
| d. Prevent untoward reactions or complications while client is in cast and after its removal. | Proper casting procedures prevent damage to underlying musculoskeletal tissues, reduction in joint mobility, and impaired circulation to extremity. |
| 2. Assemble and prepare equipment (may all be assembled already on "cast cart"): | |
| a. Plaster rolls (sizes include 2-, 3-, 4-, and 6-in rolls). Depending on purpose of cast or specific client condition, other cast materials such as fiberglass, cast tape, or plastic may be used instead of plaster. | Plaster serves to hold tissues rigidly. |
| b. Padding material (may use felt, stockinette, sheet wadding, Webril, or other material; various thicknesses and lengths are available) | Provides protection over bony prominences. |
| c. Plastic-lined pail filled three-fourths full with warm water. | Warm water facilitates plaster setting. |
| d. Gloves and aprons | Used to protect hands and clothing of persons applying cast. |
| e. Scissors | Used to cut plaster rolls if needed. |
| f. Paper or plastic sheets | Used to protect floor. |
| g. Cast saw (if old cast is to be removed) | |
| h. Cart, chair, fracture table | Used to position properly and comfortably. |
| 3. Continue to instruct client, parent, other assistants how they can facilitate application of cast by maintaining desired positions. | Cast will hold tissues in position in which they are held. Client teaching reduces anxiety and increases cooperation. |
| 4. Administer analgesic 20 to 30 min before cast application. | Reduces pain during cast application. Provides optimal analgesia effect. |
| **Implementation** | |
| 1. Wash hands. | Reduces transmission of microorganisms. |
| 2. Position client as desired by professional applying cast; client may be lying, sitting, standing, depending on type of cast and tissues to be casted. | Parts to be put in cast must be supported and in optimal position for cast application. |
| 3. Prepare skin for cast if necessary; may involve cleansing with soap and water, changing dressing, trimming long hair. Use gentle strokes to maintain skin integrity. | Reduces complications to underlying tissues after casting. Gentle manipulation prevents pain or additional injury. |
| 4. Depending on type of cast material being applied, do *one* of the following: | |
| a. Hold plaster roll under water until bubbles stop, then squeeze slightly and hand roll to person applying cast. | Dampened plaster rolls are unrolled and molded to fit part being put in cast. Some have resin for easy moldability. |
| b. Hold part or parts to be put in cast in position requested by person applying cast. | Support of part may involve applying slight manual traction, if desired, to maintain optimal position. |
| c. Hold parts while casting tape is applied and molded. Allow time for casting tape to dry or set. | Casting tape is impregnated with synthetic adhesive or fiberglass materials, which dry quickly and are lightweight. |
| 5. Continue to supply dampened rolls of plaster or to hold parts as necessary until cast is finished. | Plaster must be of sufficient thickness to give strength to cast. |
| 6. Supply walking heel, brace, bar, or other stabilizing material as requested by physician. | Ambulation may be permitted with partial weight bearing, which is facilitated by walking heel or sole. Bars stabilize spica cast, or "posts" (metal poles) stabilize "four-poster" cast. Brace can be incorporated into cast to aid in maintaining joint motion and mobility. |

| Steps | Rationale |
|---|---|
| 7. Assist with "finishing" cast by folding stockinette or other padding down over outer edge of cast to provide smooth edge to cast. Damp plaster is then unrolled over padding to hold it securely outside cast. | Smooth edges lessen possible skin irritation. By finishing cast with stockinette, later "petaling" is not required when cast is dry. |
| 8. Supply scissors to trim plaster rolls around thumb, fingers, toes as necessary. | Cast should be snug but not constrict joint movement or circulation. |
| 9. Depending on tissues casted, do *one* of the following: | |
| a. Place damp cast on pillows to prevent deformation or pressure points as it sets. | Pillows or soft areas prevent cast from hardening in undesirable position. |
| b. Place casted tissues in sling, making sure sling just holds, and does not encase, cast. | Covering (encasing) delays air movements and delays drying. |
| c. Cover client or reclothe as needed, leaving damp, casted areas uncovered. | Covering blocks air movements and delays drying. |
| 10. Assist with transfer of client to cart or wheelchair, to responsible person for return to nursing unit, to prepare client for discharge. | Safety in transfer requires use of pillows to support cast, side rails, restraints, sufficient personnel to support client and cast. |
| 11. May accompany client to room and assist with transfer to bed if necessary. | Safety requires more than one person to accompany client in body, spica, long-arm, long-leg, Minerva jacket cast. |
| 12. Clean equipment used (pail, scissors, cast saw, etc.), return to usual places; discard used materials. Wash hands. | Facilitates use of equipment and area for next client. Reduces transmission of infection. |
| 13. Explain purposes of exposure for fast drying, use of elevation if pertinent, application of ice bags if ordered, use of fans or lights to facilitate drying. | Casts must dry from inside out for thorough drying. Elevation and use of ice decreases edema formation. Fans should not be used to open areas or under cast; organisms may be blown in to cause infection. Synthetic casts are dry or set by time of transfer because they set in 7 to 15 min. Soft tissues around affected area may swell from processes of "reducing" or manipulating before cast was applied. |

### *Evaluation*

| Steps | Rationale |
|---|---|
| 1. Reassess client to determine response to casting. | Clients in spica or body cast may experience claustrophobic feelings. |
| 2. Observe client for signs of pain or anxiety: hyperventilation, swallowing air (aerophagia), tachycardia, blood pressure increases. | These are signs of development of "cast syndrome"—severe claustrophobia from snugness of cast. |
| 3. Assess neurovascular status by performing neurovascular checks: | Neurovascular status determines circulation and oxygenation of tissues. |
| a. Observe color of tissues distal to cast (may be pink, whitish, bluish). Older clients may have bluish color normally; however, no other signs of circulatory compromise should be present. | Pink indicates arterial pressure is normal, whitish signifies decreased arterial supply, bluish signifies venous statis. |
| b. Observe for edema distal to cast. Older persons may have concurrent dependent edema because of health state. | Edema results from trauma or venous stasis. Rarely, heat of plaster drying may contribute to development of edema. |
| c. Feel temperature of tissues above and below or around cast. Older clients frequently have cooler-than-usual extremities because of decreased peripheral circulation. | Warmth of tissues distal or proximal to cast usually indicate adequate perfusion. If tissues are cold or cool, *compare* with similar unaffected tissues, such as opposite fingers, toes, or foot, to determine if coolness is excessive, which would indicate decreased arterial perfusion. |
| d. Ask client to move parts in ROM if possible; note if client is unable to do active ROM of uncasted areas. Older clients may have stiffness of joints or edema because of other health conditions. | Range of motion should be performed within limitations, imposed by cast. Only tissues out of cast can, or *should,* be moved. |
| e. If client cannot do *active* ROM to contiguous tissues, perform *passive* ROM to these joints, noting responses or complaints of increased pain. | Passive movements decrease edema and demonstrate ability of part to be moved. However, inability to perform active ROM and increased pain during passive movement may signify development of compartment syndrome and should be reported. |
| f. Ask client to describe sensations or feelings of tissues in cast; listen for descriptions of "pins and needles," "asleep," "numb," "burning," or "throbbing"; Do *not* prompt client by using those words. Older clients may have decreased sensory response because of circulatory impairments. A child may not be able to describe sensations; use more than one neurovascular check. | May signify pressure or anoxia affecting normal transmission of nerve impulses. |
| g. Assess capillary refill by pressing on toe or fingernail (if cast is on extremity), releasing, and noting "pinking" of | "Blanching" on pressure with subsequent capillary refill is indicative of arterial perfusion. Capillary refill is too sluggish if refill |

| Steps | Rationale |
|---|---|
| nail; nail should "pink up" in 2 to 4 sec. Older clients may have slow or even poor capillary refill because of peripheral vascular conditions; use more than one neurovascular check to determine circulatory adequacy. | takes 4 to 6 sec. It takes 2 sec to say "capillary refill" slowly and 4 sec to repeat it once. |
| h. Determine amount and severity of pain if present; ask client for descriptions; avoid coaching client with words to describe pain. Older clients may have decreased pain perceptions. Babies or children may signify pain through crying or restlessness. | Manipulation and reduction may produce dull, aching pain as results of pressure on nerve endings. Clients vary in perception and tolerance of pain. Sudden increase in pain should be investigated further because it may signify thrombus formation. |
| i. Compare tissues in cast with contralateral tissues to determine current condition. | Comparison with normal tissues assists in forming judgment of neurovascular status. |
| ***Expected outcomes*** | |
| 1. Client experiences slight edema, soreness, mild pain, some limitation of active ROM from being in cast. | Cast is unnatural encumbrance to normal functions of affected tissues. |
| 2. Skin of tissues below cast is of normal color, warm, with normal capillary refill. | Circulation to body part is maintained. |
| 3. Client is able to do limited ROM actively. | Other joints should move without impairment. |
| 4. Client had some impaired function in mobility initially. | Casts may be heavy or impair mobility because of size or area of body in cast. |
| 5. Client needs assistance with usual ADL if head, neck, or upper extremity is in cast. | Cast can hamper ability to dress, feed, or bathe oneself. |
| ***Unexpected outcomes*** | |
| 1. Client experiences malunion or malposition of affected parts. | May be caused by insufficient reduction (placement) in cast. |
| 2. Client experiences nonunion. | May result from local or systemic factors, such as infection, foreign objects in area, diabetes, or malnutrition. |
| 3. Client experiences osteomyelitis if open wound is present at casting. | Causes of osteomyelitis may be bacterial, fungal, tubercular, or other and may not develop for years after injury and cast. |
| 4. Client develops decubitus ulcer over bony prominence. | May result from inward pressure of cast on tissues. |
| 5. Client experiences muscle weakness. | May result from prolonged immobility. |
| 6. There is decreased circulation or sensation distal to cast, as indicated by cold extremity, decreased capillary refill, numbness, and tingling. | Indicates cast is constricting circulation to extremity. If constriction remains, extremity can be permanently damaged. |

## Recording and Reporting

| Steps | Rationale |
|---|---|
| 1. Record application of cast and report abnormal or untoward findings from neurovascular checks; report following immediately: bluish color to distal parts, marked increase in edema or pain, delayed capillary refill (longer than 6 sec), inability to palpate distal peripheral pulses if originally could palpate pulse, increased numbness or tingling, cold tissues, inability to move tissues actively. | All are signs of circulatory compromise, stasis, and, possibly, development of compartment syndrome. |
| 2. Report signs of increasing anxiety, restlessness, aerophagia to oncoming personnel. | May signify claustrophobic feelings or beginning of "cast syndrome." |
| 3. Record elevated temperature if rising. | May signify infection in body. |
| 4. Record all responses to strategies to relieve symptoms (e.g., elevation and application of ice bags to decrease edema, change of position to relieve pain, cutting of cast to relieve pressure or increase circulation). | Elevation increases venous return; ice aids vasoconstriction; changing position eases sore or painful muscles; cutting cast restores circulation. |
| 5. Record all findings of neurovascular checks performed initially every 1 to 2 hr and gradually extending to every 3 to 4 hr. | Checks are performed to detect signs as soon as possible. |
| 6. Record client's ability or inability to perform ADL and specific requirements for care. | Independence is valued for continuity of care and self-care. |

## Follow-up Activities

| Steps | Rationale |
|---|---|
| 1. Edges of cast begin to fray. | |
| a. Apply "petals" to further protect cast. Small pieces of adhesive tape 2.5-5.0 cm (1 to 2 inches) are cut and taped over edge of cast (optional). | Petaling protects cast from further disintegration, and smooth cast edges decrease possibility of skin irritaiton. If edges of cast are too broken down entire cast may need to be replaced. |

| Steps | Rationale |
|---|---|
| 2. Odor and drainage from cast is noted. | Indicates infectious process and should be investigated by physician. |
| a. Contact physician. | |
| b. Draw circle on cast around drainage site. Record time and date on circle (optional). | Documents drainage and allows nursing and medical personnel to quantify amount of drainage. Some drainage should be expected in postoperative orthopedic clients. |
| 3. If circulation to extremity is compromised: | Pressure must be relieved to restore circulation. |
| a. Call physician. | |
| b. Anticipate splitting or removing case. | |

### Special Considerations

- Casts are removed earlier in babies, children, older persons to facilitate muscle and joint function.
- If cast is applied for clubfoot, person applying cast can usually mold cast in desired position.
- Plaster of paris casts on babies or children and older persons may have less plaster to aid in moving or lifting.
- Clients in casts may be more comfortable than when not in cast if deformity or crepitation (ends rubbing against each other with fracture) is present.
- Client with wet large-limb or wet spica cast require three people to assist in turning. Proper assistance prevents undue pressure on cast.
- Realign pillows to promote cast drying when client is repositioned.

### Teaching Considerations

- Clients must be taught to care for casts in home to protect it from moisture and unnecessary wear.
- If child has clubfoot, parents and child should be taught that frequent cast changes are necessary. Cast changes accomodate normal bone and tissue growth and correction of abnormality.
- Babies in casts for treatment of clubfoot have limited maneuverability.
- Teach client about effects of pressure from cast on underlying skin and tissue.
- Prepare client for itching sensations under cast. Client should avoid sticking objects down or in casts to scratch because these objects can cause break in underlying skin and subsequent infections.
- If client must use crutches instruct in crutch walking techniques (Skill 36-5).
- Teach client proper ROJM and isometric exercises for affected extremity.

### Home Care Considerations

- Client must inspect cast and petal rough edges to reduce risk of trauma to underlying skin and need for cast changes.
- Client must inspect cast daily for foul odor, which indicates skin excoriation or infection under cast.
- Client must inspect skin daily for pressure or friction areas.
- Client must inspect cast daily for cracks or changes in alignment.
- Client must keep plaster of paris cast dry. When bathing, casted extremity must not be submerged because cast absorbs water. If cast becomes wet, dry immediately.
- Synthetic casts may be cleaned with warm water and mild soap.
- Some synthetic casts, those applied with polypropylene stockinette, may be emersed in water. Thorough drying with blow dryer on cool or warm is essential. Complete drying prevents skin maceration.

## *SKILL 34-2 Assisting with Cast Removal*

Cast removal consists of removing the cast and padding with a mechanical device such as a cast saw. The nurse must prepare for this procedure so the client remains still and cooperates during cast removal. The removal of a cast is painless but can be noisy. A child or confused client may need to be gently restrained during the procedure to prevent injury by the equipment.

### Purposes

1. Facilitate removal of the cast.
2. Provide appropriate skin care after cast removal.

## Procedure 34-2

| Steps | Rationale |
|---|---|
| **Assessment** | |
| 1. Assess client's understanding of upcoming cast removal. | Assists in developing a teaching plan that aids in reducing anxiety. |
| 2. Assess client's readiness for cast removal (client's physical findings, physician's orders, x-ray results). | Determines level of healing and readiness to remove cast. |
| 3. Ask client if any itching or irritation under cast is felt. | Indicates healing and accumulation of dried skin layers. |
| **Nursing Diagnosis** | |
| 1. Cluster data to reveal actual or potential nursing diagnoses: | Use of case provides rest of affected tissues to permit healing. |
| a. Impaired mobility: related to fractured bone (see Table 35-1 for types of fractures). | Fractured bones must be held in contact and immobile for union of bone to occur. |
| b. Impaired skin integrity: related to cast application. | Skin encased in cast may become dry, flaky, irritated. |
| **Planning** | |
| 1. Develop individualized goals for client based on nursing diagnoses: | |
| a. Remove cast safely. | Proper positioning techniques prevent accidental injury to skin when cast saw is used. |
| b. Promote skin integrity. | Dry, irritated skin will require special care. |
| 2. Assemble equipment: | |
| a. Cast saw | Cast is cut off slowly and carefully to avoid injury to underlying tissues. |
| b. Plastic sheets or papers | |
| c. Cold water enzyme wash | Removes dead skin cells. |
| d. Skin lotion | |
| e. Basin, water, washcloths, towels | Used to cleanse tissues |
| f. Scissors | Used to cut padding next to skin. |
| 3. Explain procedure to client, including noise made by cast saw. | Cients may be frightened by noise of cast saw. |
| **Implementation** | |
| 1. Assist person removing cast by positioning, turning, holding cast and tissues in cast. | Prevents injury from saw. |
| 2. After removal of cast and padding, inspect tissues for general condition, redness, heat, drainage. | May signify inflammation or infection of tissues. |
| 3. If skin is intact, gently apply cold water enzyme wash to skin; let stay on skin 15 to 20 min. | Helps dissolve or emulsify dead cells and fatty deposits on tissues. |
| 4. After elapsed time, gently wash off enzyme wash; if possible, immerse tissues in basin or tub to aid in removal of tissue debris without undue rubbing or pressure. | Removes as much debris as possible. |
| 5. After patting tissues dry (avoid rubbing), apply generous coating of skin lotion, gently massaging into pores. | Rubbing could traumatize tender tissues. Lotion lubricates skin. |
| 6. Gently put tissues through active and passive ROM. | Joints and muscles will be stiff and weak. |
| 7. Assist in transfer of client for return to room or for discharge if anticipated. | Home recovery is preferable when possible. |
| **Evaluation** | |
| 1. Reassess client to determine response to cast removal. Observe for discomfort and assess condition of skin. | Provides for modification of nursing care plan. |
| ***Expected outcome*** | |
| 1. After removal of cast, client experiences transient (from 24 to 48 hr) return of edema, pain, limited use and mobility. | Return of ability to use affected limb results in temporary alteration in circulation and pain perception. |

| Steps | Rationale |
|---|---|
| ***Unexpected outcomes*** | |
| 1. Client experiences extensive edema, pain, limited use of affected tissues. | Patterns may be related to malunion, nonunion, extreme muscle weakness. |
| 2. Client is unable to perform ADL. | May be related nonunion or pain. |
| **Recording and Reporting** | |
| 1. Record cast removal and person removing cast in nurses' notes. | Provides for completeness of care and documentation for legal concerns. |
| 2. Record client's responses to cast removal and feelings of insecurity. | Insecurity is common after cast is gone. |
| 3. Record condition of tissues formerly in cast. | Provides baseline data to ensure continuity of care. |
| 4. Record instructions given to client, parent, relatives. | Provides for safety and documentation for legal concerns. |
| 5. Record transfer of client to room or preparations for discharge. | Documents discharge teaching. |
| **Follow-up Activities** | |
| 1. Client may have transient symptoms after cast removal. Physician or nurse should instruct client to deal with these symptoms by: | |
| a. Elevating part if edema returns. | Elevation aids in venous return. |
| b. Using nonnarcotic analgesics every 4 hr for up to 24 hr if needed. | |
| c. Slowly performing ROM exercises every 4 hr. (If marked weakness exists, physician may order client to receive physical therapy or to use sling for 1 to 2 days for continued rest.) | Gradual return of muscle strength should occur over time. |
| 2. Report changes in movement, severe swelling, increased pain to physician. | May signify insufficient healing, muscle atrophy, weakness, nonunion of bone. |

## Special Considerations

- Amount of cellular debris under client's cast depends on length of time tissues are in cast and overall skin integrity.
- Use caution with tender skin areas or joints.
- Older person's skin is drier, thinner, more fragile than that of a baby, child, younger adult.
- Babies, children, older clients may experience marked stiffness or weakened muscles, depending on length of time in cast.

## Teaching Considerations

- Instruct client to call physician if unable to perform ADL, if excessive edema occurs, if client experiences limited use of joints or muscles, if mobility is affected. If client is treated for congenital deformity with repeated cast changes, instruct when next cast change is due; give client written appointment.
- Provide client with scheduled exercises to increase mobility and muscle strength.

## Home Care Considerations

- Client should have chair or bed with pillows to elevate extremity for intermittent edema.
- Suggest regular use of moisturizers for dry, scaly skin of casted extremity.
- Inspect client's environment for potential safety risks.

# *SKILL 34-3 Assisting With Application of Skin Traction*

Skin traction is one of the two basic types of traction used for the treatment of fractured bones and correction of orthopedic abnormalities. Skin traction applies pull to an affected body structure by straps attached to the skin around the structure. There are eight major forms of skin traction with some variation within some of the types:

1. Bryant's traction—vertically held type of bilateral traction to the legs (Fig. 34-2, *A*). This type of traction can be used for children weighing under 40 lb. Adhesive strips are applied to the lateral surfaces of each leg and wrapped with elastic bandages to secure them in place. A spreader bar is attached to the strips and then

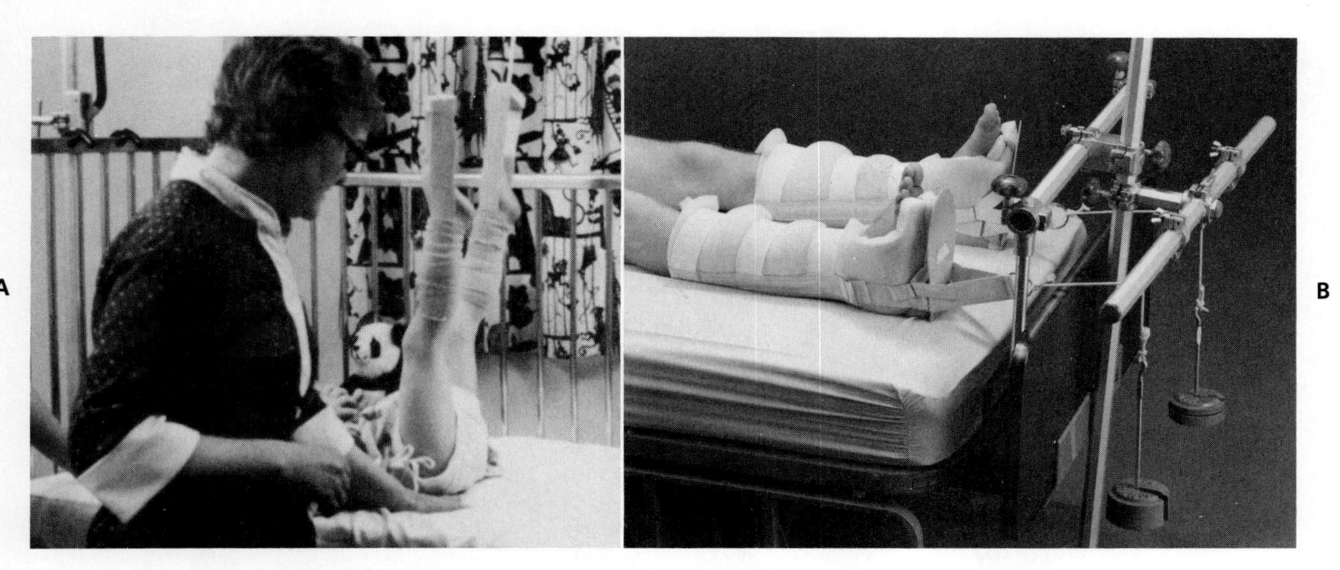


***Fig. 34-2*** Types of skin traction. **A,** Bryant's traction. **B,** Buck's extension.

to ropes, pulleys, and weights. Bryant's traction, called Gallow's traction in England, is used for children with fractures of the femur. After the muscle spasms are overcome and the fragments are aligned with some evidence of union, the child is removed from traction and placed in a spica cast to continue recovery and for callus formation to progress. Children may remain in Bryant's traction for only 7 to 10 days.

2. Buck's extension—horizontally applied unilateral or bilateral traction (Fig. 34-2, *B*). Adhesive strips are applied to the lateral surfaces of the limb or limbs (usually one leg or forearm) and wrapped with elastic bandages. A spreader bar is attached to the adhesive strips as in Bryant's traction and then to ropes, pulleys, and weights. Buck's extension is used before repair of hip fractures, to reduce muscles spasms and contractures in client with arthritic conditions, and occasionally as an interim treatment for lumbosacral muscle spasms causing low back pain.
3. Cotrel's traction—skin traction consisting of two separate forms: head halter and pelvic belt (Fig. 34-2, *C*). Cotrel's traction is used occasionally as a preoperative treatment to help to straighten spinal curvatures before insertion of skeletal rods for correction of scoliosis. The pull in opposite directions on the head and pelvis helps to overcome the deforming muscle pull causing the curvature. Head halter traction and pelvic belt traction are explained later in this section.
4. Dunlop's traction—simultaneous horizontal form of Buck's extension to the humerus with an accompanying vertical Buck's extension to the forearm (Fig. 34-2, *D*). The horizontal Buck's extension is the "treating" traction for fractures of the humerus, whereas the vertical Buck's extension is primarily used to maintain the forearm in the desired position relative to the humerus.
5. Head halter—traction involving a specially shaped halter with cutout areas for the ears, face, and top of the head (Fig. 34-2, *E*). The halter cups the chin and has straps leading from the occipital skull area that attach to the chin portion and then connect to one or two spreader bars on either side of the head; the bar or bars are then attached to ropes, pulleys, and weights. Head halter traction should be used only for degenerative or arthritic conditions of the cervical vertebrae, not for fractures of the vertebrae. Because head halter traction must be removed occasionally for client safety and care, because this traction doesn't result in total spinal immobilization, it is unsafe and potentially dangerous for a client with a fracture of cervical vertebrae. Release of the weights in such a situation could lead to paralysis.
6. Pelvic belt—traction consisting of a girdlelike belt that fits around the lumbosacral and abdominal areas, fastening in the middle of the abdomen with pressure-sensitive straps or buckles (Fig. 34-2, *F*). The belt has long straps that hook to a wide spreader bar beyond the feet; the bar is then attached to ropes, pulleys, and weights. This pelvic belt, or lumbosacral traction, is used for clients with low back pain, muscle spasms, and a ruptured nucleus pulposus (herniated or ruptured disk). Basically, this traction serves to keep the client in bed, thus relieving inflammation and irritation of the injured nerves or muscles. It does not overcome the herniation of the nucleus pulposus. Additional treatments, including diathermy, use of muscle relaxant drugs, and physical therapy are used in conjunction with this traction.

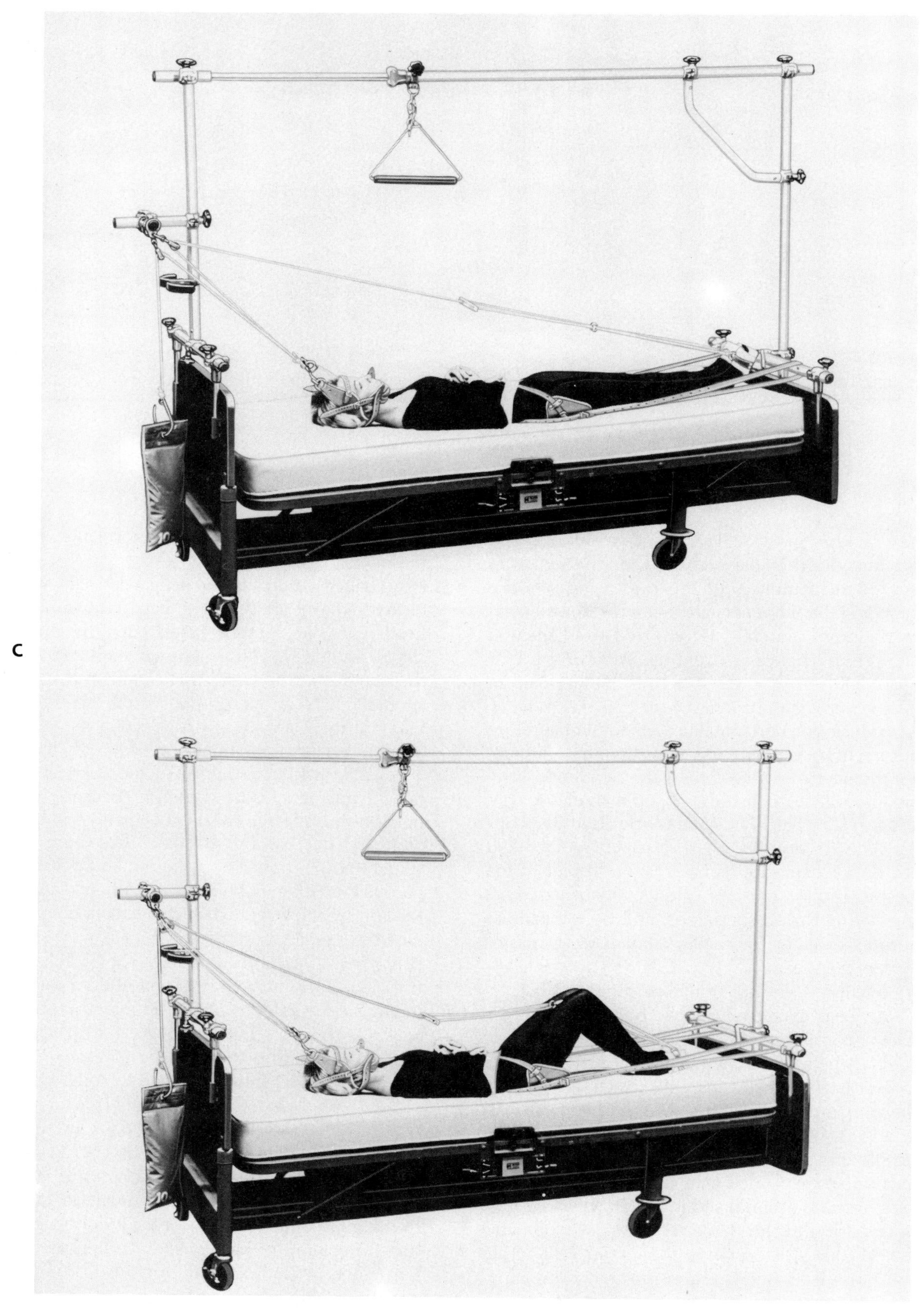


***Fig. 34-2, cont'd.*** **C,** Cotrel's traction.

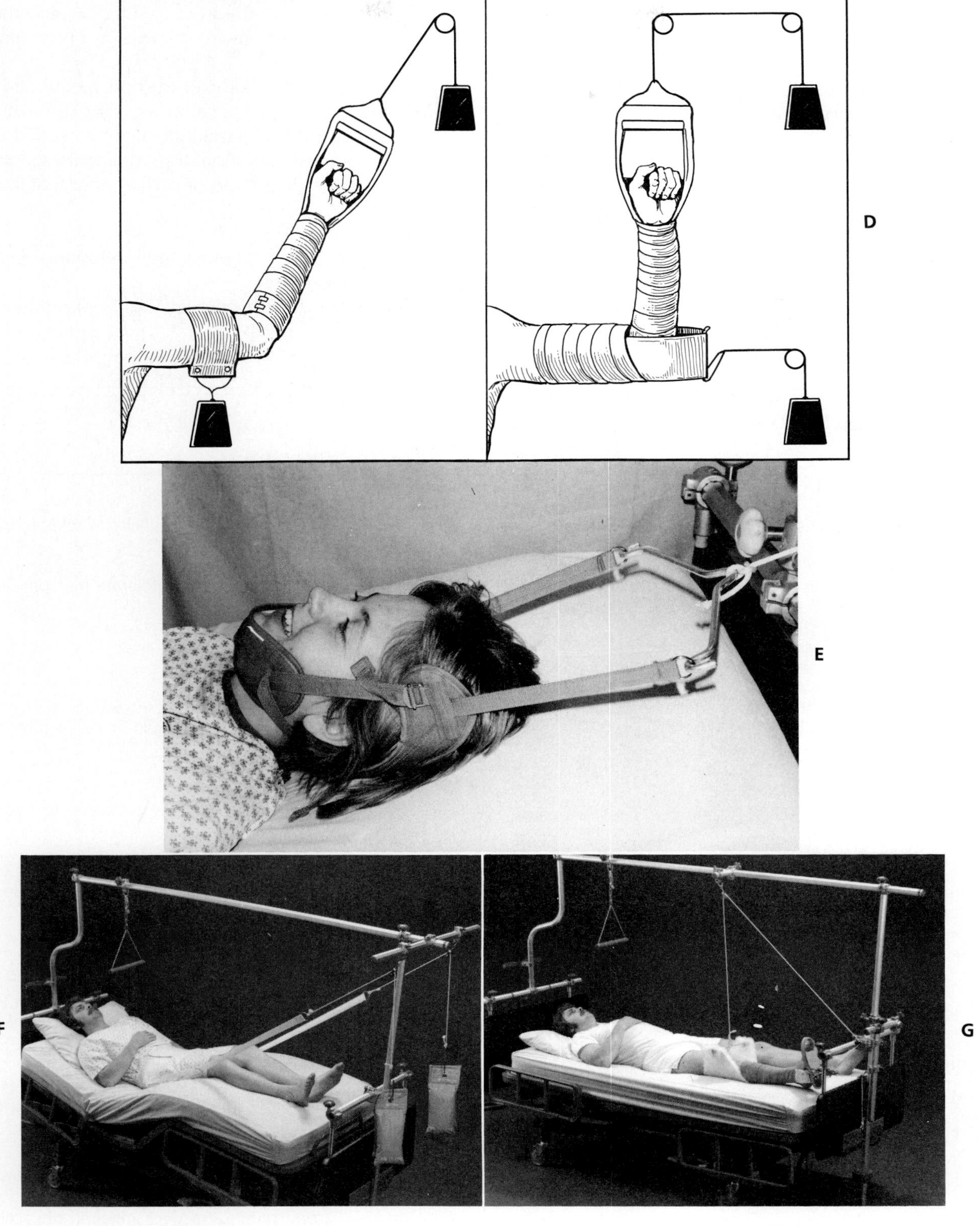


***Fig. 34-2, cont'd.*** **D,** Dunlop's traction. **E,** Head halter. **F,** Pelvic belt. **G,** Russell's traction.
From Thompson JM, et al: Mosby's manual of clinical nursing, ed 2, St Louis, 1989, The CV Mosby Co.

7. Pelvic sling (Weil sling)—"traction" consisting of a hammocklike belt wherein the sling cradles the pelvis in its boundaries for treatment of one or more fractures of the pelvic bones. The sling is attached on each side to a pin threaded through a sewn tunnel; each pin is then placed in a grooved spreader bar attached to ropes, pulleys, and weights. The sling applies gentle inward pressure to the injured tissues, thereby providing much comfort and security to the client.
8. Russell's traction—modification of Buck's extension using Newton's second law of thermodynamics to double the amount of pull through the arrangement of ropes, pulleys, and weights (for each force in one direction there is an equal force in the opposite direction) (Fig. 34-2, *G*).

Because skin tissues and subcutaneous attachments cannot tolerate great amounts of weight without losing strength and continuity, skin traction forms use amounts of weights varying from 1 to 2 lb for children in Bryant's traction to 7 to 10 lb for head halter traction. Average weights are 5 to 7 lb for Buck's extension, 7 to 10 lb for Dunlop's traction, 10 to 15 lb for pelvic belt traction (weight is distributed over the entire pelvis and lower back), and 10 to 20 lb for a pelvic sling because the sling is really a form of hammock suspension rather than traction.

Basically, each form of skin traction mentioned above has a usual or "classic" position used for the majority of clients in that traction. Variations may be needed to treat a specific injury or condition. If pertinent, these variations are noted in the discussion of each type of traction.

## Purposes

1. Facilitate recovery through immobilization and alignment of body parts.
2. Provide safe care through skillful application of traction.

## *Procedure 34-3*

| Steps | Rationale |
|---|---|
| **Assessment** | |
| 1. Assess condition of client for overall health. Ask parents for child's health state. Older persons may have one or more health alterations. | Determines client's health state and ability to tolerate traction. |
| 2. Assess specific tissues to be placed in traction; note skin condition, excessive hair, bruises, rash, other lesions. | Determines ability of local tissues to tolerate traction. |
| a. Head halter: assess head, ears, chin, neck. | |
| b. Bryant's traction: assess both legs. | |
| c. Buck's extension: assess one or both legs. | |
| d. Dunlop's traction: assess arm and forearm. | |
| e. Pelvic belt: assess lower back and abdomen. | Pain and spasms should be relieved by traction. |
| f. Pelvic sling: assess back and abdomen. | Bruises may indicate trauma that would be relieved by traction. |
| g. Russell's traction: assess lower limbs. | |
| NOTE: Cotrel's traction includes head halter and pelvic belt and is not considered separately. | |
| 3. Assess client's understanding of reason for traction. | Determines concerns, acceptance, and response to traction. |
| **Nursing Diagnosis** | |
| 1. Cluster data to reveal actual or potential nursing diagnoses: | |
| a. Impaired physical mobility, related to: | |
| ▪ Injury to musculoskeletal tissue. | Traction requires bed rest and relative immobility. |
| ▪ Pain or trauma and muscle spasms. | Discontinuity of bone or other musculoskeletal tissue causes painful ambulation and mobility. Traction helps to restore function to overcome pain and trauma. |
| b. Pain: related to immobility of injury. | Amount of pain varies with specific condition or injury of client. |
| **Planning** | |
| 1. Develop individualized goals for client based on nursing diagnoses: | |
| a. Ensure that client will regain mobility and independence when traction is discontinued (or ended). | Unless instructed to do so, client in traction should not keep other body parts immobile. |
| b. Ensure that client's skin remains intact. | Impaired physical mobility increases client's risk for skin breakdown. |
| c. Relieve client's pain. | Pain can result from trauma, traction, impaired physical mobility. |

| Steps | Rationale |
|---|---|
| 2. Prepare or assemble following equipment: | |
| a. Ropes, pulleys, weights, weight holder (ropes are nylon for strength; weights vary from 1-5 lb—have several of each weight). (Babies, children, and older persons require less weight than do young adults.) | Pull of traction comes from attachment of ropes and weights to specific apparatus or sling. |
| b. Bed frame for attachment of traction, or portable frames that attach to bed | |
| c. One of more spreader bars | Attach to ropes and weights. |
| d. Adhesive-backed moleskin | Attaches to skin for traction. |
| e. Elastic bandages | Hold strips to skin. |
| f. Heel or elbow protectors (optional) | Reduce skin breakdown on bony prominences. |
| g. Knee sling for Russell's traction | |
| h. Wastebasket with plastic bag liner | |
| 3. Explain procedure to client. | Promotes cooperation and reduces anxiety. |

## Implementation

| Steps | Rationale |
|---|---|
| 1. Prepare client and area of body to be in traction. | |
| a. Head halter: cleanse face and neck; shave man unless he has beard. | Lessens irritation under head halter. |
| b. Bryant's traction: cleanse both legs gently if necessary (change diaper if necessary for baby.) | |
| c. Buck's traction: wash affected leg (or legs) very gently and dry carefully. Do no shave legs. | Shaving may create micronicks that could become inflamed under traction strips. |
| d. Dunlop's traction: cleanse arm and forearm gently if needed. | |
| e. Pelvic belt: check back and iliac crests for lesions. | |
| f. Pelvic sling: ask female client to void before being placed in sling if no catheter is in place. | Sling must be removed for placement of bed pan. Male client can use urinal with no change in position of sling. |
| g. Russell's traction: cleanse lower extremity to knee as needed. | |
| 2. Position client as requested by physician. | Position varies with part of body to be placed on traction, plus effects of weight and gravity. |
| a. Head halter: client flat on back. | |
| b. Bryant's traction: child flat on back. | |
| c. Buck's traction: client on back; head of bed flat or elevated 30 degrees. | |
| d. Dunlop's traction: client flat on back. | |
| e. Pelvic belt: client flat on back. | |
| f. Pelvic sling: client flat on side or back. | |
| g. Russell's traction: client on back; head of bed slightly elevated. | |
| 3. Assist with application of specific head halter, adhesive strips and elastic bandages, pelvic belt or sling as needed. Nurse may be asked to hold client in desired position or apply halter, strips, elastic bandages while physician and other assistants hold client's tissues in desired positions. | For lower extremity, adhesive strips are applied beginning below head of fibula on lateral surface of leg to avoid pressure over peroneal nerve. Ensures proper alignment of body parts under traction. Elastic bandages are applied from distal to proximal to promote venous return. |
| 4. Assist with attachment of spreader bars, ropes, pulleys. Ropes are tied securely in knots and passed in grooves of pulleys to weights. | Provides proper weighted traction for extremity alignment. |
| 5. When all traction materials and spreader bars are in place, weights are placed on weight holder and hooked to loop in rope and *lowered slowly and gently* until rope is taut. Physician determines exact amount of weight to be applied and position to be maintained for majority of time by client (clients should have written orders for specific traction weights, bed position, turning regimen when pertinent). | Traction is slowly established to avoid involuntary muscle spasms or pain for client. Weight should be sufficient to create enough pull to overcome muscle spasms but not to cause distraction or marked increase in pain. |
| 6. Before physician leaves, check client's position and ask about additional permissible positions for client and bed: | Ensures safety of care and position for effective traction. |
| a. Head halter: client stays flat on back, or head of bed may be elevated 15 to 20 degrees if ordered. | Angle of pull may allow head to be up to use body weight as countertraction. |
| b. Bryant's traction: baby or child must stay on back at all times; buttocks are held slightly off bed if traction weight is correct amount. | Child cannot turn to side or abdomen because traction would be ineffective and reinjury could occur. |

| Steps | Rationale |
|---|---|
| c. Buck's traction: client is primarily on back; may be allowed to turn to unaffected side for brief periods (10 to 15 min). Pillow placed under leg in traction may be used only when client is on side. | Positioning on side permits back care and rest to tissues. Pillows under leg or legs in traction create friction and should not be used because they lessen traction's effectiveness. |
| d. Dunlop's traction: client must lie on back. Bed may be tilted on low shock blocks toward side opposite traction. Head of bed is kept flat. | Tilting uses body for some countertraction. |
| e. Pelvic belt: client lies on back; knee gatch and head of bed may be raised so hips and knees are flexed at 45-degree angles (so-called Williams' position). | Flexion of hips and knees relaxes lumbosacral muscles to lessen spasms. |
| f. Pelvic sling: client lies on back when in sling; sling should have enough weight attached to raise buttocks slightly off bed. If sling is off, it can be used carefully as turning sheet if client's fractures permit side lying. | Hammock effect of sling is most effective with client on back. Sling must be removed for placement of bedpan. |
| g. Russell's traction: client lies on back; head of bed may be elevated 30 to 45 degrees, depending on injury. | Low Fowler's position on back creates most effective traction pull. |
| h. Cotrel's traction: client must lie flat on back. | |
| 7. Ask client how traction is affecting injured tissues if client is able to respond (ask parents of baby or child how client has been responding since traction has been on). Babies or young children may cry when weights are initially applied but soon cease crying and appear more comfortable. | Initial reaction may be slight increase in soreness or pain until client is able to relax and allow traction to perform as designed. |
| 8. For safety, raise side rails as appropriate. Clients in Bryant's traction should always have someone in attendance. | Promotes client's safety. |
| 9. Gather unused materials and return to storage areas. | Promotes safety and cleanliness. |
| 10. Wash hands. | Reduces transmission of microorganisms. |

## Evaluation

| Steps | Rationale |
|---|---|
| 1. Observe entire traction setup and functioning: check all knots, ropes in pulleys, weights on weight holder; whether apparatus is hanging freely; position of halter, sling, belt, other material for specific traction. | Reassessment is necessary to determine if traction is functioning as designed or desired, or to make needed adjustments. |
| 2. Assess condition of skin around traction straps or bandages. | Ensures early identification of irritation or breakdown. |
| 3. Ask if client is experiencing muscle pain or burning. | Indicates presence of muscle spasms. |
| 4. Conduct neurovascular checks every 1 to 2 hr initially, then every 4 hr if client is stabilizing. | Provides objective data concerning peripheral perfusion to tissues. |

### *Expected outcomes*

| Steps | Rationale |
|---|---|
| 1. As result of being in one specific type of skin traction, one of the following occurs: | Each type of traction is designed to relieve muscle spasms; restore alignment or lessen shortening, overriding, rotation; relieve pain; increase comfort. |
| a. Head halter: client notes relief of spasms and pain in neck and back of neck and head (may require administration of muscle relaxant and narcotic medications while in traction). | |
| b. Buck's traction: client is able to maintain leg in alignment. Older clients with severe hip pain noticeably relax. | Narcotic use may be required for 1 to 3 days for acute pain. |
| c. Dunlop's traction: same result occurs as for Buck's traction (used for upper extremity). | Clients may require narcotics for 1 to 3 days for acute pain of fractured humerus. |
| d. Pelvic belt: client notes lessening of spasms of lumbrosacral muscles, possibly slight lessening of sensory signs of pressure on sciatic nerve (numbness, tingling, or "pins and needles" radiating down back of leg to toes), and possibly less pressure in vertebral area at site of injury. Client is usually ordered to be in traction for 2 hr, out of traction for 2 hr, and out of traction at night, plus have orders for muscle relaxant medications, narcotic analgesics, physical therapy. | Pull may lessen pressure on spinal or peripheral nerves, thereby alleviating symptoms. |
| e. Pelvic sling: client experiences almost immediate comfort and relief from pelvic and abdominal discomfort, pain, and feeling of "coming apart"—sling compresses tissues together. | Clients are very comfortable in sling and develop sense of security while in it. |
| f. Russell's traction: client notes lessening of pain in hip area (if traction is for hip trauma), relief of muscle | Russell's traction exerts double pull with less weight than Buck's traction because of pulley arrangement. |

| Steps | Rationale |
|---|---|
| spasms, ease in ability to maintain more normal anatomical position of leg and thigh. | |
| g. Cotrel's traction: client experiences some straightening of curvature of spine. | Surgical correction may be required for marked curvature. |
| 2. X-ray studies confirm satisfactory alignment of fracture fragments with or without evidence of beginning callus formation (evidence of callus may not become apparent for 7 to 10 days or longer) if client is in traction for fracture. | Objective evidence is required for comparison with subjective relief of symptoms. |
| 3. Anatomical position of injured tissues is easily maintained by client in specific traction without rotation or shortening. | Pull of traction facilitates maintenance of more anatomical position. |
| 4. Sufficient time in traction (varying from 1 to 10 or more days) elicits symptom relief. | Time is required for inflammation to abate and tissues to regain more normal functions. |
| 5. Skin around straps and moleskin remains intact without irritation. | Skin free of pressure and/or pulling. |
| ***Unexpected outcomes*** | |
| 1. Client experiences increased pain, soreness, stiffness. | Pull on injured tissues may cause pressure on injured nerve endings, increasing pain. |
| 2. Client suffers more frequent or severe muscle spasms. | Pull may indicate muscle irritation to greater extent. |
| 3. Client experiences displaced alignment (evident on x-ray film) if fracture is present. | Too much weight may pull fragments too far apart, altering alignment. |
| 4. Client experiences sense of claustrophobia or being "held down" in one or another type of traction. | Restraint and position required may cause client to experience such feelings. |
| 5. Specific unexpected outcomes: | |
| a. Head halter: client has pain in temporomandibular joint and chin or may develop headaches. | Pull of head halter is incorrect; straps need to be shortened between chin and occipital part of halter to direct pull from occipital area and away from chin and jawline. |
| b. Bryant's traction: baby or child develops edema of feet. Peripheral pulses are not palpable. | Plastic bandages may be too snugly applied. Bandages can be removed and reapplied with two persons performing rewrapping; one person holds limb in vertical position as other rewraps bandage. |
| c. Buck's traction: client develops pressure area on heel, or client is unable to dorsiflex or evert foot in traction if traction boot, adhesive straps, or elastic bandages exert pressure over head of fibula. | Pressure area is related to lack of circulation and insufficient position changes. Pressure on peroneal nerve results in inability to dorsiflex or evert foot. Peroneal nerve courses over head of fibula down anterolateral surfaces of leg. |
| d. Dunlop's traction: client experiences pressure on elbow, or client is unable to approximate thumb to rest of fingers and may complain of numbness of thumb or tingling along sides of thumb and index finger. | Pressure sores may develop because of bony prominence of olecranon (use of elbow pad relieves pressure). Inability to approximate thumb to fingers and numbness of thumb signifies that elastic bandage is too tight over radial nerve at wrist. Elastic bandage should be removed from forearm *only* and rewrapped more loosely; symptoms should then be rechecked for alleviation or continuance. |
| e. Pelvic belt: client experiences marked increase in pain or numbness or other sensory pressure signs when in belt. | Pull of belt may increase pressure on edematous or injured nerves, causing untoward reaction. Removal of traction should ease complaints. |
| f. Pelvic sling: client becomes very dependent on sling and refuses to allow its discontinuance or becomes anxious when out of sling. | Security felt in sling leads to anxiety and concern for comfort when sling is removed. Weaning may be required and involves releasing sling for short to longer periods of time to permit adjustment to being out of sling. |
| g. Russell's traction: client has pain behind knee or nonpalpable popliteal pulse. | Knee sling may cause knee to be flexed in too acute angle, causing pressure signs. Knee sling can be adjusted for proper size and rope pulled down at knee to permit proper position and pull to relieve symptoms. |
| 6. Client experiences burning, weeping, drainage under adhesive strips or moleskin. | Reactions may be caused by allergic reactions, skin hypersensitivity, too much weight causing loss of skin attachments to subcutaneous tissues. Loss of skin continuity necessitates removal of traction. |
| **Recording and Reporting** | |
| 1. Record type of traction, site to which applied, amount of weight, person applying traction, time, client response, other pertinent data in nurses' notes. | Ensures continuity of care and provides documentation for legal considerations. |
| 2. Report untoward findings to nurse in charge immediately. If adjustments to particular traction do not relieve complaints, | Increases in pain may signify development of compartment syndrome (Skill 34-1). |

| Steps | Rationale |
|---|---|
| traction should be released (*except* Bryant's traction) if ordered by physician. Physician should be notified of marked increase in pain, muscle spasm, marked anxiety. | |
| 3. Record all steps of neurovascular checks (Skill 34-1, Evaluation, Step 3). Perform neurovascular checks every 1 to 2 hr initially, then every 4 hr if client stabilizes. If edema appears to be increasing, measure both extremities. | Bilateral comparison provides objective evidence for assessing edema. |
| 4. Record traction functioning every shift: observe all ropes, pulleys, weights, slings at beginning of shift and after turning or other position changes or if traction is removed for care or eating (head halter). | Safety, continuity of care, and legal factors require recording over time or after removal. |
| 5. Record length of time client is in or out of specific traction. NOTE: Clients in head halter and pelvic belt tractions are to be in 2 hr, out 2 hr, and out to sleep. Babies and children in Bryant's traction must sleep in traction; it is rarely removed once established, except to loosen elastic bandages for marked edema of feet. | Skin traction can be removed for care (with specific orders or based on institutional policies) for brief periods unless orders give specific directions. Clients in head halter or pelvic belt must sleep out of traction because muscle tone required for traction would prevent muscle relaxation and thus sleep. |
| 6. Record responses to narcotic or other analgesic and muscle relaxant. | Documents administration of analgesic and client's response. Older persons metabolize drugs more slowly and thus may require less narcotic administration over time. |

## Follow-up Activities

| | |
|---|---|
| 1. After final discontinuance of specific traction, one of following may occur. | |
| a. Head halter: client may be taught to apply traction for home care. | Arthritic or degenerative conditions may require prolonged treatment. |
| b. Bryant's traction: client may be placed in spica cast. | Skin traction is only initial treatment for femoral fractures in babies or children. |
| c. Buck's traction: client may have hip nailing, prosthesis, or muscle-lengthening procedures. | Buck's traction provides safety and comfort while preparations are made for surgical repair. |
| d. Dunlop's traction: client may be placed in hanging cast to humerus (Skill 34-1). | Hanging long-arm casts permit callus to form while maintaining immobility of fractured bones. |
| e. Pelvic belt: client may be discharged or may undergo outpatient physical therapy. Surgical repair may involve laminectomy, spinal fusion, chemonucleolysis. | Skin traction for lumbrosacral pain and conditions is only one part of overall treatment. |
| f. Pelvic sling: client is ambulatory with walker, crutches, cane. Occasionally, client with multiple fractures may have external fixation with Hoffman or other apparatus. | Pelvic fractures generally heal without major surgical repair. |
| g. Russell's traction: client may have surgical correction of hip fracture or release of muscle contractures. | Traction is preliminary treatment for client being prepared for surgery. |
| h. Cotrel's traction: client may be placed in brace or undergo surgery. | |

## Special Considerations

- Babies and children have immature musculoskeletal tissues and are almost constant "movers."
- Older adults may have keratoses, rashes, other lesions that could become irritated in skin traction.
- Older persons may have long-standing condition of musculoskeletal tissues such as arthritis or gout.
- Older and chronically ill clients may have increased need for position changes resulting from limitations from osteoporosis, osteomalacia, weakened muscles, increased risk of skin breakdown.
- If institutional policies of physician's orders specify, clients are removed from traction for skin care or as ordered. If removed for skin care, client is out of traction only for 10 to 15 min before it is reapplied.
- Clients in traction are more susceptible to hazards of immobility.
- Muscles and joints may be weakened from bed rest or traction and need time to regain strength.

## Teaching Considerations

- Explain procedure to parents, who can clarify for child.
- Disoriented clients may need repeated explanations.
- Traction may increase muscle weakness, spasms, pain in older clients.
- Client should be taught to ambulate slowly, gradually increasing length of time out of bed and distance walked.
- Client should be taught to nofity physician of undesirable signs, such as marked increase in pain, muscle spasms, increased numbness. Symptoms may signify reinjury or insufficient healing.

## Home Care Considerations

- If client is to be discharged to home, relatives or care givers should be instructed of care needs (including home traction) and mode of ambulation.
- Home environment must be assessed and adapted to accomodate hospital bed and traction.
- Integrity of traction should be inspected daily.

## *SKILL 34-4* Assisting with Insertion of Pins or Nails for Skeletal Traction

Skeletal traction is the second kind of traction used for the treatment of fractures or correction of orthopedic abnormalities. Skeletal traction is applied to the affected structure by a metal pin or wire inserted in the tissue of the structure and attached to traction ropes. Skeletal traction is often used when continuous traction is desired to properly immobilize, position, and align a fractured bone during the healing process.

As with skin traction, skeletal traction may be applied to one or several bones. Skeletal traction begins externally but continues internally directly through the bones. Common forms of skeletal traction include:

1. Balanced suspension to the femur—traction used for displaced, overriding, or comminuted fractures of the femur. Balanced suspension brings about relief of muscle spasms, realignment of the fracture fragments, and callus formation (Fig. 34-3). This form of traction is used less frequently because of the length of time required for hospitalization when used as the major form of treatment. It is now used primarily before surgical implantation of an internal fixation pin, plate, or nail until the client's condition or other injuries stabilize to permit surgery. Balanced suspension involves the use of splints under the thigh and leg to suspend them off the bed, with a pin or wire supplying the traction. The pin or wire is drilled through the upper tibia and attached to a spreader, which is then attached to ropes, pulleys, and weights. Sufficient weights are hung to overcome the quadriceps and hamstring muscle spasms; sometimes weights of 30 to 40 lb or more may be required initially. Suspension weights may be 7 to 8 lb, balanced by 7 to 8 lb of countertraction.
2. Dunlop's traction—skeletal form of side-arm traction similar to Dunlop's skin traction. The difference consists mainly of a pin drilled through the lower humerus (instead of the horizontal Buck's extension mentioned previously) and attached to a spreader, ropes, pulleys, and weights. The forearm is held in vertical Buck's extension, as it would be in Dunlop's skin traction. Dunlop's skeletal traction is used for severe fractures wherein the greater pull permitted with the skeletal pin is required to overcome muscle spasms to cause effective alignment and union.
3. External fixation—commonly used form of skeletal traction involving the use of one of a variety of frames of apparatuses to hold pins drilled into or through bones (Fig. 34-4). External fixation frames have been used for skull and facial fractures, ribs, all bones of the

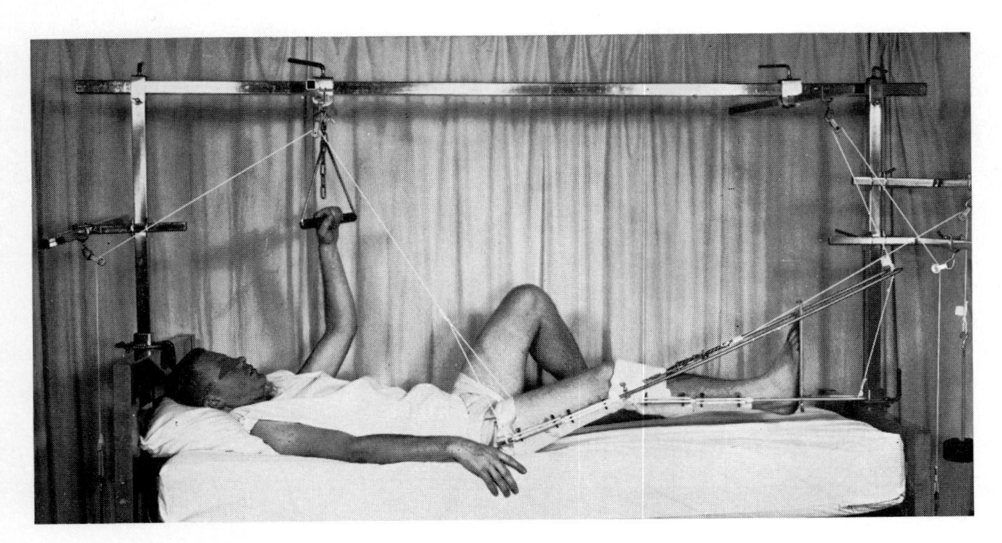

***Fig. 34-3*** Balanced skeletal traction. Traction in long axis of right thigh is applied by means of Kirschner wire through proximal portion of tibia. Limb is supported by Thomas splint beneath thigh and Pearson attachment beneath leg. Additional attachment prevents foot-drop. Weights apply counteraction to upper end of Thomas splint and suspend its lower end. By using the left arm and leg as shown , client can shift position of the hips without change in amount of traction.

From Brashear HR Jr, Raney RB Sr: Handbook of orthopaedic surgery, ed 10, St Louis, 1986, The CV Mosby Co.

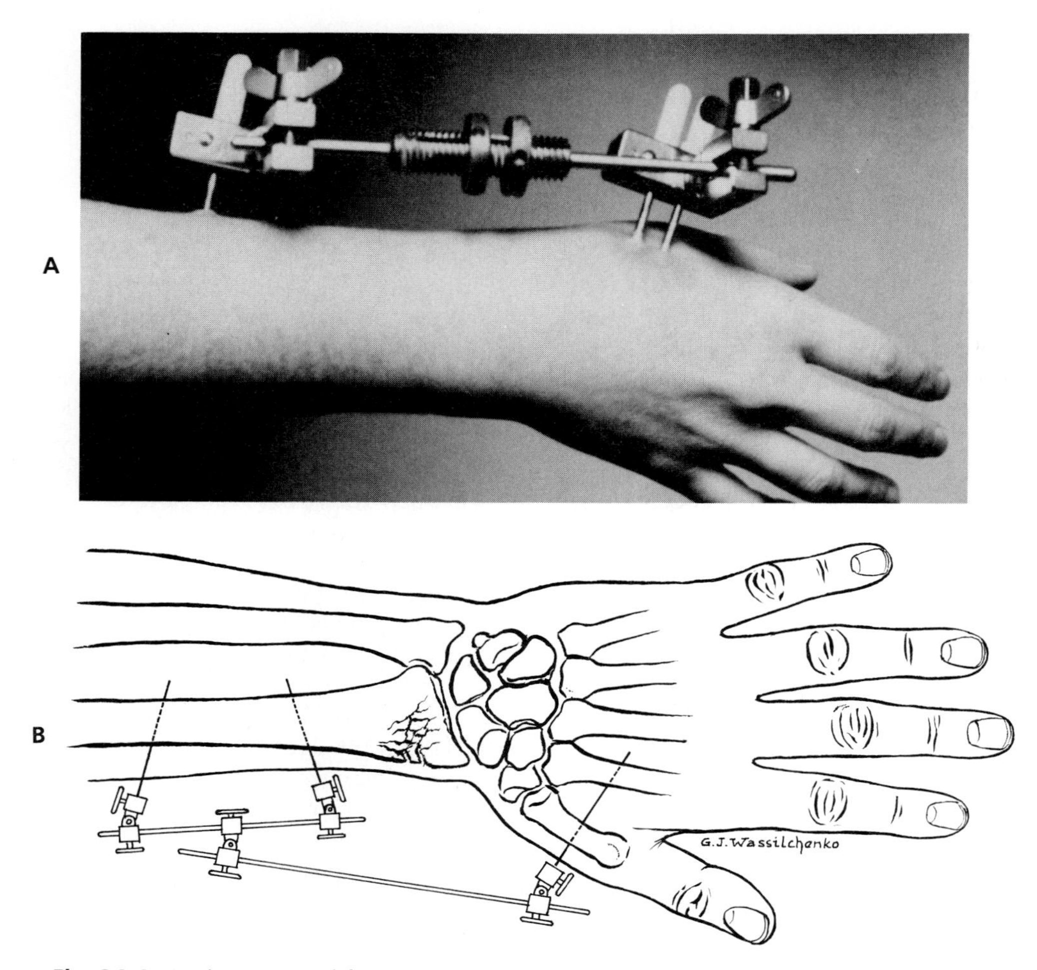


***Fig. 34-4*** Various external fixators. **A,** Hoffman. **B,** Roger Anderson.
From Thompson JM, et al: Mosby's manual of clinical nursing, ed 2, St Louis, 1989, The CV Mosby Co.

upper and lower extremities, and pelvic bones. Frames may fit on one side of a bone or bones or may be attached to pins on either side of an injured limb.

4. Skull tong traction—traction involving the use of one of a variety of tongs (Crutchfield, Vinke, Gardner-Wells, or Barton) drilled into the skull or placed below the scalp and attached to ropes, pulleys, and weights. This type of traction is used for fractures of cervical vertebrae and involves the use of special beds or turning frames to facilitate nursing care.

Amounts of weights for skeletal traction vary from 10 lb for Dunlop's skeletal traction to 20 to 25 lb for cervical traction, to 30 to 40 lb for balanced suspension to the femur. Amounts of weights used are also dictated by age and overall condition of the client in traction plus the purpose of the traction.

### Purposes

1. Foster the recovery of clients with fractured bones.
2. Provide safe care through skillful application of traction.

## *Procedure 34-4*

| Steps | Rationale |
|---|---|
| **Assessment** | |
| 1. Assess overall health condition of client. Ask parents about child's health. Older persons may have concurrent health alterations (e.g., diabetes or peripheral vascular disease) that may complicate use of skeletal traction. | Determines client's health state and ability to tolerate bed rest and skeletal traction. |

| Steps | Rationale |
|---|---|
| 2. Carefully assess specific tissues to be placed in skeletal traction. Note marked edema, rash, other open lesions. | Determine ability of tissues to tolerate traction. Skeletal pin goes through skin to bone and out through skin. |
| 3. Assess client's knowledge of upcoming traction, application, purposes. | Determines willingness to participate in care. |

## Nursing Diagnosis

| Steps | Rationale |
|---|---|
| 1. Cluster data to reveal actual or potential nursing diagnoses: | |
| a. Impaired physical mobility, related to: | Bed rest is required for traction. |
| ▪ Injury and traction. | |
| ▪ Pain, muscle spasms, and severity of trauma. | Skeletal traction may lead to complications of bed rest for older clients. |
| b. Pain: related to traction equipment. | Initial pin placement and tension on fractures cause discomfort. |

## Planning

| Steps | Rationale |
|---|---|
| 1. Develop individualized goals for client based on nursing diagnoses: | |
| a. Prevent complications from traction or bed rest. | Individualized goals are directed toward promoting comfort and wound healing and reducing hazards of immobility. |
| b. Help client regain independence and ability to perform ADL. | |
| c. Help client regain pain-free mobility when treatment is concluded. | |
| 2. Assemble the following equipment: | |
| a. For balanced-suspension skeletal traction (BSST): | |
| ▪ Sterile tray for insertion of Kirschner wire or Steinman pin (secure from operating suite) | Maintains sterile asepsis during pin insertion. |
| ▪ Skin preparaton solutions as desired | |
| ▪ Local anesthetic of physician's choice, usually 1% to 2% lidocaine | Used to anesthetize skin at pin entrance and exit sites. |
| ▪ Sterile gloves | |
| ▪ Thomas or Harris splint | BSST creates "unit or system" with suspension of thigh and leg and traction through bone. |
| ▪ Pearson attachment | |
| ▪ Foot support | |
| ▪ Ropes, pulleys, weights, weight holders | Maintains traction counterbalance. |
| ▪ Towels, felt, stockinette | |
| ▪ Drill and extension cord if needed | |
| ▪ Antiseptic ointment | |
| ▪ Adhesive tape | |
| ▪ Wastebasket with plastic liner | |
| b. For Dunlop's skeletal traction: | |
| ▪ Sterile tray with Kirschner wire or Steinman pin (secure from operating room) | |
| ▪ Adhesive strips or moleskin | |
| ▪ Elastic bandages | |
| ▪ Hand grip bar | |
| ▪ Ropes, pulley, weights, weight holders | |
| ▪ Low-shock blocks (optional) | |
| ▪ Local anesthetic of physician's choice, usually 1% to 2% lidocaine | |
| ▪ Antiseptic ointment | |
| ▪ Skin preparaton materials as desired | |
| ▪ Wastebasket with plastic liner | |
| c. For external fixation: | Fixators may be placed through skin to one bone cortex only or entirely through bone to exit on opposite side of injured tissues. Four, six, eight pins may be used. |
| ▪ External fixator, usually Hoffman or Roger Anderson apparatus, Vital fixator, or other fixator | |
| ▪ Sterile tray with pins for insertion (secure from operating room | |
| ▪ Antiseptic ointment | |
| ▪ Skin preparation materials | |
| ▪ Wastebasket with plastic liner | |
| d. Skull tong traction: | Placement of skull tongs is a surgical procedure. Placement of these tongs through the scalp or cranium maintains spinal alignment after cervical or thoracic spinal cord injury. |
| ▪ Tongs: Crutchfield, Vinke, Gardner-Wells, or Barton | |
| ▪ Sterile tray: usually traction is applied in operating room | |

| Steps | Rationale |
|---|---|
| ▪ Antiseptic ointment<br>▪ Skin preparation materials<br>▪ Wastebasket and plastic liners | |
| 3. Explain procedure to client. | Reduces anxiety and increases cooperation. |

## Implementation

| Steps | Rationale |
|---|---|
| 1. Position client according to physician's request. Nurse or other assistant may be asked to support tissues to be placed in traction. Client will most often be on back with head of bed slightly elevated. Client will be flat in bed for Dunlop's skeletal traction. | Ensures proper alignment during and after traction application. |
| 2. Physician performs skin preparation and discards materials in wastebasket. | Reduces possibility of wound infection. |
| 3. Physician injects local anesthetic into sites desired. Nurse and other assistants support client, limb, other tissues to be placed in traction. | Anesthetic acts quickly to create painless area. Client will feel pressure of pin being drilled through or into bones and will hear drill but should feel no pain. |
| 4. Assist (usually by holding spreader bar, splint, Pearson attachment) while physician continues to use drill to insert number of pins or nails desired for traction. Support area of joints not at injury site. Do not move distal portion unnecessarily. | Movement can cause severe pain or additional trauma. |
| 5. Complete traction setup: | |
| a. BSST: | |
| ▪ Assist with placement of Thomas or Harris splint, Pearson attachment, foot support, ropes, pulleys, weights. Apply antiseptic ointment to pin exit sites. | Splint and attachment are usually previously prepared for use quickly. Ointment is applied to close open pores to prevent infection. |
| ▪ Assist with application of Buck's extension to forearm (see Skill 34-3 for Buck's extension), place hand grip, and establish skin traction by *slowly* lowering weights until rope is taut. | Skin traction allows forearm to remain in vertical position without undue effort from client. |
| ▪ Assist with application of spreader to hold skeletal pin; tie rope to spreader and thread through pulleys to weight holder and weights. Slowly lower weights until rope is taut. Place shock blocks if requested. Apply antiseptic ointment to pin exit sites. | Amount of weight depends on severity of client's injury. Amounts vary from 5 to 10 or more lb. Shock blocks allow one side of bed to be raised to help client maintain desired position. Ointment is applied to prevent infection. |
| c. External fixation:<br>▪ Hold affected tissues or limb while physician attaches and tightens fixator screws or clamps. Apply antiseptic ointment to pin exit sites. | Proper tension or tightness to pins is vital to prevent twist or "torque," which would delay healing. Ointment is applied to prevent infection. |
| d. Skull tong traction:<br>▪ Client's cervical vertebrae is maintained in proper alignment with a Thomas cervical collar. Collar remains in place until skull tong traction is surgically placed. Traction is applied by weights ordered by physician. | Maintains proper cervical vertebrae alignment, thus reducing further injury and/or paralysis to the cervical segment of the spinal cord. |
| 6. cific traction before physician leaves. | Client in BSST or Dunlop's skeletal traction must lie in recumbent position. Client with external fixator may be confined to bed or be ambulatory depending on tissues involved. |
| 7. Assess client's initial reaction or response to traction before physician leaves. | Adjustments may be required immediately. |
| 8. Gather equipment and supplies and return to proper storage places. | Provides for safety and cleanliness. |
| 9. Raise side rails if appropriate. | Provides for client's safety. |

## Evaluation

| Steps | Rationale |
|---|---|
| 1. Observe entire traction set-up and functioning: check all knots, ropes, pulleys, weights. | Determines if traction is functioning as desired. |
| 2. Determine client's response to traction; client should begin to note lessening of muscle spasms, relief of pain, sense or comfort. | Skeletal traction takes longer for client to note abatement of symptoms because of more involvement of tissue trauma. |
| 3. Determine response to or continued need for narcotic analgesics. | Reducing need is common because pain is markedly lessened from effects of traction and relief of inflammation. |

| Steps | Rationale |
|---|---|
| 4. Perform neurovascular checks (Skill 34-1). | Checks peripheral perfusion to tissues. |
| 5. Perform motor assessment. | Checks for status of client's voluntary motor activity. |
| ***Expected outcomes*** | |
| 1. As result of specific skeletal traction, client notices decreased muscle spasms, lessening of pain, relief of inflammation, reduction of numbness, tingling, other sensory signs of pressure | Realignment of fractured bones and wound healing promotes comfort; as client's level of comfort continues, mobility increases. |
| 2. With bone healing, increased client mobility results. | |
| ***Unexpected outcomes*** | |
| 1. Client experiences delayed union, malunion, nonunion. | Too much weight may cause distraction or pulling of fragments. |
| 2. Client has severe edema, marked increase in pain, inability to actively move joints, increased pain on passive movement. | Indicate compartment syndrome, which leads to increased venous stasis, decreased arterial perfusion; tissue anoxia may be developing. |
| 3. Client develops infection at pin site or at fracture site with development of osteomyelitis. | Interruption in skin continuity may lead to infection being carried into fracture site. |
| 4. Client experiences prolonged bleeding or frank hemorrhage. Chronically ill or older persons may have preexistent iron deficiency anemia made worse by bleeding or hemorrhage. | Bleeding into joints, soft tissues, cavities is common with bone fractures; as much as 2 to 3 units of blood loss is common in fractures of hip, femur, humerus, pelvis. Replacement of blood loss may be required. |
| 5. Client experiences nerve damage: | |
| a. Peroneal nerve: foot drop with inability to evert and dorsiflex foot. | There may be excessive pressure or pin trauma to nerve at head of fibula. |
| b. Radial or median nerve at wrist with inability to approximate thumb and fingers (radial), and numbness and tingling of thumb, index, middle fingers (median) with wrist drop. | Elastic bandage may be too tight at wrist. Median nerve pressure can result in carpal tunnel syndrome. Volkmann's contracture can occur from compartment syndrome, causing claw hand and wrist drop. |
| 6. Client experiences fat embolism (more common in fractures of long bones) with symptoms of anoxia: restlessness, mental changes, tachycardia, tachypnea, dyspnea, low blood pressure, petechial rash over upper chest and neck. | Fat molecules are released in bloodstream and travel to lungs. Fifty percent of persons with fat emboli die. Emboli occur most frequently in first 24 to 72 hours after long bone fractures. |
| 7. Client experiences posttraumatic arthritis. | Arthritis may be result of decreased exercises, bed rest, decreased joint circulation, injury itself. |
| 8. Client experiences declining voluntary motor responses. | There may be some edema or further injury to the spinal cord (skull tong traction only). |

## Recording and Reporting

| Steps | Rationale |
|---|---|
| 1. Record type of traction applied, persons applying traction, site to which traction applied, time of application, amount of weights, client's initial response in nurses' notes. | Provides for continuity of care and documentation for legal concerns. |
| 2. Report client's responses to specific traction. | Provides for safety and continuity of care. |
| 3. Immediately report untoward reactions or unexpected outcomes with specific signs or symptoms to nurse in charge and physician. Immediacy of care may prevent progression of symptoms, development of infection, loss of life. | Emergency procedures and care should be well understood by nurses to prevent delay in care. |
| 4. Record all findings of neurovascular checks (Skill 34-1, Evaluation, Step 3) every 1 to 2 hr or as ordered. | Enables nurse or physician to note beginning changes in patterns as soon as they develop. |
| 5. Record client's episodes of pain, narcotic analgesic need and use, changes in pain over time. | Provides safety and continuity of care and enables nurse or physician to note resolution of inflammation. Children and older clients metabolize drugs differently than young adults. |

## Follow-up Activities

| Steps | Rationale |
|---|---|
| 1. Following discontinuance of specific form of skeletal traction, client may be treated with: | |
| a. Open reduction and internal fixation of fracture. | Permits mobility and discharge from hospital. |
| b. Application of cast. | Permits union to occur over time and permits discharge from hospital. |
| 2. Client should be assisted in dangling at bedside and in ambulating. Older clients adjust more slowly to upright positions and may experience postural hypotension. | Allows circulatory and musculoskeletal tissues to adjust to effects of gravity. |

## Special Considerations

- Parents should be present to divert and support child.
- Clients need frequent encouragement and praise during drilling periods.
- After traction procedure, nurse must institute "pin care," which includes routine cleaning of pin entrance and exit sites with sterile applicator soaked in hydrogen peroxide, followed by cleansing with sterile water. Last, thin coat of povidone-iodine or neomycin is applied at site.
- Client may complain of heaviness of entire apparatus, depending on number of pins used and whether bilateral fixators are applied.
- All clients are at risk for fat embolization.

## Teaching Considerations

- Parents are taught that babies may cry when traction is established.
- Client should be taught use of ambulatory aid (cane, walker, crutches); instructions in writing should be given to client and significant others.
- Client should have written instructions for home cast maintenance.
- Clients should have dietary instructions if necessary.
- Client should be taught to notify physician of undesirable signs, including increase in pain, muscle spasms, increased numbness or tingling, appearance of drainage, redness, soreness at operative or traction pin sites.

---

### BIBLIOGRAPHY

Baird SE: Development of a nursing assessment tool to diagnose altered body image in immobilized patients, Orthop Nurs 4(1):47, 1985.
Benz J: The adolescent in a spica cast, Orthop Nurs 5(3):22, 1986.
Birdsall C: How do you use the continuous passive motion device? Am J Nurs 86(6):657, 1986.
Brashear HR Jr, Raney RB Sr: Handbook of orthopaedic surgery, ed 10, St Louis, 1986, The CV Mosby Co.
Callahan J: Compartment syndrome, Orthop Nurs 4(4):11, 1985.
Ceccio CM: Rx: Home care. Keeping pin sites problem-free, RN 51(2):70, 1988.
Cuddy CM: Caring for the child in a spica cast: a parent's perspective, Orthop Nurs 5(3):17, 1986.
Farrell J: Illustrated guide to orthopedic nursing, ed 2, Philadelphia, 1982, JB Lippincott Co.
Farrell J: The trauma patient with multiple fractures, RN 48(6):22, 1985.
Farrell NA: Cast syndrome, Orthop Nurs 4(4):61, 1985.
Hines NA, Bates MS: Discharging the patient in skeletal traction, Orthop Nurs 6(4):21, 1987.
Hogt NJ: Infections following orthopaedic injury, Orthop Nurs 5(5):15, 1986.
Iverson ID, Clawson DK: Manual of acute orthopaedic therapeutics, Boston, 1977, Little, Brown & Co.
Johnston RM, editor: Advances in external fixation, Chicago, 1980, Year Book Medical Publishers, Inc.
Lewis R Handbook of traction, casting and splinting techniques, Philadelphia, 1977, JB Lippincott Co.
Mears DC: External skeletal fixation, Baltimore, 1983, Williams & Wilkins.
Mercien L: Practical orthopedics, Chicago, 1980, Year Book Medical Publishers, Inc.
Morris L, Kraft S, Tessem S, Reinisch S: Nursing the patient in traction, RN 51(1):26, 1988.
Mourad L: Nursing care of adults with orthopedic conditions, New York, 1980, John Wiley & Sons, Inc.
Rowe JW, Dyer L: Care of the orthopedic patient, London, 1977, Blackwell Scientific Publications, Inc.
Scoles PV: Pediatric orthopedics in clinical practice, Chicago, 1982, Year Book Medical Publishers, Inc.
Thompson JM, et al: Mosby's manual of clinical nursing, ed 2, St. Louis, 1989, The CV Mosby Co.
The Traction Handbook, Warsaw, Ind, 1975, Zimmer Manufacturing Co.
Wells DL: The elderly orthopaedic patient with Alzheimer's disease, Orthop Nurs 5(1):11, 1986.

# 35

# BEDS, FRAMES, AND MATTRESSES

### OBJECTIVES

*Mastery of content in this chapter will enable the nurse to:*

- Define key terms.
- Identify the different types of support surfaces used to prevent pressure sore formation.
- Explain why preventive nursing care is still essential when using special beds, turning frames, or support surface mattresses.
- Describe guidelines to follow when placing clients on special beds, frames, or mattresses.
- Describe the two mechanisms by which skin breakdown can occur in an air-suspension, Rotokinetic treatment table, or air-fluidized bed.
- Correctly place a client on a Rotokinetic treatment table, air-fluidized bed, air-suspension bed, or support surface mattress.

### KEY TERMS

*Air fluidization*
*Decubitus ulcer*
*Flotation device*
*Friction*
*Immobility*
*Kinesthetic*
*Neurological*
*Orthopedic*
*Rotokinetic treatment table*
*Shearing*

### SKILLS

**35-1** Placing a Client on a Support Surface Mattress
**35-2** Placing a Client on an Air-Suspension Bed
**35-3** Placing a Client on an Air-Fluidized Bed
**35-4** Placing a Client on a Rotokinetic Treatment Table
**35-5** Placing a Client on a CircOlectric Bed

A variety of conditions can confine a client to bed. Multiple trauma, spinal cord injury, severe burns, or seriously debilitating illnesses are just a few examples. Other clients, not actually immobilized by an illness or injury, are prescribed bed rest for therapeutic reasons. Their conditions require nursing care measures that maintain proper body alignment and minimize the physiologic effects of immobility.

Special beds, frames, and mattresses have been designed to help the nurse care for bedridden clients and their special needs. There are beds and frames that help to turn immobilized clients and that are designed to maintain correct body alignment at all times. They also make it easier for nurses to lift, turn, or position clients with reduced strain on their back muscles. Certain beds also have specially designed mattresses or surfaces that reduce the risk of pressure sore formation. Many mattresses or support devices can be applied to an ordinary bed mattress to help reduce pressure on dependent body parts by dispersing it over a larger area.

However, no bed, frame, or mattress totally eliminates the need for meticulous nursing care. Turning devices can still injure soft tissues, requiring a nurse to be especially observant for signs of pressure sore formation. A soft surface, such as a bed mattress or special flotation pad, does not totally eliminate pressure on dependent body parts; routine turning and positioning are still essential to the client's care. No single nursing study has identified the best type of device to reduce the soft tissue and musculoskeletal complications of immobility. However, special beds, frames, and mattresses have proven very helpful to nurses' efforts to reduce the complications of immobility.

## GUIDELINES

1. Know the reason for the client's reduced mobility. A totally immobilized client will benefit from support devices different than those used for a partially immobile client.
2. Continue to provide basic preventive care measures against the hazards of immobility, for example, turning, correct positioning, skin care, or range of motion exercises (when allowed).
3. Use proper body mechanics when positioning or working with clients.
4. Follow all safety measures to prevent accidental falls or improper positioning when clients are placed on special beds or frames.

5. Encourage clients to remain as mobile as possible within the limits of their physical conditions.
6. Educate family members about the advantages and disadvantages of all support devices to ensure their proper use in the home care setting.

### PREREQUISITE KNOWLEDGE

1. Hazards of physical immobility.
2. Factors influencing pressure ulcer formation.
3. Normal body alignment positioning.
4. Principles of fluid and electrolyte balance (Skill 35-3 only).

### PREREQUISITE SKILLS

1. Techniques of proper body mechanics (Chapter 32).
2. Proper positioning techniques (Chapter 33).
3. Physical assessment (Chapter 13).

## SKILL 35-1 Placing a Client on a Support Surface Mattress

Numerous support surfaces are available that are designed to reduce pressure on tissues overlying bony prominences. The wide acceptance of these devices has led many nurses to recommend their use as common preventive measures for clients with reduced mobility and at risk for developing pressure sores. Most of the devices are easy to apply and keep clean. The extent to which the devices actually relieve pressure and prevent skin breakdown is highly variable. Few systematic studies exist that point consistently to one support surface being better than all others.

The types of support surfaces can be classified as flotation pads, foam mattresses, air mattresses with and without continuous pressure cycling, water mattresses, and sheepskin. A flotation pad is constructed of a silicone or polyvinyl chloride gel encased in a vinyl-covered square. The pad serves as an artificial layer of fat to protect bony surfaces such as the sacrum and greater trochanters.

Foam mattresses are pads that rest on top of a regular bed mattress. Some foam mattresses have a flat smooth surface while others (egg crate variety) have foam rubber peaks that help to disperse and evenly distribute the client's weight (Fig. 35-1). Usually the nurse places a sheet over foam mattress pads to prevent soiling and provide ease of cleaning.

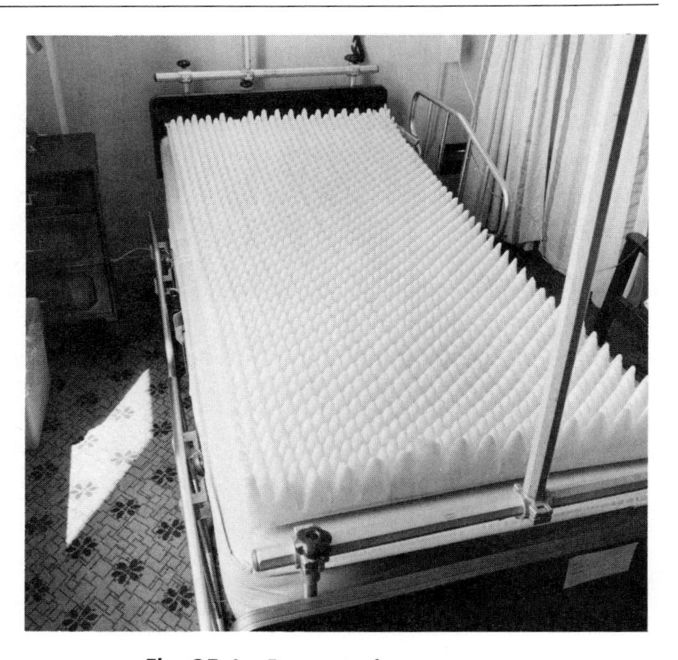

***Fig. 35-1*** Egg crate foam mattress.

Several types of air mattresses are used to reduce pressure on skin surfaces. The standard type is made of vinyl plastic and contains a series of undulating tubes running the entire length of the device. More complex air mattresses contain several layers of tubes or support cells. A mattress may be inflated once with a simple air blower and then applied to a bed or it may connect with a pressure cycling device that intermittently inflates and deflates it to create a cycling effect to minimize pressure (Fig. 35-2). A sheet is always used to cover air mattresses to prevent the client's skin from contacting the plastic surface.

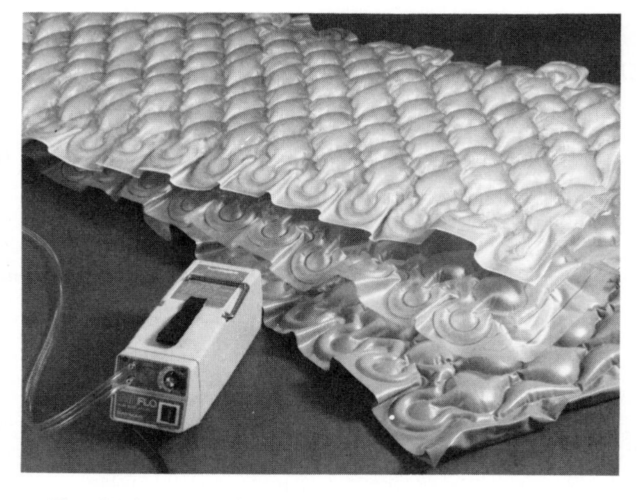

***Fig. 35-2*** Intermittent pressure inflated air mattress. Courtesy Gaymar Industries, Inc, Orchard Park, NY.

Water mattresses are available in a variety of configurations. The mattress may be a complete unit with or without a heating unit, similar to those available for home use, or it may be a mattress that rests on top of a regular bed mattress. When a water mattress is used, the filling may be completed by the nurse *or,* when supplied by a rental agency, by the company service representative. A sheet is always used to cover the water mattress to protect the client's skin from the plastic surface.

The sheepskin pad consists of a thick density layer of synthetically made 1-in long fibers. The pads can vary in length to fit the size of a chair or bed mattress. The sheepskin should rest directly against a client's skin and not be covered by a sheet. The pad is soft and resilient and thus reduces friction and shearing when a client moves in bed. Clients often use sheepskins at home because they are economical and easy to launder. The disadvantage of the pad is that it causes the client's skin to become warm and perspire. Retained moisture can cause fibers on the pad to mat and become less effective.

When using any support surface it is still necessary that the nurse turn clients regularly, position them properly, and administer proper skin care to effectively minimize the risk of pressure sore formation.

### Purposes

1. Help to reduce pressure to skin and soft tissues.
2. Promote client's comfort.

## *Procedure 35-1*

| Steps | Rationale |
|---|---|
| **Assessment** | |
| 1. Determine client's risk for pressure ulcer formation, i.e., immobility, diaphoresis, poor nutrition, reduced sensation. | Nurse can recommend to physician use of support surface as preventive measure against pressure sores. |
| 2. Inspect condition of skin, especially over dependent sites and skin overlying bony prominences. | Data provide baseline to determine change in skin integrity or change in existing pressure sores. |
| 3. Assess client's understanding of purpose of support surface. | Misconceptions can affect client's cooperation in use of mattresses. |
| 4. Check physician's order for type of support surface. | Physician's order required for mattress to be covered by third-party payment. |
| **Nursing Diagnosis** | |
| 1. Cluster data to reveal actual or potential nursing diagnoses: | |
| a. Impaired skin integrity: related to pressure ulcer formation. | Mattresses are used in cases of existing ulcers to prevent formation of new ulcers and to aid healing of existing ulcers. |
| b. Potential impaired skin integrity: related to immobility. | Mattresses are used as preventive measures for clients at risk for developing pressure sores. |
| **Planning** | |
| 1. Develop individualized goals for client based on nursing diagnoses: | |
| a. Skin remains intact. | Mattresses relieve pressure against skin. |
| b. Client achieves sense of comfort. | Relief of pressure can minimize localized discomfort. |
| 2. Explain purpose of mattress and method of application to client. | Relieves any anxiety client may experience and promotes cooperation. |
| 3. Prepare necessary equipment and supplies: | |
| a. Mattress support surface of choice: flotation pad; foam mattress; air mattress; water mattress; sheepskin. | |
| b. Two bed sheets. | Used to cover certain types of support surfaces and bed mattress. |
| c. Pillowcases (optional). | To cover flotation pads only. |
| d. Air flow pumping unit. | Used only with alternating air-flow mattresses. |
| e. Hose or tubing and water source. | Used only with water mattresses. |
| **Implementation** | |
| 1. Wash hands. | Reduces transmission of microorganisms. |
| 2. Close room door or bedside curtain. | Provides client privacy during application of mattress to bed. |
| 3. Be sure bed mattress surface is clean and dry. | Prevents soiling of support surface. Moisture can move by capillary action through foam pads and sheepskin. |
| 4. Apply clean sheet to bed mattress. | Protects bed mattress from possible soiling. Provides clean surface against client's skin in cases where support device does not cover entire bed mattress. |
| 5. Apply support surface to bed (bed may be occupied or unoccupied). | |

| Steps | Rationale |
|---|---|
| *Flotation pad/mattress* | |
| a. Apply foam pad over bed mattress by unrolling it fully. | Pad should lie flat to ensure smooth surface against skin. |
| b. Apply sheet over foam pad. | Sheet minimizes soiling. |
| c. Place flotation pad in center cut-out portion of foam pad. | Pad designed to distribute pressure along greater trochanters of hip and sacrum. |
| d. Flotation mattress would replace bed mattress. | Alternate to gel pad is the flotation (gel) mattress. |
| *Foam mattress* | |
| a. Unroll foam mattress and apply over surface of bed mattress. | Pad should lie flat to ensure smooth surface against skin. |
| b. With egg crate variety, foam peaks should point up. | Peaks distribute client's weight to more effectively relieve pressure. |
| c. Apply bed sheet over mattress, being careful to avoid wrinkles. | Prevents soiling. |
| *Air mattress* | |
| a. Apply deflated mattress flat over surface of bed mattress. (There may be directions on pad indicating which side to place up.) | Provides smooth, even surface. |
| b. Bring any plastic strips or flaps around corners of bed mattress. | Secures air mattress in place. |
| c. Attach connector on air mattress to inflation device. | Mattresses vary as to requiring one-time or continuous inflation cycle. |
| d. Inflate mattress to proper air pressure determined by air pump or blower. | Manufacturer's directions indicate desired air pressure designed to distribute client's body weight evenly. Directions are included with each mattress. |
| e. Place sheet over air mattress, being sure to eliminate all wrinkles. | Prevents soiling of mattress and reduces direct contact of skin against plastic surface. |
| f. Check air pumps to be sure pressure cycle alternates. | Alternating air flow mattress produces intermittent cycling, inflating only parts of mattress at any one time. Intermittent cycle continually alternates pressure against skin and soft tissue. |
| *Water mattress* | |
| a. Apply unfilled mattress flat over the surface of bed mattress. (Self-contained water mattresses would replace bed mattress. | Provides a smooth, even surface. |
| b. Bring any plastic strips or flaps around corners of bed mattress. | Secures water mattress in place. |
| c. Attach connector on water mattress to water source. | Mattress should be filled in close proximity to water source. |
| d. Fill mattress to level recommended by manufacturer. | Manufacturer's directions (enclosed with mattress) indicate desired water level designed to distribute client's body weight evenly. (Usually determined by client weight or height and weight.) |
| e. Place sheet over water mattress, being sure to eliminate all wrinkles. | Prevents soiling of mattress and reduces direct contact of skin against plastic surface. |
| *Sheepskin* | |
| a. Apply sheepskin flat over desired area of bed mattress. | Provides smooth, even surface. |
| 6. Position client comfortably as desired over support surface. Reposition routinely. | Location of existing decubiti might influence type of positioning. Support surfaces do not replace need for regular turning. |

## Evaluation

| | |
|---|---|
| 1. Reinspect condition of client's skin routinely. | Determines if pressure sores develop or if condition of existing sores change. |
| 2. Evaluate client's level of comfort. | If pressure relief mattress is effective, client experiences less discomfort. |

### ***Expected outcomes***

| | |
|---|---|
| 1. Skin remains clear and intact without evidence of erythema or swelling. Existing pressure sores begin to heal. | Skin remains free of new pressure sores. Support surface does not interfere with circulation to dependent areas. |
| 2. Client expresses sense of comfort. | Localized areas of discomfort have been eliminated by equalized pressures. |

### ***Unexpected outcomes***

| | |
|---|---|
| 1. Skin develops localized areas of erythema, swelling, and tenderness with evidence of skin breakdown. Existing pressure sores will fail to heal or increase in size. | Support surface fails to relieve pressure over dependent sites and bony prominences; method and frequency of positioning, client's weight, and exposure of skin to moisture may cause pressure sore formation. |

| Steps | Rationale |
|---|---|
| 2. Client expresses inability to achieve a sense of comfort. Demonstrates restlessness, difficulty sleeping, agitation. | Support surface fails to optimize level of comfort. May require change in air/water level to appropriate level or the selection of a different surface. |

## Recording and Reporting

| | |
|---|---|
| 1. Record type of support surface applied to bed and condition of client's skin in nurses' notes. | Documents therapy initiated; provides data for other nurses to compare in determining changes in condition of skin. |
| 2. Report evidence of pressure sore formation to nurse in charge or physician. | Onset of pressure sore may require different type of therapy. |

## Follow-up Activities

| | |
|---|---|
| 1. Keep client's skin clean and dry. | Moisture and exposure to microorganisms increase risk of skin maceration and breakdown. |
| 2. Remove and replace any foam pad or sheepskin that becomes soiled with feces, urine, or wound drainage. | Reduces transfer of microorganisms. |

## Special Considerations

- Risk factors for pressure ulcer formation include reduced physical mobility, inadequate nutrition, anemia, moist skin, and reduced tactile sensation, resulting in less independent turning.
- *Foam pad/mattresses*
  a. Should be replaced when wet or soiled (determine wetness by placing hand between standard bed mattress and the foam mattress).
  b. Washing removes fire retardant chemicals.
  c. Replace at regular intervals (refer to hospital policy or manufacturer's recommendations), since foam compresses over time and no longer acts as a pressure-relieving device.
- *Air mattresses*
  a. Keep sharp objects away from air mattresses. Tears can cause loss of air, making mattress ineffective.
  b. Assist client with transferring in and out of bed as surface may be slippery.
  c. Surface may be wiped clean with disinfectant solution.
- *Water mattresses*
  a. Keep sharp objects away from water mattresses. Tears and punctures will result in loss of water, making mattress ineffective.
  b. Surface may be wiped clean with disinfectant solution.
  c. Filled mattresses are heavy, move beds with water mattresses with assistance.

## Teaching Considerations

- Explain risks of immobility to client and family members.
- Instruct in positioning and pressure relief.
- Explain risks for pressure ulcers.

## Home Care Considerations

- Most of the devices covered in this section may be used at home with relative ease.
- Selection should be driven by client needs and environmental audit. For example:
  a. The client on total bed rest who smokes heavily would not be an ideal candidate for a foam mattress because of the potential for fire.
  b. The client with pets who sleep with the client may not be suited for a water- or air-filled mattress because of the risk of puncture.

# *SKILL 35-2 Placing a Client on an Air-suspension Bed*

As with the air-fluidized beds, air-suspension beds are indicated for clients who are immobile or otherwise confined to the bed. The air-suspension bed supports a client's weight on air-filled cushions. The bed minimizes pressure and reduces shear in a low air loss system.

For clients requiring high air loss under a given body part, e.g., under the buttocks, high air loss cushions may be substituted. This provides for selective drying while not having the effect of substantially increasing insensible losses.

It is also possible to adapt the air-suspension beds to individual client needs with specialty cushions for proning, foot support, and lateral arm supports. Pediatric air suspension beds are also now available.

## Purposes

1. Prevent formation of pressure ulcers.
2. Eliminate further tissue breakdown of existing skin lesions.
3. Maintain immobilization.
4. Manage pain.

## Procedure 35-2

| Steps | Rationale |
|---|---|
| **Assessment** | |
| 1. Identify clients, i.e., immobilized or burn clients, who would benefit from air-suspension therapy. | Selected for clients who require pressure relief for treatment of or prevention of pressure ulcers. |
| 2. Review client's medical orders. | Physician's order is needed to receive third-party reimbursement for the cost of the bed. |
| 3. Assess condition of client's skin with particular attention to potential pressure sites and any existing skin lesions. | Data provide baseline to determine any change in client's condition while on bed. |
| 4. Assess client's level of consciousness. | Baseline used to detect change while client is on bed. |
| 5. Assess client's and family members' understanding of purpose of bed. | Bed inflation is maintained by one or two blowers, which make a sound that may create anxiety for client. |
| 6. Review client's serum electrolyte levels in medical record, if available. | Baseline data used to compare with subsequent laboratory results to determine electrolyte imbalances. |
| **Nursing Diagnosis** | |
| 1. Cluster data to reveal actual or potential nursing diagnoses: | |
| a. Impaired physical mobility: related to musculoskeletal injury or weakness. | Traumatic or debilitating conditions place clients at risk for immobilization problems. |
| b. Impaired skin integrity: related to burns, decubiti, or wound grafts. | Bed surface designed not to worsen condition of existing skin lesions. |
| c. Sensory perceptual alteration: related to immobilization. | Continuous suspension creates sense of floating that may cause disorientation. |
| **Planning** | |
| 1. Develop individualized goals for client based on nursing diagnoses: | |
| a. Skin remains intact. | Bed's surface exerts minimum pressure on client's skin; nurse must still monitor client's skin and keep it dry and clean. |
| b. Client achieves sense of comfort. | Bed's surface is very soft and conforms readily to body parts, minimizing pain stimulation. |
| c. Client has minimal anxiety. | Client usually remains supine and is thus dependent on nurse for all care; he can become anxious about use of bed as well as his general condition. |
| 2. Explain procedure and purpose of bed to client and family. | Reduces anxiety and promotes client's cooperation. |
| 3. Prepare the necessary equipment and supplies: | |
| a. Air-suspension bed (KinAir, Therapulse, Flexicare, Medisceus). | |
| b. Gortex sheet. | Permeable to rising airflow from mattress and downward flow of fluids, e.g., sweat, urine, or wound drainage. |
| 4. Obtain any additional personnel needed to transfer client to bed. | Ensures client's safety by having sufficient personnel to assist in transferring. |
| 5. Review instructions supplied by bed manufacturer. | Promotes safe and correct use of bed. |
| **Implementation** | |
| 1. Wash hands. | Reduces transmission of microorganisms. |
| 2. Close client's room door or bedside curtain. | Maintains client's privacy during transfer. |
| 3. For clients with severe to moderate pain, premedicate approximately 30 min before transfer. | Promotes client's comfort and ability to cooperate during transfer to bed. |
| 4. Transfer client to bed using appropriate transfer techniques (Chapter 33). | Appropriate transfer techniques maintain alignment and reduce risk of injury during procedure. |
| 5. Turn bed on by depressing switch, regulate temperature. | Fluidization minimizes pressure against skin's surface and reduces friction and shear force when client moves. Company representative will adjust bed to client's height and weight. |
| 6. Position client and perform range of motion (ROM) exercises as appropriate. | Promotes comfort and reduces contracture formation: The bed reduces pressure on skin but clients must still be turned and exercised to avoid joint deformity or contractures. |
| 7. To turn clients, position bed pans, or perform other therapies, set instaflate. Once procedure is completed release instaflate. | Instaflate firms the bed surface to facilitate turning and handling client. Client will not receive pressure relief while bed is in this mode. |

| Steps | Rationale |
|---|---|
| 8. In emergencies when resuscitation is required, touch button to deflate bed immediately. | Creates firm surface against which cardiopulmonary resuscitation can be performed. |
| 9. Wash hands. | |

## Evaluation

| | |
|---|---|
| 1. Inspect condition of client's skin periodically while he is on bed. | Evaluates healing progress of any existing lesions. Determines if any new pressure areas are forming. |
| 2. Ask client to rate sense of comfort. | Flotation effects of bed minimize pain stimuli. |
| 3. Measure client's level of consciousness. | To determine onset of perceptual changes. |

### *Expected outcomes*

| | |
|---|---|
| 1. Skin remains warm, clean, and intact or existing lesions show evidence of healing. | Skin free from pressure effects of immobility. |
| 2. Client rates comfort level as acceptable. | Bed's surface is soft, minimizing pain stimulation. |
| 3. Client remains alert and oriented or shows no change in level of consciousness. | Client does not experience sensory perceptual changes from flotation. |

### *Unexpected outcomes*

| | |
|---|---|
| 1. Areas of existing skin breakdown worsen. | Continued advancement of decubitus ulcer can indicate deep tissue necrosis and need for surgical debridement of wound. |
| 2. Client is restless/agitated. | Low pressure floatation devices may cause a sense of "lack of support," which some clients find unacceptable. |
| 3. Client becomes disoriented and complains of nausea. | Constant flotation causes dizziness and sensory perceptual changes. |

## Recording and Reporting

| | |
|---|---|
| 1. Record transfer of client to bed, tolerance to procedure, and condition of skin in nurses' notes. | Documents therapy initiated and records baseline data for other nurses to compare findings. |
| 2. Report changes in condition of skin and electrolyte levels to nurse in charge or physician. | Changes may indicate need for additional therapies. |

## Follow-up Activities

| | |
|---|---|
| 1. Disorientation and nausea: periodically turn unit to instaflate. | Reduces sensation of floating and decreases subsequent disorientation and nausea. |
| 2. Debridement of pressure areas. | Removes necrotic tissue and promotes wound healing. |
| 3. Increase of fluid intake. | Promotes proper hydration and assists in lowering body temperature. |

## Special Considerations

- Scales are available in some air-suspension beds and available as under-bed units for client's who require frequent weights or for those who cannot be moved for weighing.
- Some beds are equipped with a seat deflate to assist with transferring clients in and out of bed.
- Air-suspension beds are equipped with a CPR switch to instantly deflate for CPR.
- Gortex sheet may cause pressure from hammocking if applied too tightly to bed. Check lateral client surfaces for reddening, e.g., lateral ankles, thighs, shoulders.
- Transport units are available to maintain inflation during interruption of primary power source.
- Experience has shown less analgesia is usually required by clients while on the bed.
- Specialty cushions are available to permit lying prone.
- Beds are usually rented and must be cleaned and disinfected between clients.
- Gortex sheets should be changed at regular intervals. The company renting the beds will supply and launder the sheets.
- Bed surface may be slippery and transfers should not be attempted without assistance.

## Teaching Considerations

- Explain function and purpose of air-suspension therapy.
- Explain the need to continue to change position at intervals to diminish the effects of immobility.

## Home Care Considerations

- A less sophisticated version of the bed is available for home use for rental or purchase.

# SKILL 35-3 Placing a Client on an Air-fluidized Bed

When a client is confined to bed, tissue between the skeleton and supporting bed surface becomes compressed. Blood vessels within the tissues become occluded. A client lying supine on a hospital bed may exert as much as 150 mm Hg pressure (2.9 lb/sq in) on skin and soft tissue. Usually once pressure reaches above 78 mm Hg for a period of time a person feels discomfort and changes position. However, the client with altered sensation or one who cannot move independently will sustain pressure sores of superficial and deep tissues unless pressure is significantly reduced. Pressures in excess of 20-40 mm Hg for prolonged periods can cause tissue injury.

Beds are designed with special types of support surfaces to reduce contact pressure against skin surfaces and to minimize shearing and friction forces that can also contribute to pressure ulcer formation. The Clinitron bed is an example.

An air-fluidized bed (Fig. 35-3) is designed to distribute a client's weight evenly over its support surface. The bed minimizes pressure and reduces shear force and friction through the principle of fluidization. Fluidization is created by forcing a gentle flow of temperature-controlled air upward through a mass of fine ceramic microspheres. The microspheres fluidize and take on the appearance of boiling milk and all the properties of a fluid. The client lies directly on a polyester filter sheet that allows air to pass through but does not allow the microspheres to escape. The client feels as though he is floating on a surface like a warm waterbed. The contact pressure of the client's body against the filter sheet stays at 11-16 mm Hg.

Air-fluidized beds are useful in the care of clients who are immobilized, either by their condition or nature of therapy, and by clients who experience significant pain when being turned or positioned. Clients who can benefit from the bed include burn clients, those who have undergone extensive skin grafts or who have existing pressure ulcers, and multiple trauma victims. One primary problem nurses and physicians must be alert for when using air-fluidized therapy is the tendency for clients to perspire and lose body fluids while on the bed. The surface of the filter sheet warms and as clients perspire, moisture

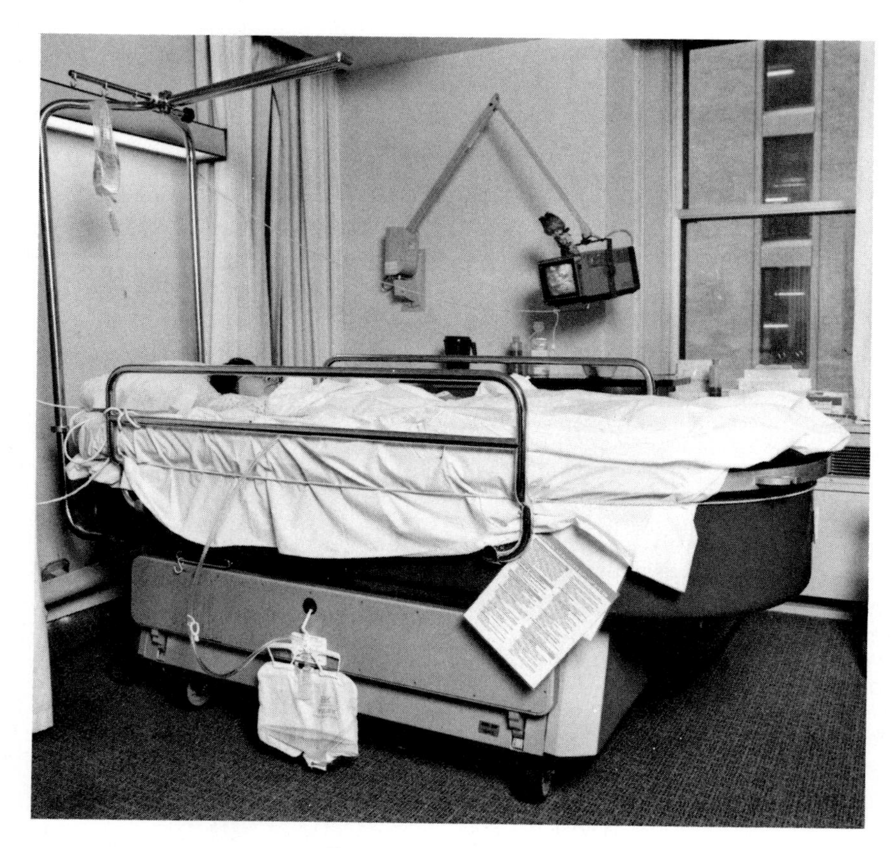

***Fig. 35-3*** Clinitron bed.

is quickly absorbed into the circulating microspheres. Diaphoresis can go undetected and thus insensible fluid loss may not be noticed until a client develops fluid and electrolyte imbalances.

### Purposes

1. Prevent formation of pressure ulcers.
2. Eliminate further tissue breakdown of existing skin lesions.
3. Maintain immobilization.
4. Manage pain.

## *Procedure 35-3*

| Steps | Rationale |
|---|---|
| **Assessment** | |
| 1. Identify clients who would benefit from air-fluidized therapy. | Selected for clients who must not move because of risk of increased pain or trauma. |
| 2. Review client's medical orders. | Physician's order is needed to receive third-party reimbursement for cost of bed. |
| 3. Assess condition of client's skin; pay particular attention to potential pressure sites and any existing skin lesions. | Data provide baseline to determine any change in client's condition while on bed. |
| 4. Assess client's level of consciousness. | Baseline used to detect change while client is on bed. Flotation effect may cause altered sensory perceptions. |
| 5. Assess client's and family members' understanding of purpose of bed. | Bed is large and makes sound when air blower is operating, may create anxiety for client. |
| 6. Review client's serum electrolyte levels in medical record (if available). | Baseline data used to compare with subsequent laboratory results to determine electrolyte imbalances. |
| 7. Identify clients at risk for complications of air-fluidized therapy. | |
| a. Elderly clients. | Air flow may increase insensible fluid losses leading to dehydration. |
| b. Clients with enteric tube feedings. | Ability to elevate head of bed is limited to placing foam wedges under client's head/shoulders. |
| c. Clients with pulmonary secretions. | Limited ability to change position and potential dehydration effect may render secretions tenacious and difficult to remove. |
| d. Client with specific positioning requirements. | Elevation of head of bed is limited to foam wedges; proning should not be attempted. |
| **Nursing Diagnosis** | |
| 1. Cluster data to reveal actual or potential nursing diagnoses: | |
| a. Impaired physical mobility: related to pain and muscular impairment. | Traumatic or debilitating conditions place clients at risk for immobilization problems. |
| b. Impaired skin integrity: related to immobility. | Bed surface designed not to worsen condition of existing skin lesions. |
| c. Potential fluid volume deficit: related to diaphoresis. | Diaphoresis occurring while on bed can cause fluid and electrolyte changes. |
| d. Potential sensory perceptual alteration: related to immobilization. | Continuous fluidization creates sense of floating that may cause disorientation. |
| **Planning** | |
| 1. Develop individualized goals for client based on nursing diagnoses: | |
| a. Prevent further disruption of skin. | Bed's surface exerts minimum pressure on client's skin; nurse must still monitor client's skin and keep it dry and clean. |
| b. Client achieves sense of comfort. | Bed's surface is very soft and conforms readily to body parts, minimizing pain stimulation. |
| c. Maintain adequate fluid volume and electrolyte balance. | Air flow may increase insensible losses leading to dehydration. |
| d. Maintain baseline level of orientation. | Client usually remains supine and is thus dependent on nurse for all care; he can become anxious about use of bed as well as his general condition. |

| Steps | Rationale |
|---|---|
| 2. Explain procedure and purpose of bed to client and family. | Reduces anxiety and promotes client's cooperation. |
| 3. Prepare the necessary equipment and supplies: | |
| a. Air-fluidized bed (Clinitron, Skytron, Fluidair) | |
| b. Filter sheet | Permeable to rising airflow from mattress and downward flow of fluids, e.g., sweat, urine, or wound drainage. |
| 4. Obtain any additional personnel needed to transfer client to bed. | Ensures client's safety by having sufficient personnel to assist in transferring. |
| 5. Review instructions supplied by bed manufacturer. | Promotes safe and correct use of bed. |

## Implementation

| Steps | Rationale |
|---|---|
| 1. Wash hands. | Reduces transmission of microorganisms. |
| 2. Close client's room door or bedside curtain. | Maintains client's privacy during transfer. |
| 3. For clients with severe to moderate pain, premedicate approximately 30 min before transfer. | Promotes client's comfort and ability to cooperate during transfer to bed. |
| 4. Transfer client to bed using appropriate transfer techniques (Chapter 33). | Appropriate transfer techniques maintain alignment and reduce risk of injury during procedure. |
| 5. Turn fluidization cycle on by depressing switch, regulate temperature. | Fluidization minimizes pressure against skin's surface and reduces friction and shear force when client moves. |
| 6. Position client and perform range of motion (ROM) exercises as appropriate. | Promotes comfort and reduces contracture formation: The bed reduces pressure on skin but clients must still be turned and exercised to avoid joint deformity or contractures. |
| 7. To turn clients, position bed pans, or perform other therapies, stop fluidization. Once procedure is completed set to continuous fluidization. | Stopping fluidization provides firm, molded support that facilitates turning and handling client. Continuous fluidization provides permanently fluid support. |
| 8. In emergencies when resuscitation is required, touch button and unplug to defluidize bed immediately. | Creates firm surface against which cardiopulmonary resuscitation can be performed. Unplugging bed prevents automatic start of fluidization, which occurs 30 min after cycle is stopped. |
| 9. Wash hands. | |

## Evaluation

| Steps | Rationale |
|---|---|
| 1. Ask client to rate ability to sleep/rest. | Bed's surface is soft and conforming, minimizing pain stimulation. |
| 2. Inspect condition of client's skin periodically while on bed. | Evaluates healing progress of any existing lesions. Determines if any new pressure areas are forming. |
| 3. Review client's serum electrolyte levels, monitor body temperature, and note hydration status of skin and mucous membranes. | Factors may reveal fluid and electrolyte losses. |
| 4. Measure client's level of consciousness. | To determine onset of perceptual changes. |

### *Expected outcomes*

| Steps | Rationale |
|---|---|
| 1. Client is able to sleep without disturbance. | Client achieves sense of comfort. |
| 2. Skin remains warm, clean, and intact or existing lesions show evidence of healing. | Skin free from pressure effects of immobility. |
| 3. Skin remains well hydrated with good turgor, mucous membranes are moist, and electrolytes are in normal range. | Client's fluid and nutrient intake balances insensible fluid loss on bed. |
| 4. Client remains alert and oriented or shows no change in level of consciousness. | Clients does not experience sensory perceptual changes from flotation. |

### *Unexpected outcomes*

| Steps | Rationale |
|---|---|
| 1. Client becomes restless, agitated with increased somatic complaints. | Sense of constant floatation may not be universally acceptable. Complaints of sinking or inability to adjust to bed may necessitate transfer to another surface. |
| 2. Areas of existing skin breakdown worsen. | Continued advancement of decubitus ulcer can indicate deep tissue necrosis and need for surgical debridement of wound. |
| 3. Client's skin and mucous membranes are dehydrated with abnormal electrolyte levels. | Temperature and evaporative effects of bed's surface causes fluid and electrolyte loss. |
| 4. Client becomes disoriented and complains of nausea. | Constant flotation causes dizziness and sensory perceptual changes. |

## Recording and Reporting

| Steps | Rationale |
|---|---|
| 1. Record transfer of client to bed, tolerance to procedure, and condition of skin in nurses' notes. | Documents therapy initiated and records baseline data for other nurses to compare findings. |

| Steps | Rationale |
|---|---|
| 2. Report changes in condition of skin and electrolyte levels to nurse in charge or physician. | Changes may indicate need for additional therapies. |

### Follow-up Activities

| | |
|---|---|
| 1. Disorientation and nausea: periodically turn unit off. | Reduces sensation of floating and decreases subsequent disorientation and nausea. |
| 2. Increase of fluid intake. | Promotes proper hydration and assists in lowering body temperature. |

### Special Considerations

- Use foam wedges as positioning aids.
- Beds weigh between 1700 and 2100 pounds and are not recommended for clients who require frequent transport in bed.
- Some beds allow nurse to adjust fluidization cycle.
- Beds are usually rented and must be cleaned and disinfected between clients.
- Experience has shown less analgesia is usually required by clients during air-fluidized therapy.
- May not provide stable surface for clients requiring skeletal traction.
- *Never* attempt to place a client in a face-down position on an air-fluidized bed.
- Beds are equipped with special loose-fitting filter sheets that allow for optimal fluidization and pressure relief. Sheets should be inspected for tears, which allow the escape of microspheres contained in tank. Tears may be mended with adhesive tape as temporary measure until sheet can be replaced. Use of additional sheets, pads, etc., should be discouraged, since they will interfere with optimal bed operation.
- Sheets are available that will control high air loss normally observed with air-fluidized therapy.
- When stopping fluidization, allow client to settle without disturbance onto surface of bed. Surface will mold to dependent surfaces of client and pressures will be equalized with no points of pressure. (Similar to laying in sand at the beach.)
- Company renting bed is responsible for cleaning tank of microspheres (usually by sieving) at regular intervals. Interval will vary from 1 to 4 weeks depending on need as body fluids (i.e., wound drainage, perspiration, urine, etc.) drain into the bed.

### Teaching Considerations

- Explain function and purpose of air-fluidized therapy.
- Explain client will require assistance to change positions.

### Home Care Considerations

- Beds weigh between 1700 and 2100 pounds; therefore company leasing bed will need to inspect home for accessibility and structural support.

## *SKILL 35-4 Placing a Client on a Rotokinetic Treatment Table*

The Rotokinetic treatment table is a bed that can rotate a client up to 124 degrees continuously every 3 min from the extreme left lateral position to the extreme right lateral position. Turning ranges are adjustable so that the bed may rotate a minimum of 20 degrees each direction up to the maximal rotation of 62 degrees each direction. A client's physical condition dictates the range of turning. For example, if weight-bearing on the client's right side is undesirable, the bed can be set to rotate from the flat position to 62 degrees to the left side.

The bed is most useful for clients who have experienced multiple trauma, spinal cord injuries, and who are severely immobilized with orthopedic traction devices. The bed maintains a constant slow rotation that reduces certain physiologic hazards of immobility and still provides for easy access to the client. One distinct disadvantage is the Rotokinetic table's surface, which is very hard and firm. The bed must stay in motion, otherwise clients can develop pressure sores very quickly. If the client's extremities and body are not positioned securely with support packs, the resultant friction of skin surfaces can cause tissue damage from shearing.

The constant rotation of the bed can cause special sensory problems for clients. Frequently, after a client has been on the table for several days, confusion and disorientation develop. The specific cause of these problems has not been identified. However, constant kinesthetic sensory stimulation, visual disorientation with the horizontal plane, and inner ear disequilibrium may be contributing factors. The nurse should be constantly alert for this complication so as to maintain meaningful sensory stimulation for the client.

### Purposes

1. Maintain skeletal alignment.
2. Reduce pulmonary, renal, and gastrointestinal complications of immobility.
3. Maximize stability of fracture sites.

## *Procedure 35-4*

| Steps | Rationale |
|---|---|
| **Assessment** | |
| 1. Identify clients who may benefit from or require use of Rotokinetic treatment table. | Table is selected for clients who must maintain skeletal alignment and who require complete immobilization and thus would benefit from rotation to reduce hazards of immobility. |
| 2. Assess condition of client's skin. Pay particular attention to potential pressure sites. | Provides baseline observations to determine changes in condition of skin. Table has hard surface that can cause pressure, and rotation can cause shearing of tissues if table is used improperly. |
| 3. Assess client's level of consciousness, including orientation. | Provides baseline data to determine changes in client's consciousness or responsiveness. Sensory alterations can occur once client is on table for several days. |
| 4. Assess client's blood pressure. | Serves as baseline to detect orthostatic changes once table rotation begins. |
| 5. Assess client's and family's understanding of purpose of treatment table. | Appearance of table and its rotation can frighten client and family. |
| 6. Determine client's height and weight. | Table can accommodate clients ranging in height from 4'10" (145 cm) to 6'3" (187 cm). Adjustments may be made to accommodate overweight clients. (A pediatric kinetic bed is now available.) |
| 7. Check medical record for physician's order for kinetic therapy. | Physician's order is required to receive third-party reimbursement for cost of bed. |
| **Nursing Diagnosis** | |
| 1. Cluster data to reveal actual or potential nursing diagnoses: | |
| a. Impaired physical mobility: related to traumatic injuries | Client's condition causes need to immobilize to prevent further tissue trauma. |
| b. Impaired skin integrity: related to tissue abrasion. | Multiple trauma victims often suffer skin and soft tissue injury. |
| c. Potential impaired skin integrity: related to shearing effect and pressure. | If client is positioned improperly on table, shearing against skin surfaces can occur. Failure to rotate bed continually can cause pressure on dependent body parts. |
| d. Potential sensory perceptual alteration: related to constant rotation of bed. | Clients who remain on treatment table for several days often develop symptoms of sensory overload. |
| e. Anxiety: related to use of treatment table. | Client and family can be anxious over way table rotates, requiring much explanation and support. |
| **Planning** | |
| 1. Develop individualized goals for client based on nursing diagnoses: | |
| a. Maintain correct body alignment at all times. | Prevents further tissue injury. |
| b. Maintain rotation of treatment table as constantly as possible. | The need to stop rotation of table to administer care results in client's skin being exposed to pressure of hard surface. |
| c. Keep skin dry and well lubricated. | Moisture on skin surface can increase risks for breakdown. |
| d. Keep all body parts well supported by support packs. | Sliding of body parts on table surface can cause skin breakdown. |
| e. Promote normal sensory stimulation. | Familiar sights and explanations from nurse help to reduce disorientation. |
| f. Client's anxiety is minimized. | Frequent explanations of use of bed and related procedures will minimize anxiety. |
| 2. Explain procedure and its purpose to client and family. | Helps to minimize anxiety and misunderstanding. |
| 3. Prepare necessary equipment and supplies: | |
| a. Rotokinetic treatment table with support packs and bolsters and straps | Bolsters and straps maintain alignment and reduce sliding of body parts on table surface during rotation. |
| b. Top sheet | |

| Steps | Rationale |
|---|---|
| c. Pillowcases for bolsters (optional) | Keeps bolsters clean. Bolsters are usually covered in Gortex, which can be easily wiped off. |
| d. Equipment representative | Certified to position client correctly on table. |
| 4. Obtain additional personnel needed to place client on table. | Ensures client safety by having sufficient personnel to assist with transfer, so as to maintain client's body alignment at all times. Clients with spinal cord injuries or skeletal traction should be moved with a physician in attendance. |
| 5. Review instructions supplied by manufacturer. | Ensures safe and correct use of table and attachments. |
| **Implementation** | |
| 1. Wash hands. | Reduces transmission of microorganisms. |
| 2. Close client's room door or bedside curtains. | Provides privacy during transfer to treatment table. |
| 3. Place Rotokinetic treatment table in horizontal position and remove all bolsters, straps, and pillows and close posterior hatches. | Provides smooth, flat surface for transfer. |
| 4. Unplug electrical cord and be sure gatch is locked. | Keeps bed from rotating during transfer. |
| 5. Position any catheters, tubes, or intravenous (IV) solutions on client or in hands of person transferring client. | Prevents accidental extubation when client is transferred to Rotokinetic treatment table. |
| 6. Use three-person carry technique to transfer client to treatment table. Keep injured parts in straight anatomical alignment. | Reduces risk of further tissue injury during transfer. |
| 7. Secure side panels, bolsters, and extremity supports as recommended by manufacturer's representative. | Body parts must be in straight alignment; client must be positioned so as to not slide on table surface during rotation. |
| 8. Cover with top sheet. | Provides warmth and privacy. |
| 9. Plug bed in. | Bed is electrically powered for rotation. |
| 10. Have manufacturer's representative set degree of rotation as ordered by physician and turn bed on (may begin with gradual rotation by degrees). | Orders must be specific and geared to considerations, such as need to maintain movement, prevent weight bearing on specific injured parts, and prevent worsening of motion sickness or orthostatic changes. |
| 11. If client tolerates rotation, be sure full rotational direction is set. | Provides for optimal benefits of bed to reduce immobility complications. |
| 12. When there is need to stop bed to administer care, wait until table rotates to desired position and release gatch to turn table off *or* stop bed, release gatch while holding bed firmly, and slowly manually rotate bed to desired position. | Prevents need to manually rotate bed. Manual rotation may result in the client experiencing nausea and/or dizziness if done too rapidly. Reserve the use of manual rotation for emergency situations. |
| **Evaluation** | |
| 1. Measure client's level of consciousness routinely while on table. | Clients often become disoriented or confused after several days on table. |
| 2. Determine if client feels nauseated or dizzy, especially when rotation first begins. | Symptoms of motion sickness often occur and may result from inner ear changes or visual perceptions. Orthostatic hypotension may also occur. |
| 3. Assess client's blood pressure when rotation begins. | Rotational changes may cause drop in baseline blood pressure. |
| 4. Monitor skin surfaces for pressure sites when table is not rotating: | Inspection during rotation of table can cause displacement of bolsters and pads. |
| a. Open position gatches *one at a time* to inspect back of trunk and extremities. | Client could slip through table if both gatches are opened simultaneously. |
| b. Look at sides of thorax and abdomen. | Sites at risk to develop shearing pressure. |
| c. Inspect shoulders, ears, axilla, and groin. | Body sites in contact with bolsters and packs that can cause pressure if malpositioned. |
| 5. Periodically check timer at foot of bed. | Manufacturer recommends bed stay in rotation majority (greater than 20 hr) of every 24 hr. Periodic monitoring ensures continued rotation. |
| 6. Assess lung and bowel sounds routinely every shift. | Determines status of airways and intestinal peristalsis. |
| ***Expected outcomes*** | |
| 1. Client remains alert, oriented, and cooperative. | Sensory alterations do not cause perceptual changes. |
| 2. Client denies symptoms of nausea or orthostatic hypotension. | Rotational changes are tolerated. |
| 3. Blood pressure remains within client's normal baseline. | Rotation of table fails to cause cardiovascular alterations. |
| 4. Skin remains dry and intact or pressure areas begin to heal. | No pressure or shear force to cause skin breakdown. |
| 5. Lung sounds remain clear and bowel sounds are active. | Rotation of bed effective in preventing atelectasis and accumulation of pulmonary secretions. Intestinal peristalsis remains normal. |

| Steps | Rationale |
|---|---|
| ***Unexpected outcomes*** | |
| 1. Client becomes confused, disoriented, or combative. | Symptoms result from sensory perceptual distortion. |
| 2. Client is nauseated or dizzy. | Constant rotation may cause inner ear or visual perception changes to create nausea. |
| 3. Blood pressure falls. | Result of orthostatic hypotension. |
| 4. Areas of pressure sores develop on skin's surface or existing areas of skin breakdown worsen or fail to heal. | Bed is kept out of rotation, resulting in pressure on skin. Client positioned improperly with shearing effect against skin. |
| 5. Lung sounds become abnormal with evidence of crackles or gurgles. | Atelectasis developing or accumulation of airway secretions. |
| 6. Bowel sounds reduced or absent. | Peristalsis slowed. |
| **Recording and Reporting** | |
| 1. Record placement of client on table, degree of rotation set, and client's tolerance in nurses' notes. | Documents initiation of therapy. Degrees of rotation cannot be changed without physician's order. |
| 2. Record condition of client's skin, vital signs, lung and bowel sounds in nurses' notes. | Provides data for other nurses to measure client's response to therapy. |
| 3. Report client's intolerance to procedure and any signs of immobility complications to nurse in charge or physician. | May indicate need for additional therapies or discontinuation of table. |

### Special Considerations

- Company providing kinetic treatment table will assist with placing client on the bed. Keep company representative's phone number available.
- Bed has a timer that will assist in documenting hours of client use. Using a daily flowsheet, such as used for measuring intake and output, may be helpful.
- Clients having cervical spine injuries, neurological injuries, or orthopedic injuries should have physician in attendance when placing client on or removing from the kinetic treatment table.
- Rotation may be gradually increased to prescribed rotation to allow client time to adjust to continual movement.
- Television viewing may be difficult for client; a small television may be mounted on the bed to rotate with the client.
- Nurses should plan care measures to minimize number of times needed to stop rotation.
- To reduce client's disorientation, minimize "clutter" of objects within the client's visual field while in rotation (e.g., suspended IV solutions, suction equipment, etc.).

### Teaching Considerations

- Explain purpose of kinetic treatment table to client and family members.
- Explain any manipulation (including taking table out of rotation) of the table to client prior to performing.
- Explain risks of prolonged periods of stopping rotation to client and family members. If client/family visits are impaired by rotation, set up a schedule to stop rotation for short (10-15 min) intervals to facilitate communication. When rotation is stopped for family visits, table should be at midpoint of cycle (e.g., 30° to the right, never completely on side or flat).

## *SKILL 35-5 Placing a Client on a CircOlectric Bed*

There are special devices, consisting of a bed frame and turning mechanism, that allow for turning of severely immobilized clients. The CircOlectric bed is an example. This is an electronically controlled circle-shaped bed frame that rotates vertically 210 degrees (Fig. 35-4). The bed turns a client from prone to supine without any effort on the part of the client. Clients with healing spinal injuries whose vertebrae must remain in straight alignment and clients with severe burns who must be completely turned for adequate exposure during dressing changes are examples of clients who can benefit from use of these beds. However, this bed is contraindicated for clients with acute spinal cord injury because of pressure exerted on the injury site during position changes.

The CircOlectric bed can still create pressure against the client's bony prominences while maintaining a set position. However, pressure points can be protected and the bed position can be adjusted frequently enough so that sustained pressure should not develop. The bed has a relatively narrow frame that limits the placement of the client's extremities but provides nurses with easy access to the client.

Client safety is a prime concern when the CircOlectric bed is used. The bed should always be unplugged when a client is not being turned. A client who has the use of his hands could easily manipulate the bed controls, causing him to be turned completely over and out of bed. Because the bed frame is so narrow, safety belts should be secured around the client at all times. During turning it is important to always have two nurses in attendance. The nurse is responsible for the client's safety and the correct operation of the bed.

As soon as a client's condition stabilizes to a point where he is free to move, the nurse should recommend to the physician that a more comfortable bed or flotation device be used. The CircOlectric bed is not the best choice for preventing pressure sores.

## Purposes

1. Maintain proper body alignment in clients who are severely immobilized.
2. Provide an easy mechanism for turning clients who must remain in proper alignment.

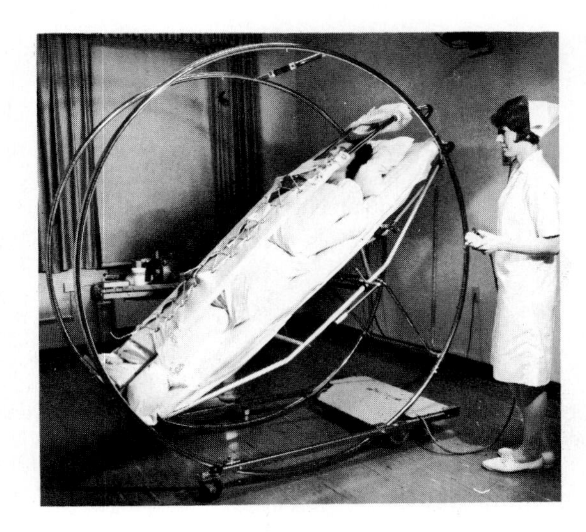

***Fig. 35-4*** CircOlectric bed.
From Larson CB, Gould M: Orthopedic nursing, ed 9, St Louis, 1978, The CV Mosby Co.

## *Procedure 35-5*

| Steps | Rationale |
|---|---|
| **Assessment** | |
| 1. Assess client's risks for developing pressure ulcers, e.g., moisture on skin, inadequate nutrition, anemia, infection. | Will create need to turn bed more frequently and to be observant for early signs of pressure sores. |
| 2. Determine which body part must remain immobilized by conferring with physician or reading client's medical history. | Bed allows for some movement and positioning of extremities. Clients placed on bed usually have body part that must be immobilized to prevent further injury to tissues. |
| 3. Determine client's level of alertness and ability to cooperate. | Bed frame is very narrow. Restless, combative, or confused clients must be securely restrained at all times. |
| 4. Assess client's blood pressure and pulse in supine position. | Data serve as baseline to detect occurrence of postural hypotension when client is positioned upright. |
| 5. Assess client's respiratory rate and character while in supine position. | Client can develop respiratory distress while lying in flat prone position. Data serve as baseline to note changes. |
| 6. Determine client's understanding of purpose of bed. | Indicates need for explanation or emotional support. |
| **Nursing Diagnosis** | |
| 1. Cluster data to reveal actual or potential nursing diagnoses: | |
| a. Alteration in skin integrity: related to immobilization. | Some clients may be placed on bed to treat existing decubiti. |
| b. Impaired physical mobility: related to musculoskeletal injury. | Most clients who use bed have injuries requiring immobilization of body parts. |
| c. Anxiety: related to turning procedure. | Turning completely over from prone to supine position can make client feel powerless. |
| d. Potential alteration in breathing pattern: related to impaired chest excursion | Frame can restrict chest wall movement with client in prone position. |
| e. Potential for injury: related to falling. | Significant risk of client falling unless safety precautions are followed. |
| **Planning** | |
| 1. Develop individualized goals for client based on nursing diagnoses: | |
| a. Promote normal skin integrity. | Nurse must initiate measures to prevent pressure sores. Bed frame provides easy means for turning and thus directly removing pressure on bony prominences. |
| b. Protect affected body part(s). | Provides rest and support for injured body parts. |
| c. Reduce anxiety level. | Design of frame helps prevent twisting and improper positioning of body parts. |

| Steps | Rationale |
|---|---|
| d. Breathing pattern is normalized. | Chest wall movement is not restricted |
| e. Maintain client's safety. | Precautions used during actual turning reduce risk of falls from bed. |
| 2. Explain to client direction bed rotates, need for safety belts, and method for turning. | Reduces client's anxiety and anticipation during turning. |
| 3. Prepare following equipment and supplies: | |
| a. CircOlectric bed | |
| b. Hand crank | Used to adjust bed if electricity is turned off. |
| c. 2 canvas sheets with laces | Sheets come with bed to fit over frame and serve as mattresses. |
| d. Two safety belts | To secure client in bed. |
| e. Pillows | Used to cushion and position body parts |
| f. Additional bath blankets or foam rubber supports (optional) | To protect bony prominences against rough canvas surface. |
| 4. Obtain any additional personnel needed to transfer client to bed. | Ensures client safety during transfer. |

## Implementation

| Steps | Rationale |
|---|---|
| 1. Wash hands. | Reduces transmission of microorganisms. |
| 2. Close client's room door or bedside curtain. | Provides privacy during transfer. |
| 3. Transfer client to CircOlectric bed using three-person carry (Chapter 33). | Maintains straight alignment of client during transfer. |
| 4. Apply safety belt over client's lower extremities and at waist. | Prevents accidental falls. |
| 5. Place call light within client's reach. | Client is immobilized and requires means to call for assistance. |
| 6. Turn client on bed by: | |
| a. Explain to client direction in which he is to be turned. | Helps client to cooperate during procedure. |
| b. Place small pillow over both lower legs. | This elevates toes off canvas frame once client is turned prone. |
| c. Place small pillows over upper chest and upper legs. | Provides more cushion and comfort once client is turned. |
| d. With another nurse assisting, apply anterior frame on top of client as thought client were sandwiched between both frames; bring frame through large rings of bed. | Proper frame placement ensures immobilization of client during turning. |
| e. Be sure canvas bands support client's forehead and chin as client looks straight up. | Bands will prevent neck from flexing, rotating, or extending. |
| f. Secure anterior frame at head of bed with metal pin or bolt. | Pin placement prevents accidental slippage of frame during turning. |
| g. Be sure footboard is placed firmly against soles of client's feet. | Prevents client from sliding down during turning. |
| h. Secure anterior frame at foot of bed with metal pin or bolt. | Prevents accidental slippage of frame. |
| i. Place client's arms through slings at side of frame or have client hold anterior frame. | Prevents client's arms from dropping off sides of frame during turning. |
| j. Apply safety belts to encircle anterior and posterior frames. | Helps reduce chance of client slipping between frames. |
| k. Plug in electrical cord and check to be sure area within turning radius is clear of equipment. | Bed should be plugged in only when ready for turning. |
| l. Remove safety belts and raise posterior frame up by removing pin or bolt. Pull support bar in frame outward and lift frame until it locks in place. | Raising frame releases pressure on chest, head, and abdominal areas, minimizing risk of pressure ulcer formation and improving client's ventilation and comfort. |
| m. Raise gatch of posterior frame at client's feet. | Removes pressure from heels. |
| n. Replace safety belts around client. | Minimizes risk of falls. |
| o. Attach side boards to frame and position client's arms comfortably. | Allows for slight flexion and abduction of arms. |
| p. Unplug electrical cord; place call light in reach. | Ensures client's safety. |
| q. Wash hands. | |

## Evaluation

| Steps | Rationale |
|---|---|
| 1. Inspect areas of skin previously lying against canvas frame for redness, warmth, edema. | Pressure against sheets or canvas mattress can cause decubiti formation. |
| 2. Ask client how he feels during and after turning. | Measures client's tolerance to postural changes. |
| 3. Measure client's respiratory rate, blood pressure, and pulse after turning. | Detects any respiratory or cardiovascular changes resulting from postural changes. |

### *Expected outcomes*

| Steps | Rationale |
|---|---|
| 1. Client's skin remains clear, normal color, and intact (especially around bony prominences). | No pressure sore formation. |

| Steps | Rationale |
|---|---|
| 2. Client expresses no discomfort during turning. | Postural changes fail to cause discomfort. |
| 3. Client's vital signs remain within normal baseline after position change. | Upright or prone positions do not create respiratory or cardiovascular changes. |
| ***Unexpected outcomes*** | |
| 1. Areas of redness, edema, and skin breakdown are noted. | Pressure or rubbing of skin against canvas frame caused pressure ulcer formation. |
| 2. Client complains of dizziness, nausea, or lightheadedness during turning. | Result of hypotensive changes. |
| 3. Client's blood pressure falls and pulse rises when in upright position. | Symptoms of postural hypotension. |
| 4. Client's breathing becomes more rapid and labored when placed in prone position. | Prone position interferes with chest wall movement, causing respiratory distress. |

## Recording and Reporting

| | |
|---|---|
| 1. Record in nurses' notes when client is placed on CircOlectric bed. | Documents initiation of therapy. |
| 2. Record condition of skin, vital sign changes, and client's tolerance to turning in nurses' notes and flow sheets. | Documents client's response to therapy. |
| 3. Report unusual vital sign changes or signs of skin breakdown to nurse in charge or physician. | Client may need to be transferred to different type of bed or mattress device. |

## Follow-up Activity

| | |
|---|---|
| 1. Debridement of pressure areas. | Removes necrotic tissue and promotes wound healing. |

## Special Considerations

- CircOlectric bed should not be plugged in except when turning client.
- Frame is limited to clients weighing less than 300 pounds. Refer to manufacturer's guidelines or institution policy and procedure manual.
- Potential pressure areas include all bony prominences, forehead, chin, under security straps.

## Teaching Considerations

- Explain function and purpose of CircOlectric bed.
- Explain frame is narrow and limits movement.
- Explain process of turning the CircOlectric bed.
- Instruct in the risks of immobility and the need for position changes.

### BIBLIOGRAPHY

Adelstein W, et al.: Cervical spine injuries: the use of the Roto-Rest kinetic treatment table, J Neurosurg Nurs 15:65, 1983.

Baier RE, et al.: Pressure relief characteristics of various support surfaces for human tissue, Arvin-Calspan Advanced Technology Center, Buffalo, NY, May 14, 1982.

Berjian RA, et al.: Skin pressure measurements on various mattress surfaces in cancer patients, Am J Phys Med 62:217, 1983.

Breen BA, et al.: Acute spinal cord injury: current concepts, Clin Orthop 154:125, 1981.

Dudas S, Stevens KA: Central cord injury: implications for nursing, J Neurosurg Nurs 16:84, 1984.

Fowler EM: Equipment and products used in management and treatment of pressure ulcers, Nurs Clin Nor Am 22(7):449, 1987.

Maguire CA: Using Clinitron therapy, Nurs 84 14:14, 1984.

Sanchez DG, et al.: How air-fluidized beds revolutionize skin care, RN 46:46, 1983.

Shannon ML: Five famous fallacies about pressure sores, Nurs 84 14:34, 1984.

Whitney JD, et al.: Do mattresses make a difference, J Gerontol Nurs 10:20, 1984.

Wills P, et al. Paraplegic body support pressure on convoluted foam, water bed, and standard mattresses, Res Nurs Health, 7:127, 1984.

Winkler JB, et al.: Use of air-fluidized therapy in the postoperative care of burned children—the Clinitron bed, Crit Care Nurs 4:92, 1984.

# 36

# EXERCISE AND AMBULATION

### OBJECTIVES

*Mastery of content in this chapter will enable the nurse to:*

- Define key terms.
- Discuss indications for assisting with ambulation or utilizing devices to assist ambulation.
- Discuss indications for performing range of motion and isometric exercises.
- Describe measures to take when trying to minimize orthostatic hypotension.
- Identify significant assessment data to be noted before assisting with ambulation.
- Identify significant assessment data to be noted before assisting with range of motion and isometric exercises.
- Demonstrate the following skills on selected clients: assisting with ambulation, assisting ambulation with the use of an ambulation aid, assisting with range of motion exercises, assisting with isometric exercises, applying elastic stockings, and instituting measures to minimize orthostatic hypotension.
- Develop teaching plans for selected clients for: safety precautions to take at home while using an ambulation aid, applying and monitoring effects of elastic stockings at home, and performing range of motion and isometric exercises at home.

### KEY TERMS

*Abduction*
*Activity tolerance*
*Adduction*
*Atrophy*
*Bed rest*
*Body mechanics*
*Circumduction*
*Contracture*
*Crutch gait*
*Crutch palsy*
*Decubitus ulcer*
*Dorsal*
*Dorsiflexion*
*Eversion*
*Exercise*
*Extension*
*External rotation*
*Flexion*
*Footboard*
*Gait*
*Hyperextension*
*Immobility*
*Internal rotation*
*Inversion*
*Isometric contraction*
*Isotonic contraction*
*Joints*
*Plantar flexion*
*Posture*
*Pronation*
*Rigidity*
*Spasm*
*Supination*
*Thrombus*
*Ventral*
*Walking belt*

### SKILLS

**36-1** Performing Range of Motion Exercises
**36-2** Performing Isometric Exercises
**36-3** Applying Elastic Stockings
**36-4** Changing Client's Position to Minimize Occurrence of Orthostatic Hypotension
**36-5** Assisting with Ambulation

Mobility refers to a person's *ability* to move about freely, and immobility refers to the *inability* to move about freely. Mobility and immobility are best understood as the endpoints of a continuum, with many degrees of partial immobility in between. Some clients move back and forth on the mobility-immobility continuum, but for other clients, immobility is absolute and continues for an indefinite period.

Being able to move body parts independently is a function most people take for granted. This function, however, has a significant impact on an individual's physiological, psychosocial, and developmental dimensions. When there is an alteration in mobility, each body system is at risk for impairment (see box). The severity of the impairment depends on the client's age and overall health and the degree of immobility experienced. For example, elderly clients with chronic illnesses develop pronounced effects of immobility more quickly than younger clients. Alterations in mobility can have profound psychosocial and developmental effects. For adults, immobility may alter employment, family decision-making functions, and social interactions. Such changes can lead to altered self-concept and lowered self-esteem. Children also are greatly affected by immobility. Activity for them is a way of releasing energy and expressing themselves. When deprived of physical activity, children become restless and may even show signs of anger and aggression.

Changes in a client's mobility can result from any type of health problems. Examples of medical conditions that can alter mobility are musculoskeletal conditions, such as fractured extremities or muscle sprains; neurological conditions, such as spinal cord trauma; degenerative neuro-

### *PHYSIOLOGIC, PSYCHOSOCIAL, AND DEVELOPMENTAL EFFECTS OF IMMOBILITY*

**Physiologic effects**

Metabolic
- Fluid and electrolyte changes
- Bone demineralization
- Altered exchange of nutrients and gases
- Altered gastrointestinal functioning

Respiratory
- Decreased lung expansion
- Pooling of secretions

Cardiovascular
- Orthostatic hypotension
- Increased cardiac workload
- Thrombus formation

Musculoskeletal
- Decreased endurance
- Decreased muscle mass
- Atrophy
- Decreased stability
- Contracture formation
- Osteoporosis

Skin
- Pressure ulcer formation
- Elimination
- Renal calculi
- Stasis of urine
- Kidney infection
- Fecal impaction

**Psychosocial effects**

Depression
Behavioral changes
Change in sleep-wake cycles
Decreased coping abilities
Decreased problem-solving abilities
Decreased interest in surroundings
Increased isolation
Sensory deprivation

**Developmental effects**

In the young
- Retardation of developmental stages

In the elderly
- Increased rate of dependence
- Increased rate of loss of system functions

logical conditions, such as myasthenia gravis; and head injuries. Some clients may not actually be immobilized by an injury or musculoskeletal problem but are prescribed bed rest or restricted ambulation for therapeutic reasons, for example, for a cardiovascular condition or infectious problem. Nursing measures are taken to attempt to restore optimal mobility and decrease the hazards associated with immobility. Frequent repositioning, deep breathing and coughing exercises, increased fluid intake, and dietary intake of fiber foods are measures that aid in reducing the hazards of immobility.

## GUIDELINES

1. Check the physician's order sheet to determine the client's activity level and type of exercises or assistive device to be used. This must be done to protect the physician and nurse legally, as well as to determine the frequency of intervention and type of ambulation or exercise to be used.
2. Know the client's normal range of vital signs. Vital signs vary. Exercise and mobility can be fatiguing and stressful, so a set of baseline vital signs is needed.
3. Assess baseline muscle strength. The client may need muscle strengthening exercises before ambulation.
4. Assess baseline joint function. This will help the nurse determine whether range of motion exercises are needed and will provide a baseline for comparison following range of motion exercises.
5. Know the client's past medical history. The nurse should know why the client needs assistance with ambulation and any contraindication or limits to exercise.
6. Obtain and become familiar with the type of assistive device to be used. There are various assistive devices available. Nurses need to know proper preparation and use of devices to be able to teach clients to use them correctly.
7. Prepare client. The client may be afraid of falling. Schedule other activities so the client is not fatigued. Obtain extra personnel or safety device and hard flat shoes for the client.
8. Determine the type and frequency of intervention. This is based on assessment findings. Activity that is appropriate for one day or one shift can change, resulting in an increased or decreased need for assistance with ambulation or change in the type of intervention.
9. Know the client's home care plan. The client may need to continue the exercise regimen or use of an assistive device at home.

***TABLE 36-1*** Incorporating Active Range of Joint Motion Exercises into Activities of Daily Living

| Joint Exercised | Activity of Daily Living | Movement |
|---|---|---|
| Neck | Nodding head yes | Flexion |
| | Shaking head no | Rotation |
| | Moving right ear to right shoulder | Lateral flexion |
| | Moving left ear to left shoulder | Lateral flexion |
| Shoulder | Reaching to turn on overhead light | Extension |
| | Reaching to bedside stand for book | Extension |
| | Scratching back | Hyperextension |
| | Rotating shoulders toward chest | Abduction |
| | Rotating shoulders toward back | Adduction |
| Elbow | Eating, bathing, shaving, grooming | Flexion, extension |
| Wrist | Eating, bathing, shaving, grooming | Flexion, extension, hyperextension, abduction, adduction |
| Fingers and thumb | All activities requiring fine motor coordination, e.g., writing, eating, hobbies | Flexion, extension, abduction, adduction, opposition |
| Hip | Walking | Flexion, extension, hyperextension |
| | Moving to side-lying position | Flexion, extension, abduction |
| | Moving from side-lying position | Extension, adduction |
| | Rolling feet inward | Internal rotation |
| | Rolling feet outward | External rotation |
| Knee | Walking | Flexion, extension |
| | Moving to and from a side-lying position | Flexion, extension |
| Ankle | Walking | Dorsiflexion, plantar flexion |
| | Moving toe toward head of bed | Dorsiflexion |
| | Moving toe toward foot of bed | Plantar flexion |
| Toes | Walking | Extension, hyperextension |
| | Wiggling toes | Abduction, adduction |

# *SKILL 36-1 Performing Range of Motion Exercises*

Regardless of whether the cause of immobility is permanent or temporary, the immobilized client must receive some type of exercise to prevent excessive muscle atrophy and joint contractures. The total amount of activity required to prevent physical disuse syndrome is only about 2 hr for every 24-hr period, but this activity must be scheduled throughout the day to prevent the client from remaining inactive for long periods.

Exercises done in bed can help promote both joint mobility and muscle strength. Exercise will prevent some of the complications of immobility and help prepare a client for ambulation. Three types of exercises the nurse may use to help the client maintain muscle and joint function are range of motion (ROM), isometric (Skill 36-2), and resistive isometric exercises.

ROM exercises put each joint through as full a range of motion as possible without causing discomfort. ROM exercises may be *active, passive,* or *active-assisted.* They are *active* if the client is able to perform the exercises independently and *passive* if the exercises are performed for the client by someone else. *Active-assisted* exercises are done by a client with some assistance. A client who is weak or partially paralyzed may be able to move a limb partially through its range of motion. In this case the nurse can help the client perform active-assisted range of motion exercises by assisting him in finishing the full range. Another form of active-assisted exercise is when a client uses his strong arm to exercise a weaker or paralyzed arm.

ROM exercises remain the same regardless of the degree of assistance required by the client. Active ROM exercises should be encouraged if the client's health status allows because this involves the client in self-care and increases independence and self-esteem. Active and active-assisted ROM exercises help prevent muscular atrophy and joint contracture. *Passive ROM exercises help maintain joint function but do not exert enough muscle tension to maintain muscle tone.* Active ROM exercises can be incorporated into activities of daily living (Table 36-1), as well as into children's play activities. Examples of exercise through play include having the child act like a butterfly or throw a bean bag or wadded piece of paper into a trash can or at a target.

## PREREQUISITE KNOWLEDGE

1. Anatomy and physiology of the musculoskeletal system.

### PREREQUISITE SKILLS

1. Correct body mechanics (Chapter 32).
2. Proper positioning (Chapter 33).
3. Physical assessment (Chapter 13).
4. Vital signs (Chapter 12).
5. Proper handwashing techniques (Chapter 37).

### Purposes

1. Maintain joint mobility.
2. Maintain muscle strength and prevent muscle atrophy.
3. Provide stress for maintenance and growth of bones.
4. Increase client's strength in preparation for ambulation.
5. Increase client's independence by maintaining joint function and muscular strength.

## *Procedure 36-1*

| Steps | Rationale |
|---|---|
| **Assessment** | |
| 1. Review client's chart to determine client's medical history. | Any type of joint problem, cardiac problem, or other conditions that may be aggravated by energy expenditure or joint movement indicates need to discuss ROM exercises with client's physician. Therefore nurse must use some judgment in deciding whether to institute exercises independently or to consult physician before beginning exercises. |
| 2. Assess baseline joint function: | |
| a. Observe client's ability to perform ROM during normal activities of daily living. | Assessment of baseline ROM capabilities is important for evaluating later ROM capabilities. |
| b. During ROM exercises assess for the following: | |
| ▪ Any limitation in normal ROM or any unusual increase in mobility of joint | Decreased ROM may indicate arthritis, inflammatory process, or contracture. |
| ▪ Any signs of redness or increased heat noted in skin overlying joint | May indicate joint problem that contraindicates ROM exercises. May indicate septic arthritis. |
| ▪ Tenderness in or around joint | |
| ▪ Crepitation produced by motion of joint | Crepitation suggests roughening of articular cartilages and is also felt in stenosis tenosynovitis. |
| ▪ Deformities | Suggests bony enlargement, such as degenerative joint disease, or contracture. |
| 3. Assess client's or care giver's understanding of ROM exercises to be utilized. | Allows client to verbalize concerns and identifies educational needs of client or care giver. |
| **Nursing Diagnosis** | |
| 1. Cluster data to reveal actual or potential nursing diagnoses: | |
| a. Impaired physical mobility: related to joint inflammation. | Decreased joint mobility and contractures can occur after brief period of immobility. |
| b. Potential hygiene/feeding self-care deficit: related to decreased joint function. | Clients with decreased joint mobility may not be able to perform activities of daily living. This may be extremely significant because client may live alone. Degree of self-care deficit will depend on degree of joint immobility. |
| c. Self-esteem disturbance: related to difficulty performing self-care activities. | Being dependent on someone else to help with self-care activities can be depressing and embarrassing. Person may feel like a burden. This is significant for children, as well as adults. Children take pride in their degree of independence in activities, such as feeding and dressing themselves. |
| **Planning** | |
| 1. Develop individualized goals for client based on nursing diagnoses: | |
| a. Minimize client's discomfort during ROM exercises. | Client's maximal ROM is reached at point of resistance or pain. ROM exercises should be stopped if client complains of discomfort because this could cause trauma and is very painful for client. |
| b. Maintain joint mobility. | If joint contracture occurs, it will alter client's self-image and affect ability to care for himself independently. May also affect mobility status. |

**Steps** | **Rationale**

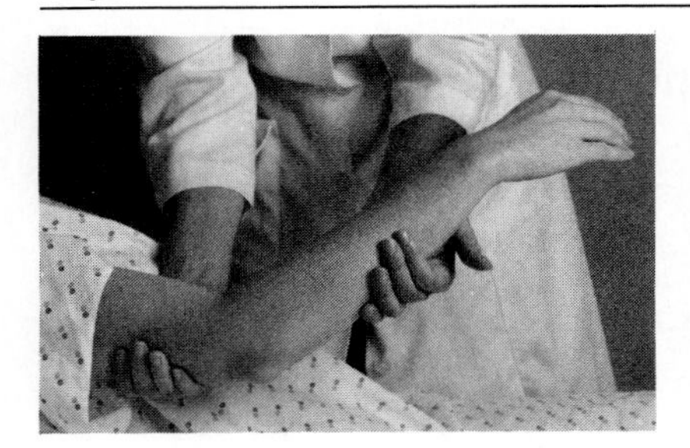

*Fig. 36-1*

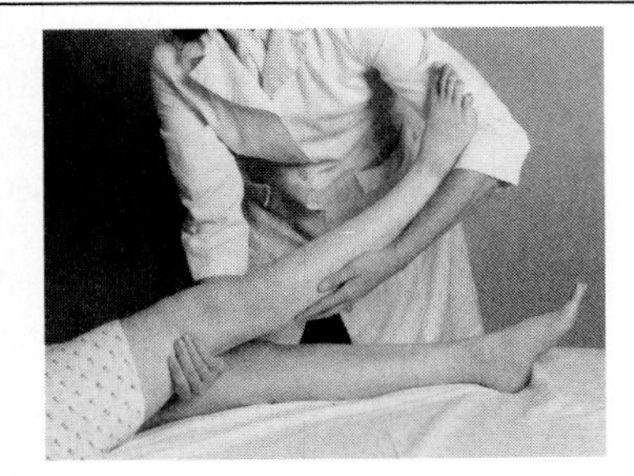

*Fig. 36-2*

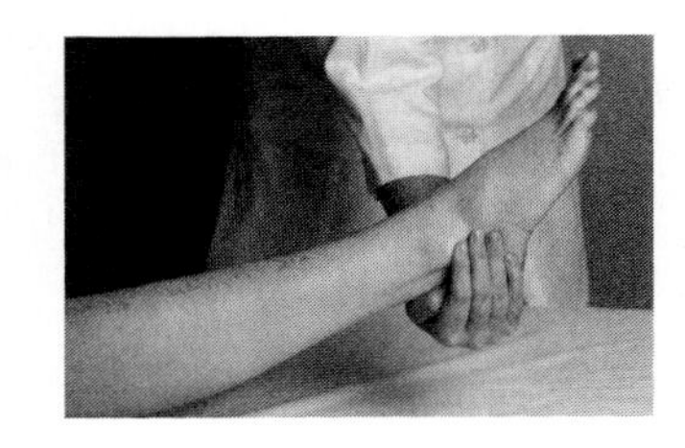

*Fig. 36-3*

c. Have client perform ROM exercises independently.

Client can take active role in treatment. Also, client may be able to exercise more frequently since he will not have to wait for nurse's assistance.

2. No actual equipment is necessary except bed.
3. Prepare client for procedure by explaining reason for performing ROM exercises to client or client's parent.

Relieves client's anxiety and encourages cooperation.

4. Assist client to comfortable position.

Positioning for easy access to joints for complete ROM.

## Implementation

1. Wash hands.

Reduces transmission of microorganisms.

2. Expose only limb to be exercised.

Provides privacy and avoids embarrassing client.

3. Raise bed to comfortable position.

Maintains proper body mechanics to prevent back strain as exercises are carried out.

4. Stand on side of bed of joints to be exercised.

Maintains proper body mechanics.

5. Be sure ROM exercises are performed slowly and gently.

Rapid, jerky movements may cause muscle spasms with resulting discomfort.

6. When performing ROM exercises, support joint by holding distal and proximal areas adjacent to joint (Fig. 36-1); by cradling distal portion of extremity (Fig. 36-2), or by using cupped hand to support joint (Fig. 36-3).

Provides support while performing ROM exercises.

7. Begin following exercises in sequence outlined. Each movement should be repeated 5 times during exercise period.
   NOTE: Discontinue exercise if client complains of discomfort or if there is resistance or muscle spasm.

It is easiest to perform exercises in head-to-toe format.

   a. **Neck:**
      - *Flexion:* Bring chin to rest on chest (ROM: 45*) (Fig. 36-4).
      - *Extension:* Return head to erect position (ROM: 45) (Fig. 36-4).
      - *Hyperextension:* Bend head as far back as possible (ROM: 10) (Fig. 36-4).
      - *Lateral flexion:* Tilt head as far as possible toward each shoulder (ROM: 40-45) (Fig. 36-5).
      - *Rotation:* Rotate head in circular motion (ROM: 360) (Fig. 36-6).

If flexion contracture of neck occurs, client's neck is permanently flexed with his chin to or actually touching his chest. Ultimately, client's total body alignment is altered, visual field is changed, and overall level of independent functioning is decreased.

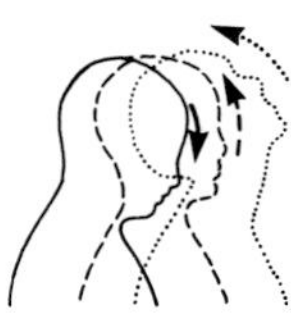

*Fig. 36-4*

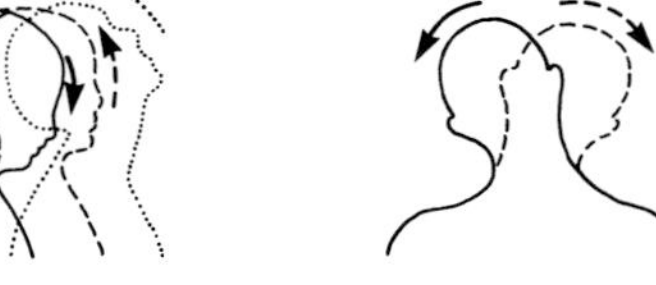

*Fig. 36-5*

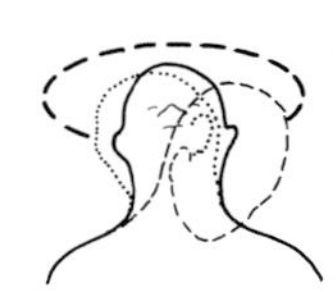

*Fig. 36-6*

   b. **Shoulder:**
      - *Flexion:* Raise arm from side position forward to above head (ROM: 180) (Fig. 36-7).
      - *Extension:* Return arm to position at side of body (ROM: 180) (Fig. 36-7).
      - *Hyperextension:* Move arm behind body, keeping elbow straight (ROM: 45-60) (Fig. 36-7).
      - *Abduction:* Raise arm to side to position above head with palm away from head (ROM: 180) (Fig. 36-8).
      - *Adduction:* Lower arm sideways and across body as far as possible (ROM: 320) (Fig. 36-8).

Exercising shoulder effectively increases power of deltoid muscle. This will aid client if he needs to use an ambulation device, such as crutches, later.

A frozen shoulder makes it impossible to reach overhead.

*Ranges are measured in degrees.

| Steps | Rationale |
|---|---|

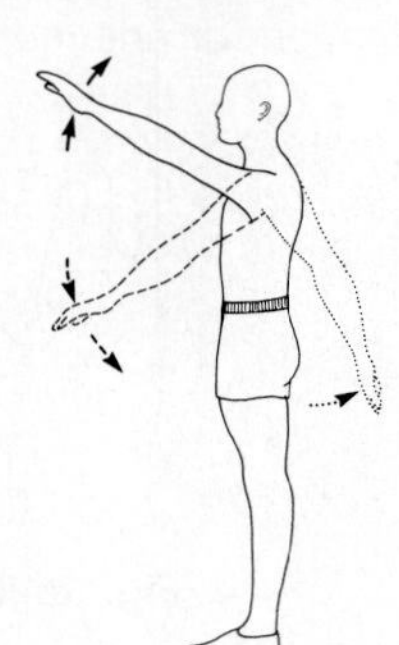

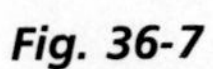

Fig. 36-7 Fig. 36-8

- *Internal rotation:* With elbow flexed, rotate shoulder by moving arm until thumb is turned inward and toward back (ROM: 90) (Fig. 36-9).
- *External rotation:* With elbow flexed, move arm until thumb is upward and lateral to head (ROM: 90) (Fig. 36-9).
- *Circumduction:* Move arm in full circle. Circumduction is a combination of all movements of ball-and-socket joint (ROM: 360) (Fig. 36-10).

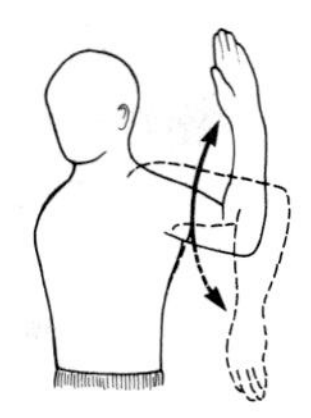

Fig. 36-9

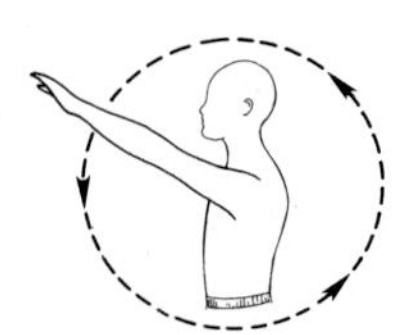

Fig. 36-10

c. **Elbow:**
- *Flexion:* Bend elbow so that lower arm moves toward its shoulder joint and hand is level with shoulder (ROM: 150) (Fig. 36-11).
- *Extension:* Straighten elbow by lowering hand (ROM: 150) (Fig. 36-11).
- *Hyperextension:* Bend lower arm back as far as possible (ROM: 10-20).

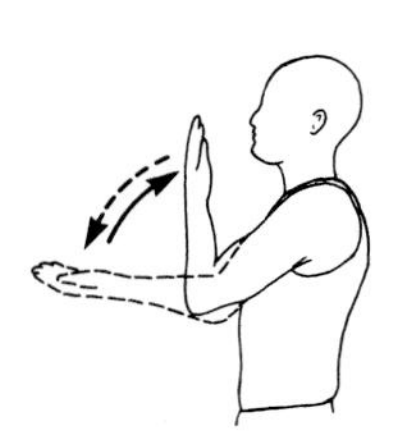

Fig. 36-11

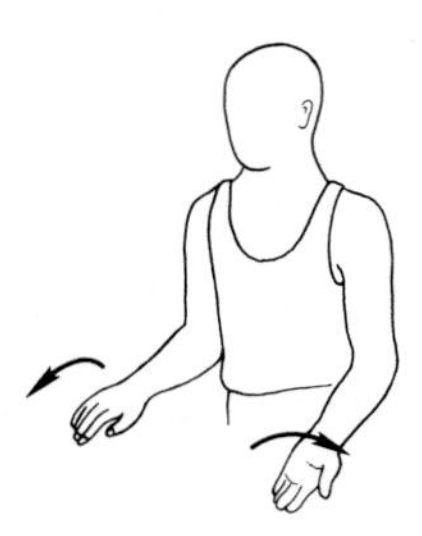

Fig. 36-12

Elbow fixed in full extension is very disabling and limits client's independence.

d. **Forearm:**
- *Supination:* Turn lower arm and hand so palm is up (ROM: 70-90) (Fig. 36-12).
- *Pronation:* Turn lower arm so palm is down (ROM 70-90) (Fig. 36-12).

For optimal functioning forearm must be able to rotate from supination to pronation.

e. **Wrist:**
- *Flexion:* Move palm toward inner aspect of forearm (ROM: 80-90) (Fig. 36-13).
- *Extension:* Move fingers so fingers, hands, and forearm are in same plane (ROM: 80-90) (Fig. 36-13).
- *Hyperextension:* Bring dorsal surface of hand back as far as possible (ROM: 80-90) (Fig. 36-13).
- *Abduction (radial flexion):* Bend wrist medially toward thumb (ROM: Up to 30) (Fig. 36-14).
- *Adduction (ulnar flexion):* Bend wrist laterally toward fifth finger (ROM: 30-50) (Fig. 36-14).

If wrist becomes fixed in even slightly flexed position, person's grasp is weakened. Wrist strength is necessary to be able to use crutches.

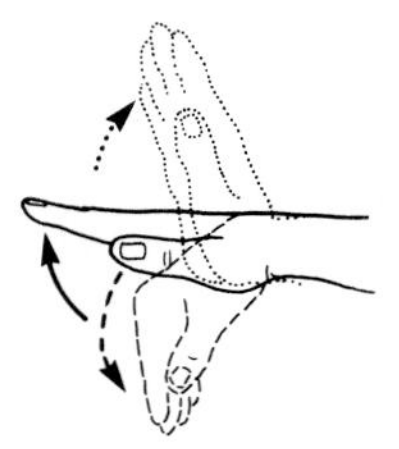

Fig. 36-13

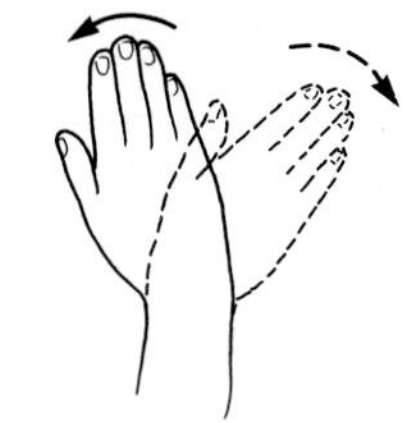

Fig. 36-14

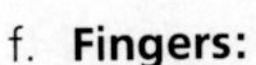

f. **Fingers:**
- *Flexion:* Make fist (ROM: 90) (Fig. 36-15).
- *Extension:* Straighten fingers (ROM: 90) (Fig. 36-16).
- *Hyperextension:* Bend fingers back as far as possible (ROM: 30-60) (Fig. 36-16).
- *Abduction:* Spread fingers apart (ROM: 30) (Fig. 36-17).
- *Adduction:* Bring fingers together (ROM: 30) (Fig. 36-17).

Flexibility of fingers and thumb are necessary to grasp items, i.e., holding onto crutch.

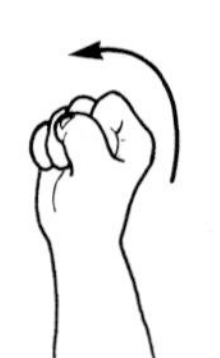

Fig. 36-15

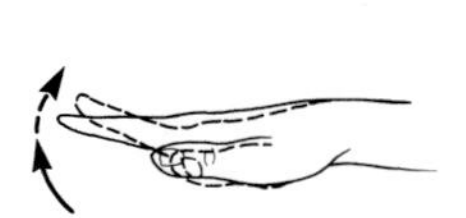

Fig. 36-16

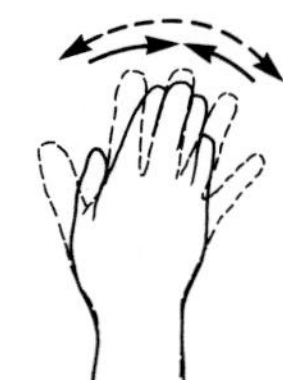

Fig. 36-17

| Steps | Rationale |
|---|---|
| g. **Thumb:** | Flexibility of thumb maintains coordination for fine motor activities. |
| ▪ *Flexion:* Move thumb across palmar surface of hand (ROM: 90) (Fig. 36-18). | |
| ▪ *Extension:* Move thumb straight away from hand (ROM: 90). | |
| ▪ *Abduction:* Extend thumb laterally (usually done when placing fingers in abduction and adduction) (ROM: 30). | |
| ▪ *Adduction:* Move thumb back toward hand (ROM: 30). | |
| ▪ *Opposition:* Touch thumb to each finger of same hand (Fig. 36-19). | |

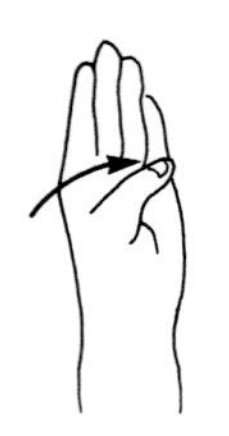

**Fig. 36-18**

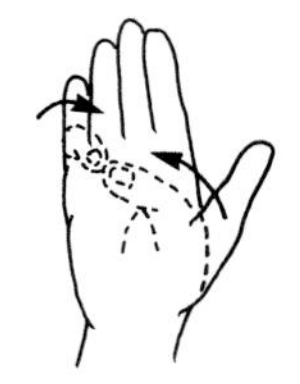

**Fig. 36-19**

| Steps | Rationale |
|---|---|
| h. **Hip:** | Contracture of hip can cause unsteady gait or difficulty ambulating. |
| ▪ *Flexion:* Move leg forward and up (ROM: 90-120) (Fig. 36-20). | |
| ▪ *Extension:* Move leg back beside other leg (ROM: 90-120) (Fig. 36-20). | |
| ▪ *Hyperextension:* Move leg behind body (ROM: 30-50) (Fig. 36-21). | |
| ▪ *Abduction:* Move leg laterally away from body (ROM: 30-50) (Fig. 36-22). | |
| ▪ *Adduction:* Move leg back toward medial position and beyond if possible (ROM: 30-50) (Fig. 36-22). | |
| ▪ *Internal rotation:* Turn foot and leg toward other leg (ROM: 90) (Fig. 36-23). | |
| ▪ *External rotation:* Turn foot and leg away from other leg (ROM: 90) (Fig. 36-23). | |
| ▪ *Circumduction:* Move leg in circle (ROM: 360) (Fig. 36-24). | |

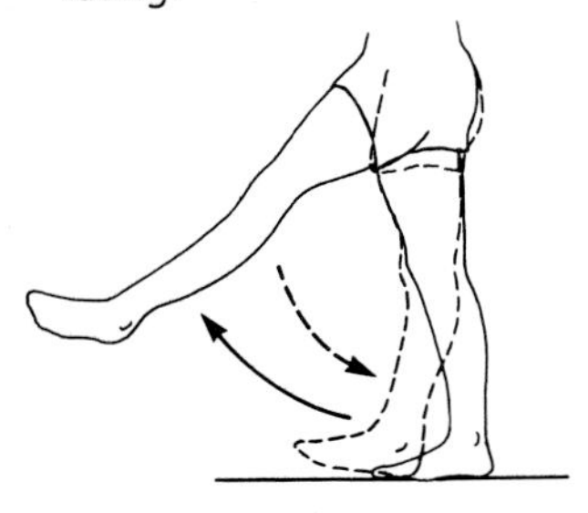

**Fig. 36-20**

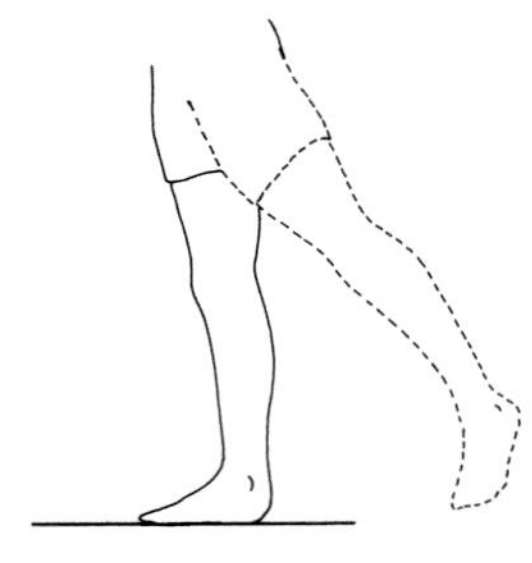

**Fig. 36-21**

| Steps | Rationale |
|---|---|
| i. **Knee:** | Stiff knee can result in severe disability, degree of which depends on position in which knee is stiffened. If knee is fixed in full extension, person must sit with leg thrust straight out in front. If knee is fixed in flexed position, person limps when walking. |
| ▪ *Flexion:* Bring heel toward back of thigh (ROM: 120-130) (Fig. 36-25). | |
| ▪ *Extension:* Return leg to floor (ROM: 120-130) (Fig. 36-25). | |
| j. **Ankle:** | Deformity of ankle can impair client's ability to walk. |
| ▪ *Dorsal flexion:* Move foot so toes are pointed upward (ROM: 20-30) (Fig. 36-26). | |
| ▪ *Plantar flexion:* Move foot so toes are pointed downward (ROM: 45-50) (Fig. 36-26). | |
| k. **Foot:** | Adequate ROM in lower extremities allows client to walk. |
| ▪ *Inversion:* Turn sole of foot medially (ROM: 10 or less) (Fig. 36-27). | |
| ▪ *Eversion:* Turn sole of foot laterally (ROM: 10 or less) (Fig. 36-27). | |
| ▪ *Flexion:* Curl toes downward (ROM: 30-60) (Fig. 36-28). | |
| ▪ *Extension:* Straighten toes (ROM: 30-60) (Fig. 36-28). | |
| ▪ *Abduction:* Spread toes apart (ROM: 15 or less) (Fig. 36-29). | |
| ▪ *Adduction:* Bring toes together (ROM: 15 or less) (Fig. 36-29). | |
| 8. Reposition client to position of comfort. | |
| 9. Wash hands. | |

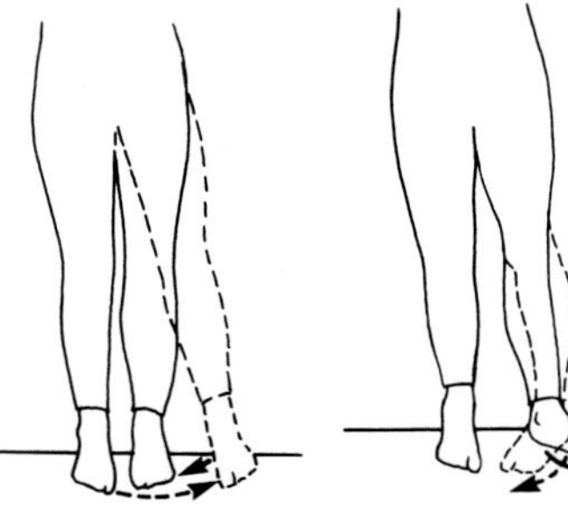

**Fig. 36-22**

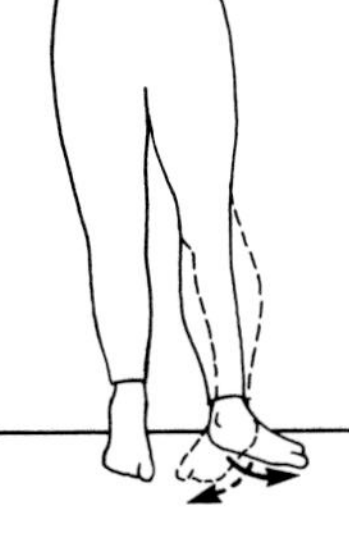

**Fig. 36-23**

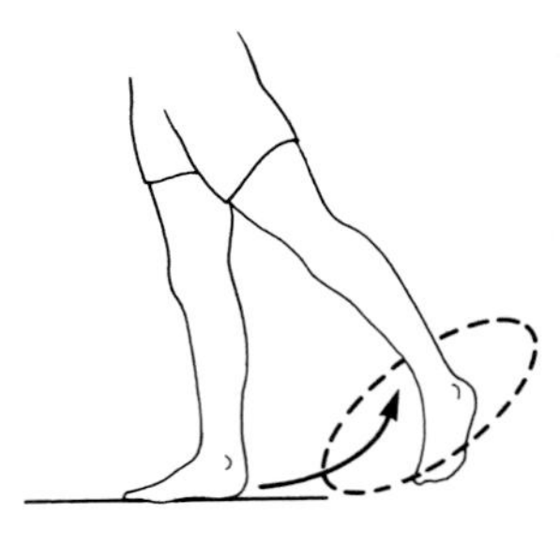

**Fig. 36-24**

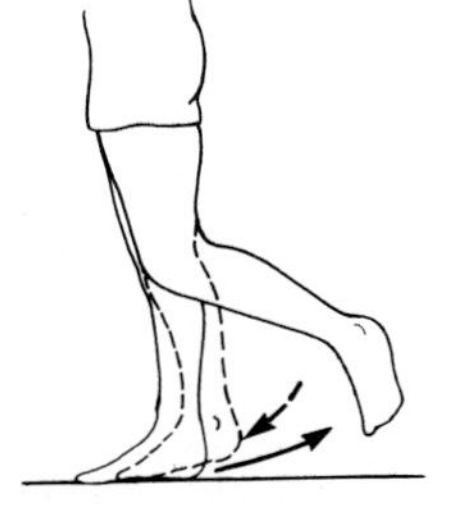

**Fig. 36-25**

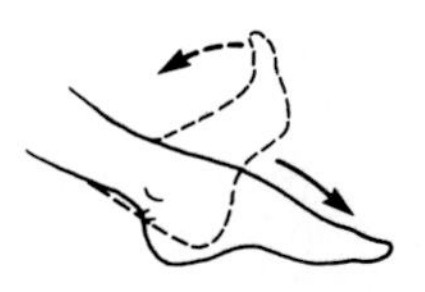

**Fig. 36-26**

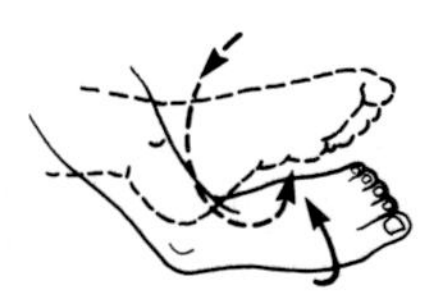

**Fig. 36-27**

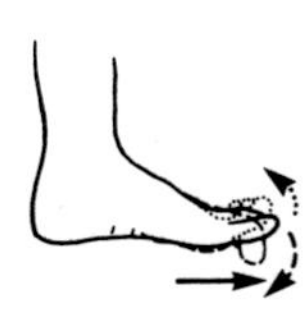

**Fig. 36-28**

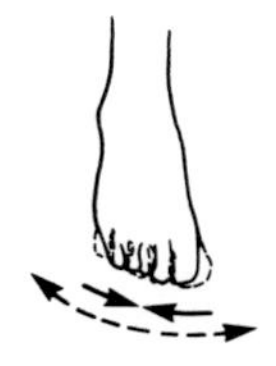

**Fig. 36-29**

| Steps | Rationale |
|---|---|
| **Evaluation** | |
| 1. Reassess client to determine response to ROM exercises. | |
| a. Observe range of various joints as compared to baseline range of those joints. | Determines whether exercises have had desired effect of increasing or maintaining joint mobility. |
| b. Ask for client's subjective statements regarding experience (e.g., complaints of discomfort, level of fatigue). | Evaluates client's tolerance to exercise. |
| c. Determine degree of assistance required to perform exercises. | Establishes guidelines to maximize self-care ability. |
| ***Expected outcomes*** | |
| 1. Range of joint motion is within normal limits for each joint. | Indicates full joint mobility and decreases risk of contracture formation. |
| 2. Client denies discomfort during exercises. | Joints exercised safely. |
| ***Unexpected outcomes*** | |
| 1. Client experiences discomfort on ROM exercise. | Could indicate inflammation, infection, or contracture of joint. |
| 2. Resistance is encountered when performing ROM exercise. | Could indicate beginning of joint contracture or joint disease. |
| 3. Client develops spastic muscle contraction during ROM exercises. | Could indicate muscle fatigue. Movement of affected part is stopped, and continuous gentle pressure is placed on muscle group until it relaxes. Exercises are then restarted, using slower steady movement. |
| **Recording and Reporting** | |
| 1. Record in nurse's notes: joints exercised; extent to which joints can be moved; any joint abnormalities; and client's subjective statements regarding tolerance of activity, along with your objective observation of tolerance. | Documents performance and subsequent effect of ROM exercises. |
| 2. Report immediately to nurse in charge or physician if there is resistance on performance of ROM exercises, if client complains of pain on movement of joint, or if there are signs of swelling, redness, or heat in joint. | Notifies physician of alteration so necessary treatment can be started. |
| **Follow-up Activities** | |
| 1. Instruct client and care giver as follows: | |
| a. Demonstrate performance of ROM exercises. | Exercises are performed safely. |
| b. Provide opportunity for return demonstration. | Assists client in learning how to perform exercises. |

## Special Considerations

- It is essential to maintain joint flexibility. Contracted or immobile joints make protective positioning of a client difficult or impossible. It is hard to relieve pressure over bony prominences and to protect the client from pressure sores. Adequate skin care is difficult because it is hard to separate the skin folds adequately. If the client is in a curled or fetal position, chest expansion is restricted, and changes in abdominal pressure makes elimination difficult.
- Contractures can begin shortly after onset of immobility. ROM exercises should be started as soon as possible. However, not all clients will require ROM exercises. Assess to determine which joints will get full ROM during client's normal activities and which will not and will require intervention.
- Some clients may need ROM exercises several times a day. Frequency depends on individual client's medical diagnosis, present health condition, and willingness and ability to perform ROM exercises. At a minimum, try to perform exercises once a shift. Schedule exercises when it is convenient for nurse and client. Bath time is a good time because bath water relaxes muscles, and joints are exposed so they are easy to manipulate and observe.
- When a person is immobile, the hip joint may become affected because full extension of the hip is difficult in all positions except relaxed standing. Partial flexion of the hip may occur. Elevation of the headrest, use of pillows under the knee, or elevation of the legs all increase flexion of the hip (Milde, 1988).
- Full extension of the knee while in bed seldom occurs without conscious effort. All positions, except prone, favor flexion. The dominant muscle of the lower leg, the hamstring muscle group, tends to draw the knee up into flexion. Other factors contributing to flexion of the knee include use of pillows under the knee, painful disabilities, and stationary positions (Milde, 1988).
- The ankle has a high risk for the development of flexion contractures (drop foot) because of gravity and the strength of the plantar flexion group. Plus, the weight of bedclothes contributes to the fatigue of the dorsal flexor muscles. Along with instituting ROM exercises of the ankle, a footboard or pillow may be useful in the prevention of footdrop. The client is instructed to place the feet against a pillow or footboard and to flex and extend the ankles against a pillow or footboard frequently throughout the day.

### Teaching Considerations

- Instruct client or care giver in performing exercises slowly.
- Teach care giver how to provide adequate support to joint being exercised.
- Instruct to exercise only to point of resistance and to stop if client expresses pain.

### Home Care Considerations

- Assess family/primary care giver's ability, availability, and motivation to assist client with exercises client is unable to perform independently.
- Assist family/primary care giver to arrange home environment to promote exercise program, e.g., space allocation, lighting, temperature.
- Consult physical therapist for additional assistance or exercises and client's response to exercise program.
- Develop schedule for recording the performance of the exercise program.

## *SKILL 36-2 Performing Isometric Exercises*

In addition to ROM exercises, some immobilized clients may be able to perform some muscle conditioning exercises. These include *isotonic, isometric,* and *resistive* exercises. *Isotonic* exercises cause muscle contraction, as well as change in muscle length. Examples of isotonic exercises are walking, aerobics, and moving arms and legs against light resistance. Isotonic exercises increase circulation and respiratory rate and have beneficial effects on the entire body. Some individuals, however, are unable to tolerate such increases in activity. For these individuals, *isometric* exercises are more appropriate. Isometric exercises involve tightening or tensing of muscles without moving body parts. They increase muscle tension but do not change the length of muscle fibers. Isometric exercises are easily accomplished by an immobilized client in bed. Both isotonic and isometric exercises help prevent muscular atrophy and combat osteoporosis.

Isometric exercises may also be resistive. *Resistive* exercises are those in which the individual contracts the muscle while pushing against a stationary object or resisting the movement of an object (Brill, 1980). Examples of resistive exercises are locking hands and attempting to pull them apart, attempting to lift the trunk of your body off the bed by means of an overhead trapeze, and pushing against a footboard. Resistive exercises help promote muscular strength as well as providing the necessary stress for bone maintenance and growth. Without sufficient stress against bone, osteoclastic activity (cells responsible for bone tissue absorption) increases over osteoblastic activity (bone-forming cells). The result is demineralization of the bone and eventual osteoporosis.

### Purposes

1. Maintain and improve muscle strength.
2. Increase client's strength in preparation for ambulation.
3. Increase client's independence by maintaining muscle strength.

## *Procedure 36-2*

| Steps | Rationale |
|---|---|
| **Assessment** | |
| 1. Review client's chart for contraindications for isometric exercises. | Isometric exercises raise blood pressure and pulse and temporarily obstruct flow around tensed muscle. Client's medical condition, especially if history of cardiac problems is present, may be a contraindication. |
| 2. Assess client's baseline vital signs. | Isometric exercises may raise blood pressure so documentation of baseline vital signs is necessary to determine whether exercises cause an elevation. |
| 3. Assess client's baseline muscle strength. | Enables nurse to compare muscle strength before and after exercise. |
| a. Ask client to perform task against resistance, e.g., to push his foot against palm of your hand. | |
| b. Assess grasp strength by having client grasp your hands. Note whether hand grasps are equal. | |
| c. Have client grasp two fingers of your right hand with his left hand and two fingers of your left hand with his right hand. | |

| Steps | Rationale |
|---|---|
| d. Observe client's abilities to do daily activities, e.g., whether client has adequate strength to bathe self, pull self up in bed, move from bed to chair. | |
| e. Obtain client's subjective statements related to muscle strengths. Does client feel weaker? | |
| 4. Assess client's or care giver's understanding of isometric exercises to be utilized. | Allow client to verbalize concerns and identify educational needs of client or care giver. |

## Nursing Diagnosis

| Steps | Rationale |
|---|---|
| 1. Cluster data to reveal actual or potential nursing diagnoses: | |
| a. Activity intolerance: related to immobility. | Muscle weakness and atrophy can result from immobility and client's ability to tolerate activity decreases. Decreased mobility can lead to increased weakness. |
| b. Knowledge deficit concerning exercises: related to inexperience. | Client may be unfamiliar with isometric exercises. |

## Planning

| Steps | Rationale |
|---|---|
| 1. Develop individualized goals for client based on nursing diagnoses: | |
| a. Client will be able to perform the various exercises correctly. | Achieves optimum effect from exercises. |
| b. Client will gradually increase number of repetitions of each exercise. | Increases strength. |
| c. Client will have increased muscle strength following exercises. | Isometric exercises increase muscle tone. |
| 2. No supplies necessary. | |
| 3. Prepare client for procedure. | Relieves anxiety and encourage client's cooperation. |
| a. Explain rationale for and describe exercises. | |
| b. Assist client to position of comfort. | |
| c. All of these exercises can be done while in bed and some can be done while sitting or standing. | Useful for immobilized clients who cannot get out of bed. |

## Implementation

| Steps | Rationale |
|---|---|
| 1. Provide privacy. | Prevents client embarrassment. |
| 2. Instruct client to perform following exercises daily and gradually increase repetitions. Muscle groups used for walking should be exercised isometrically 4 times per day until client is ambulatory. Muscle group is tightened (contracted) for 8 secs, then completely relaxed for several seconds. Repeated 10 times for each muscle group during each exercise session. Exercises are as follows: | |
| a. Quadriceps isometrics<br>▪ Assist to supine recumbent position.<br>▪ Instruct client to press back of the knee against mattress while trying to lift heel from bed (Fig. 36-30).<br>▪ Hold muscles tightly contracted for 8 sec and then relax completely for several seconds.<br>▪ Repeat. Perform on each extremity 10 times. | For person to ambulate and get out of chair large muscles of thigh (quadriceps) must be strong enough for him to extend his knees and stabilize them.<br>Nurse can assist client in learning this exercise by placing her hand between client's knee and mattress and asking client to press hand against mattress with the knee (Beyers and Dudas, 1977). |
| b. Gluteal muscle isometrics<br>▪ Assist client to recumbent position. | Improves client's balance when sitting. |

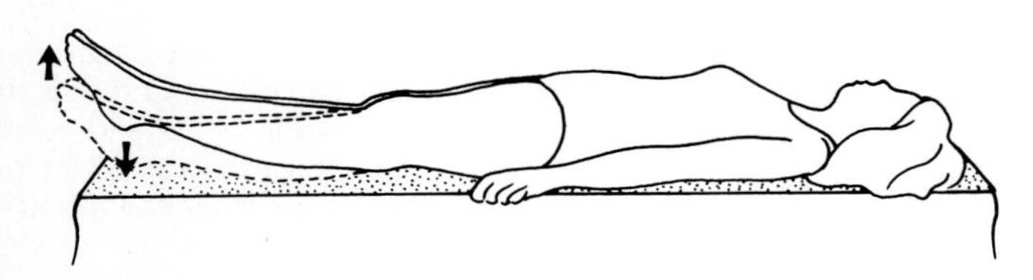

*Fig. 36-30*

| Steps | Rationale |
|---|---|
| ▪ Instruct client to pinch buttocks muscles together and hold for 8 sec and then relax completely for several seconds (Fig. 36-31, *A*). ▪ Repeat 10 times. | |
| c. Abdominal muscle isometrics (Fig. 36-31, *B*) ▪ Pull abdominal muscles in as tightly as possible. ▪ Hold for 8 sec. ▪ Release muscles gradually. ▪ Repeat 10 times. | Improves trunk stability. |

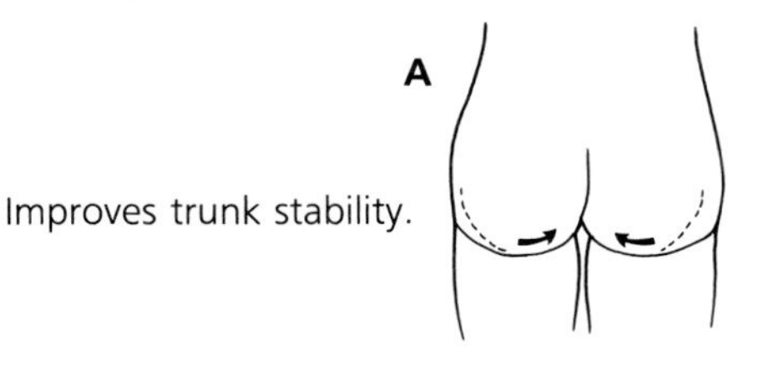


***Fig. 36-31***

| Steps | Rationale |
|---|---|
| d. Foot muscle isometrics ▪ Instruct client to move his foot in a circle in all directions and flex foot toward and away from knee. | Increases muscle activity in leg and thereby promotes venous return to heart. |
| e. Hand muscle isometrics ▪ Obtain sponge rubber ball. (Size of ball depends on size of client's hand.) ▪ Grip ball with entire hand 5-10 times. ▪ Dig each fingertip, one at a time, into ball 5-10 times each. ▪ Gradually increase exercise until client can grip ball and exercise once or twice a day. | Strengthens grip to hold onto crutch or walker more effectively. |

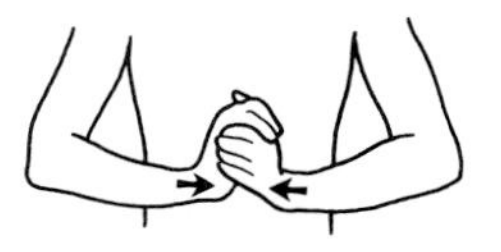

***Fig. 36-32***

| Steps | Rationale |
|---|---|
| f. Biceps isometrics ▪ Raise arms to shoulder height and interlock fingertips of both hands. ▪ Try to pull hands apart using arm muscles. ▪ Hold for 6 sec. ▪ Relax for 2 min. ▪ Repeat 10 times. | Strengthens biceps and so helps with ambulation if ambulation device is used. |
| g. Triceps muscle isometrics (Fig. 36-32) ▪ Raise arms to shoulder height. ▪ Make fist with one hand and place against palm of other hand. ▪ Push hands together as hard as possible for 6 sec. ▪ Relax and repeat after 2 min. | Strengthens triceps to assist with transfer techniques and use of crutches or walker. |
| 3. Instruct client in the following resistive exercises: | |
| a. Triceps muscle isometrics (Fig. 36-33) ▪ Assist client to sitting position on edge of bed or in chair. ▪ Instruct client to try to lift his buttocks off bed or seat of chair by pressing down on mattress or chair seat with his hands. ▪ Hold muscle tight for 8 sec; then release. ▪ Repeat 10 times. | To use crutches or walker effectively, client must have enough strength in the triceps to extend and stabilize the elbows while lifting or shifting body weight. |

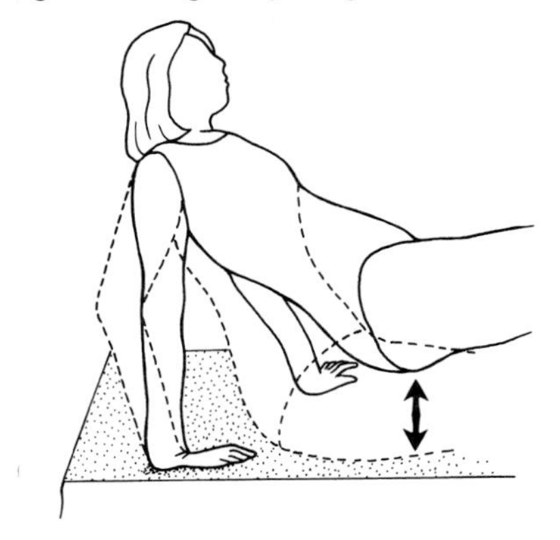

***Fig. 36-33***

| Steps | Rationale |
|---|---|
| b. Quadriceps muscle isometrics ▪ Push feet against footboard. ▪ Repeat several times a day. | Builds strength, size, and shape of leg muscles and provides stress against bone that is needed to maintain a balance between osteoblasts and osteoclasts. Without sufficient stress the osteoclastic activity increases over the osteoblastic activity and bone demineralization takes place. If mattress is soft, blocks or books are placed on bed under client's hands (Lewis and Timby, 1988). |

| **Steps** | **Rationale** |
|---|---|
| **Evaluation** | |
| 1. Reassess client to determine response to isometric and resistive exercises. | |
| a. Observe client's ability to perform exercises. | Assesses whether client is performing exercises accurately and whether they are increasing muscle strength. |
| b. Determine client's level of energy and muscular strength following exercises. | |
| c. If client appears unusually fatigued or short of breath, reassess vital signs. | Assesses tolerance to activity. |
| ***Expected outcomes*** | |
| 1. Client will gradually increase number of exercise repetitions. | Client will gradually become stronger and able to increase number of repetitions. |
| 2. Muscle strength will increase. | Isometric exercises increase muscle tone. |
| 3. Vital signs remain stable. | Documents client's ability to tolerate activity. |
| ***Unexpected outcomes*** | |
| 1. Client is unable to perform exercises. | Client may be too weak. Continue ROM exercises and repositioning client to try to increase strength. Make sure nutrition and rest are adequate. |
| 2. Client is unwilling to perform exercises. | Lack of understanding of significance of exercises. Stress importance. |
| 3. Muscular strength is not increasing. | May not be performing exercises as described or as often as instructed. Stress importance. |
| 4. Client's blood pressure and heart rate increase significantly during exercises. | May not be able to tolerate procedure. Discontinue exercises and consult physician. |
| **Recording and Reporting** | |
| 1. Record in nurse's progress notes: type of isometric exercises used; length of time contractions held; number of repetitions of each exercise that was performed; assessment of client's muscular strength following exercises; and client's subjective statements regarding muscular strength. | To provide documentation of client's progress using isometric exercises. |
| 2. Report client's tolerance or untoward effect to nurse or physician. | Notifies appropriate personnel of untoward effects and modification of exercise plan. |
| **Follow-up Activities** | |
| 1. Assess client's ability to perform isometric exercises. | Ensures that client is performing exercises accurately. |
| 2. Assess client's understanding of significance of exercises. | Ensures that client will comply with exercise plan. |
| 3. Notify physician if having difficulty performing exercises or if muscle strength is not improving. | Indicates need for further evaluation. |

## Special Considerations

- It may be more effective to instruct client to perform exercises before each meal and at bedtime instead of 4 times per day.
- Clients doing isometric exercises should be taught to exhale while exerting effort. Many persons will hold their breath when exerting effort (valsalva maneuver). This increases intrathoracic pressure, causing decrease in venous return to heart. When breath is released, intrathoracic pressure decreases, causing large surge of blood to return to the heart and increase cardiac work load (Long and Phipps, 1989).
- Shorter regular periods of exercise cause less fatigue to client and maintain better ROM and muscle tone than infrequent, long periods of exercise.
- Proper nutrition is essential if client is to be able to perform exercises. The promotion of protein anabolism involves conservation and replenishment of energy stores. Energy conservation results from a decrease in stressors, such as anxiety or increased temperature. Replenishment of energy stores involves adequate intake of protein and calories. Primary indicator of adequate intake is maintenance or increase of weight (Milde, 1988).

## Teaching Considerations

- Instruct client to gradually increase exercises each day and to exhale on exertion to avoid valsalva maneuver.

# SKILL 36-3 Applying Elastic Stockings

One hazard of attempting ambulation following a period of immobility is the potential for orthostatic hypotension. Orthostatic or postural hypotension is a drop in blood pressure of 15 mm Hg or more when the client rises from a sitting to a standing position. As a result of the decrease in blood pressure the client becomes dizzy on rising and may even faint. Immobilized clients and those undergoing prolonged bed rest are at risk for orthostatic hypotension. This is thought to be caused by two factors. The first factor is loss of muscle tone. Contraction of muscles in the legs assist venous return to the heart. Decreased muscle tone in the legs reduces muscular action on the great veins in the lower extremities, and venous return to the heart is decreased.

The second factor leading to orthostatic hypotension in immobilized clients is the diminished ability of the autonomic nervous system to equalize blood supply in the client when he sits up. Normally the baroreceptor reflexes elicit an immediate sympathetic response to the decreased arterial blood pressure that occurs when a person stands up. This sympathetic response causes peripheral vasoconstriction, which prevents pooling of blood in the lower extremities and maintains arterial blood pressure. In an immobilized client the absence or reduction of peripheral vasoconstriction allows pooling of blood in the lower extremities and thus decreases venous return to the heart. This in turn leads to a decrease in cardiac output and lowered blood pressure.

Although orthostatic hypotension cannot be prevented, its effects can be minimized. Interventions are directed toward maintaining muscle tone to increase venous return to the heart and decrease stasis of blood in the lower extremities. Two interventions to assist clients in maintaining muscle tone are range of motion and isometric leg exercises (Skill 36-1 and Skill 36-2) and the application of elastic stockings. Elastic stockings promote venous return by maintaining pressure on superficial veins and muscles of the lower extremities. This compression increases flow through deep veins and thereby prevents venous pooling and reduces the risk for clot formation in the lower extremities.

## Purposes

1. Decrease venous pooling in the extremities.
2. Prevent injury to the client.
3. Increase mobility status.

## Procedure 36-3

| Steps | Rationale |
|---|---|
| **Assessment** | |
| 1. Observe client to determine need for elastic stockings. | Clients who are immobile, who have problems with varicose veins, or who are experiencing lower extremity edema are potential candidates for elastic stockings. |
| 2. Observe for signs, symptoms, and conditions that might contraindicate use of elastic stockings. Signs and symptoms include: | |
| a. Dermatitis or open skin lesion. | Elastic socks may aggravate skin condition or cause it to spread. Also, physician may want medication and dressing applied to lesion. |
| b. Recent skin graft. | Continuous pressure is necessary to keep graft adherent to recipient bed, but pressure should not be so firm as to cause death of graft (Long and Phipps, 1985). |
| c. Severe atherosclerosis. | Persons with atherosclerosis should not wear clothing that constricts and further impedes circulation and so should avoid rolled garters and socks with tight bands. |
| d. Pulmonary edema. | Elastic socks promote venous return. Treatments for pulmonary edema (diuretics, rotating tourniquets, and phlebotomy) are to decrease venous return and circulating blood volume to decrease workload on heart. |
| e. Decreased circulation in lower extremities as evidenced by cyanotic, cool extremities. | Elastic stockings may further impede circulation. |
| 3. Assess client's or care giver's understanding of application of elastic socks. | Identifies potential educational needs of client or client's care giver. |
| 4. Assess the condition of the client's skin and circulation to the legs. | Identifies a baseline for skin integrity and quality of peripheral pulses in the lower extremities. |

| Steps | Rationale |
|---|---|
| **Nursing Diagnosis** | |
| 1. Cluster data to reveal actual or potential nursing diagnoses: | |
| a. Impaired physical mobility: related to prolonged bedrest. | Immobility can lead to venous stasis and thrombus formation. |
| b. Altered tissue perfusion: related to immobility. | Venous stasis can result from immobility. |
| c. Knowledge deficit regarding application of elastic stockings: related to inexperience. | Client and other care givers need instruction in application of elastic stockings. Some clients may have allergic reaction to stocking material. |
| **Planning** | |
| 1. Develop individualized goals for client based on nursing diagnoses: | |
| a. Teach client the rationale for use of elastic stockings. | Client's compliance with therapy will increase. |
| b. Have client or care giver demonstrate procedure for applying stockings. | Ensures client or care giver can apply stockings properly and avoid complications. |
| c. Instruct client in proper method of caring for stockings. | Ensures that socks will last as long as possible before needing to be replaced. |
| d. Promote client's understanding of rationale for inspecting lower extremities daily and knowledge of symptoms of thrombophlebitis. | Detects and treats complications as early as possible. |
| 2. Obtain physician's order. | Protects nurse, physician, and client. May be needed for legal reimbursement reasons. |
| 3. Prepare client for procedure. | |
| a. Explain reason for and technique of applying stockings. | Relieves anxiety and encourages cooperation. |
| 4. Measure stockings for proper size. | If too large, stockings will not adequately support extremities. If too small, they may impede blood flow. Compare your measurements with the manufacturer's sizing chart. |
| 5. Prepare needed equipment: | |
| a. Tape measure | Stockings must be measured according to directions of specific manufacturer. |
| b. Elastic support stockings in correct size | Elastic socks come in two lengths, knee-high and thigh-high. Choice depends on physician's specifications. |
| c. Talcum powder | Eases application of stockings. |
| **Implementation** | |
| 1. Wash hands. | Reduces transmission of microorganisms. |
| 2. Elevate head of bed to comfortable level. | Promotes good body mechanics for nurse. |
| 3. Position client in supine position. | Eases application. Also, the stockings should be applied before standing up in order to prevent stagnation of blood in lower extremities. If client has been standing, client should sit in chair for 15 min with legs elevated before applying elastic stockings (Beyers and Dudas, 1977). |
| 4. Apply small amount of talcum powder to legs and feet, provided client doesn't have sensitivity to talcum powder. | Talcum powder reduces friction and allows for easier application of stockings. |
| 5. Apply stockings. | |
| a. Turn elastic stocking inside out by placing one hand into sock, holding toe of sock with your other hand, and pulling (Fig. 36-34). | Allows easier application of stocking. |
| b. Place client's toes into foot of elastic stocking making sure that sock is smooth (Fig. 36-35). | Wrinkles in sock can impede circulation to lower region of extremity. |
| c. Slide remaining portion of sock over client's foot, being sure that the toes are covered. Sock will now be right side out (Fig. 36-36). | If toes remain uncovered, they will become constricted by elastic and their circulation can be reduced. |
| d. Slide sock up over client's calf until sock is completely extended. Be sure sock is smooth and no ridges are present (Fig. 36-37). | Ridges impede venous return and can counteract overall purpose of elastic stocking. |
| e. Instruct client not to roll socks partially down. | Rolling sock partially down will have a constricting effect and impede venous return. |
| 6. Reposition client to position of comfort. | Maintains proper body alignment and promotes comfort. |
| 7. Wash hands. | Reduces transmission of microorganisms |

**Steps** | **Rationale**

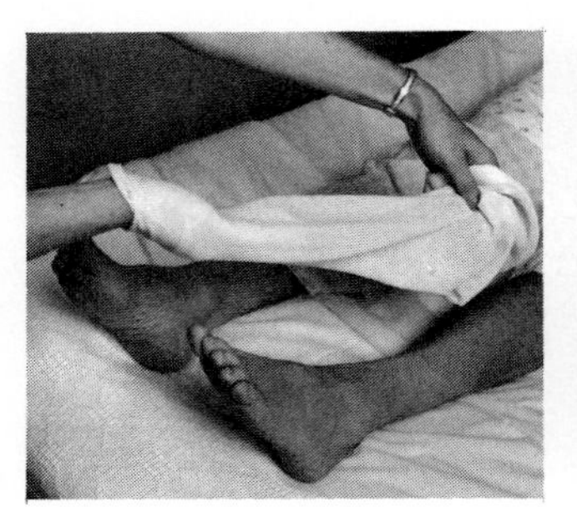

*Fig. 36-34*

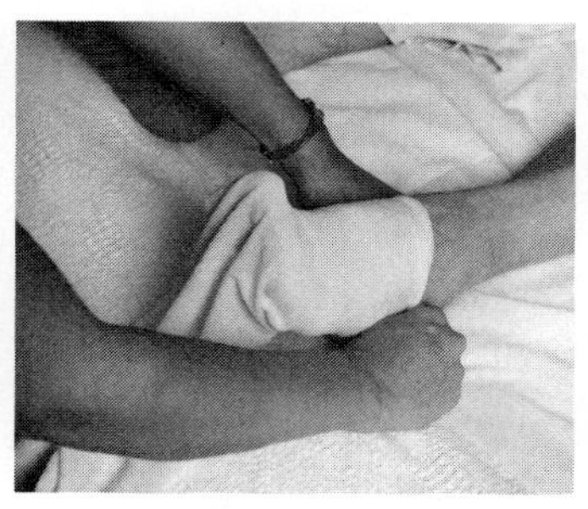

*Fig. 36-35*

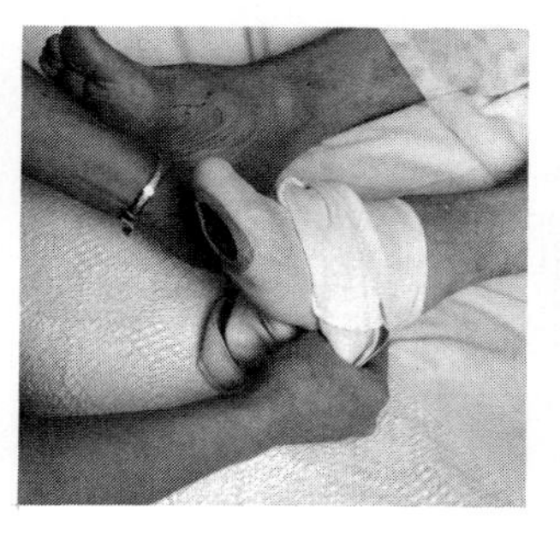

*Fig. 36-36*

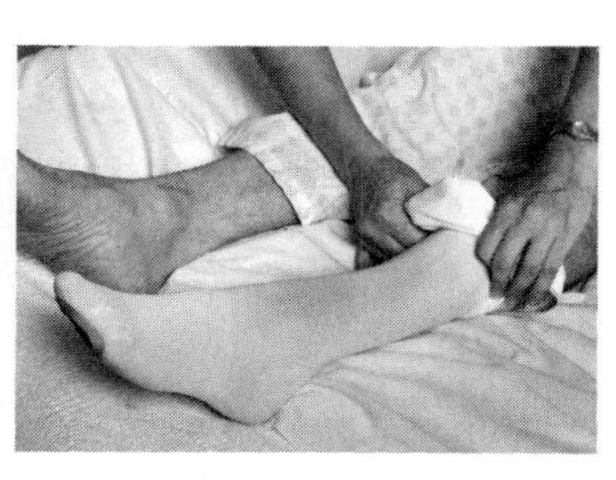

*Fig. 36-37*

## Evaluation

1. After approximately 1 hr reassess client to determine response to application of elastic stockings.
   a. Check stocking to make sure there are no wrinkles or binding at top of stocking. — Leads to increased pressure and alters circulation.
   b. Observe circulatory status of lower extremities. Observe color, temperature, and condition of skin. — Ensures circulatory status in lower extremities has not been compromised.
   c. Assess client's reaction to stockings. — Ensures client is adapting to and is not experiencing any discomfort from stockings.

### *Expected outcomes*

1. Client is able to demonstrate application of elastic stockings. — Verifies correct psychomotor learning.
2. Client has reduction in edema in lower extremities. — Elastic stockings decrease venous pooling in lower extremities.
3. Client shows no evidence of skin irritation or thrombophlebitis. — Ensures that there are no side effects to the circulatory system or client's skin.

### *Unexpected outcomes*

1. Client develops skin reaction to elastic stockings. Observe for evidence of redness, skin lesions, and client's subjective complaint of itching or burning. — Some clients may have skin reaction to material used in elastic socks. May indicate allergic reaction.
2. Client develops decrease in circulation in lower extremities. Assess for coolness in lower extremities; cyanosis; decrease in pedal pulses; decrease in blanching; and numbness or tingling sensation. — Elastic stockings may be too small or have wrinkles or folds that impede circulation. Signs and symptoms may indicate obstruction of arterial blood flow.
3. Client develops thrombophlebitis in lower extremity. Clinical manifestations of thrombophlebitis vary according to size and location of thrombus. Signs and symptoms of *superficial thrombosis* include palpable vein, area surrounding vein is tender to touch, reddened, and warm. There may be slight temperature elevation. Edema of extremity may or may not occur. Signs and symptoms of *deep thrombosis* include swollen extremity, pain, warm cyanotic skin, and temperature elevation. If calf is involved, positive Homan's sign (Fig. 36-38) (pain in calf on dorsiflexion of foot). — Venous stasis with resultant clot formation may have occurred even though stockings were in place. Other causes could be injury to vein or hypercoagulability. Extremity with phlebitis will be larger. Area over inflamed vein may be reddened and skin may be warmer in area of phlebitis.

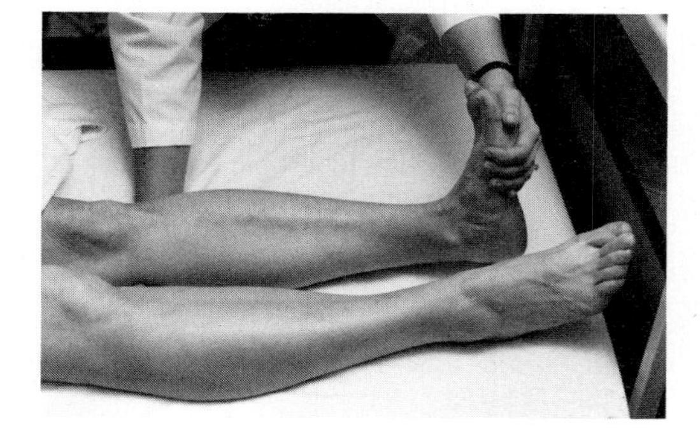

***Fig. 36-38*** Assessing Homan's sign.

## Recording and Reporting

1. Record in nurse's progress notes:
   a. Date and time of stocking application and condition of skin before application. — Documents condition of lower extremities before and after application of elastic stockings.
   b. Circulatory status of lower extremities before stocking application.

| Steps | Rationale |
|---|---|
| c. Stocking length and size. | |
| d. Date and time stockings are removed. | |
| e. Condition of skin and circulatory status after removal. | |
| f. Calf or thigh circumferences (daily if client is at risk for thrombophlebitis). | Unexplained increase in circumferences of the calf or thigh could indicate thrombophlebitis. |
| 2. Immediately report signs of thrombophlebitis or impeded circulation in lower extremities to charge nurse or physician. (Signs and symptoms in Unexpected Outcomes, 2 and 3.) | Institutes prompt therapy to restore circulation. Remove stockings and elevate leg until given further orders. |
| 3. Report any signs of skin irritation to physician. | |

## Follow-up Activities

| Steps | Rationale |
|---|---|
| 1. Remove stockings at least once a shift. | Provides for observation of skin and circulatory status. |
| 2. Demonstrate application of elastic stockings. | Enhances learning. |
| 3. If any signs of thrombophlebitis, or skin irritation are noted remove stockings and contact physician. | Ensures treatment as soon as possible. |

### Special Considerations

- Lower extremity should not be massaged if client complains of pain, swelling, or if it is red.
- Clients may require two pair of elastic stockings, one for wear and one for laundering.

### Teaching Considerations

- Have client demonstrate stocking application.
- Instruct client to remove stockings twice daily.
- Instruct client to launder stockings as follows:
  —every 2 days with mild detergent.
  —lay flat to dry as dryer heat weakens elastic and hanging stockings causes elastic to stretch out of shape.

### Home Care Considerations

- Assess and evaluate proper fit and application of stockings at regularly scheduled intervals.
- Measure leg and compare findings with base-line measurements, reporting findings to client's physician.
- Document assessment findings including skin temperature, color, and changes in measurements.

# *SKILL 36-4 Changing Client's Position to Minimize Occurrence of Orthostatic Hypotension*

Another intervention to reduce the effects of orthostatic hypotension is helping the client become mobile as soon as possible, whether ambulating or transferring to a chair. Before getting a client out of bed, certain safety measures must be taken and assessments made (Chapter 33).

### Purposes

1. Minimize orthostatic hypotension.
2. Increase mobility status.

## *Procedure 36-4*

### Assessment

| Steps | Rationale |
|---|---|
| 1. Review client's chart to assess previous activity level. | Determines how long client has been on bed rest and current activity order. The longer a client has been immobile the greater the risk for orthostatic hypotension. |
| 2. Obtain set of client's vital signs in supine position. | Provides baseline for comparison when client changes from supine to upright position; dizziness and/or a decrease of 15 mm Hg in blood pressure when upright is indicative of postural hypotension. |

| Steps | Rationale |
|---|---|
| **Nursing Diagnosis** | |
| 1. Cluster assessment data to reveal actual or potential nursing diagnoses: a. Impaired physical mobility: related to bedrest. b. Decreased cardiac output: related to decreased sympathetic tone. c. Potential for injury: related to dizziness and instability. | Immobility can lead to decreased venous return to the heart because of decreased muscle tone in the lower extremities. As a result cardiac output is lowered and when changing position the client may become dizzy and faint due to decreased blood supply to the brain. |
| **Planning** | |
| 1. Develop individualized goals for client based on nursing diagnoses: | |
| a. Client will be able to sit up or ambulate without symptoms of dizziness or decrease in blood pressure greater than 15 mm Hg. | Client is able to tolerate position changes better when there are no symptoms of orthostatic hypotension. |
| 2. Prepare needed equipment: | |
| a. Elastic stockings (optional) | Decreases venous stasis in lower extremities. |
| b. Safety belt (optional) | Ensures safety of client if unsteady on feet. |
| c. Shoes/slippers | Provide additional support and prevent client from slipping. |
| d. Robe | To ensure modesty. Clothing should be nonrestrictive. |
| 3. Prepare client for procedure by explaining rationale for getting client out of bed and describing procedure for accomplishing this. | Relieves anxiety and encourages cooperation. |
| **Implementation** | |
| 1. Wash hands. | Reduces transfer of microorganisms. |
| 2. Place bed in low position. | Have bed as close to floor as possible in case client becomes dizzy and falls. |
| 3. Slowly raise head of bed to high Fowler's position and obtain blood pressure. | Raising slowly allows body to adjust to change in position. Note whether blood pressure decreases or client complains of dizziness when changing from supine to upright position. |
| 4. Observe client for signs of orthostatic hypotension: dizziness; seeing spots; or lightheadedness. | Indicates orthostatic hypotension. Procedure may need to be postponed until client is able to tolerate high Fowler's position without signs and symptoms of orthostatic hypotension. |
| 5. Assist client to sit on side of bed for a few minutes while continuing to assess client for signs of orthostatic hypotension. | Allows autonomic nervous system to adapt to postural change. |
| 6. If there are no signs of dizziness or lightheadedness assist client to ambulate or to sit in chair. | Absence of dizziness or lightheadedness indicates that it is safe to attempt to transfer client to chair or assist with ambulation. |
| 7. Wash hands. | |
| **Evaluation** | |
| 1. While assisting client to chair or to ambulate continue to assess for signs of orthostatic hypotension. | Dizziness can indicate reduced blood pressure and the nurse must safely guide client into chair or back to bed. |
| ***Expected outcomes*** | |
| 1. Client will have no symptoms of orthostatic hypotension. | Client is able to maintain a stable blood pressure during transfer. |
| ***Unexpected outcomes*** | |
| 1. Client becomes lightheaded and begins to fall. | Results from orthostatic hypotension. |
| **Recording and Reporting** | |
| 1. Record in nurses' progress notes: | |
| a. Supine and upright blood pressures. b. Any changes in respiratory rate, skin color, or temperature noted when client placed in upright position. | Documents client's tolerance of increased activity level. |
| c. Client's subjective statements regarding upright position. | Documents any symptom client perceived during transfer. |
| d. If client sat in chair, note length of time client was able to sit and how well procedure was tolerated. May want to recheck blood pressure while client is sitting up. | Documents client's activity tolerance when transferring to a chair or ambulating. |

| Steps | Rationale |
|---|---|
| e. If client ambulates, note distance walked; stability of gait; any assistance needed; and how procedure was tolerated. | |
| 2. Report immediately if client sustains injury or is unable to tolerate procedure. | Provides prompt follow up care of any injuries sustained. |

### Follow-up Activities

| Steps | Rationale |
|---|---|
| 1. Have client rise from supine to upright position slowly. | Allows stabilization of blood pressure. |
| 2. Have client sit for a few moments to gain balance. Instruct client not to rise if symptoms of lightheadedness are present. | Reduces the risk of falling or fainting if orthostatic hypotension is present. |
| 3. If client experiences dizziness, instruct client to sit down and lower the head or lie down. | This will help restore blood pressure immediately. |
| 4. If client starts to fall as you walk together, put your arms around client's waist and stand with your feet apart to provide broad base of support. Extend your leg and let client slide against it to floor. As client slides, bend your knees to lower your body. | Attempting to catch adult who is falling is usually not successful and may injure person. Assisting client to floor decreases risk of injury. When safely on floor, assess client and decide whether to help client to stand, or wait for additional personnel. |

### Special Considerations

- Attempt to gradually increase client's mobility status as soon as possible to decrease effects of immobility.
- Before attempting to get person out of bed be sure you have adequate assistance. When assisting child be sure you have assessed weight accurately; looks can be deceiving.

### Home Care Considerations

- Safety belt can be made from cotton webbing, wrapping it around client's waist over clothing and tie it into square knot. Belt can be made at home or purchased commercially and is used by primary care giver to provide secure grip on client while changing client's position.
- When changing client's position, allow adequate time for client to regain balance before another movement.
- Assess client's skin for pressure areas or skin abrasions.

## *SKILL 36-5 Assisting with Ambulation*

Clients who have been immobile for even a short period of time may require assistance with ambulation. Assistance may mean walking alongside the client while providing support, or the client may require the use of an assistive device to aid ambulation. Various devices are available to assist ambulation. These range from standard canes, which provide minimal support, to crutches and walkers, which can be used by clients who are unable to bear complete weight on their lower extremities. Selection of the appropriate device depends on the client's age, diagnosis, muscular coordination, and ease of maneuverability. Use of assistive devices may be temporary, such as during recuperation from a fractured extremity or orthopedic surgery, or permanent, as in the case of a client with paralysis or permanent weakness of the lower extremities.

*Canes* are lightweight, easily movable devices that reach about waist high and are made of wood or metal. Canes help maintain balance by widening the base of support. They are indicated for clients with hemiparesis and are used to ease strain on weight-bearing joints. Canes are not recommended for clients with bilateral leg weakness; crutches or a walker are more appropriate. There are three types of commonly used canes. The *standard* cane provides the least support and is used by clients requiring only slight assistance to walk. It has a half-circle handle, which allows it to be hooked over chairs. The *T-handle* cane has a bent shaft and a straight, shaped handle with grips, which makes it easier to hold. It provides greater stability than the standard cane and is especially useful for clients with hand weakness. The *quad* cane has three or four legs that provide a wide base of support. It is useful for clients with unilateral partial or complete leg paralysis.

A *crutch* is a wooden or metal staff that reaches from the ground almost to the axilla. Crutches are used to remove weight from one or both legs. There are three types of crutches: the *axillary* crutch, the *Lofstrand* (or Canadian) crutch, and the *Platform* crutch. The *axillary* crutch is used frequently by clients of all ages, usually for a short-term basis. The *Lofstrand* crutch has a hand grip and a metal band that fits around the client's forearm. Both the metal band and the hand grip are adjusted to fit the client's height. This type of crutch is useful for clients who have a permanent disability, such as a paraplegic client. The metal arm band stabilizes and assists in guiding the crutch. The *Canadian* crutch is like the Lofstrand, only it has an additional cuff for the upper arm to give added support. The *Platform* crutch is used by clients who are unable to bear weight on their wrists.

*Walkers* are extremely light, movable devices, about waist high, consisting of a metal frame with handgrips, four widely placed, sturdy legs, and one open side. Because it has a wide base of support, the walker provides great stability and security. Walkers can be used by clients who are weak or who have balance problems (Fig. 36-39).

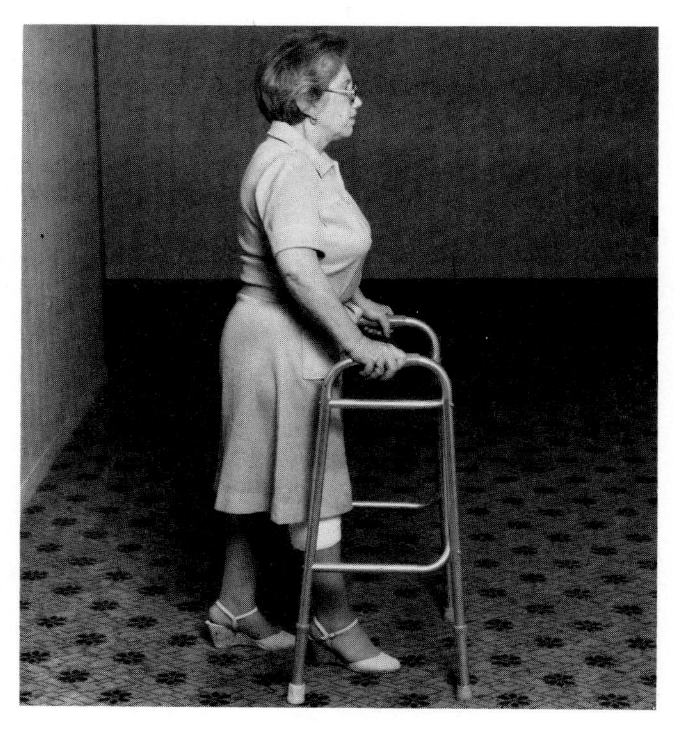

*Fig. 36-39*

### Purposes

1. Increase muscle strength and joint mobility, thereby decreasing some potential complications of immobility.
2. Increase the client's sense of independence.
3. Increase the client's self-esteem.

## Procedure 36-5

| Steps | Rationale |
|---|---|
| **Assessment** | |
| 1. Review client's chart. Note medical diagnosis, e.g., arthritis; fractures that decrease ambulation; medical orders for ambulation; ambulation aides. | Identifies client's previous activity level. Client may tire easily or be prone to orthostatic hypotension if bed rest has been prolonged. Medical diagnosis, type of ambulation to be attempted, and whether ambulating device is to be used will all be included in client's chart. Therapy may also be coordinated with physical therapy. |
| 2. Observe client's physical readiness to attempt ambulation. | |
| a. Determine baseline vital signs. | Ambulation following immobility can be fatiguing and stressful. Baseline vital signs offer means for comparison following exercises. |
| b. Assess range of motion of joints and muscle strength (Procedure 36-1). | Determines whether client has enough flexibility and muscle strength to ambulate safely. Determines if client needs muscle strengthening exercises before ambulation. |
| c. Assess client for discomfort. | Client may be in pain or may fear pain will result from exercise. If necessary, administer pain medication before ambulation. |
| 3. Explain rationale and benefit of exercise. | To reassure client and increase compliance. |
| 4. Assess client's or caregiver's understanding of technique of ambulation to be used. | Allows client to verbalize concerns. Clients who have been immobile for a while may be hesitant to ambulate. Caregiver may be hesitant to learn how to assist with ambulation. It also helps identify education needs of client or caregiver. |
| 5. Determine optimum time schedule for exercise sessions. | To be successful, client's personal habits and circadian rhythms should be taken into consideration. |
| 6. Assess degree of assistance client needs. | For safety purposes, another person may be needed to assist with ambulation initially. Do allow the client as much independence as possible. |
| **Nursing Diagnosis** | |
| 1. Cluster data to reveal actual or potential nursing diagnoses: | |
| a. Potential for injury: related to instability or use of ambulation device. | Weakness or inaccurate use of ambulation aid increases client's risk of injury. |

| Steps | Rationale |
|---|---|
| b. Activity intolerance: related to attempting ambulation following immobility. | Clients become weak following immobility. Ambulating, especially if an ambulation aid must be used, can be fatiguing. |
| c. Knowledge deficit regarding use of ambulation device: related to unfamiliarity with device. | Client may be unfamiliar with ambulation aid to be used. |
| d. Social isolation: related to immobility. | Clients who are not mobile may not be able to attend social activities or visit friends as they used to. |
| e. Impaired home maintenance management: related to altered mobility. | Client may need assistance when he returns home. |

## Planning

| Steps | Rationale |
|---|---|
| 1. Develop individualized goals for client based on nursing diagnoses:<br>a. Enable client to ambulate without episode of injury.<br>b. Minimize client's fatigue following period of ambulation.<br>c. Instruct client in assigned ambulation gait and safety precautions to take.<br>d. Maintain client's contact with friends and family.<br>e. Allow client to openly discuss concerns and fears with medical personnel, family, and friends.<br>f. Increase client's ambulation tolerance gradually.<br>g. Enable client to ambulate without use of ambulation aid.<br>h. Enable client to assume all self-care activities.<br>i. Enable client to resume previous social activities. | Ultimate goal is to assist client to regain as much mobility, and therefore independence, as possible. In order to do this client must be able to accurately use an ambulation device if one is needed, to be aware of safety precautions when ambulating, and to feel free to ask questions or discuss difficulties with family, friends, or medical personnel. |
| 2. Prepare following equipment and supplies: | |
| a. Ambulation device (crutch, walker, or cane) | By widening the base of support these devices help maintain balance and ease ambulation. |
| b. Safety device, e.g., walking belt | Clients may feel more secure if safety belt is used. |
| c. Well-fitting, flat shoes | For added support and to prevent injury. |
| d. Robe | To ensure modesty. Clothing should remain nonrestricting. |
| 3. Prepare client for procedure. | |
| a. Explain reason for, and demonstrate specific gait technique to client or care giver. | Demonstration enhances learning. Also relieves anxiety and encourages cooperation. Teach ambulation technique preoperatively if possible. |
| b. Decide with client how far to ambulate. | Determines mutual goal. |
| c. Schedule ambulation around client's other activities. | Space activities so client does not become too fatigued. |
| d. Place bed in low position and slowly assist client to upright position. Let client sit or stand for a few min. until balance is gained. | Prevents orthostatic hypotension and potential injuries. If client becomes dizzy when position is changed from supine to upright, refer to Procedure 36-4 for measures to minimize orthostatic hypotension. |
| e. Check client's height and weight before attempting to assist client in ambulating. | Nurse must be proper height in order to supply adequate support. |
| f. If ambulation device is used, make sure it is appropriate height: | If crutch is too long, it can cause pressure on axilla. |
| ▪ Crutch measurement includes 3 areas: client's height, distance between crutch pad and axilla, and angle of elbow flexion. Use 1 of 2 methods: *Standing*—Position crutches with crutch tips at point 4-6 in (14-15 cm) to side and 4-6 in front of client's feet and crutch pads 1½-2 in (4-5 cm) below axilla. *Supine*—Crutch pad should be 3-4 finger widths under axilla with crutch tips positioned 6 in (15 cm) lateral (Fig. 36-40) to client's heel. | Radial nerve passes under axillary area superficially. Injury to nerve causes paralysis of elbow and wrist extensors, commonly called crutch palsy. Also, if crutch is too long shoulders are forced upward and client cannot push his body off ground. If ambulation device is too short client will be bent over and uncomfortable.<br>Instruct client to report any tingling or numbness in the upper torso. This may mean crutches are being used incorrectly or that they are wrong size. |

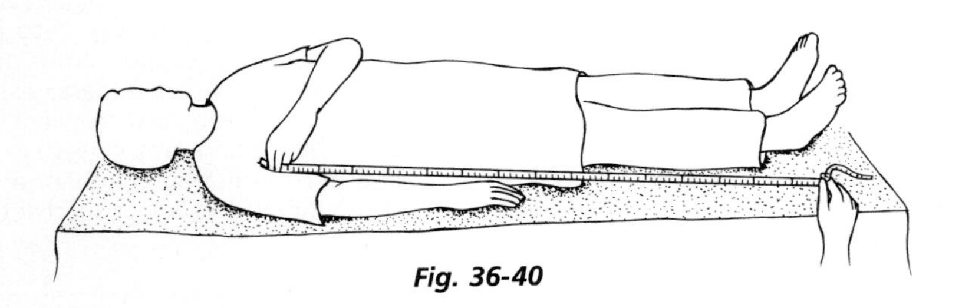

***Fig. 36-40***

| Steps | Rationale |
|---|---|
| 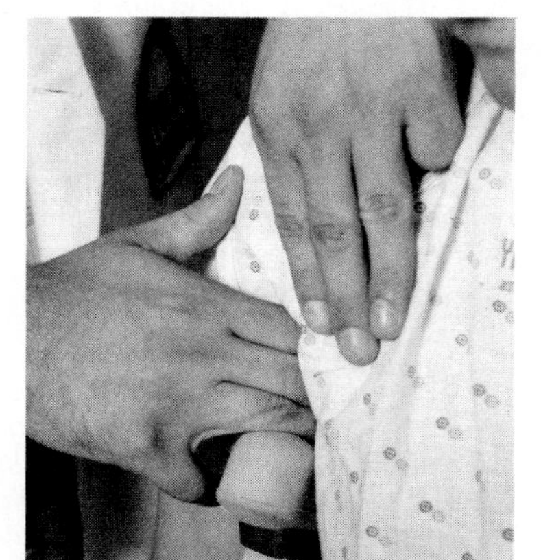 *Fig. 36-41* | 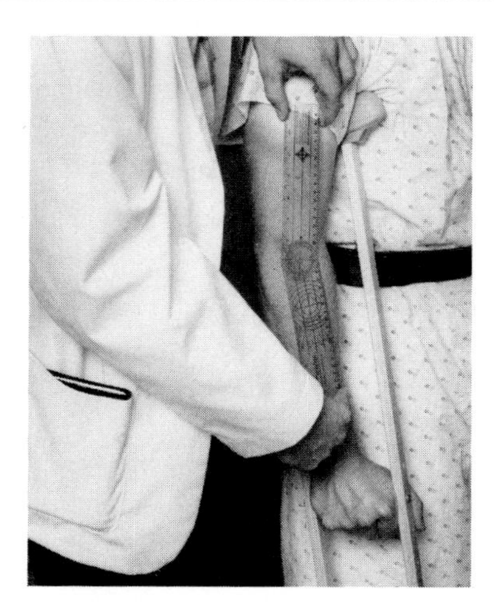 *Fig. 36-42* |
| | Following correct crutch measurement, you should be able to place two or three fingers between top of crutch and axilla (see Fig. 36-41). |
| ▪ With either method elbows should be flexed 15-30 degrees. Elbow flexion is verified with goniometer (Fig. 36-42). | In addition to overall *length* of axillary crutch, *height* of handgrip is important. Both dimensions are adjustable on well-made crutch, and this is an important feature for a growing child. Handgrip should be adjusted so that patient's elbow is *slightly flexed.* If handgrip is too low, radial nerve can be damaged even if overall crutch length is correct because extra length between handgrip and axillary bar can force bar up into axilla as patient stretches down to reach handgrip. If handpiece is too high, patient's elbow is sharply flexed, and strength and stability of arms are decreased. |
| ▪ Cane measurement: Client should hold cane on uninvolved side 4-6 in. to side of foot. Cane should extend from greater trochanter to floor. Allow approximately 15-30 degrees elbow flexion. | Offers most support when on stronger side of body. Cane and weaker leg work together with each step. If cane is too short client will have difficulty supporting his weight and be bent over and uncomfortable. As weight is taken on by hands and affected leg is lifted off floor, complete extension of elbow is necessary. |
| ▪ Walker measurement: Elbows should be flexed at approximately 15-30 degrees when standing within walker with hands on handgrips. | As weight is taken on by hands and legs are lifted off floor, complete extension of elbow is necessary. |
| g. Make sure the ambulation device has rubber tips. | Rubber tips increase surface tension and prevent device from slipping. |
| h. Make sure surface client will walk on is clean, dry, and well lighted. Remove any objects that might obstruct pathway. | Prevents injuries. |

## Implementation

***Assisted ambulation with one nurse***

| Steps | Rationale |
|---|---|
| 1. Review how to minimize effects of orthostatic hypotension (Procedure 36-4). | Helps client gain balance before attempting ambulation and ensures that client will not become faint while walking. |
| 2. Apply safety belt if unsure of client's stability. | Prevents injury. Safety belt encircles client's waist and has space for nurse to hold while client walks. |
| 3. Assist client to standing position and observe his balance. | If client appears weak or unsteady, return him to bed. |
| 4. Have client take a few steps while nurse positions herself behind client. | Standing behind client will prevent nurse from possibly obstructing client's pathway. Also prevents client from leaning to one side for support from nurse. However, if client has hemiplegia (one-sided paralysis) or hemiparesis (one-sided weakness), stand next to client's affected side and support client by placing arm closest to client around client's waist and other arm around inferior aspect of client's upper arm. |
| 5. Grasp safety belt in middle of client's back or place hands at client's waist if no safety belt is used. | Provides support at waist so client's center of gravity remains midline. |

| Steps | Rationale |
|---|---|
| 6. Take a few steps forward with client. Then assess for strength and balance. | Ensures client has satisfactory strength and balance to continue. |
| 7. Gradually increase distance walked. | Prevents client from becoming too fatigued. |
| 8. If client becomes weak or dizzy return to bed or chair, whichever is closer. | Allows client to rest. |
| 9. If client begins to fall, use procedure in Skill 36-4, Unexpected Outcomes, 2, for lowering client to floor. | Can cause more damage to self and client by trying to catch client. |
| ***Assisted ambulation with two nurses*** | |
| 1. Follow Steps 1-3, "assisted ambulation with one nurse." | |
| 2. Stand on either side of client. | |
| 3. Place arms nearest client around client's waist and other arms so that both nurses' hands support client's axillas. | Provides secure grip for each nurse. |
| 4. Step forward in unison with client, keeping speed and step size same as client's. | Ensures stability of client. |
| 5. Gradually increase distance walked. | Prevents client from becoming too fatigued. |
| 6. Follow Steps 8-9, "assisted ambulation with one nurse." | |
| ***Ambulation with assistive devices*** | |
| 1. Assist client in crutch-walking by choosing appropriate gait. | To use crutches, client supports himself with his hands and arms; therefore strength in arm and shoulder muscles, ability to balance body in upright position, and stamina are necessary. Type of gait client uses in crutch walking depends on amount of weight he is able to support with one or both legs. |
| a. Four-point gait | Most stable of crutch gaits because it provides at least three points of support at all times. Requires weight bearing on both legs. Often used when there is paralysis as in spastic children with cerebral palsy (Whaley and Wong, 1987). May also be used for arthritic clients. |
| ▪ Begin in tripod position (Fig. 36-43). Crutches are placed 6 in (15 cm) in front and 6 in to side of each foot. | Improves client's balance by providing wider base of support. Posture should be erect head and neck, straight vertebrae, and extended hips and knees. |
| ▪ Move right crutch forward 4-6 in. (Fig. 36-44) | Crutch and foot position are similar to arm and foot position during normal walking. |
| ▪ Move left foot forward to level of left crutch. | |
| ▪ Move left crutch forward 4-6 in. | |
| ▪ Move right foot forward to level of right crutch. | |
| ▪ Repeat above sequence. | |
| b. Three-point gait | Requires client to bear all weight on one foot. Weight is borne on uninvolved leg, then on both crutches. Affected leg does not touch ground during early phase of three-point gait. May be useful for client with broken leg or sprained ankle (Narrow and Buchle, 1987). |
| ▪ Begin in tripod position. | Improves client's balance by providing wide base of support. |
| ▪ Advance both crutches and affected leg (Fig. 36-45). | |
| ▪ Move stronger leg forward. | |
| ▪ Repeat sequence. | |
| c. Two-point gait | Requires at least partial weight bearing on each foot. Is faster than the four-point gait. Requires more balance because only two points support body at one time. |
| ▪ Begin in tripod position. | Improves client's balance by providing wider base of support. |
| ▪ Move left crutch and right foot forward (Fig. 36-46). | Crutch movements are similar to arm movement during normal walking. |
| ▪ Move right crutch and left foot forward. | |
| ▪ Repeat sequence. | |
| a. Assist client in swing-to-gait and swing-through-gait. | Frequently used by clients whose lower extremities are paralyzed or who wear weight-supporting braces on their legs. |
| *Swing-to-gait:* | |
| a. Move both crutches forward. | This is the easier of the two swinging gaits. |

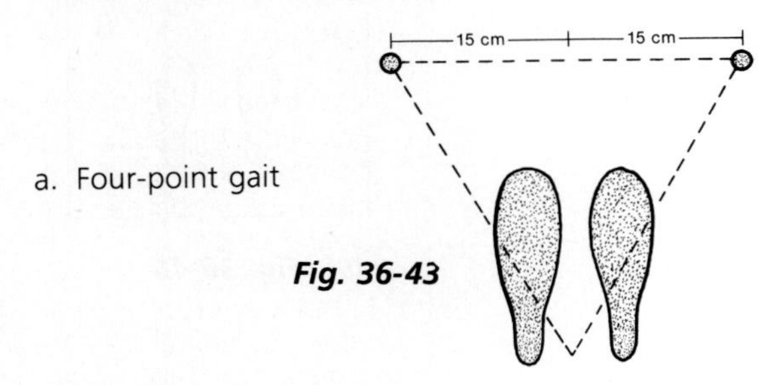

***Fig. 36-43***

| Steps | Rationale |
|---|---|

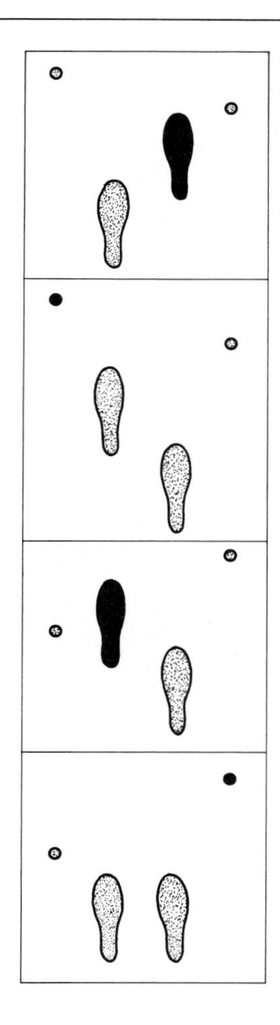

*Fig. 36-44*

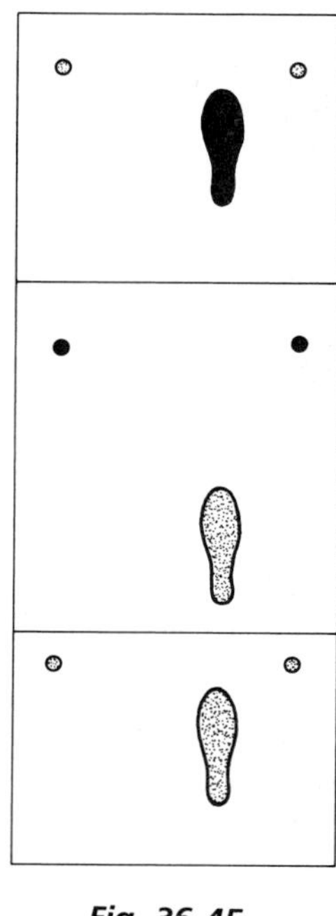

*Fig. 36-45*

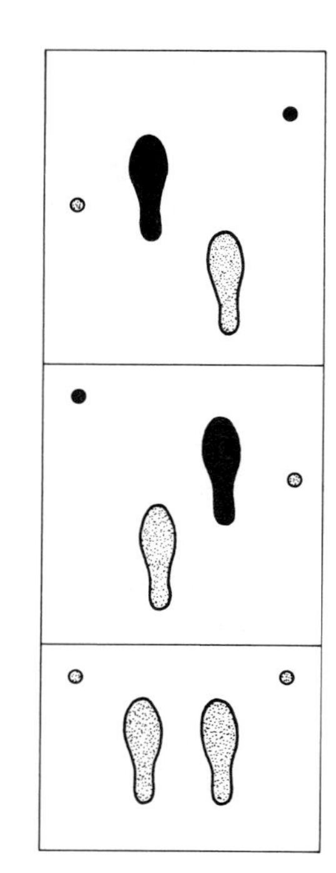

*Fig. 36-46*

| Steps | Rationale |
|---|---|
| b. Lift and swing legs to crutches letting crutches support body weight. | |
| c. Repeat Steps 1 and 2. | |
| *Swing-through gait:* | Align in middle of 2 swinging gaits. |
| a. Move both crutches forward. | Initial placement of crutches is to increase the client's base of support so that when the body swings forward the client is moving the center of gravity toward the additional support provided by the crutches. |
| b. Lift and swing legs through and beyond crutches. | |
| 2. Assist client in climbing stairs with crutches. | |
| a. Begin in tripod position. | Improves client's balance by providing wider base of support. |
| b. Transfers body weight to crutches (Fig. 36-47). | Prepares client to transfer weight to unaffected leg when ascending first stair. |
| c. Advance unaffected leg to stair (Fig. 36-48). | Crutch adds support to affected leg. Client then shifts weight from crutches to unaffected leg. |
| d. Align both crutches and unaffected leg on stairs (Fig. 36-49). | Maintains balance and provides wide base of support. |
| e. Repeat sequence until client reaches top of stairs. | |
| 3. Assist client in descending stairs with crutches. | |
| a. Begin in tripod position. | Improves client's balance by providing wider base of support. |
| b. Client transfers body weight to unaffected leg (Fig. 36-50). | Prepares client to release support of body weight maintained by crutches. |
| c. Move crutches to stair and instruct client to begin to transfer body weight to crutches (Fig. 36-51) and move affected leg forward. | Maintains client's balance and base of support. |
| d. Move unaffected leg to stair and align with crutches (Fig. 36-52). | Maintains balance and provides base of support. |
| e. Repeat sequence until stairs are descended. | |

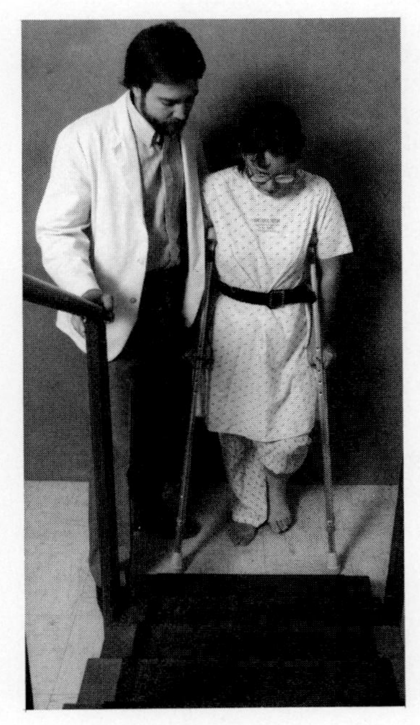

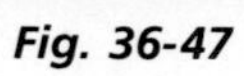

*Fig. 36-47*

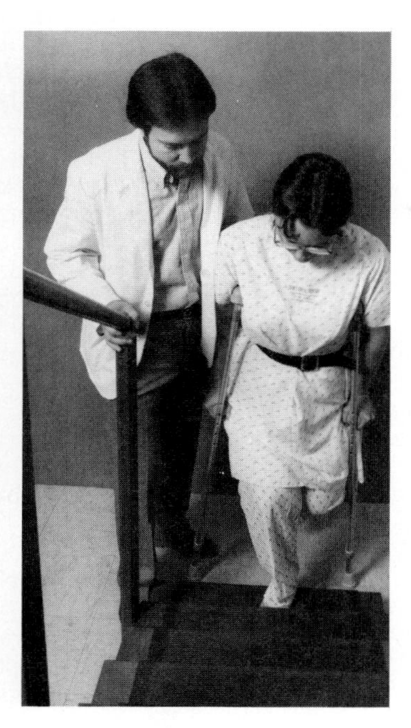

*Fig. 36-48*

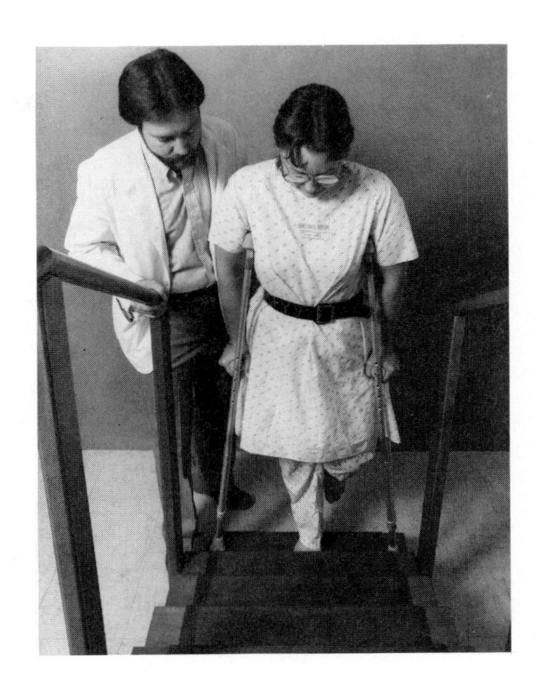

*Fig. 36-49*

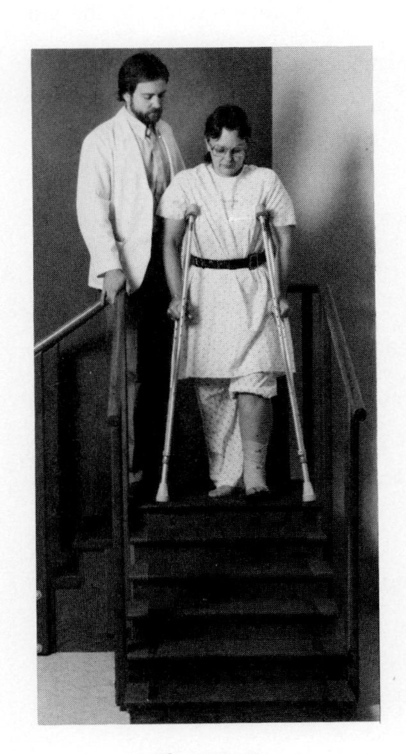

*Fig. 36-50*

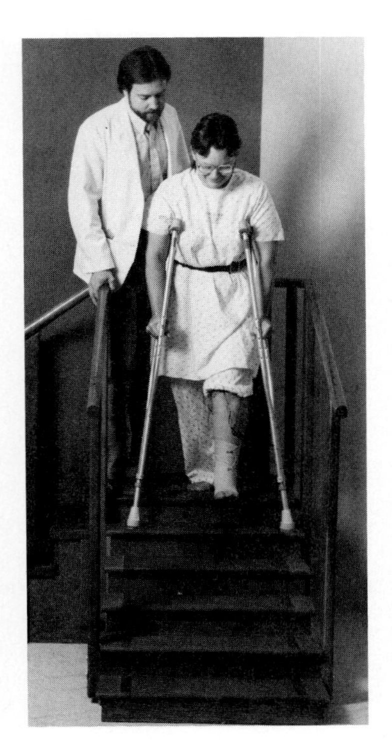

*Fig. 36-51*

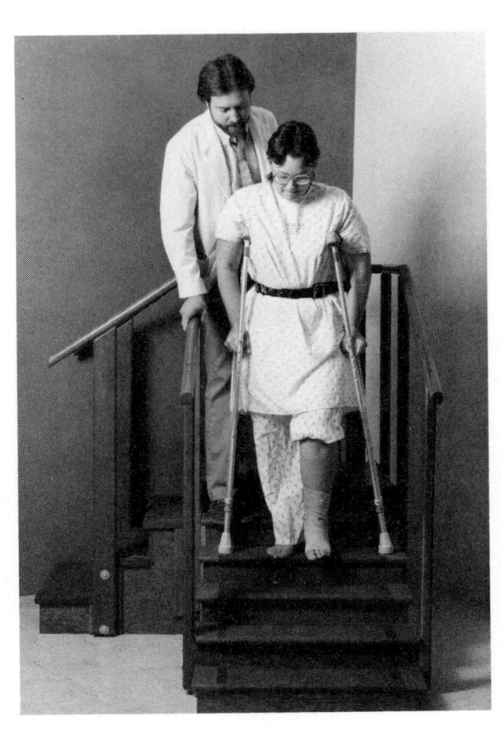

*Fig. 36-52*

| Steps | Rationale |
|---|---|
| 4. Assist client in ambulating with walker. | Walker is used by clients who are able to bear partial weight. Walkers do need to be picked up, so client does need sufficient strength to be able to pick up walker. Four-wheeled model, which does not need to be picked up, is not as stable. |
| a. Stand in center of walker and grasp handgrips on upper bars. | Client balances self before attempting to walk. |
| b. Take step forward into walker. | Aligns client's center of gravity with walker. |
| c. Move walker 6-8 in forward and take another step forward with either leg. | Provides broad base of support between walker and client. Client then moves his center of gravity toward the walker. If there is one-sided weakness, instruct the client after advancing walker to step forward with uninvolved leg, support self with the arms, and follow through with involved leg. If unable to bear weight on one leg, after advancing walker have the client swing on to it, supporting weight on hands. |
| d. Repeat steps. | |
| 5. Assist client in ambulating with cane. (Same steps are taught to client whether standard cane or quad cane is used.) | |
| a. Begin by placing cane on weaker side. | Provides added strength to side with impairment or weakness. Increases client's base of support. |
| b. Place cane forward 6-10 in (15-25 cm), keeping body weight on both legs. | |
| c. Move weaker leg forward. | In this way, body weight is divided between cane and stronger leg. Instruct client to always look straight ahead, to prevent injuries, and to use good posture. |
| d. Advance stronger leg past cane. | Weaker leg and body weight are supported by cane and weaker leg. |
| e. Move weaker leg forward, even with stronger leg. | Aligns client's center of gravity. |
| f. Repeat steps. | |

## Evaluation

| | |
|---|---|
| 1. Reassess client to determine response to ambulation. | |
| a. Assess client's energy level, heart rate, respiratory rate, skin color, and temperature following ambulation. | Assesses how client tolerated procedure and evaluate whether there was progress in ambulation. Assess stage of client's illness and degree of convalescence when evaluating the process. |
| b. Assess client's subjective statements regarding experience. | |
| c. Assess gait of client, observing body alignment in standing position and balance. | Determines if client is correctly using supportive aids for ambulation. Keep in mind the client's previous manner of ambulating when assessing gait. |

### *Expected outcomes*

| | |
|---|---|
| 1. Client's ambulatory ability will gradually increase as evidenced by ability to ambulate increasing distances without excessive fatigue. | Progressive ambulating activities increases client's endurance and independence. |

### *Unexpected outcomes*

| | |
|---|---|
| 1. Client will be unable to ambulate. | Possible reasons include fear of falling, physical discomfort, upper body muscles that are too weak to use ambulation device, and lower extremities that are too weak to support body. |
| 2. Client sustains injury. | Obstacles were in client's path, incorrect technique was used, or proper safety precautions were not taken. |

## Recording and Reporting

| | |
|---|---|
| 1. Record in nurse's progress notes type of gait client used; amount of assistance required; distance walked; and client's tolerance of activity. | Documents technique used and client's progress using technique. |
| 2. Immediately report any injury sustained during attempts to ambulate, alteration in vital signs, or inability to ambulate to nurse in charge or physician. | |

| Steps | Rationale |
| --- | --- |
| **Follow-up Activities** | |
| 1. Inspect rubber tips on bottom of ambulation device frequently. | If tips are worn they should be replaced. If tips become wet, dry them off because water decreases surface friction and increases risk of client slipping. |
| 2. If wooden crutch is used, examine it for cracks. | Cracks in wood decrease support afforded by crutches. |
| 3. Remove obstacles from pathways, including throw rugs, and wipe up any spills immediately. | Prevents slippage and potential injury. |
| 4. Avoid large crowds. | Ambulation device may get jarred in large crowd. |
| 5. If client begins to fall do not try to catch client, but follow technique mentioned in Skill 36-4, Follow-up Activities, 4, on p. 791. | Reduces risk to client or nurse if client is gently guided to the floor or bed. |
| 6. Notify medical personnel if there are symptoms of tingling or numbness when client uses crutches. | Indicates client is using crutches incorrectly or that they are too long. |
| 7. Continue muscle strengthening exercises at home. | |

## Special Considerations

- It is important to remember that children and adolescents are also subject to potential problems of immobility.
- When client is ambulating, with or without assistive device, emphasize need to always look ahead, to prevent injuries, and to use good posture. Slouching and looking down at floor will cause client to tire more easily.
- For habilitating small child who has not yet learned to walk or who is unsteady, special crutches stabilized with three or four legs provide needed stability for child to maintain upright position and learn to walk (Whaley and Wong, 1987).
- Whenever possible, promise to honor client's request to stop when more activity cannot be tolerated, then keep promise. In some situations, exercise or activity is essential for prevention or treatment of potentially disabling condition and must not be cut short. If so, explain to client why exercise must be completed in face of pain and discomfort.
  Try to understand what exercise or ambulation means to client. It may represent the return to an uncertain future, inability to deny any longer reality of situation, or pressure to do something that seems far too difficult. Client's feelings, such as frustration at being weak, anger over an amputated leg, or denial that paralysis is permanent, may create reluctance to try to exercise or ambulate.
- Walkers have disadvantage of being difficult to maneuver in small spaces and on stairs.
- When walking with clients using crutches, stand on affected side and grasp safety belt in midspine area at small of back. Position free hand at shoulder area so you can pull client toward you in event client falls.

## Teaching Considerations

- Instruct client to inspect rubber tips on bottom of crutch or walker daily. Worn or wet tips decrease surface friction and increase risk of falling.
- If wooden crutch is used, client is taught to examine for cracks daily. Cracks decrease support of crutch.

## Home Care Considerations

- Rearrange home to remove obstacles from walk areas. These include throw rugs.

**BIBLIOGRAPHY**

Barnes B, et al.: Functional outcomes after hip fracture, Phys Therap 67(11):1675, 1987.

Bates B: A guide to physical examination, ed. 4, Philadelphia, 1987, JB Lippincott Co.

Beyers M, Dudas S: The clinical practice of medical-surgical nursing, Boston, 1977, Little, Brown, & Co.

Bornar JA, et al.: Exercise and osteoporisis: a critique of the literature, Physiother Canada 40(3):146, 1988.

Brill E, Kilts D: Foundations for nursing, New York, 1980, Appleton-Century-Crofts.

Brown SP, et al.: Exercise, aging and longevity, Health Education 19(2):4, 1988.

Brunner and Suddarth D: Textbook of medical-surgical nursing, ed 6, Philadelphia, 1988, JB Lippincott Co.

Fochtman D, Raffensperger J: Principles of nursing care for the pediatric surgery patient, Boston, 1976, Little, Brown, & Co.

Freed MM, et al.: Choosing ambulatory aids, Patient Care 21(16):20, 1987.

Gvoich B: Equipping a home gym, Vibrant Life 3(8):24, 1987.

Hirschberg G, et al.: Promoting patient mobility and preventing secondary disabilities, Nursing '77 7:42, 1977.

Jones D, Dunbar C, Jirovec M: Medical-surgical nursing: a conceptual approach, New York, 1978, McGraw-Hill Book Co.

Kerr KM: Exercise and health related fitness, Physiotherapy 74(8):411, 1988.

Larson C, Gould M: Orthopedic nursing, ed 9, St. Louis, 1978, The CV Mosby Co.

Lewis S, Collier I: Medical-surgical nursing: assessment and management of clinical problems, ed. 2, New York, 1987, McGraw-Hill Book Co.
Long B, Phipps W: Medical-surgical nursing: a nursing process approach, ed. 2, St. Louis, 1989, The CV Mosby Co.
Milde F: Impaired physical mobility, J Gerontol Nurs 14(3):20, 1988.
Potter PA, Perry AG: Fundamentals of nursing, ed 2, St. Louis, 1989, The CV Mosby Co.
Seidel HM, et al.: Mosby's guide to physical examination, St. Louis, 1987, the CV Mosby Co.
Selcher D: When your patient needs a cane, walker or wheelchair, RN 50(12):60, 1987.
Smith M, Goodman J, Ramsey N, Pasternak S: Family-centered concepts of nursing practice, New York, 1982, McGraw-Hill Book Co.
Walsh J, Persons C, Wieck L: Manual of home health care nursing, Philadelphia, 1987, JB Lippincott Co.
Whaley L, Wong D: Nursing care of infants and children, ed. 3, St. Louis, 1987, The CV Mosby Co.

# UNIT XI

# INFECTION CONTROL

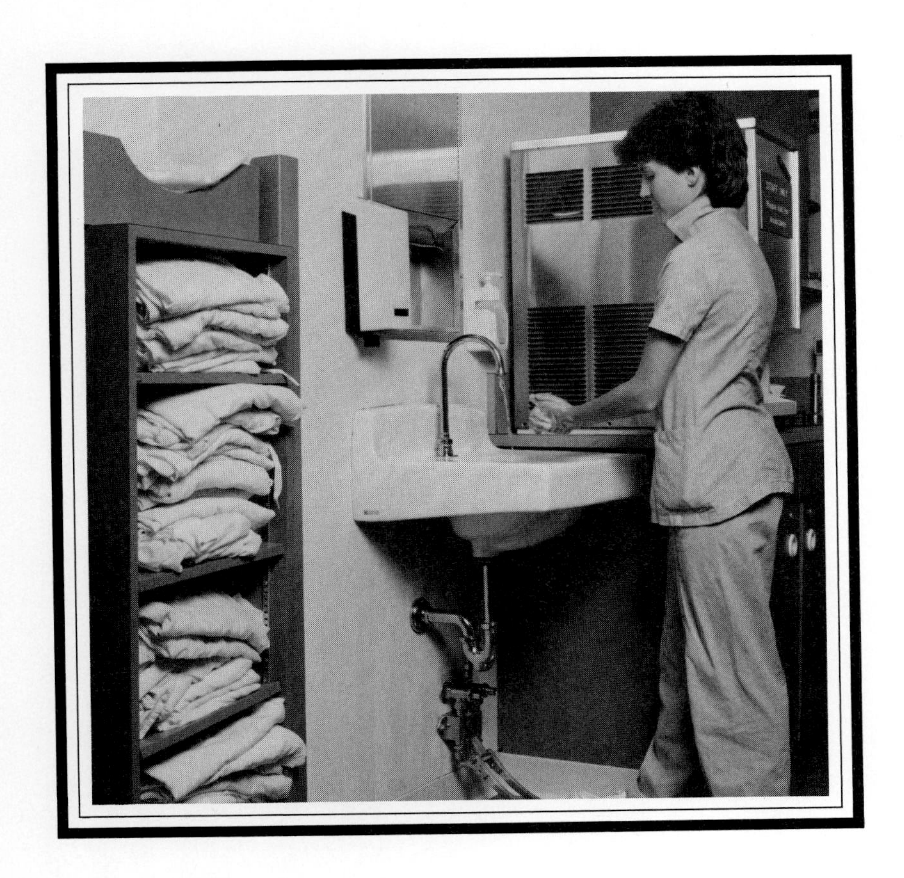

One of the foremost concerns for health care workers is maintaining aseptic conditions. It is impossible to ensure that the client's environment is free of microorganisms. However, there are steps a nurse can take to reduce microorganism spread and thus promote safety for both clients and staff. Chapter 37, "Medical Asepsis," focuses on basic measures to reduce occurrence of the infectious process. Skills of basic handwashing and care of the client under protective asepsis are discussed. Chapter 38, "Surgical Asepsis," presents skills needed to promote sterile conditions in an operating room or treatment area. Included here are proper donning of masks, caps, and gloves; surgical handwashing; preparing a sterile field; and applying sterile drapes.

# 37

# MEDICAL ASEPSIS

### OBJECTIVES

*Mastery of content in this chapter will enable the nurse to:*

- Define key terms.
- Identify elements of the infection chain.
- Discuss nursing care measures intended to break the infection chain.
- Describe guidelines for maintaining medical asepsis.
- Identify appropriate situations for handwashing.
- Correctly wash hands.
- Describe appropriate apparel necessary for each type of protective isolation.
- Describe universal blood and body fluid precautions.
- Correctly apply a gown, mask, and gloves before entering an isolation room
- Correctly care for a client in isolation.

### KEY TERMS

| | |
|---|---|
| *Asepsis* | *Medical asepsis* |
| *Contamination* | *Microorganism* |
| *Immunosuppresive* | *Nosocomial infection* |
| *Infection* | *Pathogen* |
| *Invasive* | *Phlebotomy* |
| *Isolation* | *Surgical asepsis* |

### SKILLS

***37-1*** Handwashing
***37-2*** Caring for a Client Under Protective Asepsis

Infection control practices, which control or eliminate sources of infection, help protect clients from disease. Clients in health care settings are particularly vulnerable to infection because of lowered resistance, increased exposure to numbers and types of disease-causing organisms, and invasive procedures performed. It is important to know the general principles of medical asepsis, or infection control, as they relate to the infection chain, since the nurse plays a key role in controlling infection and thus ensuring the safe care of clients.

Nosocomial infections result from delivery of health services in a health care setting. Microorganisms of every kind can usually be found in a health care setting because of both the types of clients being treated and environmental factors. The number of workers caring for clients, the type and number of invasive procedures, and the length of hospitalization all influence the chance of infection.

The development of an infection depends on six elements (Table 37-1). These include the infection agent, a reservoir for its growth, a portal of exit from the reservoir, a means of transmission, a portal of entry into the host, and a susceptible host. If the chain of infection is uninterrupted, an infection develops. Medical asepsis, as practiced by the nurse, is intended to break the infection chain (Fig. 37-1).

It is important for nurses to understand the principles of infection control thoroughly. Nurses can never be too cautious in their efforts to control and prevent the spread of infection. These efforts are based on the principles of aseptic technique. The two types of aseptic technique the nurse practices are medical and surgical asepsis.

Asepsis is a term referring to the absence of germs or pathogens. Medical asepsis consists of techniques used to reduce the number of microorganisms and help reduce or prevent their spread. It is also known as clean technique. Washing hands between client contact, changing bed linen daily, and maintaining a neat, clean environment for the client are examples of medical asepsis.

The elimination of microorganisms from an area is known as surgical asepsis (Chapter 38) or sterile technique. Any object free of all microorganisms is sterile. Surgical aseptic techniques are practiced in the operating, labor, and delivery rooms and at the bedside during procedures such as central intravenous line placement, urinary catheter placement, and suturing of wounds. The techniques used in maintaining surgical asepsis are more rigid than those performed under medical asepsis.

***TABLE 37-1*** Breaking the Chain of Infection

| Element of Infection Chain | Medical Aseptic Practices |
|---|---|
| Infection agent | Cleanse contaminated objects.<br>Perform disinfection and sterilization. |
| Reservoir | ***Eliminate sources of body fluids and drainage***<br>Bathe with soap and water.<br>Change soiled dressings.<br>Remove standing water on bedside tables.<br>Cover bottles of used solutions.<br>Maintain patency of surgical wound drains.<br>Empty and rinse suction bottles.<br>Empty drainage bags every shift.<br>Place syringes and uncapped needles in moisture-resistant, puncture-proof containers. |
| Portal of exit | ***Respiratory***<br>Avoid talking, sneezing, or coughing directly over wound or sterile dressing field.<br>Cover nose and mouth when sneezing or coughing.<br>Wear mask if suffering respiratory tract infection.<br>***Blood and wound drainage***<br>Wear gloves.<br>Handle blood and wound drainage carefully.<br>Dispose of soiled dressings appropriately.<br>***Urinary and gastrointestinal***<br>Handle urine, feces, and emesis carefully.<br>Dispose of soiled linen in linen bag.<br>Wear disposable gloves when necessary. |
| Transmission | ***Reduce microorganism spread***<br>Wash hands.<br>Use personal set of care items for each client.<br>Avoid shaking bed linen or clothes.<br>Avoid contact of soiled item with uniform.<br>Discard any item that touches floor. |
| Portal of entry | ***Skin and mucosa***<br>Maintain skin and mucous membrane integrity.<br>Clean wound sites thoroughly.<br>Use proper hygiene measures.<br>Dispose of used needles in proper receptacles.<br>***Urinary***<br>Keep all drainage systems closed and intact. |
| Host | ***Reduce susceptibility to infection***<br>Provide adequate nutrition.<br>Ensure adequate rest.<br>Promote body defenses against infection.<br>Provide immunization. |

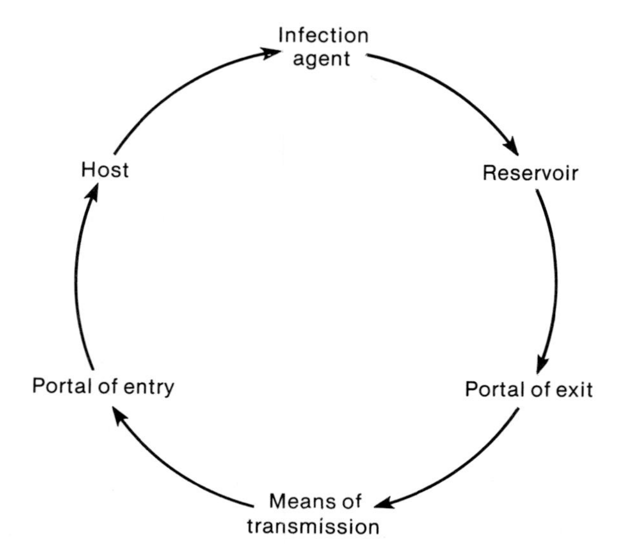


***Fig. 37-1*** Chain of infection.

## GUIDELINES

1. Remember that thorough handwashing is the most important and basic technique for infection control.
2. Always know a client's susceptibility to infection. Age, nutritional status, stress, disease processes, and forms of medical therapy can place clients at risk.
3. Recognize the elements of the infection chain and initiate measures to prevent the onset and spread of infection.
4. Never practice aseptic techniques haphazardly. Rigid adherence to aseptic procedures is the only way to ensure that a client is at minimal risk for infection.
5. Protect fellow health care workers from exposure to infectious agents. Nosocomial infections occur with greater frequency when clients become exposed to health care workers who are carriers of infection.
6. Be aware of body sites where nosocomial infection is most likely to develop, including the urinary tract, respiratory tract, bloodstream, and wounds of the skin. This enables the nurse to direct preventive measures at infection control.

## PREREQUISITE KNOWLEDGE

1. Principles of medical asepsis.
2. Elements of the infection chain.
3. Categories of isolation (Skill 37-2).

## PREREQUISITE SKILLS

1. Proper handwashing (Skill 37-2 only).
2. Application of a mask (Chapter 38).
3. Assessment of vital signs (Chapter 12).
4. Administration of medications (Chapter 19, 20, 21).
5. Hygiene measures (Unit III).

# SKILL 37-1 Handwashing

Handwashing is the most important measure in controlling the transmission of microorganisms. Handwashing is a vigorous, brief rubbing together of all surfaces of lathered hands, followed by rinsing under a stream of water (Garner and Farero, 1985). The need for handwashing depends on the type, intensity, duration, and sequence of activity. The Centers for Disease Control (CDC) recommends that nurses should routinely wash their hands in the following situations:

1. Before contact with a client (particularly those with high susceptibility to infection).
2. After caring for an infected client.
3. After touching organic material.
4. Before performing invasive procedures, such as parenteral injections or tracheal suctioning.
5. Before and after handling dressings or touching open wounds.
6. After handling contaminated equipment.
7. Before preparing medications.
8. Between contact with different clients in high-risk units, e.g., critical care and nursery units.

The ideal duration of handwashing is not known. The CDC and Public Health Service note that washing times of at least 10 to 15 seconds (Garner and Favero, 1985) will remove most transient microorganisms from the skin. If hands are visibly soiled, more time may be needed. Agency policies often recommend staff to wash hands for 1 to 2 minutes after working in high-risk areas. Routine handwashing may be performed with bar, liquid, or granule soap, or soap-impregnanted tissue.

## Purposes

1. Reduce the numbers of transient and resident bacteria residing on the hands.
2. Prevent transmission of infection to a client and family members.
3. Prevent transmission of infection to other health care workers or personal contacts.
4. Prevent transmission of infection to oneself.

## Procedure 37-1

| Steps | Rationale |
|---|---|
| **Assessment** | |
| 1. Consider whether unclean object or another client has been touched. | Wash hands whenever there is potential for transmission of microorganisms. |
| 2. Assess need to repeat handwashing if hands have become contaminated during procedure. | Contact with contaminated items requires additional 1-2 min handwashing. |
| 3. Inspect surface of hands for breaks or cuts in skin or cuticles. Report such lesions when caring for highly susceptible clients. | Open cuts or wounds can harbor high concentrations of microorganisms and may serve as portals of exit, increasing client's exposure to infection, or as portals of entry, increasing nurse's risk of acquiring infection. |
| **Nursing Diagnosis** | |
| 1. All clients are cared for with nurse using good handwashing practices. Examples of nursing diagnoses that necessitate meticulous medical aseptic technique include: | |
| a. Impaired skin integrity. | Provides a portal of entry for infection. |
| b. Altered nutrition: less than body requirements. | Client's resistance to infection can be impaired. |
| c. Potential for infection. | Client highly susceptible to infection. |
| **Planning** | |
| 1. Goals for handwashing procedure include: | |
| a. Cleanse all skin surfaces thoroughly. | Nurse should take care to wash all sides of fingers and hands. |
| b. Prevent contact with contaminated objects. | During handwashing nurse avoids touching sink or portion of faucet. |
| 2. Prepare following equipment and supplies: | |
| a. Sink with warm running water | Helps loosen dirt and debride skin. |
| b. Soap or disinfectant | Breaks down lipid chains and removes oil and dirt from hands. |
| c. Paper towels | |
| d. Orange stick (optional) | |

## Implementation

| Steps | Rationale |
|---|---|
| 1. Push wristwatch and long uniform sleeves up above wrists. Remove jewelry, except a plain band, from fingers and arms. | Provides complete access to fingers, hands, and wrists. Jewelry may harbor microorganisms. |
| 2. Keep fingernails short and filed. | Dirt and secretions under fingernails contain microorganisms. Long fingernails can scratch a client's skin. |
| 3. Stand in front of sink, keeping hands and uniform away from sink surface. Use sink with easily accessible faucet. If hands touch sink during handwashing, repeat the process. | Inside of sink is contaminated. Reaching over sink increases risk of touching contaminated edge. |
| 4. Turn on water. Press foot pedals to regulate flow and temperature (Fig. 37-2). Push knee pedals laterally to control flow and temperature. Turn on hand-operated faucets by covering faucet with paper towel. | When hands contact faucet, they are considered contaminated. Organisms spread easily from hands to faucet. |
| 5. Avoid splashing water on uniform. | Microorganisms travel and grow in moisture. |
| 6. Regulate flow of water, so temperature is "warm." | Warm water is more comfortable than hot water, which opens skin pores, causing irritation. |
| 7. Wet hands and lower arms thoroughly under running water. Keep hands and forearms lower than elbows during washing. | Hands are most contaminated parts to be washed. Water flows from least to most contaminated areas, rinsing microorganisms into the sink. |
| 8. Apply 1 ml of regular or 3 ml of antiseptic liquid soap to the hands, lathering thoroughly. If bar soap is used, hold it throughout handwashing. Soap granules, leaflets, and liquid preparations may be used. | Bar soap should be rinsed before returning to soap dish. A soap dish that allows water to drain keeps the soap firm. Jellylike soap permits growth of microorganisms. |
| 9. Wash hands, using plenty of lather and friction, for 10-15 sec for each hand. Interlace fingers and rub palms and backs of hands with circular motion at least 5 times (Fig. 37-3). | Soap cleanses by emulsifying fat and oil and lowering surface tension. Friction and rubbing mechanically loosen and remove dirt and transient bacteria. Interlacing fingers and thumbs ensures that all surfaces are cleansed. |
| 10. If areas underlying fingernails are soiled, clean with fingernails of other hand and additional soap or clean with orangewood stick. Do not tear or cut skin under or around nail. | Mechanical removal of dirt and sediment under nails reduces microorganisms. |
| 11. Rinse hands and wrists thoroughly, keeping hands down and elbows up (Fig. 37-4). | Rinsing mechanically washes away dirt and microorganisms. |
| 12. Repeat steps 8 through 11 but extend the actual period of washing for 1, 2, and 3 minute handwashings. | The greater likelihood of hands being contaminated, the greater need for thorough handwashing. |
| 13. Dry hands thoroughly, from fingers up to wrists and forearms. | Dry from cleanest area (fingertips) to least clean (wrists) to avoid contamination. Drying hands prevents chapping and roughened skin. |
| 14. Discard paper towel in proper receptacle. | Proper disposal of contaminated objects prevents transfer of microorganisms. |
| 15. Turn off water with foot or knee pedals. Turn off hand faucet with clean, dry paper towel. | Wet towel and wet hands allows transfer of pathogens by capillary action. |

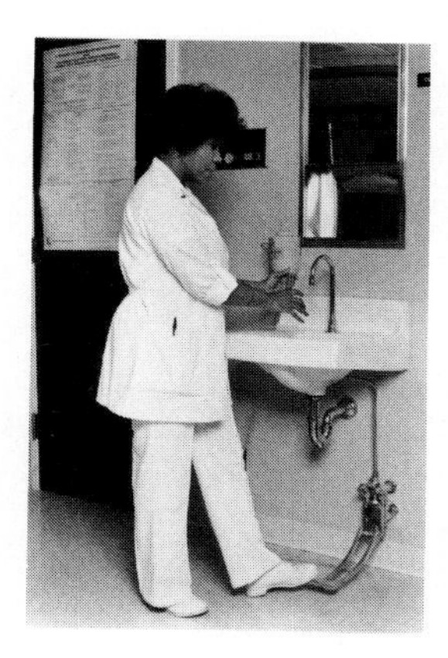

***Fig. 37-2***

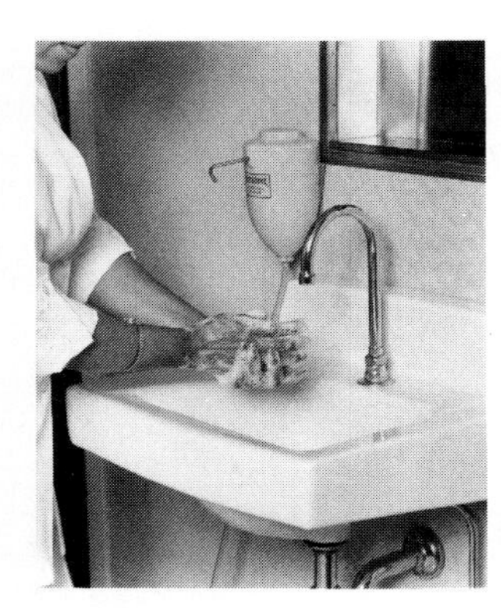

***Fig. 37-3***

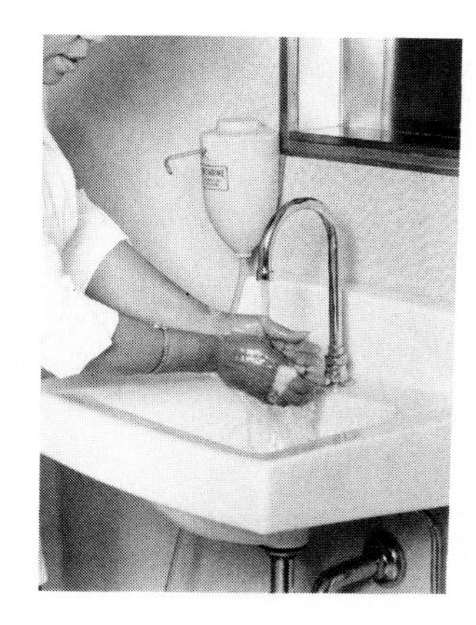

***Fig. 37-4***

| Steps | Rationale |
|---|---|
| **Evaluation** | |
| 1. Inspect surface of hands for obvious signs of dirt or other contaminants. | Determines if handwashing is adequate. |
| ***Expected outcomes*** | |
| 1. Hands and areas under fingernails are clean and free of debris. | Procedure effective. |
| ***Unexpected outcomes*** | |
| 1. Hands or areas under fingernails remain soiled. | Requires nurse to repeat handwashing. |
| **Recording and Reporting** | |
| 1. It is not necessary to record or report this procedure. | |
| **Follow-up Activities** | |
| 1. Keep hands and cuticles well lubricated with hand lotion or moisturizer. | Dry, chapped skin cracks easily, creating portal of entry for infection. |

### Special Considerations

- When preparing for sterile procedure, use antimicrobial scrub rather than simple hand soap.
- Timing of hand scrub varies, depending on purpose of wash.

### Teaching Considerations

- Instruct the client and primary caregiver in proper techniques for handwashing.

### Home Care Considerations

- Evaluate client and primary caregiver to determine their understanding of the transmission of microorganisms and their ability and motivation to perform handwashing according to medical asepsis.
- Evaluate the handwashing facilities in the home to determine the possibility of contamination, the proximity of the facilities to the client, and the ability to maintain supplies and equipment in the area.

## *SKILL 37-2 Caring for a Client under Protective Asepsis*

Often clients acquire infections that can easily be transmitted to other clients, family members, or health care personnel. Protective aseptic techniques or isolation precautions are used to control transmission of pathogens. Environmental barriers, such as a private room, a closed door, a mask, or a protective gown and gloves, keep pathogens in a confined area. The CDC has guidelines for isolating clients within a controlled environment (Table 37-2).

There are two systems for protective asepsis: disease-specific isolation and category-specific isolation. The category-specific precautions listed in Table 37-2 group diseases or disorders by transmission of organisms. An additional category, no longer officially acknowledged by the CDC, is protective or reverse isolation. Clients with compromised immunity, such as those with lymphoma, bone marrow suppression, or organ transplantation, are isolated from other clients or personnel who may transmit infection.

Isolation precautions for prevention of the transmission of human immunodeficiency virus (HIV), hepatitis B virus, and other blood-borne pathogens are the most recent revisions. These guidelines, also called universal blood and body fluid precautions, are intended to prevent parenteral mucous membrane and skin exposures of health care workers to blood-borne pathogens. These precautions are intended to supplement rather than replace recommendations for routine infection control, such as handwashing. The nurse should view all clients as potentially infected and adhere strictly to universal precautions (Table 37-3).

The nurse working in a protective isolation room must carefully plan a client's care. Reducing the number of times a room is entered or exited will help reduce the

***TABLE 37-2*** Isolation Categories

| Type of Isolation (Specific Category) | Purpose | Example of Disease or Condition | Room |
|---|---|---|---|
| Strict | Prevents transmission of highly contagious or virulent infections spread by air and contact. | Chickenpox; diphtheria. | Private room with door closed. |
| Contact | Prevents transmission of highly transmissible infections spread by close or direct contact, which do not warrant strict precautions. | Acute respiratory infections in infants and young children; impetigo; herpes simplex; infections by multiple resistant bacteria. | Private room; clients infected with same organism may share a room. |
| Respiratory | Prevents transmission of infectious diseases over short distances via air droplets. | Measles; meningitis; mumps; pneumonia; *Haemophilus* influenza (in children). | Private room; clients infected with same organism may share a room. |
| Enteric precautions | Prevents infections transmitted by direct or indirect contact with feces. | Cholera; diarrhea of an infectious cause; hepatitis A; gastroenteritis caused by highly infectious organism. | Private room if client's hygiene is poor (does not wash hands, shares contaminated items); clients with same organism may share a room. |
| Tuberculosis isolation | Special category for clients with pulmonary tuberculosis who have positive results on sputum or chest x-ray examination indicating active disease. | Laryngeal tuberculosis. | Private room with special ventilation preferred; door closed. |
| Drainage/secretion precautions | Prevents infections transmitted by direct or indirect contact with purulent material or drainage from an infected body site. | Abscess; burn infection; infected wound; minor infections not included in contact isolation. | Private room not indicated. |
| Universal blood and body fluid precautions* | Transmitted by direct or indirect contact with infective blood or body fluids. | Acquired immune deficiency syndrome (AIDS); hepatitis B; syphillis. | Private room indicated if client's hygiene is poor. |
| Care of severely compromised clients† | Protects an uninfected client with lowered immunity and resistance from acquiring infectious organisms. | Leukemia; lymphoma; aplastic anemia. | Private room with door closed. |

*Formerly blood and body fluid precautions.
†Formerly protective or reverse isolation.

possibility of transmitting infection. Careful assessment of the client's needs, preliminary preparation of equipment and supplies, and coordination of all care measures will give the client a higher quality of care. The skills for caring for clients under protective asepsis outline a variety of separate tasks the nurse often performs in an isolation room.

## Purposes

1. Minimize the transmission of infection while entering or leaving the client's room.
2. Protect the nurse from exposure to microorganisms while in the client's room.
3. Minimize the susceptible client's exposure to microorganisms in the environment.

| Gown | Gloves | Mask | Precautions |
|---|---|---|---|
| Required of all persons entering room. | Required of all persons entering room. | Required of all persons entering room. | Discard or bag and label articles contaminated with infective materials. Send reusable articles for disinfection and sterilization. |
| Indicated if soiling or contact is likely. | Indicated for persons touching infective material. | Indicated for persons coming close to client. | Discard or bag and label articles contaminated with infective material. Send reusable items for disinfection and sterilization. |
| Not indicated. | Not indicated. | Indicated for persons who come close to client. | Discard or bag and label articles contaminated with infective material. Send reusable items for disinfection and sterilization. Bathroom should not be shared by clients. |
| Indicated if soiling is likely. | Indicated when touching infective material. | Not indicated. | Discard or bag and label articles contaminated with infective material. Send reusable items for disinfection and sterilization. Bathroom should not be shared by clients. |
| Indicated only if needed to prevent gross contamination of clothing. | Not indicated. | Indicated only if client is coughing and does not reliably cover mouth. | Articles are rarely involved in transmission of tuberculosis. Articles should be thoroughly cleansed, disinfected, or discarded. |
| Indicated if soiling or contact with infective material is likely. | Indicated for touching infective material. | Not indicated. | Discard or bag and label articles contaminated with infective material. Send for disinfection or sterilization. |
| Indicated during procedures that are likely to generate splashes of blood or body fluids. | Indicated for touching blood or body fluids, mucous membranes or nonintact skin of all clients; indicated for touching soiled items. | Indicated during procedures likely to generate droplets of blood. | Discard or bag and label articles contaminated with blood or body fluids. Disinfect and sterilize articles. Avoid needle stick injuries. Dispose of used needles in properly labeled, puncture-resistant container. Clean blood spills promptly with 5.25% solution of sodium hypochloride diluted 1:10 with water. |
| Required of all persons entering room. | Required of all persons entering room. | Indicated for persons coming in contact with client. | For open wound or burns, use sterile gloves. |

***TABLE 37-3*** Universal Blood/Body Fluid Precautions

| Exposure | Recommendations | Exposure | Recommendations |
|---|---|---|---|
| Contact with blood, body fluids containing visible blood, mucus membranes, nonintact skin, items soiled by blood or fluids containing blood. | Disposable gloves should be changed after each client contact. | Needles, syringes, scalpel blades, intravenous catheters. | Do not recap or break, place in puncture resistant container near work area.<br>Disposable gloves reduce incidence of blood contamination of hands during phlebotomy. |
| Invasive procedures or procedures that may generate droplets or splashes of blood or body fluids.<br>CPR/Artificial respiration. | Masks, goggles, face shields, barrier gowns (gowns with plastic or nonabsorbent backing).<br>Pocket mask, resuscitation bags, or other ventilator devices. | Hands, skin, surfaces contaminated with blood/body fluids. | Wash immediately and thoroughly after removing gloves. |

## *Procedure 37-2*

| Steps | Rationale |
|---|---|
| **Assessment** | |
| 1. Refer to physician's orders for type of isolation. | Type of isolation category influences type of protective clothing worn and precautions followed. |
| 2. Refer to policy and procedure manual or infection control policy of institution for precautions to follow. | Institution may have guidelines that vary from CDC recommendations. |
| 3. Review laboratory test results to determine type of microorganisms for which client is being isolated. | Allows nurse to know what microorganisms is infecting client and media in which it was identified, e.g., sputum, blood, wound. This allows nurse to be appropriately cautious when handling infected exudate or drainage. |
| 4. Consider types of care measures or procedures to be performed while in client's room. | Enables nurse to anticipate needs for supplies, time organization while in room, and coordination of activities. |
| **Nursing Diagnosis** | |
| 1. Cluster data to reveal actual or potential nursing diagnoses: | |
| a. Potential for infection: related to immunosuppression. | Susceptible client is at risk for serious infection. |
| b. Impaired social interaction: related to isolation status. | Client confined to room for several days experiences loneliness and depersonalization. |
| **Planning** | |
| 1. Develop individualized goals for client based on nursing diagnoses: | |
| a. Provide normal meaningful sensory stimulation. | During delivery of care nurse should interact actively with client and offer comfort measures that provide physical stimulation, such as setting client in a chair, repositioning, backrub, or tepid sponge bath. |
| b. Maintain organized approach to care. | Reduces unnecessary trips outside client's room. |
| c. Avoid contamination of articles brought into and removed from room. | Nurse uses techniques that prevent contamination of articles and equipment transferred in and out of room. |
| 2. Prepare following equipment and supplies: | |
| a. Personal care items | |
| ▪ Linen | |
| ▪ Isolation linen bag (usually colored red or labeled) | Contaminated linen is placed in impervious bag with ties to prevent exposure to personnel. |
| ▪ Clean gown | |
| ▪ Water for water pitcher | |
| ▪ Drinking cups | |
| b. Vital signs measurement | |
| ▪ Stethoscope | Can be worn into room if risk of contamination is minimal. Otherwise used only when vital signs are measured. Disposable stethoscopes can stay in room; however, are not as accurate in auscultating blood pressure. |
| ▪ Thermometer (optional) | Nursing divisions using electronic thermometers usually do not have one for each client. When mercury in glass thermometers are used, each client has one. |
| ▪ Manometer and blood pressure cuff (optional) | |
| ▪ Extra pair of disposable gloves | Used to handle stethoscope just before taking vital signs. |
| ▪ Wristwatch | |
| c. Specimen collection | |
| ▪ Appropriate collection container (Chapter 45) | Specimens must be placed in proper containers for preservation before reaching laboratory. |
| ▪ Brown paper bag | All specimens removed from isolation room are bagged and labeled to protect health care workers from body excretions or exudate. |
| ▪ Laboratory requisition | Needed to be sure proper laboratory test is performed. |

| Steps | Rationale |
|---|---|
| ▪ Isolation labels | Warns laboratory workers that specimen came from isolated client. Particularly important if client has communicable infection. |
| ▪ Client identification label | |
| d. Medications | |
| ▪ Oral medication in individual wrappers or cup | All medications are prepared in medication room before being taken to client's room. |
| ▪ Prepared disposable syringe | |
| ▪ Alcohol swab | |
| e. Isolation cart | |
| ▪ Gown | |
| ▪ Mask | |
| ▪ Gloves | |
| ▪ Paper bags | |

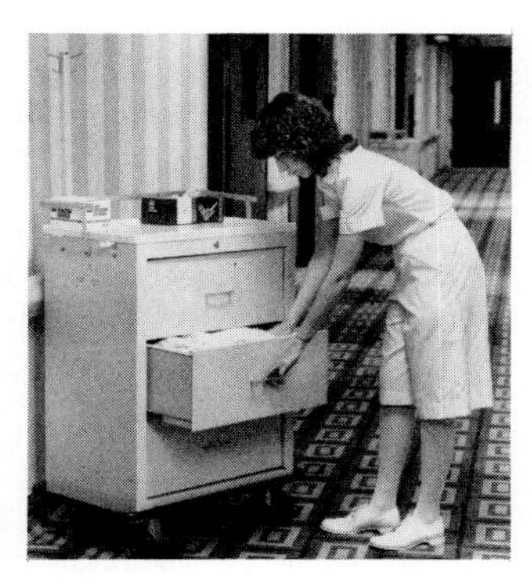

*Fig. 37-5*

## Implementation

### *Donning protective clothing*

| Steps | Rationale |
|---|---|
| 1. Wash hands. | Reduces transmission of microorganisms. |
| 2. Remove isolation gown from cart (Fig. 37-5). Apply so cuffed sleeves cover wrists and shoulders are enclosed by gown. Tie securely at neck and waist. | Long sleeves and tightfitting cuffs prevent exposure of arms to microorganisms. Uniform is completely covered to avoid contamination |
| 3. Apply clean disposable gloves, being sure edge of glove covers cuff of gown. | Prevents transmission of pathogens by direct and indirect contact. |
| 4. Apply mask securely over face and mouth (see Skill 38-1). | Protects nurse from inhaling large particle aerosols and small particle droplets. Also protects susceptible clients from organisms nurse can spread. |

### *Preparing to enter room*

| Steps | Rationale |
|---|---|
| 1. Leave medication cart or tray outside of room. | Prevents contamination of cart or medication tray. |
| 2. Leave brown paper bag and isolation label for specimen collection on isolation cart. | Specimen will eventually be placed in bag so that outer surface of bag remains clean. This allows anyone to transport specimen without fear of contamination. |
| 3. Place stethoscope on inside handle of door or on paper towel away from bedside work area. | Stethoscope should remain free of contamination as nurse performs care. |
| 4. Avoid taking into room any reusable equipment or supplies that are absolutely essential for use with other clients or by other personnel. | Equipment exposed to infected material is contaminated and must be disinfected or sterilized before reuse. |

### *Entering room*

| Steps | Rationale |
|---|---|
| 1. Take all necessary equipment and supplies into room. Avoid placing on contaminated surfaces.<br>Items such as bed linen or medications can be placed away from immediate bedside areas until used. | Minimizes transfer of microorganisms. |
| 2. Lower glove cuff, remove watch, and place on clean paper towel, within easy view.<br>If gown or gloves are not required in room, nurse may wear wristwatch. | Wristwatch is used for vital sign measurement and should remain uncontaminated since it is later removed from room. |
| 3. Place specimen containers on clean paper towel in client's bathroom.<br>Blood tubes may be kept outside on isolation cart. Second nurse assists with specimen transfer. | Specimen containers will be handled by laboratory personnel. Contamination should be kept to minimum. Urine and feces should be transferred in bathroom. |

| Steps | Rationale |
|---|---|
| ***Taking vital signs*** | |
| 1. Vital signs can be taken at any time while in isolation room; however, nurse should always have clean pair of disposable gloves to handle equipment. | Reduces contamination of equipment that may be leaving the room and used for other clients, i.e., electronic thermometer, portable blood pressure cuff. |
| 2. Place stethoscope around neck. During its use be sure it has minimal contact with contaminated material, e.g., drainage, excretions. | If stethoscope will be reused with other clients, it should not contact contaminated material. |
| 3. Measure client's temperature according to Skill 12-1 using client's thermometer. | Mercury thermometer remains in room to prevent infection transfer.<br>If you take electronic thermometer in room, remove it immediately after use. |
| 4. Measure client's blood pressure according to Skill 12-6. (Wrap cuff around thin gown sleeve, above antecubital fossa.) | Minimizes soiling of cuff. |
| 5. With watch in view on towel, assess pulse and respirations according to Skills 12-4 and 12-5. | If gloved hand touches client or any contaminated object, watch should not be touched. |
| 6. Record results of vital signs on a clean paper towel at bedside. | Chart and flow sheets cannot be taken into client's room. Nurse will transcribe results onto form outside room once all care is completed. |
| 7. Place stethoscope on clean surface in room. Wash off diaphragm or bell, if soiled, with alcohol swab. | Stethoscope will be removed from room once nursing care is completed. Alcohol helps to disinfect soiled surfaces. |
| ***Administering medications*** | |
| 1. Take medications to bedside and administer medications following the appropriate skills (Chapters 18, 19, or 20). | Techniques maintain asepsis. |
| 2. After administering injection, discard contaminated needle and syringe in appropriate containers in client's room. Dispose of cups and wrappers in container in room. | Prevents exposure of personnel to contaminated objects by avoiding transport of equipment to medication room. |
| ***Collecting specimens*** | |
| 1. Collect necessary specimens following procedures in Chapter 45. Transfer specimen to appropriate container, minimizing contact of gloved hands with outer surface of container. Blood specimens can easily be transferred to clean blood tubes held by another nurse outside client's door. | Each type of body excretion or exudate must be collected in a specific manner to prevent contamination by resident flora. Containers will be handled by laboratory personnel and should remain clean on outside. |
| 2. Be sure specimen container is tightly sealed. | Prevents spillage and contamination of outer surface of container. |

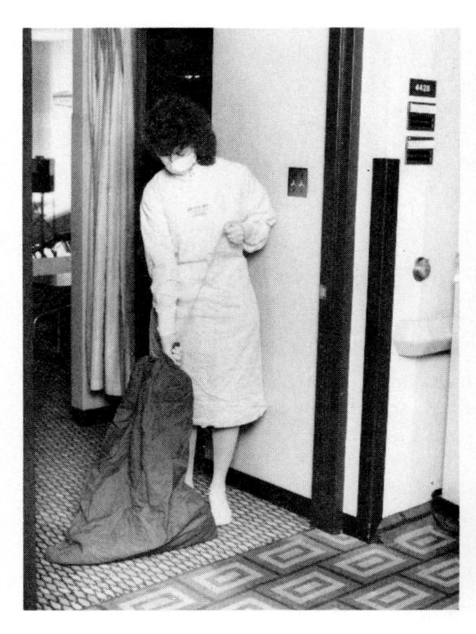

*Fig. 37-6*

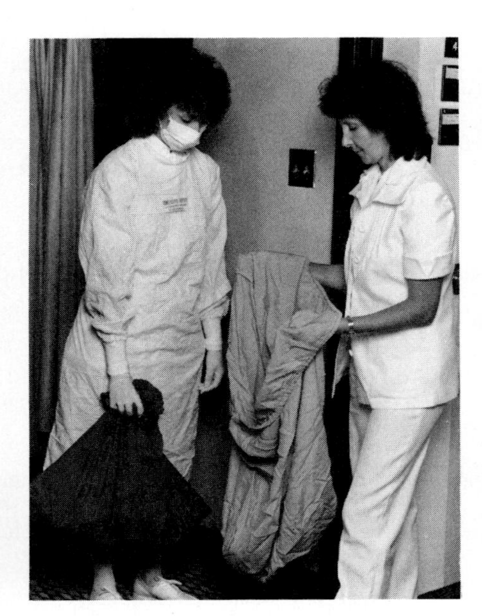

*Fig. 37-7*

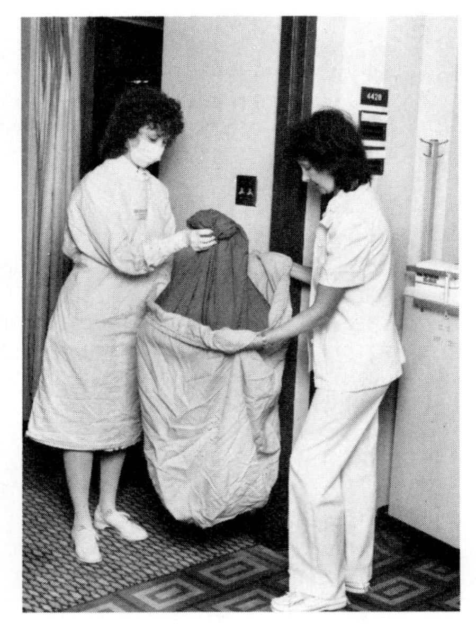

*Fig. 37-8*

| Steps | Rationale |
|---|---|
| 3. Label specimen container with client's name. | Properly labeled specimens are essential to be sure correct laboratory results are reported for the correct client. |
| 4. Have another nurse stand outside client's room holding brown paper bag. Place specimen into bag without contaminating bag's outer surface. | Outer surface of bag is considered clean and can be touched by other personnel. |
| 5. Ask second nurse to place isolation label on bag and have specimen transported. | Specimens should be transported to laboratory immediately for proper preparation. |
| ***Performing hygiene measures*** | |
| 1. Perform necessary hygiene measures according to skills in Unit III. Avoid wetting gown. | Moisture on gown provides path for microorganisms to spread to uniform. |
| 2. Discard soiled linen into special isolation linen bag in client's room. | Isolation linen bag must be impervious and sturdy to reduce infection spread. |
| ***Bagging articles*** | |
| 1. If linen bag is filled be sure all soiled linen is contained and tie top of bag securely (Fig. 37-6). | Contaminated linen should be well-contained to prevent exposure to health care personnel. |
| 2. Have second nurse stand outside client's room and hold clean linen bag (Fig. 37-7). | Double bagging is practiced to prevent exposure of personnel to contaminated outer surface of soiled linen bag. Maki (1986) suggests double bagging offers no aseptic technique. |
| 3. Nurse outside room holds clean bag by folding its top edges back to form cuff over hands. | Cuff protects nurse from contacting soiled linen bag. |
| 4. As bag opening separates, place your hand inside clean bag and pull opening out fully. | Inside of bag will be considered contaminated. Outer bag should be opened so contaminated bag can be easily dropped in. |
| 5. Drop contaminated linen bag into clean receiving bag without touching receiving bag's sides (Fig. 37-8). | Contaminated bag is contained and now can be transported outside client's room. |
| 6. Have second nurse discard linen into appropriate hamper. | Reduces transmission of microorganisms. |
| 7. Take any contaminated reusable objects, such as suction bottles or instruments, and carefully place in paper or plastic bag held by second nurse outside room. Suction bottles or equipment that has been rinsed should not be contained in single paper bag. | CDC recommends single bag is adequate to discard items if bag is impervious and sturdy and article can be placed inside bag without contaminating its outer surface. Otherwise follow double bag procedure. |
| 8. Second nurse seals bag with tape or according to agency policy. | Contains contaminated item safely. |
| ***Preparing to leave room*** | |
| 1. Be sure client's needs have been attended. | Nurse attempts to control number of visits into isolation room particularly when strict precautions are followed. Nurse may not return to room for some time. |
| 2. Remove gloves by grasping cuff of one glove and pulling it off, turning glove inside out. With ungloved hand tuck finger inside cuff of remaining glove and pull off, turning inside out. Dispose in proper receptacle. | Gloves are removed first because they are most likely to be contaminated and should not be used to touch hair around mask. |
| 3. Untie or pull off mask from around ears and dispose in receptacle. | Reduces transmission of infection. Masks are disposable. |
| 4. Untie gown at neck and waist (Fig. 37-9). Keeping hand inside one cuff, pull opposite sleeve down from arm (Fig. 37-10). Do same for other arm (Fig. 37-11). | Keeping hands inside gown minimizes contact with microorganisms. |
| 5. Pull gown off by turning it inside out (Fig. 37-12). Fold so that contaminated sides face one another. Discard in proper receptacle. | Gown is turned inside out so hands and clothing do not come in contact with outer contaminated surface. |
| 6. Wash hands thoroughly. | Mechanically removes any transient microorganisms contacted. |
| 7. Pick up wristwatch and stethoscope taking care not to touch a contaminated surface. Note vital sign recordings made in room. | Clean hands may touch watch and stethoscope without risk of contamination. |
| 8. Leave client's room, closing door securely. | Room should remain closed, especially when airborne infection is being isolated. |

## Recording and Reporting

| | |
|---|---|
| 1. Document in nurse's notes: | |
| a. Type of isolation status being maintained. | Assures that proper procedures are followed by all nursing staff. |

| Steps | Rationale |
|---|---|

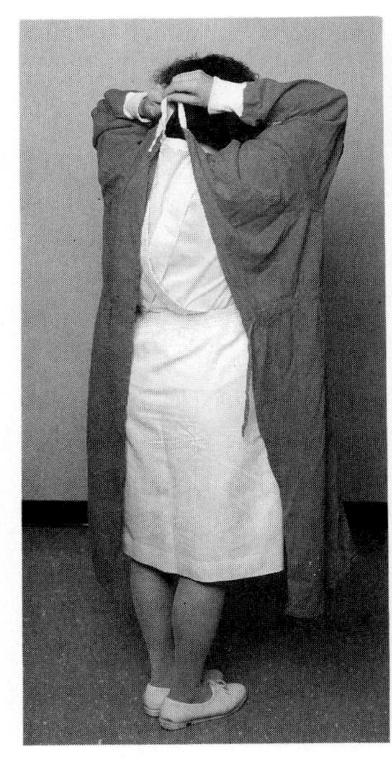

*Fig. 37-9*

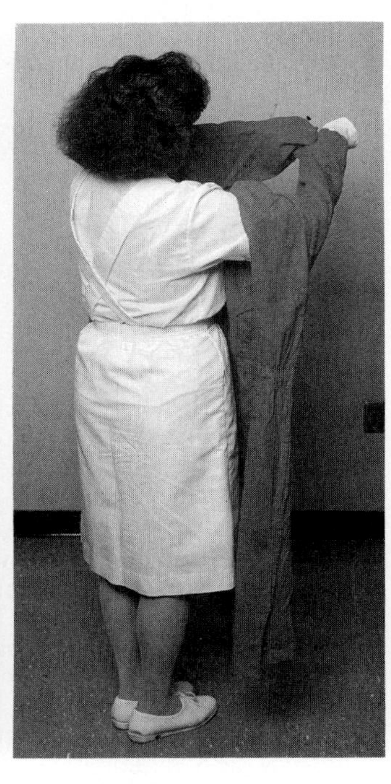

*Fig. 37-10*

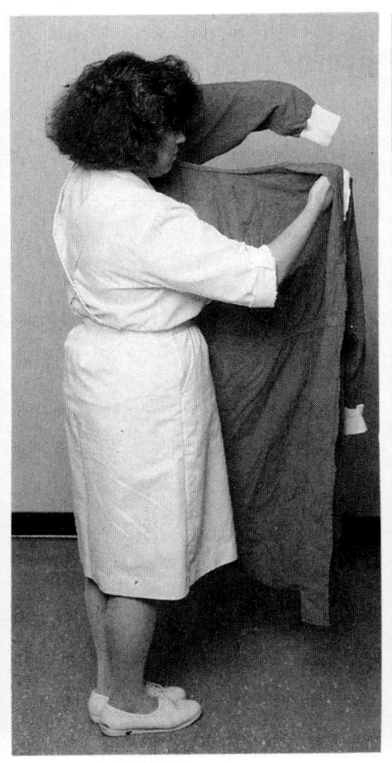

*Fig. 37-11*

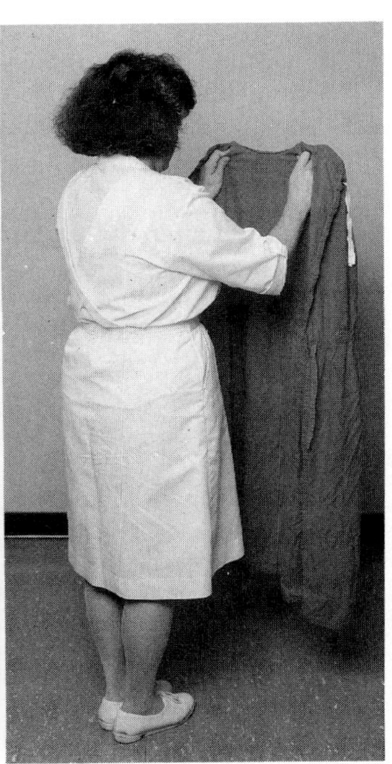

*Fig. 37-12*

| Steps | Rationale |
|---|---|
| b. Client's psychologic response to isolation | Monitoring client's psychologic status directs nursing staff to initiate supportive care. |
| 2. Record vital signs and other procedures according to guidelines for each skill. | Documents care provided. |

### Follow-up Activities

| Steps | Rationale |
|---|---|
| 1. Instruct family members and friends on isolation precautions, techniques for applying and removing protective clothing, and handwashing. | Family or friends visiting client often make close contact and should be protected against organism spread. Family should understand purpose of precautions so as not to avoid or act differently toward client. |

## Special Considerations

- A nurse progresses with isolation procedures by moving from cleanest to dirtiest procedures.
- In hospital settings infection control nurse may confer with physician in selecting proper isolation category.
- Topical creams or lotions usually can be left at client's bedside.
- Client's chart is never taken into isolation room.
- Immunosuppressed clients should not receive fresh flowers or fresh fruit, and the use of black pepper should be limited. These harbor microorganisms that can infect the client.

## Teaching Considerations

- Client should be able to verbalize the reasons for isolation.
- Instruct client about responsibilities for infection control, such as properly discarding facial tissues or dressings.
- Have client demonstrate proper handwashing techniques.
- Ensure client and family understand and are compliant with infection control measures, such as gowning, gloving, and application of masks.
- Caution family to restrict visitors to client.

## Home Care Considerations

- If client will need continued infection control measures at home, such as the immunosuppressed client, instruct the family in proper procedures.
- Instruct primary care giver to wash soiled linens and eating utensils in hot water.
- Instruct primary care giver to disinfect bathroom with household bleach and water.
- Caution family to restrict visitors to client.

## BIBLIOGRAPHY


Barrick B: Caring for AIDS patients: a challenge you can meet, Nurs '88 18(11):50, 1988.

Centers for Disease Control: Recommendations for prevention of HIV transmission in health care settings, MMWR 36:(25) 2, 1987.

Centers for Disease Control: Update: Universal precautions for prevention of transmission of HIV, hepatitis B, and other blood borne pathogens in health care settings, MMWR 37:377, 1988.

Garner JS, Simmons BP: CDC guidelines for isolation precautions in hospitals, Infect Control 4(4):249, 1983.

Garner JS, Favero MS: Guidelines for handwashing and hospital environmental control, 1985, Hospital infection program, CDC, DPH, and U.S. Department of Health and Human Services.

Garrett J: The AIDS patient: helping him and his parents to cope, Nurs '88 18(9):50, 1988.

Hargins CO, Larson E: Infection control guidelines for prevention of hospital acquired infections, Am J Nurs 81:2175, 1981.

Kim MJ, McFarland GK, McLane AM: Pocket guide to nursing diagnoses, ed 2, St. Louis, 1987, The CV Mosby Co.

Larson EL, et al.: Physiological and microbiologic changes in skin related to frequent handwashing, Infect Control 7:59, 1986.

Larson EL, et al.: Quantity of soap as a variable in handwashing, Infect Control 8:371, 1987.

Maki DG, et al.: Double bagging of items from isolation rooms is unnecessary as an infection control measure: a comparative study of surface contamination with single and double bagging, Infect Control 7(11):535, 1986.

Marchiondo K: The very fine art of collecting culture specimens, Nurs '79 9(4):34, 1979.

Potter PA, Perry AG: Fundamentals of nursing: concepts, process, and practice, St. Louis, ed 2, 1989, The CV Mosby Co.

Roth MK, et al.: How to prevent infection in a home care patient, RN 50(11):61, 1987.

Schietinger H: A home care plan for AIDS, Am J Nurs 9:1021, 1986.

Simmons BP: Guidelines for prevention of surgical wound infections, Am J Infect Control 11(4):133, 1983.

Walsh J, Persons C, Wieck L: Manual of home health care nursing, Philadelphia, 1987, JB Lippincott Co.

Williams WW: CDC guidelines for infection control in hospital personnel, Infect Control 4(4):325, 1983.

# 38

# SURGICAL ASEPSIS

### OBJECTIVES

*Mastery of content in this chapter will enable the nurse to:*

- Define key terms
- Discuss settings where surgical aseptic techniques may be used.
- Describe conditions when surgical asepsis should be used.
- Identify principles of surgical asepsis.
- Explain importance of organization and caution when using surgical aseptic techniques.
- Apply and remove a cap and mask correctly.
- Perform surgical handwashing correctly.
- Apply sterile gloves using open glove method.
- Prepare a sterile field.
- Apply a sterile drape correctly.

### KEY TERMS

*Asepsis*
*Autoclave*
*Broad spectrum antibiotic*
*Contaminated*
*Flora*
*Pathogen*
*Sterile*
*Sterile field*
*Surgical asepsis*

### SKILLS

**38-1** Donning and Removing Cap and Mask
**38-2** Surgical Handwashing
**38-3** Preparing a Sterile Field
**38-4** Applying Sterile Gloves (Open Gloving)

Surgical asepsis or sterile techniques require a nurse to use greater precautions than with medical asepsis. The aim is to eliminate all microorganisms, including pathogens and spores, from an object. The nurse working with a sterile field or with sterile equipment must understand that the slightest break in technique results in contamination. The nurse also practices surgical asepsis in an effort to keep microorganisms away from an area, e.g., when changing a dressing on a wound.

Although surgical asepsis is commonly practiced in the operating room, labor and delivery areas, and major diagnostic rooms, the nurse may also use sterile technique at the client's bedside. This would include, for example, inserting IV or urinary catheters. A nurse in an operating room will follow a series of steps to maintain sterile technique, including donning a mask and cap, performing a surgical handwash, and donning a sterile gown and gloves. In contrast, a nurse performing a dressing change may only wash hands and don sterile gloves. A mask may be optional at the bedside, depending on whether the nurse is affected by a respiratory infection or whether agency policy requires a mask. If there is a risk for body fluids to splash into the nurse's eyes, only goggles or the pulldown fiberglass masks offer protection to the eyes. Indications for the use of sterile technique include:

- During procedures that require intentional perforation of a client's skin (e.g., insertion of IV catheters and administration of injections).
- When the skin's integrity is broken due to trauma, surgical incision, or burns.
- During procedures that involve insertion of catheters or surgical instruments into sterile body cavities.

Strict aseptic technique is essential in the above situations to prevent exposing a client to the risk of infection. A nurse cannot be too cautious when performing procedures under sterile technique. Any procedure should be well-organized, with client, environment, and supplies prepared so that the nurse's actions will not be interrupted. Clients should understand the purpose and steps of any sterile procedure and know the importance of not contaminating sterile objects. The nurse should warn clients to avoid sudden movements of body parts covered by sterile drapes. Clients should never touch sterile supplies, drapes, or the nurse's sterile gloves or gown. The client should also be warned against coughing, sneezing, or talking over a sterile area.

Sterile procedures often require much time. The nurse anticipates a client's needs in advance so that procedures are not interrupted. The client's elimination and comfort needs are met to enhance his ability to cooperate during procedures.

The room in which a procedure is to be performed should be neat so that it is easy to arrange sterile supplies. Windows should be closed and drafts reduced to lessen chances of contaminating sterile objects by airborne microorganisms. Closing the room door and posting a sign warning that a procedure is in progress can also help prevent interruptions. There should be a minimal number of people in a room during a sterile procedure.

## GUIDELINES

1. Equipment and supplies used in surgical aseptic procedures are sterile. Reusable objects are sterilized after each use with either dry or moist heat, radiation, ethylene oxide gas, or chemicals. All sterile items are stored in special properly labeled sterile wrappers. Wrappers are impervious to microorganisms as long as they are dry and intact. All sterile items should be stored in clean, dry areas. Some specially wrapped pieces of equipment have chemical indicator tapes applied to the outside of the package in addition to a date indicating when the package is no longer sterile. When the equipment is gas autoclaved the tapes change color to indicate sterility of contents. Whenever the color change is not evident the package and enclosed item are considered contaminated.
2. A sterile object remains sterile when touched only by another sterile object. The following points guide the nurse in where to place sterile objects and how to handle them:
   a. Sterile touching sterile remains sterile. Thus sterile gloves are worn to handle objects on a sterile field.
   b. Sterile touching clean becomes contaminated; for example, if the tip of a syringe or needle touches the surface of a clean disposable glove, the syringe or needle is contaminated.
   c. Sterile touching contaminated is contaminated; e.g., when the nurse touches a sterile object with an ungloved hand, the object is contaminated.
   d. Sterile touching questionable is contaminated. When a tear in the covering of a sterile package is found, the item is automatically discarded.
3. Only sterile objects may be placed on a sterile field. The following points apply:
   a. Sterile objects are kept in clean and dry storage areas for only a prescribed time; thereafter they are considered unsterile.
   b. Check all sterile packages for sterilization dates or time periods before use.
   c. A package that is torn, punctured, wet, or open is unsterile.
4. A sterile object or field out of the range of vision or held below a person's waist is contaminated. The following points apply:
   a. Never turn your back on a sterile tray or leave it unattended. Keep sterile objects in view.
   b. Never hold any objects, including hands, below waist level since they cannot be viewed and are thus contaminated.
   c. Sterile objects should be kept in front with hands as close together as possible.
5. A sterile object or field becomes contaminated by microorganisms transported to it through the air. The following points apply:
   a. Avoid activities that create air currents, for example, excessive movement or rearranging linen once sterile objects are exposed.
   b. When opening sterile objects, minimize the number of people walking into the area.
   c. Avoid talking, coughing, sneezing, or laughing when working with sterile equipment.
   d. Wear a mask when opening a tray and adding sterile equipment or while working over a sterile area.
   e. Do not perform sterile procedures unless wearing a double mask when experiencing even mild respiratory ailments.
   f. Never reach over a sterile field.
   g. When opening sterile packages, hold items or pieces of equipment, without touching surfaces, as close as possible to the sterile field.
   h. Keep all work areas in a client's room reasonably free of microorganisms by damp dusting with appropriate germicide.
   i. Keep your hair clean and short or covered with a cap while performing a sterile procedure.
   j. Keep doors closed and drafts minimal in areas where sterile procedures are performed.
6. A sterile object or field becomes contaminated by capillary action when a sterile surface comes in contact with a wet contaminated surface. Moisture can seep through protective wrappings or coverings to allow microorganisms to enter. The following points apply:
   a. Discard or recycle for sterilization any stored sterile package that becomes wet.
   b. Be sure the underlying surface is sterile and unpenetrable by moisture when pouring sterile solutions over a tray or field. Many prepackaged kits, such as a catheterization tray, contain plastic containers into which solutions can be poured.
   c. Replace sterile drapes that become moist.
7. Fluid flows in the direction of gravity. A sterile object becomes contaminated if gravity causes a contaminated liquid to flow over the object's surface. The following points apply:
   a. When handling objects with sterile transfer forceps always keep tips of the forceps pointed downward. Forceps may be stored in sterile liquid disinfectant.

If forcep tips are raised upward, disinfectant may flow toward the nurse's hands and become contaminated. Once the tips are again lowered, the forceps will then be contaminated. Dry disposable forceps are preferred.

b. Keep hands above elbows during surgical hand scrub. Water will flow downward without contaminating hands and fingers.

8. The edges of a sterile field or container are considered to be contaminated. The following points apply:
   a. Since the edges of sterile drapes touch unsterile surfaces, a 2.5 cm (1-inch) border around the drape is considered contaminated.
   b. Place all sterile objects at least 2.5 cm (1 inch) away from edge of a sterile field.
   c. The edges of a sterile container are contaminated once exposed to air. For example, do not allow a sterile needle, once it has been uncapped, to touch the edge of the cap.
   d. The lip of an opened bottle of solution is contaminated when exposed to air. Pour out a small amount of sterile solution to wash microorganisms away from the lip of a bottle and discard solution. Then pour desired amount of solution.

**PREREQUISITE KNOWLEDGE**

1. Principles relating to the chain of infection
2. Principles of medical and surgical asepsis.

**PREREQUISITE SKILLS**

1. Proper handwashing techniques (Skill 37-1).

# *SKILL 38-1 Donning and Removing Cap and Mask*

For sterile procedures on a general nursing division, the nurse may wear a surgical mask without a cap. For sterile procedures in the operating room or labor and delivery room the nurse first applies a clean paper or cloth cap that covers all of the hair and then the surgical mask.

Surgical caps, made of paper or cloth, prevent loose hair from hanging down over a sterile area. Microorganisms are abundant in hair and thus can easily contaminate sterile objects. If the nurse's hair is kept short and clean, a cap may not be necessary. Masks reduce accidental contamination of the nurse's hands and all sterile objects by airborne droplet nuclei. Even when performing simple sterile procedures, nurses should wear masks if they have colds or respiratory infections. After a mask is worn for several hours, the area over the mouth and nose often becomes moist. Nurses in the operating room must thus apply a second mask over the first, since removing a mask in a surgical area results in immediate contamination of surrounding objects.

**Purposes**

1. Prevent transfer of airborne microorganisms from the nurse's respiratory tract to a sterile area.
2. Prevent transfer of microorganisms that reside on the nurse's hair onto a sterile area.
3. Prevent transfer of microorganisms to exposed layers of the client's skin.

## *Procedure 38-1*

| Steps | Rationale |
|---|---|
| **Assessment** | |
| 1. Consider type of sterile procedure to be performed and consult institutional policy for use of cap and mask. | Not all sterile procedures will require cap and mask. |
| 2. If you have symptoms of cold or respiratory infection, either avoid participating in procedure or apply two masks. | Greater number of pathogenic microorganisms reside within respiratory tract when infection is present. |
| **Planning** | |
| 1. Goal of procedure is to: | |
| a. Minimize transfer of microorganisms. | Cap and mask must fit snugly. |
| 2. Prepare the following supplies: | |
| a. Paper or cloth cap (may be optional) | |
| b. Hair pins (optional) | |
| c. Paper mask | |

| Steps | Rationale |
|---|---|

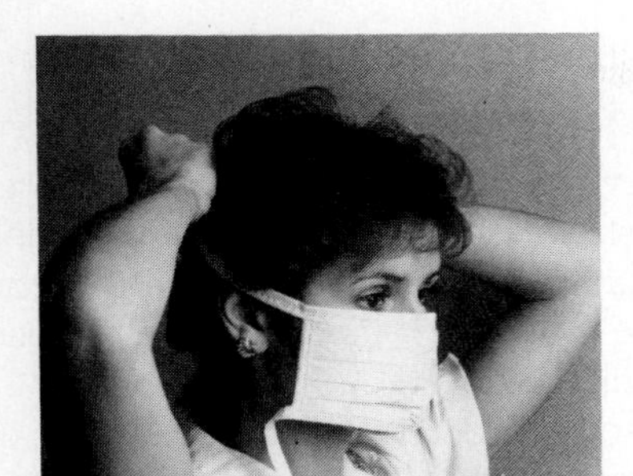
*Fig. 38-1*

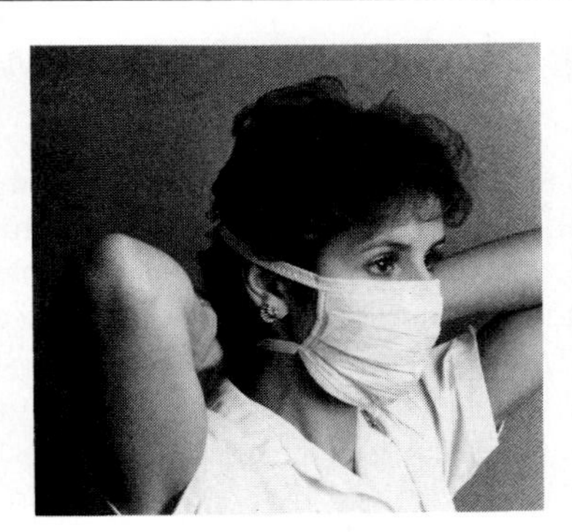
*Fig. 38-2*

## Implementation

### *Donning cap (OR and labor and delivery procedures)*

| Steps | Rationale |
|---|---|
| 1. If hair is long, comb back behind shoulders and arrange on crown of head. | Cap must cover all hair entirely. |
| 2. Secure hair in place with pins. | Long hair should not fall down or cause cap to slip and expose hair. |
| 3. Apply cap over head as you would apply hairnet. Be sure all hair fits under cap's edges. | Loose hair hanging over sterile field results in contamination of objects on field. |

### *Donning mask*

| Steps | Rationale |
|---|---|
| 1. Find top edge of mask (usually has thin metal strip along edge). | Pliable metal fits snugly against bridge of nose. |
| 2. Hold mask by top two strings or loops, keeping top edge above bridge of nose. | Prevents contact of hands with clean facial portion of mask. Mask will cover all of nose. |
| 3. Tie two top strings at top of back of head, with strings above ears. (Alternative: slip loops over each ear) (Fig. 38-1). | Position of ties at top of head provides tight fit. Ties over ears may cause irritation. |
| 4. Tie two lower ties snugly around neck with mask well under chin (Fig. 38-2). | Prevents escape of microorganisms through sides of mask as nurse talks and breathes. |
| 5. Gently pinch upper metal band around bridge of nose. | Prevents microorganisms from escaping around nose. |

### *Disposing of cap and mask*

| Steps | Rationale |
|---|---|
| 1. Untie lower strings of mask first. (Alternative: lift side loops up from ears.) | Prevents top part of mask from falling down over nurse's uniform. Contaminated surface of mask could then contaminate uniform. |
| 2. Untie top strings and remove mask from face, holding ties securely. | Avoids contact of nurse's hands with contaminated portion of mask. |
| 3. Hold top strings or loops of mask. Fold mask in half with inner surfaces together. | Avoids contact with area of mask that has become moistened. |
| 4. Grasp outer surface of cap and lift from hair. | Minimizes contact of hands with hair. |
| 5. Discard cap and mask together in proper receptacle and wash hands. | Reduces transmission of infection. |

## Special Considerations

- Procedures that usually require cap and mask include major dressing changes; wound debridement; assistance to physician when inserting central line intravenous catheters; major invasive diagnostic procedures (Chapter 46); surgical procedures; delivery of infant.
- When cap is worn, ties fit over cap at top of head.

# SKILL 38-2 Surgical Handwashing

The procedure for surgical handwashing requires greater effort than does medical aseptic practice. Since strict surgical procedures are to be carried out, the nurse must use extra precautions to rid hand surfaces of microorganisms. The skin can never be rendered sterile; however, it can be made surgically clean through scrubbing. Surgical handwashing is necessary for nurses working in operating (Chapter 40) or delivery rooms and in special diagnostic test areas. Regular handwashing is satisfactory before routine sterile procedures on a general nursing division.

Surgical handwashing or scrubbing should take at least 5 minutes before the first procedure of the day (Garner, 1985). The CDC does not recommend a duration for surgical scrubs performed between procedures. However, 2 to 5 minutes is probably acceptable (check agency policy). For maximum elimination of bacteria, the nurse removes all jewelry and keeps fingernails short, clean, and free of polish. Brushes are used during scrubbing. Some experts caution that too much brushing removes outer layers of the epidermis, thereby exposing bacterial flora in the deeper skin layers.

If harsh soaps are used, the nurse's skin can become irritated, providing an environment for additional microorganism growth. Antiseptic solutions such as iodophor and chlorhexidine improve removal of bacteria from the hands and lower arms.

## Purposes

1. Thoroughly remove transient and resident bacteria from the surfaces of hands, nails, and forearms.
2. Leave an antimicrobial residue on skin to prevent growth of microbes for several hours.

## Procedure 38-2

| Steps | Rationale |
|---|---|
| **Assessment** | |
| 1. Consult institutional policy regarding required length of time for handwash. | Guidelines vary regarding ideal time needed for surgical scrub. |
| 2. Be sure fingernails are short and free of polish. | Long nails and polish increase number of bacteria residing on nails. Long fingernails can puncture gloves causing contamination. |
| 3. Inspect condition of hands for presence of abrasions, cuts, or open lesions. | Conditions increase likelihood of more microorganisms residing on skin surfaces. |
| **Planning** | |
| 1. Develop appropriate goals for procedure: | |
| a. Ensure thorough cleansing of all surfaces of hands and forearms. | In surgical scrub, fingers, hands, and forearms are viewed as having four sides that must be thoroughly scrubbed. |
| 2. Prepare following equipment and supplies: | |
| a. Deep sink with foot, knee, or elbow controls for dispensing soap and controlling water temperature and flow; faucets of sink positioned high enough for hands and forearms to fit below | |
| b. Antiseptic detergent such as chlorhexidine or triclosan | Antiseptics maximally reduce the number of microorganisms on the hands. |
| c. Surgical scrub brushes | Used to clean under nails. |
| d. Orange stick or nail file | |
| e. Sterile towel | Prevents exposing hands to airborne microorganisms. |
| f. Paper mask and cap | |
| 3. Remove all jewelry, including rings, watch, and bracelets. | Jewelry harbors microorganisms and interferes with access to all surfaces of skin to be cleaned. |
| 4. Be sure sleeves are above elbows and uniform is fitted or tucked at waist. | Scrubbed hands and arms can become contaminated by brushing against loose garments. |
| **Implementation** | |
| 1. Apply cap and face mask (Skill 38-1). | Prevents escape into air of microorganisms that can contaminate hands. |

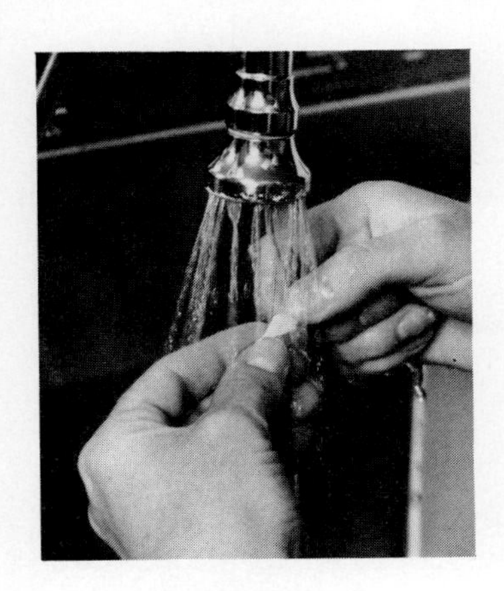

Fig. 38-3

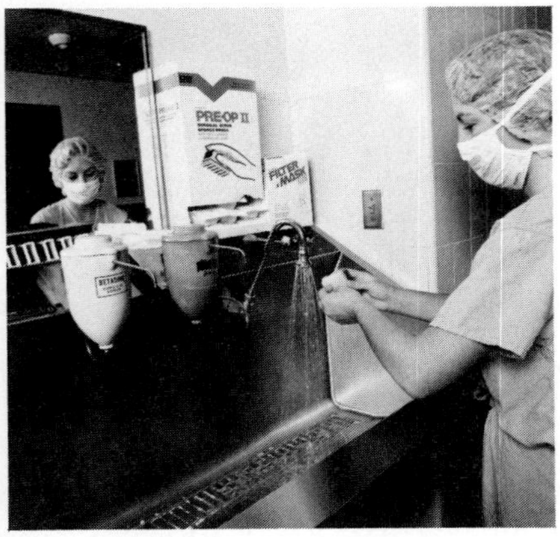

Fig. 38-4

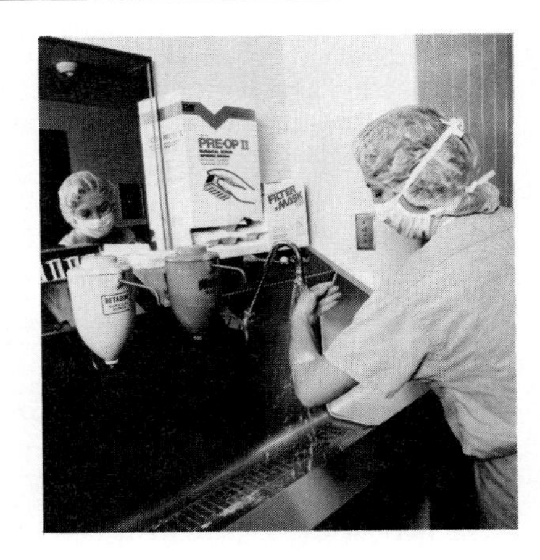


Fig. 38-5

| Steps | Rationale |
|---|---|
| 2. Turn on water and adjust to comfortable lukewarm temperature. | Hot water removes protective oils from skin and increases skin sensitivity to soap. |
| 3. Wet hands and forearms liberally, keeping hands above level of elbows during entire procedure. NOTE: Nurse's scrub dress or uniform must be kept dry. | Water runs by gravity from fingertips to elbows. Hands become cleanest part of upper extremity. Keeping hands elevated allows water to flow from least to most contaminated area. |
| 4. Dispense liberal amount of soap (2-5 ml) into hands. Lather hands and forearms for a few minutes to a level 5 cm (2 in) above elbows. | Washing a wide area reduces risk of contaminating overlying gown nurse later applies (Chapter 40). |
| 5. With hands under running water, clean under nails with orange stick or file. Discard after use (Fig. 38-3). | Removes dirt and organic material that harbor large numbers of microorganisms. Antiseptic soap remains on hands and arms to provide continuous antimicrobial action. |
| 6. Rinse hands and arms thoroughly under running water. *Remember to keep hands above elbows.* | Rinsing removes transient bacteria from fingers, hands, and forearms. |
| 7. Apply soap, and lather hands and arms. Scrub each hand with brush for 45 sec. Holding brush perpendicular to fingers, scrub all sides of each digit, including web spaces between, and palm and back of hand (Fig. 38-4). | Scrubbing loosens resident bacteria that adheres to skin surfaces. Holding brush perpendicular ensures coverage of all surfaces. |
| 8. Then using the same brush, scrub each arm to 5 cm (2 inches) above the elbow dividing the arm into thirds: scrub each lower forearm 15 seconds, each upper forearm 15 seconds, and 5 cm above each elbow 15 seconds. | Scrubbing is performed from cleanest area (hands) to marginal area (upper arms). |
| 9. Discard brush and rinse hands and arms thoroughly. | After touching skin, brush is considered contaminated. Rinsing removes resident bacteria. |
| 10. Using a second brush, scrub each hand for 30 seconds. Then use the same brush to scrub each arm up to the elbow by dividing the arm in half: scrub each lower forearm 15 seconds and each upper forearm 15 seconds. | A second scrubbing ensures thorough cleansing of hands and forearms. The number of resident microorganisms remaining on skin will be minimal. |
| 11. Discard brush and rinse hands and arms thoroughly (Fig 38-5). Turn off water with foot pedal. | Removes transient bacteria. |
| 12. Use a sterile towel to dry one hand thoroughly moving from fingers to elbow. Dry in a rotating motion. NOTE: Nurses wishing to apply sterile gloves for use in a regular clinical area need not use brushes or dry hands with sterile towels. Thorough lathering and friction performed twice according to procedure will ensure clean hands. In this situation the nurse may use clean paper towels for drying. | Dry from cleanest to least clean area. Drying prevents chapping and facilitates donning of gloves. |
| 13. Repeat drying method for other hand, using a different area of the towel or a new sterile towel. | Prevents accidental contamination. |
| 14. Keep hands higher than elbows and away from the body. | Prevents accidental contamination. |
| 15. Proceed into operating room, labor and delivery area, or treatment room. | |

### Special Considerations

- Cuts or abrasions of the hands can contraindicate nurse's participation in procedure.
- Nurses often pin rings or watches to uniforms to prevent loss.
- Nurses in operating room and labor and delivery wear special scrub suits (Chapter 40).

# *SKILL 38-3 Preparing a Sterile Field*

When performing sterile aseptic procedures, the nurse must have a work area in which objects can be handled with minimal risk of contamination. A sterile field serves such a purpose. It is an area considered free of microorganisms and may consist of a sterile tray or a surface draped with a sterile towel or wrapper.

A sterile drape establishes a sterile field around a treatment site, such as a surgical incision, venipuncture site, or site for introduction of a catheter. The drape provides a larger work surface for placing sterile supplies and for manipulating items with sterile gloves. It also allows the nurse to manipulate body parts underlying the drape, without contaminating sterile gloves. Drapes are available in cloth, paper, and plastic. They may be wrapped in individual sterile packages or be included within sterile kits or trays. Many styles, shapes, and sizes are available to accommodate different areas or body parts to be covered. For example, a drape with a slitlike hole in the center is used to cover the perineal area during urinary catheter insertion.

Many sterile items come prepackaged within containers that also serve as sterile fields. For example, bladder catheterization kits and tracheal suction kits contain sterile items that can be moved within the tray and containers into which sterile solutions can be poured. The kits serve as work areas for the nurse.

The following skill of preparing a sterile field incorporates skills of opening sterile packages, preparing a sterile drape, adding sterile supplies to a field, pouring sterile solutions, and transferring items with a forceps.

### Purposes

1. Provide a large enough work space to perform a sterile procedure without risk of contaminating sterile items.
2. Add needed supplies to a field when supplies in prepackaged kits are insufficient.

## *Procedure 38-3*

| Steps | Rationale |
|---|---|
| **Assessment** | |
| 1. Assess client's comfort, oxygen requirements, and elimination needs before preparing for procedure. | Certain procedures for which sterile field is prepared may last a long time. The nurse anticipates client's needs so that client can relax and avoid any unnecessary movement that might disrupt procedure. |
| 2. Anticipate number and variety of supplies needed for procedure. | Not all sterile kits contain sufficient amounts or types of supplies. Failure to have necessary supplies will cause nurse to leave sterile field, increasing risk of contamination. |
| **Planning** | |
| 1. Develop goal for procedure: | |
| a. Maintain sterility of all items added to sterile field | During transfer of items onto sterile field items cannot contact anything that is unsterile. |
| 2. Prepare following equipment and supplies: | |
| a. Large package containing sterile item or kit onto which items are to be added | Inside of package wrapper or kit serves as sterile field. The larger the work area the greater the ease of handling sterile supplies. |
| b. Supplies specific to procedure, e.g., dressings, sterile needles, catheter, or instrument sets | |

| **Steps** | **Rationale** |
|---|---|
| c. Sterile container | Used to hold sterile solutions. |
| d. Sterile solutions specific to procedures, e.g., alcohol or povidone-iodine (Betadine) solution | |
| e. Paper towel | |
| f. Sterile gloves | |
| 3. Check dated labels or chemical tapes for date when sterilization period expires. | Supplies considered contaminated once expiration date is reached. |
| 4. Position client comfortably for specific procedure to be performed. If a body part is to be examined or treated, position client so part is accessible. | Client should be able to lie still in one position comfortably during procedure. Movement can cause contamination of sterile items. |
| 5. Explain to client purpose of procedure and importance of sterile technique. | Ensures client's ability to cooperate. |

## Implementation

| Steps | Rationale |
|---|---|
| 1. Apply cap and mask. (May be optional; consult institutional policy.) | Controls spread of airborne microorganisms. |
| 2. Select a clean work surface above waist level. | A sterile object held below a person's waist is contaminated. |
| 3. Assemble equipment at bedside. | Preparation of equipment in advance prevents break in technique. |
| 4. Wash hands thoroughly. | Prevents transmission of infection. |
| ***Preparing sterile work surface*** | |
| 1. Place sterile kit or package containing sterile items on clean, flat work surface above waist level. | Items placed below waist level are considered contaminated. |
| 2. Open sterile kit or package containing sterile items. | |
| a. Sterile kit: Grasp or separate edge of paper wrapper on sterile kit and slowly tear it pulling away from your body. Do not touch inside of wrapper. | Prevents nurse from reaching over sterile field. Once inside of wrapper is contaminated, it can contaminate sterile item if wrapper accidentally slips backward over item. |
| b. Package: Remove tape or seal with expiration date. | |
| ▪ Grasp outer surface of tip of outermost flap. | Outer surface of package is considered unsterile. There is a 2.5-cm (1-in) border around any sterile drape or wrap that is considered contaminated. |
| ▪ Open outermost flap away from body, keeping arm outstretched and away from sterile field (Fig. 38-6). | Reaching over sterile field contaminates it. |
| ▪ Grasp outside surface of edge of first side flap. | Outer surface is considered unsterile. |
| ▪ Open side flap pulling to side, allowing it to lie flat on table surface. Keep your arm to side and not over sterile surface (Fig. 38-7). | Drape or wrapper should lie flat so it will not accidentally raise up and contaminate inner surface or sterile contents. |
| ▪ Repeat steps for second side flap (Fig. 38-8). | |
| ▪ Grasp outside border of last and innermost flap (Fig. 38-9). | Outer surface is considered unsterile. |
| ▪ Stand away from sterile package and pull flap back, allowing it to fall flat on table (Fig. 38-10). | Never reach over a sterile field. |
| 3. Use opened kit or package wrapper as sterile field. | Inner surface of kit and wrapper are considered sterile. |

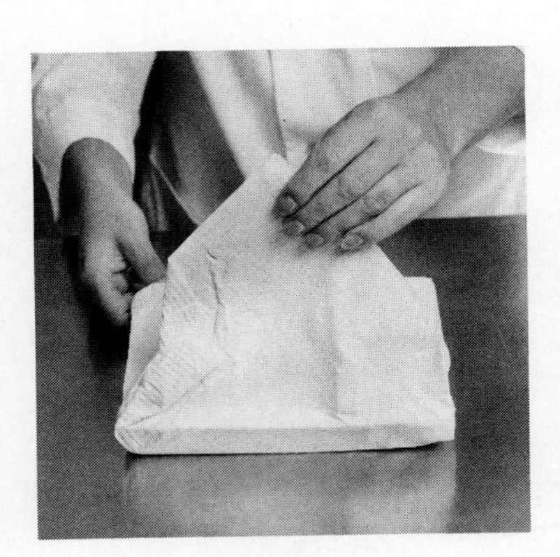

**Fig. 38-6**

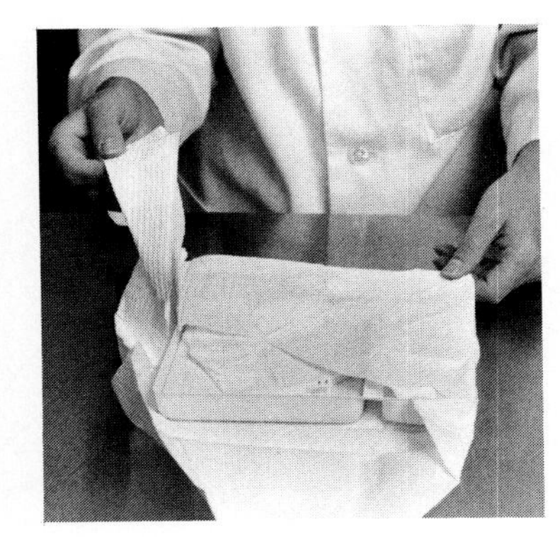

**Fig. 38-7**

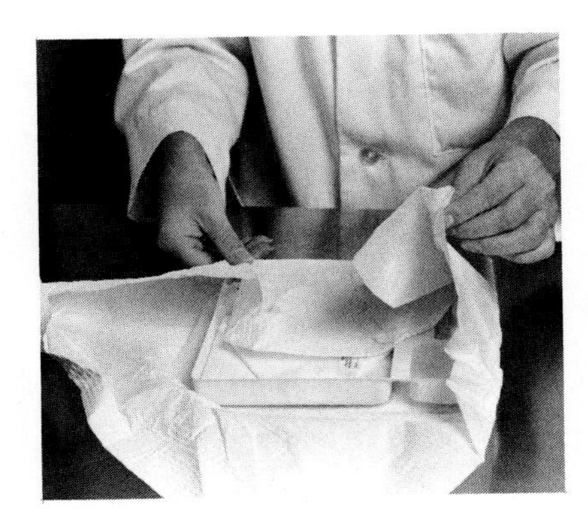

**Fig. 38-8**

| Steps | Rationale |
|---|---|

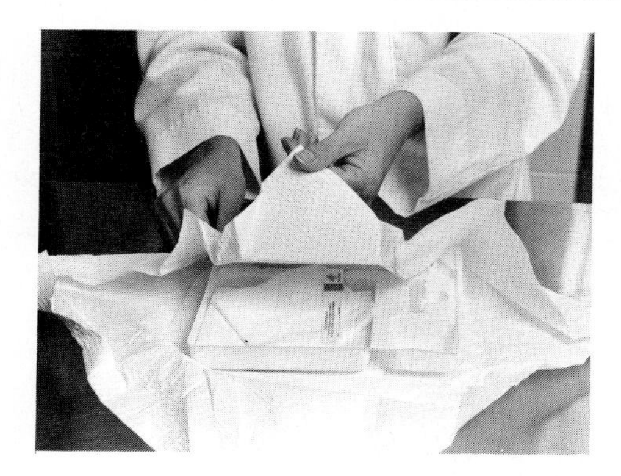

Fig. 38-9

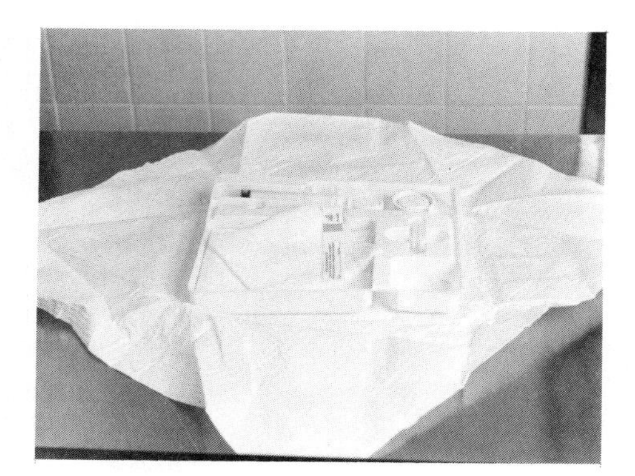

Fig. 38-10

***Preparing a sterile drape*** *(This technique may be optional but is useful when a large work surface is desirable.)*

| Steps | Rationale |
|---|---|
| 1. Place pack containing sterile drape on flat surface and open as described above for package. | Assures sterility of packaged drape. |
| 2. With fingertips of one hand pick up the folded top edge of the sterile drape (Fig. 38-11). | One-inch border around drape is unsterile and may be touched. |
| 3. Gently lift the drape up from its outer cover and let it unfold by itself without touching any object. Discard the outer cover with your other hand. | If a sterile object touches any other nonsterile object it becomes contaminated. |
| 4. With the other hand grasp an adjacent corner of the drape and hold it straight up and away from your body. | Drape can now be properly placed while using two hands. Drape must be held away from unsterile surfaces. |
| 5. Holding the drape, first position the bottom half over the intended work surface (Fig. 38-12). | Prevents nurse from reaching over sterile field. |
| 6. Allow the top half of the drape to be placed over the work surface last (Fig. 38-13). | Creates flat sterile work surface. |

***Adding sterile items***

| Steps | Rationale |
|---|---|
| 1. Open the sterile item (following package directions) while holding the outside wrapper in the nondominant hand. | Frees dominant hand for unwrapping outer wrapper. |
| 2. Carefully peel the wrapper onto the nondominant hand. | Item remains sterile. Inner surface of wrapper covers hand, making it sterile. |
| 3. Being sure the wrapper does not fall down on the sterile field, place the item onto the field at an angle (Fig. 38-14). Do not hold arm over the sterile field. | Prevents reaching over field and contaminating its surface. |
| 4. Dispose of outer wrapper. | Prevents accidental contamination of sterile field. |

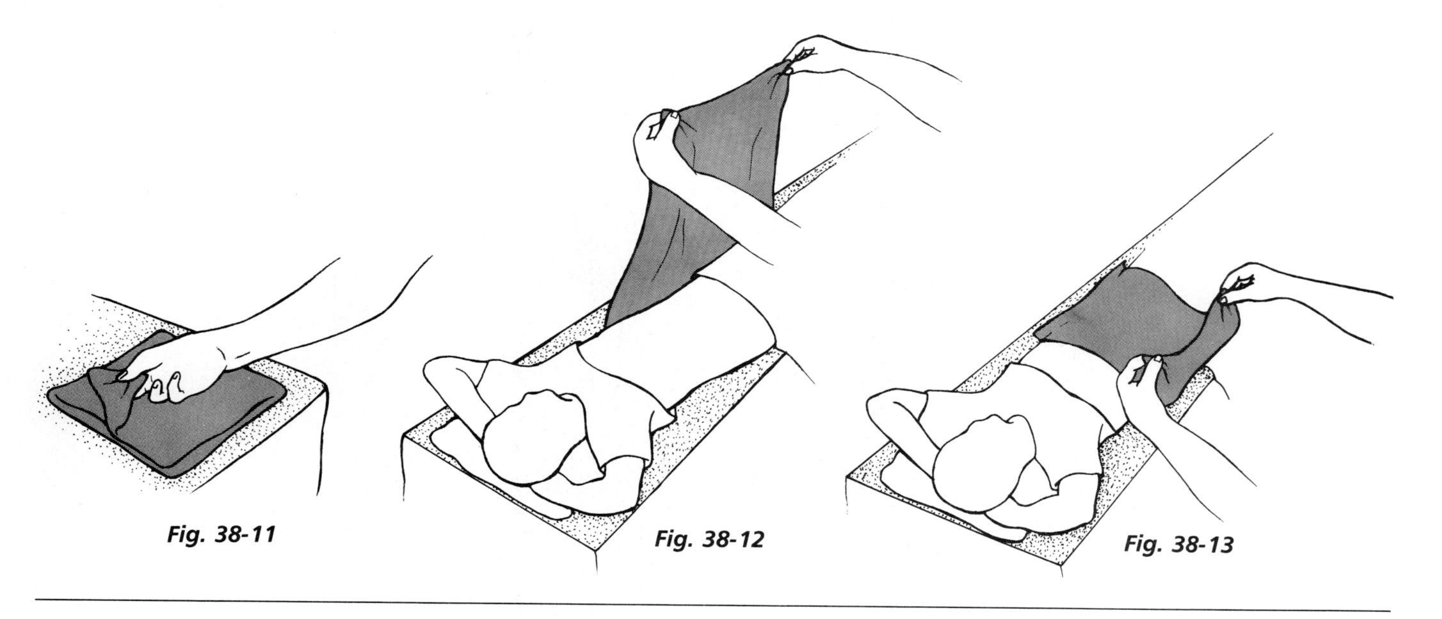

Fig. 38-11 Fig. 38-12 Fig. 38-13

| Steps | Rationale |
|---|---|

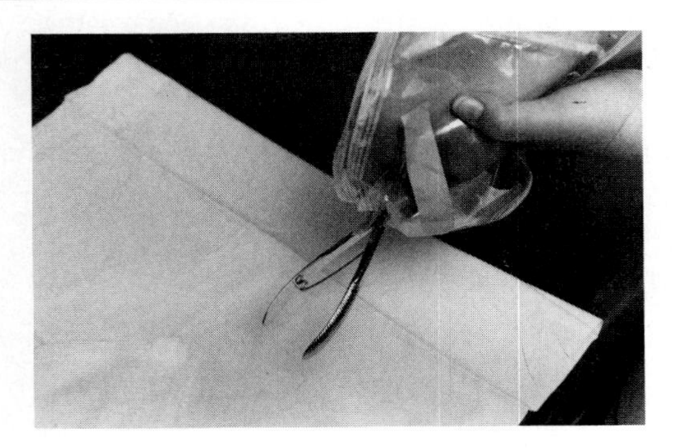

*Fig. 38-14*

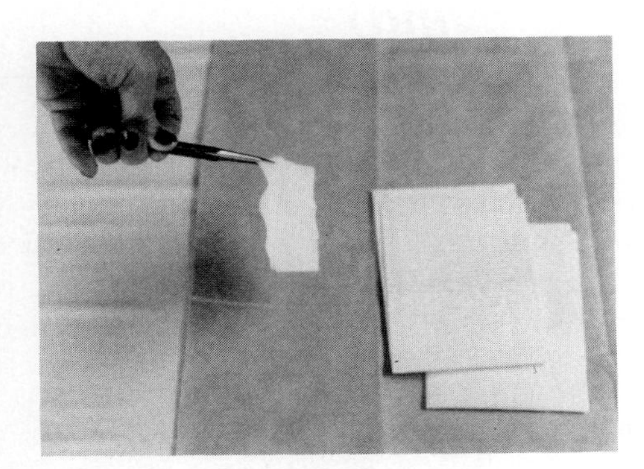

*Fig. 38-15*

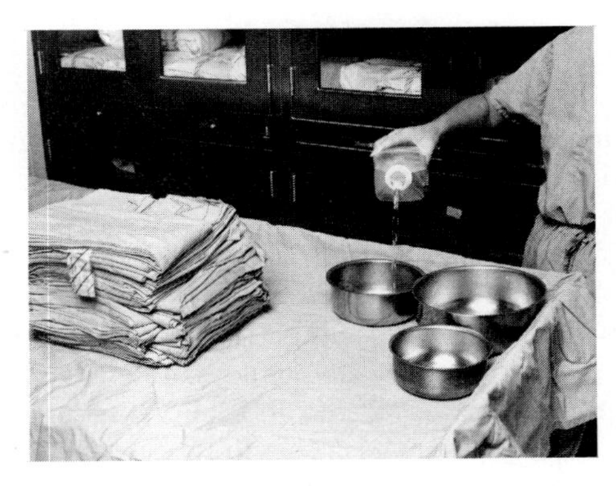

*Fig. 38-16*

### *Transferring items with a forcep*

| Steps | Rationale |
|---|---|
| 1. Open package containing sterile forceps, allowing forceps to lie on surface of inner sterile cover. | Inner cover of package creates temporary sterile field. |
| 2. Open the sterile item (following package directions) that is to be placed on sterile field. | Keeps contents sterile. |
| 3. Carefully grasp handle of forceps and raise them above the waist and away from your body. (Only handles of forceps are considered contaminated). | Keeping ends of forceps in sight and above waist level prevents their contamination. |
| 4. With the ends of the forceps, grasp the sterile item to be placed on the sterile field. (Do not let forceps touch edge of wrapper.) | If sterile portion of forceps touches any object that is unsterile, the forceps becomes contaminated. |
| 5. Raise the sterile item straight up and lift it over and onto the sterile field. Keep the handles of the forceps outside the sterile area (Fig. 38-15). | Reaching over a sterile field with an unsterile object contaminates the field. |

### *Pouring sterile solutions*

| Steps | Rationale |
|---|---|
| 1. Remove cap from bottle of solution and place on clean surface with sterile side (inside) up. | Prevents inside of cap from becoming contaminated. |
| 2. Hold bottle with label in palm of hand. | Prevents solution that may drip down side of bottle from wetting or fading label. |
| 3. Before pouring solution into sterile container, pour small amount (1-2 ml) into disposable cup or plastic lined waste receptacle. | Discarded solution cleans lip of bottle. |
| 4. With edge of bottle held away from edge and above inside of sterile receiving container, slowly pour solution (Fig. 38-16). | Edge of bottle is considered contaminated. Slow pouring prevents splashing that can contaminate underlying sterile field. |
| 5. Wipe off outer edge of bottle with paper towel and replace cap. | Surplus solution on outer edge may cause cap to stick. |

### Special Considerations

- It is always helpful to have another nurse stand by to offer assistance and collect supplies should you overlook an item.
- Many sterile kits have cups or plastic molded sections into which fluids can be poured.
- Do not flip or throw objects onto a sterile field.

### Teaching Considerations

- Instruct the client, family member, or primary care giver on the principles of creating a sterile environment.

### Home Care Considerations

- In the home setting, most care will be performed in a clean environment. In the event that a sterile environment is ordered, the client and family need to be aware of the principles that apply to the sterile environment.
- Assess the client and family's ability and understanding to provide for a sterile environment when needed for the performance of a specific procedure.

---

# SKILL 38-4 Applying Sterile Gloves (Open Gloving)

Wearing sterile gloves allows the nurse to handle and manipulate sterile objects freely. Once thorough handwashing is completed, sterile gloves act as an additional barrier to bacterial transfer. Bacteria can multiply rapidly under gloves and contaminate a wound or sterile object through a puncture in a glove. Thus the nurse is careful to keep glove surfaces intact while handling sharp instruments, pointed needles, and other equipment.

There are two gloving methods: open and closed. Nurses commonly use the open method in clinical areas before changing dressings, inserting urinary catheters, or suctioning airways. Both methods are acceptable in the operating or delivery rooms; however, closed gloving is more often used for initial gloving. Skill 40-1 describes the method for closed gloving.

Sterile gloves are prepackaged with labels indicating glove size. Each nurse should learn the glove size that is most comfortable and fits best. The proper glove size should not stretch so tightly that the glove can easily tear, however, the glove should be tight enough that objects can be picked up easily. Loose rubber may snag or tear. Common glove sizes range from small (size 6-6½) to large (size 8-8½).

### Purpose

1. Provide an additional barrier against microorganisms between the nurse's hands and sterile objects
2. Allow the nurse to handle sterile objects directly without risk of contamination
3. Protect an open wound or body cavity from microorganisms residing on the nurse's hands

---

## Procedure 38-4

| Steps | Rationale |
|---|---|
| **Assessment** | |
| 1. Examine glove package to determine whether it is dry and intact. | Torn or wet package is considered contaminated. |
| 2. Inspect condition of hands for presence of cuts, open lesions, or abrasions. | Lesions harbor microorganisms. When strict surgical asepsis is to be used, presence of such lesions may prevent nurse from participating in procedure. |
| **Planning** | |
| 1. Develop goals for procedure: | |
| a. Maintain sterility of glove surfaces. | Nurse applies gloves carefully so that sterile surfaces remain sterile. |
| 2. Prepare equipment and supplies: | |
| a. Package of sterile gloves in proper glove size | |
| b. Flat working surface, e.g., table above waist level | Sterile items below waist level are considered contaminated. |
| c. Cap and mask (optional) | May not be required in simple procedures using sterile gloves. |
| 3. Explain use of sterile gloves to client (when appropriate). | Explanation helps client understand what he can do to avoid contaminating gloves during procedure. |

| Steps | Rationale |
|---|---|
| **Implementation** | |
| ***Applying gloves*** | |
| 1. Apply mask and cap as needed. | Prevents spread of airborne microorganisms to nurse's hands. |
| 2. Perform thorough handwashing. | Reduces numbers of microorganisms residing on nurse's hands. |
| 3. Arrange glove package on flat surface. | Provides easy opening of package and prevents accidental contamination of gloves. |
| 4. Remove outer package wrapper by carefully peeling apart sides. | Prevents inner glove package from opening accidentally and touching contaminated objects. |
| 5. Grasp the inner package and lay it on a clean, flat surface above waist level. Open package, keeping gloves on wrapper's inside surface. | Sterile object held below waist is considered contaminated. Inner surface of glove package is considered sterile. |
| 6. If gloves are not prepowdered, take packet of powder from package and apply lightly to hands held over wastebasket or sink. | Powder allows gloves to slip on easily. |
| 7. Identify right and left glove. Each glove has cuff approximately 5 cm (2 in) wide. Glove dominant hand first. (Example in figures is of a left-handed person.) | Proper identification of gloves prevents contamination caused by improper fit. Gloving of dominant hand first improves nurse's dexterity with procedure. |
| 8. With thumb and first two fingers of nondominant hand, grasp edge of cuff of glove for dominant hand. Touch glove's inside surface only (Fig. 38-17). | Inner edge of cuff will lie against skin of hand and thus is not considered sterile once applied. |
| 9. Carefully pull glove over dominant hand leaving a cuff and being sure cuff does not roll up wrist. Be sure thumb and fingers are in proper spaces (Fig. 38-18). | If glove's outer surface touches hand or wrist, it is contaminated. |
| 10. With gloved dominant hand, slip fingers underneath second glove's cuff (Fig. 38-19). | Cuff protects gloved fingers. Sterile touching sterile prevents glove contamination. |
| 11. Carefully pull second glove over nondominant hand. Do not allow fingers and thumb of gloved dominant hand to touch any part of exposed nondominant hand. Keep thumb of dominant hand abducted (Fig. 38-20). | Contact of gloved hand with exposed hand results in contamination. |
| 12. Once second glove is on, interlock fingers. Cuffs usually fall down after application. Be sure to touch only sterile sides (Fig. 38-21). | Ensures smooth fit over fingers. |

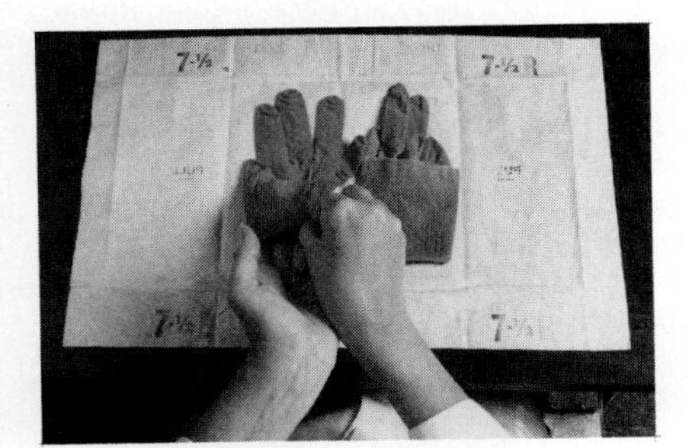

*Fig. 38-17*

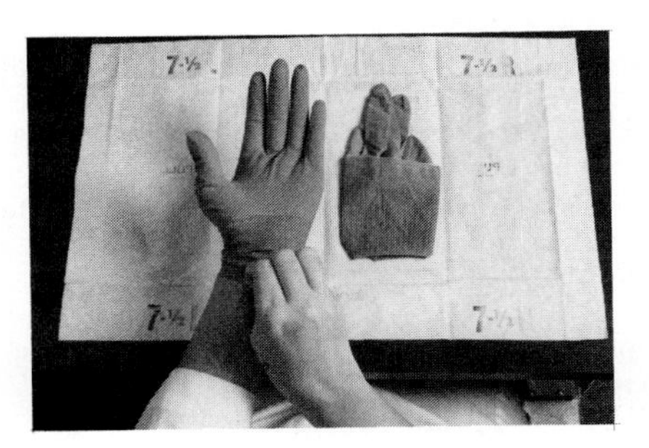

*Fig. 38-18*

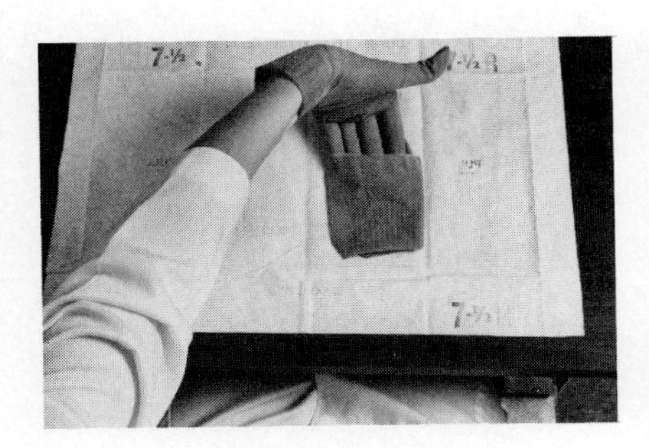

*Fig. 38-19*

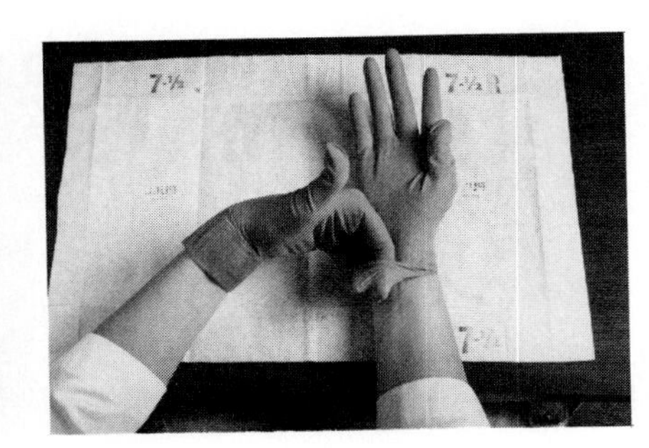

*Fig. 38-20*

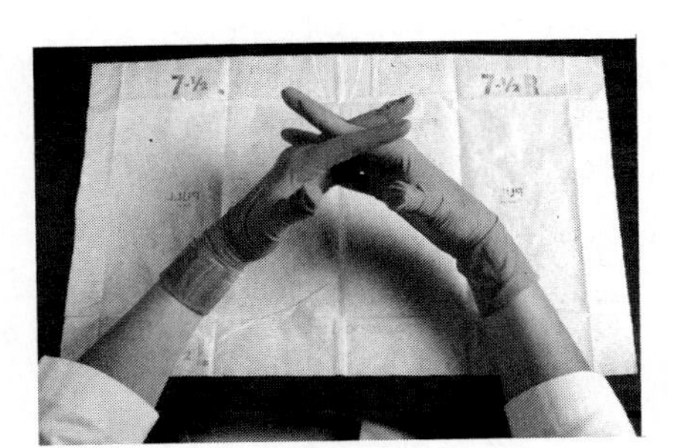

*Fig. 38-21*

| Steps | Rationale |
|---|---|
| ***Removing gloves*** | |
| 13. Take dominant gloved hand and grasp palmar surface of other glove. Do not touch exposed wrist. | After use, outer surface of gloves may contain contaminated material and should not touch surface of hands or wrist. |
| 14. Lift and pull glove straight back off nondominant hand, hold inverted glove in dominant hand, and discard in receptacle. | Minimizes contact with microorganisms. |
| 15. With ungloved nondominant hand, slide fingers just under cuff of gloved hand. Grasp undersurface of cuff and pull glove straight off. Discard in receptacle. | Prevents contact of fingers with any contaminated material that may be on glove's outer surface. |
| 16. Wash hands. | Reduces transfer of microorganisms. |

## Special Considerations

- In operating and delivery rooms, once nurse scrubs hands, an assistant has gloves open, ready to be applied.
- Use of powder is optional. Powder may promote growth of microorganisms on hands.

## Teaching Considerations

- Explain the procedure for opening packages and gloving while performing the procedure.
- Observe the client, family member and/or primary care giver in the performance of the sterile gloving.
- Instruct on the difference between a clean surface, a sterile surface, and a contaminated surface.

**BIBLIOGRAPHY**


Garner JS: Guidelines for prevention of surgical wound infections, 1985, Hospital Infections Program, DCD, PHS, and U.S. Department of Health and Human Services.

Garner JS, Favero MS: Guidelines for handwashing and hospital environmental control, 1985, Hospital Infections Program, CDC, PHS, and U.S. Department of Health and Human Services.

Jacobson G, et al.: Handwashing: ring wearing and number of microorganisms, Nurs Res 34:186, 1985.

Kneedler JA, Dodge GH: Perioperative patient care, Boston, 1983, Blackwell Scientific Publications.

Larson EL, et al.: Physiologic and microbiologic changes in skin related to frequent handwashing, Infect Control 7:54, 1986.

Larson EL: Effects of handwashing agent, handwashing frequency, and clinical area on hand flora, Am J Infect Control 12:76, 1984.

Long B, Phipps W: Medical-surgical nursing, ed 2, St. Louis, 1989, The CV Mosby Co.

Miller B, Keane C: Encyclopedia and dictionary of medicine, nursing, and allied health, Philadelphia, 1987, WB Saunders Co.

Potter PA, Perry AG: Fundamentals of nursing: concepts, process, and practice, St. Louis, ed 2, 1989, The CV Mosby Co.

Nursing Procedures: Nursing reference library, Springhouse, Pa, 1985, Springhouse Corp.

Roth MK, et al.: How to prevent infection in a home care patient, RN 50(11):61, 1987.

Simmons BP: Guidelines for prevention of surgical wound infections, Am J Infect Control 11(4):133, 1983.

Smith S, Duell D: Clinical nursing skills, Los Altos, Calif, 1985, National Nursing Review.

Thompson JM, et al.: Mosby's manual of clinical nursing, ed 2, St. Louis, 1989, The CV Mosby Co.

Walsh J, Persons C, Wieck L: Manual of home health care nursing, Philadelphia, 1987, JB Lippincott Co.

Williams WW: CDC guidelines for infection control in hospital personnel, Infect Control 4:325, 1983.

# UNIT XII

# CARE OF THE SURGICAL CLIENT

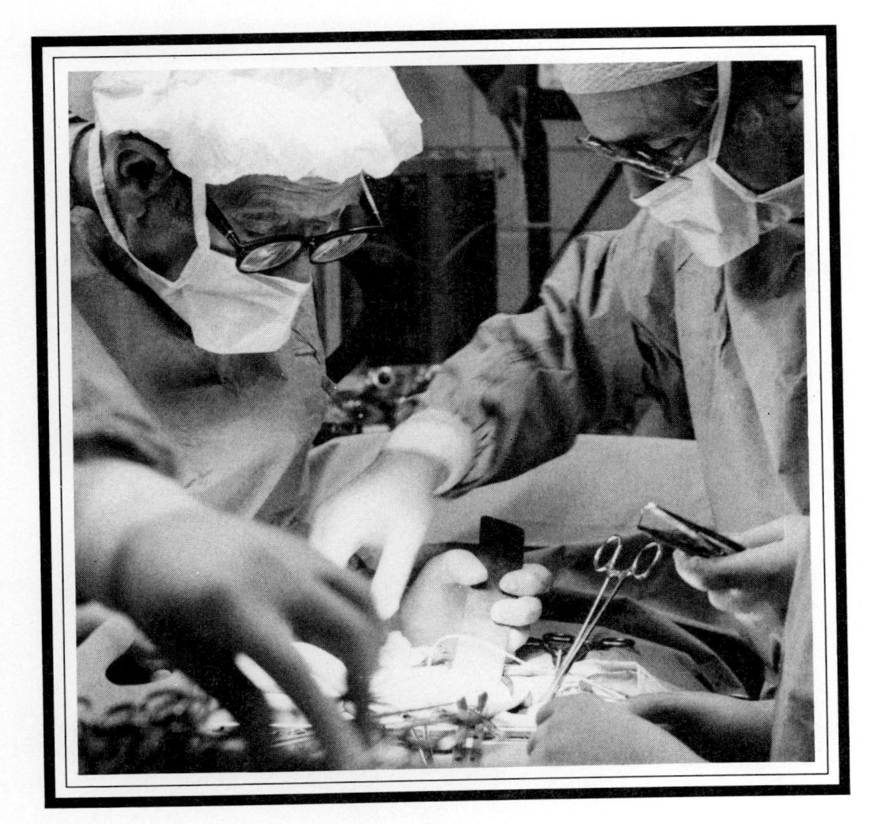

*Surgical procedures represent special challenges for the nurse in providing optimal care for clients. Both emotional and physical factors related to such invasive procedures place stress on the client and demand special skills from the nurse. The nurse must be involved with physically preparing the client for surgery, as well as anticipate the client's needs after surgery.*

*Chapter 39, "Preoperative and Postoperative Care," includes preparatory skills for the surgical procedure, such as shaving and preparing the skin and inserting a nasogastric tube; a teaching skill for the recovery period; and assessment of the postoperative client.*

*Chapter 40, "Intraoperative Care," features assistive skills in the intraoperative phase, including donning a sterile gown and closed gloving.*

# 39

# PREOPERATIVE AND POSTOPERATIVE CARE

## *OBJECTIVES*

*Mastery of content in this chapter will enable the nurse to:*

- Define key terms.
- Describe the benefits of structured preoperative teaching.
- Explain the rationale for each of the four postoperative exercises.
- Successfully instruct a client in performing postoperative exercises.
- Identify the benefits and risks associated with shaving a surgical site.
- Correctly perform a dry and wet shave of a surgical site.
- Describe purposes for nasogastric tube insertion.
- Discuss techniques used to ensure correct tube placement.
- Explain potential complications resulting from a nasogastric tube.
- Correctly insert, check placement, irrigate, and discontinue a nasogastric tube.
- Discuss the differences in nursing assessment during the immediate postoperative period and the convalescent phase of recovery.
- Conduct an assessment of a postoperative client.

## *KEY TERMS*

*Anesthesia*
*Aspiration*
*Atelectasis*
*Dehiscence*
*Decompression*
*Hypovolemic shock*
*Paralytic ileus*
*Postoperative*
*Preoperative*

## *SKILLS*

**39-1** Demonstrating Postoperative Exercises
**39-2** Shaving the Surgical Site
**39-3** Inserting and Maintaining the Nasogastric Tube
**39-4** Performing Postoperative Care of the Surgical Client

Any form of surgery can be a stressful event, whether it is a major surgical procedure occurring in a large medical center or a minor procedure taking place in an outpatient center. The client must frequently make the decision to undergo a procedure that is associated with pain, possible disfigurement, dependence, and even the threat of loss of life. Physiologically, the more complex the surgery the more likely a client is to undergo changes in most major body systems. The surgical client requires a variety of skills from the nurse to adequately prepare for the physiologic and psychologic stressors that surgery imposes.

During the preoperative phase the nurse performs a thorough assessment of the client's physical and emotional status (Table 39-1). Coordination of a variety of diagnostic tests ensures that the surgeon will have the information needed to determine the client's risks during surgery. In preparation for surgery, the nurse instructs the client on postoperative exercises so that the client can actively participate in the recovery process. Certain procedures such as the surgical shave or insertion of a nasogastric tube may be performed to protect the client from risks associated with surgery. The nurse also communicates pertinent information to all members of the health care team so that the client receives the comprehensive care required.

During the postoperative phase, when the client returns from the operating room, the nurse is initially responsible for assessing the client's physical status to monitor any changes during the recovery process. Once the client's condition stabilizes the nurse focuses efforts on returning the client to a functional level of wellness as soon as possible within the limitations created by surgery. The speed of a client's recovery depends on how effectively the nurse can anticipate potential complications, initiate necessary supportive and preventive therapies, and actively involve client and family in the recovery process. Each client's plan of care is individualized to provide an improved state of wellness and to maximize an ultimate level of independence.

## GUIDELINES

1. Know the type and nature of any previous surgery. Anatomical and physiological alterations may affect the client's health care needs.
2. Identify the factors and conditions that may increase a client's risks during surgery. Preoperative preparation and postoperative care will depend upon these risks.
3. Know the rationale for and extent of impending surgery. Each type of surgical procedure requires different types of nursing care.
4. Administer pain relief therapies according to the client's needs postoperatively. Pain can become a significant barrier to the surgical client's recovery.
5. Encourage the client's independence as soon as possible during the postoperative period. This will minimize the occurrence of postoperative complications.
6. Anticipate how surgery will affect the client's ability to return home to a functional life-style. Early discharge planning, client education, and rehabilitation measures are needed to prepare the client to return home.

## PREREQUISITE KNOWLEDGE

1. Principles of teaching and learning.
2. Principles of medical asepsis.
3. Principles of oxygenation and thrombus formation (Skill 39-1).
4. Anatomical structure and function of the gastrointestinal tract (Skill 39-3).
5. Principles of medication administration (Skill 39-4).
6. Principles of fluid and electrolyte balance (Skill 39-4).

***TABLE 39-1*** Assessment of the Surgical Client

| Assessment Category | Key Criteria |
|---|---|
| Nursing history | Past experience with surgery<br>Client's and family's perceptions and understanding of surgery<br>Medication history<br>Allergies<br>Previous surgeries<br>Smoking habits<br>Alcohol ingestion<br>Family support<br>Occupation<br>Emotional health |
| Physical examination | General surgery<br>Head and neck<br>Integument<br>Thorax and lungs<br>Heart and vascular<br>Abdomen<br>Neurological |
| Risk factors | Age<br>Nutrition<br>Radiotherapy<br>Fluid and electrolyte balance<br>Preexisting infection |

## PREREQUISITE SKILLS

1. Physical assessment (Chapter 13).
2. Basic handwashing techniques (Chapter 37).
3. Assessment of vital signs (Chapter 12) (Skill 39-4).
4. Pain relief measures (Chapter 5) (Skill 39-4).
5. Administering intravenous therapy (Chapter 23) (Skill 39-4).

# *SKILL 39-1 Demonstrating Postoperative Exercises*

Structured preoperative teaching has a positive influence on a surgical client's recovery. The nurse provides information and skills that will help clients understand the surgical experience and participate actively in the recovery process. Ideally a client should have adequate time to learn about the surgical experience. Often teaching occurs the evening before surgery when clients are most anxious. However, more and more health care institutions are realizing the value of preparing clients well in advance so that clients gain the knowledge and skills needed to participate in their own care. Clients now frequently receive instruction before admission to a hospital or an outpatient surgical clinic. Teaching booklets and videotapes are available to supplement any instruction a nurse provides. Ultimately a well-designed preoperative teaching program can improve a client's physical functioning and sense of well-being, and shorten the length of hospital stay. A detailed discussion and demonstration of postoperative exercises is vital to any preoperative teaching plan.

The postoperative exercises included in the teaching plan are diaphragmatic breathing, effective coughing, turning, and leg exercises. During the discussion of these exercises, the nurse explains the relationship between the exercises and the physiological principles that make them important. Through specific explanations and guided practice the nurse helps develop client commitment to the recovery process. The nurse provides demonstration of the exercises and then continues to coach the client through several return practice sessions. Commitment to the exercise regimen is evidenced by the client's independent practice.

Whenever possible the nurse includes family members or other significant persons in the practice sessions. Frequently, these individuals are with the client during the postoperative period and can thus serve as coaches. The nurse also provides the client with information about the sensations typically experienced after surgery, such as incisional pain and tightness of dressings. The information helps the client interpret realistically the events that occur in the postoperative period. As a result, the client is able to conserve his energies and attend to performing the exercises that will assist in his recovery.

**Purposes**

1. Improve lung expansion and oxygen delivery with minimum expenditure of energy.
2. Facilitate expectoration of mucus that accumulates in the airways following general anesthesia.
3. Improve blood flow in the lower extremities so as to reduce venous stasis.
4. Reduce incidence of postoperative complications.
5. Provide clients a means to actively participate in the recovery process.

## *Procedure 39-1*

| Steps | Rationale |
|---|---|
| **Assessment** | |
| 1. Assess client's risk for postoperative respiratory complications. Review client's medical history to identify presence of chronic pulmonary condition (e.g., emphysema or asthma), any condition that affects chest wall movement, history of smoking, and presence of reduced hemoglobin. | General anesthesia predisposes client to respiratory problems because lungs are not fully inflated during surgery; cough reflex is suppressed and mucous collects within airway passages.<br>Postoperatively, client may have reduced lung volume and require greater efforts to cough and deep breathe; inadequate lung expansion can lead to atelectasis and pneumonia; client is at greater risk to develop respiratory complications if other chronic lung conditions are present; smoking damages ciliary clearance and increases mucous secretion. |
| 2. Assess client's ability to cough and deep breathe by having him take a deep breath and observing movement of shoulders and chest wall. Measure chest excursion during deep breath. Ask client to cough after taking a deep breath. | Reveals maximum potential for chest expansion and ability to cough forcefully; serves as baseline to measure client's ability to perform exercises postoperatively. |
| 3. Assess client's risk for postoperative thrombus formation (elderly, immobilized clients are most at risk). | Following general anesthesia, circulation is slowed and when rate of blood flow is slowed, there is greater tendency for clot formation. Immobilization results in decreased muscular contraction in lower extremities, which promotes venous stasis. |
| 4. Assess client's willingness and capability to learn exercises; note factors such as attention span, level of consciousness, language level. | Ability to learn depends on three conditions: readiness, ability, and learning environment. Readiness to learn implies that client has accepted fact that surgery is treatment of choice. |
| 5. Assess family members' willingness to learn and to support client postoperatively. | Family's presence postoperatively can be potential motivating factor for client's recovery; family member can coach clients on exercise performance. |
| 6. Assess client's medical orders preoperatively and postoperatively. | May require adaptations in way exercises are performed. |
| **Nursing Diagnosis** | |
| 1. Cluster data to reveal actual or potential nursing diagnoses: | |
| a. Ineffective airway clearance: related to ineffective cough. | Ineffective cough, pain, and fatigue related to surgery can interfere with client's ability to clear airway. |
| b. Impaired physical mobility: related to bed rest. | Immobility will increase risk of pulmonary and circulatory complications unless exercises are performed. |
| c. Anxiety: related to impending surgery. | Will influence amount of information client is willing and able to learn. |
| d. Altered thought processes: related to pain. | Number of factors can interfere with client's ability to attend to nurse's instructions e.g., pain, anxiety. |
| **Planning** | |
| 1. Develop individualized goals for the client based on nursing diagnoses: | |
| a. Promote full lung expansion postoperatively. | Successful deep breathing will maintain ventilation. |
| b. Maintain clear airways postoperatively. | Effective coughing will clear airways of mucus. |

| Steps | Rationale |
|---|---|
| c. Promote mobility and range of motion of lower extremities postoperatively. | Leg exercises will reduce risk of venous stasis. |
| d. Provide opportunity for practice and return demonstration of exercises. | Necessary to ensure client's learning. |
| e. Encourage client's active participation in care. | Exercises can be independently performed by client. |
| 2. Prepare following supplies: | |
| a. Pillow (optional) | Client may prefer to use a pillow to splint incision when coughing to reduce discomfort. |
| 3. Explain postoperative exercises to the client, including their importance to recovery, and physiological benefits. | Information can motivate client to attend and learn. Persons tend to learn new skills when benefits can be gained. |

## Implementation

### *Teaching diaphragmatic breathing*

| Steps | Rationale |
|---|---|
| 1. Assist client to comfortable sitting or standing position. If client chooses to sit, assist to side of bed or to upright position in chair. | Upright position facilitates diaphragmatic excursion. |
| 2. Stand or sit facing client. | Client will be able to observe breathing exercise performed by nurse. |
| 3. Instruct client to place palms of hands across from each other, down, and along lower borders of anterior rib cage; place tips of third finger lightly together (Fig. 39-1). Demonstrate for client. | Position of hands allows client to feel movement of chest and abdomen as diaphragm descends and lungs inside chest wall expand. |
| 4. Have client take slow, deep breaths, inhaling through nose. Tell client to feel middle fingers separate as client inhales. Demonstrate for client. | Slow, deep breath prevents panting or hyperventilation. Inhaling through nose warms, humidifies, and filters air. |
| 5. Avoid using chest and shoulders while inhaling and instruct client in same manner. | Using auxiliary chest and shoulder muscles during breathing increases useless energy expenditures. |
| 6. Hold slow, deep breath for count of 3, and then slowly exhale through mouth as if blowing out a candle. Explain that client will feel middle finger tips touch as chest wall contracts. | Allows for gradual expulsion of all air. |
| 7. Repeat breathing exercise three to five times. | Allows client to observe slow, rhythmical breathing pattern. |
| 8. Have client practice exercise. Client is instructed to take 10 slow, deep breaths every 2 hr while awake during postoperative period until mobile. Another option is to use incentive spirometry (Chapter 14). | Repetition of exercise reinforces learning. Regular deep breathing will prevent postoperative complications. |

### *Controlled coughing*

| Steps | Rationale |
|---|---|
| 1. Explain importance of maintaining an upright position. | Position facilitates diaphragm excursion and enhances thorax expansion. |
| 2. Demonstrate coughing. Take two slow, deep breaths, inhaling through nose and exhaling through mouth. | Deep breaths expand lungs fully so that air moves behind mucus and facilitates effects of coughing. |
| 3. Inhale deeply a third time and hold breath to count of 3. Cough fully for two to three consecutive coughs without inhaling between coughs. (Tell client to push all air out of lungs.) | Consecutive coughs help remove mucus more effectively and completely than one forceful cough. |
| 4. Caution client against just clearing throat instead of coughing. | Clearing throat does not remove mucus from deep in airways. |
| 5. If surgical incision is to be either abdominal or thoracic, teach client to place pillow over incisional area and place hands over pillow to splint incisional area. During breathing and coughing exercises, client splints incision with pillow to reduce discomfort. | Surgical incision cuts through muscles, tissues, and nerve endings. Deep breathing and coughing exercises place additional stress on suture line and cause discomfort. Splinting incision with pillow provides firm support and reduces incisional pulling. |
| 6. Client continues to practice coughing exercises, splinting imaginary incision. The client is instructed to cough two to three times every 2 hr while awake (Fig. 39-2). | Value of deep coughing with splinting is stressed to effectively expectorate mucus with minimal discomfort. |

### *Turning*

| Steps | Rationale |
|---|---|
| 1. Instruct client to assume supine position to right side of bed. Side rails on both sides of bed should be in up position. | Positioning begins on right side of bed so that turning to left side will not cause client to roll toward bed's edge. |
| 2. Have client place the left hand over incisional area to splint it. | Splinting incision supports and minimizes pulling on suture line during turning. |
| 3. Instruct client to keep left leg straight and flex right knee up and over left leg. | Straight leg stabilizes the client's position. Flexed right leg shifts weight for easier turning. |

| Steps | Rationale |
|---|---|

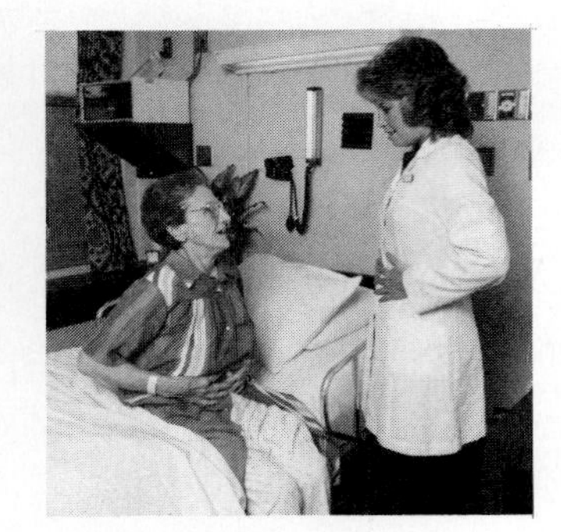

Fig. 39-1

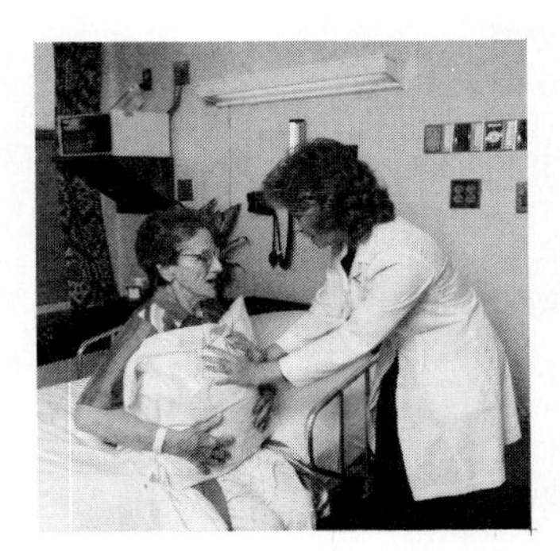

Fig. 39-2

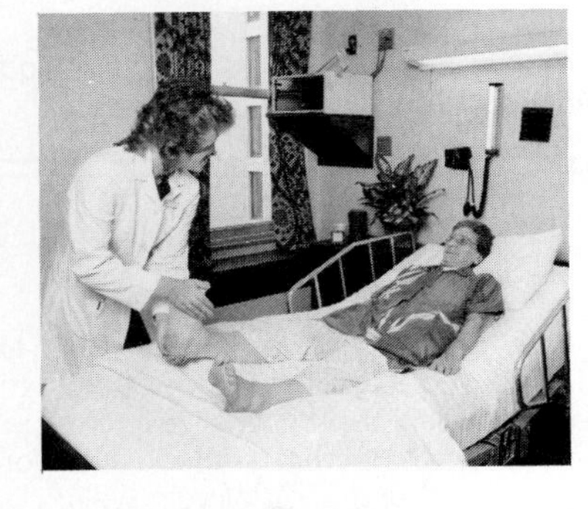

Fig. 39-3

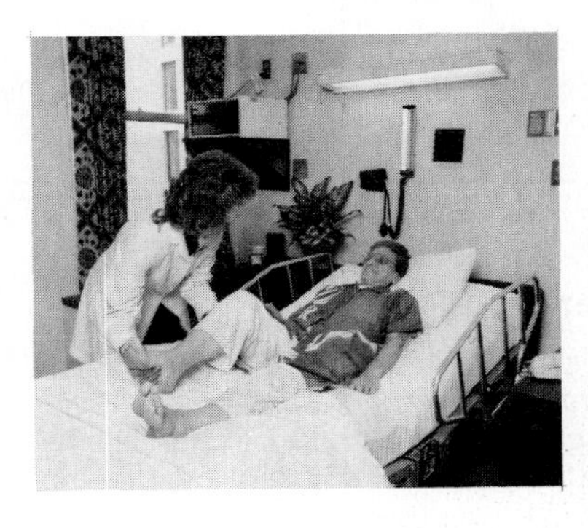

Fig. 39-4

| Steps | Rationale |
|---|---|
| 4. Have client grab left side rail with right hand, pull toward left, and roll onto left side. | Pulling toward side rail reduces effort needed for turning. |
| 5. Instruct client to turn every 2 hours while awake. | Reduces risk of vascular and pulmonary complications. |
| ***Leg exercises*** | |
| 1. Have client assume supine position in bed. Demonstrate leg exercises by performing passive range of motion exercises and simultaneously explaining exercise. | Provides normal anatomical position of lower extremities. |
| 2. Rotate each ankle in complete circle. Instruct client to draw imaginary circles with big toe. Repeat five times. | Leg exercises maintain joint mobility and promote venous return. |
| 3. Alternate dorsiflexion and plantar flexion by moving both feet up and down. Direct client to feel calf muscles contract and relax alternately (Fig. 39-3). | Stretches and contracts gastrocnemius muscles. |
| 4. Client continues leg exercises by alternately flexing and extending knees. Repeat five times (Fig. 39-4). | Contracts muscles of upper legs and maintains knee mobility. |
| 5. Client alternately raises each leg straight up from bed surface, keeping legs straight. | Promotes contraction and relaxation of quadriceps muscles. |
| 6. Have client continue to practice exercises at least every 2 hr while awake. Client is instructed to coordinate turning and leg exercises with diaphragmatic breathing and coughing exercises. | Repetition of sequence of performing exercises reinforces learning. Establishes routine for exercises that develops habit for performance. Sequence of exercises should be leg exercises, turning, breathing, and coughing. |

## Follow-up Activities

| | |
|---|---|
| 1. Instead of diaphragmatic breathing client can also benefit from use of incentive spirometer (Skill 14-6). | Incentive spirometer causes forced inspiration against resistance, maximizing ventilation. |

## Evaluation

| | |
|---|---|
| 1. Observe client's ability to perform all four exercises independently. | Ensures client has learned correct technique. |
| 2. Observe family members' ability to coach client. | Family member can assist positively or interfere with correct technique. |
| ***Expected outcomes*** | |
| 1. Client is able to correctly deep breathe, cough, turn, and perform leg exercises throughout postoperative period. | Client's ability to perform exercises should be ensured by return demonstration. |

| Steps | Rationale |
|---|---|
| ***Unexpected outcomes*** | |
| 1. Client is unable to perform exercises correctly. | Additional instruction needed. Anxiety, pain, complications, or fatigue alter client's performance. |
| 2. Client will develop pulmonary and circulatory complications postoperatively. | Atelectasis and venous stasis develop. |

## Recording and Reporting

| | |
|---|---|
| 1. Record which exercises have been demonstrated to client and whether client can perform exercises independently. | Documents client education and provides data for instructional follow-up. |
| 2. Report any problems client has in practicing exercises to nurse assigned to client on next shift. | Provides consistency and follow-up with teaching. |

## Follow-up Activities

| | |
|---|---|
| 1. Increase frequency of observation of exercises if client has difficulty practicing exercises. | Nurses' judgment determines need for additional teaching or additional demonstration of exercises. |

## Special Considerations

- Observe and report to physician if client has had a cold or upper respiratory infection within past week.
- Surgery involving thorax will impair client's ability to effectively deep breathe or cough because of incisional pain.
- Highly anxious clients or those in severe pain will have difficulty learning and performing postoperative exercises.
- Encourage client to ask for pain medication ½ hour before performing exercises postoperatively.
- Clients at risk for post-operative thrombus formation include elderly and those immobilized by preexisting medical conditions or treatments applied postoperatively.
- Client may usually be positioned upright with head of bed elevated initially postoperatively. If client must remain flat in bed, stress that exercises can still be performed.
- Coughing may be contraindicated following brain, spinal, or eye surgery. Some clients may be restricted from flexing their legs postoperatively, e.g., back surgery or aortic or femoral repair.
- If client's surgery involves one or both extremities, surgeon must order leg exercises in postoperative period. Legs unaffected by surgery can be safely exercised unless client has preexisting phlebothrombosis (blood clot formation) or thrombophlebitis (inflammation of vein wall).

## Teaching Considerations

- Teach client/primary caregiver about surgical procedure, healing process, sutures, dressing, drains, feeding tubes, pain control, and diet. State rationale for each.

## Home Care Considerations

- Review coughing, deep breathing, and relaxation exercises before admission to hospital or surgical clinic and after discharge.

# *SKILL 39-2 Shaving the Surgical Site*

The body's first line of defense against infection is intact skin. A break in the integrity of the skin as a result of a surgical incision can become a potential source of infection. Before surgery, the skin overlying the proposed surgical site is thoroughly cleansed to minimize skin contamination and the risk of postoperative wound infection. Preparation of the incisional area often begins the evening before surgery and involves washing the skin and shaving the skin around the incisional site.

The skin is cleansed by scrubbing with an antimicrobial soap, e.g., chlorhexidine, two or more times. The client can perform the scrubbing during either a bath or shower. If an enema is given in preparation for surgery, the final shower or bath should be given after the enema. The client may also shampoo hair if surgery involves the head, neck, or even the upper chest.

Shaving the surgical site removes hair that serves as a reservoir for infection, although evidence shows that wound infections due to small cuts made by a razor occur more often in clients who are shaved preoperatively than clients who are not shaved. Shaving today is usually done immediately before the operation to reduce the time for potential bacterial growth. The procedure may be done by a nurse or surgical technician. The CDC recommends clippers or a depilatory to remove hair to minimize skin abrasions and cuts.

**Purposes**

1. Prevent infection of the surgical site by removing hair that holds bacteria
2. Improve the surgeon's view of the surgical site by removing thick or coarse hair

## Procedure 39-2

| Steps | Rationale |
|---|---|
| **Assessment** | |
| 1. Inspect general condition of skin. | If lesions, irritations, or signs of skin infection are present, shaving should not be done. These conditions increase chances for postoperative wound infections. |
| 2. Review physician's order or the facilities' procedure book for specific area to be shaved. | Ensures correct area is shaved. |
| **Nursing Diagnosis** | |
| 1. Cluster data to reveal actual or potential nursing diagnoses: | |
| a. Impaired skin integrity: related to presence of lesions, irritations, etc. | Shaving may be deferred. |
| b. Anxiety: related to exposure of body part. | Nurse must take care to avoid embarrassing client. |
| c. Body image disturbance: related to hair loss. | Male clients may lose sense of manliness from loss of hair. |
| d. Potential impaired skin integrity: related to shaving. | Nurse takes care to avoid nicks in skin. |
| **Planning** | |
| 1. Develop individualized goals for client based on nursing diagnoses: | |
| a. Prevent skin irritation and infection. | Use of proper aseptic and shaving techniques will prevent skin injury. |
| b. Skin clear of body hair. | Exposes site for surgical incision. |
| c. Client remains comfortable. | Incorrect shaving technique can cause discomfort. |
| 2. Prepare following equipment and supplies: | |
| a. Portable lamp | Needed if room light is not sufficient. Good lighting important to inspect skin condition. |
| b. Bath blanket | Used for draping client to provide privacy. |
| c. Towel or waterproof pad | |
| *Clipping:* | |
| a. Electric clippers | Used to remove short hair. |
| b. Scissors | Used to cut long body hair. |
| c. Towel | |
| d. Cotton balls, applicators, and antiseptic solution (optional) | |
| *Wet shave:* | |
| a. Razor with extra blade | Sharp blade minimizes skin abrasion. |
| b. Clean basin with warm water | Used to cleanse skin in body crevices. |
| c. Gauze sponges | |
| d. Basin with liquid antiseptic soap mixed with water (avoid using iodophor for clients with allergies) | |
| e. Washcloth | |
| f. Cotton balls, cotton applicators, and antiseptic solution (optional) | |
| 3. Explain procedure and rationale for removal of hair over large surface area. | Promotes cooperation and minimizes anxiety because client may think incision will be as large as shaved site. |
| **Implementation** | |
| 1. Wash hands. | Reduces transmission of microorganisms. |
| 2. Close room doors or bedside curtains. | Provides client privacy. |
| 3. Raise bed to high position. | Avoids need to bend over for long periods of time. |
| 4. Position client comfortably with surgical site accessible. | Shave and skin preparation can take several minutes. Nurse should have easy access to hard to reach areas. |
| 5. Hair clipping: | |
| a. Lightly dry area to be clipped with towel. | Removes moisture, which interferes with clean cut of clippers. |

| Steps | Rationale |
|---|---|
| b. Hold clippers in dominant hand, about 1 cm above skin, and cut hair in direction it grows. Clip small area at a time. | Prevents pulling on hair and abrasion of skin. |
| c. Rearrange drapes as necessary. | Prevents unnecessary exposure of body parts. |
| d. Lightly brush off cut hair with towel. | Removes contaminated hair and promotes client's comfort. Improves visibility of area being clipped. |
| e. When clipped area is over body crevices, (for example, umbilicus or groin), clean crevices with cotton-tipped applicators or cotton ball dipped in antiseptic solution, then dry. | Removes secretions, dirt, and any remaining hair clippings, which harbor microorganisms. |
| 6. Wet shave | |
| a. Place towel or waterproof pads under body part to be shaved. | Prevents soiling of bed linen. |
| b. Drape client with bath blanket, leaving only area to be shaved at one time (10-20 cm [4-8 in]) exposed. | Prevents unnecessary exposure of body parts and reduces client's anxiety. |
| c. Adjust lamp. | Provide maximum skin illumination. |
| d. Lather skin with gauze sponges dipped in antiseptic soap. | Softens hair and reduces friction from razor. |
| e. Shave small area at a time. With nondominant hand hold gauze sponge to stabilize skin. Hold razor at 45-degree angle in dominant hand and shave hair in direction it grows. Use short, gentle strokes (Fig. 39-5). | Shaving small areas minimizes cutting skin; shaving in direction hair grows prevents pulling. 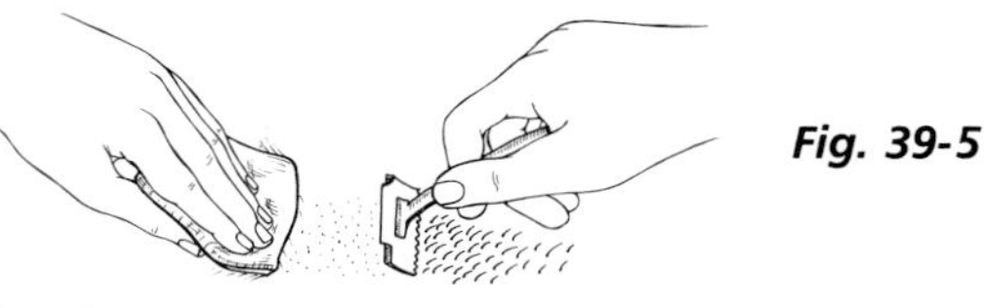 ***Fig. 39-5*** |
| f. Rinse razor in basin of water as soap and hair accumulate on the blade. Change and discard blades as they become dull. | Maintains clean, sharp razor edge to promote client's comfort. |
| g. Rearrange bath blanket as each portion of shave is completed. | Maintains client's comfort and privacy. |
| h. Use washcloth and warm water to rinse away remaining hair and soap solution. Change water as needed. | Reduces skin irritation and allows good visualization of skin. |
| i. If shaved area is over body crevices, e.g., umbilicus or groin, cleanse with cotton-tipped applicators or cotton balls dipped in antiseptic solution. | Removes secretions, dirt, and other remaining hair clippings, which harbor microorganisms. |
| j. Dry crevices with cotton balls or applicators. | Reduces maceration of skin from retained moisture. |
| k. Discard waterproof towel or pad. | Reduces spread of microorganisms. |
| l. Observe skin closely for any nicks or cuts. | Any break in skin integrity increases risk of wound infection. |
| m. Tell client that procedure is completed. | Relieves client's anxiety. |
| n. Clean and dispose of equipment according to policy. | Reduces spread of infection and reduces risk of injury from razor blades. |
| 7. Wash hands. | Reduces spread of microorganisms. |

## Evaluation

| | |
|---|---|
| 1. Inspect condition of skin after completion of hair removal. | Determines if there is remaining hair or if skin was cut. |
| 2. Question if clients feels burning or discomfort. | Indicates presence of skin cut or irritation. |

### *Expected outcomes*

| | |
|---|---|
| 1. Client's skin is free of all hair over shaved area. | Skin has received initial preparation for surgical incision to eventually be made. |
| 2. Skin is free of visible cuts or nicks. | Less likelihood of skin infections developing. |
| 3. Client denies burning or discomfort. | Skin intact without abrasions or cuts. |

### *Unexpected outcomes*

| | |
|---|---|
| 1. Client's skin is not totally clear of all hair. | Exceptionally thick hair difficult to cut first time. Another shave is necessary. |
| 2. Client's skin becomes cut or nicked. | Blade may be dulled. Risk of postoperative wound infection. |
| 3. Client experiences burning over shaved site. | Local nicks or cuts cause burning. |

## Recording and Reporting

| | |
|---|---|
| 1. Record procedure, area clipped or shaved, and condition of skin before and after in nurses' notes. | Documents procedure performed and condition of skin before surgery. |

| Steps | Rationale |
|---|---|
| 2. Report any skin alterations or nicks or cuts in skin to surgeon. | Skin problems may cause cancellation of surgery. |

### Follow-up Activities

| | |
|---|---|
| 1. Following shave, client should be checked to be sure that sheets are dry, bath blanket is removed, hospital clothing is being worn, and client is placed in comfortable position. | Make client comfortable and provide a period of rest before transfer to operating room. |

### Special Considerations

- Most operating room departments have manual describing areas to be shaved for each type of surgery. Eyebrows are never shaved because hair does not grow back over scar tissue. Usually the face and neck of females and children are not shaved. Usually preparation for head and neck surgery does not occur until after client is anesthetized.
- During emergencies, client may be shaved in operating room to save critical time. If this is the case, heavy lather should be used to help control hair clippings removed by the razor. Following shave, carefully remove loose hair so that it does not remain on linen and possibly get into surgical wound.
- Most hospitals use disposable razors to prevent transmission of serum hepatitis from a contaminated razor. If disposable razor is not available, an autoclaved razor and new blade should be used for each client.
- Many nurses begin by trying to shave too slowly, but this can pull hair.
- If client's skin becomes nicked or cut, some institutional policies and procedures may require an incident report to be completed.
- Razor blades are discarded into contaminated syringe and needle holders.
- Scissors may be used to trim especially long hair. Never dispose of client's scalp hair without permission, since this is considered personal property. Some client's use hair for wig.

## *SKILL 39-3 Inserting and Maintaining the Nasogastric Tube*

A nasogastric (NG) tube is a pliable plastic tube that is inserted through the client's nasopharynx and into the stomach. The tube is hollow and allows for removal of gastric contents and the introduction of liquids into the stomach. The primary use of the NG tube in the surgical client is for decompression or removal of flatus and fluids from the stomach. The NG tube helps prevent postoperative vomiting and distention caused by reduced peristalsis resulting from general anesthesia, manipulation of the viscera during surgery, or obstruction of the operative site by edema. When used for decompression, it is usually connected to an intermittent gastric suction device. The nurse routinely measures contents of the suction container to monitor intake and output.

The tubes most commonly used for decompression are the Levin and Salem sump tubes. The Levin tube is single-lumen and has several holes near the tip. The Salem sump tube is a double-lumen tube; one provides an air vent and the other is for removal of gastric contents.

The client with an NG tube presents several nursing care problems. One of the greatest problems is maintaining a client's comfort. Some clients state that the discomfort from the tube exceeds the pain from the surgical incision. The tube is a source of constant irritation to the nasal mucosa. To lessen this discomfort, the tube should be secured with tape to the nose and then to the client's gown with a pin to prevent unnecessary movement. Other comfort measures include removing excess secretions from around the nares and lubricating the nostrils and tube with a water-soluble lubricant to avoid crusting of secretions. With one nostril occluded, the client tends to breathe through the mouth, and the lips and tongue may become dry and cracked. Mouth care should be provided at least every 2 hours to minimize dehydration. Frequent mouth rinses with cool water are helpful, although the nurse should caution the client not to swallow the water. The client may be allowed to chew gum to increase salivation or suck on small ice chips, which helps relieve the dryness in the throat. Sometimes an ice bag applied externally to the throat provides relief.

Another nursing care problem is maintaining patency of the tube. The tip of the tube may become occluded because the tube rests against the stomach wall or because it becomes blocked with thick secretions. The NG tube should be irrigated regularly with normal saline and an Asepto or cone-tipped syringe. Turning the client facilitates draining the stomach. If necessary, the nurse should reposition the tube by advancing or withdrawing it slightly. However some surgical procedures require that only a physician may reposition the tube. For example, a nurse should not reposition an NG tube for a client who has had gastric or esophageal surgery.

**Purposes**

1. Remove secretions and gas from the gastrointestinal tract to prevent or relieve abdominal distention.
2. To irrigate the stomach because of active bleeding, poisoning, or gastric dilation.

## *Procedure 39-3*

| Steps | Rationale |
|---|---|
| ***Assessment*** | |
| 1. Inspect condition of client's oral cavity. | Determines baseline condition of oral cavity so as to determine need for special nursing measures for oral hygiene following tube placement. |
| 2. Palpate client's abdomen. | Baseline determination of level of abdominal distention will later serve as comparison once tube is inserted. |
| 3. Assess client's level of consciousness and ability to follow instructions. | Determines client's ability to assist in procedure. |
| ***Nursing Diagnosis*** | |
| 1. Cluster data to reveal actual or potential nursing diagnoses: | |
| a. Ineffective breathing pattern: related to placement of NG tube in the nares. | May lead to mouth breathing because of feeling of stuffiness in nostrils from NG tube. |
| b. Pain: related to presence of NG tube. | Presence of tube in nasopharynx causes local discomfort, causing client to complain of lump in the throat, hoarseness, earache, and nostril irritation. |
| c. Altered oral mucous membrane: related to mouth breathing and increase of mucous secretions. | Oral hygiene measures helpful in maintaining integrity of oral mucosa. |
| d. Anxiety or fear: related to constant irritation of nares by NG tube. | Some clients, even after careful teaching and explanation, may remain apprehensive and fearful. Client needs assistance to adapt to presence of this stressor. |
| ***Planning*** | |
| 1. Develop individualized goals for client based on nursing diagnoses: | |
| a. Assist client to breathe through nose. | Achieved through routine cleansing of nares. |
| b. Promote client's comfort. | Cleansing, retaping, or repositioning can help relieve discomfort. |
| c. Prevent injury to oral mucosa. | Mouth breathing dries mucosa. |
| 2. Check medical record for surgeon's order, type of NG tube to be placed, and whether tube is to be attached to suction or drainage bag. | Procedure requires physician's order. Adequate decompression depends on suction. |
| 3. Prepare following equipment and supplies: | |
| a. #14 or #16 Fr NG tube (smaller lumen for child) | For decompression, smaller lumen catheters are not used because they must be able to remove thick secretions. |
| b. Water-soluble lubricating jelly | Lubricates tube for insertion. If aspirated, will not cause aspiration pneumonia. |
| c. Stethoscope | Determines tube placement. |
| d. Tongue blade | |
| e. Flashlight | |
| f. Asepto bulb or cone tip syringe, or catheter tip syringe | Irrigate or instill fluid into tube. |
| g. 1 in (2.5 cm) wide hypoallergenic tape | Hypoallergenic tape prevents loss of skin on nose. |
| h. Safety pin and rubber band | |
| i. Clamp, drainage bag, or suction machine | NG tube may be open or closed to drainage. |
| j. Disposable gloves | |
| k. Bath towel | |
| l. Emesis basin with ice (optional) | |
| m. Glass of water with straw | |
| n. Facial tissues | |
| o. Normal saline | For irrigation of tube. |
| p. Tincture of Benzoin (optional) | Increases adhesion of tape to nose. |
| 4. Identify client and explain procedure. | Identification prevents error and gains client's cooperation to facilitate passage of tube and lessen possibility that client will remove tube. |

| Steps | Rationale |
|---|---|
| 5. Position client in high Fowler's position with pillows behind head and shoulders. Raise bed to its highest horizontal level. | Promotes client's ability to swallow during procedure. Good body mechanics prevents injury to nurse or client. |
| ***Implementation*** | |
| 1. Wash hands. | Reduces transmission of infection. |
| 2. Assemble equipment at bedside and place on side of bed nearest nurse. | Procedure should be organized to limit client's discomfort. |
| 3. Pull curtain around the bed or close room door. | Provides privacy. |
| 4. Stand on client's right side if right-handed; left side if left-handed. | Allows easiest manipulation of tubing. |
| 5. If NG tube is too pliable, place in emesis basin and cover with ice. (optional) | Stiffens tube for easier insertion. (Do not ice plastic tube.) |
| 6. Place bath towel over client's chest; give facial tissues to client. | Prevents soiling of client's gown. Tube insertion through nasal passages may cause tearing. |
| 7. Apply disposable gloves. | Prevents contact with body fluids. |
| 8. Instruct client to relax and breathe normally while occluding one naris. Then repeat this action for other naris. Select nostril with greater air flow. | Tube passes more easily through naris that is more patent. |
| 9. Measure distance to insert tube by placing tip of tube at client's nose and extending tube first to tip of earlobe and then from earlobe down to xiphoid process of sternum (Fig. 39-6). | Tube should extend from nares to stomach; distance varies with each client. |
| 10. Mark length of tube to be inserted with piece of tape or note distance of point from next tube marking. | Marks amount of tube to be inserted from nares to stomach. |
| 11. Curve 4-6 in (10-15 cm) of end of tube tightly around index finger; then release. | Curving tube tip aids insertion. |
| 12. Lubricate 3-4 in (7.5-10 cm) of end of tube with water-soluble lubricating jelly. | Minimizes friction against nasal mucosa. |
| 13. Initially instruct client to extend his neck back against pillow; insert tube slowly through naris with curved end pointing downward. | Facilitates initial passage of tube through naris and maintains clear airway for open naris. |
| 14. Continue to pass tube along floor of nasal passage aiming down toward ear. When resistance is felt, apply gentle downward pressure to advance tube (do not force past resistance). | Minimizes discomfort of tube rubbing against upper nasal turbinates. Resistance is caused by posterior nasopharynx. Downward pressure helps tube curl around corner of nasopharynx. |
| 15. If resistance is met, withdraw tube, allow client to rest, relubricate tube and insert into other naris. | Forcing against resistance can cause trauma to mucosa. Helps relieve client's anxiety. |
| 16. Continue insertion of tube until just past nasopharynx by gently rotating tube toward opposite nares. | |
| a. Stop tube advancement, allow client to relax, and provide tissues. | Relieves client's anxiety; tearing is natural response to mucosal irritation. |
| b. Explain to client that next step requires him to swallow. | Tube about to enter esophagus. |
| 17. With tube just above oropharynx, instruct client to flex head forward and dry swallow or suck in air through straw. Advance tube 2.5-5 cm (1-2 in) with each swallow. If client has trouble swallowing and is allowed fluids, offer glass of water. Advance tube with each swallow of water. | Flexed position closes off upper airway to trachea and opens esophagus. Swallowing closes epiglottis over trachea and helps move the tube into the esophagus. Swallowing water reduces gagging or choking. |
| 18. If client begins to cough, gag, or choke, withdraw slightly and stop tube advancement. Instruct client to breathe easily and take sips of water. | Tubing may accidently enter larynx and initiate cough reflex. Gagging is eased by swallowing water. |
| 19. If client continues to cough during insertion, pull tube back slightly. | Tube may enter larynx and obstruct airway. |
| 20. If client continues to gag, check back of pharynx using flashlight and tongue blade. | Tube may coil around itself in back of throat. |
| 21. After client relaxes, continue to advance tube desired distance. | Tip of tube should be within stomach to decompress properly. |
| ***Checking tube placement*** | |
| 1. Ask client to talk. | Client would be unable to talk if NG tube has passed through vocal cords. |
| 2. Check posterior pharynx for presence of coiled tube. | Tube is pliable and can coil up in back of pharynx instead of advancing into esophagus. |

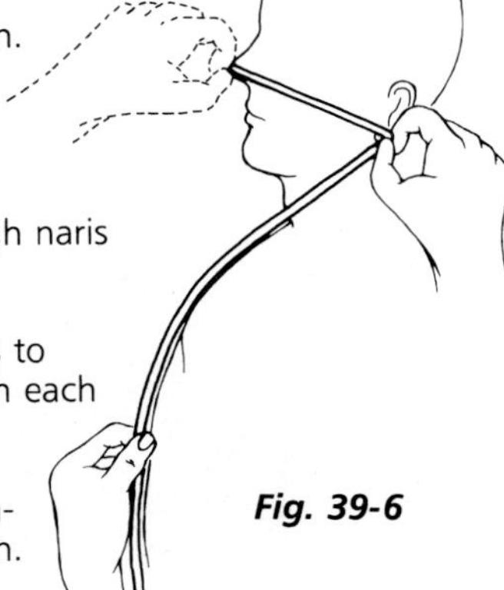

***Fig. 39-6***

| Steps | Rationale |
|---|---|

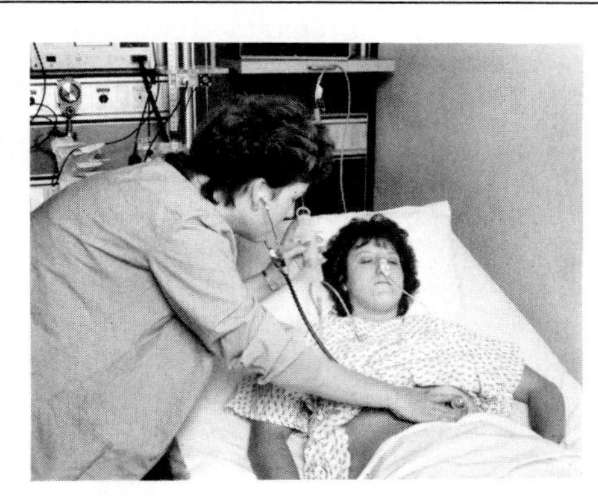

*Fig. 39-7*

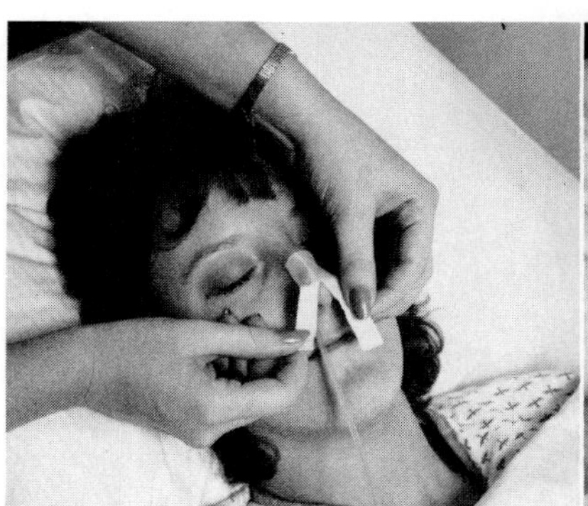

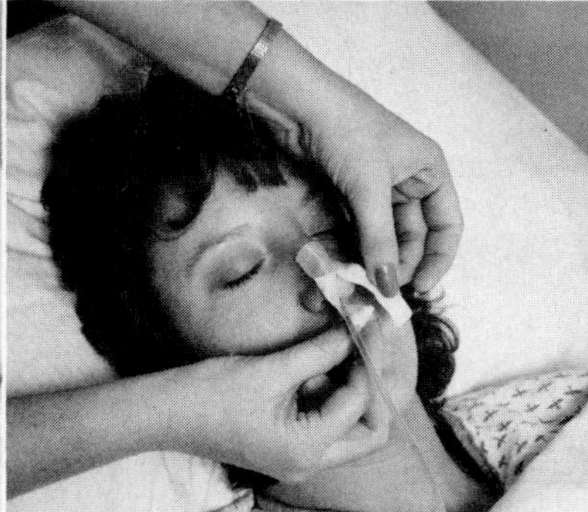

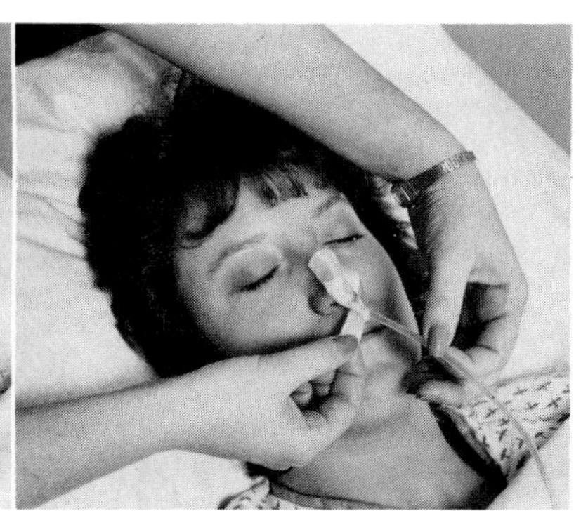

*Fig. 39-8*

| Steps | Rationale |
|---|---|
| 3. Attach syringe to end of NG tube. Place diaphragm of stethoscope over upper left quadrant of abdomen just below costal margin. Inject 10-20 cc of air while auscultating abdomen (Fig. 39-7). | Air entering stomach creates "whooshing" sound and confirms tube placement in stomach. Absence of sound may indicate tip of tube is still in esophagus. |
| 4. Aspirate gently back on syringe to obtain gastric contents. (optional—check pH of gastric contents) | Placement of tube in stomach should result in return of gastric contents. Gentle suction prevents collapse and closure of tube tip. (Gastric contents are acidic and intestinal contents are basic). |
| 5. If tube is not in stomach, advance another 2.5-5 cm (1-2 in) and repeat Steps 3 and 4 to check tube position. | NG tube must be in stomach to provide decompression. |
| ***Anchoring tube*** | |
| 1. After tube is properly inserted, either clamp end or connect it to drainage bag or suction machine. | Drainage bag is used for gravity drainage: Intermittent suction is most effective for decompression. Client going to operating room often will have tube clamped. |
| 2. Tape NG tube to client's nose; avoid putting pressure on nares. Cut 4 in (10 cm) long piece of tape. Apply small amount of tincture of benzoin to lower end of nose and allow to dry (optional). Place one end of tape over nose and wrap opposite split ends around tube as it exits nose (Fig. 39-8). | Prevents tissue necrosis.<br>Tape anchors tube securely. |
| 3. Fasten end of NG tube to client's gown by looping rubber band around tube in slip knot. Pin rubber band to gown (provides slack for movement). | Reduces pressure on the nares if tube moves. |
| 4. Unless physician orders otherwise, head of bed should be elevated 30 degrees. | Helps prevent esophageal reflux and minimizes irritation of tube against posterior pharynx. |
| 5. Explain to client that sensation of tube will decrease somewhat. | Adaptation to continued sensory stimulus. |
| 6. Wash hands. | |

| Steps | Rationale |
|---|---|
| ***Tube irrigation*** | |
| 1. Check tube placement by auscultation while injecting air. | Prevents accidental entrance of irrigating solution into lungs. |
| 2. Draw up 30 ml of normal saline into Asepto or catheter-tipped syringe. | Use of saline minimizes loss of electrolytes from stomach fluids. |
| 3. Clamp connection tubing proximal to connection site for drainage or suction apparatus. Disconnect tubing and lay end on towel. | Reduces backflow of secretions and soiling of client's gown and bed linen. |
| 4. Insert tip of irrigating syringe into end of NG tube. Hold syringe with tip pointed at floor and inject saline slowly and evenly. (Do not force solution.) | Position of syringe prevents introduction of air into vent tubing, which could cause gastric distention. Solution introduced under pressure can cause gastric trauma. |
| 5. If resistance occurs, check for kinks in tubing. Turn client onto left side. Repeated resistance should be reported to surgeon. | Tip of tube may lie against stomach lining. Buildup of secretions will cause distention. |
| 6. After instilling saline, immediately aspirate or pull back slowly on syringe to withdraw fluid. Subtract amount instilled from amount withdrawn and record difference as output. | Irrigation clears tubing so stomach should remain empty. Fluid remaining in stomach is measured as intake. |
| 7. Reconnect NG tube to drainage or suction. (If solution does not return, repeat irrigation.) | Reestablishes drainage collection; may repeat irrigation or repositioning of tube until NG tube drains properly. |
| ***Discontinuation of NG tube*** | |
| 1. Verify order to discontinue NG tube. | Physician's order required for procedure. |
| 2. Apply disposable gloves. | Prevents contact with body fluids. |
| 3. Turn off suction and disconnect NG tube from drainage bag or suction. Remove tape from bridge of nose and unpin tube from gown. | Have tube free of connections before removal. |
| 4. Explain procedure to client and reassure that removal is less distressing than insertion. | Minimize anxiety and increase cooperation. Tube passes out smoothly. |
| 5. Hand the client facial tissue; place clean towel across his chest. Instruct him to take and hold deep breath. | Airway will be temporarily obstructed during tube removal. Client may wish to blow nose after tube removed. |
| 6. Clamp or kink tubing securely and then pull tube out steadily and smoothly while client holds breath. | Reduces trauma to mucosa and minimizes client's discomfort. Clamping prevents tube contents from draining into oropharynx. |
| 7. Dispose of tube and drainage equipment. Measure unit of drainage. | Reduces transfer of microorganisms. Provides accurate measure of fluid output. |
| 8. Clean nares and provide mouth care. | Promotes comfort. |
| 9. Position client comfortably and explain procedure for drinking fluids. | Depends on physician's order; usually begins with small amount of ice chips each hour and increases as client is able to tolerate more. |
| 10. Clean equipment and return to proper place. Place soiled linen in "dirty" utility room or proper receptacle. | Proper disposal of equipment prevents spread of microorganisms and ensures proper exchange procedures. |
| 11. Remove gloves and wash hands. | Reduces spread of microorganisms. |
| **Evaluation** | |
| 1. Observe amount and character of contents draining from NG tube. | Determines if tube is decompressing stomach of contents. |
| 2. Palpate client's abdomen periodically, noting any distention. | Determines success of abdominal decompression. |
| 3. Inspect condition of nares and nose. | Evaluates onset of skin and tissue irritation. |
| 4. Observe position of tubing. | Determines if tension is being applied to nasal structures. |
| 5. Ask client if he feels sore throat or irritation in pharynx. | Evaluate level of client's discomfort. |
| ***Expected outcomes*** | |
| 1. NG tube drains light, green-colored gastric contents. | If tube is patent and in correct position gastric contents will drain easily. |
| 2. Abdomen remains soft and flat. | Indicative of abdominal decompression. |
| 3. Nares and surface of nose remain clear, without abrasions or excoriation, and nares remain moist. | Absence of mucosal and skin irritation. |
| 4. Tubing hangs loosely from nose and remains secured to gown. | No tension applied to nares. |
| 5. Client describes feeling of irritation in throat but not of severe nature. | Presence of tube causes some pharyngeal irritation. |

| Steps | Rationale |
|---|---|
| ***Unexpected outcomes*** | |
| 1. NG tube fails to drain fluid. | Tubing occluded, kinked, or malpositioned in upper stomach or esophagus. |
| 2. Client experiences vomiting. | Symptomatic of distention and/or reduced peristalsis. |
| 3. Abdomen becomes distended and tight. | Symptomatic of distention. |
| 4. Redness, tenderness, and excoriation of naris are present. Surface of nose is reddened and tender. | Result of tube rubbing against surface of nares and tape irritating skin on nose. |
| 5. Tube is pulling on naris. | Tube has inappropriate slack. |
| 6. Client complains of severe sore throat and irritation in swallowing. | Symptomatic of pharyngeal irritation. |

## Reporting and Recording

| | |
|---|---|
| 1. Record time and type of NG tube inserted, client's tolerance to procedure, confirmation of placement, character of gastric contents, and whether tube is changed or connected to drainage device in nurses' notes. | Documents procedure performed correctly. Description of gastric contents provides baseline to determine any change. |
| 2. Record each irrigation, type and amount of solution used, character and volume of aspirate in nurses' notes or flow sheet. | Documents procedure and results. |
| 3. Record balance of fluid instilled and aspirated on intake and output sheet. | Balance reflects fluid gained or lost. |
| 4. Record time NG tube discontinued. | Documents termination of therapy. |
| 5. Report failure of tube to drain, abdominal distention, and unusual character of drainage, e.g., blood, to physician. | Findings indicate need to reposition tube or administer additional therapies. |

## Follow-up Activities

| | |
|---|---|
| 1. Increase frequency of NG tube irrigations or tube repositioning if client vomits or abdomen becomes hard or distended. | Nurse's continuous assessment determines need for frequency of irrigations or repositioning of tube to prevent obstruction and increased abdominal distention. |
| 2. Continue to provide nursing measures for mouth care and client comfort. | Assisting client to remain comfortable will also help reduce anxiety and unnecessary irritation from NG tube. |

## Special Considerations

- If client is confused or disoriented, obtain assistance from another nurse to insert tube. After NG tube insertion, client's hands should be safely restrained because confused clients are at risk for removing NG tubes.
- Comatose or semiconscious clients have reduced or absent gag reflex, making it difficult to determine if tube has passed correctly. If tube is in esophagus, client may often belch when air is instilled to check tube's placement.
- If no contents are aspirated when checking tube placement, ask client to roll onto left side. This maneuver brings gastric contents into greater curvature of stomach.
- Periodically, check to be sure surface of tube is not taped against inside surface of nares. This will cause tissue erosion. Change tape at least daily or whenever soiled to minimize irritation.
- To provide additional comfort for client, apply vaseline to nostrils to prevent crusting of secretions. When tube is in nostril, client tends to breathe through mouth, causing lips and tongue to become dry and crusted. Vaseline applied to lips helps prevent dryness. Physician may allow sucking on small ice chips, gargling solution, throat lozenges, or chewing gum to increase saliva and decrease irritation. Sometimes frequently changing client's position helps relieve pressure from tube on one area in throat.
- Never use the air vent or pigtail on tubing of Salem sump tube for irrigation.
- If NG tube has problems draining, nurse should reposition tube by advancing it or withdrawing it slightly (only with a physician's order). After changing NG position, nurse should reassess tube placement.
- Unless otherwise ordered, NG tube should be irrigated every 2 hours. Sometimes after instilling fluid, large amounts of air are aspirated. Continue to aspirate air and check client's abdomen to determine if hardness or distention is reduced.
- If gastric bleeding occurs, saline solution for irrigation should be iced.
- To prevent leakage of fluid from airway vent of Salem sump tubes, nurse should introduce 30 cc of air into airway lumen to clear tube, maintain patency of NG tube by checking drainage from main lumen, secure airway lumen above stomach level to avoid siphoning effect, and keep collection apparatus below client's midline to prevent reflux.

## Teaching Considerations

- Explain purpose of tube and rationale for each technique, such as irrigation and confirming tube placement.

# SKILL 39-4 Performing Postoperative Care of the Surgical Client

Nursing care of the postoperative surgical client is divided into two phases. During both phases the nurse must make comprehensive and detailed assessments of the client's condition. The effects of anesthesia and the physiological stressors imposed by surgery can place the client at risk for a variety of physiologic alterations. It is also important for the nurse to facilitate communication among all members of the health care team, the client, and the client's family.

The first phase of postoperative care takes place during the immediate recovery period, which extends from the time the client leaves the operating room to the time he has stabilized in the recovery room (RR) or postanesthesia room (PAR) and has been transferred to the nursing division. For an ambulatory surgical client, recovery normally lasts 1 to 2 hr before discharge home. This is the most critical postoperative phase for assessing aftereffects of anesthesia, airway clearance, cardiovascular complications, temperature control, and neurological function. The client's condition can change rapidly. The nurse in the recovery area must make timely, intelligent, and accurate assessments to select the most appropriate measures of care for the client.

Each hospital has its own policies directing the process for recovering clients during the immediate postoperative period. Frequently, for example, clients transfer from the operating room to an intensive care unit. In this situation the client is not sent to the recovery room area. The conditions of these clients are potentially so unstable as to require the monitoring available only in an intensive care unit.

The second phase of recovery is the postoperative convalescent period. This period extends from the time the client is discharged from the recovery room to the time he is discharged from the hospital. Outpatient surgical clients undergo convalescence at home. Clients who have undergone surgical procedures have similar postoperative needs. However, nursing care becomes very individualized depending on the nature of the client's surgery, his preexisting medical conditions, the onset of complications, and the speed with which he recovers. Not all surgical clients recover at the same rate. During the convalescent period the nurse begins preparation for discharge and actively includes both the client and his family in the process. The nurse promotes the client's independence, educates him about any limitations imposed by surgery, and provides resources needed for the client to assume an improved state of wellness.

## Purposes

Nursing care is provided to the postoperative surgical client to:

1. Reduce surgical complications.
2. Promote healing of the surgical wound.
3. Provide rest and comfort.
4. Return the client to his preoperative level of functioning.
5. Maintain the client's self-concept.
6. Prepare the client for discharge from the hospital.

## Procedure 39-4

| Steps | Rationale |
|---|---|
| **Assessment** | |
| ***Immediate recovery period*** | |
| 1. Assess client's condition during operative procedure. | Determines client's general status and allows nurse to anticipate need for special equipment, nursing care, and activities in recovery room. |
| 2. Upon client's arrival at recovery room, obtain report from surgeon and anesthesiologist. | Review provides detailed analysis of client's physiological status, allowing nurse to make appropriate observations and interventions. Provides baseline data to determine any change in condition. |
| 3. Consider type of surgery client underwent and anesthesia used. | Influences type of assessments nurse initiates, type of complications to observe for, and specific nursing interventions. |
| ***Convalescent period*** | |
| 1. Collect report from nurse in recovery room by phone. | Preliminary report allows nurse to prepare hospital room with necessary supplies and equipment for client's special needs. |
| 2. Upon client's arrival at division, collect more detailed report from nurse accompanying client. | Detailed report helps nurse plan appropriate assessment and nursing care measures. Data provide baseline to detect any change in client's condition. |

| Steps | Rationale |
|---|---|
| 3. Review client's chart for information pertaining to type of surgery, preoperative medical risks, baseline vital signs. | Nature of surgery and presence of medical risks dictate complications to observe for. Vital signs provide means to measure postoperative changes. |
| 4. Review surgeon's postoperative orders. | Offers additional guidelines for type of care to provide. |
| **Nursing Diagnosis** | |
| 1. Cluster data to reveal actual or potential nursing diagnoses: | |
| a. Pain: related to surgical incision. | Client in immediate recovery period will not perceive pain as readily as one in convalescent period. General anesthesia prevents pain perception. |
| b. Impaired physical mobility: related to activity restrictions, pain, etc. | Client undergoing major surgery is restricted in activity postoperatively. As client recovers, activity should increase. |
| c. Ineffective breathing pattern: related to pain, effects of anesthesia or analsegia. | Respirations depressed until effects of anesthesia disappear. Pain of surgical incision can reduce ventilatory movement. |
| d. Ineffective airway clearance: related to increased mucous secretions, reduced cough reflex. | General anesthesia and dependent position during surgery cause increased mucous collection. Anesthesia depresses cough reflex. |
| e. Impaired skin integrity: related to immobility, wound drainage. | Client is in dependent position and immobilized immediately postoperatively. Wound drainage can macerate skin layers. |
| f. Sensory perceptual alteration: related to anesthetic effects. | Anesthesia dulls client's sensations. |
| **Planning** | |
| 1. Develop individualized goals for client based on nursing diagnoses: | |
| a. Physiologic responses remain normal during recovery phase. | Frequent vital sign assessment is needed immediately postoperatively. During convalescence frequency of assessment declines as client's condition improves. |
| b. Prevent onset of medical complications throughout recovery. | Certain complications, e.g., hemorrhage or airway obstruction, are more common early postoperatively. Complications such as wound infection or thrombophlebitis tend to occur later. |
| c. Client attains rest and comfort. | Pain control affects client's ability to participate in recovery activities. |
| d. Skin remains intact. | Nurse protects skin from exposure to irritants. |
| e. Client returns to a functional state of health. | Each type of surgery poses specific limitations on client's physical functioning. |
| 2. Prepare following equipment and supplies: | |
| *Recovery room:* | |
| a. Stethoscope, sphygmomanometer, thermometer | Frequent vital sign assessment. |
| b. Intravenous fluid poles | |
| c. Oxygen equipment, e.g., mask, tubing, oxygen regulator | |
| d. Continuous suction equipment | To maintain patency of client's airway. |
| e. Dressing supplies | Used to reinforce soiled dressings. |
| f. Intermittent suction | To connect to nasogastric (NG) or wound drainage tubes. |
| g. Warmed blankets | Promotes warmth and return to normal body temperature. |
| h. Additional equipment for physical assessment | |
| *Nursing division:* | |
| a. Stethoscope, sphygmomanometer, thermometer | Vital signs continue to be monitored. |
| b. IV fluid poles | |
| c. Emesis basin | As client awakens, effects of anesthesia can cause nausea. |
| d. Wash cloth and towel | |
| e. Waterproof pads | Placed under client to absorb wound drainage. |
| f. Equipment for oral hygiene (Chapter 8) | Early complaint made as client awakens is dry mouth. |
| g. Pillows | Used for positioning. |
| h. Facial tissue | |
| i. Oxygen equipment | |
| j. Continuous suction equipment | To suction airway. |
| k. Intermittent suction | To connect to NG or wound drainage tubes. |
| l. Orthopedic appliances (if traction needed) | |
| 3. Explain to client all procedures you are to perform and rationale for each. On nursing division include family members in explanations. | Involves client in plan of care and minimizes anxiety. As recovery progresses, client is able to make more choices regarding how procedures should be performed. |

| Steps | Rationale |
|---|---|

## Implementation

### *Immediate recovery period*

| Steps | Rationale |
|---|---|
| 1. Wash hands. | Reduces transmission of infection |
| 2. Check equipment setup in cubicle of recovery room. | All equipment must be operational and ready to use on client's arrival. |
| 3. As client enters recovery room on stretcher, immediately attach oxygen tubing to regulator, hang IV fluids, and check IV flow rates. Connect any drainage tubes to intermittent suction. | Maintaining oxygenation and circulation are two priorities during critical recovery period. Inhaled oxygen improves percentage delivered to alveoli. IV fluids maintain circulatory volume and provides route for emergency drugs. Drainage tubes must remain patent to allow fluid to drain from wound bed. |
| 4. Conduct complete assessment of all vital signs. Compare findings with client's normal baseline. Continue assessing vital signs every 15 min or more often until client stabilizes. | Vital signs can reveal onset of postoperative complications, e.g., respiratory depression, hypo- or hyperthermia, pulse irregularity, or hypotension. |
| 5. Be sure client has patent airway. | |
| a. Position client on the side with face down and neck slightly extended. | Extension prevents occlusion of airway at pharynx. Downward position of head moves tongue forward and mucus can drain out of mouth. |
| b. Place small folded towel under client's head. | Supports head in extended position. |
| c. If client is restricted to supine position, elevate head of bed slightly, extend neck, and turn head to side. | Prevents aspiration. |
| d. Encourage client to cough and deep breathe on awakening. | Promotes lung expansion and expectoration of mucous secretions. |
| e. Suction artificial airway and oral cavity as secretions accumulate. | Clears airway of secretions. |
| f. Once gag reflex returns, have client spit out oral airway. | Indicates client can clear airway independently. |
| 6. Call client by name in moderate tone of voice. If there is no response, attempt to arouse the client by touching or gently moving a body part. Explain that the client is in a recovery room. | Determines client's level of consciousness and ability to follow commands. |
| 7. Assess circulatory perfusion by inspecting color of nail beds and skin. Palpate for skin temperature. | Pink or normal skin color indicates adequate perfusion. Warm extremities reveal adequate circulation. |
| 8. Observe condition of dressing and drains for any evidence of bright red blood. Also look underneath client for any pooling of bloody drainage. | Hemorrhage from a surgical wound usually occurs within first few hours, indicating that blood vessel was improperly tied or cauterized during surgery. When a dressing becomes saturated, blood will ooze down client's side and collect under bedclothes. |
| 9. Inspect surgical area for swelling or discoloration. | Symptomatic of internal hemorrhage. |
| 10. Note condition of surgical dressing, including amount, color, odor, and consistency of drainage. | Determines extent of fluid loss and condition of underlying wound. |
| 11. Refer to physician's order and reinforce or change dressing as indicated. | Dressing helps to maintain hemostasis and absorb drainage. |
| 12. Inspect condition and contents of any drainage tubes and collecting devices. Note character and volume of drainage (Fig. 39-9). | Determines drainage tube patency and extent of wound drainage. |
| 13. Observe patency, intactness, volume, and character of urine from indwelling Foley catheter (if present). | Patent drainage system prevents bladder distention. Urine volume monitored to measure renal function. |

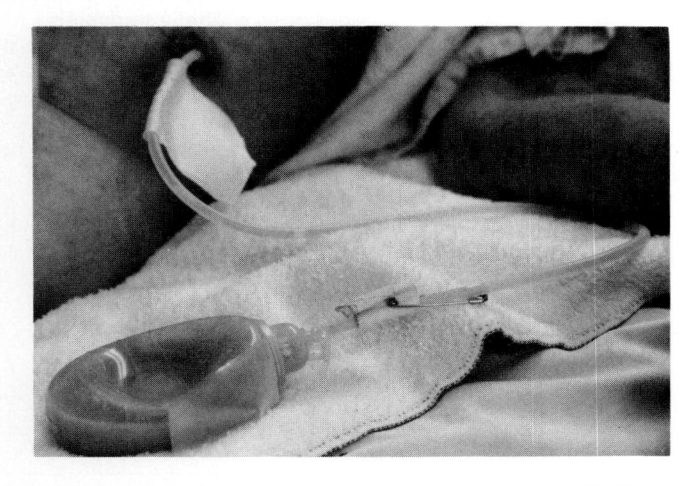

***Fig. 39-9***

| Steps | Rationale |
|---|---|
| 14. If NG tube is present, irrigate periodically (Skill 40-3) with normal saline. | Maintains patency of tube to ensure gastric decompression. |
| 15. Continue monitoring of IV fluid rates. Observe IV site for signs of infiltration. | Continuous regular infusion of IV fluids maintains client's fluid intake to maintain adequate hydration and circulatory function. |
| 16. As client awakens, provide mouth care by placing moistened washcloth to lips, swabbing oral mucosa with dampened swab, or apply Vaseline jelly to lips. | Client still at risk for aspirating and should not be given fluids to rinse mouth. Moist cloth or swab can be soothing to dry mucosa. |
| 17. Assess level of pain as client awakens. Provide pain medication as ordered and when vital signs have stabilized. | Pain can interfere with postoperative exercises. Pain medication can further depress vital signs if anesthetic's effect still present. |
| 18. Explain how client is progressing and that plans for transfer to a nursing division are being made. | Helps client remain oriented to surroundings and recovery activities. |
| 19. Once all physiological signs have stabilized, contact physician for order to release client to floor. | Physician responsible for dictating level of observation and care required by client. |
| ***Convalescent period*** | |
| 1. Make final check of equipment set up in client's room. Be sure bed is placed in high horizontal position and to side so that stretcher can easily be moved beside bed. | During transfer, client's status may change, necessitating quick interventions upon his arrival. Availability of equipment ensures smooth transfer process. |
| 2. Assist recovery room staff and use three-person carry to transfer client to bed. | Technique avoids strain on nurse's back muscles and maintains client's safety. |
| 3. Once client is transferred to bed, immediately attach any existing oxygen tubing, hang IV fluids, and check IV flow rate. | Maintains client's oxygenation and circulation. |
| 4. Conduct complete assessment of all vital signs. Compare findings with vital signs in recovery area as well as client's baseline values. Continue monitoring as ordered. | Client should be stabilized once transferred to nursing division. Change in vital signs can reveal early onset of postoperative complications. |
| 5. Maintain client's airway. | |
| a. If artificial airway is still present, suction any secretions. | During transfer period, secretions can accumulate within airway. |
| b. Position client on side (if allowed); if client remains sleepy or lethargic, keep head extended. | Positioning minimizes chances of aspiration. |
| c. Encourage coughing and deep breathing. | Promotes lung expansion and expectoration of mucus. |
| 6. Be sure any drainage tubes are connected to proper suction of drainage device. If NG tube is present, irrigate as ordered and connect to proper drainage device. | Maintains drainage tube patency so that wound beds remain dry for healing. Occlusion of NG tube can lead to abdominal distention. |
| 7. Assess client's surgical dressing for intactness and presence and character of drainage. Reinforce as ordered. If no dressing present, inspect condition of wound. | Wound can hemorrhage quickly during early postoperative period. Observations of wound and dressings provides data to measure progress of wound healing. |
| 8. Assess client for bladder distention. Offer bedpan if client senses urge to void. | Anesthetics and analgesics depress sensation of bladder fullness. |
| 9. Measure all sources of fluid intake and output. | Assists in monitoring client's fluid and electrolyte balance. |
| 10. Position client for comfort, maintaining correct body alignment. Avoid positioning on surgical wound site. | Good positioning reduces stress on suture line. Comfortable position helps client relax. |
| 11. Explain to client that you have completed all observations and that you will ask family members to enter room. Place call light within reach and raise side rails. | Promotes client's orientation and sense of well-being. Call light and side rail positioning ensure client's safety as effects of anesthesia continue to diminish. |
| 12. Explain to family client's general status, describe purpose of any equipment in room, and explain reason for frequent observations and procedures. | Family is normally anxious to learn about client's status. Unfamiliar sights (equipment, client's appearance) can be anxiety provoking. Family's understanding can promote their participation in client's care. |
| 13. Refer to recovery record to determine if pain medication administered. Administer analgesic if vital signs remain stable. | Pain relief is essential for client to be able to begin postoperative exercises. |
| 14. Provide oral hygiene and repeat as needed. | Maintenance of moist mucous membranes facilitates expectoration of secretions and promotes client's comfort. |
| 15. As client stabilizes over the next hours or days, perform the following measures. | |
| a. Have client participate in postoperative exercises. | Promotes pulmonary and circulatory function to minimize onset of postoperative complications. |
| b. Encourage use of incentive spirometer as ordered. Watch client use spirometer first few times to judge efficacy of breathing. | Promotes lung expansion. |

| Steps | Rationale |
|---|---|
| c. Begin activity orders (assess vital signs first time client sits or stands to judge tolerance). | Promotes circulation, lung expansion, peristalsis (sudden positional changes can cause postural hypotension). |
| d. Begin dietary orders slowly according to client's tolerance. | Promotes normal fluid and electrolyte balance, restores nutritional intake, and promotes normal gastrointestinal function. |
| e. Assist client in assuming normal urinary voiding pattern. | Promotes normal urinary elimination. |
| f. Closely monitor progress of wound healing and change dressings as ordered. | Wound infection occurs most often within 3-6 days postoperatively. Wound dehiscence occurs most often 3-11 days postoperatively. |
| 16. Gradually increase client's involvement in decision making and in any explanations about surgery and related implications. | Promotes client's sense of control and independence. Encourages feeling of self-esteem. |
| 17. Discuss with client and family plans for discharge. | Discharge planning is continuous process, beginning with client's admission. |

## Evaluation

| Steps | Rationale |
|---|---|
| 1. Compare all vital sign assessment measurements with client's baseline and expected normals. | Evaluates client's respiratory, cardiovascular, and thermoregulatory status throughout recovery. |
| 2. Evaluate effects of pain relief measures, e.g., positioning, use of analgesia. | Determines level of comfort achieved. |
| 3. Monitor lung sounds following postoperative exercises. | Determines status of airways. |
| 4. Auscultate bowel sounds at least each shift. | To evaluate return of peristalsis and diet tolerance. |
| 5. Monitor intake and output balance for each shift. | Can reveal onset of fluid imbalances. |
| 6. Hold discussion with client regarding general level of comfort and progress toward recovery. | Gives client sense of participation in care. Client's perceptions can also be helpful in noting onset of complications. Reveals readiness to learn about discharge. |
| 7. Conduct physical assessments according to client's unique type of surgery. | Monitors course of recovery. |
| ***Expected outcomes*** | |
| 1. Client's vital signs remain within previous baseline or normal expected range. | No cardiovascular, pulmonary, or thermoregulatory changes except those expected from effects of anesthesia or analgesia. |
| 2. Client reports relief of discomfort following analgesia or other pain relief measures. | Measures effectively alter client's reception or perception of pain. |
| 3. Breath sounds remain clear. | Postoperative exercises and activity promote lung expansion and alveolar stability. |
| 4. Normal bowel sounds present following bowel surgery or general anesthesia within 48-72 hr. Normal bowel sounds are heard within 24 hours in cases of minor surgery. | Return of intestinal peristalsis. |
| 5. Intake and output remain relatively in balance. | Adequate urinary elimination maintained. Fluid intake maintained. |
| 6. Client is able to discuss recovery and discharge plans. Verbalizes no specific physical complaints. | Client coping with stress of surgery. |
| ***Unexpected outcomes*** | |
| 1. Vital signs are above or below client's baseline or expected range. | Alterations may result from anesthetic effects or surgical complications such as hypovolemic shock, airway obstruction, fluid and electrolyte imbalances or hypothermia. |
| 2. Client continues to experience incisional pain. | Factors may heighten client's pain perception, such as anxiety, isolation, fatigue. Analgesic ordered may be of insufficient dosage. |
| 3. Abnormal breath sounds are auscultated. | Result of atelectasis or mucous secretions in larger airways. |
| 4. Bowel sounds are absent or decreased. | Paralytic ileus can develop as common complication following bowel surgery. Intestinal motility may return slowly depending on anesthetic effects. |
| 5. Intake and output measurements reflect imbalance. | Client suffering fluid volume excess or deficit and is at risk for electrolyte imbalance. |
| 6. Client is unable to discuss discharge plans or has negative view of recovery. | Coping poorly with stress of surgery. |

| Steps | Rationale |
| --- | --- |
| **Recording and Reporting** | |
| 1. Document client's arrival to recovery room or nursing division; describe vital signs, assessment findings, and all nursing measures initiated in nurse's notes. | Documents care provided. Data provide baseline to compare changes in client's condition. Information ensures continuity of care among health team members. |
| 2. Record vital signs and intake and output on appropriate flow sheet. | Provides means to record repetitive types of data over frequent time intervals. Provides graphic view of trends. |
| 3. Report any abnormal assessment findings and signs of complications to nurse in charge or physician. | Certain physiological changes may require emergency measures. |
| **Follow-up Activities** | |
| 1. Increase frequency of monitoring should complications arise. | Surgical client's condition can change quickly, especially during first 24 hr postoperatively. |
| 2. Increase frequency of supportive care, e.g., postoperative exercises, ambulation, if signs of complications develop. | Many nursing care measures are preventive in nature. |

## Special Considerations

- Clients under spinal anesthesia may benefit from being placed in quiet area of recovery room.
- Client with spinal anesthesia is unable to feel sensation below level of spinal cord.
- Report between surgeon and nurse should include level of anesthesia, vital signs, IV fluids or blood products used in surgery, presence of drains under surgical dressing, special concerns, e.g., risk for hemorrhage or arrythmias, and incidence of complications during surgery.
- Examples of specific surgeries requiring special interventions: craniotomy—detailed neurological assessment; neck surgery—special attention to airway status; vascular surgery—need to observe for bleeding complications; orthopedic surgery—special positioning techniques.
- Postoperative orders usually include frequency of vital signs and special assessments, types of IV fluids and infusion rate, postoperative medications, fluids or foods allowed by mouth, level of activity or type of positioning, intake and output, laboratory tests or x-ray studies to be done, and special directions, e.g., dressing changes, care of traction, use of incentive spirometers.
- Client is usually asleep upon arrival in recovery room. Factors influencing consciousness include anesthesia, medications, electrolyte and metabolic changes, pain, and emotions.
- In early postoperative phase, client tends to be lethargic and less responsive because of lingering effects of general anesthesia.
- Respiratory depression can result from anesthetic. Client may have endotracheal tube or airway in place when arriving in recovery room. Each requires special oxygen adaptor. Do not elicit gag reflex because client may vomit secretions that could be aspirated. Never position client with hands over the chest (reduces chest expansion).
- Hypotension may result from anesthesia or acute blood loss. Acute blood loss may lead to hypovolemic shock with signs of reduced blood pressure, elevated heart and respiratory rates, pale skin, and restlessness. Clients who suffer severe blood loss postoperatively may receive blood products.
- Lowered level of metabolism causes hypothermia. Rare complication of anesthesia is hyperthermia.
- Size, location, and depth of wound influence amount of drainage. Nurse can estimate drainage by counting number of saturated gauze sponges. Appearance of bright red blood should be reported to physician immediately, except where chest tubes are used. Some bloody drainage is expected through tube. Changing dressings immediately postoperatively can disrupt wound edges and aggravate drainage. Most physicians prefer reinforcement with additional dressings only. First dressing changes most often occur 24 hours postoperatively and are usually done by the physician. Minor surgical wounds may not have dressings but simply skin closure.
- Typical postoperative assessment of vital signs includes measurements every 15 min first hour followed by measurements every 30 min for 1-2 hours, then every hour for 4 hours or more. Measurement is then adjusted to desired daily observations. Frequency depends on the client's condition and physician's preferences. Nurse can judge need for more frequent vital signs.
- Male client may need assistance to stand to void. If client is unable to void within 8 hr after surgery, it may be necessary to insert urinary catheter. Fewer clients have urinary catheters placed postoperatively because of risk of infection. Normal kidney function is revealed by urinary output of at least 30 ml/hr. Bloody urine is common following surgery of genitourinary tract.
- In some cases, client is placed in bed in recovery room. Transfer is unnecessary when client reaches nursing division. Nature of client's surgery may restrict type of position he can assume.
- Many nurses are hesitant to administer pain medications until client requests them. Nurse is best judge to provide pain control independently during time when patient is at high risk for discomfort. Client with spinal anesthesia usually feels no pain. Remember that pain can sometimes lower blood pressure, thus analgesia may restore vital signs to normal. Use with caution.
- Clients who had abdominal surgery usually resume their diet with clear liquids. If these are tolerated, diet is advanced to full liquids, soft, or regular diet. Some clients have surgeries that allow them to advance to regular diet once nausea subsides.
- Signs of wound infection include fever, tenderness, and pain at wound site; increased white blood cell count; or purulent drainage. Signs of dehiscence: client reports feeling that something in wound "gave way," and increased serosanguinous wound drainage. Obese clients are more at risk for this.

- Clients are usually ordered to sit in chair evening of surgery or next day. Activity progresses to walking in room and then in hallways. Allow clients to use toilet facilities as soon as activity allows.

## Teaching Considerations

- Thorough preoperative teaching should prepare family for frequent observations that will occur postoperatively.
- If client had spinal anesthesia, remind family that loss of extremity movement is normal for several hours.
- Instruct client and primary care giver to identify signs and symptoms of infection; respiratory, circulatory, or gastrointestinal difficulties; and wound disruptions.
- Instruct client and primary care giver actions to take in event of any abnormal postoperative events.
- Set up important phone numbers in readily available location for client and primary care giver to use in event of emergency.

## Home Care Considerations

- Teach primary care giver about any postoperative restrictions, home modifications, or activity limitations.
- If client is discharged with dressing changes, bedroom or bathroom is usually ideal for procedure.

---

**BIBLIOGRAPHY**

Aish A, et al.: How to use risk factors and assessment skills to individualize patient care, Can Nurse 78:46, 1982.

American Nurses' Association and Association of Operating Room Nurses: Standards of perioperative nursing care, Kansas City, Mo, 1982, The Associations.

AORN: Recommended practices for preoperative skin preparation of patients, AORN J 37:244, 1983.

Ayliffe GAJ, et al.: A comparison of preoperative bathing with chlorhexidine detergent and nonmedicated soap in the prevention of wound infection, J Hosp Infect 237, 1983.

Breslin EF: Prevention and treatment of pulmonary complications in patients after surgery of the upper abdomen, Heart Lung 10:511, 1981.

Croushove TM: Postoperative assessment: the key to avoiding the most common nursing mistakes, Nurs '79 9:47, 1979.

Fortin F, Kirovac S: A randomized controlled trial of preoperative patient education, Int J Nurs Stud 13:11, 1976.

Garner JS: Guidelines for prevention of surgical wound infections, 1985, Hospital Infections Program, CDC, PHS, and US Department of Health and Human Services.

Golden S: Nursing a loved one at home, Philadelphia, 1988, Running Press.

Gruendemann BJ, Meeker MH: Alexander's care of the patient in surgery, ed 8, St. Louis, 1987, The CV Mosby Co.

Horsley J, Crane J: Structured preoperative teaching, New York, 1981, Grune & Stratton, Inc.

Hughes JM: Postoperative pulmonary care: past, present, and future, Crit Care Q 6:67, 1983.

King I, Tarsitano B: The effect of structured and unstructured preoperative teaching: a replication, Nurs Res 31:324, 1982.

Kleinbeck SVM: Simplifying postoperative assessment, AORN J 38:344, 1983.

Krause DH: Postoperative hypothermia, Focus Crit Care 10:48, 1983.

Lindeman C, Van Aernam B: Nursing intervention with the presurgical patient—the effects of structured and unstructured preoperative teaching, Nurs Res 20:319, 1971.

McHugh NG, et al.: Preparatory information: what helps and why, Am J Nurs 82:780, 1982.

Nursing Photobook: Caring for surgical patients, Springhouse, Pa, 1984, Springhouse Corp.

Podjasek JH: Which postop patient faces the greatest respiratory risk? RN 48:44, 1985.

Potter P, Perry A: Basic nursing: theory and practice, St. Louis, 1987, The CV Mosby Company.

Volden C, Grinde J: Taking the trauma out of nasogastric intubation, Nurs '80 10:64, 1980.

Walsh J, Persons C, Wieck L: Manual of home care nursing, Philadelphia, 1987 JB Lippincott Co.

Wells N: The effect of relaxation on postoperative muscle tension and pain, Nurs Res 31:236, 1982.

# 40

# INTRAOPERATIVE CARE

### OBJECTIVES

*Mastery of content in this chapter will enable the nurse to:*

- Define key terms.
- Describe the roles of the circulating and scrub nurse.
- Identify guidelines for use of sterile technique in the operating room.
- Correctly don a sterile surgical gown.
- Correctly apply sterile gloves using the closed technique.

### KEY TERMS

*Asepsis*
*Aseptic technique*
*Chemical indicator*
*Contaminated*
*Don*
*Scrubbed team members*
*Sponge*
*Spores*
*Sterile*
*Sterile field*
*Sterilization*
*Surgical scrub*
*Terminal disinfection and sterilization*
*Unscrubbed team members*

### SKILLS

***40-1*** Donning a Sterile Gown and Gloves

The registered nurse in the operating room (OR) is one member of the team that cares for the client during the surgical experience. Nursing in the operating room encompasses the client's surgical experience from the preoperative throughout the intraoperative period, and into the postoperative phase. This is called the perioperative role of the operating room nurse. The activities that the nurse performs as part of the perioperative role are carried out using the nursing process.

The preoperative phase begins when the decision for surgical intervention is made and ends when the client is transferred onto the operating room table. Activities during this phase can include a preoperative visit to the client by the OR nurse in the clinic, at home, on the patient care area, in the holding area of the OR, or elsewhere in the surgical suite. A preoperative assessment can decrease the fears and anxieties of the client and family by providing information about the surgical experience, to collect data that will assist the OR staff to provide individualized quality care, and to decrease feelings of depersonalization for the client and family.

The intraoperative phase begins with the client's transfer to the OR table and ends with admission to the recovery area. The OR nurse provides support, safety, and comfort for the client during the intraoperative phase.

In the intraoperative phase the nurse assumes one of two roles during the surgical procedure: scrub nurse or circulating nurse (see box). The scrub nurse provides the surgeon with instruments and supplies, disposes of soiled sponges, and accounts for sponges, needles, and instruments on the surgical field. The circulating nurse is an assistant to the scrub nurse and surgeon. When a client enters the operating room, the circulating nurse helps position the client and applies necessary equipment and drapes. During the procedure the circulating nurse works with the scrub nurse to be sure aseptic technique is followed and that the client receives necessary supportive care.

During the postoperative phase the operating room nurse assists in transferring the client to the recovery room or postanesthesia room. Information about the client's status, including a review of IV fluids, medications, and blood products administered, the surgical dressing, the nature of any complications in the OR, and unusual risks for hemorrhage or cardiac irregularities are reviewed with the recovery room staff. The OR nurse is an important resource in planning the client's postoperative care.

## ASEPTIC TECHNIQUE IN THE OR

Principles of aseptic technique must be strictly followed to maintain the safety and welfare of clients in the operating room. The overall goal of asepsis is to minimize contamination of the surgical wound. Principles of surgical asepsis apply before the client even reaches the operating room. Supplies, instruments, and equipment must be thoroughly sterilized to remove all microorganisms. Members of the surgical team follow specific guidelines when donning surgical attire and performing a surgical scrub before handling sterile items. The special preparation of the client's skin before application of sterile drapes helps reduce the numbers of microorganisms around the surgical incision. The scrub nurse and surgeons create a sterile field around the surgical wound and maintain its integrity throughout the procedure in accordance with strict aseptic principles. The surgical procedure itself finally ends with sterile application of dressings.

All members of the health care team in the operating room must develop a surgical conscience. Surgical conscience means that each individual must assume responsibility for monitoring aseptic practices. It requires discipline, integrity, honesty, and outspokenness concerning any shortcomings in aseptic practice. Development of a surgical conscience requires knowledge of the principles of asepsis, self-discipline regarding personal hygiene and nursing practices, good communication skills to identify and correct any breaks in technique, and maturity to overcome personal preferences. A surgical conscience is a special commitment to providing optimal care to the client.

## GUIDELINES

1. All items used within a sterile field must be sterile (see Chapter 39).
2. Gowns used by scrub persons must be sterile. The entire gown is sterile before donning. Once donned, gowns are considered sterile in front from the chest to table level and on the sleeves to 2 inches (5 cm) above the elbow.
3. Sterile persons must keep hands in sight and above the waist level to avoid contamination.
4. When wearing a sterile gown, arms should not be folded with hands tucked in axillary region.
5. Draped tables should be considered sterile only at table level. Sides of the drape extending below table level are unsterile.
6. All personnel moving around or within a sterile field must do so in a manner consistent with maintaining the sterility of that field. Scrubbed persons move from sterile areas to other sterile areas, contacting a sterile field only with sterile gowns and gloves. Unscrubbed persons should stay at least 1 foot away from the sterile field and contact only unsterile areas.
7. All sterile supplies and equipment should be grouped around the client.
8. Unsterile persons should avoid reaching over the sterile field.
9. Scrubbed persons should remain close to the sterile field. When changing position, they should turn face to face or back to back.

### *NURSE'S ROLES IN THE OPERATING ROOM*

#### CIRCULATING NURSE

- Prepares operating room with necessary equipment and supplies and ensures that equipment is functional.
- Arranges sterile and nonsterile supplies; opens sterile supplies for scrub nurse.
- Sends for client at proper time.
- Visits with client preoperatively; explains role, verifies operative permit, identifies client, and answers any questions.
- Confirms client's allergies.
- Checks medical record for completeness.
- Assists in safe transfer of client to operating room table.
- Positions client on operating room table in accordance with type of procedure and surgeon's preference.
- Places conductive pad on client if electrocautery is to be used.
- Counts sponges, needles, and instruments with scrub nurse before surgery.
- Assists scrub nurse and surgeons by tying gowns and preparing client's skin.
- Assists scrub nurse in arranging tables to create sterile field.
- Maintains continuous astute observations during surgery to anticipate needs of client, scrub nurse, surgeons, and anesthesiologist.
- Provides supplies to scrub nurse as needed.
- Observes sterile field closely for any breaks in aseptic technique and reports accordingly.
- Cares for surgical specimens.
- Documents operative record and nurses' notes.
- Counts sponges, needles, and instruments when closure of wound begins.
- Transfers client to stretcher for transport to recovery area.
- Accompanies client to the recovery room and provides a report.

#### SCRUB NURSE

- Performs surgical hand scrub.
- Dons sterile gown and gloves aseptically.
- Arranges sterile supplies and instruments in manner prescribed for procedure.
- Checks instruments for proper functioning.
- Counts sponges, needles, and instruments with circulating nurse.
- Gowns and gloves surgeons as they enter operating room.
- Assists with surgical draping of client.
- Maintains neat and orderly sterile field.
- Recognizes and corrects breaks in aseptic technique.
- Observes progress of surgical procedure.
- Hands surgeon instruments, sponges, and necessary supplies during procedure.
- Identifies and handles surgical specimens correctly.
- Watches sponges, needles, and instruments so none will be misplaced or lost in wound.

**PREREQUISITE KNOWLEDGE**

1. Principles of surgical asepsis.

**PREREQUISITE SKILLS**

1. Surgical handwashing (Skill 38-2).
2. Donning a mask and cap (Skill 38-1).

## *SKILL 40-1 Donning a Sterile Gown and Gloves*

Attiring oneself correctly for the operating room begins with personal hygiene. Potentially pathogenic bacteria are present on the skin, hair, and in the respiratory tract of all persons. Daily bathing and clean hair are necessary to minimize numbers of microorganisms. Because they harbor bacteria, fingernails should be well trimmed, clean, and free from polish. Hands should always be washed before and after contact with a client and after handling equipment or potentially contaminated items. Anyone with a transmittable bacterial infection such as an upper respiratory tract infection, draining or unhealed wound, or infection of the mouth, eye, and ear should be excluded from the surgical suite.

All persons entering a surgical suite must wear OR apparel. A clean scrub suit (pants and top) is worn to contain bacterial shedding. If scrub suits become visibly soiled or wet, they should be changed. Sleeves should be short enough to allow adequate scrubbing above the elbow, and the top should be tucked in to prevent brushing against sterile areas and to decrease the amount of bacteria shed from the thoracic and abdominal skin.

OR apparel should be worn only within the surgical suite. If it is worn outside the OR, it should be covered or changed before the person reenters the area. Street clothes should never be worn in the restricted areas of the surgical suite.

All possible head and facial hair should be covered when one is in the surgical suite. The cap or hood should be the first piece of OR attire that is donned to prevent hair from collecting on the scrub clothes. A clean hat should be worn each day and should not be worn outside the surgical suite.

Shoe covers should be worn inside the OR. They should be removed on leaving the restricted areas of the suite and new shoe covers should be put on when returning to the OR. Clean shoe covers should be worn each day and should be changed if they become soiled. Clogs and sandals are not recommended in the OR because they are not considered safe.

Masks must be worn in specified restricted areas of the surgical suite. The surgical mask should completely cover the mouth and nose since its purpose is to filter organisms from exhaled air. The mask should be secured over the nose, along the sides of the face, and under the chin to keep air from escaping around it (see Chapter 38). As a mask becomes moist, its effectiveness decreases since bacteria can pass through it. Therefore, a moist mask should be changed if possible. Surgical masks should be changed between procedures so that a clean dry mask is used for each client. Masks should either be on or off and should not be allowed to hang around the neck. Masks that hang around the neck harbor bacteria from the nasopharyngeal airway. Only mask strings should be touched when removing a mask in order to reduce contamination of hands by bacteria from the airway.

Jewelry should not be worn in the surgical suite. Rings, watches, and necklaces serve as reservoirs for bacteria. Dangling earrings that hang outside the cap can fall onto the sterile field.

Before a nurse dons a sterile gown and gloves in the operating room, a complete surgical scrub must be performed. The purpose of the scrub (see Chapter 38) is to remove soil, debris, skin oil, and microorganisms so as to reduce the microbial count to as near zero as possible on the hands. A thorough scrub leaves an antimicrobial residue on the skin to prevent growth of microbes for several hours.

**PURPOSES**

1. Permit members of the surgical team to come in contact with the sterile field during a surgical procedure.
2. Provide a barrier to microorganisms.

### *Procedure 40-1*

| Steps | Rationale |
|---|---|
| **Assessment** | |
| 1. During handwashing procedure check hands and fingers for cuts, abrasions, or areas of inflammation. Nails should be trimmed (for gloving). | Microorganisms will reside in inflamed and opened areas of skin. |

| Steps | Rationale |
|---|---|
| **Planning** | |
| 1. Establish goal for procedure. | |
| a. Prevent contamination of gown's outer surface. | Nurse may touch sterile surgical field with sterile surface of gown. |
| b. Prevent contamination of gloves outer surface. | Technique of gloving maintains sterility of surface so that sterile items on surgical field can be handled. |
| 2. Have circulating nurse in the OR prepare gown and gloves: | |
| a. Open sterile pack containing gown on waist-high table, keep inner wrapping sterile. | Scrub nurse will be able to don gown without contaminating scrubbed hands. |
| b. Open outer glove wrapper and transfer sterile inner wrapper and gloves to sterile field (Chapter 38). | Gloves are ready for application immediately following gowning. |
| 3. Before entering the operating room (OR) or treatment area, apply a cap and face mask. Foot covers are also required in the OR. | Prevents hair and air droplet nuclei from contaminating sterile work areas. Foot covers are paper or cloth and fit over work shoes. |
| 4. Perform a thorough surgical handwash (Skill 38-2). | Removes transient and resident bacteria from fingers, hands, and forearms. |
| 5. Dry hands according to Steps 12-14 in Procedure 38-2. | Prevents chapping, facilitates application of gloves, and prevents transmission of microorganisms through moisture. |
| **Implementation** | |
| 1. Pick up the gown, grasping the inside surface of the gown at the collar. | The hands are not completely sterile. The inside surface of the gown will contact the skin's surface and is thus considered contaminated. |
| 2. Stand away from the sterile pack and table. Hold the gown at arm's length away from your body and allow the gown to unfold by itself. Be careful not to allow the gown to touch the floor or nearby table (Fig. 40-1). | Contact of the outer surface or front of the gown with a dirty or clean surface would result in gown contamination. Shaking of the gown can cause air currents that increase the risk of contamination. |
| 3. Hold the gown by the inside, open shoulder seams, and insert each hand through the armholes. | The inside of the gown is considered contaminated. |
| 4. Keeping your upper arms in front of you at shoulder height, extend the hands toward the gown cuff. (Do not push the hands through the cuffs if using the closed glove method) (Fig. 40-2). | Extension of the arms straight ahead keeps the sterile surface of the gown in view and reduces the risk of touching the floor or a portion of the body. |
| 5. Have a circulating nurse (considered unsterile) tie the collar securely from behind and pull the sleeves onto your arms for proper fit and comfort (Fig. 40-3). | Working from behind the gowned person prevents contamination by the circulating nurse. The back of the gown is unsterile. |
| 6. If the waist ties or snaps fall in front of the gown, enclose them within a sterile towel (with hands inside sleeves) and hand the sterile towel to the circulating nurse. (Disposable paper gowns have a special tag the circulating nurse may grasp.) | The towel provides a surface the circulating nurse can grasp without contaminating the gown. |

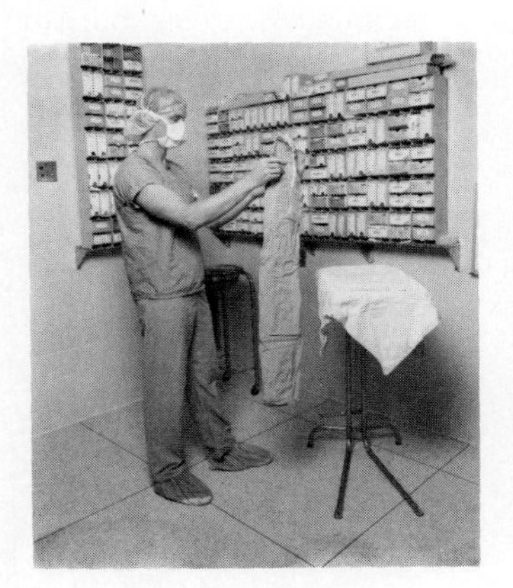

*Fig. 40-1*

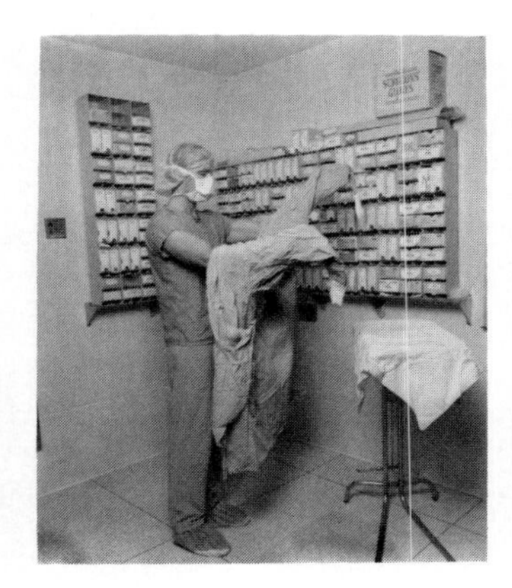

*Fig. 40-2*

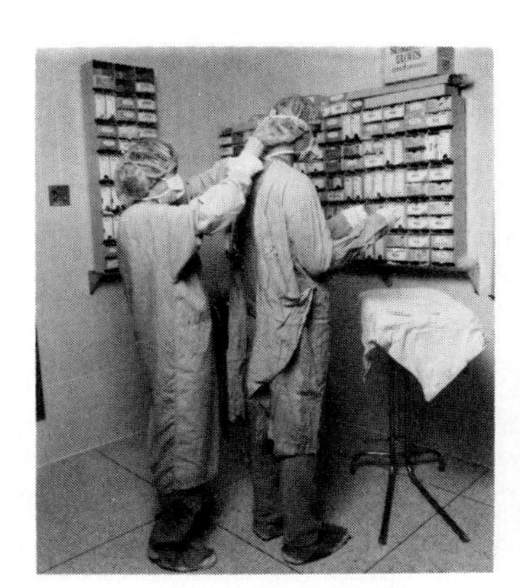

*Fig. 40-3*

| Steps | Rationale |
|---|---|

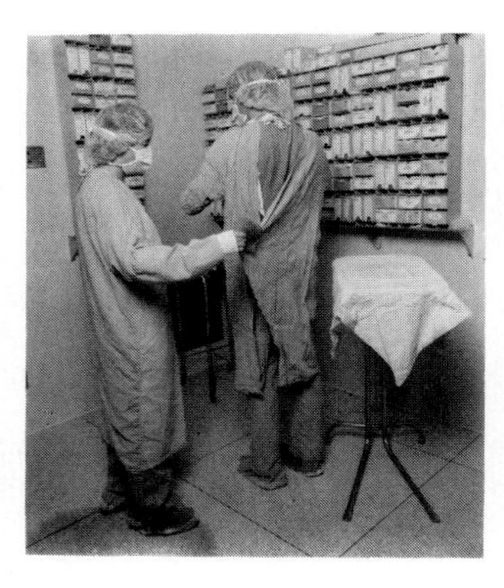

*Fig. 40-4*

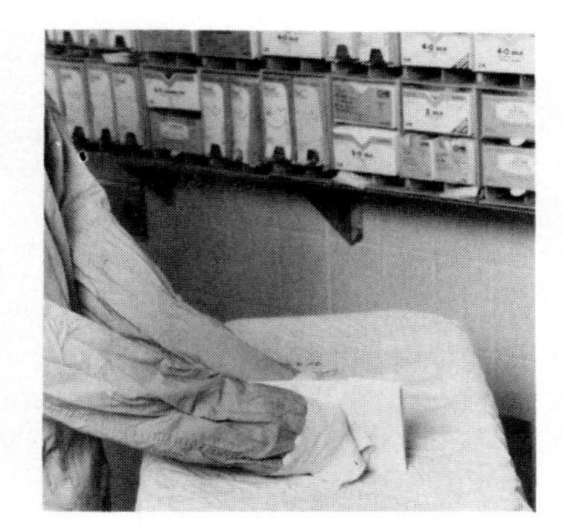

*Fig. 40-5*

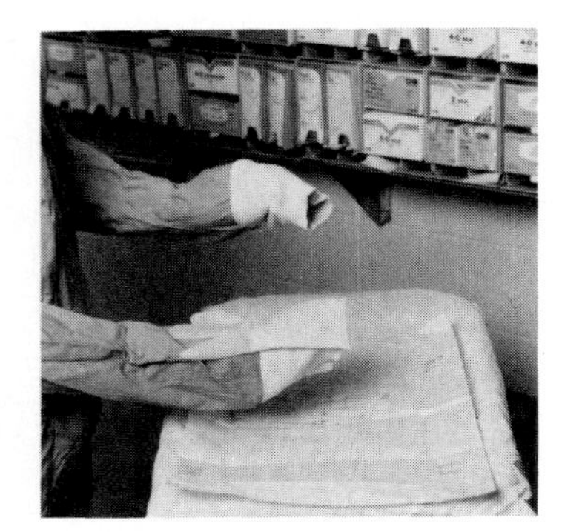

*Fig. 40-6*

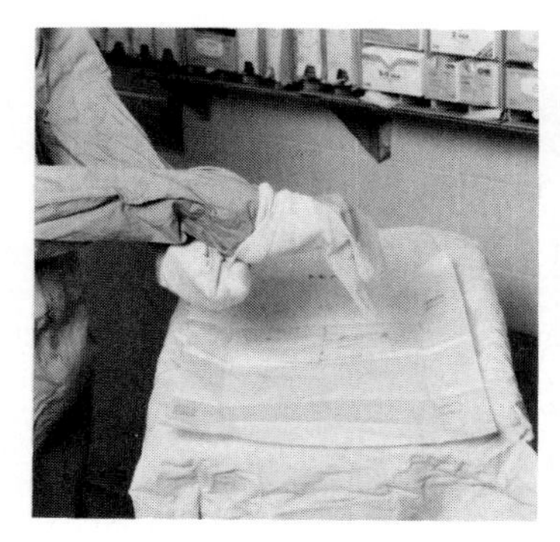

*Fig. 40-7*

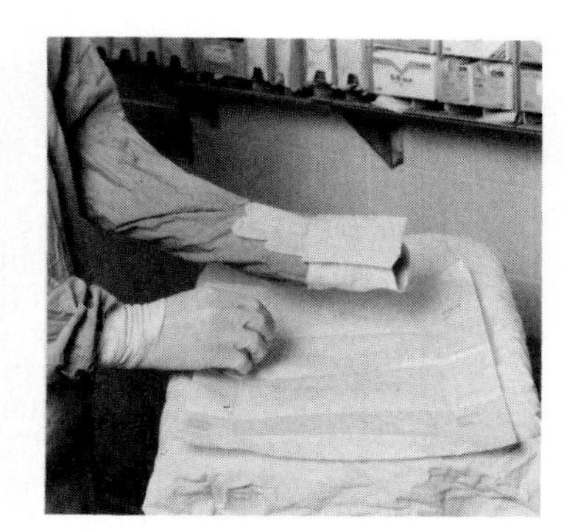

*Fig. 40-8*

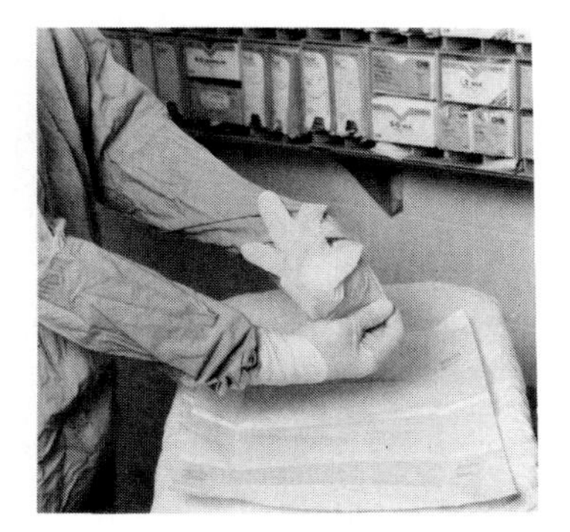

*Fig. 40-9*

7. Make a three-quarter turn away from the circulating nurse, then grasp the sterile tie and secure it in front of the gown (Fig. 40-4),

   Back side of gown is considered unsterile. Prevents gown from loosening and touching unsterile objects.

   or

   have the circulating nurse, who is wearing sterile gloves, tie or wrap waistband from behind, making certain gown is completely closed.

   Reduces air currents and risk of contamination.

## Closed Gloving

1. With the hands covered by the gown sleeves, open the inner sterile glove package (Fig. 40-5).

   Keeps hands clean. Sterile gown touches sterile glove package.
2. Grasp the inside of the cuff sleeve covering the nondominant hand. With the same hand pick up the glove for the dominant hand. Place the glove palm side down on the palm of the covered dominant hand, with the glove fingers pointing toward the elbow of the dominant arm (Fig. 40-6).

   The gown protects the nurse's fingers. Sterile touching sterile is sterile. Positioning of the glove will allow the nurse to slip it over the gown cuff.
3. The fingers of the covered dominant hand pinch the underside of the glove's cuff. With the covered nondominant hand, grasp the topside of the glove's cuff for the dominant hand. Pull the glove over the gown cuff and fingers of the dominant hand simultaneously (Fig. 40-7).

   Since the fingers do not exit through the gown's cuff, gown and glove contamination is prevented.
4. Carefully push the fingers into the glove and be sure the glove's cuff covers the gown's cuff.

   This ensures proper fit. The glove fits over the gown cuff to provide extra protection against contamination.
5. With the gloved dominant hand, place the opposite glove palm side down over the palm of the covered nondominant hand with the glove fingers pointing toward the elbow (Fig. 40-8).

   Sterile touching sterile is sterile.

| Steps | Rationale |
|---|---|
| 6. Repeat steps 10 and 11 for the nondominant hand (Fig. 40-9). | |
| 7. Interlock the gloved hands. | This ensures smooth fit over the fingers. |
| 8. Remove powder from gloves with sterile wet gauze sponge or sterile towel. | Powder on gloves can irritate client's skin at surgical site. Powder can also be a vehicle for microorganism transport and cause wound adhesions. |

## Evaluation

| | |
|---|---|
| 1. Inspect gloves for holes or tears. | Tear or hole provides route for microorganisms to travel. |
| ***Expected outcome*** | |
| 1. Gloves are intact. | Ensures sterility. |
| ***Unexpected outcome*** | |
| 1. Gloves are torn. Discard glove and don another pair. | Gloves considered contaminated. |

## Special Considerations

- Nurse with cut or lesions on hands may not be allowed to assume role of scrub nurse.

### BIBLIOGRAPHY

Association of Operating Room Nurses, Inc: AORN standards and recommended practices for perioperative nursing AORN, Jan. 24, 1983.

Ganner JS: Guidelines for prevention of surgical wound infections, 1985, Hospital Infections Program, CDC, PHS, and U.S. Department of Health and Human Services

Groah LK: Operating room nursing: the perioperative role, Reston, Va, 1983, Reston Publishing Company, Inc.

Gruendemann BJ, Meeker MH: Alexander's care of the patient in surgery, ed 8, St. Louis, 1987, The CV Mosby Co.

Kneedler JA, Dodge GH: Perioperative patient care, Boston, 1983, Blackwell Scientific Publications.

Potter PA, Perry AG: Fundamentals of nursing: concepts, process, and practice, ed 2, St. Louis, 1989, The C.V. Mosby Co.

# UNIT XIII

# DRESSINGS AND WOUND CARE

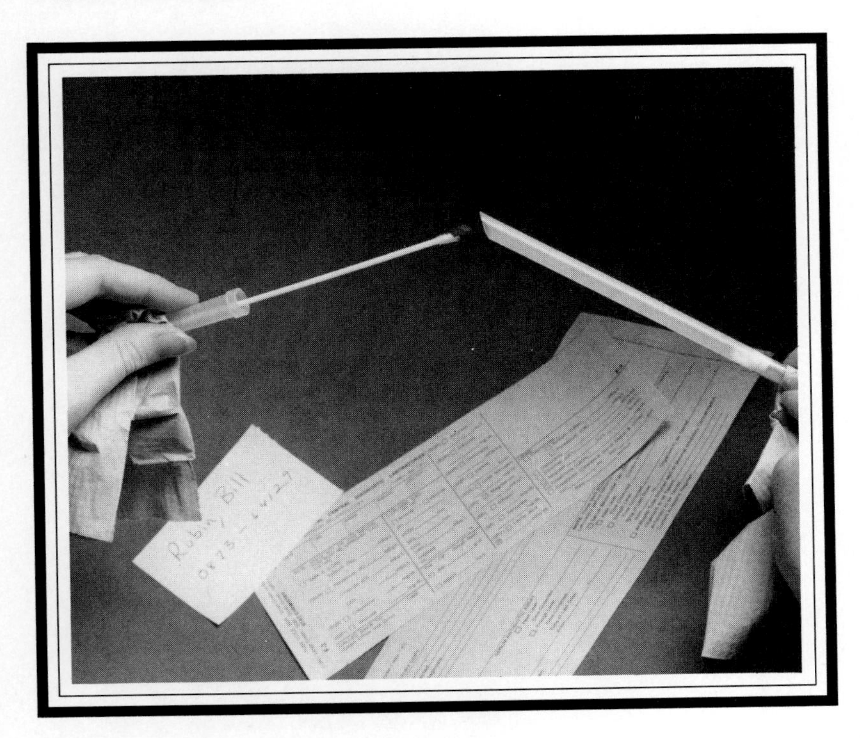

Caring for a surgical, traumatic, thermal, or abrasive wound is necessary to promote wound homeostasis, prevent transmission of infection to the wound site, prevent further wound injury, prevent transmission of infection from an infected wound to clients or health care personnel, support the process of wound healing, maintain skin integrity, or promote a return to normal function. Dressings, binders, hot and cold therapies, and irrigations are measures directed at achieving one or more of the objectives of wound care.

This unit explores dressing and wound care measures in four chapters. Chapter 41, "Dressings," details different skills the nurse uses to change and reapply various dressings that are ordered by the physician. Chapter 42, "Binders and bandages," describes the types of bandages that are used to support an abdominal incision or a sprained or strained extremity. Hot and cold therapies, discussed in Chapter 43, are used to reduce swelling from an injury or to promote circulation and healing. Last, Chapter 44 describes irrigations used to cleanse a wound of necrotic tissue to promote healthy tissue growth and wound healing.

# 41

# DRESSINGS

## OBJECTIVES

*Mastery of content in this chapter will enable the nurse to:*

- Define key terms.
- Properly assess wound healing.
- Choose the correct dressing for a wound.
- Understand the technique of a dressing application.
- State advantages and disadvantages of the types of dressings used.
- Correctly apply a dry, pressure, wet-to-dry, and synthetic dressings.

## KEY TERMS

*Debride*
*Erythema*
*Excoriated*
*Exudate*
*Granulation*
*Macerate*
*Pseudomonas*

## SKILLS

**41-1** Applying a Dry Dressing
**41-2** Applying a Pressure Bandage
**41-3** Applying a Wet-to-Dry Dressing
**41-4** Applying a Transparent Dressing
**41-5** Applying a Hydrocolloid Dressing
**41-6** Applying a Hydrogel Dressing

The properly applied dressing can decrease pain, enhance healing, and improve cosmetic results. The exudate absorbed by the dressing can provide valuable diagnostic information. Dressings serve several functions including protection from outside contaminants, protection from further injury, prevention of the spread of microorganisms, increased client comfort, and the control of bleeding. The ideal dressing should be easy to apply; able to conform to body contours; durable, but flexible; cost effective; able to absorb or contain exudate; easily removed without damage to the healing surface; and acceptable in appearance.

When performing a dressing change the nurse must be knowledgeable about wound healing in order to differentiate a normal or expected appearance from abnormal changes. Primary healing takes place when tissue is cleanly cut and the margins are reapproximated. Repair should occur without complication. New capillary circulation will bridge the wound in 3 to 4 days, and once normal tissue oxygenation is achieved, the wound is considered to be healed. A wound closed for primary healing is most susceptible to infection during the first 4 days. Healing by secondary intention occurs with a wound left open. Healing results through the formation of granulation tissue and eventual epithelialization to close the defect made by the wound. Burns, infected wounds, and deep pressure ulcers heal in this manner. There are various types of dressings applied to wounds. Gauze dressings, the most common type, do not interact with wound tissues and thus cause little wound irritation. Gauze comes in a variety of sizes and shapes. The nurse applies gauze either wet or dry; dry dressings are ideal for wounds with minimal drainage. Wet dressings are preferred for wounds requiring debridement. The nurse moistens the contact dressing layer that touches the wound surface. The moistened gauze increases the absorptive ability of the dressing to collect all exudate and wound debris. The second or absorbent dressing layer is a dry dressing. This wet-to-dry dressing is very effective in cleansing infected and necrotic wounds.

Telfa gauze dressings contain a shiny, nonadherent surface on one side. When used as a contact layer the Telfa gauze does not stick to incisions or wound openings. Drainage passes through the nonadherent surface to the softened gauze above.

The hydrocolloid dressings (DuoDerm, Comfeel, etc.), represent a category of hydroactive dressings. These dressings provide a moist environment for wound healing while facilitating the softening and subsequent removal of wound debris. The dressing promotes wound healing by providing an occlusive protective barrier which absorbs drainage from the wound into the dressing. In addition, the dressing stays in place through an adhesive backing, reduces local pain, and may be used with wound exudate absorbers (e.g., DuoDerm granules) to increase wear time.

Hydrogel dressings (e.g., Vigilon) are useful over clean, moist, or macerated tissues. The dressing provides a nonadherent, protective barrier with the ability to absorb wound drainage.

Dressings are also available as thin, self-adhesive elastic films (e.g., Op-site). The dressing is a synthetic permeable membrane that acts as a temporary second skin. This type of dressing has several advantages: (1) it adheres to undamaged skin to contain exudate and minimize wound contamination, (2) it serves as a barrier to external fluids and bacteria but still allows the wound surface to "breathe," (3) it promotes a moist environment that speeds epithelial cell growth, and (4) it can be removed without damaging underlying tissues. The disadvantage of such a dressing is that it cannot debride an infected or necrotic wound. Op-site is ideal for small, superficial wounds or those that do not require debridement. It is also useful as a dressing over an intravenous catheter site. The transparent film allows the nurse to assess the wound without removing the dressing.

### GUIDELINES

1. Know the expected wound drainage. Wounds that have large amounts of drainage require more frequent dressing changes. Such wounds include fresh postoperative sites, open wounds, and fistulae.
2. Know the type of dressing ordered by the physician. Wet-to-dry dressings require more equipment than do dry dressings. Pressure dressings require elastic bandages to maintain the pressure.
3. Determine if wound drainage tubes are present. This prevents accidental dislocation of a wound drainage tube when the old dressing is removed.
4. Determine the presence of any further break in skin integrity adjacent to the wound. Breaks in skin integrity further increase the client's risk for infection and further skin breakdown due to excoriation from wound drainage or pressure.

### PREREQUISITE KNOWLEDGE

1. Principle of wound healing.
2. Medial asepsis.
3. Surgical asepsis.
4. Signs, symptoms, and treatment of hemorrhagic shock (Skill 41-2 only).

### PREREQUISITE SKILLS

1. Basic handwashing techniques (Chapter 37).
2. Prepare a sterile field (Chapter 38).
3. Perform sterile open gloving (Chapter 38).
4. Monitor vital signs (Chapter 12 for Skill 41-2 only).

## *SKILL 41-1 Applying a Dry Dressing*

A dry dressing may be chosen for management of a wound with little drainage. The dressing protects the wound from injury, prevents introduction of bacteria, reduces discomfort, and speeds healing. A dry dressing also prevents deeper tissues from drying out by keeping the wound surface moist.

Dry dressings are most commonly used for abrasions and nondraining postoperative incisions. The dry dressing does not debride the wound and should not be selected for wounds requiring debridement. If a dry dressing adheres to a wound, the nurse should moisten the dressing with normal saline before removing the gauze. Moistening the dressing in this manner decreases the adherence of the dressing to the wound and reduces the risk of further trauma to the wound.

### Purposes

1. Protect a wound from injury.
2. Protect a wound from introduction of bacteria.
3. Promote wound healing.
4. Reduce discomfort from the wound.

### *Procedure 41-1*

| Steps | Rationale |
|---|---|
| **Assessment** | |
| 1. Assess size of wound to be dressed. | Assists nurse to plan for proper type and amount of supplies needed. |
| 2. Assess location of wound. | Wound location alerts nurse when assistance is needed to hold dressings in place. |
| 3. Assess client's level of comfort. | Removal of dry dressing can be painful; client may require pain medication. |

| Steps | Rationale |
|---|---|
| 4. Assess client's knowledge of purpose of dressing change. | Determines level of support and explanation required by client. |
| 5. Assess need for client or family member to participate in dressing wound. | Prepares client or family member if dressing must be changed at home. |
| 6. Review medical orders for dressing change procedure. | Indicates type of dressing or applications to use. |
| 7. Identify clients at risk for wound healing problems including: | |
| a. Elderly. | Physiological changes of aging alter the immune system, resulting in decreased resistance to pathogens. |
| b. Obesity. | Subcutaneous tissue has diminished vascularity. |
| c. Diabetes. | Vascular changes associated with diabetes reduces blood flow to peripheral tissues, also leukocyte malfunction secondary to hyperglycemia. |
| d. Compromised circulation. | Results in inadequate supply of nutrients, blood cells, and oxygen to wound. |
| e. Poor nutritional state. | Impairs stages of inflammation and collagen formation states. |
| f. Immunosuppressive drugs. | Decreases inflammatory response and decreases collagen synthesis. |
| g. Irradiation in area of wound. | Decreases blood supply to tissues. |
| h. High levels of stress. | Increased cortisol levels reduces number of lymphocytes and decreases inflammatory response. |
| i. Steroids. | Slows rate of epithelialization, neovascularization, and inhibits contraction. |

## Nursing Diagnosis

| Steps | Rationale |
|---|---|
| 1. Cluster data to reveal actual or potential nursing diagnoses: | |
| a. Impaired skin integrity: related to surgical wound. | Wound is a potential entry site for infection. |
| b. Pain: related to incisional inflammation. | Swelling and inflammation related to healing cause discomfort. |
| c. Impaired physical mobility: related to incisional pain. | Clients tend to splint incision and avoid movement |
| d. Knowledge deficit regarding wound healing and care: related to inexperience. | Dressing change procedure takes several minutes and is an excellent time for client/family teaching. |

## Planning

| Steps | Rationale |
|---|---|
| 1. Develop individualized goals for client based on nursing diagnosis: | |
| a. Wound healing progresses without complication. | Nurse uses techniques to minimize pain. Proper application promotes healing process. Clean dressings minimize risk of infection. |
| b. Client has minimal pain. | |
| c. Client increases activity to baseline level. | Proper healing allows for return of mobility. |
| d. Client verbalizes understanding of wound care. | Verbalization of steps of wound care indicates learning is taking place. |
| 2. Explain procedure to client. | Decreases client's anxiety. |
| 3. Assess need for pain medication. | Dressing change will be better tolerated by client if pain medication has been administered before dressing change. |
| 4. Prepare necessary equipment and supplies: | |
| a. Sterile gloves | |
| b. Dressing set (sterile); scissors; forceps | Used to apply dressing and cut gauze to size. |
| c. Sterile drape (optional) | |
| d. Gauze dressings | |
| e. Sterile basin | For antiseptic or cleansing solution. |
| f. Antiseptic ointment (optional) | Prescribed by physician. |
| g. Cleansing solution | |
| h. Sterile saline or water | |
| i. Clean disposable gloves | |
| j. Tape, ties, or bandage as needed | |
| k. Waterproof bag | For disposal of old dressing and supplies. |
| l. Extra gauze dressings | |
| m. Surgi-pads or ABD pads | |
| n. Bath blanket | |
| o. Adhesive remover (optional) | |
| p. Clean, dry work area to place supplies. | |
| 5. Instruct client not to touch wound area or sterile supplies. | Sudden unexpected movement on client's part could result in contamination of wound and supplies. |

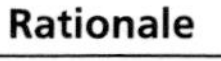

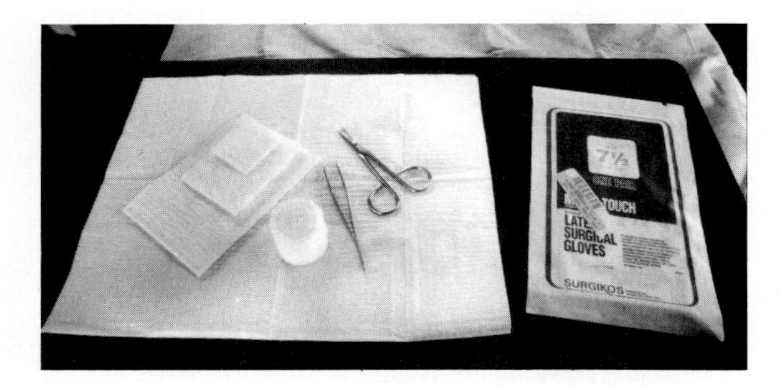


*Fig. 41-1*

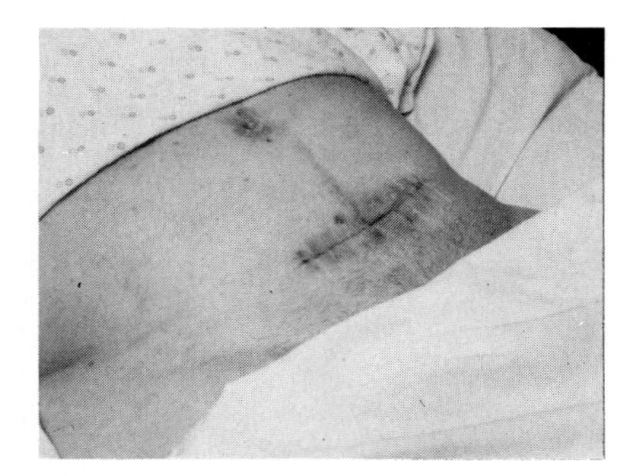

*Fig. 41-2*

## Implementation

| Steps | Rationale |
|---|---|
| 1. Close room or cubicle curtains; close any open windows. | Provides for privacy and reduces airborne microorganisms. |
| 2. Position client comfortably and drape with bath blanket to expose only wound site. | Draping provides access to the wound yet minimizes unnecessary exposure. |
| 3. Wash hands. | Reduces transmission of pathogens to exposed tissues. |
| 4. Place disposable bag within reach of work area. Fold top of bag to make cuff. | Ensures easy disposal of soiled dressings. Prevents soiling of bag's outer surface. |
| 5. Put on clean disposable gloves. | Prevents transmission of infectious organisms from soiled dressings to nurse's hands. |
| 6. Remove tape: pull parallel to skin; pull toward dressing; remove remaining adhesive from skin. | Pulling tape toward dressing reduces stress on suture line or wound edges. |
| 7. With gloved hand remove dressings. Keep soiled undersurface out from client's sight. | Appearance of drainage may be upsetting to client. |
| 8. Observe appearance and amount of drainage on dressing. | Provides estimate of drainage amount and assessment of wound's condition. |
| 9. Dispose of soiled dressings in disposable bag. | Reduces transmission of microorganisms to other persons. |
| 10. Remove gloves by pulling them inside out. Dispose in bag. | Prevents contact of nurse's hands with material on gloves. |
| 11. Open sterile dressing tray or individually wrapped sterile supplies. Place on bedside table (Fig. 41-1). | Sterile dressings remain sterile while on or within sterile surface. Preparation of all supplies prevents break in technique during dressing change. |
| 12. Open bottle of antiseptic solution and pour into sterile basin or over sterile gauze. | Keeps supplies sterile. |
| 13. If sterile drape or gauze packages become wet from solution, repeat preparation of supplies. | Microorganisms move from unsterile environment thorugh dressing package to dressing itself. |
| 14. Put on sterile gloves. | Sterile gloves allow handling of sterile supplies without contamination. |
| 15. Inspect wound for appearance, drains, drainage, and integrity (Fig. 41-2). Measure wound if indicated. Avoid contact with contaminated material. | Indicates status of healing. |
| 16. Cleanse wound with antiseptic solution: | |
| a. Use separate swab for each cleansing stroke. | Prevents contaminating previously cleaned area. |
| b. Clean from least contaminated area to most contaminated. | Cleansing in this direction prevents introduction of organisms into wound. |
| 17. Use dry gauze to swab in same manner in step 16 to dry wound. | Drying reduces excess moisture, which could eventually harbor microorganisms. |
| 18. Apply antiseptic ointment if ordered, using same technique as for cleansing. | Helps reduce growth of microorganisms. |
| 19. Apply dry sterile dressings to incision or wound site | |
| a. Apply loose woven gauze as contact layer. | Promotes proper absorption of drainage. |
| b. Cut 4 × 4 gauze flat to fit around drain if present or use precut drain flat. | Secures drain and promotes drainage absorption at site. |
| c. Apply second layer of gauze. | Layering ensures proper coverage and optimal absorption. |
| d. Apply thicker woven pad (surgi-pad). | Protects wound from external environment. |
| 20. Secure dressing with tape, Montgomery ties (Figs. 41-3) or binder. | Supports wound and ensures placement and stability of dressing. |
| 21. Remove gloves and dispose in bag. | Reduces transmission of microorganisms. |
| 22. Dispose of all supplies. | Clean environment enhances client comfort. |
| 23. Assist client to comfortable position. | Promotes client's sense of well-being. |
| 24. Wash hands. | Reduces transmission of microorganisms. |

| Steps | Rationale |
|---|---|

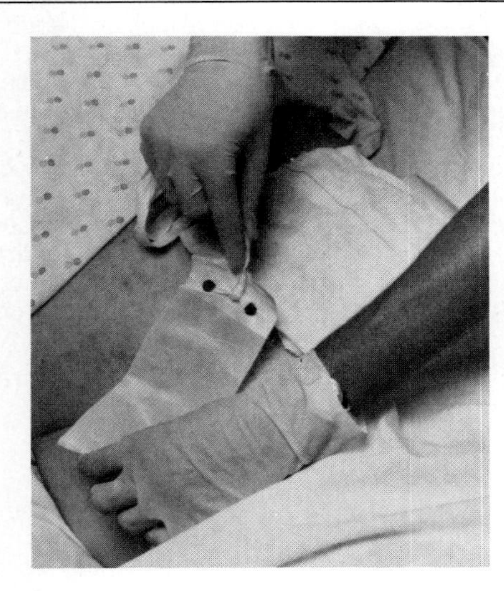

*Fig. 41-3*

## Evaluation

| Steps | Rationale |
|---|---|
| 1. Assess condition of wound. | Determines rate of healing. |
| 2. Ask if client notes discomfort during procedure. | Pain may be early indication of wound complication or result of dressing pulling tissue. |
| 3. Inspect condition of dressing at least every shift. | Determine status of wound drainage. |
| 4. Ask client to describe steps and techniques of dressing change. | Evaluates client's understanding of procedure. |
| ***Expected outcome*** | |
| 1. Client's wound is free of infection; drainage begins to diminish in amount. | Indicates wound is healing appropriately. |
| 2. Client reports minimal discomfort. | Indicates dressing procedure and choice is appropriate. |
| 3. Client explains method of dressing application. | Indicates learning has occurred. |
| ***Unexpected outcomes*** | |
| 1. Wound drainage increases resulting in frequent dressing changes. | May indicate disruption of incision, hemorrhage, or onset of infection. |
| 2. Wound bleeds after removal of dry dressing. | Indicates disruption of epidermal surface. |

## Recording and Reporting

| Steps | Rationale |
|---|---|
| 1. Report: | |
| a. Change in drainage amount to physician on rounds | Change may indicate need for different plan for management. |
| b. Tolerance of client to dressing change during shift change | Allows nurses to provide continuity in pain control. |
| c. Unexpected appearance of wound or drainage or accidental removal of drain within an hour to physician | Unless client shows evidence of wound dehiscence, notification of physician of unexpected findings within an hour is adequate. |
| 2. Record appearance of wound and drainage, client's tolerance, and type of dressing applied in nurses' notes. | Documents progress of wound healing and promotes continuity in dressing change techniques. |
| 3. Record frequency of dressing change and supplies needed on Kardex. | Alerts staff members to dressing change times and supplies needed. |
| 4. Write date and time dressing applied on tape. | Maintains record of time dressing changed for reference should condition change. |

## Follow-up Activities

| Steps | Rationale |
|---|---|
| 1. If teaching self-wound care or family participation, provide feedback to client and family regarding their ability to perform dressing change. | Alerts client and family members to their ability to perform dressing change and provides reinforcement of skill. |
| 2. Provide comfort measures, including positioning, relaxation exercises, analgesics. | Promotes relaxation |

### Special Considerations

- Circumferential wounds may require assistance to cover.
- Administer pain medication to allow drug's peak effect during dressing change.
- Fresh postoperative dressings are usually changed by physician. Subsequent changes are done by staff.
- Tape located over hairy areas should be removed in direction of hair growth to reduce irritation and discomfort.
- If drains are present, remove dressings one layer at a time to avoid accidental removal of drain.
- Wounds requiring a dressing change more often than every 4 hr may indicate need for drain placement or alternate dressing procedure.
- Adherent dressing should be loosened with sterile water or saline before removal.
- Wound dehiscence, evisceration, or unexplained pulsatile bleeding should be reported immediately.
- Personnel resources to assist in wound care include enterostomal therapist, clinical nurse specialist—surgery or oncology, and infection control nurse.

### Teaching Considerations

- Wounds out of client's reach and vision will require a family member's assistance.
- Explain risks of improper wound care.
- Explain expected wound appearance and what should be reported.
- After demonstrating wound care, allow client or family member to perform dressing change with supervision.
- Teach client and primary caregiver method of holding and applying dressing without contamination.
- Allow for return demonstration from the client and primary caregiver on dressing change technique.

### Home Care Considerations

- At home, supplies for wound care should be kept together at convenient location.
- Assess extent of wound or incision in relation to client's level of activity to determine type of dressing that will achieve desired purpose.
- Assess area where procedure will be performed for adequate lighting. Determine if there is table or cabinet on which sterile supplies may be placed with reasonable security.

---

# *SKILL 41-2 Applying a Pressure Bandage*

A pressure bandage is a temporary treatment for the control of excessive bleeding. The bleeding is usually sudden and not anticipated. It may follow surgical intervention, or it may be a life-threatening occurrence related to accidental trauma, stabbing, suicide attempt, or other injury.

An adult weighing 70 kg has a total volume of 5 liters of circulating blood. All nursing actions must be rapidly and effectively executed when excessive blood loss occurs. Once pressure has been applied, it *must* continue until definitive actions can be executed by the health care team. Surgical repair is most often the option of choice.

### Purposes

1. Control bleeding from hemorrhage.
2. Support skin grafts.
3. Support underlying structures following "apron" surgery.
4. Control bleeding from arterial puncture sites.

## *Procedure 41-2*

| Steps | Rationale |
|---|---|
| **Assessment** | |
| 1. Identify clients at risk for unexpected bleeding:<br>a. Traumatic injury.<br>b. Donor graft site.<br>c. Arterial puncture sites.<br>d. Postoperative wounds.<br>e. Wounds after surgical debridement. | Nurse should be familiar with conditions associated with unexpected bleeding to rapidly respond to bleeding. |
| ***Phase I: Immediate action—first nurse "on the scene"*** | |
| 1. Identify client with sudden hemorrhage:<br>a. Locate external bleeding site.<br>b. Apply direct pressure immediately. | Maintaining asepsis and privacy are considered only if time and severity of blood loss permit inclusion of these activities.<br>Hemostasis maintained as supplies are prepared. |
| 2. Seek assistance. | Bandage must be quickly secured. |

| Steps | Rationale |
|---|---|
| ***Phase II: Applying pressure bandage—second nurse "on the scene"*** | |
| 1. Quickly observe location of bleeding. | Bleeding source determines method and supplies needed for applying pressure bandage. |
| 2. Quickly assess client's pulse; blood pressure; skin; anxiety/restlessness. | Findings of tachycardia, hypotension, diaphoresis, restlessness, and diminished urinary output indicate impending hypovolemic shock. |

## Nursing Diagnosis

| Steps | Rationale |
|---|---|
| 1. Nursing diagnoses representative of a problem that requires application of a pressure bandage may include: | |
| a. Altered tissue perfusion: related to hypovolemia. | Uncontrolled bleeding is not compatible with life. |
| b. Decreased cardiac output: related to circulating volume loss. | |

## Planning

| Steps | Rationale |
|---|---|
| 1. Develop individualized goals for client based on nursing diagnosis: | |
| a. Control bleeding. | Pressure bandage controls blood loss until surgical control can be achieved. |
| b. Prevent hypovolemic shock while awaiting definitive intervention. | |
| 2. Explain application of pressure bandage procedure and related goals. | This step may reduce client's stress and anxiety level and is integrated as nurse carries out implementation phase. |
| 3. Quickly prepare necessary equipment and supplies: | Dressing supplies are selected to provide thickness and maintain pressure. |
| a. 6-8 sterile gauze compresses (size $4 \times 4$ or $4 \times 6$) | |
| b. 2- or 3-in roller bandage | |
| c. 2-in adhesive tape | |
| 4. Position client. | |
| a. Elevate bleeding body part. | May diminish vascular flow to part. |
| b. Lower head of client if bleeding is on torso or extremities. | Increases oxygen supply to brain. |

## Implementation

| Steps | Rationale |
|---|---|
| 1. If client's condition permits, wash hands and provide privacy. | Maintaining asepsis and privacy are considered only if time and severity of blood loss permit inclusion of these activities. |
| 2. First person presses on site of bleeding. Second person unwraps roller bandage and places within easy access. | Hemostasis maintained as supplies are prepared. |
| 3. Second person quickly cuts 3-5 lengths of adhesive tape and places them within easy reach | Bandage must be quickly secured. |
| 4. In *simultaneous coordinated actions:* | |
| a. Rapidly cover bleeding area with many thicknesses of gauze compresses. First person slips fingers out as other nurse exerts adequate pressure to continue controlling bleeding. | Gauze is absorbent. Layers provide bulk against which local pressure can be applied to bleeding site. |
| b. Adhesive strips are placed with even pressure on both sides of nurse's fingers as close as possible to central bleeding source. Secure tape on distal end, pull tape across dressing, and maintain firm pressure as proximate end of tape is secured. | Tape exerts downward pressure, promoting hemostasis. |
| c. Remove fingers and quickly cover center of area with third strip of tape. | Provides pressure to source of bleeding. |
| d. Continue reinforcing area with tape as each successive strip is overlapped on alternating sides of center strip. | Prevents tape from loosening. |
| e. When pressure bandage is on extremity, apply roller gauze: apply 2 circular turns tautly on both sides of fingers that are pressing gauze. Compress over bleeding site. Simultaneously remove finger pressure and apply roller gauze pressure over center. Continue with figure-eight turns. Secure end with 2 circular turns and strip of adhesive. | Roller gauze acts as pressure bandage, exerting more even pressure over extremity. To ensure blood flow to distal tissues and prevent tourniquet effect, adhesive tape must not be continued around entire extremity. |

| Steps | Rationale |
|---|---|
| **Evaluation** | |
| 1. Immediately evaluate client to determine response to pressure dressing. Assess: | |
| a. Control of bleeding. | Effective pressure bandage will control bleeding without blocking distal circulation. |
| b. Adequacy of circulation (distal pulse, skin characteristics). | Determines level of perfusion to distal body parts. |
| c. Estimated volume of blood loss. | Determines blood and fluid replacement needs. |
| d. Monitor vital signs. | Identifies early stages of hypovolemic shock. |
| ***Expected outcomes*** | |
| 1. Bleeding is temporarily controlled. | Source of bleeding controlled with pressure. |
| 2. Fluid loss is minimal. | |
| 3. Client is not in state of hypovolemic shock. | Minimal volume of blood lost. |
| 4. Circulation to distal parts is adequate. | Blood flow to periphery maintained. |
| ***Unexpected outcomes*** | |
| 1. Excessive pressure is exerted that results in pain; weak or absent pulses; edema of distal body part; tissue necrosis. | Impaired distal circulation. |
| 2. Uncontrolled hemorrhaging progresses to fluid and electrolyte imbalance; tissue hypoxia; confusion; hypovolemic shock; cardiac arrest; death. | Source of bleeding too large to control by local pressure or bleeding was extensive before care giver arrived. |
| **Recording and Reporting** | |
| 1. Report immediately to physician present status of client's bleeding control, time bleeding was discovered, estimated blood loss, nursing interventions (including effectiveness of applied pressure bandage), apical and distal pulses, blood pressure, sensorium level, signs of restlessness, and need for physician to administer to client without delay. | Provides physician with data describing client's status and type of therapies indicated. |
| 2. Record and implement physician's verbal orders in response to above reporting. (NOTE: Institutional policy on telephone/verbal orders varies). | Nurse must act quickly on basis of client's status. |
| 3. Between-shift report includes emergency situation, intervention and evaluation as reported to physician, and need for continuous bedside monitoring of bleeding control; distal pulse; vital signs; IV; consciousness level; oxygenation or hypoxia; anxiety level. | Provides nurses with data regarding client's status and types of interventions needed to maintain continuity of care. |
| 4. Record on progress note exact findings and care administered in relation to application of pressure bandage. | Documents therapy administered. |
| **Follow-up Activities (Immediate)** | |
| 1. Initiate IV therapy (physician's order is required). | This will replace fluids and is started before onset of hypovolemic shock whenever possible. |
| 2. Initiate NPO order. | Prepares client for definitive surgical intervention and prevention of aspiration. |
| 3. Apply pressure to pressure point PRN; place client in Trendelenburg position; provide warmth. | Reduces surge of blood through arterial vessel. Lowering head and elevating feet maintains oxygenation of brain and vital organs. Maintaining peripheral warmth enhances vital organ perfusion/oxygenation. |
| 4. Monitor vital signs q15min (apical, distal rate, BP). | Indicates bleeding control or continuation of bleeding. |
| 5. Monitor dressing for signs of bleeding. | Provides evaluation of extent of continuing blood loss. |
| a. Reinforce dressing with tape as needed to prevent seepage. | |
| b. If dressing is saturated, remove top layers only and replace. | Prevents disturbing primary layer should a clot have begun forming. |
| **Follow-up Activities (After Definitive Intervention)** | |
| 1. Assess client's emotional status. | Client in shock can suffer neurologic symptoms. |

### Special Considerations

- *Arterial bleeding* is bright red and gushes forth in waves; related to hearth rhythm; if vessel is very deep, flow will be steady. *Venous bleeding* is dark red and flows smoothly. *Capillary bleeding* is oozing of dark red blood; self-sealing controls this bleeding. *Hemorrhage* is loss of a large amount of blood either externally or internally in short period of time.
- Pressure dressing will provide interim control of bleeding while preparing client for definitive intervention by physician.
- If client is in shock, level of consciousness may be diminished.
- Establish IV line quickly if signs and symptoms of hypovolemic shock are present.
- Adhesive tape should extend 3-4 in beyond width of dressing. If bleeding is from incision, adhesive tape should extend from one side to other, pulling edges of incision together.
- Outside pressure does not exclude possibility of extended bleeding into tissues and body cavities.

### Teaching Considerations

- Explain purpose of pressure bandage.
- Explain need to monitor vital signs.
- Explain need for client to remain quiet and stay in position to reduce bleeding.
- Teach primary care giver how to apply a pressure dressing if client is at risk of hemorrhage.

### Home Care Considerations

- At home client may apply pressure with clean towels or linen.
- Emergency system (911) should be activated.
- Client should be positioned to promote elevation of affected body part (if extremity) and promote relaxation.
- Apply pressure dressing with clean towel or piece of linen if gauze is unavailable.
- Contact physician immediately with information about cause, size, and status of the wound.

## SKILL 41-3 Applying a Wet-to-Dry Dressing

The primary purpose of wet-to-dry dressings is to mechanically debride a wound. The moistened contact layer of the dressing increases the absorptive ability of the dressing to collect exudate and wound debris. As the dressing dries, it adheres to the wound and debrides it when the dressing is removed. These dressings are most appropriate for wounds that do not have significant amounts of ischemic or necrotic tissue or large amounts of drainage. One must take care not to apply a dressing so wet that it remains wet continuously (Table 41-1). A too-wet dressing may cause tissue maceration and bacterial growth.

Commonly used wetting agents include normal saline and lactated Ringer's solution, which are isotonic solutions that aid in mechanical debridement. Hydrogen peroxide may be used to irrigate a wound, and varying strengths of acetic acid may be used to treat a *Pseudomonas* infection. Providone-iodine, usually one-half strength, is a rapid-acting antimicrobial agent. Other antibiotic solutions may be ordered, although their use is controversial. Wetting solutions should be discarded 24 hr after opening and replaced with fresh solution because they can harbor microorganism growth.

### Purposes

1. Debride a wound.
2. Promote wound healing.

**TABLE 41-1 PROBLEMS ASSOCIATED WITH WOUNDS REQUIRING DEBRIDEMENT**

| Problem | Nursing Activities |
|---|---|
| Solutions used are irritating to healthy skin around wound, i.e., Dakin's solution, acetic acid, povidone-iodine, etc. | Protect healthy skin with protective barrier, such as stomahesive, or apply topical ointments, such as zinc oxide. If zinc oxide is used, it should be removed with mineral oil. |
| Wound becomes excessively dry. | Continually moist dressing (with a physician's order) might be tried. Eliminate fine mesh gauze and lightly pack wound with fluffy gauze dampened with prescribed solution. |
| Wound is deep and retention of dressing in cavity is suspected. | Irrigate wound copiously with prescribed solution to remove. Use continuous "ribbon" of gauze to dress deep wounds. |
| Wound drainage is damaging healthy tissue. | Protect healthy tissue with skin barrier, such as stomahesive. Wounds with large amounts of drainage may benefit from occlusive drainage collection device. |
| Client's skin is irritated by tape. | Use stomahesive under tape, use Montgomery ties as needed, use fabric tape that has multidirection stretch, secure dressing with binder, or wrap with roll gauze if on extremity. |

## *Procedure 41-3*

### Assessment

| Steps | Rationale |
|---|---|
| 1. Assess location and size of wound to be dressed. | Allows nurse to determine supplies needed and if assistance is required. |
| 2. Review nurses' notes and care plan for description of wound. | Provides baseline for previous wound appearance and drainage characteristics. |
| 3. Review physician's orders for frequency of dressing change and solution to be used. | Physician will order frequency of dressing changes and solutions needed. |
| 4. Assess clients' level of comfort, administer pain medication as needed. | For dressing changes known to be painful, medications may be ordered specifically timed to peak during procedure. |
| 5. Assess client's knowledge of purpose of dressing change. | Determines level of support and explanation required by client. |
| 6. Assess need for client or family member to participate in dressing wound. | Prepares client or family member if dressing must be changed at home. |
| 7. Identify clients at risk for wound healing. Risks include: a. Elderly. b. Obesity. c. Diabetes, especially when not under good control. d. Compromised circulation. e. Poor nutritional state. f. Immunosuppressive drugs. g. Irradiation in area of wound. h. High level of stress. i. Steroids. | Influences type of observations made by nurse during dressing changes because such clients are at risk for wound healing complications. |

### Nursing Diagnosis

| Steps | Rationale |
|---|---|
| 1. Cluster data to reveal actual or potential nursing diagnoses: | |
| a. Impaired skin integrity: related to pressure ulcer, abdominal wound, etc. | Wound provides potential entry site for infection. |
| b. Pain: related to incisional swelling. | During healing process wounds may be inflamed and tender. |
| c. Potential for infection related to surgical incision. | Wound provides potential entry site for infection. |
| d. Impaired physical mobility: related to incisional pain. | Clients tend to splint incision and avoid movement. |
| e. Knowledge deficit regarding wound healing and care: related to inexperience. | Dressing change procedure takes several minutes and is an excellent time for client/family teaching. |

### Planning

| Steps | Rationale |
|---|---|
| 1. Develop individualized goals for client based on nursing diagnoses: | |
| a. Wound heals. | Proper dressing technique keeps wound clean. |
| b. Control pain. | Dressing technique should minimize manipulation of tissues. |
| c. Freedom from infection. | Wet-to-dry dressing debrides tissue to allow for healing. |
| d. Increase knowledge of wound care. | During procedure nurse explains techniques and rationale. |
| 2. Explain procedure to client. Instruct client not to touch sterile supplies. | Relieves anxiety and promotes understanding of dressing change. Prevents contamination of supplies. |
| 3. Prepare necessary equipment and supplies: a. Sterile gloves b. Dressing set (scissors and forceps) c. Sterile drape (optional) d. Thin fine mesh gauze e. Gauze dressings and pads f. Basin for antiseptic or cleaning solution g. Sterile solution prescribed to moisten dressing h. Waterproof pad i. Sterile saline or water j. Clean disposable gloves k. Tape, ties, or bandage as needed l. Waterproof bag for disposal m. Extra gauze dressings and surgi-pads or ABD pads n. Bath blanket o. Adhesive remover p. Clean, dry work area | Reduces risk of break in sterile technique. |
| 4. Position client to allow access to area to be dressed. | Facilitates application of dressing. |

| Steps | Rationale |
|---|---|
| **Implementation** | |
| 1. Close room or cubicle curtains. Close any open windows. | Provides for client privacy and reduces air currents that may transmit microorganisms. |
| 2. Expose wound site and cover client with bath blanket. | Provides access to wound while minimizing exposure. |
| 3. Take disposable waterproof bag and make cuff at top. Place bag within reach of work area. | Cuff prevents accidental contamination of top of outer bag. Nurse should not reach across sterile field. |
| 4. Place waterproof pad under client where dressing is to be changed. | Prevents soiling of bed linens. |
| 5. Wash hands thoroughly. | Removes microorganisms from skin surface. |
| 6. Put on clean disposable gloves and remove tape or bandage or untie Montgomery ties. | Prevents transmission of infectious organisms. |
| 7. Remove tape by loosening end and pulling gently, parallel to skin and toward dressing. | Reduces tension against wound edges. |
| 8. With gloved hand or forceps, lift dressings off, keeping soiled undersurface away from client's sight. If dressing adheres to underlying tissues, do not moisten it. Gently free dressing and warn client about possible discomfort. | Appearance of drainage may be upsetting to client. Purpose of dressing is to remove necrotic tissue and exudate. |
| 9. Observe character and amount of drainage on dressings. | Provides estimate of amount of drainage lost and assessment of wound's condition. |
| 10. Dispose of soiled dressings in prepared waterproof bag. | Reduces transmission of microorganisms to other persons. |
| 11. Remove disposable gloves by pulling them inside out and dispose of them properly. | Reduces risk of microorganisms transmission to others. |
| 12. Prepare sterile dressing supplies. | Reduces risk of break in sterile technique resulting in contamination. |
| 13. Pour prescribed solution into sterile basin and add fine mesh gauze. | Contact layer must be totally moistened to increase dressing's absorptive abilities. |
| 14. Put on sterile gloves. | Allows handling of sterile supplies without contamination. |
| 15. Inspect wound for color, character of drainage, presence and type of sutures, presence of any drains. | Provides assessment of wound healing. |
| 16. Cleanse wound with prescribed antiseptic solution or normal saline. Clean from least to most contaminated area. | Assists in debridement and cleanses wound of debris. |
| 17. Apply moist fine-mesh gauze directly onto wound surface in a single layer. If wound is deep, gently pack gauze into wound with forceps until all wound surfaces are in contact with moist gauze (Fig. 41-4). | Moist gauze absorbs drainage and adheres to debris. Wound should be loosely packed to facilitate wicking of drainage into absorbant outer layer of dressing. |

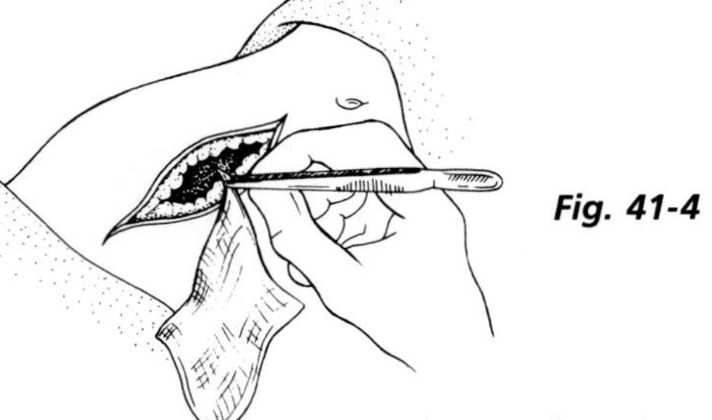

***Fig. 41-4***

| Steps | Rationale |
|---|---|
| 18. Apply dry sterile gauze fluffs over wet gauze. | Dry layer pulls moisture from wound. |
| 19. Cover with ABD pad, surgi-pad, or gauze. | Protects wound from the entrance of microorganisms. |
| 20. Apply tape over dressing, roll gauze (for circumferential dressings), or Montgomery ties. For application of Montgomery ties: | Secures dressing in place. |
| a. Expose adhesive surface of tape end. | Montgomery tie allows for frequent dressing changes without removal of adhesive tape. |
| b. Place ties on opposite sides of dressing. | |
| c. Adhesive may be placed directly on client's skin or skin barrier may be used. | |
| d. Secure dressing by lacing ties across dressing. | |
| 21. Remove and dispose of gloves. | Restores client's sense of well-being. |
| 22. Assist client to comfortable position. | |
| 23. Wash hands thoroughly. | Reduces transfer of microorganisms. |
| **Evaluation** | |
| 1. Assess if client indicates pain during procedure. | Determines client's comfort level. |
| 2. Monitor status of dressing at least every shift. | Evaluates extent of drainage and integrity of dressing. |
| 3. Ask client to describe wound care method. | Evaluates level of client's understanding of procedure. |

| Steps | Rationale |
|---|---|
| ***Expected outcomes*** | |
| 1. Wound is clean; granulation tissue is present; exudate and necrotic debris are decreased. | Indicates progress in wound healing. |
| 2. Client experiences minimal discomfort. | Pain medication and positioning effective. |
| 3. Client explains procedure correctly. | Indicates learning has occurred. |
| ***Unexpected outcomes*** | |
| 1. Wound eschar toughens. | Eschar may require surgical debridement before resumption of wet-to-dry dressing changes. |
| 2. Character of wound drainage changes (increases, purulent). | May indicate infection or dehiscence. |
| 3. Skin around wound margins becomes red and excoriated. | May indicate solution in contact with skin or acidity of wound drainage. |
| **Recording and Reporting** | |
| 1. Report brisk bright red bleeding or evidence of wound dehiscence to physician immediately. | Requires immediate intervention. |
| 2. Report wound appearance and characteristics of drainage at shift change. | Ensures continuity of care by nursing staff. |
| 3. Record wound appearance, color, presence and characteristics of exudate, type and amount of dressings used, and tolerance of client to procedure. | Documents client's progress and therapy provided. |
| 4. Write date and time dressing applied on tape. | Maintains record of time dressing changed for reference should condition change. |
| **Follow-up Activities** | |
| 1. Instruct client to observe wound for change in drainage. | Client may be first to observe change. |
| 2. Encourage client or significant other to participate in dressing changes (if it is anticipated that dressings will need changing after discharge). | Involvement of client or family member while in hospital will give client encouragement that he can manage dressing change at home. |

### Special Considerations

- Saturated dressing will remain wet, and bacteria will grow.
- If drains are present, remove dressings one layer at a time.
- Physician will specify type of solution to be used for cleansing.
- Rapid removal of adherent gauze layer may cause unnecessary discomfort and bleeding.
- If dressing is to be changed twice a day or more frequently, Montgomery ties reduce skin irritation from adhesives.
- Resources to assist in wound care include enterostomal therapist, clinical nurse specialist—surgery or oncology, infection control nurse, and home health nurse.

### Teaching Considerations

- Explain risks of improper wound care.
- Explain expected appearance of wound and what should be reported.
- Wounds out of client's reach and vision will require family member's assistance.
- After demonstrating wound care, allow client or family member to perform dressing change with supervision.

## *SKILL 41-4* Applying a Transparent Dressing

Polyurethane moisture-vapor permeable film dressings were developed for the management of superficial wounds. Pain and discomfort are diminished with the use of a transparent dressing, and the film conforms well to different body contours. Therefore bodily movement is less restricted.

With the use of a transparent dressing, a moist exudate forms over the wound surface, which prevents tissue dehydration and allows for rapid, effective healing.

For best results these dressings should be used on clean, debrided wounds that are not actively bleeding. The film should be applied wrinkle free but not stretched over the skin. Should the fluid accumulation take on a white, opaque appearance with erythema of the surrounding tissue, one must assume an infectious process, the dressing should be removed, and a wound culture obtained.

## Purposes

1. Promote wound healing.
2. Prevent entrance of bacteria into the wound.
3. Provide for easy visualization of a wound.
4. Reduce discomfort from wound.

# *Procedure 41-4*

| Steps | Rationale |
|---|---|
| **Assessment** | |
| 1. Assess location and size of wound to be dressed. | Allows nurse to determine supplies and assistance needed. |
| 2. Review physician's orders for frequency and type of dressing change. | Physician will order frequency of dressing changes and special instructions. |
| 3. Assess client's level of comfort. | If client is comfortable during procedure, he is less likely to move suddenly causing wound or supply contamination. |
| 4. Assess client's knowledge of purpose of dressing. | Identifies client's learning needs. |
| **Nursing Diagnosis** | |
| 1. Cluster data to reveal actual or potential nursing diagnoses: | |
| a. Impaired skin integrity: related to abraded tissue. | Dressing used for superficial wounds that are entry site for infection. |
| b. Pain: related to wound irritation. | Process of healing causes inflammation and tenderness. |
| **Planning** | |
| 1. Develop individualized goals for client based on nursing diagnoses: | |
| a. Control pain. | Proper application minimizes discomfort. |
| b. Prevent skin breakdown. | Dressing avoids use of tape. |
| c. Enhance wound healing. | Proper use of dressing promotes healing. |
| 2. Explain procedure to client. | Relieves anxiety and promotes understanding of healing process. |
| 3. Prepare following equipment and supplies:<br>a. Sterile gloves<br>b. Dressing set (optional)<br>c. Basin for cleansing solution<br>d. Sterile saline<br>e. Clean disposable gloves<br>f. Waterproof bag for disposal<br>g. Transparent dressing (size as needed)<br>h. Bath blanket (optional)<br>i. Sterile gauze pads (4 × 4s)<br>j. Clean, dry work area | Reduces risk of break in sterile technique. |
| 4. Position client to allow access to dressing site. | Facilitates application of dressing. |
| **Implementation** | |
| 1. Close room or cubicle curtains. | Provides for client privacy and reduces air currents that may transmit microorganisms. |
| 2. Expose wound site and cover client with bath blanket. | Draping provides access to wound while minimizing exposure. |
| 3. Cuff top of disposable waterproof bag and place within reach of work area. | Cuff prevents accidental contamination of top of outer bag. Nurse should not reach across sterile field. |
| 4. Wash hands. | Removes microorganisms present on skin surface. |
| 5. Put on clean disposable gloves. | Reduces transmission of infectious organisms from soiled dressings to nurse's hands. |
| 6. Remove old dressing. For easier removal soak area with water, ease off using cotton swab soaked in mineral oil, or secure piece of tape to corner of dressing and pull back slowly across dressing in direction of hair growth. | Reduces excoriation or irritation of skin following dressing removal. |
| 7. Dispose of soiled dressings in waterproof bag. | Reduces transmission of microorganisms. |
| 8. Remove disposable gloves by pulling them inside out and dispose of them in waterproof bag. | Reduces transmission of microorganisms. |
| 9. Prepare sterile dressing supplies. | Reduces risk of break in sterile technique. |
| 10. Pour saline or prescribed solution into basin and soak 4 × 4s. | Maintains sterility of dressing. |

| Steps | Rationale |
|---|---|

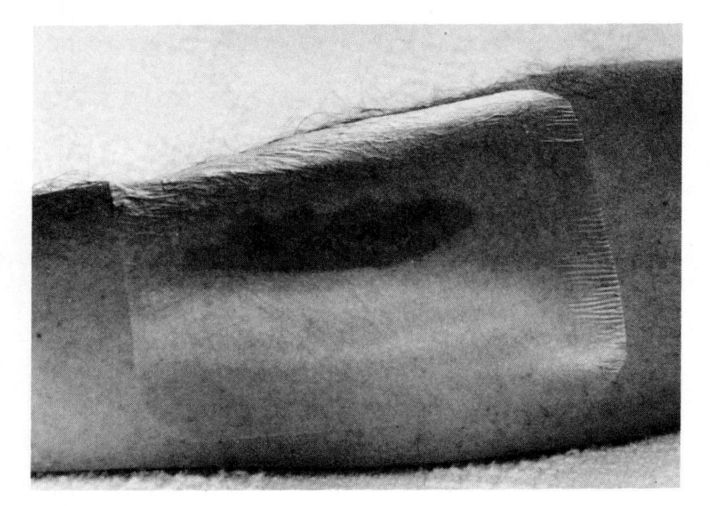

*Fig. 41-5*

| Steps | Rationale |
|---|---|
| 11. Put on sterile gloves. | Allows nurse to handle sterile dressings. |
| 12. Cleanse area gently with soaked 4 × 4s, swabbing toward area of most exudate. | Reduces introduction of organisms into wound. |
| 13. Dry area thoroughly with dry 4 × 4s. | Dressing will not adhere to damp surface. Transparent dressing has adhesive backing. |
| 14. Inspect wound for color, odor, and drainage. | Appearance indicates state of wound healing. |
| 15. Apply transparent dressing according to manufacturer's directions (Fig 41-5). | Film should not be stretched during applications. Avoid wrinkles in film that would provide tunnel for exudate drainage. |
| 16. Remove sterile gloves by pulling inside out and discard in prepared bag. | Reduces risk of microorganism transfer. |
| 17. Assist client to comfortable position. | Enhances client comfort and relaxation. |
| 18. Discard soiled dressing change materials properly. | Reduces transmission of microorganisms. |
| 19. Wash hands. | Reduces risk of microorganism transmission. |

## Evaluation

| | |
|---|---|
| 1. Inspect condition of wound on ongoing basis. | Determines status of wound healing. Wound can easily be viewed. |
| 2. Evaluate client's level of comfort. | Determines if pain resulted from procedure. |

### *Expected outcomes*

| | |
|---|---|
| 1. Wound heals rapidly with little pain and mobility restriction for client. | Dressing effective in preventing infection and promoting healing. |

### *Unexpected outcomes*

| | |
|---|---|
| 1. Wound becomes infected. | Dressing changes may need to be done more frequently, or different type of dressing may be required. |
| 2. Dressing does not stay in place. | Evaluate size of dressing used for adequate (1-1½ in) margin, or dry skin more thoroughly before reapplication. |

## Recording and Reporting

| | |
|---|---|
| 1. Report unusual observations immediately, then chart what reported and when. | Change in wound's condition may require new therapy. |
| 2. Record characteristics of wound, color, odor, viscosity, and amount of drainage, and application of dressing in nurse's notes. | Documents status of wound and ensures continuity of care. |

## Follow-up Activities

| | |
|---|---|
| 1. Observe wound, without disturbing dressing, every shift. | Transparency of dressing allows for easy evaluation of wound appearance. |

### Special Considerations

- Evaluate wound appearance after cleansing.
- Measure wound using greatest and smallest dimensions after cleansing.
- Transparent dressings may be used over "island" dressing, such as Telfa, cut to fit area of wound.
- Transparent dressings may stay in place up to 7 days, if complete occlusion is maintained.
- Appearance of wound may not be tolerated by client. Cover transparent dressing with dry gauze dressing taking care not to place tape directly on transparent dressing.
- If wound exudate builds up to cause bulge in dressing, either change dressing or aspirate fluid using small-gauge needle; patch hole with small piece of film.

### Teaching Considerations

- Explain wound healing process with film dressing.
- Explain need to change dressing should edges loosen.
- Allow client or family member to demonstrate dressing change should need be identified.

### Home Care Considerations

- Wound cleansing may be accomplished in shower, if approved by physician.
- Client may shower/bathe with dressing in place.
- Many types of transparent dressings exist on market. Explore types with client and recommend type client finds easy to work with and has access to.

## *SKILL 41-5 Applying a Hydrocolloid Dressing*

Hydrocolloid dressings were developed for the management of primarily stage 1, 2, and 3 wounds. Pain and discomfort are diminished with the use of a hydrocolloid dressing, and the adhesive-backed dressing conforms well to different body contours.

With the use of a hydrocolloid dressing, wound exudate will be absorbed into the dressing, forming a gel next to the wounded surface. The dressing maintains a moist, insulated environment that promotes rapid, effective healing.

The hydrocolloid dressings are used frequently over venous stasis ulcers, arterial ulcers, and pressure ulcers (Chapter 7). When used in combination with wound exudate absorbers, these dressings are useful over stage 3 ulcers.

### Purposes

1. Promote wound healing.
2. Prevent entrance of bacteria into the wound.
3. Reduce discomfort from wound.
4. Reduce the frequency of dressing changes.

## *Procedure 41-5*

| Steps | Rationale |
|---|---|
| **Assessment** | |
| 1. Assess location and size of wound to be dressed. | Allows nurse to determine supplies and assistance needed. |
| 2. Review physician's orders for frequency and type of dressing change. | Physician orders mode of therapy. |
| 3. Assess client's level of comfort. | If client is comfortable during procedure, he is less likely to move suddenly causing wound or supply contamination. |
| 4. Assess client's knowledge of purpose of dressing. | Identifies client's learning needs. |
| **Nursing Diagnosis** | |
| 1. Cluster data to reveal actual or potential nursing diagnoses: | |
| a. Impaired skin integrity: related to tissue ulceration. | Dressing used for superficial wounds that are entry site for infection. |
| b. Pain: related to wound irritation. | Process of healing causes inflammation and tenderness. |
| **Planning** | |
| 1. Develop individualized goals for client based on nursing diagnoses: | |
| a. Control pain. | Proper analgesia before dressing change minimizes discomfort. |
| b. Prevent skin breakdown. | Dressing avoids use of tape. |
| c. Enhance wound healing. | Proper use of dressing promotes healing. |

| Steps | Rationale |
|---|---|
| 2. Explain procedure to client. | Relieves anxiety and promotes understanding of healing process. |
| 3. Prepare following equipment and supplies:<br>a. Sterile gloves<br>b. Dressing set (optional)<br>c. Basin for cleansing solution<br>d. Sterile saline<br>e. Clean disposable gloves<br>f. Waterproof bag for disposal<br>g. Hydrocolloid dressing (size as needed)<br>h. Bath blanket (optional)<br>i. Sterile gauze pads (4 × 4s)<br>j. K-Y jelly (optional)<br>k. Clean, dry work area | Reduces risk of break in sterile technique. |
| 4. Position client to allow access to dressing site. | Facilitates application of dressing. |

## Implementation

| Steps | Rationale |
|---|---|
| 1. Close room door or cubicle curtains. | Provides for client privacy and reduces air currents that may transmit microorganisms. |
| 2. Expose wound site and cover client with bath blanket. | Draping provides access to wound while minimizing exposure. |
| 3. Cuff top of disposable waterproof bag and place within reach of work area. | Cuff prevents accidental contamination of top of outer bag. Nurse should not reach across sterile field. |
| 4. Wash hands. | Removes microorganisms present on skin surface. |
| 5. Put on clean disposable gloves. | Reduces transmission of infectious organisms from soiled dressings to nurse's hands. |
| 6. Remove old dressing. For easier removal, ease off with K-Y jelly and pull back slowly across dressing in direction of hair growth. | Reduces irritation and possible injury to skin with removal of adhesive dressing. |
| 7. Dispose of soiled dressings in waterproof bag. | Reduces transmission of microorganisms. |
| 8. Remove disposable gloves by pulling them inside out and dispose of them in waterproof bag. | Reduces transmission of microorganisms. |
| 9. Prepare sterile dressing supplies. | Reduces risk of break in sterile technique. |
| 10. Pour saline or prescribed solution into basin and soak 4 × 4s. | Maintains sterility of dressing. |
| 11. Put on sterile gloves. | Allows nurse to handle sterile dressings. |
| 12. Cleanse area gently with soaked 4 × 4s, swabbing exudate away from wound. | Reduces introduction of organisms into wound. |
| 13. Dry area thoroughly with dry 4 × 4s. | Dressing will not adhere to damp surface. Hydrocolloid dressing has adhesive backing. |
| 14. Inspect wound for color, odor, and drainage. | Appearance indicates state of wound healing. |
| 15. Apply hydrocolloid dressing according to manufacturer's directions. Apply hydrocolloid granules or paste to deeper wounds. | Dressing should not be stretched during applications. Avoid wrinkles that would provide tunnel for exudate drainage. Edges may be notched to help mold around wound. Hydrocolloid granules assist in absorbing drainage to increase wearing time of dressing. |
| 16. Remove sterile gloves by pulling inside out and discard in prepared bag. | Reduces risk of microorganism transfer. |
| 17. Assist client to comfortable position. | Enhances client comfort and relaxation. |
| 18. Discard soiled dressing change materials properly. | Reduces transmission of microorganisms. |
| 19. Wash hands. | Reduces risk of microorganism transmission. |

## Evaluation

| Steps | Rationale |
|---|---|
| 1. Inspect condition of wound on ongoing basis. | Determines status of wound healing. Wound can easily be viewed. |
| 2. Evaluate client's level of comfort. | Determines if pain resulted from procedure. |

### *Expected outcomes*

| Steps | Rationale |
|---|---|
| 1. Wound heals rapidly with little pain and mobility restriction for client. | Dressing effective in preventing infection and promoting healing. |

### *Unexpected outcomes*

| Steps | Rationale |
|---|---|
| 1. Wound becomes infected. | Dressing changes may need to be done more frequently, or different type of dressing may be required. |

| Steps | Rationale |
|---|---|
| 2. Dressing does not stay in place. | Evaluate size of dressing used for adequate (1-1½ in) margin, or dry skin more thoroughly before reapplication. |
| 3. Wound develops more necrotic tissue and increases in size. | In rare instances, wounds do not tolerate hypoxia induced by hydrocolloid dressings. In these clients use should be discontinued. |

### Recording and Reporting

| | |
|---|---|
| 1. Report unusual observations immediately, then chart what reported and when. | Change in wound's condition may require new therapy. |
| 2. Record characteristics of wound, color, odor, viscosity, and amount of drainage, and application of dressing in nurse's notes. | Documents status of wound and ensures continuity of care. |

### Follow-up Activities

| | |
|---|---|
| 1. Observe dressing for adhesion every shift. | Proper adhesion reduces the risk of wound contamination by microorganisms. |
| 2. Document wound appearance with dressing changes. | Most hydrocolloid dressings do not allow visualization of the wound. |

### Special Considerations

- Evaluate wound appearance after cleansing.
- Hydrocolloid dressings may be left in place as long as 7 days, if complete occlusion is maintained.
- Hydrocolloid dressings may be used over wound exudate absorbers.
- Some hydrocolloid dressings swell as dressing absorbs wound exudate, change when dressing has changed or swollen to within ½ in of dressing edge.
- Edge of dressing may be "picture-framed" with hypoallergenic tape to prevent accidental pulling on edge of dressing.
- Hydrocolloid dressings should be left in place at least 48 hr. If wound appearance must be evaluated more frequently, alternative dressing should be used.

### Home Care Considerations

- See transparent dressings (Skill 41-4).

## *SKILL 41-6 Applying a Hydrogel Dressing*

Hydrogel dressings are a type of colloid that will expand in water but will not dissolve in it. The gel is available in a "sheet" form or a fluid, which can be placed in the wound.

Hydrogel dressings facilitate wound debridement by rehydrations; they will absorb exudate and encourage healing by maintaining a moist wound healing environment. The gel dressings are nonadherent and must be covered with a secondary dressing.

The hydrogels may be used over leg ulcers, pressure ulcers, minor burns, protection of skin before radiation, and extravasation injuries.

### Purposes

1. Promote wound healing.
2. Reduce discomfort from the wound.
3. Promote wound debridement.
4. Absorb wound exudate.

## *Procedure 41-6*

| Steps | Rationale |
|---|---|
| **Assessment** | |
| 1. Assess location and size of wound to be dressed. | Allows nurse to determine supplies and assistance needed. |
| 2. Review physician's orders for frequency and type of dressing change. | Physician will order frequency of dressing changes and special instructions. |

| Steps | Rationale |
|---|---|
| 3. Assess client's level of comfort. | If client is comfortable during procedure, he is less likely to move suddenly causing wound or supply contamination. |
| 4. Assess client's knowledge of purpose of dressing. | Identifies client's learning needs. |

## Nursing Diagnosis

| Steps | Rationale |
|---|---|
| 1. Cluster data to reveal actual or potential nursing diagnoses: | |
| a. Impaired skin integrity: related to thermal injury. | Dressing used for superficial wounds that are entry site for infection. |
| b. Pain: related to wound irritation. | Process of healing causes inflammation and tenderness. |

## Planning

| Steps | Rationale |
|---|---|
| 1. Develop individualized goals for client based on nursing diagnoses: | |
| a. Control pain. | Proper application minimizes discomfort. |
| b. Prevent skin breakdown. | Dressing avoids use of tape. |
| c. Enhance wound healing. | Proper use of dressing promotes healing. |
| 2. Explain procedure to client. | Relieves anxiety and promotes understanding of healing process. |
| 3. Prepare following equipment and supplies:<br>a. Sterile gloves<br>b. Dressing set (optional)<br>c. Basin for cleansing solution<br>d. Sterile saline<br>e. Clean disposable gloves<br>f. Waterproof bag for disposal<br>g. Hydrogel dressing<br>h. Bath blanket (optional)<br>i. Sterile gauze pads (4 × 4s)<br>j. Clean, dry work area | Reduces risk of break in sterile technique. |
| 4. Position client to allow access to dressing site. | Facilitates application of dressing. |

## Implementation

| Steps | Rationale |
|---|---|
| 1. Close room door or cubicle curtains. | Provides for client privacy and reduces air currents that may transmit microorganisms. |
| 2. Expose wound site and cover client with bath blanket. | Draping provides access to wound while minimizing exposure. |
| 3. Cuff top of disposable waterproof bag and place within reach of work area. | Cuff prevents accidental contamination of top of outer bag. Nurse should not reach across sterile field. |
| 4. Wash hands. | Removes microorganisms present on skin surface. |
| 5. Put on clean disposable gloves. | Reduces transmission of infectious organisms from soiled dressings to nurse's hands. |
| 6. Remove old dressing. | Hydrogel sheet dressing may be lifted off. Fluid gels will need to be irrigated from wound. |
| 7. Dispose of soiled dressings in waterproof bag. | Reduces transmission of microorganisms. |
| 8. Remove disposable gloves by pulling them inside out and dispose of them in waterproof bag. | Reduces transmission of microorganisms. |
| 9. Prepare sterile dressing supplies. | Reduces risk of break in sterile technique. |
| 10. Pour saline or prescribed solution into basin and soak 4 × 4s. | Maintains sterility of dressing. |
| 11. Put on sterile gloves. | Allows nurse to handle sterile dressings. |
| 12. Cleanse area gently with soaked 4 × 4s, swabbing exudate away from wound. | Reduces introduction of organisms into wound. |
| 13. Inspect wound for color, odor, and drainage. | Appearance indicates state of wound healing. |
| 14. Apply hydrogel dressing according to manufacturer's directions. | Fluid gells will take form of cavity-type wounds. |
| 15. Remove sterile gloves by pulling inside out and discard in prepared bag. | Reduces risk of microorganism transfer. |
| 16. Assist client to comfortable position. | Enhances client comfort and relaxation. |
| 17. Discard soiled dressing change materials properly. | Reduces transmission of microorganisms. |
| 18. Wash hands. | Reduces risk of microorganism transmission. |

| Steps | Rationale |
|---|---|
| **Evaluation** | |
| 1. Inspect condition of wound on ongoing basis. | Determines status of wound healing. |
| 2. Evaluate client's level of comfort. | Determines if pain resulted from procedure. |
| ***Expected outcomes*** | |
| 1. Wound heals rapidly with little pain and mobility restriction for client. | Dressing effective in preventing infection and promoting healing. |
| ***Unexpected outcomes*** | |
| 1. Wound becomes infected. | Dressing changes may need to be done more frequently, or different type of dressing may be required. |
| **Recording and Reporting** | |
| 1. Report unusual observations immediately, then chart what reported and when. | Change in wound's condition may require new therapy. |
| 2. Record characteristics of wound, color, odor, viscosity, and amount of drainage, and application of dressing in nurse's notes. | Documents status of wound and ensures continuity of care. |
| **Follow-up Activities** | |
| 1. Observe dressing for containment of exudate every shift. | Dressing should be changed when absorptive capacity has been reached. |

## Special Considerations

- Hydrogel dressings must be used with secondary dressing.
- Hydrogel dressings may be used as carrier for topical medications.
- Hydrogel dressings should not be used in infected wounds.
- Frequency required for dressing changes will be dependent on amount of exudate produced by wound. Fluid gels should not be left in place more than 3 days.

### BIBLIOGRAPHY

Barnett A, et al.: Comparison of synthetic adhesive moisture vapor permeable and fine mesh gauze dressings for split-thickness skin graft donor sites, Am J Surg 145:379, 1983.

Bauman, B: Update your technique for changing dressings: dry-to-dry, Nurs '82, January, p. 64.

Bauman, B: Update your technique for changing dressings: wet-to-dry, Nurs '82, February, p. 68.

Choosing the right wound dressing, Patient Care, July 15, 1984, p. 149.

Cuzzell JZ: Artful solutions to chronic problems, Am J Nurs 85(2):162, 1985.

Flynn ME, Rovee DT: Wound healing mechanisms, Am J Nurs 82(10):1544, 1982.

Hunt TK: Wound healing in current surgical diagnosis and treatment, ed 6, Los Altos, Calif, 1983, Lange Medical Publications.

Jeter K, Tintle T: Principles of wound cleaning and wound care, J Home Health Care Prac 1:1, 1988.

Lawrence JC: What materials for dressings? Injury 13(6):500, 1982.

Lobe TE, et al.: An improved method of wound management for pediatric patients, J Pediat Surg 15(6):886, 1980.

May SR, and Still JM: Contemporary wound management with natural and synthetic dressings, Ostomy/Wound Management 15:14, 1987.

Meyer D: Client teaching guides for home health care, Rockville, Md, 1989, Aspen Publishing Company (1989)

Neuberger G, Reckling J: A new look at wound care, Nurs '85 15(2):34-41, 1985.

Neuberger GB, Reckling JB: Preventing wound complications in an age of DRGs, Ostomy/Wound Management 17:20, 1987.

Strauss MB: Wound hypoxia, Curr Conc Wound Care 9(4):16, 1986.

# 42

# BINDERS AND BANDAGES

### OBJECTIVES

*Mastery of content in this chapter will enable the nurse to:*

- Define key terms.
- Discuss the purposes of binders, bandages, and slings.
- Describe the precautions for binders, bandages and slings.
- Demonstrate correct application of turned bandages.
- Demonstrate correct application of binders.
- Demonstrate correct application of a sling.

### KEY TERMS

*Approximate*
*Binder*
*Compress*
*Elastic bandage*
*Scultetus bandage*
*Sling*
*T binder*

### SKILLS

**42-1** Applying an Elastic Bandage
**42-2** Applying an Abdominal Binder, T Binder, or Breast Binder
**42-3** Applying a Sling

Binders and bandages are applied to specific areas of the body to enhance the healing process in a variety of ways, including:

1. Providing support to a specific area.
2. Maintaining immobilization.
3. Maintaining or improving circulation.
4. Securing placement of dressings.
5. Reducing tension in the area of a wound or suture line.
6. Providing physical comfort.
7. Maintaining the position of special equipment for applying traction (e.g., Buck's extention).
8. Enabling the client to participate in effective respiratory functions of deep breathing, coughing, and expectoration of secretions.

Binders and bandages are made of a variety of cotton fabrics ranging from thin, porous gauze to medium-thickness elasticized webbing and other knitted bandage to heavier muslin and flannel bandage. Thin gauze bandage is inexpensive and disposable after a single use. Because of its porous nature the circulation of air in the area of the wound is enhanced. Gauze bandage is available in 1 in (2.5 cm), 2 in (5.0 cm), and 3 in (7.5 cm) widths. The width selected is determined by the size of the body part to be covered. One-inch gauze is appropriate for bandaging an adult's fingers or a child's forearm. Select wider width gauze for larger body parts.

Elastic bandages simply follow the shape of the part being bandaged. They are lightly stretched and applied with even pressure. Elastic bandages are used to secure dressings on extremities, stumps, and the hand (Table 42-1).

Muslin and flannel bandages and binders provide strength and support and maintain body warmth. Included in this category are triangular muslin slings for upper extremity support, flannel bandages for providing support and warmth of inflamed joints, muslin and elastic abdominal binders, and muslin breast binders.

Binders are especially designed for the body part to be supported. The most common types are breast binders, abdominal (scultetus and straight) binders, and T binders.

*Breast binders* provide support after breast surgery or reduce lactation after childbirth. A breast binder looks like a tight-fitting, sleeveless vest, which should conform to the chest wall. It is essential that excess pressure be avoided. Chest wall expansion should not be impeded.

*Abdominal binders* provide protection and support for suture lines that are vulnerable to tension or stress as the client moves or coughs. They are rectangular pieces of muslin or elasticized material that have many tails attached to the longer sides (Fig. 42-1, *A*), or have long extensions on each side to surround the abdomen (Fig. 42-1, *B*).

*T binders* look like the letter T (Fig. 42-2). The single T is for female clients and the double T fits male clients. The belt of the binder fits securely around the client's

***TABLE 42-1*** Basic Bandage Turns

| Basic Bandage Turns | Use |
|---|---|
| **Circular turns**<br>1. Unroll 3-4 in of bandage from back of roll.<br>2. Place flat bandage surface on anterior surface of portion of body to be covered and hold end in place with thumb of nondominant hand.<br>3. Continue rolling bandage around same area until two overlapping layers of bandage cover part. Remove excess bandage roll.<br>4. Secure end of bandage with safety pin or clip if it is attached to end of bandage. If end of bandage has raw edge, fold ½-1 in under before securing bandage. Gauze bandage may be secured with strip of adhesive tape. | Circular turns are used to cover small body regions such as a digit or wrist.<br>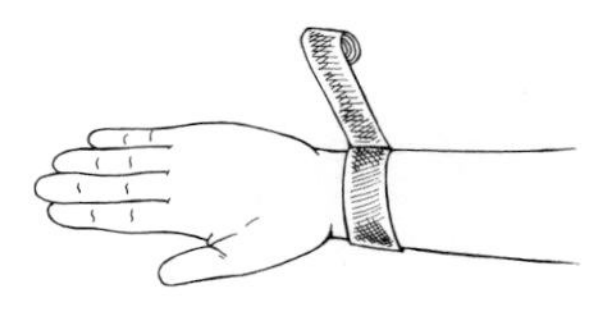 |
| **Spiral turns**<br>1. Anchor bandage at distal end of body part with two circular turns (note Steps 1-3 above).<br>2. Advance bandage on ascending angle overlapping each preceding turn by ½ to ⅔ width of bandage roll until proximal border of area is covered.<br>3. Secure end of bandage. | Used to cover cylindrical body parts where contour of part does not vary significantly in size, (e.g., slender wrist and forearm) |
| **Spiral-reverse turns**<br>1. Anchor bandage at distal border of area to be covered (note 1-3 circular turns).<br>2. Advance bandage on ascending angle of approximately 30 degrees.<br>3. Halfway through each turn fold bandage toward nurse and continue around part in downward stroke.<br>4. Continue advancing bandage as in Steps 2 and 3 until desired proximal point is reached.<br>5. Secure bandage. | Used to cover inverted cone-shaped body parts such as forearm or calf.<br>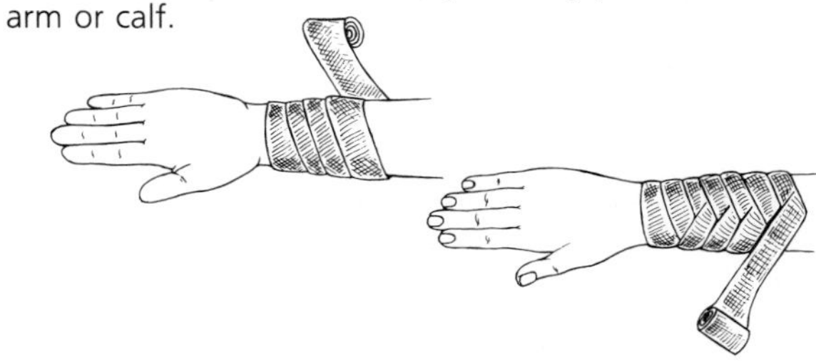 |
| **Figure-eight turns**<br>1. Anchor bandage at center of joint (Steps 1-3, Circular Turns).<br>2. Ascend obliquely around upper half of circular turn above joint followed by turn that descends obliquely below joint.<br>3. Continue in same manner, overlapping half of previous turn until desired immobilization is attained.<br>4. Secure end of bandage. | Designed to cover joints and provide immobilization. Outer surface of fabric is against skin during ascending application of bandage. Each reverse turn places alternate side of bandage toward skin.<br>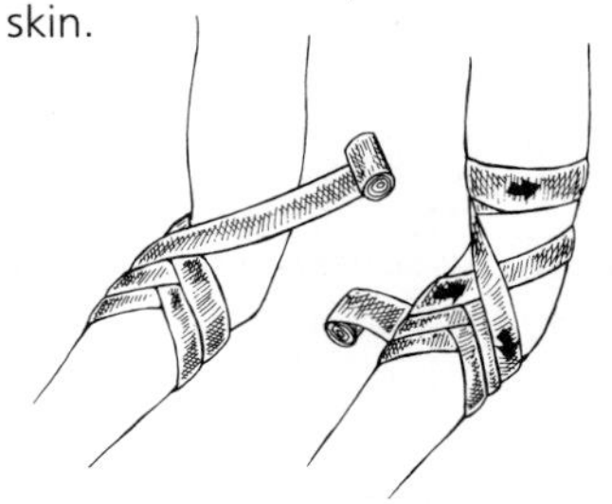 |
| **Recurrent turns**<br>1. Anchor bandage with two circular turns (note Steps 1-3 circular turns) at *proximal* end of body part to be covered.<br>2. Make reverse turn at center front, advance fabric over distal end of the body part to center back, forming covering perpendicular to first circular turns.<br>3. Make reverse turn at back and bring bandage forward, overlapping ½ of perpendicular bandage on one side. Make reverse turn at front and overlap opposite side of center as nurse continues on to back. Repeat these steps, overlapping each previous strip of bandage until entire area is covered.<br>4. Anchor bandage with two circular turns.<br>5. Secure end of bandage. | Provides caplike coverage for scalp or amputation stump.<br>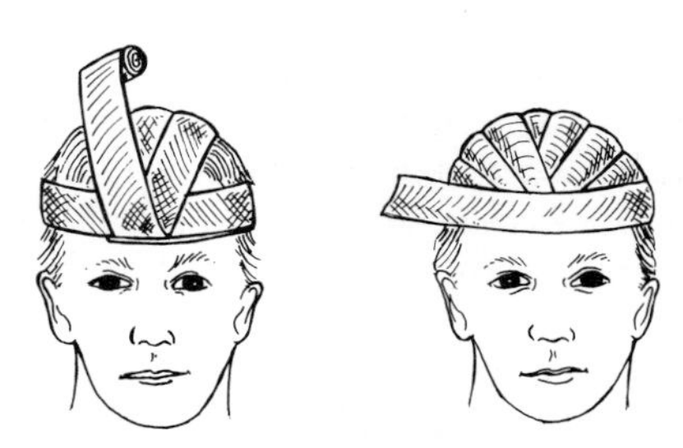 |

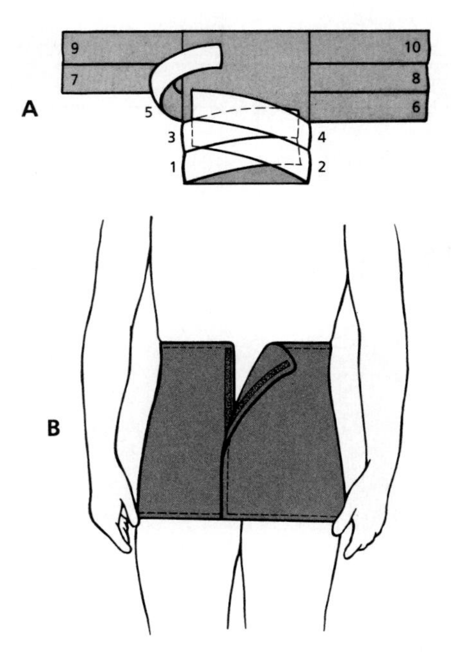


***Fig. 42-1*** Abdominal binders. **A,** Scultetus binder. **B,** Straight.

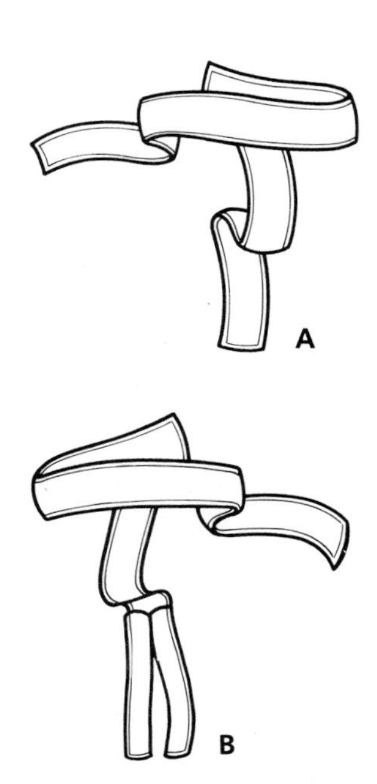


***Fig. 42-2*** Spiral bandage turn. **A,** T binder (female). **B,** Double-T binder (male).

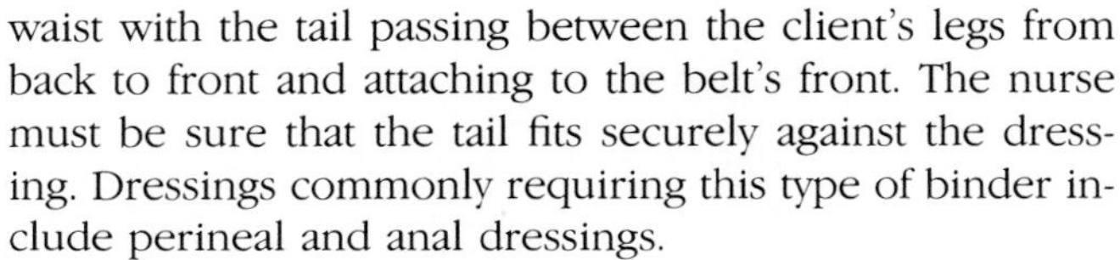

waist with the tail passing between the client's legs from back to front and attaching to the belt's front. The nurse must be sure that the tail fits securely against the dressing. Dressings commonly requiring this type of binder include perineal and anal dressings.

*Slings* are made of strong muslin or lightweight canvas and used primarily to support, limit movement, enhance circulation, and prevent edema of the arm, hand, or wrist. Other uses include assuring placement of dressings and preventing the gravitational pull of the arm while healing injuries to the shoulder. The lower arm is positioned above the level of the elbow to reduce the risk of dependent edema. The bandage is fashioned from a 36 in (90.0 cm) to 42 in (105.0 cm) square fabric that is cut in half diagonally to form two triangular bandages (Fig. 42-3). One or two safety pins complete the support at the angle near the elbow. Soft padding may be desired in axillary and cervical areas and under the square knot to reduce the risk of skin irritations.

## GUIDELINES

1. Inspect the skin for abrasions, edema, discoloration, or exposed wound edges to provide base line data before applying the binder or bandage.
2. Cover exposed wounds or open abrasions with a sterile dressing. This prevents further trauma to the wound from friction caused by the binder or bandage.
3. Inspect condition of underlying dressings. If dressings are soiled or nonadherent, change before binder application.
4. Inspect the skin of underlying body parts and parts distal to the bandage for signs of circulatory impairment (coolness, pallor or cyanosis, diminished or absent pulses, swelling, numbness, or tingling). Provides base line data to compare changes in circulation after bandage application.

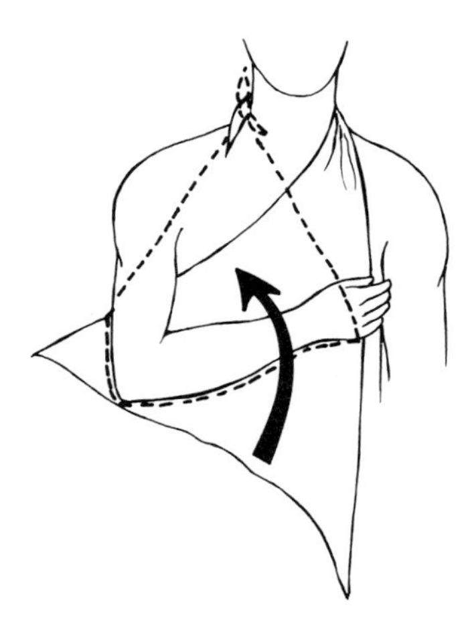

***Fig. 42-3*** Triangular sling.

## PREREQUISITE KNOWLEDGE

1. Risks of venous stasis.
2. Normal thoracic, abdominal, and perianal anatomy.
3. Normal respiratory functioning.
4. Medical and surgical asepsis.

## PREREQUISITE SKILLS

1. Basic handwashing techniques (Chapter 37).
2. Physical assessment (Chapter 13).
3. Range of joint motion exercises (Chapter 36).

# *SKILL 42-1 Applying an Elastic Bandage*

The elastic bandage is used to apply compression to an area. It is used most often on the lower extremities to prevent edema and support varicosities. Other uses include support of the knee, ankle, elbow, and wrist in conditions such as strains and sprains. On rare occasions the elastic bandage may be used as a chest support for a client with fractured ribs.

When fully stretched the elastic bandage extends to 3 yards (270 cm). Shorter lengths are available for bandaging the wrist or a child's foot or knee. Bandages are available in widths of 2 in (5.0 cm), 3 in (7.5 cm), 4 in (10 cm), 6 in (15.0 cm) and 8 in (20 cm). The elastic bandage is washable and is placed in large folds over a line to dry. The bandage is always rolled loosely, without any tension, in preparation for application. When fully rolled the outside is placed next to the skin as a starting point. Even tension is applied and the bandage is started at the site furthest from the heart (distal) and proceeds toward the heart (proximal).

The type of bandage turn and selected width are determined by the size and shape of the body part to be bandaged. Three- and four-inch bandages are most commonly used for the adult leg.

### Purposes

1. Apply pressure to a specific area.
2. Support a strained or sprained extremity.

## *Procedure 42-1*

| Steps | Rationale |
|---|---|
| **Assessment** | |
| 1. Inspect skin for alterations in integrity as indicated by presence of abrasion; discoloration; chafing; edema. (Look carefully at bony prominences.) | Altered skin integrity contraindicates the use of elastic bandage. |
| 2. Inspect dressing for cleanliness and dryness. Does dressing cover wound edges? | Reduces nosocomial infection. |
| 3. Observe adequacy of circulation by noting surface temperature; skin color; and sensation of body parts to be wrapped. | Comparison of area before and after application of bandage is necessary to assure continued adequate circulation. Impairment of circulation may result in coolness to touch when compared with opposite side of body; cyanosis or pallor of skin; diminished or absent pulses; edema or localized pooling; numbness and or tingling of part. |
| 4. Review client's medical record and nursing prescriptions for specific orders related to application of elastic bandage. Note area to be covered; type of bandage required; frequency of change; previous response to treatment. | Specific prescription may direct procedure including such factors as: extent of application, (i.e., toe to knee, toe to groin) or duration of treatment. |
| 5. Identify client's present knowledge level of skill if bandaging will be continued at home. | Ensures that planning and teaching are individualized. |
| **Nursing Diagnosis** | |
| 1. Cluster data to reveal actual or potential nursing diagnoses: | |
| a. Impaired tissue integrity: related to venous stasis in extremity. | Venous stasis is responsible for development of thrombophlebitis, potential for emboli, joint and peripheral edema. |
| b. Impaired physical mobility: related to muscular strain. | Immobilization of body part, with or without bandage, is desired to prevent further damage and promote healing following injury to musculoskeletal system. |
| c. Pain: related to unsupported wound. | Unsupported wounds produce unnecessary discomfort. Anchoring of dressings after injury or operative procedure will minimize pain. |
| **Planning** | |
| 1. Develop individualized goals for client based on nursing diagnoses: | |
| a. Promote healing. | Immobilization reduces pain and permits healing of sprained or strained extremities. |
| b. Reduce pain. | |

| Steps | Rationale |
|---|---|
| c. Prevent clot formation and development of thrombi. | Elastic bandages to lower extremities promotes venous stasis. |
| d. Maintain circulation. | Monitoring of distal pulses evaluates the adequacy of circulation. |
| 2. Obtain necessary equipment and supplies (determine if present bandage to be reused or replacement to be obtained): | |
| a. Correct widths and number of bandages. ▪ Elastic bandages are available in 2 in (5 cm), 2½ in (6.25 cm), 3 in (7.5 cm), 4 in (10.0 cm), 6 in (15.0 cm), and 8 in (20.0 cm) and in lengths of 3 yd (270 cm) and 1½ yd (135 cm) length. 3- and 4-in width bandages are most often appropriate. | Use increasingly wider bandages as size of body part increases (e.g., 3-in, 4-in, and 6-in bandages may be used to cover foot, calf, and thigh.) |
| b. Safety pins, tape | Secure bandage in place. |
| 3. Explain procedure to client. Reinforce teaching that smooth, even, light pressure will be applied to improve venous circulation; prevent clot formation; reduce or prevent swelling; immobilize arms; secure surgical dressings; provide pressure. | Promotes cooperation and reduces anxiety. Improves client's knowledge level regarding the need for elastic bandages. |

## Implementation

| Steps | Rationale |
|---|---|
| 1. Wash hands. | Reduces transmission of microorganisms. |
| 2. Close room door or curtains. | Maintains client's comfort and dignity. |
| 3. Assist client to assume comfortable, anatomically correct position. | Maintains alignment. Prevents musculoskeletal deformity. |
| 4. Hold roll of elastic bandage in dominant hand and use other hand to lightly hold beginning of bandage at distal body part. Continue transferring roll to dominant hand as bandage is wrapped. ▪ Toes or finger tips should be visible for follow-up assessment. | Maintains appropriate and consistent bandage tension. |
| 5. Apply bandage from distal point toward proximal boundary using variety of turns to cover various shapes of body parts (Table 42-1). | Bandage applied in manner that conforms evenly to body part and promotes venous return. |
| 6. Unroll and very slightly stretch bandage. | Maintains uniform bandage tension. |
| 7. Overlap turns. | Prevents uneven bandage tension and circulatory impairment. |
| 8. Secure first bandage before applying additional rolls. ▪ Apply additional rolls without leaving any uncovered skin surface. | To prevent wrinkling or loose ends. |

## Evaluation

| Steps | Rationale |
|---|---|
| 1. Assess distal circulation as bandage application is complete and at least twice during 8-hr period. | Early detection and management of circulatory difficulties will assure healthy neurovascular status. |
| a. Observe skin color for pallor or cyanosis. b. Palpate skin for warmth. c. Palpate pulses. | Steps a-c are indicators of circulatory status. |
| d. Ask if client is aware of pain, numbness, tingling or other discomfort. | Neurovascular changes indicate impaired venous return. |
| e. Observe mobility of extremity. | |

### *Expected outcomes*

| Steps | Rationale |
|---|---|
| 1. Client is comfortable. | All are indicators of proper application of the elastic bandage. |
| a. No tingling or numbness is noted by client. | |
| b. Distal parts (toes, fingers) feel warm (symmetrically to the touch), there is no cyanosis or blanching, and motion is not unnecessarily impaired. | Indicates adequate circulation to distal regions. |
| 2. Bandage is properly anchored; completely covers body part; is wrinkle-free; shows no looseness or stricture; ends are secured. | Maintains adequate support to extremity. |

### *Uexpected outcomes*

| Steps | Rationale |
|---|---|
| 1. Tingling or numbness is present in portions distal to wrap. | Indicates impaired circulation because wrap was applied too tightly. |
| 2. Extremity distal to wrap is cool, cyanotic, or blanched. | Wrap was applied too tightly. |
| 3. Dressing is loose or improperly wrapped. | Improper support to area. |
| 4. Extremity has decreased range of joint motion | |

| Steps | Rationale |
|---|---|
| **Recording and Reporting** | |
| 1. Document treatment and response on the client's record. | Assures continuity of care and meets legal requirements regarding documentation of care given and client's response. |
| **Follow-up Activities** | |
| 1. Remove and reapply elastic bandage: | Inspection of area is integral factor in on-going assessment. |
| a. Once every 8 hr unless otherwise directed by physician | |
| b. PRN for wrinkles; looseness or tightness; client discomfort or itchiness; changes, including drainage; tingling or numbness; cool, cyanotic, or blanched extremity | Inadequately applied elastic bandage does not maintain support to area and compromises circulation. |

### Special Considerations

- Heels, elbows, and ankles are subject to edema due to pooling if circulation is impaired or restricted.
- Preexisting vascular problems, copious wound drainage, client comfort level and presence of pulses will determine need for additional nursing interventions.
- Use adhesive tape rather than loose clips or pins to fasten bandage on small child or infant. Safety pins are more effective than clips and do not fall out of bandage.
- Bandages applied to lower extremities are applied before client sits or stands. Elevation of dependent extremities before bandage application for 20 min will enhance venous circulation.
- Unless total immobilization is medically prescribed, range of motion exercises are continued.

### Teaching Considerations

- Applying elastic bandage to oneself is difficult. Teach significant other if treatment will continue after hospitalization.

### Home Care Considerations

- Assess client and primary care giver's ability and motivation to participate in bandaging procedure.
- Assess client's understanding of bandaging and willingness to leave bandage in place.
- Assess client's environment to determine potential for permitting bandaged area to remain free from contaminants.

## *SKILL 42-2 Applying an Abdominal Binder, T Binder, or Breast Binder*

Binders are indicated for the support of underlying muscles and large incisions. The muscles and viscera surrounding an operative site may require support during the postoperative period. This promotes healing and permits a client to move more freely without additional discomfort. Assorted binders are available with the basic shape being a rectangle that is wide enough to extend from the groin to the waistline and long enough to encircle the area with an overlap for closure.

### Purposes

1. Support underlying muscles and viscera.
2. Support an operative incision.
3. Support a strained visceral muscle.

### *Procedure 42-2*

| Steps | Rationale |
|---|---|
| **Assessment** | |
| 1. Identify client in need of abdominal, breast, or T binder. | Identifies when support is needed to thoracic, abdominal, or perineal structures. |
| 2. For client with need for support of thorax or abdomen, observe ability to breathe deeply; cough effectively. | Baseline assessment determines client's ability to breathe and cough. Impaired ventilation of lung can lead to alveolar atelectasis and inadequate arterial oxygenation. |
| 3. Inspect skin for actual or potential alterations in integrity. Observe for irritation, abrasion; skin surfaces that rub against each other; allergic response to adhesive tape used to secure dressing. | Actual impairments in skin integrity can be worsened with application of a binder. Binder can cause pressure and excoriation. |

| Steps | Rationale |
|---|---|
| 4. Inspect any surgical dressing. | Dressing replacement or reinforcement precedes application of any binder. |
| a. Dressing should be clean and dry. | Prevents nosocomial infection. |
| b. Incision/wound should be entirely covered by dressing. | Avoids soiling of bandage and irritation of wound. |
| 5. Identify client's comfort level. Expect client in moderate to severe pain to have diaphoresis, tachycardia, and elevated blood pressure reading. | Data will determine effectiveness of binder placement. |
| 6. Identify learning needs of client related to self-care and discharge planning. | Use of supportive binders may continue after discharge. |
| 7. Assess level of anxiety. | Body image issues, self-inspection of surgical incision and/or anatomical changes requiring emotionally supportive nursing intervention should be integrated into holistic client care. |
| 8. Review client's medical record if medical prescription for particular binder is required and reasons for binder application. | Application of supportive binders may be based on nursing judgment. In some situations physician input is required. |
| 9. Gather necessary data regarding size of client and appropriate binder. | Ensures proper fit of binder. |

## Nursing Diagnosis

| Steps | Rationale |
|---|---|
| 1. Cluster data to reveal potential nursing diagnoses related to application of binder: | |
| a. Ineffective breathing pattern: related to constricted chest expansion. | Tightness of binder can interfere with client's ability to fully expand lungs. |
| b. Potential impaired skin integrity: related to friction of bandage. | Maintains decreased tension on suture line to promote healing. Snug support helps maintain intact suture line. Wrinkle-free application of binder encourages healthy skin response. Skin irritations progress rapidly in presence of consistent pressure or rubbing of skin against skin. |
| c. Pain: related to incisional trauma. | Support of incision and surrounding body parts permits client compliance with planned postoperative activities of lung expansion, coughing, and expectoration, mobilization, and ambulation. |
| d. Impaired tissue integrity: related to surgical incision. | Snugly applied binder provides support for surgically traumatized tissues; complications are prevented by improving circulation. |

## Planning

| Steps | Rationale |
|---|---|
| 1. Develop individualized goals for client based on nursing diagnoses: | |
| a. Maintain adequate gas exchange. | Bandage applied too tightly may restrict ventilation. |
| b. Promote healing process. | Support to incisional area promotes comfort during postoperative exercises of coughing, turning, and ambulating. |
| c. Minimize extent and duration of pain. | |
| d. Reduce skin impairment. | Careful application avoids pressure or friction against skin. |
| 2. Prepare necessary equipment and supplies: | |
| a. Abdominal binder: | |
| ▪ Correct size cloth/elastic straight binder or scultetus binder | Binder must be large enough to surround client's abdomen and overlap to secure closure. |
| ▪ Safety pins (unless Velcro closure is attached): 6-8 safety pins are usually adequate for abdominal binders. | |
| b. T and double-T binder: | |
| ▪ Correct size | |
| ▪ Safety pins: 2 pins for T binder; 3 pins for double-T binder | One pin secures horizontal waistband. One pin secures each tail, placing pin through all thicknesses at horizontal level. |
| c. Breast binders: | After securing front closure with pins it may be necessary to form darts (and secure them with safety pins) in order to shape binder to snugly fit client's contour. |
| ▪ Correct size binder | |
| ▪ Safety pins (approximately 12) unless velcro closure is attached. | |
| 3. Explain procedure to client. | Promotes client's understanding. |

## Implementation

| Steps | Rationale |
|---|---|
| 1. Wash hands. | Maintains medical asepsis and infection control. |
| 2. Close curtains or room door. | Provides privacy. |

| Steps | Rationale |
|---|---|
| ***Abdominal binder (straight and scultetus)*** | |
| 1. Apply abdominal binder as follows: | |
| a. Position client in supine position with head slightly elevated and knees slightly flexed. | Minimizes muscular tension on abdominal organs. |
| b. Fanfold far side of binder toward midline of binder. | Reduces time client remains in uncomfortable position. |
| c. Instruct and assist client to roll away from nurse toward raised side rail while firmly supporting abdominal incision and dressing with hands. | Reduces pain and discomfort. |
| d. Place fanfolded ends of binder under client. | Permits placement and centering of binder with minimal discomfort. |
| e. Instruct/assist client to roll over folded ends. | |
| f. Unfold and stretch ends out smoothly on far side of bed. ▪ Binders extend from just above symphysis pubis to just below costal margins. | Maintains skin integrity and comfort. |
| g. Instruct client to roll back into supine position. | Facilitates chest expansion and adequate wound support when the binder is closed. |
| h. Adjust binder so that supine client is centered over binder using symphysis pubis and costal margins as lower and upper landmarks. | Centers support from binder over abdominal structures. |
| i. Close binder. ▪ *Straight binder:* Pull distal end of binder over center of client's abdomen. While maintaining tension on that end of binder, pull opposite end of binder over center and secure with Velcro closure tabs or safety pins. | Provides continuous wound support and comfort. |
| ▪ *Scultetus binder:* With left hand bring bottom tail at client's left side over center of abdomen. Maintain tension on that tail and overlap it with bottom right tail. Repeat procedure with each successive pair of tails, moving toward top of binder. Secure each end of top set of tails with safety pin. | Provides continuous wound support and comfort. |
| j. Assess client's ability to breathe deeply and cough effectively. | Determines ventilation and clears the airways of pulmonary secretions. |
| k. Ask client about comfort level. | |
| l. Adjust binder as necessary. | |
| ***T and double-T binders*** | |
| 1. Apply T or double-T binder as follows: a. Assist client to dorsal recumbent position. | To facilitate placement of perineal dressings position client on back with lower extremities slightly flexed and rotated slightly outwardly. |
| b. Have client raise hips and place horizontal band around client's waist (or above iliac crests) with vertical tails extending past buttocks. Overlap waistband in front and secure with safety pins. | Minimizes muscular tension on perineal organs. Secures binder around client. |
| c. Complete binder application: ▪ *T binder:* Bring remaining vertical strip over perineal dressing and continue up and under center front of horizontal band. Bring ends over waistband and secure all thicknesses with safety pin. ▪ *Double-T binder:* Bring remaining vertical strips over perineal or suprapubic dressing with each tail supporting one side of scrotum and proceeding upward on either side of penis. Continue drawing ends behind and then downward in front of horizontal band. Secure all thicknesses with one safety pin. | Single-T and double-T binders provide support to perineal muscles and organs. |
| d. Assess client's comfort level with client in lying, sitting, and standing positions. Readjust front pins as necessary. Increase padding if any area rubs against surrounding tissues. ▪ Binder should hold perineal dressings in place as the client ambulates. | Determines efficacy of binder to maintain dressings and support perineal structures. |
| e. Instruct client regarding removal of binder before defecating or urinating and need to replace binder after these bodily functions. | Cleanliness of binder reduces infection risk. |

| Steps | Rationale |
|---|---|
| ***Breast binder*** | |
| 1. Apply breast binder as follows: | |
| a. Assist client in placing arms through binder's armholes. | Eases binder placement process. |
| b. Assist client to supine position in bed. | Supine positioning facilitates normal anatomical situation of breasts. Maintains normal anatomical alignment of breasts, facilitates healing and comfort. |
| c. Pad area under breasts if necessary. | Prevents skin contact with undersurface. |
| d. Using Velcro closure tabs or horizontally placed safety pins secure binder at nipple level first. Continue closure process above and then below nipple line until entire binder is closed. | Horizontal placement of pins may reduce risk of uneven pressure or localized irritation. |
| e. Make appropriate adjustments including individualizing fit of shoulder straps; pinning waistline darts to reduce binder size. | Maintains support to client's breasts. |
| f. Instruct and observe skill development in self-care related to reapplying breast binder. | Self-care is integral aspect of discharge planning. Skin integrity and comfort level goals are assured. |
| g. Wash hands. | Prevents cross-infections. |
| **Evaluation** | |
| 1. Observe site for skin integrity, circulation, characteristics of the wound. | Determines that binder has not resulted in complication to skin or underlying organs. |
| 2. Note comfort level of client. | Binders should not impede breathing or increase discomfort. |
| 3. Assess client's ability to ventilate properly including deep breathing and coughing. | Identifies any impaired ventilation and potential pulmonary complications. |
| 4. Identify client's need for assistance with activities such as hair combing, dressing, ambulating. | Mobility of upper extremities may be limited depending on severity and location of incision. |
| ***Abdominal binder—expected outcomes*** | |
| 1. Respirations are normal. | Indicates adequate respiratory function. |
| 2. Pain is absent. | Denotes comfort and support have been achieved by binder. |
| 3. Skin is intact. | Notes absence of any trauma to the skin. |
| 4. Pulse distal to binder is normal. | Indicates adequate circulation distal to the binder. |
| ***Abdominal binder–unexpected outcomes*** | |
| 1. Lung expansion is reduced. | Binder too tight, restricting ability to deep breathe. |
| 2. Pain is present. | Binder may be exerting too much or too little support of suture line. |
| 3. Fresh bleeding or separation of sutured incision occurs. | Continued suture-line tension and poorly applied supportive binder can result in incisional separation. |
| 4. Circulation is decreased. | Binder restrictive. Local pressure can cause circulatory impairment. |
| ***T binder, double-T binder—expected outcomes*** | |
| 1. Dressing placement is secured. | Binder is supporting perineal dressings and organs. |
| 2. Scrotal support provided (perineal/suprapubic). | |
| 3. Client is comfortable. | Absence of friction or pressure from binder. |
| 4. Client either asks for help or is able to remove and replace binder for bowel and bladder elimination. | Level of self-care is appropriate. |
| ***T binder, double-T binder—unexpected outcomes*** | |
| 1. Chafing and irritation of area are present. | Improper application of binder, resulting in pressure and irritation to underlying structures. |
| 2. Containment of dressing is inadequate. | Improperly applied binder, insufficient support to perineal area. |
| ***Breast binder—expected outcomes*** | |
| 1. Comfort level is satisfactory. | Rubbing of fabric against skin may require padding. Tension of binder must be supportive and not restrictive. |
| 2. Suture-line tension is reduced. | Binder supports incisional area. |
| 3. Client is able to cope with postpartum physiological changes. | Effective application of binder will optimize healing process of wound and/or provide support for breasts in the post-partum client. |
| 4. Respirations are unrestricted. Coughing and expectoration of secretions are effective. | The ability to fully expand the lungs and cough must continue after application of the binder to enhance oxygenation and avoid pulmonary complications. |

| Steps | Rationale |
|---|---|
| ***Breast binder—unexpected outcomes*** | |
| 1. Impaired breathing leads to ineffective oxygenation. | Restrictive application of binder with too much tension inhibits client's ability to fully expand lungs. |
| 2. Tight binder causes impaired circulation. | Postoperative risks of venous stasis, clot formation, and embolization can result from restrictive application of binder. |
| 3. Skin integrity is impaired. | Uneven pressure occurs in presence of wrinkles and leads to irritation. Rubbing together of skin surfaces causes excoriation of area. |
| 4. Pain and discomfort are increased. | Incorrect application of binder increases discomfort. |
| **Recording and Reporting** | |
| 1. Report ineffective lung expansion to physician immediately. | Loosening of tight binder should permit client to fully expand lungs. Rapid reporting and appropriate intervention may prevent change from becoming serious emergency or irreversible complication. |
| 2. Report any skin irritation at lower end of binder to nurse at between-shift report. | Promotes continuity of care and prevention of complications. |
| 3. Record application of binder, condition of skin and circulation, integrity of dressings, and client's comfort level. | Promotes continuity of care. |
| **Follow-up Activities** | |
| 1. Assess client immediately and readjust binder as necessary. | Assures correct application. |
| 2. Every 4 hr observe: a. Ability to deep breathe. b. Cough effectiveness. | Adequate lung expansion and expectoration of bronchial secretions will permit proper alveolar expansion and exchange of gases in capillary beds. |
| c. Objective and subjective symptoms of pain/unnecessary discomfort. | Pain should be reduced with binder application. |
| 3. Every 8 hr and PRN remove binder and inspect dressing; skin condition. | Determines presence of trauma or irritation to underlying surfaces. |
| 4. Bathe area daily and PRN. | Promotes wound healing and maintains skin integrity. |
| 5. Reapply binder or assist client with skill. | |

## Special Considerations

- Before applying breast binder for management of engorgement and suppression of lactation, note condition of nipples and physiologic changes. Pad nipple areas with soft dressings to prevent seepage of fluid.
- Cover any exposed areas of incision or wound with sterile dressing.
- Advanced age, general health, nutrition, and condition of tissues surrounding surgical area affect healing process.
- Placing pins in cake of soap while applying or changing binder will prevent loss or danger to client and facilitate ease in gliding pin through thicknesses of cloth.
- Innermost tails of scultetus binder are always at lowest part of binder and lowest portion of the buttocks.
- In the extremely thin client, padding of iliac prominences will prevent excessive pressure and skin irritation.
- For postsurgical application of scultetus abdominal binders precede upward from bottom to minimize pull on suture line.
- T binders are easily soiled and require frequent replacement.
- Properly fitting brassiere that extends to lower rib cage and has front closure may be substituted for breast binders for postsurgical and postpartum clients.
- Elastic thoracic binders designed to provide support to area below breasts are commercially manufactured. This binder may be used for bruised and cracked ribs (in good alignment) on both male and female clients.
- Shallow respirations, continuing after tight binder has been loosened, may indicate beginning of serious respiratory problems including alveolar atelectasis, pulmonary embolus, etc.

## Teaching Considerations

- Instruct client or care giver on application of binder. Consider extent of incision; client's dexterity in reapplying binder to self, opportunities to practice skill, and need to teach significant other.

## Home Care Considerations

- Assess primary care giver's understanding, ability, and motivation to participate in application of binder.
- Assess client's understanding of purpose of binder and willingness to permit binder to remain in place.
- Assess client's environment to determine level of compliance with procedure.

# *SKILL 42-3 Applying a Sling*

A commercially made sling consists of a long sleeve that fits around the client's lower arm and a strap that fits around the neck. In the home setting a large triangular piece of cloth can be used as a sling.

When a sling is being applied the client may sit or lie supine. The nurse instructs the client to bend the affected arm, bringing the forearm straight across the chest. The open sling fits under the client's arm and over the chest, with the base of the triangle under the wrist and the triangle's point at the client's elbow. One end of the sling fits around the back of the client's neck. The nurse brings the other end up over the affected arm while supporting the extremity. The nurse ties the two ends at the side of the neck so that the knot does not press against the cervical spine. The loose fold at the elbow can be folded evenly around the elbow and pinned to provide optimal support. The lower arm should always be supported at a level above the elbow to prevent the formation of dependent edema.

### Purposes

1. Support the arms injured from muscular sprain or skeletal fracture.
2. Reduce excessive pressure on shoulder and neck structures.

## *Procedure 42-3*

| Steps | Rationale |
|---|---|
| **Assessment** | |
| 1. Identify client with impairment of upper extremity or shoulder who would benefit from support of sling. | Sling may be applied to prevent unnecessary pull on shoulder related to paralysis or cast application; prevent dependent edema; support or immobilize any or all parts of upper extremity; maintain placement of dressing; limit movement of upper extremity in presence of fracture, muscle strain or sprain, or joint dislocation. |
| 2. Assess client's presenting condition (stroke; fracture; dislocation; surgery; injury). | Determines client's motor and sensory level of affected extremity. |
| 3. Observe condition of client's upper extremity (mobility/immobility; presence of suture line; presence of paralysis; presence of cast; level of comfort/pain). | Objective and subjective symptoms are indicators of expected outcomes/client goals. |
| 4. Review client's medical record for physician's prescription in relation to desired angle of forearm and time determinants. | Venous return, prevention of edema, and maintenance of functional alignment result from properly applied sling. Slings may be ordered around clock or whenever client is sitting or out of bed. |
| 5. Identify client's learning needs regarding condition; correct application of sling. | Identifies areas for client teaching for increasing client's self-care ability. |
| **Nursing Diagnosis** | |
| 1. Cluster data to reveal actual or potential nursing diagnoses: | |
| a. Impaired physical mobility: related to sling placement. | Immobilization of extremity with sling is designed to permit healing, reduce gravitational pull on shoulder. |
| b. Potential impaired skin integrity: related to irritation of sling. | Skin irritations of the back of the neck are prevented by carefully padding the area. |
| c. Pain: related to muscular injury. | Expected outcome of sling is a decrease in pain. |
| d. Self-care deficit in activities of daily living (ADL) related to extended limitation of one arm. | Presence of a sling reduces client's ability for self-care. |
| e. Knowledge deficit regarding self-application of sling: related to inexperience. | Development of skill of application of sling will expedite self-care and early discharge. |
| **Planning** | |
| 1. Develop individualized goals for client based on nursing diagnoses: | |
| a. Maintain tolerable comfort level. | Adequate physical support facilitates maintenance of comfort. |
| b. Develop self-care skills including application of sling, eating, dressing, maintaining balance while walking. | Loss of use of one arm impinges on many aspects of client's daily activities. |

| Steps | Rationale |
|---|---|
| c. Prevent venous stasis. | Proper elevation of hand prevents stasis. |
| d. Immobilize upper extremity. | Prevents gravitational pull on shoulder. |
| 2. Prepare necessary equipment and supplies: | |
| a. Triangular bandage | |
| b. Safety pins | |
| c. Padding (fluffed gauze squares) | Neck and axillary area may require padding to prevent irritation. |
| 3. Prepare client. | |
| a. Position client sitting or supine with forearm at angle with fingers higher than hand, hand higher than wrist, and wrist higher than forearm, all in anatomically correct alignment. | Ensures client cooperation facilitating rapid application of sling. |
| b. Explain procedure. | Reduces anxiety. |
| c. Teach skill to client or significant other. | Promotes coping abilities and reduces stress. |

## Implementation

| Steps | Rationale |
|---|---|
| 1. Wash hands. | Prevents cross-infections. |
| 2. Provide privacy. | Reduces anxiety and maintains personal dignity. |
| 3. Open sling. | Prepares sling for application. |
| 4. Place open sling over client's torso with binder centered under arm. Place longest side at wrist and triangle's apex extending beyond arm at elbow. | Facilitates placement of closure beyond center of neck. Ensures support of forearm. |
| 5. Bring top binder point upward over neck on unaffected side of body, continuing around client's neck to affected side. At this point longest side of triangle will extend straight down in vertical line on unaffected side of body. | Provides support to the client's affected side as the sling is applied. |
| 6. Bring lower binder point over forearm and hand up to neck on affected side. | Prepares sling to maintain optimum support to affected arm. |
| 7. Reassess angle of forearm and adjust position if needed. | Proper positioning facilitates venous return and reduction of edema of digits. |
| 8. Secure closure of sling at shoulder level on unaffected side using square (reef) knot. | Prevents pressure from knot on affected shoulder, which may be without sensation. |
| 9. Fold remaining loose area of binder around elbow and maintain fold with safety pin. | Provides support to elbow and maintains appropriate alignment. |
| 10. Apply padding as needed (under knot; at cervical vertebral area; between skin surfaces of axilla; between cast and skin surfaces). | Reduces localized skin pressure; prevents cervical flexion related to pressure; avoids excoriation of skin. |
| 11. Inspect applied sling in relation to adequacy of support; position of lower arm above level of elbow; avoidance of pressure on cervical vertebra. | Maintains proper alignment of affected arm. |
| 12. Integrate teaching process while applying sling. | Reduces skill deficit. |
| 13. Wash hands. | Prevents cross-infections. |
| 14. Arrange client's environment to facilitate use of healthy arm. | Promotes client's independence in activities of daily living. |

## Evaluation

| Steps | Rationale |
|---|---|
| 1. Evaluate circulation to hand and condition of skin. | Determines adequacy of neurovascular status to distal area. |
| 2. Inspect alignment of shoulder and extremity. | Determines adequacy of support and alignment provided by the sling. |
| 3. Question client regarding level of comfort. | Identifies presence of any pain or discomfort. |
| ***Expected outcomes*** | |
| 1. Comfort level is tolerable. | Support and immobilization facilitate reduction in pain. |
| 2. Circulation of extremity is adequate. | Proper positioning with hand higher than forearm and properly aligned will facilitate venous return and reduce swelling. |
| 3. Skin integrity is maintained. | Absence of pressure or irritation from sling or knot. |
| ***Unexpected outcomes*** | |
| 1. Pain increases. | Multiple causes are possible including position, presence of sling, shoulder dislocation. |
| 2. Edema persists or increases. | Positioning hand and arm improperly may promote venous stasis. |
| 3. Cervical discomfort or flexure is present. | Sling places too much pressure on cervical vertebra. |
| 4. Skin is irritated. | Presence of abrasion from the sling. |

| Steps | Rationale |
|---|---|
| 5. Severe emotional distress related to reduced ability to function at usual level. | Impact on personal and business activity can cause anger, depression, withdrawal. |

## Recording and Reporting

| | |
|---|---|
| 1. Report between shift client responses to application of sling. | Maintains continuity of care and denotes client's response to sling application. |
| 2. Record alignment, circulation, and skin integrity of the affected extremity. | Denotes the presence or absence of complications related to application of sling. |

## Follow-up Activities

| | |
|---|---|
| 1. Continue assisting client or significant other with application of sling procedure. | Mastery of skill by significant other will permit early discharge. |
| 2. Initiate discharge planning according to individual needs. | Maintains continuity of care into the home environment. |

## Special Considerations

- Sling is placed outside usual clothing to reduce risk of skin irritation.
- For application of sling on child, fold standard triangular sling in half and use it doubled or cut along fold to form 2 slings.

## Teaching Considerations

- Significant others may need instruction if condition prevents skill mastery by client.
- Comprehensive, early discharge planning with follow-up after discharge is imperative.
- Significant other may need to be involved to facilitate care during recovery period.
- Maintain awareness of time limitations. Outpatients and significant others may need to learn how to apply sling at time of first application:
- Consider dominant handedness of client, severity of injury, pain, paralysis, age. Discharge planning will vary according to client responses and availability of significant other.
- Instruct client regarding range of motion exercises.

## Home Care Consideration

- Assess client's ability and motivation to comply with use of sling.

### BIBLIOGRAPHY


Brunner LS, Suddarth DS: Lippincott manual of nursing practice, Philadelphia, 1982, JB Lippincott Co.

Bruno P: The nature of wound healing: implications for nursing practice, Nurs Clin North Am 14:667, 1979.

Bruno P, Craven RF: Age challenges to wound healing, J Gerontol Nurs 8:686, 1982.

Bulau J. Clinical policies and procedures for home health care, Rockville, Md, 1986, Aspen Publishers Co.

Creighton H: Law every nurse should know, ed 2, Philadelphia, 1981, WB Sanders Co.

Golden S: Nursing a loved one at home Philadelphia, 1988, Running Press.

Gordon M: Nursing diagnosis: process and application, ed 2, New York, 1982, McGraw-Hill Book Co.

Kim MJ, et al.: Pocket guide for nursing diagnosis, ed 2, St Louis, 1988, The CV Mosby Co.

Potter P, Perry A: Fundamentals of nursing, ed 2, St Louis, 1989, The CV Mosby Co.

Smith S, Duell D: Clinical nursing skills, Los Altos: Calif, 1985, National Nursing Review

Thompson JM, et al.: Mosby's manual of clinical nursing, ed 2, St Louis, 1989, The CV Mosby Co.

Walsh J, Persons C, Wieck L: Manual of home health care nursing, Philadelphia, 1987, JB Lippincott Co.

# 43

# HOT AND COLD THERAPY

### *OBJECTIVES*

*Mastery of content in this chapter will enable the nurse to:*

- Define key terms.
- Identify the effects of heat and cold on the skin.
- Differentiate the types of injuries or conditions that benefit from hot and cold applications.
- Identify the risks to clients related to hot and cold applications.
- Explain common guidelines used to protect clients who receive hot and cold applications.
- Correctly apply the following: dry heat applications, hot moist compresses to an open wound, dry cold applications, moist cold applications.
- Correctly administer a warm sitz bath or soak.

### *KEY TERMS*

| | |
|---|---|
| *Compress* | *Neuropathy* |
| *Conduction* | *Piloerection* |
| *Evaporation* | *Sitz bath* |
| *Insulation* | |

### *SKILLS*

**43-1** Applying a Moist Hot Compress to an Open Wound
**43-2** Assisting with Warm Soaks and Sitz Baths
**43-3** Using a Heat Lamp and Heat Cradle
**43-4** Applying Aquathermia and Heating Pads
**43-5** Applying a Moist Cold Compress
**43-6** Applying an Ice Pack, Bag, or Collar

The local application of heat and cold to body parts can have a beneficial effect. To use heat and cold therapies safely the nurse must understand how the body normally responds to temperature variations and what risks clients are exposed to during such applications.

Exposure to heat or cold causes both systemic and local responses. The hypothalamus acts as the thermostat of the body to maintain body temperature at 37° C, or 98.6° F. Systemically, when the skin is exposed to warm or hot temperatures vasodilation and perspiration occur to promote heat loss. As perspiration evaporates from the skin, cooling occurs. When the skin is exposed to cool or cold temperatures, the systemic response includes vasoconstriction and piloerection to conserve heat. Shivering also occurs in response to cooler temperatures. Shivering produces heat through muscular contraction.

The local response to heat and cold results from changes in blood vessel size, which affect blood flow to the exposed area. This physiological response is the major basis for the use of hot and cold therapies. Heat causes vasodilation; cold causes vasoconstriction. The resulting changes in blood flow affect the extent to which nutrients reach damaged tissues and metabolic wastes escape from the injured site. Table 43-1 outlines the therapeutic effects of heat and cold applications.

When receptors for heat or cold are stimulated, sensory impulses travel via somatic afferent fibers to the hypothalamus and cerebral cortex. The cerebral cortex makes a person aware of temperature sensations. The person can then adapt as necessary to maintain normal body temperature; if cold, he can put on additional clothing. The hypothalamus simultaneously controls physiologic reflexes needed to regulate normal body temperature. The body also has a protective reflex response for exposure to temperature extremes. Exposure to an extremely hot or cold stimulus sends impulses traveling to the spinal cord, synapsing at the cord, and returning by way of motor nerves to cause withdrawal from the stimulus. The person becomes aware of the discomfort as withdrawal occurs.

Sensory adaptation to local temperature extremes can occur quickly within the body. A person initially feels a temperature extreme, but once the sensory receptors adapt he may become unaware of any temperature variation. Eventually excessive heat causes a burning sensation; excessive cold causes a numbing sensation before pain is sensed. Because of this physiologic phenomenon the risk of tissue injury from hot and cold applications is great. Certain clients are also more at risk than others for injury from hot and cold applications (Table 43-2) because of the nature of underlying disease processes and the status of their skin integrity. The nurse plays an important role in maintaining the client's safety. The nurse must always have an order for a hot or cold application, and the order should include the desired temperature to be used (Table 43-3). Heat and cold must be used without inducing injury or causing further damage to previously injured tissues. The nurse must also instruct clients in the proper use of heat and cold applications because many of the therapies can be used at home.

When using hot and cold therapy, the nurse will apply either dry or moist applications. The selection of dry or moist applications is affected by the nature of temperature conduction as well as the result desired from therapy. Temperature travels from an external source such as a compress, waterpad, or ice bag to the skin's surface. A substance that conducts temperatures poorly is a good in-

**TABLE 43-1** Therapeutic Effects of Heat and Cold Applications

| Therapy | Physiologic Response | Therapeutic Benefit | Examples of Conditions Treated |
|---|---|---|---|
| Heat | Vasodilation | Improves blood flow to injured body part, promotes delivery of nutrients and removal of wastes, lessens venous congestion in injured tissues. | Inflamed or edematous body part; new surgical wound; infected wound; arthritis, degenerative joint disease; localized joint pain, muscle strains; low back pain, menstrual cramping; hemorrhoidal, perianal, and vaginal inflammation; local abscesses. |
| | Reduced blood viscosity | Improves delivery of leukocytes and antibiotics to wound site. | |
| | Reduced muscle tension | Promotes muscle relaxation and reduces pain from spasm or stiffness. | |
| | Increased tissue metabolism | Increases blood flow; provides local warmth. | |
| | Increased capillary permeability | Promotes movement of waste products and nutrients. | |
| Cold | Vasoconstriction | Reduces blood flow to injured body part, prevents edema formation, reduces inflammation. | Immediately after direct trauma, e.g., sprains, strains, fractures, muscle spasms; superficial laceration or puncture wound; minor burn; when malignancy is suspected in area of injury or pain; after injections; arthritis, joint trauma. |
| | Local anesthesia | Reduces localized pain. | |
| | Reduced cell metabolism | Reduces oxygen needs of tissues. | |
| | Increased blood viscosity | Promotes blood coagulation at injury site. | |
| | Decreased muscle tension | Relieves pain. | |

**TABLE 43-2** Conditions That Increase Risk of Injury from Heat and Cold Application

| Condition | Risk Factors |
|---|---|
| Very young; elderly | Thinner skin layers in children increase risk of burns; elderly have reduced sensitivity to pain. |
| Open wounds, broken skin, stomas | Subcutaneous and visceral tissues more sensitive to temperature variations; also contain no temperature and fewer pain receptors. |
| Areas of edema or scar formation | Reduced sensation to temperature stimuli because of thickening of skin layers from fluid buildup or scar formation. |
| Peripheral vascular disease (e.g., diabetes or arteriosclerosis) | Body's extremities less sensitive to temperature and pain stimuli because of circulatory impairment and local tissue injury; cold application would further compromise blood flow. |
| Confusion or unconsciousness | Reduced perception of sensory or painful stimuli. |
| Spinal cord injury | Alterations in nerve pathways preventing reception of sensory or painful stimuli. |
| Abscessed tooth or appendix | Infection highly localized; application of heat may cause rupture with spread of microorganisms systemically. |

sulator. For example, cloth placed over an ice bag insulates the skin from cold temperature extremes. Rubber, which is the external covering for most commercial water flow pads, conducts heat well. Air tends to not conduct heat as well as water. There are, however, distinct advantages to using both dry and moist applications (Table 43-4). The nurse should be familiar with the effects of each application type.

## GUIDELINES

1. Protect damaged skin layers. Exposed layers of skin are more sensitive to temperature variations than intact skin layers.
2. Time all applications carefully. A person tolerates temperature extremes better when the duration of exposure is short. Prolonged exposure can injure tissue. Keep a timer or clock close by so that the client can help the nurse time applications.
3. Know the temperature of the application being used. Many devices, such as heating pads or water flow pads, have thermostats to regulate temperature. The nurse always checks the temperature of moist compresses applied directly to the skin.
4. Certain body parts are more sensitive than others to temperature extremes. The nurse can modify the intensity of heat and cold when sensitive skin areas are being treated.
5. Check a client frequently during a hot or cold application. The condition of the skin indicates whether tissue injury is occurring.
6. Know a client's risk for injury from heat or cold. Certain clients are more predisposed than others to injury because of sensory alterations or changes in skin integrity.
7. Do not allow a client to adjust temperature settings. It is common for the client to adapt to a temperature extreme and then think that the temperature should be adjusted.
8. Never position a client so that he is unable to move away from the temperature source. This avoids the risk of injuries from temperature exposure. The client should always have a call light within reach.
9. Do not leave unattended a client who is unable to sense temperature changes or move away from the temperature source. The nurse is responsible for this client's safety.
10. Discourage a client from moving an application. This may result in injury to an unprotected area of the body.

**TABLE 43-3** Temperature Ranges for Hot and Cold Applications

| Temperature | Centigrade Range | Fahrenheit Range |
|---|---|---|
| Very hot | 41-46°C | 105-115°F |
| Hot | 37-41°C | 98-105°F |
| Warm | 34-37°C | 93-98° F |
| Tepid | 26-34°C | 80-93° F |
| Cool | 18-26°C | 65-80° F |
| Cold | 10-18°C | 50-65° F |

## PREREQUISITE KNOWLEDGE

1. Principles of medical asepsis.
2. Physiologic effects of heat and cold applications to the skin.
3. Extent of client's physiologic condition or injury.

## PREREQUISITE SKILLS

1. Basic handwashing techniques (Chapter 37).
2. Donning sterile gloves by the open method (Chapter 38).
3. Application of dressings (Chapter 41).
4. Physical assessment of skin and sensory function (Chapter 13).
5. Assessment of vital signs (Chapter 12).

**TABLE 43-4** Choice of Dry or Moist Applications

| Type | Advantages | Disadvantages |
|---|---|---|
| Moist applications | Moist application reduces drying of skin and softens wound exudate.<br>Moist compresses conform well to body area being treated.<br>Moist heat penetrates deeply into tissue layers.<br>Warm moist heat does not promote sweating and insensible fluid loss. | Prolonged exposure can cause maceration of the skin.<br>Moist heat will cool rapidly because of moisture evaporation.<br>Moist heat creates a greater risk for burns to the skin since moisture conducts heat. |
| Dry applications | Dry heat is less likely to burn skin than moist applications.<br>Dry application does not cause skin maceration.<br>Dry heat retains temperature longer, since it is not influenced by evaporation. | Dry heat increases body fluid loss through sweating.<br>Dry applications do not penetrate deep into tissues.<br>Dry heat causes increased drying of skin. |

# *SKILL 43-1 Applying a Moist Hot Compress to an Open Wound*

A hot compress is a section of sterile or clean gauze moistened in a prescribed heated solution and applied directly to the skin's surface or an open wound. A sterile compress is necessary only when there is a break in skin integrity. Commercially packaged sterile, premoistened compresses are available in some agencies. The nurse uses a special infrared lamp to heat the packaged compress. Plain sterile or clean gauze can be heated by adding the gauze to a container of warmed solution. Often the nurse will apply an aquathermic heating pad over a compress to deliver a continuous source of heat and thus improve the application's therapeutic effects.

### Purposes

1. Improve circulation to injured tissues.
2. Relieve edema.
3. Promote consolidation of pus and drainage in a wound.
4. Promote comfort.

## *Procedure 43-1*

| Steps | Rationale |
|---|---|
| **Assessment** | |
| 1. Inspect condition of exposed skin and wound on which compress is to be applied. | Provides baseline to determine changes in skin during heat application. Very thin or damaged skin is more susceptible to injury from heat. |
| 2. Assess client's extremities for sensitivity to temperature and pain by measuring light touch, pin prick, and temperature sensation tests. | Determines if client is insensitive to heat and cold extremes. |
| 3. Refer to medical record to identify any systemic contraindications to heat application, e.g., area of active bleeding, inflammation. | Heat causes vasodilation, which will aggravate active bleeding. Heat applied to localized area of acute inflammation or tumor may cause rupture or activate cell growth. |
| 4. Refer to physician's order for type of compress, location and duration of application, desired temperature, and institutional policies regarding temperature of compress. | Ensures likelihood of safe application. |
| 5. Assess client's understanding of application and its purpose. | Determines need for health teaching. |
| **Nursing Diagnosis** | |
| 1. Cluster data to reveal actual or potential nursing diagnoses: | |
| a. Impaired skin integrity: related to surgical incision. | Compresses can be used over wounds to improve healing. |
| b. Potential for injury: related to risk of burns. | Risk of burns is significant. Sterile petrolatum jelly can be used to protect intact skin areas. |
| c. Knowledge deficit regarding moist heat: related to misinformation. | Nurse will explain procedure and its purpose thoroughly. |
| d. Sensory/perceptual alteration: related to reduced tactile sensation. | Extra precaution is needed to protect client from injury. |
| **Planning** | |
| 1. Develop individualized goals for client based on nursing diagnoses: | |
| a. Prevent local tissue injury. | |
| b. Promote wound healing. | Frequent observation and use of proper techniques will protect client from injury and promote physiological responses for healing. |
| c. Improve client's understanding of therapy. | Client may require instruction for home care. |
| 2. Prepare following equipment and supplies: | |
| a. Prescribed solution warmed to proper temperature, approximately 43-46° C (110-115° F). | Correct temperature prevents accidental burns. |
| b. Sterile gauze dressings | |
| c. Sterile container for solution | |
| d. Commercially prepared compresses (optional) | |
| e. Sterile gloves | |
| f. Petrolatum jelly | Protects untreated skin surface. |
| g. Sterile cotton swabs | |
| h. Waterproof pad | Prevents soiling of bed linen. |

| Steps | Rationale |
|---|---|
| i. Tape or ties | |
| j. Dry bath towel | |
| k. Aquathermic or heating pad (optional) | Provides continuous source of heat. |
| l. Disposable gloves | |
| m. Bath thermometer | Measures solution temperature |
| n. Bath blanket | |
| 3. Explain steps of procedure and purpose to client. Describe sensation to be felt, e.g., feeling of warmth and wetness. Explain precautions to prevent burning. | Minimizes client's anxiety and promotes cooperation during procedure. |

## Implementation

| Steps | Rationale |
|---|---|
| 1. Assist client in assuming comfortable position in proper body alignment. | Compress remains in place for several minutes. Limited mobility in uncomfortable position causes muscular stress. |
| 2. Place waterproof pad under area to be treated. | Prevents soiling of bed linen. |
| 3. Expose body part to be covered with compress and drape client with bath blanket. Close bedside curtains. | Prevents unnecessary cooling and exposure of body part. |
| 4. Wash hands. | Reduces transmission of infection. |
| 5. Assemble equipment.<br>▪ Pour warmed solution into sterile container.<br>▪ Check immersed bath thermometer for desired temperature.<br>▪ If using portable heating source, keep solution warm. Commercially prepared compresses may remain under infrared lamp until just before use. Open sterile packages and drop gauze into container to become immersed in solution. Turn aquathermia pad (if desired) to correct temperature. | Compresses must retain warmth for therapeutic benefit. |
| 6. Don disposable gloves. Remove any existing dressing covering wound. Dispose of gloves and dressings in proper receptacle. | Reduces transmission of microorganisms. |
| 7. If wound was covered, assess condition of it and surrounding skin.<br>▪ Inflamed wound will appear reddened but surrounding skin will be less red in color. | Provides baseline to determine skin changes following compress application. |
| 8. Don sterile gloves. | Allows nurse to manipulate sterile dressing and touch open wound. |
| 9. Apply sterile petrolatum jelly with cotton swab to skin surrounding wound. Do not apply jelly on broken areas of skin. | Jelly protects skin from possible burns and maceration. |
| 10. Pick up one layer of immersed gauze and wring out any excess water. | Excess moisture macerates skin and increases risk of burns and infection. |
| 11. Apply gauze lightly to open wound. Watch client's response and ask if client feels discomfort. In few seconds lift edge of gauze to assess for redness. | Skin is sensitive to sudden change in temperature. Redness indicates burn. |
| 12. If client tolerates compress, pack gauze snugly against wound. Be sure all wound surfaces are covered by hot compress. | Packing of compress prevents rapid cooling from underlying air currents. |
| 13. Wrap or cover moist compress with dry bath towel. If necessary, pin or tie in place. | Towel insulates compress to prevent heat loss. |
| 14. Change hot compress every 5 min or as ordered. | Prevents cooling and maintains therapeutic benefit of compress. |
| 15. Apply aquathermic or waterproof heating pad over towel (optional). Keep it in place for desired duration of application (approximately 20-30 min). | Provides constant temperature to compress. Local application of heat for greater than 60 min often results in reflex vasoconstriction. Removing hot compress after 30 min and then reapplying in 15 min, if desired, maintains vasodilation and positive therapeutic effects. |
| 16. Ask client periodically if there is any discomfort or burning sensation. Observe area of skin not covered by actual compress. | Continued exposure to heat can cause burning of skin. |
| 17. Remove pad, towel, and compress in 30 min. Again assess wound and condition of skin. | Continued exposure to moisture will macerate skin. |
| 18. Replace dry sterile dressing as ordered. | Prevents entrance of microorganisms into wound site. Maintains client's comfort. |
| 19. Assist client to preferred comfortable position. | Maintains client's comfort. |
| 20. Dispose of equipment and soiled compress. Wash hands. | Reduces transmission of microorganisms. |

| Steps | Rationale |
|---|---|
| **Evaluation** | |
| 1. Inspect affected area covered by compress and heating pad. | Assists in determining effects of application. |
| 2. Ask if client notices any unusual burning sensation not felt before application. | It may be difficult to assess burn merely by color changes if wound is inflamed or drainage is present. |
| ***Expected outcomes*** | |
| 1. Affected site is pink and warm to touch immediately following application. | Vasodilation increases blood flow to site. |
| 2. After multiple applications wound shows signs of healing, e.g., granulation, reduced inflammation, drainage. | Moist heat increases blood flow, enhances white blood cell infiltration, and removes wastes of metabolism. |
| 3. Client denies burning sensation. | |
| 4. Client able to safely apply therapy. | Measures level of learning. |
| ***Unexpected outcomes*** | |
| 1. There is redness and tenderness at affected site. | Temperature of compress too extreme for condition of skin. Redness and tenderness are signs of first-degree burn. |
| 2. Client complains of burning and discomfort. | Extreme temperature for client to tolerate. |
| **Recording and Reporting** | |
| 1. Record type, location, and duration of application. Note temperature used in nurses' notes. | Documents therapy administered. |
| 2. Describe condition of wound, skin, and client's response. | Documents client's response to therapy. |
| 3. Report unusual findings to nurse in charge or physician. | Burn or other change may require different therapies. |
| **Follow-up Activities** | |
| 1. If heat applications are to be continued after discharge, allow client or family member to provide return demonstration before discharge. | Ensures safe treatment at home. |

### Special Considerations

- Clients receiving long-term steroid therapy develop thin fragile skin.

### Teaching Considerations

- Teach client to gently pack wound to avoid discomfort.
- Care givers and clients need to be taught that careful assessment is needed for clients with reduced sensation to determine if temperature of compress is too hot.

### Home Care Considerations

- Assess availability of primary care giver to assist client in application of compress, their understanding of purpose of procedure, their willingness to comply with procedure and not leave client with compress in place.
- Assess physical environment to determine existence of adequate facilities with which to prepare hot compress.

## *SKILL 43-2 Assisting with Warm Soaks and Sitz Baths*

Another form of moist heat application is the use of warm baths, soaks, and sitz baths. A warm bath or soak simply involves immersion of a body part into a warmed solution. A physician usually orders a soak for a body extremity. If a body part is too large to immerse, a soak can be accomplished by wrapping the part in dressings and saturating them with the prepared solution.

A sitz bath is a special tub or chair basin that allows a client to sit in water without immersing the legs, feet, and upper trunk (Fig. 43-1). Sitz basins are disposable and especially easy to use in the home. Clients who have had rectal surgery or an episiotomy during childbirth or who have painful hemorrhoids or perineal inflammation may benefit from a sitz bath.

When preparing a soak or bath, the nurse should remember that the heated solution is in direct contact with the client's skin. It is very important to check water temperature carefully to prevent the risk of burns. It is also desirable to keep the solution temperature constant so as to enhance the moist heat's therapeutic effects. Whenever heated solution is added to a soak basin or bath the client's body part should be removed and then reimmersed once the solution has mixed.

### Purposes

1. Promoting circulation.
2. Reducing edema and inflammation.
3. Increasing muscle relaxation.
4. Debriding wounds.
5. Applying medicated solutions.

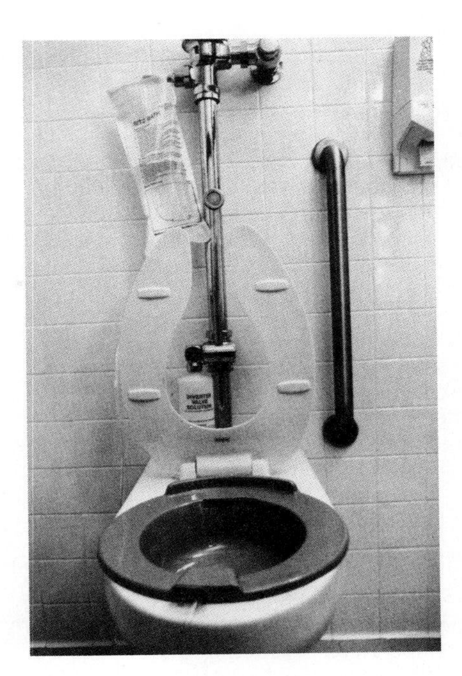

***Fig. 43-1*** Disposable sitz bath.

## *Procedure 43-2*

| Steps | Rationale |
| --- | --- |
| **Assessment** | |
| 1. Assess condition of skin of body part to be immersed. | Identifies thin or sensitive skin that is prone to injury from temperature extremes. Provides baseline to determine changes in skin during therapy. |
| 2. Assess client's level of comfort. | Inflamed or injured body parts may be soothed by soak or bath. |
| 3. Determine client's risk for having reduced temperature sensation by referring to medical record. | Certain conditions alter conduction of sensory impulses that transmit temperature and pain stimuli. |
| 4. Identify any systemic contraindications to immersion in warm baths by referring to medical record. | Certain cardiovascular conditions place clients at risk for sudden changes in blood pressure and blood flow caused by vasodilation. |
| 5. Assess client's understanding of therapy and its purpose. | Determines need for health teaching. |
| 6. Check physician's order for desired solution, body part to be soaked, and desired temperature, as per institutional policy. | Ensures safe use of moist heat. |
| **Nursing Diagnosis** | |
| 1. Cluster data to reveal actual or potential nursing diagnoses: | |
| a. Impaired skin integrity: related to inflamed incision. | Soaks and baths are used commonly for incisions and open wounds. |
| b. Potential for injury: related to risk of burns. | Improper use of soaks can cause burns. Nurse uses correct techniques to prevent injury. |
| c. Decreased cardiac output: related to heart failure. | This diagnosis may contraindicate use of baths or large extremity soaks. |
| d. Knowledge deficit regarding moist heat therapy: related to inexperience. | Nurse explains procedure and provides instruction for possible home care. |
| **Planning** | |
| 1. Develop individualized goals for client based on nursing diagnoses: | |
| a. Prevent local tissue injury.<br>b. Promote wound healing.<br>c. Promote relaxation and comfort. | Frequent observation, monitoring, and use of proper techniques will protect client from injury and promote physiological responses of healing. |

| Steps | Rationale |
|---|---|
| d. Improve client's understanding of therapy. | |
| e. Maintain adequate cardiac output. | |
| 2. Prepare following equipment and supplies: | |
| a. Clean basin, tub, or sitz bath (basin may need to be sterile if part to be soaked has an open wound). | To soak or immerse body part. |
| b. Bath thermometer. | To measure solution temperature. |
| c. Prescribed solution warmed to proper temperature approximately 37-41° C (98-105° F). (Tap water is commonly used for sitz baths.) | Correct temperature prevents accidental burns. |
| d. Bath towel | |
| e. Bath blanket or sheet | Prevents over-exposure during immersion. |
| f. Absorbent gauze or cloth rolls (optional) | If body part too large to immerse, used to cover part for soaking. |
| g. Prescribed medicated solution (optional) | |
| h. Waterproof pad for soak | |
| 3. Explain procedure and type of sensations client will feel. | Helps reduce client's anxiety and promote cooperation. |
| 4. Close all room doors, windows, or curtains. | Controls for drafts that can cause cooling. Provides client privacy. |

## Implementation

| Steps | Rationale |
|---|---|
| 1. Wash hands. | Reduces transmission of microorganisms. |
| 2. Fill basin or tub with warmed solution. Use thermometer to check temperature. | Checking for correct temperature reduces risk of burns. |
| 3. For soaks, position client comfortably and place waterproof pad under area to be treated. | Prevents soiling of bed linen or clothing. |
| 4. Assist client in immersing body part in tub or basin. | Prevents risk of falls. |
| 5. Cover client with bath blanket or towel as desired. | Prevents chilling and enhances client's ability to relax. |
| 6. Maintain temperature constant throughout soak for 15-20 min. | Therapeutic effects of soak can only be obtained from constant temperature. |
| a. Keep large sheet or blanket over container or basin. | |
| b. After 10 min, remove body part, empty cooled solution, add newly heated solution, and reimmerse body part. | Adding warmed solution to basin with body part immersed can cause burn. |
| 7. After 15-20 min remove client from soak or bath; dry body parts thoroughly. | Avoids chilling. Enhances client's comfort. |
| 8. Assist client to bed or chair. | Maintains comfortable environment for client. |
| 9. Drain solution from basin or tub. Clean and place in proper storage area. Dispose of soiled linen and wash hands. | Reduces transmission of microorganisms. |

## Evaluation

| Steps | Rationale |
|---|---|
| 1. Inspect condition of body part immersed. | Evaluates effects of treatments. |
| 2. Question client regarding presence of burning sensation, pain, and general response to therapy. | Determines if client was exposed to temperature extreme resulting in burn. Evaluates client's subjective response to therapy. |
| 3. Assess vital signs if client complains of dizziness or lightheadedness. | Determines if vascular response to vasodilation has occurred. |
| 4. Ask client to explain purpose of soak/sitz bath. | Measures level of learning. |

### *Expected outcomes*

| Steps | Rationale |
|---|---|
| 1. Client's skin is pink and warm to touch immediately following soak. | Result of local vasodilation. |
| 2. Client has decreased muscle tension. | Relaxation results from effect of warmth on muscle fibers. |
| 3. Client has less pain at affected site. | Moist heat reduces edema and inflammation. Heat applications lower pain perception by activating large diameter sensory fibers that block painful stimuli. |
| 4. Blood pressure and pulse are normal. | No vascular changes occurred. |
| 5. Client correctly uses sitz bath. | Documents learning. |

### *Unexpected outcomes*

| Steps | Rationale |
|---|---|
| 1. Client's skin is reddened and sensitive to touch. | Extreme warmth caused burning of skin layer. |
| 2. Client experiences hypotension and complains of dizziness, nausea, lightheadedness. | Result of systemic vasodilation. |

| Steps | Rationale |
|---|---|
| **Recording and Reporting** | |
| 1. Record procedure, including temperature and duration of soak in nurse's notes. | Documents therapy delivered to the client. |
| 2. Describe condition of body part immersed and client's response. | Documents response to therapy. |
| 3. Report client's intolerance to procedure or any unusual observations to nurse in charge or physician. | Provides guidelines for repeating therapy. Change in client's condition may require different therapy. |

### Special Considerations

- Clients with thin skin include children and those receiving long-term steroid therapy. These clients may have impaired skin integrity and therapy may be contraindicated.
- Caution must be used in applying baths or soaks for certain clients, e.g., those with a history of myocardial infarction, angina pectoris, or hypotension.
- Geriatric clients tolerate somewhat cooler temperature better because of less stable temperature regulation mechanisms.
- In some clients, e.g., frail, elderly cardiac clients, it may be necessary to monitor vital signs throughout procedure.

### Teaching Considerations

- Client may resume therapy at home and should understand risks of burns. Explain risks of using warm baths and methods to ensure safety.

### Home Care Considerations

- Assess availability of primary care giver to assist client. If care giver is not available, evaluate client as to ability, willingness, and understanding of preparing soaks or baths.
- Assess home environment to determine adequacy of facilities for use by client. Medical equipment companies may be contacted for assistance in determining best product for client.

## *SKILL 43-3 Using a Heat Lamp and Heat Cradle*

Dry heat is less likely than moist heat to injure the skin, because there is less skin maceration from moisture and dry heat is not conducted as well to the deeper tissue layers. Two forms of dry heat therapy, heat lamps and heat cradles, have an added advantage of nothing directly touching the client's skin. This is important for clients with sensitive or painful skin conditions or wounds.

Heat lamps use infrared or regular (40-75 watt) light bulbs to expose superficial layers of the skin to heat. The lamp is used primarily to increase circulation to the wound.

A heat cradle is a long, metal, half-circle frame that fits over a large body part such as a leg or lower trunk. The client remains in bed while using the heat cradle. A series of small (25-watt) light bulbs emits heat over a broad exposed area. Because of the bulbs' low wattage it is generally safer to use a heat cradle longer than a heat lamp. However, in both cases one of the nurse's main responsibilities is to prevent prolonged exposure to the lamp's heat.

### Purposes

1. Increase circulation to injured tissues.
2. Promote drying of weeping or draining wounds.

## *Procedure 43-3*

| Steps | Rationale |
|---|---|
| **Assessment** | |
| 1. Inspect skin for presence of scars or stomas. Note condition of ulcer or wound to be warmed. | Scars and stomas are insensitive to heat and thus can easily burn. Inspection provides baseline to determine response to therapy. |

| Steps | Rationale |
|---|---|
| 2. Assess area to be treated for sensitivity to temperature and pain by measuring light touch, pin prick, and temperature sensation. | Determines if client is insensitive to heat and cold extremes. |
| 3. Be sure lamps are electrically safe; check for frayed cords, broken sockets. | Ensures safe environment for both nurse and client. |
| 4. Check physician's order for area to be treated and duration of therapy. | All dry heat applications require physician's order. |
| 5. Assess client's understanding of procedure and its purpose. | Determines extent of need for health teaching. |
| **Nursing Diagnosis** | |
| 1. Cluster data to reveal actual or potential nursing diagnoses: | |
| a. Impaired skin integrity: related to pressure ulcer. | Heat lamp therapy used for existing skin alterations and not when skin is intact. |
| b. Potential for injury related to burns. | Prolonged use of heat lamps and placement of lamp too close to skin can cause burns. |
| c. Knowledge deficit regarding heat applications: related to misinformation. | Nurse will include explanations during procedure. |
| **Planning** | |
| 1. Develop individualized goals for client based on nursing diagnoses: | |
| a. Protect client from injury. | Frequent monitoring during heat application helps minimize risk of burns. |
| b. Promote wound healing. | Heat improves circulation to wound. |
| c. Improve client's understanding of therapy. | Procedure lasts several minutes and requires client's cooperation. |
| 2. Prepare following equipment and supplies:<br>a. Heat lamp or cradle<br>b. Sheet or bath blanket<br>c. Bath towel | |
| 3. Explain procedure and caution client against touching lamp's surface. | Surface of lamp can become very warm. Understanding of procedure promotes client's cooperation. |
| **Implementation** | |
| 1. Close room door and cubicle curtains. | Provides client privacy |
| 2. Wash hands. | Reduces transmission of infection. |
| 3. Position client comfortably with area to be heated exposed. | Maintenance of position of comfort helps client tolerate procedure for necessary period of time. |
| 4. Wipe off any moisture noted on area to be heated. | Moisture conducts heat. |
| 5. Use bed sheet or bath blanket to drape as much of area not to be exposed as possible. | Enhances client's level of comfort. |
| 6. If using heat lamp, place it an appropriate distance above area exposed: 40-60 watts, 50 cm or 24 in; 60 watts 75 cm or 30 in. | Allows heat to radiate skin with minimal risk of burning. |
| 7. If using heat cradle, place it over area to be warmed with 25-watt bulbs at least 40-45 cm (16-18 in) away. | Provides for radiation of skin with minimal risk of burning. |
| 8. Turn lamp/cradle on and adjust light to illuminate affected area. | Heat should be applied to localized area. Sensitive body parts should be protected. |
| 9. Heat cradle: Place bed sheet over cradle frame. Do not allow sheet to touch light bulbs. | Reduces exposure of body parts and prevents cooling from air currents. |
| 10. Assess client's skin every 5 min during duration of procedure (20 min). Ask if client notes burning or hot sensation. | Determines change in skin condition during procedure. Burns can occur easily in clients with reduced sensation. |
| 11. Turn lamp/cradle off and move it to side of room. | Client should not be able to turn lamp back on without supervision. |
| 12. Assist client to assume comfortable position. | Maintains relaxing environment. |
| 13. Dispose of any soiled linen and wash hands. | Reduces spread of infection. |
| **Evaluation** | |
| 1. Inspect condition of skin and/or wound that was heated. | Evaluates response to heat exposure. |
| 2. Ask if client feels any localized discomfort or burning that was not present before therapy. | Dry radiated heat can cause burns. |
| 3. Ask client to describe heat lamp procedure. | Measures level of learning. |

| Steps | Rationale |
|---|---|
| ***Expected outcomes*** | |
| 1. Client's skin is pink and warm to touch immediately following therapy. | Vasodilation from local heat application increases blood flow to affected part. |
| 2. Exudate at open wound is dry. | Heat promotes drying effect that increases healing. |
| 3. Client can correctly use heat lamp. | Documents learning. |
| ***Unexpected outcomes*** | |
| 1. Client's skin is reddened and sensitive to touch. | Prolonged exposure under lamp can result in burns. Redness and tenderness are symptoms of first degree burn. |

### Recording and Reporting

| Steps | Rationale |
|---|---|
| 1. Record procedure including duration of therapy, area heated, and client's response in nurses' notes. | Documents therapy administered and results of care. |
| 2. Report any unusual findings such as burn to nurse in charge or physician. | Other therapies may be indicated. |

### Follow-up Activities

| Steps | Rationale |
|---|---|
| 1. Apply moisturizing lotion to skin surrounding actual ulcer or wound. | Dry heat causes drying of skin. |

### Special Considerations

- If client is unable to tolerate heat after only few minutes exposure, move lamp farther back and continue monitoring response.

### Teaching Considerations

- *Never* place sheet over heat lamp to form tent. This creates greater hazard for fire because of light bulb's higher wattage.
- Instruct primary caregiver not to leave disoriented client alone during procedure.

### Home Care Considerations

- Assess client and primary caregiver's understanding of purpose of procedure and ability and willingness to follow proper procedures for implementation.
- Assess home environment for adequacy of facilities with which to implement procedure.

## *SKILL 43-4 Applying Aquathermia and Heating Pads*

Aquathermia and heating pads are common forms of dry heat therapy used in health care settings as well as in the home (Fig 43-2). Both are applied directly to the skin's surface and for this reason extra precautions are needed to prevent burns. The aquathermia (water flow pad) consists of a waterproof rubber or plastic pad connected by two hoses to an electrical control unit that has a heating element and motor. Distilled water circulates through hollowed channels in the pad to the control unit where water is heated (or cooled). The temperature setting is adjusted by a plastic key that inserts into the control unit. In most health care institutions the central supply department sets the temperature regulators to the recommended temperature, approximately 40.5°-43° C (110°-115° F). Because of the constant temperature control, aquathermia pads tend to be safer than heating pads. If distilled water within the unit runs low, the nurse simply

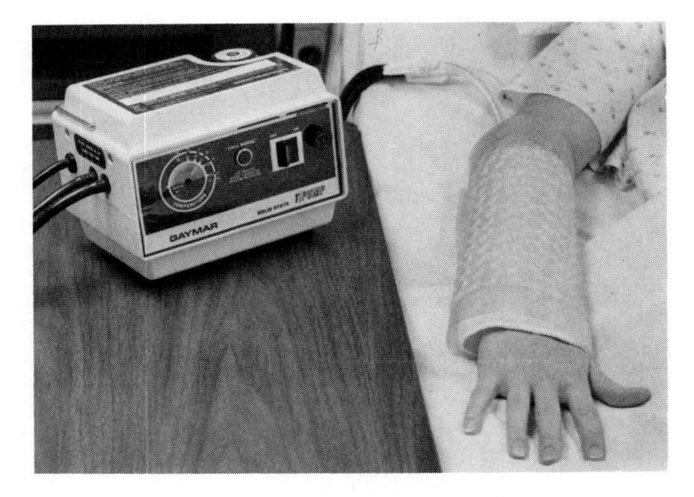


***Fig. 43-2*** Aquathermia pad.

adds water to the reservoir at the top of the control unit. Rubber and plastic conduct heat, so the pad should be encased in a towel or pillow case to avoid direct exposure to the skin.

The conventional heating pad consists of an electric coil enclosed in a waterproof covering. A cotton or flannel cloth covers the outer pad. The pad connects to an electrical cord that has a temperature regulating unit for high, medium, or low settings. Because it is so easy to readjust temperature settings on heating pads, clients should be advised not to turn the setting higher once they have adapted to the temperature. It is wise to avoid ever using the highest setting.

### Purposes

1. Reduce localized areas of edema and inflammation.
2. Relieve discomfort of muscle sprains and cramping.

## *Procedure 43-4*

| Steps | Rationale |
|---|---|
| **Assessment** | |
| 1. Assess condition of skin over which pad is to be applied. | Provides baseline to determine change in skin condition following heat application. |
| 2. Assess level of discomfort and range of motion if client is being treated for muscle sprain. | Baseline to determine if pain relief achieved. |
| 3. Assess area to be treated for sensitivity to temperature, light touch, and pain. | Determines if client is insensitive to heat extremes. |
| 4. Check electrical plugs and cords for obvious fraying or cracking. | Prevents injury from accidental electrical shock. |
| 5. Check physician's order for location of application and duration of therapy. Institutional policy usually sets recommended temperature. | Order required to help ensure client's safety. |
| 6. Determine client or family members' knowledge of procedure including steps for application and safety precautions. | Heating pads are frequently used in home. Assessment determines extent of health teaching required. |
| **Nursing Diagnosis** | |
| 1. Cluster data to reveal actual or potential nursing diagnoses: | |
| a. Impaired skin integrity: related to inflammation. | Aquathermia pads are used frequently for treating phlebitis at intravenous sites. |
| b. Pain: related to muscular strain. | Heat can relieve edema and relax muscles so as to reduce pain. |
| c. Impaired physical mobility: related to muscle sprain. | Clients with muscle strains may be unable to carry out normal physical activity. |
| d. Potential for injury related to burns. | Nurse must follow safety precautions as well as educate clients about safe use of heating pads. |
| e. Knowledge deficit regarding heat applications: related to inexperience. | |
| **Planning** | |
| 1. Develop individualized goals for client based on nursing diagnoses: | |
| a. Promote healing of injured tissues. | Proper application of pads will ensure delivery of warm heat to injured tissues. Heat will reduce edema and relax stiff muscles. |
| b. Improve muscle range of motion. | |
| c. Promote client's comfort. | Heat relaxes strained muscles. |
| d. Prevent local tissue injury. | Safe application avoids burns to skin. |
| e. Improve client's understanding of therapy. | Ensures cooperation during procedure. |
| f. Provide client with skills needed to administer therapy at home. | If repeated use of heating pad is required, client should give demonstration of its proper use. |
| 2. Prepare following equipment and supplies: | |
| a. Aquathermia or heating pad | |
| b. Distilled water | Used to refill aquathermia pad as needed. |
| c. Bath towel or pillowcase | Used to prevent pad's rubber surface from touching client's skin. |
| d. Tape, ties, or gauze roll. | Used to secure pad in place. |
| ▪ *Never use safety pins.* Pins can cause leaks in aquathermia pads and electrical shock in heating pads. | |
| 3. Explain procedures and precautions to client. | Improves likelihood of client's compliance with therapy. |

| Steps | Rationale |
|---|---|
| **Implementation** | |
| 1. Close bedside curtain or room door. | Provides for client's privacy. |
| 2. Wash hands. | Reduces transfer of infection. |
| 3. Position client comfortably so area to be treated is exposed. | Client must be able to assume position for several minutes during application. |
| 4. For aquathermia or uncovered heating pad, cover or wrap affected area with bath towel or enclose pads with pillowcase. | Prevents heated surface from touching client's skin. |
| 5. Place pad over affected area (see Fig. 43-2, p. 903) and secure with tape, tie, or gauze as needed. | Pad delivers dry warm heat to injured tissues. Pad should not slip onto different body part. |
| 6. Turn heating pad on to low or medium setting and check temperature of aquathermia pad. | Prevents exposure of client to temperature extremes. |
| 7. Monitor condition of skin every 5 min during application and question client regarding sensation of burning. | Determines if heat exposure is resulting in burn. |
| 8. After 20-30 min remove pad and store. | Continued exposure will result in burns. Client should not have access to pad without supervision. |
| 9. Assist client in returning to preferred comfortable position. | Promotes relaxing environment. |
| 10. Dispose of soiled linen and wash hands. | Reduces spread of infection. |
| **Evaluation** | |
| 1. Inspect condition of skin exposed to heat. | Evaluates response of skin to heat exposure. |
| 2. Ask client if strained muscle or inflamed area continues to be painful. | Heat relieves pain from muscle stiffness and spasm. |
| 3. Note if client is able to move strained muscle with less discomfort. | Heat relaxes strained muscle. |
| 4. Observe client apply aquathermia. | Measures level of learning. |
| ***Expected outcomes*** | |
| 1. Skin is pink and warm to touch following application. | Vasodilation from heat exposure increases blood flow to affected part. |
| 2. Client reports less discomfort of inflamed tissues or strained muscles. | Heat applications lower pain perception by stimulating large diameter sensory nerve fibers and blocking pain impulses of smaller nerve fibers. |
| 3. Client may be able to move strained muscles more freely. | Reduced stiffness improves range of motion. |
| 4. Client correctly applies aquathermia. | Documents learning. |
| ***Unexpected outcomes*** | |
| 1. Skin is reddened and sensitive to touch. | Symptoms indicate first-degree burn. |
| 2. Body part is painful to move. | Movement stretches burn-sensitive nerve fibers in skin. |
| **Recording and Reporting** | |
| 1. Record site of application, duration of therapy, and client's response. | Documents therapy administered and results of care. |
| 2. Report changes in skin integrity such as burns. | Further therapy may be needed to treat burn. |
| **Follow-up Activities** | |
| 1. If applications are to be done at home, have client apply pad and explain safety measures. | Ensures client's ability to safely use heat therapy. |

## Special Considerations

- Heating and aquathermia pads are rarely applied over open wounds.
- Never position client to lie directly on pads. This prevents dissipation of heat and increases risk of burns.
- Do not actively exercise muscle to evaluate results of therapy. This can aggravate muscle strain.

## Teaching Considerations

- Highlight safety precautions as you follow them during application.

## Home Care Considerations

- Assess client and primary care giver as to understanding, ability, and motivation to comply with procedure.
- Assess home environment for facilities to comply with implementation of procedure.

# *SKILL 43-5 Applying a Moist Cold Compress*

A moist cold compress or the immersion of a body part into a cold soak are forms of therapy used following the sudden onset of acute inflammation or swelling. (Table 43-1). Vasoconstriction resulting from cold application reduces blood flow to the injured part and thus limits fluid accumulation and slows bleeding. The lower temperature also suppresses inflammation and produces a local anesthetic response. When used appropriately, cold applications can significantly lessen pain and immobility by reducing swelling of injured tissues. This is an important distinction for nurses to know when deciding on the choice of heat or cold for acute injuries.

A cold compress usually consists of a gauze dressing or a washcloth and is immersed in iced or chilled solution to achieve the desired temperature. The compress may be sterile or clean; however, a clean compress is most commonly used. Any open wounds require sterile applications. A variety of sizes or thicknesses of gauze can be used depending upon the site of injury. For example, a cold compress to the eye requires a thicker gauze that fits a small area to maintain a cold temperature. Thin gauze works more effectively for larger areas such as the face.

### Purposes

1. Reduce acute local inflammation and edema.
2. Stop localized bleeding.
3. Create local anesthesia.

## *Procedure 43-5*

| Steps | Rationale |
|---|---|
| **Assessment** | |
| 1. Inspect condition of injured or affected part. Gently palpate area. During inspection keep injured part immobilized and in alignment. Movement can cause further injury to strains, sprains, or fractures. | Provides baseline for determining change in condition of injured tissues. |
| 2. Consider time in which injury occurred. | Cold should be applied quickly after an injury. |
| 3. Ask client to describe character of pain. | Provides baseline for determining pain relief with therapy. |
| 4. Assess area to be treated for sensitivity to temperature, light touch, and pain. | Determines if client is insensitive to cold extremes. |
| 5. Review physician's order for location and duration of application. | Physician's order required for all cold applications. |
| 6. Assess client's understanding of procedure. | Determines need for health teaching. |
| **Nursing Diagnosis** | |
| 1. Cluster data to reveal actual or potential nursing diagnoses: | |
| a. Pain: related to muscular sprain or burn. | Musculoskeletal injuries, burns, and insect bites can be very painful. |
| b. Impaired physical mobility: related to skeletal trauma. | Developing edema from injury can severely limit mobility of affected part. |
| c. Impaired skin integrity: related to abrasion. | Traumatic injuries may result in skin excoriation. |
| d. Potential for injury: related to cold exposure. | Prolonged exposure to cold can lead to tissue ischemia. |
| e. Knowledge deficit regarding therapy: related to inexperience. | Nurse should provide instructions during procedure. |
| **Planning** | |
| 1. Develop individualized goals for client based on nursing diagnoses: | |
| a. Promote client's comfort. | Comfort can be gained through anesthetic effect of cold and reduction in edema. |
| b. Reduce extent of tissue injury. | Cold applied quickly after injury can retard edema or bleeding. |
| c. Maintain mobility of affected part. | In certain musculoskeletal injuries damage to ligaments, tendons, or other supportive structures cannot be reversed by cold applications; in minor injuries cold helps to prevent swelling and stiffness. |
| d. Improve client's understanding of therapy. | Clients can benefit from learning about procedure including first aid tips for using cold compresses. |

| Steps | Rationale |
|---|---|
| 2. Prepare following equipment and supplies: | |
| a. Absorbent gauze (clean or sterile) folded to desired size. | Gauze should fit size of area to be covered to prevent exposure of other sensitive areas to cold. |
| b. Clean or sterile basin with ice and water at desired temperature (15° C or 59° F). | |
| c. Bath towel or absorbent pad. | |
| d. Two pair disposable or sterile gloves (according to agency policy). | Controls risk of infection even when clean technique used. |
| e. Bath thermometer. | |
| 3. Explain procedure to client including sensations he will feel; include explanation of importance of applying cold quickly after an injury. | Promotes client's cooperation; compress must be applied for several minutes. |

## Implementation

| Steps | Rationale |
|---|---|
| 1. Wash hands. | Reduces spread of infection. |
| 2. Position client, carefully keeping body part in proper alignment. | In cases of strains, sprains, or fractures extremity or body part should remain aligned to prevent further injury. |
| 3. Close room door or curtain and expose only area to be treated. | Avoid unnecessary exposure of body parts, maintaining client's comfort and privacy. |
| 4. Place towel or absorbent pad under area to be treated. | Prevents soiling of bed linen. |
| 5. Apply disposable gloves. | Reduces spread of infection. |
| 6. Check temperature of solution and submerge gauze into filled basin at bedside; wring out excess moisture. | Extreme temperature can cause tissue damage. Dripping gauze is uncomfortable to client. |
| 7. Apply compress to affected area, molding it gently over site. | Ensures cold is directed over site of injury. |
| 8. Remove gloves and dispose in proper container. | Reduces transfer of microorganisms. |
| 9. Check condition of skin every 5 min for duration of application. | Determines if there are adverse reactions to cold. |
| 10. After 15-20 minutes reapply gloves, remove compress, and gently dry off any moisture. | Drying prevents maceration of skin. Prolonged application of cold can result in diminished blood flow and tissue ischemia. |
| 11. Assist client to comfortable position. | Maintains relaxing environment. |
| 12. Empty basin, dry, and store. Dispose of soiled linen, gloves, and wash hands. | Reduces transfer of microorganisms. |

## Evaluation

| Steps | Rationale |
|---|---|
| 1. Inspect affected area for changes in condition of skin. | Determines reaction to cold compress application. |
| 2. Palpate affected area gently. | Determines level of edema. |
| 3. Question client about level of comfort. | Determines if pain relieved. |
| 4. Ask client how to use cold compress. | Measures level of learning. |

### *Expected outcomes*

| Steps | Rationale |
|---|---|
| 1. Affected area is slightly pale and cool to touch. | Result of vasoconstriction. |
| 2. Extent of edema is decreased. | Cold reduces blood flow to affected part, reducing edema formation. |
| 3. Client experiences less discomfort. | Cold creates local anesthetic effect. |
| 4. Client correctly states how to apply cold compress. | Documents learning. |

### *Unexpected outcomes*

| Steps | Rationale |
|---|---|
| 1. Skin takes on a mottled, reddened, or bluish purple appearance. | Result of prolonged exposure causing tissue ischemia. |
| 2. Client complains of burning type pain and numbness. | Symptoms of ischemia. |

## Recording and Reporting

| Steps | Rationale |
|---|---|
| 1. Record procedure including type, location, and duration of application and client's tolerance of procedure in nurses' notes. | Documents therapy provided and client's response. |
| 2. Report undesirable changes in condition of skin to nurse in charge or physician. | Injury from prolonged exposure will require different therapy. |

## Follow-up Activities

| Steps | Rationale |
|---|---|
| 1. Cold compress may be reapplied at repeated intervals. | Repeated applications control edema. |

### Special Considerations

- If there is prolonged delay in therapy, cold application will not reverse edema formation.
- If area is edematous, sensation may be reduced.
- Numbness and tingling are common sensations.

### Teaching Considerations

- Injuries occur away from health care settings. Clients should know steps to take to minimize extent of injury.

### Home Care Considerations

- Clean cloth can be used in home setting as long as there is not open wound.
- Assess client and primary care giver as to understanding, ability, and motivation to comply with procedure.
- Assess client's home environment for adequacy of facilities with which to implement procedure.

# *SKILL 43-6* Applying an Ice Pack, Bag, or Collar

An ice pack, bag, or collar is a simple way to apply cold to a small, localized area. The applications do not create moisture and thus the client is spared any discomfort from cold solutions running down a body part. Ice bags and packs come in a variety of sizes to fit different body parts (Fig. 43-3). When a person is away from home or a health care setting a plastic bag or glove can serve as an ice bag as long as a towel or cloth is also available to prevent direct exposure of the bag against the person's skin.

Dry cold applications are most useful for clients with muscle sprains, localized hemorrhage, hematomas, or dental surgical repair.

### Purposes

1. Prevent or reduce edema formation
2. Control bleeding (internally or externally)
3. Anesthetize injured body part

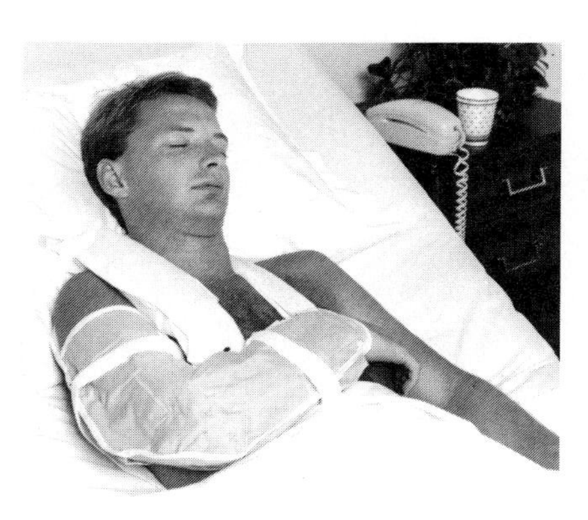

***Fig. 43-3*** Placement of ice pack (or bag) on an extremity.

## *Procedure 43-6*

| Steps | Rationale |
|---|---|
| **Assessment** | |
| 1. Examine condition of injured body part.<br>▪ During inspection keep injured part immobilized and in body alignment. | Provides baseline for determining change in condition of injured tissues. |
| 2. Consider time in which injury occurred. | Cold should be applied quickly after injury to create its therapeutic effects. |
| 3. Assess character of client's pain. | Provides baseline to determine change in client's condition. |
| 4. Assess area to be treated for sensitivity to temperature, light touch, or pain. | Determines if client is insensitive to extreme cold. |
| 5. Review physician's order for type and duration of application. | Physician's order required for cold applications. |
| 6. Assess client's understanding of procedure. | Determines extent of health teaching required. |
| **Nursing Diagnosis** | |
| 1. Cluster data to reveal actual or potential nursing diagnoses: | |
| a. Pain: related to tooth extraction. | Tissue injuries are painful. |
| b. Impaired mobility: related to muscular sprain. | Muscular sprain or strain prohibits person from placing full weight on injured part and can limit range of motion. |

| Steps | Rationale |
|---|---|
| c. Potential for injury: related to cold exposure. | Prolonged exposure can cause tissue ischemia. |
| d. Knowledge deficit: related to therapy. | Client may have no experience with procedure or not understand all precautions. |

## Planning

| Steps | Rationale |
|---|---|
| 1. Develop individualized goals for client based on nursing diagnoses: | |
| a. Promote client's comfort. | Local cold application anesthetizes underlying tissues. |
| b. Reduce extent of tissue injury. | Cold applied quickly after injury can retard edema or bleeding. |
| c. Maintain mobility of affected part. | By reducing edema and stiffness, range of motion of affected part can be preserved. |
| d. Improve client's understanding of therapy. | Will improve client's level of cooperation during procedure and will enable client to apply packs in home setting. |
| 2. Prepare following equipment and supplies: | |
| a. Ice bag or collar: | |
| ▪ Fill bag with water, secure cap and invert. | Checks for leaks. |
| ▪ Empty water, then fill bag two thirds full with small pieces crushed ice. | Bag can more easily be molded over body part. |
| ▪ Release excess air from bag by squeezing its sides before securing cap. | Excess air interferes with cold conduction. |
| ▪ Wipe bag dry of excess moisture. | Prevents skin maceration. |
| b. Ice pack | |
| ▪ Commercial packs are squeezed or kneaded | Releases alcohol-based solution to create cold temperature. |
| c. Towel or pillow case | |
| d. Cloth ties or tape | |
| 3. Explain procedure and its purpose to client. | Understanding of procedure reduces anxiety and enhances compliance. |

## Implementation

| Steps | Rationale |
|---|---|
| 1. Wash hands. | Reduces transmission of microorganisms. |
| 2. Assist client to comfortable position. Move injured part carefully. | Position must be maintained for several minutes. Keep injured parts properly aligned. |
| 3. Close room door or curtain; expose only area to be treated. | Avoids unnecessary exposure of body parts. Maintains client's comfort and privacy. |
| 4. Take prepared bag or pack and place towel or pillowcase over it. | Prevents direct exposure of cold against client's skin. |
| 5. Apply covered bag over area snugly. Secure with ties or tape as needed. | Cold should be directed over site of injury. |
| 6. Lift bag or pack and check condition of skin every 5-10 min. | Monitoring determines if there is adverse response to cold. |
| 7. After 30 min remove from client. | Prolonged exposure may cause tissue injury. |
| 8. Assist client to comfortable position. | Maintains relaxing environment. |
| 9. Empty bags of ice, dispose of used packs and soiled linen in proper receptacle. Wash hands. | Reduces transmission of infection. |

## Evaluation

| Steps | Rationale |
|---|---|
| 1. Examine mobility condition of area treated. | Evaluates effect of cold application. |
| 2. Determine comfort level. | Cold anesthetizes underlying tissues. |
| 3. Observe client apply ice collar. | Measures level of learning. |

### *Expected outcomes*

| Steps | Rationale |
|---|---|
| 1. Affected area is slightly pale and cool to touch. | Vasoconstriction reduces blood flow to affected area. |
| 2. Decreased edema over area. | Reduced blood flow slows edema. |
| 3. Client verbalizes less discomfort. | Tissues are anesthetized. |
| 4. Client safely and properly applies ice collar. | Documents learning. |

### *Unexpected outcomes*

| Steps | Rationale |
|---|---|
| 1. Affected area is reddened or bluish; numbness or burning occur. | Result of overexposure to cold that causes tissue ischemia. |

## Recording and Reporting

| Steps | Rationale |
|---|---|
| 1. Record type, location, and duration of application and client's response in nurses' notes. | Documents care provided and client's response. |

| Steps | Rationale |
|---|---|
| 2. Report any changes in skin condition to nurse in charge or physician. | Further therapy may be required. |

### Follow-up Activities

| | |
|---|---|
| 1. Do not reapply ice pack to reddened or bluish areas. | Continual use of ice pack to overexposed areas worsens ischemia. |
| 2. If skin or tissue remains undamaged ice bag or pack can be reapplied in 30 minutes. | Aids in further reducing edema and pain |

## Special Considerations

- Moisture may form on outside of bag if room temperature is warm. This does not indicate a leak.
- Some commercial packs have soft insulated coverings that can be applied directly.

## Teaching Considerations

- Ice bags are used frequently in home, necessitating safety precautions.

## Home Care Considerations

- Assess client and primary caregiver as to understanding of procedure and ability to implement procedure.
- Assess client for motivation to comply with procedure.
- Assess home environment for facilities compatible with implementation of procedure.

### BIBLIOGRAPHY


Bulau J: Clinical policies and procedures for home health care, Rockville Md, 1986, Aspen Publishers Inc.

DeCrusta T: Relieving pain: four noninvasive ways you should know more about, Nurs Life 4:28, 1984.

Francis B: Hot and cold therapy, J Nurs Care 15:18, 1982.

Golden S: Nursing a loved one at home, Philadelphia, 1988, Running Press.

Quillen WS, et al.: Initial management of acute ankle sprains with rapid pulsed pneumatic compression and cold, J Orthopedic Sports Phys Ther 4:39, Summer 1982.

Simpson CF: Adult arthritis: heat, cold, or both? Am J Nurs 83:270, 1983.

Smith S, Duell D: Clinical nursing skills, 1985, Los Altos, Calif, National Nursing Review.

Walsh J, Persons C, Wieck L: Manual of home health care nursing, Philadelphia, 1987, JB Lippincott Co.

# 44

# WOUND CARE AND IRRIGATIONS

### OBJECTIVES

*Mastery of content in this chapter will enable the nurse to:*

- Define key terms.
- Discuss the body's response during each stage of the wound-healing process.
- Differentiate between primary and secondary intention.
- Explain factors that impair or promote normal wound healing.
- Administer a wound irrigation.
- Remove sutures or staples.
- Demonstrate care of a wound drainage system.

### KEY TERMS

| | |
|---|---|
| *Granulation tissue* | *Primary intention* |
| *Hemostasis* | *Secondary intention* |
| *Irrigation* | *Staples* |

### SKILLS

**44-1** Performing Wound Irrigation
**44-2** Performing Suture and Staple Removal
**44-3** Performing Drainage Evacuation

Proper wound care is necessary to promote an intact skin layer following healing. The integumentary system is the body's first line of defense against invasion by infectious microorganisms. The skin defends the body in other ways by serving as a sensory organ for pain, touch, and temperature.

The integument has two layers: the epidermis and the dermis (Fig. 44-1). The outer layer, epidermis, has two layers. The first layer, the stratum corneum, consists of flattened dead cells. The cells of the stratum corneum originate from the stratum malpighii, the second epidermal layer. Cells of the stratum malpighii divide, multiply,

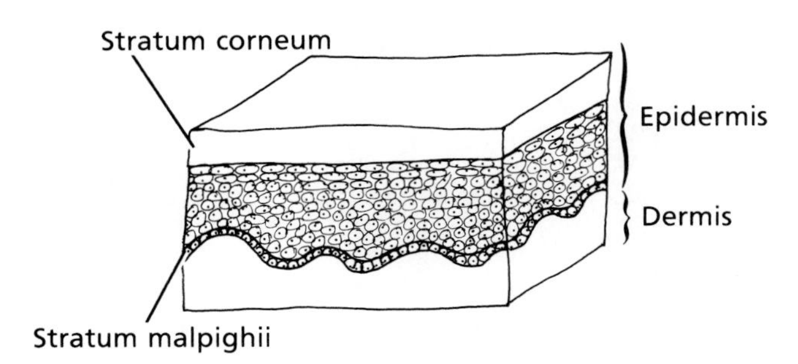


***Fig. 44-1*** Layers of the integument.

and migrate toward the epidermal surface. As they reach the stratum corneum they flatten out and die. These two strata form the epidermis. The thin layer of the stratum corneum prevents dehydration of underlying cells and is a physical barrier to the entry of certain chemicals. The barrier is selective; it does allow absorption of topical medications in paste form. Beneath the epidermis is the dermis. The dermis contains no skin cells. Collagen (a tough fibrous protein layer), blood vessels, and nerves compose the dermal layer. The dermis restores the physical properties of the skin and its structural integrity. Restoration of both the epidermal and dermal layers is necessary to promote healing. Risk of local or systemic infection, impaired circulation, and breakdown of tissue is directly influenced by the ability of the dermal layer to heal (Schummann, 1979; Bonier, 1985).

Physiologically, wound healing occurs in the same way for all clients, with skin cells and some tissues (including the vascular tissues) regenerating quickly and others regenerating slowly or not at all. The latter group includes cells of the liver, renal tubules, and central nervous system neurons (Potter and Perry, 1989).

Wound healing involves a series of physiological processes (see box). These processes can be affected by the location, severity, and extent of the injury. The ability of cells and tissues to regenerate, return to normal structure, or resume normal functioning also affects healing.

Types of healing include healing by primary intention and healing by secondary intention. Healing by primary

### STAGES OF HEALING

**Defensive Stage**

Starts when skin integrity is impaired and continues from 4-6 days.

- Hemostasis—Blood vessels constrict, gathering of platelets stops bleeding. Clots form a fibrin matrix. Scab forms, preventing entry of infectious organisms.
- Inflammatory response—Increases blood flow to wound and vascular permeability to plasma resulting in localized redness and edema.
- White blood cells arrive at wound
  *Neutrophils* ingest bacteria and small debris, then die in a few days and leave enzyme exudate, which either attacks bacteria *or* interferes with tissue repair.
  *Monocytes* become macrophages.
  *Macrophages* clean cell of debris by phagocytosis; aid in wound repair by recycling normal amino acids and sugars.
- Epithelial cells move from wound margins to base of clot or scab (for period of approximately 48 hr).

**Reconstruction Stage**

Closure begins on day 3 or 4 of defensive stage and continues for 2-3 weeks.

- Fibroblasts—Function with help of vitamins B and C; oxygen and amino acids synthesize collagen.
- Collagen—Provides strength and structural integrity to the wound.
- Epithelial cells—Differentiate to duplicate damaged cells (e.g., intestinal mucosal cells acquire their columnar appearance).

**Maturation Stage**

This final healing stage may continue for 1 yr or more as collagen scar strengthens.

intention is expected when the edges of a clean surgical incision remain close together, tissue loss is minimal or absent, the client is not at risk for developing an infection. The skin cells quickly regenerate, capillary walls stretch across under the suture line to form a smooth surface as they join, and inflammation is absent or minimized.

Healing by secondary intention is quite the opposite and accompanies an open wound with tissue loss, jagged edges, and granulation tissue gradually filling in the area of the scar. This process is typical of severe laceration or massive surgical intervention with skin loss. The risk of infection is directly related to the length of time it takes for the body surface to be covered with an intact skin covering. In secondary intention there is some gap between the edges. A thin fibrinous exudate covers the edges of the wound, prevents bacterial invasion, and coagulates surface bleeding. New capillaries are supported by connective tissue. This form of healing results in a thicker surface closure. The slowness of this process places the client at greater risk for infection and collection of body fluids that must be drained to permit healing. Some clients who heal by the secondary intention process may develop an excessive amount of connective tissue in the scar surface. This tissue is known as a *keloid.* Other developments may include the formation of a fistula in response to the presence of bacteria in the wound.

During the healing process a wound may have some type of dressing covering it. The initial dressing is not removed for direct wound inspection until a physician writes a medical order to remove the dressing. Certain situations and some institutional policies govern who changes the dressing the first time. Special attention is paid to maintaining the position of drains during dressing changes. An analgesic, as ordered, should be administered 30-45 min before changing the dressing. However, the nurse's assessment determines the best time for analgesic administration prior to wound care.

Meticulous handwashing and proper infection control procedure before and after removing soiled dressings, coupled with proper irrigation procedures, limit the risk of nosocomial infection. Basic wound cleansing is accomplished by applying antiseptic solutions with sterile gauze or by irrigation. Skin cleansing in the area of the suture line or drain site is indicated when an excessive amount of drainage occurs. The presence of wound exudate is an expected stage of epithelial cell growth.

An irrigation is gentle washing of an area with a stream of solution delivered through an irrigating syringe. This nursing intervention is used for wounds on any part of the torso or extremities. In addition to cleansing an area, prescribed medications may be introduced in solution form. Principles of basic wound irrigation include the following:

1. Cleanse in a direction from the least contaminated area to the most contaminated.
2. When irrigating, all the solution flows from the least contaminated to the most contaminated area.

When administering an irrigation be sure that the flow of irrigation moves from the area being cleansed to an area that is both distal to and lower than that area. In wound care, the area being cleansed is considered "clean" and the surrounding skin surfaces are considered "contaminated" without respect to whether or not the wound is infected. Within the wound, the flow is directed from healthy tissue toward infected tissue.

The suture line is the "least contaminated" area and is always cleansed first (Fig. 44-2). Work in straight lines moving away from the suture line with each successive stroke. Use a sterile gauze 2 × 2 containing antiseptic or an antiseptic swab for each stroke.

The tip of the irrigating syringe is placed above the area being cleansed. This prevents contamination of the

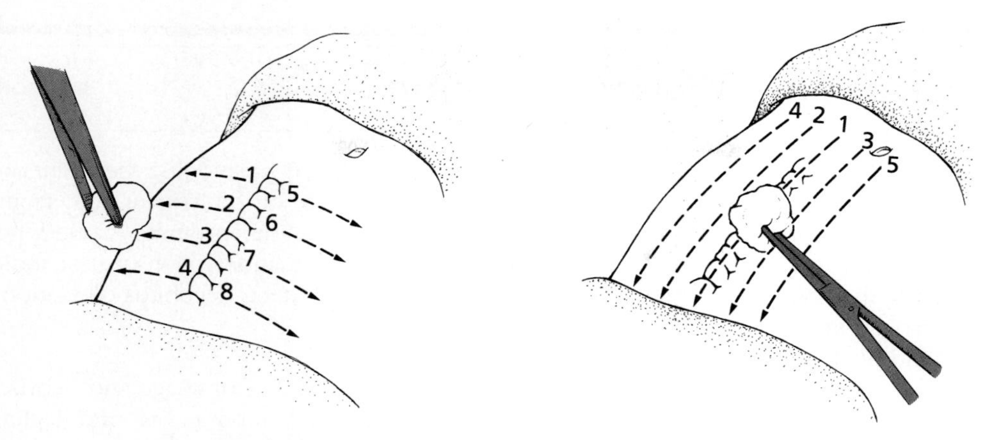


***Fig. 44-2*** Methods of cleansing the suture line area.

syringe. Careful attention to placement of the syringe also prevents unsafe pressure of the flowing solution.

Irrigating solutions are sterile. In the event that the irrigant has caustic or irritating properties, protect the skin with a film of petroleum jelly and place the collection basin close to the area of the exiting fluid.

The drain site is cleansed using a circular stroke starting with the area immediately next to the drain (Fig. 44-3). With each new swab cleanse a little further out from the drain.

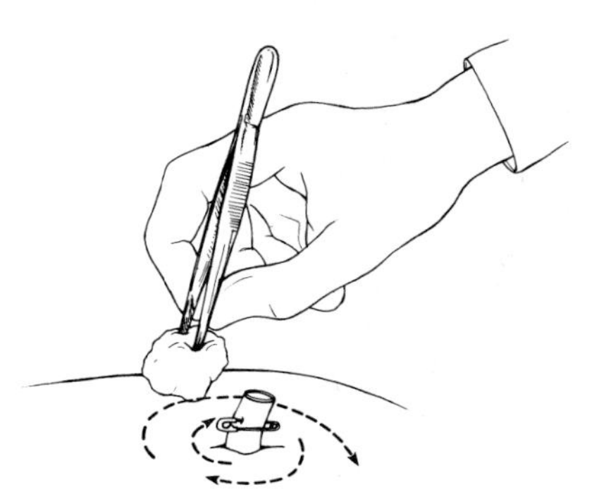

***Fig. 44-3*** Cleansing a drain site.

## GUIDELINES

1. Know the client's age. With age, there are vascular changes, collagen tissue is less pliable, and scar tissue is tighter.
2. Know the client's nutritional status. Tissue repair and infection resistance are directly related to adequate nutrition including proteins, carbohydrates, lipids, vitamins, and minerals. Nutrition requirements can double in the presence of infection.
3. Observe for obesity. Inadequate vascularization decreases delivery of nutrients and cellular elements required for healing. The obese client is at greater risk for wound infection and dehiscence or evisceration.
4. Identify factors that decrease oxygenation, such as decreased hemoglobin and smoking. Small wounds heal more quickly when exposed to air. Tissue repair is negatively influenced by a hematocrit value below 33% and a hemoglobin value below 10 g/100 ml. Hemoglobin is reduced and oxygen release to tissues is reduced in smokers.
5. Know the types of medications prescribed. Steroids reduce inflammatory response and slow collagen synthesis. Cortisone depresses fibroblast activity and capillary growth. Chemotherapy depresses bone marrow function.
6. Identify the presence of chronic diseases or chronic trauma, such as diabetes or radiation. In diabetes tissue perfusion and failure to release oxygen to tissues result from diabetes. Uncontrolled hypoglycemia interferes with phagocytosis of the leukocytes. In radiation therapy, wound healing is most effective when surgery is performed within 4-6 weeks of irradiation before the anticipated vascular scarring and fibrosis.

## PREREQUISITE KNOWLEDGE

1. Medical asepsis and infection control.
2. Surgical asepsis.
3. Principles of wound healing.
4. Complications of wound healing.

## PREREQUISITE SKILLS

1. Hand washing (Chapter 37).
2. Open gloving (Chapter 38).
3. Surgical asepsis (Chapter 38).
4. Physical assessment (Chapter 13).
5. Changing sterile dressings (Chapter 41).

## *SKILL 44-1 Performing Wound Irrigation*

Open wound irrigation requires sterile technique. Fluid is introduced directly into the wound with the tip of the syringe remaining 2.5 cm (1 in) above the wound. If the client has a deep wound with a narrow opening, a soft catheter is attached to the syringe to permit the fluid to enter the wound. Irrigation must be done gently to prevent tissue injury and avoid discomfort. Fluid retention is avoided by positioning the client on his side to encourage the flow of the irrigant away from the wound.

Wound irrigations promote wound healing in some postoperative situations. Nonsurgical indications include management of deep decubitus ulceration.

### Purposes

1. Cleanse wound of drainage and debris.
2. Promote granulation and wound healing.

## *Procedure 44-1*

| Steps | Rationale |
|---|---|
| **Assessment** | |
| 1. Review client's medical record for presence of physician's prescription for irrigation of open wound and type of solution to be used. | Open wound irrigation requires medical order including type of solution(s) to use. |
| 2. Assess recent recording of signs and symptoms related to client's open wound: | Data used as baseline to indicate change in condition of wound. |
| a. Extent of impairment of skin integrity. | |
| b. Elevation of body temperature. | May indicate response to infection. |
| c. Drainage from wound (amount, color). | Expect amount to decrease as healing takes place; serous drainage is clear; bright red drainage indicates fresh bleeding; purulent drainage is thick and yellow, pale green, or white. |
| d. Odor. | Strong odor indicates infectious process. |
| e. Consistency of drainage. | Leukocytes produce thick drainage. |
| f. Size of wound. Measure depth, length, and width. | Assesses client's stage of healing. |
| 3. Inspect dressing: dry and clean; evidence of bleeding, profuse drainage. | Provides an initial assessment of present wound drainage. |
| 4. Assess comfort level or pain. | Discomfort may be related directly to wound or indirectly to muscle tension, immobility. |
| 5. Identify symptoms of anxiety. | Anxiety results from multiple factors concerning surgery including diagnosis, awaiting pathology reports, anticipation of unknown nursing interventions (e.g., first wound irrigation). |
| 6. Identify client's history of allergies. | Known allergies suggest application of a sample of prescribed antiseptic as skin test before flushing wound with large volume of solution. |
| **Nursing Diagnosis** | |
| 1. Cluster data to reveal actual or potential nursing diagnoses: | |
| a. Impaired skin integrity: related to wound infection, dehiscence, wound drainage, evisceration. | Wound infection, evisceration, and extensive drainage may extend area of wound. |
| b. Potential for injury to soft tissues: related to surgical incision. | Soft tissues of open wound are at a slower level of healing and are subject to multiple sources of trauma including sinus and fistula formation. |
| c. Pain: related to surgical incision. | Presence of tubes (intravenous [IV], drain, nasogastric [NG] tube), tension in operative site, and infection limit comfort. |
| **Planning** | |
| 1. Develop individualized goals for client based on nursing diagnoses: | Irrigation cleans a wound to reduce inflammation and infection and to promote healing. |
| a. Promote wound healing. | |
| b. Prevent soft tissue injury. | |
| c. Reduce pain. | |
| 2. Gather equipment at bedside: | |
| a. Sterile basin | To hold sterile irrigation solution in preparation for irrigation. |

| Steps | Rationale |
|---|---|
| b. 150-500 ml prescribed irrigating solution warmed to body temperature | Maintain solution sterility during warming process. Warming adds to client comfort level. |
| c. Sterile irrigation syringe, sterile soft catheter, if needed | To prevent introduction of additional pathogens during procedure; soft catheter is used to irrigate deep wounds with small openings. |
| d. Clean basin | Basin collects contaminated irrigating solution. |
| e. Clean gloves (check policy of institution) | Gloves will protect nurse from infection while removing wound dressing. |
| f. Sterile gloves | To maintain asepsis during irrigation and redressing procedures. |
| g. Waterproof under-pad | Prevents soiling of bed linen; is both cost and time effective. |
| h. Sterile dressing tray and supplies for dressing change including packing, if ordered | Prevents infection and promotes wound healing. |
| i. Leakproof refuse bag | Used to gather soiled and contaminated dressings and prevent cross-infection. |
| j. Gown (optional) | Protects nurse's uniform from contamination. |
| k. Goggles | Body secretions can splash into nurse's eyes and increase risk of transmission of microorganisms. |
| 3. Explain procedure of wound irrigation. | Providing necessary information will reduce client anxiety. |
| 4. Administer prescribed analgesic 30-45 min before starting wound irrigation procedure. | Increased comfort level will permit client to move more easily and be positioned to facilitate wound irrigation. |
| 5. Position client comfortably to permit gravitation of flow of irrigating solution through wound and into collection basin (Fig. 44-4). Position client so that wound is vertical to collection basin. | Directing solution from top to bottom of wound and from clean area to contaminated will prevent further infection. Positioning client during planning stage provides bed surfaces for later preparation of equipment. |
| 6. Warm sterile irrigating solution to approximate body temperature. | Warmed solution increases comfort and reduces vascular constriction response in tissues. |

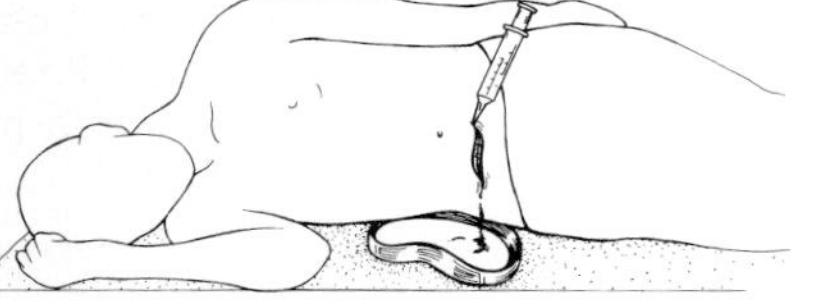

*Fig. 44-4*

## Implementation

| Steps | Rationale |
|---|---|
| 1. Form cuff on leakproof refuse bag and place it near bed. | Cuffing helps to maintain large opening, thereby permitting placement of contaminated dressing without touching refuse bag itself. |
| 2. Close room door or bed curtains. | Maintains privacy. |
| 3. Place waterproof underpad on bed surface in front of wound. | Protection of bedding eliminates need to change linens. |
| 4. Place clean basin directly under wound. | Collects contaminated irrigating solution. |
| 5. Wash hands. | Hand washing is integral to prevention of infection. |
| 6. If gown is needed, put it on now. | Protects nurse's clothing and prevents cross-infection. |
| 7. Prepare sterile field using sterile dressing set and supplies. | Maintaining sterile field reduces risk of introducing microorganisms into wound. |
| 8. Add sterile basin and pour in estimated volume of warm sterile irrigating solution and set irrigating syringe in basin with solution. | Prepares solution for wound irrigation. |
| 9. Place several strips of adhesive tape within reach and *not* on sterile field. | Provides easy access to tape for securing dressing. |
| 10. Put on clean gloves and remove soiled dressing and discard in leakproof refuse bag. | Reduces transmission of microorganisms. |
| 11. Remove and discard gloves. | |
| 12. Inspect wound and make mental note of wound size, healing process, inflammation, presence of drainage or purulent matter. | Making mental note of findings will facilitate documentation of progress in wound healing and treatment response. |
| 13. Put on sterile gloves. | |
| 14. To irrigate wound with wide opening: | Flushing wound will aid in removal of debris and facilitate healing by secondary intention. |
| a. Fill syringe with irrigating solution. | |
| b. Hold syringe tip 2.5 cm (1 in) above upper end of wound. | Prevents trauma to granulation tissue from syringe. Sterile tip can be reimmersed into basin. |
| c. Using slow, continuous pressure, flush wound; repeat Steps 14 a, b, and c until solution draining into basin is clear. | Ensures removal of all debris. |

| Steps | Rationale |
|---|---|
| 15. To irrigate deep wound with very small opening: | |
| a. Attach soft catheter to filled irrigating syringe. | Catheter permits direct flow of irrigant into wound. Expect wound to take longer to empty when opening is small. |
| b. Lubricate tip of syringe with irrigating solution; then gently insert tip of catheter and pull out about 1.2 cm (½ in) to remove tip from fragile inner wall of wound. | |
| c. Using slow, continuous pressure, flush wound; repeat Steps 15 a, b, and c until solution draining into basin is clear. | Ensures removal of debris without traumatizing new granulation tissue. |
| d. Pinch off catheter just below syringe. | To avoid contamination of sterile solution or basin. |
| e. Fill syringe and reattach to catheter; repeat process until return is clear. | |
| 16. Dry wound edges with sterile gauze. | Prevents maceration of surrounding tissue from excess moisture. |
| 17. Apply sterile dressing. | Maintains sterile protective barrier over wound. |
| 18. Remove gloves. | To facilitate handling of adhesive tape. |
| 19. Secure dressing with adhesive tape. | |
| 20. Assist client to comfortable position. | |
| 21. Dispose of equipment and refuse; retain remaining bottle of sterile solution. | Prevents cross infection. Sterile solution can be used for subsequent irrigations. |
| 22. Wash hands. | Reduces transmission of microorganisms. |

## Evaluation

| | |
|---|---|
| 1. Inspect dressing periodically. | Determines client's response to wound irrigation and need to modify plan of care. |
| 2. Evaluate skin integrity. | Determines if extension of wound has occurred. |
| 3. Observe client for signs of discomfort. | Client's pain should not increase as a result of wound irrigation. |
| 4. Observe for presence of retained irrigant. | Retained irrigant is a medium for bacterial growth and subsequent infection. |

### *Expected outcomes*

| | |
|---|---|
| 1. Client is comfortable following wound irrigation. | Premedication, gently administered irrigation, application of clean dressing, and repositioning client are designed to ensure comfort. |
| 2. Wound begins to heal: dressing clean, dry; wound free of drainage and inflammation. | Healing progresses in absence of debris and presence of protective covering. |
| 3. Skin integrity is maintained. | No further skin and tissue damage has resulted from wound irrigation. |

### *Unexpected outcomes*

| | |
|---|---|
| 1. Bleeding or serosanguinous drainage appears. | Client has increased vulnerability to hemorrhage based on fragility of capillaries, cellular nutrition, and infectious process. |
| 2. Retained fluid and debris appears. | Client is at risk for fistulization. |
| 3. Increased pain or discomfort occurs. | May indicate further wound trauma. |
| 4. Suture line opening extends. | Risk for dehiscence. |

## Recording and Reporting

| | |
|---|---|
| 1. Immediately report any evidence of fresh bleeding, sharp increase in pain, retention of irrigant, or signs of shock to attending physician. | These are presenting signs of tissue damage and fistula or sinus tract development. Shock phenomena may indicate internal bleeding or tissue damage. |
| 2. At change of shift report expected and unexpected outcomes that have actually occurred. | Continuity of care is facilitated by accurately reporting findings. |
| 3. Record wound irrigation and client response on progress notes. | Recording fulfills legal responsibility of nurse and provides information needed to ensure continuity of care. |

## Special Considerations

- Some institutional procedures include use of irrigating solutions when physician does not prescribe specific irrigant.
- Carefully and gently administer treatment, avoiding touching areas with friable capillary structure.
- Plan wound irrigation at time that permits physician and nurse to inspect wound simultaneously. This reduces number of dressing changes, limiting exposure to pathogens.

### Teaching Considerations

- Instruct primary care giver to observe procedure to be followed and then allow for repeated return demonstrations.
- Explain rationale for steps in wound irrigation and supplies/equipment being used.
- Instruct primary care giver in how to maintain sterile technique.
- Instruct primary care giver to assess for signs and symptoms of complications/wound infection to wound site.
- Instruct client to wear loose fitting clothes and to keep wound dry and covered.

### Home Care Considerations

- Assess client and primary care giver as to understanding of wound care.
- Assess client and primary care giver as to ability and willingness to comply with procedures related to wound care and irrigations.
- Assess client's home environment to determine adequacy of facilities for performing wound care, check especially for adequate lighting and running water.

## *SKILL 44-2 Performing Suture and Staple Removal*

Institutional policy determines whether *only* the physician or the physician *and* nurse may remove sutures and staples. The physician's written order is always obtained before implementing either skill. The time of removal is based on the stage of incisional healing and extent of surgery.

Sutures and staples are generally removed within 7-10 days following surgery if healing is adequate. Timing the removal of sutures and staples is important. They are left in long enough to assure initial wound closure with enough strength to support internal tissues and organs. Leaving them in too long increases the risk of infection. The physician determines and orders removal of all sutures or staples at one time or removal of every other suture or staple as the first phase, with the remainder removed in the second phase.

Sutures are threads of wire or other materials used to sew body tissues together. Sutures are placed within tissue layers in deep wounds and superficially as the final means for wound closure. The deeper sutures are usually an absorbable material that disappears in several days.

Staples are made of stainless steel wire. Their use is restricted by the location of the incision, because there must be adequate distance between the skin and structures that lie below the skin, including bone and vascular structures. The cosmetic result may not be as desirable as that obtained with finer suture material. Staples do provide ample strength. Removal requires a sterile staple extractor and maintenance of aseptic technique.

The client's history of wound healing, site of wound, tissues involved, and the purpose of the sutures determine the suture material selected. For example, a client with repeated abdominal surgeries might require wire sutures for greater strength to promote wound closure.

The nurse judges whether to remove all sutures if any sign of suture line separation is evident during the process of suture or staple removal.

### Purposes

1. Promote complete wound healing
2. Prevent infection

## *Procedure 44-2*

| Steps | Rationale |
|---|---|
| **Assessment** | |
| 1. Identify client with need for suture or staple removal: physician's order is written seventh to tenth postoperative day. | Removal of sutures or staples is dependent intervention. Adequate healing should have taken place within this time frame. |
| 2. Inspect skin integrity of suture line for uniform closure of wound edges, normal color, absence of drainage and inflammation. | These indicate adequate wound-healing progression for support of internal structures without continued assistance of sutures or staples. |
| 3. Review client's chart for: | |
| a. Specific directions related to suture or staple removal. | Indicates specifically which sutures are to be removed. |
| b. History of allergies. | Determines if client is sensitive to antiseptic. |
| c. History of conditions that may interfere with healing. | Preexisting health disorders affect speed of healing, resulting in dehiscence. |
| ▪ Conditions that place client at risk for impaired healing (partial listing): advanced age, cardiovascular disease, diabetes, immunosuppression, radiation, obesity, smoking, poor cellular nutrition, very deep wounds, infection. | |

| Skill | Rationale |
|---|---|
| 4. Identify client's needs for information and reassurance. | Anxiety level may rise in relation to new procedure, fear of pain, fear of wound opening and result of removing sutures or staples. If aseptic dressing technique will continue, client or significant other will need further instruction. |

## Nursing Diagnosis

| Skill | Rationale |
|---|---|
| 1. Cluster data to reveal actual or potential nursing diagnoses: | |
| a. Potential for infection: related to incisional wound. | Presence of sutures and staples creates portal of entry for microorganisms at each end of each suture. |
| b. Potential impaired skin integrity: related to wound healing complications. | Clients are at risk for dehiscence and evisceration during sixth to eighth postoperative day. |
| c. Pain: related to suture removal. | Some clients experience discomfort during removal of sutures or staples. Pausing momentarily will usually permit completing this skill. |
| d. Decreased activity tolerance: related to fear of wound dehiscence. | Client needs to know that there will be minimal or no reduction of strength of suture line related to this intervention. Anxiety will be reduced. |

## Planning

| Skill | Rationale |
|---|---|
| 1. Develop individualized goals for client based on nursing diagnoses: | |
| a. Avoid injury to surrounding tissue. | Correct suture or staple removal avoids injury and discomfort to surrounding tissues. |
| b. Minimize discomfort. | |
| 2. Prepare following equipment: | |
| a. Leakproof refuse disposal bag with top turned down to form cuff. | Reduces risk of cross-infections. Cuff helps hold bag open during procedure and enables full closure over contaminated materials. |
| b. Sterile suture removal set (forceps and scissors) or sterile staple extractor. | |
| c. Sterile applicators or antiseptic swabs. | For cleansing suture line. |
| d. Sterile dressing change set. | Provides sterile field as well as supplies for dressing change. |
| e. Sterile basin for antiseptic solution or impregnated swabs. | Cleansing sutures with cotton-tipped applicators is more effective than using gauze. |
| ▪ This promotes healing and is cost-effective. Povidone-iodine is an effective antiseptic and may be in prepared swabs. Note allergies before using any antiseptic. | |
| f. Butterfly adhesive strips | Reduces amount of tension on suture line. |
| 3. Ensure direct lighting on suture line. | Aids visibility and correct placement of tools during removal process, ultimately reducing soft tissue injury. |
| 4. Explain procedure. | Gains client cooperation and alleviates anxiety. |

## Implementation

| Skill | Rationale |
|---|---|
| 1. Wash hands. | Reduces risk of infection. |
| 2. Close curtains or room door. | Provides privacy. |
| 3. Position client. | Prepares area for staple or suture removal. |
| 4. Place cuffed refuse disposal bag within easy reach. | Provides for easy disposal of contaminated dressings and prevents need to pass anything over sterile work area. |
| 5. Prepare sterile field with dressing change supplies. | Maintain asepsis throughout preparation of fields and implementation of suture or staple removal. |
| a. Open sterile suture removal tray or staple extract tray and slide contents onto prepared field maintaining sterility of inside surface of wrapper or tray. | |
| b. Open sterile antiseptic swabs and place on inside surface of tray. | |
| c. Open sterile glove package, exposing cuffed ends. | |
| 6. Don clean gloves and remove dressing. | |
| 7. Discard dressing and clean gloves in prepared refuse disposal bag. | Prevents transmission of infection. |
| 8. Inspect wound (Fig. 44-5, *A*). | Determines adequacy of wound healing. |
| 9. Don sterile gloves. | Allows nurse to handle sterile supplies. |

| **Steps** | **Rationale** |
|---|---|

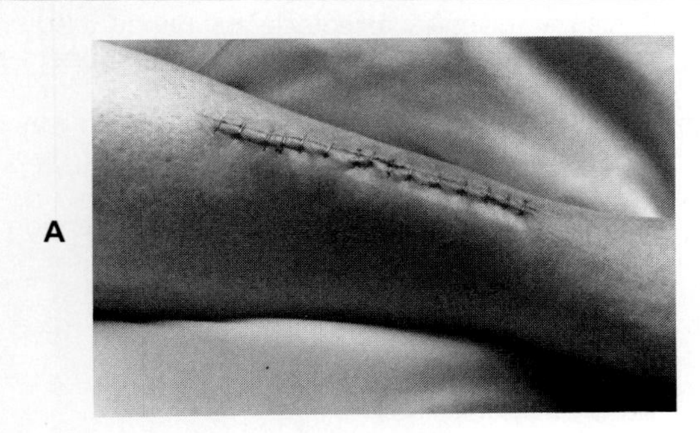


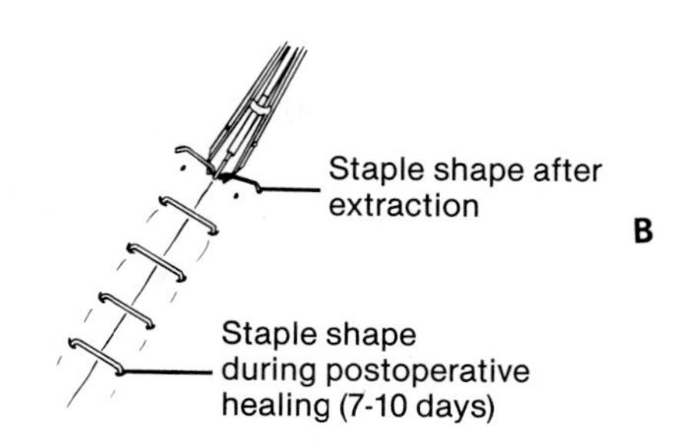


***Fig. 44-5***

10. Cleanse sutures or staples and healed incision with antiseptic swabs. — Removes surface bacteria from incision and sutures or staples.
11. Remove staples.
    a. Place lower tips of staple extractor under 1st staple. As you close handles, upper tip of extractor will depress center of staple, causing both ends of staple to be bent upward and simultaneously exit their insertion sites in the dermal layer (Fig. 44-5, *B*). — Avoids excess pressure to suture line and secures smooth removal of each staple.
    b. Carefully control staple extractor. — Avoids suture-line pressure and pain.
    c. As soon as both ends of staple are visible, move it away from skin surface and continue on until your hand is over refuse bag. — Prevent scratching tender skin surface with sharp pointed ends of staple for comfort and infection control.
    d. Release handles of staple extractor, allowing staple to drop into refuse bag. — This will avoid contaminating sterile field with used staples.
    e. Repeat Steps a-c until all staples are removed.
12. Remove intermittent sutures* (Fig. 44-6, *A*).

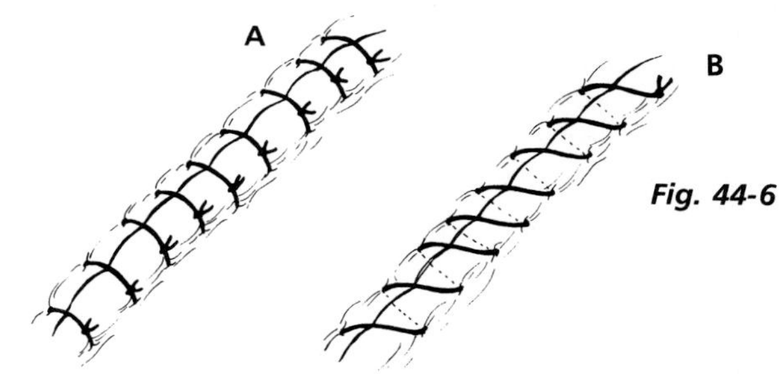


***Fig. 44-6***

    a. Place sterile gauze compress few inches from suture line. Grasp scissor in dominant hand and forceps in nondominant hand. — Sterile gauze serves as receptacle for removed sutures. Placement of scissors and forceps allows for efficient suture removal.
    b. Snip suture, close to skin surface, at end distal to knot. Be sure ends are completely severed by gently lifting exposed end away from skin. — Releases suture. *Never* snip both ends of suture; there will be no way to remove half of suture situated below surface.
    c. Grasp knotted end with forceps and in one continuous smooth action remove entire suture. Place suture on gauze compress. — Smoothly removes suture without additional tension to suture line. Exposed surface of any suture is considered contaminated and is never pulled into tissue below epidermis.
    d. Repeat Steps a-c until you have removed every other suture.
    e. Observe healing level. Based on observations of wound response to suture removal and physician's original order, determine whether or not you will remove remaining sutures at this time. If affirmative, repeat Steps a-d until all sutures have been removed. — Determines status of wound healing and if suture line will remain closed after all sutures are removed.
13. Remove continuous sutures† (Fig. 44-6, *B,* and Fig. 44-7).

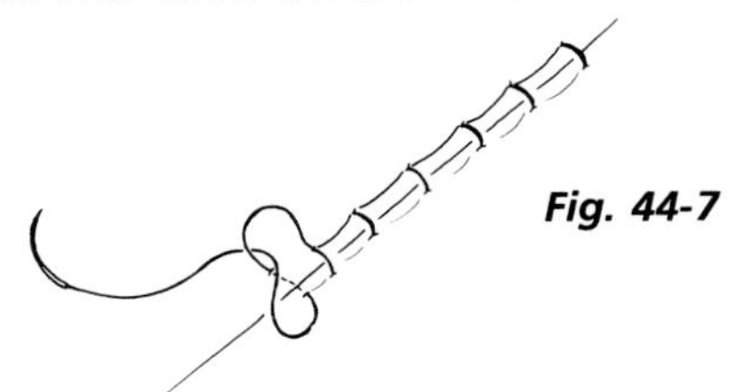

***Fig. 44-7***

*Each suture has a knot. Each interrupted suture is secured with its own knot. Knots are lined up on same side of incision.
†Including blanket stitch sutures.

| Steps | Rationale |
|---|---|
| a. Place sterile gauze compress a few inches from suture line. Grasp scissors in dominant hand and forceps in nondominant hand. | Sterile gauze serves as receptacle for removed sutures. Placement of scissors and forceps allows for efficient suture removal. |
| b. Snip first suture close to skin surface at end distal to knot. | Never snip both ends of suture; there will be no way to remove half of suture situated below surface. |
| c. Snip second "suture" on same side. | Releases interrupted sutures from knot. |
| d. Grasp knotted end and remove first line of spiral in continuous smooth action, pulling away from severed end. Place "suture" on gauze compress. | Smoothly remove sutures without additional tension to suture line. |
| e. Repeat Steps a-d in consecutive order until the entire line has been removed. | |
| 14. Inspect incision site and identify any trouble areas. If *any* separation is apparent, place supportive butterfly closures across area to maintain contact between wound edges. | Reduce risk of further incision line separation. |
| Gently wipe suture line with antiseptic swab. | To remove debris and cleanse wound. |
| 15. Apply light dressing or expose to air if no clothing will come in contact with suture line. Discard gloves. Instruct client about applying own dressing if it will be needed at home. | Healing by primary intention eliminates need for dressing. |
| 16. Note number of sutures or staples removed. | To permit documentation on client's progress note. |
| 17. Route reusable items such as staple extractor for resterilization. | To prevent cross-infections. |
| 18. Wash hands. | Reduces transmission of infection. |

## Evaluation

| | |
|---|---|
| 1. Assess site where sutures or staples were removed; inspect condition of soft tissues, including skin. | Sources of infection have been removed. |
| 2. Determine if client has pain along incision. | Determines comfort level. Can indicate if suture material remains in skin. |

### *Expected outcomes*

| | |
|---|---|
| 1. Sutures or staples have been removed. | Removes source of infection from retained sutures. |
| 2. Client is no longer restricted by bulky dressings or transient moments of incisional discomfort. | Wound is dry and intact and does not require protective dressings. |

### *Unexpected outcomes*

| | |
|---|---|
| 1. Retained suture. | On rare occasions suture may become obscured or imbedded so deeply in clotted scab formation that it is not recognized. This multiplies risk of infection. |
| 2. Wound separation secondary to healing problems. | Predisposition to wound healing problems include: diabetes; immunosuppression; radiation; wound stress; age; cellular nutrition; obesity; smoking; tissue oxygenation; depth of wound. |

## Recording and Reporting

| | |
|---|---|
| 1. Notify physician immediately of any of following findings: suture line separation; dehiscence; evisceration; bleeding; purulent drainage. | Facilitates rapid response and intervention. |
| 2. Record number of sutures or staples removed and condition of suture line. | Documents number of staples or sutures removed and status of wound healing. |
| 3. Report time sutures were removed, level of healing of wound and client's response to suture removal. | Notifies all personnel of procedure and status of wound healing. |

## Follow-up Activities

| | |
|---|---|
| 1. Discard all trash contaminated materials. | Prevent cross-infection. |
| 2. Inspect incision site every shift and PRN if client identifies change in sensation. | Assure desired healing response and deters complications early. |

### Special Considerations

- Skin testing may be advisable before use of antiseptic swabs at wound site.
- Limit amount of dressing supplies since either a very light dressing or no dressing will be needed after suture/staple removal.
- Inadequate wound healing justifies discontinuing removal of all staples. Notify physician immediately.
- If there is much tension on healing incision or if client is at risk for slow healing rate, consider removing two end sutures and every other suture as you move toward center of incision.
- Continuous suture has one knot at each end of entire incision. One long "thread" spirals around entire line at evenly spaced intervals. Surface appearance will be very similar to line of interrupted sutures, except that each section crossing incision line does not have knot (see p. 919).
- Another type of continuous stitch is "blanket continuous suture." This spirals along incision with each turn pulled over to one side. Thread is looped around thread of previous stitch before making the next turn in spiral (see p. 919).
- Dehiscence is partial or total separation of wound layers; evisceration involves protrusion of visceral organs through wound opening; it is the most serious of related emergencies because blood supply to tissues is compromised when organs protrude. Organs must be kept moist by applying sterile towels that have been saturated in warm sterile saline until surgical intervention is arranged.

### Teaching Considerations

- Teach client to observe for any sign of separation of wound edges before removing remaining sutures.
- Have client apply own dressing and inspect suture line for continued healing. Continue instruction on resumption of showering activities, prevention of abdominal strain during defecation, and provision of adequate nutrition and ambulation. Explain gradual suture line changes from red to natural color. Client with abdominal surgery or injury will need to avoid lifting heavy packages or equipment for several weeks.
- Nursing instructions should correlate with physician's orders and discharge plans.
- Instruct primary care giver and client to maintain clean technique when treating suture line and changing dressings.

## SKILL 44-3 Performing Drainage Evacuation

A wound heals only if drainage does not accumulate in the wound bed. Removal of even small amounts of drainage is accomplished by either a closed or open drain system. The drain may be inserted directly through the suture line into the wound or through a small stab-wound near the suture line into the wound.

An open drain system (for example, a Penrose drain [Fig. 44-8]) removes drainage from the wound and deposits it onto the skin surface. A safety pin is inserted through this drain, outside the skin, to prevent the tubing from moving into the wound.

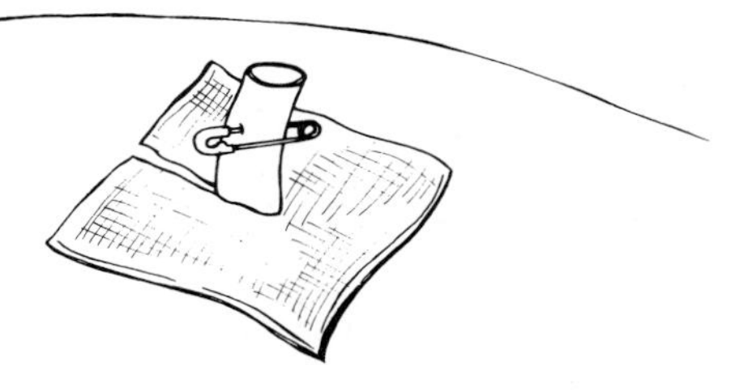

*Fig. 44-8* Penrose drain.

To remove the Penrose drain the physician advances the tubing in stages as the wound heals from the bottom up. Nursing interventions include caution to prevent inadvertent removal of the drain during dressing changes and to protect skin surfaces in direct contact with the irritating drainage.

A closed drain system (e.g., the Jackson-Pratt [Fig. 44-9], Hemovac [Fig. 44-10], VacuDrain, or Constavac) relies on the presence of a vacuum to withdraw accumulated drainage through multiple perforations in clear plastic tubing into the closed reservoir, suction bladder, or bag. The closed system ensures dry skin but only operates if the tubing is clear and a vacuum exists. Drainage is emptied periodically from the reservoir, and the vacuum is rees-

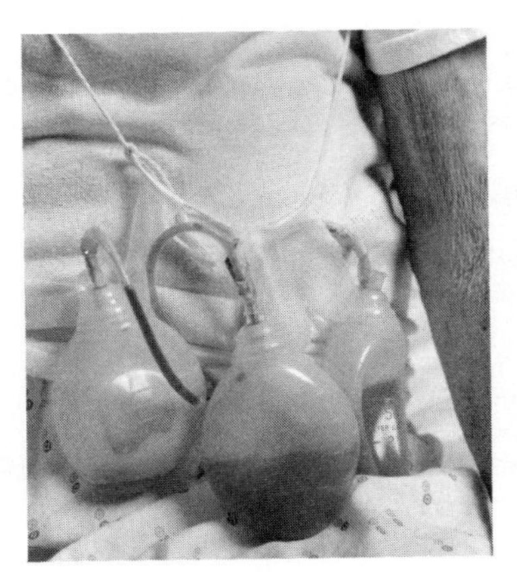

*Fig. 44-9* Jackson-Pratt wound drainage system.

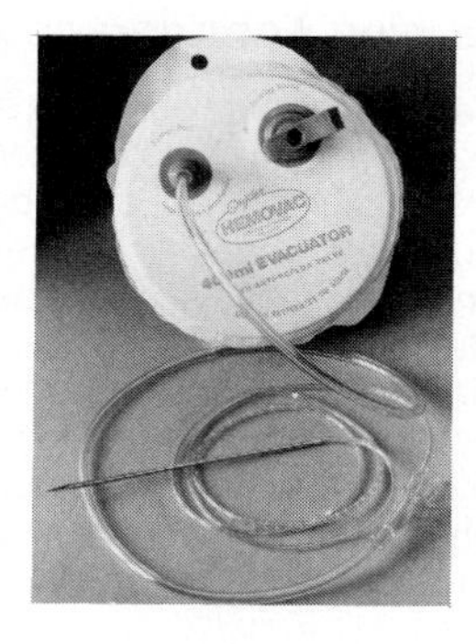


***Fig. 44-10*** Hemovac wound drainage system.

tablished by compressing the reservoir. The Constavac operates with a lightweight, battery-operated pump unit. Instead of emptying and measuring the drainage, the reservoir is discarded when full and replaced with a new reservoir. This system provides a constant vacuum and flow of drainage from the wound. The battery lasts 24 hr and is easily recharged. The Hemovac and Constavac systems both have 400 ml reservoirs. The latter has "air leak" and "no flow" indicators. It is designed to minimize occlusion of the tubing by maintaining a continuous flow of drainage. With all systems, the tubing is introduced into the client's wound by the physician and is generally sutured to the skin to avoid inadvertent removal.

The drains may be connected to portable or wall suction units with suction pressure on "low" unless otherwise ordered by physician's prescription. With all drainage evacuators nursing interventions include wound care around the insertion site of the tubing, emptying or changing the drainage collection apparatus, and being aware of the need for patent tubing. Drainage evacuation continues either until clots and debris block the tubing or until there is no more accumulation of drainage. The nurse prevents wound infection by maintaining sterile technique whenever openings to the fluid reservoirs (or "ports") are opened and by keeping the insertion site clean and covered with a sterile dressing. When the tubing is removed from the client, it is important to remember that it is held in place with a suture. Removal of the suture precedes removal of the tubing. Be aware that the suture may be obscured or imbedded in the clot formation but *must* be removed first.

A client may have more than one drain inserted. If a chest drain and wound drain are in place, mark the chest drain(s) with a "CHEST DRAIN—DO NOT REMOVE" sign on a strip of adhesive secured around that tubing. Chest drains are never removed or disconnected from the suction source by the nurse (Chapter 17). Wound drainage tubes may or may not be removed by the nurse in accordance with institutional policy. This is generally a physician's intervention.

Use of a drainage evacuator promotes healing within the wound. If drainage at the major suture line is minimized, the frequency of dressing changes is reduced. If the number of dressing changes is reduced, the client is at less risk for the development of a nosocomial infection.

### Purposes

1. Remove drainage from a surgical wound.
2. Promote wound healing.

## *Procedure 44-3*

| **Steps** | **Rationale** |
|---|---|
| **Assessment** | |
| 1. Identify presence of closed wound drain and drainage system as client returns from surgery. | Drainage tubing is placed within wound through small surgical incision near major wound. |
| 2. Inspect system to determine presence of one straight tube or Y-tube arrangement with two tube insertion sites. | To plan skin care and identify quantity of sterile dressing supplies. |
| 3. Inspect system to assure proper functioning, including: drainage moving through tubing in direction of reservoir (tubing patent), airtight connection sites. | Properly functioning system maintains suction until: reservoir is filled; drainage is no longer being produced or accumulated. |
| 4. Place and secure drainage reservoirs to prevent any pull on tubing insertion sites. | Tension on drainage tubing increases injury to skin and underlying muscle. |
| **Nursing Diagnosis** | |
| 1. Cluster data to reveal actual or potential nursing diagnoses: | |
| a. Potential for injury: related to impaired wound healing. | Epithelialization and formation of collagen take place in clean, well-drained wound site. Presence of retained debris and drainage in wound retards wound healing. |
| b. Potential for infection: related to retained wound drainage and drain site. | Presence of tubing through skin opening immediately places client at risk for hospital-acquired (nosocomial) infection. |
| c. Pain: related to wound drainage and incisional wound. | Tenderness and discomfort accompany inflammatory phase of healing process. Sutured wound and trauma that accompanied surgical procedure cause varying levels of pain or discomfort. |

| Steps | Rationale |
|---|---|
| **Planning** | |
| 1. Develop individualized goals for client based on nursing diagnoses: | |
| a. Aseptically remove drainage from evacuator. | Strict asepsis is required for removal of drainage. |
| b. Maintain drainage tube patency. | Patency of drainage tubes promotes evacuation of secretion and debris from wound. |
| c. Promote comfort. | Wounds free of secretions and debris are less painful. |
| 2. Prepare following equipment: | |
| a. Measuring graduate cylinder<br>b. Sterile alcohol<br>c. Sponges<br>d. Sterile specimen container | To measure drainage and maintain sterility at "port" containers. For culture specimen. |
| e. Sterile dressing supplies if care of sutured drain site is indicated (q 24 hr or according to institutional policy).<br>f. Gloves | For wound inspection and preventive intervention. |
| 3. Explain procedure to client. | Promotes client's cooperation. |
| **Implementation** | |
| 1. Close room door or bedside curtains. | Provides privacy. |
| 2. Wash hands and don gloves. | Reduces transmission of blood-borne microorganisms. |
| 3. Place open sterile laboratory specimen container or measuring graduate on bed between you and client. | Permits measuring and discarding of wound drainage. |
| 4. When emptying evacuator, maintain asepsis while opening port. | This will avoid entry of pathogens. |
| a. Hemovac (see Fig. 44-10) | |
| ▪ Open plug on port indicated for emptying drainage reservoir. | Vacuum will be broken and reservoir will pull air in until chamber is fully expanded. |
| ▪ Tilt evacuator in direction of plug.<br>▪ Slowly squeeze two flat surfaces together while draining into sterile laboratory specimen container and remainder into graduated cylinder. Cover specimen container. | Prevents splashing of contaminated drainage. |
| ▪ Hold uncovered alcohol sponge in dominant hand, place evacuator on flat surface with open outlet facing upward; continue pressing downward until bottom and top are in contact; hold surfaces together with one hand, quickly cleanse opening and plug with other hand, and immediately replace plug; secure evacuator on client's bed. | Compression of surface of Hemovac creates vacuum.<br>Cleansing of plug reduces transmission of microorganisms into drainage evacuation. |
| ▪ Check evacuator for reestablishment of vacuum; patency of drainage tubing; absence of stress on tubing. | Facilitates wound drainage and prevents tension on drainage tubing. |
| b. Jackson-Pratt Evacuator (Fig. 44-9): | |
| ▪ Open emptying port on opposite side of bulb-shaped reservoir.<br>▪ Compress bulb over drainage container. | Empties drainage and reestablishes vacuum. |
| ▪ Cleanse ends of emptying port with alcohol sponge. Replace cap immediately. Secure evacuator under wound site with safety pin through indicated perforation to patient's gown. | Reduces transmission of microorganisms into drainage evacuator and prevents tension on drainage tubing. |
| 5. Note characteristics of drainage; measure volume and discard. | Determines character of bacteria in wound drainage. |
| 6. Route labeled specimen to laboratory if ordered by physician *or* if purulence is noted. | Allows for culture testing to reveal infection. |
| 7. Discard soiled supplies and wash hands. | Reduces transmission of microorganisms. |
| 8. Proceed with dressing change and inspection of skin if indicated or ordered. | Prevents entrance of bacteria into surgical wound. |
| 9. Discard contaminated materials according to CDC guidelines and wash hands. | Reduces transmission of microorganisms. |
| **Evaluation** | |
| 1. Evaluate presence of drainage in drainage evacuator. | Indicates presence of vacuum, patency of tubing, and functioning of drainage evacuator. |

| Steps | Rationale |
|---|---|
| 2. Inspect wound for drainage. | Drainage should not be significant under suture line. Indicates inadequate functioning of drainage evacuator. |
| 3. Assess client's level of comfort. | Procedure should not increase client's pain. |
| ***Expected outcomes*** | |
| 1. Wound healing continues. | Client will be comfortable and epithelialization will continue in the absence of infectious pathogens or accumulated debris. |
| 2. Vacuum is reestablished. | Suction system intact. |
| 3. Tubing is patent. | Fluid draining away from wound. |
| 4. Reservoir is secured at site lower than wound. | To prevent stress on insertion site of tubing into wound and assist gravitational flow away from wound. |
| ***Unexpected outcomes*** | |
| 1. There is nosocomial infection, indicated by purulent drainage and temperature elevation. | Indicates absence of scrupulous aseptic technique by caregiver. |
| 2. There is soft tissue injury indicated by bleeding and pain. | Tension on client's drainage tube insertion site. |
| 3. Drainage evacuator system is not accumulating drainage. | Air leaks at any connection site or in reservoir. Kinks in tubing or occluded tubing prohibits drainage flow.<br>Large collections of debris may prohibit drainage flow. |
| 4. Pain. | Pain can result from infection, wound edema, increased drainage, and manipulation of drainage device. |

## Recording and Reporting

| | |
|---|---|
| 1. Quickly report to the physician:<br>a. Sudden absence of drainage flow | In presence of competent vacuum drainage system, this may indicate occlusion of openings in tubing within wound. |
| b. Pungent odor of drainage or new evidence of purulence<br>c. Severe pain. | Infectious process requires intervention. |
| 2. Report presence of functioning drainage evacuator and emptying frequency at change of shift report to nurse. | Permits continuity of care and evaluation of wound-healing progress. |
| 3. Record results of emptying wound drainage evacuator and dressing change (when performed) on progress notes and intake and output record. | Documents progress of healing and continuity of care. |

## Follow-up Activities

| | |
|---|---|
| 1. Obtain suture removal set before removal of tubing by physician. | A small suture that attaches the drain to the skin must be removed. |
| 2. Thoroughly cleanse and dry measuring graduate and store in client's bedside table. | This is to be reused for subsequent emptying of drainage. |

## Special Considerations

- Placement of drainage tubing in major suture line is avoided to promote healing. Drainage tubing has series of perforations to facilitate removal of accumulated debris and drainage.
- Drainage collection reservoir is emptied every 8 hr and PRN for large drainage volume. The nurse initiates collection of diagnostic specimen in the presence of unexpected purulence or pungent odor, reports findings to physician, and records in progress note.
- Drainage appears very red at first and later changes to lighter color. Volume will decrease after 2-3 days and as it diminishes, whole system can be removed.
- Both Hemovac and Jackson-Pratt drainage evacuators have two openings. One is attached to tubing that carries drainage from client's wound to drainage chamber or reservoir. Second port is used to empty collected drainage. Hemovac has perforation to insert safety pin to secure 400 ml drainage chamber on bed surface beside client or to pin it to client's gown.
- Attaching wall suction to Hemovac:
  a. Connect graduated adaptor to emptying port and then to wall suction tubing.
  b. Set suction level as prescribed, or on *low* if physician does not specify suction level.
- Attaching wall suction to the Jackson-Pratt:
  a. Attach connecting adaptor to suction tubing.
  b. Set suction level as prescribed, or at "low" if not specified.
  c. Attach tubing with graduated connector to open port and secure with tape.
- Drainage reservoirs fill slowly. If rapid expansion occurs after reestablishing drainage system, check all connections, wound site, and reservoir for source of air leakage.
- To prevent cross infections CDC recommendations include maintaining individualized equipment for drainage collection.

## Teaching Considerations

- Instruct client about anticipated postoperative drainage, expected progress of wound healing/drainage volume, and estimated date of removal of drain as volume diminishes.
- Unexplained dark red drainage will be major concern to any client. Being aware of what to expect will reduce anxiety.
- Instruct primary caregiver and client on how to change dressings located around drain site.
- Instruct client to wear loose fitting clothes.
- Instruct client to keep drain lower than waist level when ambulating, sitting, or lying down.

---

### BIBLIOGRAPHY


Bonier P: Wound care forum, an unusual alternative, Am J Nurs 85:418, 1985.

Briebacher CC: To heal a draining wound, RN 45:30, 1982.

Brozenec S: Caring for the postoperative patient with an abdominal drain, Nurs '85 15:55, 1985.

Bruno P: The nature of wound healing: implications for nursing practice, Nurs Clin North Am 14:667, 1979.

Creighton H: Law every nurse should know, ed 4, Philadelphia, 1981, WB Sanders Co.

Cuzzell JZ: Artful solutions to chronic problems, Am J Nurs 85:165, 1985.

Cuzzell JA: Wound care forum, a dialogue on wound care, Am J Nurs 85:715, 1985.

Gordon M: Nursing diagnosis: process and application, New York, 1982, McGraw-Hill Book Co.

Greenhalgh DG, Garnelli RA: Is impaired wound healing caused by infection or nutritional depletion, Surgery 102(2):306, 1987.

Hotter AN: Physiologic aspects and clinical implications of wound healing, Heart Lung 11:522, 1982.

Jeter K, Tintle T: Principles of wound cleaning and wound care, J Home Health Care Prac 1(1):1988.

Kim MJ, et al.: Pocket guide for nursing diagnosis, ed 2, St Louis, 1987, The CV Mosby Co.

Meyers D: Teaching guides for home health care Rockville Md, 1989, Aspen Publishing Co.

Neuberger G, Reckling J: A new look at wound care, Nurs '85 15(2):34, 1985.

Potter PA, Perry AG: Fundamentals of nursing, St Louis, ed 2, 1989, The CV Mosby Co.

Salyer J: Wound management in the home, Home Health Care Nurse 6(3):29, 1988.

Thompson JM, et al.: Mosby's manual of clinical nursing, ed 2, St Louis, 1989, The CV Mosby Co.

Schummann D: Preoperative measures to promote wound healing, Nurs Clin North Am 14:683, 1979.

Smith S, Duell D: Clinical nursing skills Los Altos: Calif, 1985, National Nursing Review.

Walsh J, Persons C, Wieck L: Manual of home health care nursing, Philadelphia, 1987, JB Lippincott Co.

# UNIT XIV

# SPECIAL PROCEDURES

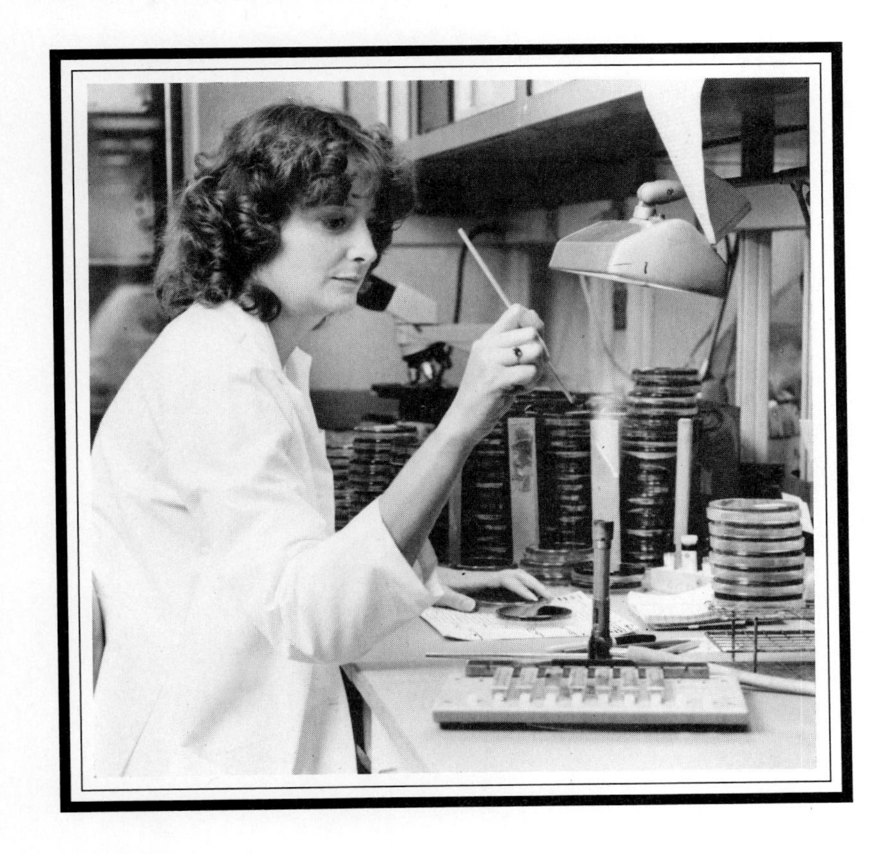

*Special procedures include laboratory studies, diagnostic tests with specimen collection, preparation of the client for the diagnostic procedure, or education of the client regarding the test. Laboratory studies and diagnostic tests provide data to assist the physician with the client's medical diagnosis and to assist the nurse with developing individualized nursing diagnoses and the subsequent nursing care plan.*

*The unit is divided into three chapters: "Specimen Collection", "Diagnostic Procedures." and "Care After Death." These chapters describe purposes of the test, pertinent nursing assessments and nursing diagnoses, and the nurse's role in planning, implementing, and evaluating the outcome of the special procedure. In addition, "Diagnostic Procedures" details the physician's responsibility because, as these are frequently invasive procedures, the physician usually completes the procedure with assistance from the nurse. "Care after Death" discusses nursing responsibilities toward the dying client and the client's family, as well as care of the body after death.*

# 45
# SPECIMEN COLLECTION

## OBJECTIVES

*Mastery of content in this chapter will enable the nurse to:*

- Define key terms.
- Explain the rationale for the collection of each specimen.
- Identify special conditions necessary for satisfactory collection of each specimen.
- Describe instructions to encourage client cooperation of successful collection of the specimen.
- Identify measures to minimize anxiety and promote safety for selected techniques.
- Discuss nursing responsibilities for processing the specimen after collection.
- Chart appropriate information in the client's record after collection of the specimen.
- Discuss precautions to prevent injury to the client during specimen collection.
- Properly collect random, clean-voided, timed, and catheterized urine specimens.
- Correctly measure specific gravity of urine.
- Correctly measure glucose and ketones in urine.
- Properly collect a stool specimen.
- Correctly measure for presence of occult blood in a stool specimen.
- Properly collect specimens for culture from the nose and throat, urethra and vagina, sputum, and wound.
- Correctly measure for pH and presence of occult blood in gastric drainage.
- Properly perform venipuncture.
- Correctly measure for blood glucose from a blood specimen collected by skin puncture.
- Properly collect an arterial blood sample.
- Perform pulse oximetry.

## KEY TERMS

*Acetest*
*Aerobe*
*Anaerobic*
*Aspiration*
*Autolet*
*Bacteremia*
*Bile*
*Clean-voided specimen*
*Clinitest*
*Culture*
*Defecation*
*Double-void*
*Ecchymosis*
*Excretion*
*Expectorant*
*Expectoration*
*Feces*
*Frequency*
*Hematemesis*
*Hematology*
*Hematoma*
*Hemoconcentration*
*Hemolysis*
*Hemostasis*
*Meatus*
*Melena*
*Midstream*
*Nebulization*
*Occult blood*
*pH*
*Platelet*
*Random-voided specimen*
*Reagent*
*Renal*
*Saliva*
*Secretion*
*Sensitivity*
*Specific gravity*
*Timed collection*
*Tourniquet*
*Urgency*
*Urinometer*
*Vacutainer tube*
*Vein lumen*
*Venipuncture*
*Void*

## SKILLS

**45-1** Collecting a Random Urine Specimen from an Adult or Toilet-Trained Child
**45-2** Collecting a Midstream (Clean-Voided) Urine Specimen
**45-3** Collecting a Timed Urine Specimen
**45-4** Collecting a Sterile Urine Specimen from an Indwelling Catheter
**45-5** Measuring Specific Gravity of Urine
**45-6** Measuring Urine Glucose and Ketones
**45-7** Collecting a Stool Specimen
**45-8** Measuring Occult Blood in Stool
**45-9** Collecting Nose and Throat Specimens for Culture
**45-10** Obtaining Vaginal or Urethral Discharge Specimens
**45-11** Collecting Sputum Specimens
**45-12** Obtaining Gastric Specimens
**45-13** Obtaining Wound Drainage Specimens
**45-14** Collecting Blood Specimens by Venipuncture
**45-15** Measuring Blood Glucose Level after Skin Puncture
**45-16** Measuring Arterial Blood Gases
**45-17** Pulse Oximetry

Nurses often assume the responsibility for collection of specimens of body secretions and excretions. Laboratory examination of specimens of urine, stool, sputum, blood, and wound drainage provides important information about body functioning and contributes to the assessment of health status. Laboratory test results can facilitate the diagnosis of health care problems, provide information about the stage and activity of a disease process, and measure the response to therapy.

Clients often experience embarrassment or discomfort when giving a sample of body excretions or secretions. Most persons believe excretions should be handled discreetly; therefore it is important to provide the client with as much comfort and privacy as possible. Anxiety is also provoked by the invasive nature of some collection procedures or by fear of unknown test results. Clients given a clear explanation about the purpose of the specimen and how it is to be obtained will be more cooperative in its collection. With proper instruction, many clients are able to obtain their own specimens of urine, stool, and sputum, thus avoiding embarrassment. Often the success of specimen collection depends on cooperation.

Laboratory tests are often expensive. The nurse can prevent unnecessary costs by using the correct procedure for obtaining and processing specimens. When there are questions about laboratory tests, the nurse should consult the institution's procedure manual or call the laboratory.

Normal values for laboratory tests can be found in reference books, but the nurse should know that each laboratory establishes its own values for each test. These values are usually readily available on the laboratory slips of the agency. Any major deviations should be immediately discussed with the physician.

## GUIDELINES

1. Consider the client's need and ability to participate in specimen collection procedures.
2. Recognize that collection of a specimen may provoke anxiety, embarrassment, or discomfort.
3. Provide support for clients who are fearful about the results of a specimen examination.
4. Recognize that children require a clear explanation of procedures and may benefit from support of parents or family members.
5. Obtain specimens in accordance with specific prerequisite conditions (e.g., fasting, npo) as required.
6. Wear gloves when collecting specimens of blood or other body fluids because it is not possible to identify all persons infected with HIV or other pathogens such as hepatitis B. (These universal precautions are advocated by the CDC.)
7. Wash hands and other skin surfaces immediately and thoroughly if contaminated with blood or body fluids; wash hands immediatley after removing gloves.
8. Collect specimens in appropriate containers, at the correct time, in the appropriate amount.
9. Properly label all specimens with the client's identification; complete laboratory requisition as necessary.
10. Deliver specimens to the laboratory within the recommended time or ensure that they are stored properly for later transport.
11. Use aseptic technique in all collections to prevent contamination, which can cause inaccurate test results.
12. Transport specimens under special conditions (e.g., iced specimens or special containers with preservatives) as required.

## PREREQUISITE KNOWLEDGE

1. Principles of medical and surgical asepsis.
2. Precautions for collecting specimens for client in protective isolation.
3. Precautions for handling body fluids.
4. Normal anatomy of appropriate systems.
5. Normal physiology of appropriate condition or process.
6. Normal test results of procedure.

## PREREQUISITE SKILLS

1. Proper handwashing techniques (Chapter 37).
2. Physical assessment of the body (Chapter 13).

# *SKILL 45-1 Collecting a Random Urine Specimen from an Adult or Toilet-Trained Child*

Urine is the most frequently collected specimen because its examination provides valuable clues about the functioning of the human body. A urinalysis can provide information about the status of kidney function, nutrition, metabolic function, and certain systemic diseases. Urine collection is part of every client's testing when admitted to an acute health care facility.

Many procedures can be used to collect urine, and many tests are performed for urine analysis. The method of urine collection depends on the type of test to be performed and the client's age, medical condition, and ability to void voluntarily. The three major types of urine specimens are single random routine specimens, timed urine collections (Skill 45-3), and specimens for culture and sensitivity (Skill 45-2).

A random routine urine specimen can be obtained with a client voiding or through a Foley catheter or urostomy collection bag. The specimen should be clean, but it need not be sterile. The specimen is generally tested for the type and amount of routine constituents such as white and red blood cells. The laboratory also performs routine screening on random specimens for constituents that normally should not be present in urine, such as protein and bacteria. The findings from a random specimen analysis may lead to additional urine testing or other types of diagnostic testing.

Before performing this procedure, the nurse must know the signs and symptoms of urinary elimination alterations and the normal characteristics of urine. The nurse should also know how to properly assist a client to a bedpan or urinal (Chapters 29 and 30) and how to provide perineal care (Chapter 6).

### Purposes

1. Quantitatively measure normal constituents of urine.
2. Screen for abnormal urine constituents.

## *Procedure 45-1*

| Steps | Rationale |
|---|---|
| **Assessment** | |
| 1. Assess client's ability to independently provide specimen: able to position self, hold container, stand or sit to void. | Determines ability to cooperate and level of assistance required. |
| 2. Assess client's understanding of need for specimen. | Determines need for health teaching. Clients understanding purpose can cooperate more fully. |
| 3. Assess for signs and symptoms of urinary tract infection: frequency, urgency, dysuria, hematuria, flank pain, fever, cloudy urine with sediment, foul odor. | Suggests bacteria in urine. |
| 4. Check agency procedures for specimen collection methods. | May vary as to proper way to collect or handle specimens. |
| **Nursing Diagnosis** | |
| 1. Cluster data to reveal actual or potential nursing diagnoses: | |
| a. Pain: related to urinary infection. | Sense of frequency, urgency and/or burning may occur with urination. |
| b. Knowledge deficit regarding collection procedure: related to inexperience. | Client may have inadequate understanding of test's purpose and steps for procedure. |
| c. Anxiety: related to unknown test results. | Findings may indicate serious health problem. |
| d. Potential for infection: related to urinary catheter. | Presence of signs and symptoms can reveal specific elimination problem. |
| **Planning** | |
| 1. Develop individualized goals based on nursing diagnoses: | |
| a. Obtain clean urine specimen, uncontaminated with feces or toilet tissue. | Ensures true determination of chemical characteristics and presence of abnormal constituents in urine. |
| b. Protect client's privacy. | Avoids client embarrassment. |
| c. Relieve client's anxiety. | |
| 2. Prepare equipment and supplies: | |
| a. Washcloth, towel, water, soap, and clean, disposable gloves | Perineum should be washed before collection of specimen. |
| b. Wide-mouth specimen container with lid. | Client may be able to void directly into container. |
| c. Clean specimen hat container to place under toilet seat (Fig. 45-1), potty chair, clean bedpan or urinal | Hat allows females to void on toilet seat in usual fashion. Young children are more likely to void in familiar receptacle. Bedpan or urinal is used for clients confined to bed. |

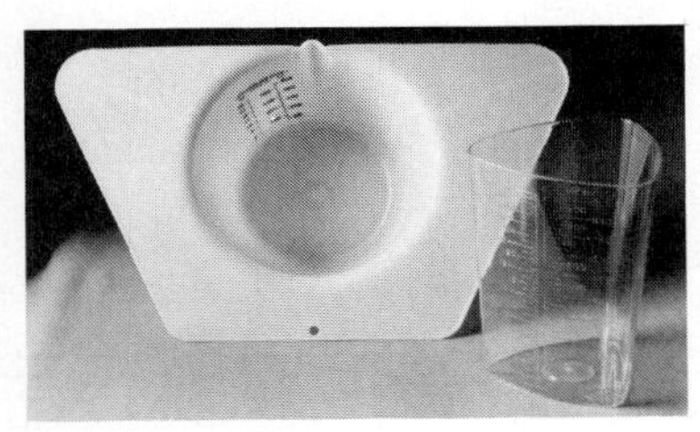

*Fig. 45-1*

| Steps | Rationale |
|---|---|
| d. Completed specimen identification label<br>e. Completed laboratory requisition with date and time of collection | Prevents confusion of specimens and allows more rapid transport to laboratory. |
| 3. Offer client fluids to drink 30 min before collecting specimen. | Improves likelihood of client being able to void. |
| 4. Explain procedure to client or family member. Discuss reason specimen is needed and how client can assist. Explain that urine must be free of feces and toilet tissue. | Client who understands procedure is more likely to cooperate and may be able to provide specimen independently. Also prevents accidental disposal of specimen. Feces change characteristics of urine and may cause abnormal values. |

## Implementation

| Steps | Rationale |
|---|---|
| 1. Wash hands and prepare equipment at bedside. | Reduces transfer of microorganisms. |
| 2. Provide privacy for client who will give specimen in bed by drawing curtain around bed or close room door. | Privacy allows client to relax and produce specimen more quickly. |
| 3. Give client or family member towel, washcloth, soap to cleanse perineal area or assist client to cleanse perineum. | Clients prefer to wash their own perineal areas when possible. Cleansing prevents contamination of specimen as urine passes urethra. |
| 4. Give male client specimen container and direct to bathroom; give female client specimen hat and direct to bathroom; assist client as needed to void into bedpan or urinal. | Maintains as much independence in client as possible. |
| 5. Put on gloves before assisting client in collection of specimen or handling urine. | Universal precautions advocated by CDC. |
| 6. If client did not void directly into specimen container, transfer 4 oz of urine into it. | Nurse should handle transfer of urine to specimen cup to avoid contamination of specimen. Proper volume of specimen ensures test can be completed. |
| 7. Place lid tightly on container. | Prevents contamination of specimen by other substances and loss due to spillage. |
| 8. If urine has been splashed on outside of container, wash it off. | Prevents spread of bacteria. |
| 9. If bedpan or urinal was used to collect specimen, cleanse and return to bedside. | Reduces transfer of microorganisms. |
| 10. Securely attach properly completed identification label and laboratory requisition to specimen. | Incorrect identification can result in diagnostic or therapeutic errors. |
| 11. Send specimen to laboratory immediately or place in specimen refrigerator. | Bacteria grow quickly in urine; therefore it should be analyzed immediately or refrigerated. |
| 12. Wash hands. | Reduces transmission of microorganisms. |

## Evaluation

| Steps | Rationale |
|---|---|
| 1. Refer to laboratory results in client's chart or appropriate record form. Compare results with normal values for routine urinalysis. | Provides complete summary of test findings. |

### *Expected outcomes*

| Steps | Rationale |
|---|---|
| 1. Urine is not contaminated with feces or toilet paper. | |
| 2. Urine has normal characteristics. | Client has no obvious alterations. |
| 3. Urine does not come in contact with nurse's skin. | |

### *Unexpected outcomes*

| Steps | Rationale |
|---|---|
| 1. Urine specimen is accidentally discarded. | Requires repeat of specimen collection procedure. |
| 2. Urine specimen is contaminated with feces or toilet paper. | |
| 3. Client is unable to urinate on demand. | May require more time, and/or more fluids to drink. |
| 4. Urine characteristics are abnormal. | May indicate a number of alterations. |

## Recording and Reporting

| Steps | Rationale |
|---|---|
| 1. Record collection of specimen in nurses' notes. Note time and date of collection, appearance and odor of urine, and abnormal signs or symptoms. | Verifies collection of specimen if report is slow to return from laboratory. |
| 2. Notify physician of significant abnormalities. | May indicate need for therapy. |

## Special Considerations

- Varying degrees of assistance will be required by clients who are seriously ill, have difficulty standing, or are confused. Some clients may need assistance in bathroom, whereas others require bedpan or urinal in bed. Elderly clients, in particular, may have difficulty in maintaining balance and raising or lowering toilet seat.
- Nurses should request feedback to assess client's understanding of purpose of test and directions for collecting specimen.
- Symptoms of urinary tract infection (UTI) in children are frequently limited to generalized symptoms such as nausea, vomiting, diarrhea, and fever, which may be accompanied by seizures.
- For infants and young children not yet potty trained, plastic urine-collecting bags with self-adhesive are attached over perineal area after it has been cleansed and dried (Fig. 45-2). In females, it is especially important that the bag adheres well to skin between vagina and rectum.
- Young children are often unable to void on request. Offer fluids they enjoy and allow them to suggest when they are ready to void.
- Children are often more cooperative when they receive positive reinforcement for their efforts; school-age children often want explanations for why things are done.
- Children may prefer assistance of parent in cleansing genitalia and collecting urine.
- In uncircumcized males, foreskin must be retracted for effective cleansing of meatus and during voiding.
- Female clients need to be instructed to discard toilet tissue into toilet or into waste bag rather than with urine because it makes analysis of urine invalid.
- If female is menstruating, nurse notes it on specimen requisition in case red blood cells appear in urine.
- Institutional policy determines type of information to include on labels and requisitions (e.g., if client is receiving antibiotics, it should be noted on laboratory requisition).
- If urine specimen is less than 1 oz, check with laboratory to see if it is enough.
- If specimen is taken from protective isolation room, it should be placed in paper bag according to hospital policy.
- Never store specimens in food refrigerator.
- Always cover specimens to prevent $CO_2$ from diffusing into the air, which will result in urine becoming alkaline and fostering bacterial growth.

## Teaching Considerations

- Discuss signs and symptoms of urinary tract infection.
- Explain reason for collecting specimen.
- Explain significance of cleansing genital area before collecting specimen.
- Explain importance of cleansing labia from front to back (in female).
- Discuss client's role in collecting specimen.
- Instruct client about procedure to use to keep urine free of feces and paper.

## Home Care Consideration

- If client is to collect urine specimen at home and bring to health care facility, client should void directly into glass jar that has been washed in the dishwasher or with boiling water, or void into a specimen container.

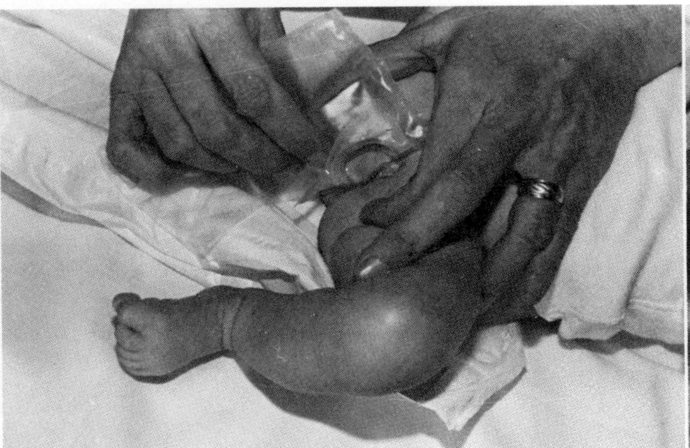

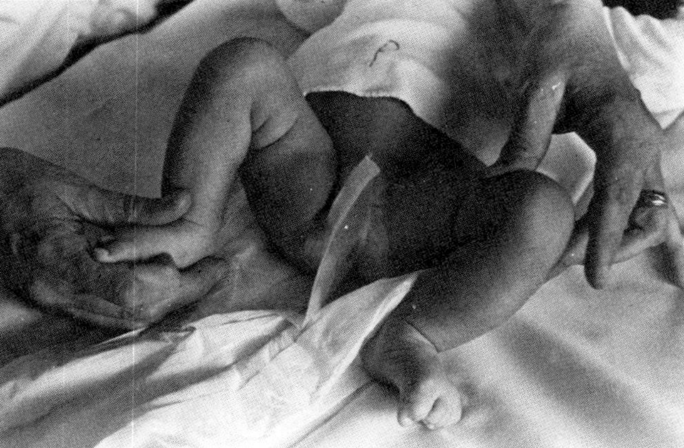

***Fig. 45-2***

From Whaley LF, Wong DL: Nursing care of infants and children, ed 3, St Louis, 1987, The CV Mosby Co.

# *SKILL 45-2 Collecting a Midstream (Clean-Voided) Urine Specimen*

A common test performed on urine is a culture and sensitivity measurement. Sterile urine is placed on a special medium to determine if bacteria are present. It takes approximately 72 hr for the laboratory to report findings. If bacteria are present, sensitivity testing reveals the antibiotics that will be effective against the microorganisms.

With clients who are able to void voluntarily, the nurse collects a midstream urine specimen for culture and sensitivity testing. A client begins the urinary stream and then during the middle portion of voiding collects a specimen. The initial stream flushes the urethral orifice and meatus of any resident bacteria. It is easiest for clients to obtain clean-voided specimens while using toilet facilities rather than a bedpan or urinal.

Before performing this procedure, the nurse should know the signs and symptoms of abnormal urinary alterations and the normal characteristics of urine. The nurse should also know how to perform perineal care (Chapter 6), open sterile packages and don sterile gloves by the open method (Chapter 38), and assist a client with a bedpan (Chapter 30).

## Purpose

1. Measure bacteria or other organisms in the urine.

## *Procedure 45-2*

| Steps | Rationale |
|---|---|
| **Assessment** | |
| 1. Assess client's mobility and balance in being able to use toilet facilities independently. | Determines level of assistance required by client. |
| 2. Refer to medical record for indications of urinary infection. | Helps nurse understand purpose of specimen procedure for client. |
| 3. Assess client's risk for urinary tract infection: poor perineal hygiene, improperly handled diagnostic instruments, previous urinary catheterization. | Allows nurse to anticipate need to test client's urine for bacteria. |
| 4. Assess for signs and symptoms of urinary tract infections: frequency, urgency, dysuria, hematuria, flank pain, fever. | Can suggest bacteria in urine. |
| 5. Assess client's level of understanding of purpose of test and method of collection. | Information allows nurse to clarify misunderstandings; promotes client cooperation. |
| 6. Refer to agency procedures for specimen collection methods. | Agency policies may vary as to proper way to collect or handle specimens. |
| **Nursing Diagnosis** | |
| 1. Cluster data to reveal actual or potential nursing diagnoses: | |
| a. Pain: related to urinary tract infection. | Burning sensation during urination is caused by inflammation of tissue in urinary tract. |
| b. Potential for infection: related to poor perineal hygiene. | Urine testing will help to diagnose specific causative organism. |
| c. Impaired physical mobility: related to arthritic joint changes. | Client will need assistance to obtain specimen. |
| **Planning** | |
| 1. Develop individualized goals based on nursing diagnoses: | |
| a. Obtain midstream specimen free from contamination of resident microorganisms. | Test will reveal bacteria in urine. |
| b. Protect client's privacy. | Procedure can be embarrassing for client. |
| 2. Prepare equipment and supplies: | Agency policy may determine type of equipment to use. |
| a. Commercial kit for clean-voided urine (Fig. 45-3), sterile cotton balls, 2 × 2 gauze pads | Used to clean, rinse, dry perineum. |

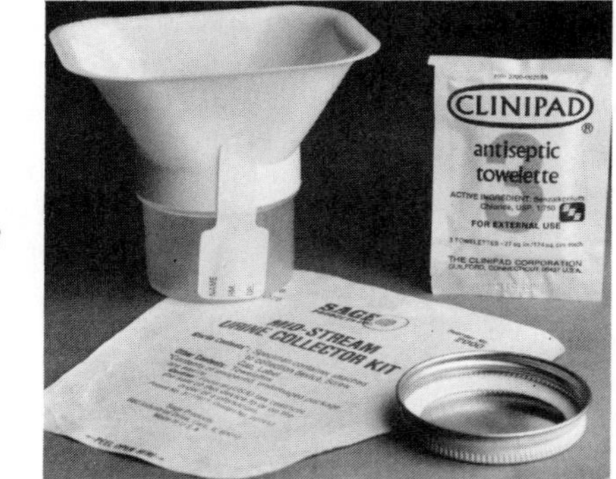


*Fig. 45-3*

| Steps | Rationale |
|---|---|
| b. Antiseptic solution (providone-iodine) | |
| c. Sterile water or saline | Rinses antiseptic solution. Solution can alter test results if allowed to enter specimen. |
| d. Sterile gloves | |
| e. Sterile specimen container | |
| f. Soap, towel, washcloth | |
| g. Bedpan (for nonambulating client), specimen hat, potty chair | Allows women to void in toilet seat in usual fashion. Children more likely to use familiar facilities. |
| h. Completed specimen identification label<br>i. Completed laboratory requisition form | Completion of label and requisition before collecting specimen prevents confusing it with other specimens and ensures more rapid transport to laboratory. |
| 3. Explain procedure to client: | |
| a. Reason midstream specimen is needed.<br>b. How client, family member can assist. | Helps client provide specimen independently. |
| c. How to obtain specimen free of feces. | Feces change characteristics of urine and may cause abnormal values. |
| 4. Use visual aides (if available) to explain procedure to client. | Because this method of urine collection is somewhat complicated, clients benefit from illustrations emphasizing correct collection techniques. |
| 5. Provide client fluids to drink ½ hr before collecting specimen. | Improves likelihood of client being able to void. |
| **Implementation** | |
| 1. Wash hands. | Reduces transfer of microorganisms. |
| 2. Provide privacy for client who will give specimen in bed by closing curtain around bed or closing room door. | Privacy allows client to relax and produce a specimen more quickly. |
| 3. Give client or family member towel, washcloth, soap to cleanse perineal area or assist client to cleanse perineum. | Clients prefer to wash their own perineal areas when possible. |
| 4. Assist bedridden client onto bedpan. | Provides easy access to perineal areas to collect specimen. |
| 5. Using surgical asepsis, open sterile kit or prepare sterile tray. | Maintains sterility of equipment. |
| 6. Don sterile gloves. | Prevents introduction of microorganisms on nurse's hands into specimen. |
| 7. Pour antiseptic solution over cotton balls unless kit contains prepared gauze pads in antiseptic solution. | Cotton ball or gauze is used to cleanse perineum. |
| 8. Open specimen container and place cap with sterile inside surface up and do not touch inside of container. | Contaminated specimen is most frequent reason for inaccurate reporting on urinary cultures and sensitivities. |
| 9. Assist or allow client to independently cleanse perineum and collect specimen: | |
| a. *Male:* | |
| ▪ Hold penis with one hand; using circular motion and antiseptic swab, cleanse end, moving from center to outside. | Cleanse from area of least contamination to area of greatest contamination to decrease bacterial levels. |
| ▪ If agency procedure indicates, rinse area with sterile water and dry with cotton balls or gauze pad. | Prevents contamination of specimen with antiseptic solution. |
| ▪ After client has initiated urine stream, pass urine specimen container into stream and collect 30 to 60 ml urine. | Initial urine flushes out microorganisms that normally accumulate at urinary meatus and prevents collection in specimen. |
| b. *Female:* | |
| ▪ Spread labia minora with thumb and forefinger of nondominant hand. | Provides access to urethral meatus. |
| ▪ Cleanse area with cotton ball or gauze, moving from front (above urethral orifice) to back (toward anus). Repeat 3 times (left side, right side, and center). Use fresh cotton ball each time. | Prevents contamination of urinary meatus with fecal material. |
| ▪ If agency procedure indicates, rinse area with sterile water and dry with cotton. | Prevents contamination of specimen with antiseptic solution. |
| ▪ While continuing to hold labia apart, client should initiate urine stream; after stream achieved, pass specimen container into stream and collect 30 to 60 ml. | Initial stream flushes out microorganisms that accumulate at urethral meatus. |
| 10. Remove specimen container before flow of urine stops and before releasing labia or penis. Client finishes voiding into bedpan or toilet. | Prevents contamination of specimen with skin flora. |
| 11. Replace cap securely on specimen container (touch only outside). | Retains sterility of inside of container and prevents spillage of urine. |

| Steps | Rationale |
|---|---|
| 12. Cleanse urine from exterior surface of container. | Prevents transfer of microorganisms to others. |
| 13. Remove gloves, dispose in proper receptacle. | Prevents transfer of microorganisms. |
| 14. Remove bedpan (if applicable) and assist client to comfortable position. | Promotes relaxation and comfort. |
| 15. Wash hands. | Reduces transmission of microorganisms. |
| 16. Label specimen and attach laboratory requisition. | Prevents inaccurate identification that could lead to errors in diagnosis or therapy. |
| 17. Take specimen to laboratory within 15 min or immediately refrigerate. | Bacteria grow quickly in urine so it should be analyzed immediately to obtain correct results, or refrigerated. |

## Evaluation

| | |
|---|---|
| 1. Refer to laboratory report for results of test. | Report shows numbers and types of bacteria present. |

### *Expected outcomes*

| | |
|---|---|
| 1. Client produces midstream urine specimen that is not contaminated with feces or toilet paper. | These substances change normal characteristics of urine. |
| 2. Urine has normal characteristics and does not reveal bacterial growth. | Provides evidence of absense of infection. |

### *Unexpected outcomes*

| | |
|---|---|
| 1. Urine specimen is accidentally discarded. | Communication regarding urine collection was ineffective. |
| 2. Urine specimen is contaminated with feces or toilet paper. | Requires repeat of specimen collection procedure. |
| 3. Client is unable to urinate on demand. | May require more time for urine to accumulate in bladder. |
| 4. Urine culture reveals bacterial growth (designated by colony count of more than 10,000 organisms/ml). | Evidence of urinary tract infection. |

## Recording and Reporting

| | |
|---|---|
| 1. Record date and time urine specimen was obtained in nurses' notes. | Documents implementation of physician's order. |
| 2. Record appearance and odor of urine and evidence of dysuria in nurses' notes. | Data can support or disclaim other evidence or urinary tract infection. |

## Follow-up Activity

| | |
|---|---|
| 1. If bacteria are in urine, physician will order antibiotic for nurse to administer. | Antibiotic chosen will be effective against organisms in urine. |

## Special Considerations

- See Procedure 45-1.

## Teaching Considerations

- See Skill 45-1.
- Use visual aides to describe collection of specimen.
- Explain importance of cleansing labia from front to back (in female).

## Home Care Consideration

- See Procedure 45-1.

# SKILL 45-3 Collecting a Timed Urine Specimen

Some tests of renal function and urine composition require urine to be collected over 2 to 72 hr. The 24 hr timed collection is most common. The tests allow for the measurement of elements such as amino acids, creatinine, hormones, glucose, and adrenocorticosteroids, whose levels change over time. Timed collections can also provide a means to measure the concentration or dilution of urine.

Timed urine collections begin after a client urinates. The nurse discards the first specimen and then collects every successive specimen until the time period has ended. Each specimen is transferred immediately to a large collection bottle kept in the client's bathroom. Any missed specimens will make test results inaccurate. The client should always void the last specimen as close as possible to the end of the collection period.

Before performing this procedure, the nurse should know the normal characteristics of urine and how to assist a client with a bedpan (Chapter 30), measure I & O (Chapter 22), and collect a random urine specimen (Skill 45-1).

## Purposes

1. Measure specific quantities of urinary constituents secreted at different rates over time.
2. Assess renal function.
3. Assess metabolic and hormonal function.

## Procedure 45-3

| Steps | Rationale |
|---|---|
| **Assessment** | |
| 1. Determine purpose of timed urine specimen collection for client and period collection is to include. | Most common collections are for 24 hr because this provides average excretion rate for substances such as hormones or proteins excreted in small, variable amounts in urine. If these substances are to be accurately measured and yield quantities of diagnostic value, urine must be collected over extended period. Challenge dose of chemical such as insulin may be given and then timed urine specimen collection may be begun to detect renal disorders. |
| 2. Determine if fluid or dietary requirements or medications need to be administered in conjunction with test. | Certain substances affect excretion and levels of urinary constituents. Glucose solution may be given for glucose tolerance test. Specific amounts of fluid may be required for concentration/dilution tests. |
| 3. Assess client's ability to collect specimens independently. | Promotes cooperation and determines level of assistance required. |
| 4. Assess client's or family members' understanding of test's purpose and need to collect urine over extended period. | Cooperation is facilitated by degree of understanding. |
| 5. Refer to agency policy for specimen collection procedure. | Agency policies may vary as to proper way to collect or handle specimens. |
| **Nursing Diagnosis** | |
| 1. Cluster data to reveal actual or potential nursing diagnoses: | |
| a. Knowledge deficit regarding specimen collection: related to inexperience. | Client may require frequent instruction and reinforcement of importance of saving all urine. |
| b. Impaired physical mobility: related to muscular stiffness. | Indicates need for nurse to assist in specimen collection. |
| c. Potential for infection. | Types of tests are indicated for specific urinary elimination alterations (e.g., infections). |
| **Planning** | |
| 1. Develop individualized goals based on nursing diagnoses: | |
| a. Collect specimen for exact period ordered. | Analysis of specimen depends on accurate timed collection of all urine. |
| b. Avoid loss of urine during period. | Loss will result in inaccurate results. |
| c. Collect specimen free of contamination by feces or toilet tissue. | Ensures accurate test results. |

| Steps | Rationale |
|---|---|
| 2. Prepare equipment and supplies: | |
| a. Large collection bottle with cap with appropriate chemical urine preservative It may be necessary to call laboratory to determine appropriate additive. | Some tests require toluene or acetic acid, whereas others require different preservatives. Often laboratory is source of specific collection bottles and preservatives. |
| b. Bedpan, urinal, specimen hat, potty chair if client does not have indwelling catheter | |
| c. Graduated measuring cup if I & O are to be measured | |
| d. Ice-filled container | For storage of urine if refrigerator is unavailable. |
| e. Completed specimen identification label | Completion before collecting specimens prevents confusing with other specimens and allows more rapid transport to laboratory. |
| f. Completed laboratory requisition with client's name, date, and time of collection | |
| g. Signs that remind client and staff of timed urine collection | Prevents accidental disposal of urine. |
| h. Clean, disposable gloves | |
| 3. Instruct client or parents to: | |
| a. Save all urine during collection period. | Loss of any urine invalidates test. |
| b. Notify nurse each time client voids. | Nurse adds urine to collection bottle. |
| c. Keep urine free of feces and toilet tissue. | These substances negatively affect test results. |
| d. Begin and end test by emptying bladder. | Ensures precise number of hours for collection period. |
| e. Begin test at precise time, usually 0700, on weekdays only. | Ensures laboratory will be open when time is completed. |
| 4. Have client drink 2 to 4 glasses of water about ½ hr before timed collection is to begin. | Enables client to void old urine (collected in bladder) at time test begins. |

## Implementation

| Steps | Rationale |
|---|---|
| 1. Provide privacy for and assist client in collecting specimen as outlined in procedure for obtaining random urine specimen (Skill 45-1). | Clients prefer collecting specimens themselves. Timed specimens are not sterile. |
| 2. Wear gloves when handling urine. | |
| 3. Discard this specimen as test begins and print time test began on laboratory requisition. | Collection period begins with empty bladder. |
| 4. When applicable, have client drink required amount of liquid or take ordered medication. | Required for specific types of tests to measure elimination of urine constituents. |
| 5. Place signs indicating timed urine specimen on client's door, bed, in bedroom, and on urinal, bedpan, potty chair, specimen hat. | Prevents uninformed staff and relatives from accidentally discarding urine specimens. |
| 6. Measure volume of each voiding if output is recorded. | Measures client's fluid balance. |
| 7. Place all voided urine into labeled specimen bottle with appropriate additive. | Preserves urine specimen and prevents deterioration. |
| 8. Unless instructed otherwise, keep specimen bottle in specimen refrigerator or in container of ice in bathroom. | Coldness prevents decomposition of urine. |
| 9. Wash hands before and after collection of each voiding. | Reduces transmission of microorganisms. |
| 10. Encourage client to drink 2 glasses of water 1 hr before timed urine collection ends. | Facilitates client's ability to void at end of period. |
| 11. Encourage client to empty bladder during last 15 min of urine collection period. | Ensures urine collected for precise amount of time. |
| 12. At end of period, send labeled specimen to laboratory with appropriate requisition. | Ensures laboratory results credited to correct client. |
| 13. Remove signs and remind client that specimen collection period is completed. | Allows client to resume usual voiding habits. |

## Evaluation

| Steps | Rationale |
|---|---|
| 1. Review laboratory report for results of tests. | May indicate specific nursing observations or procedures. |
| 2. Periodically during collection period, ask client if all urine is being saved. | Clients frequently forget about saving all voidings. |
| 3. Inspect each specimen before adding to container. | Ensures feces or toilet tissue is not present. |

### *Expected outcomes*

| Steps | Rationale |
|---|---|
| 1. All of client's urine voided during time period is saved. | Necessary for satisfactory completion of test. |
| 2. Urine specimen is not contaminated with feces or toilet tissue. | Prevents results of urine test from being adversely affected by these substances. |
| 3. Urine has normal constituency. | Client free of alterations. |

| Steps | Rationale |
|---|---|
| ***Unexpected outcomes*** | |
| 1. Urine specimen is accidentally discarded. | Results in inaccurate measurement of urinary constituents. |
| 2. Urine specimen is contaminated by feces or toilet tissue. | May cause inaccurate test results. |
| 3. Laboratory results reveal abnormal values for urine constituents. | Alteration in urinary function or metabolism. |
| **Recording and Reporting** | |
| 1. Record starting time of urine collection in client's chart. | Documents collection has begun. |
| 2. At completion of test, record time urine collection is finished, appearance, amount, odor, disposition of specimen to laboratory. | Documents completion of timed collection of urine. |
| 3. Discuss abnormal test results with physician. | Facilitates appropriate intervention. |

### Special Considerations

- See Procedure 45-1.
- If client leaves unit for test or procedure, be sure that personnel in that area collect urine.
- If client has indwelling catheter, place collection bag in ice-filled container.
- If client's physical condition warrants fluid restriction, be cautious in encouraging fluids.
- If urine is accidently discarded or contaminated, restart timed period.
- Some references call time collections "composite specimens."

### Teaching Considerations

- Explain purpose of test.
- Explain fluid or dietary requirements or medications related to test.
- Explain significance of collecting all urine for specific period.
- Explain why urine must be kept in special container, with preservative (if used) and cold.

### Home Care Consideration

- See Procedure 45-1.

## *SKILL 45-4 Collecting a Sterile Urine Specimen from an Indwelling Catheter*

It often becomes necessary to collect urine specimens from clients who are unable to void voluntarily or who have difficulty providing a clean-voided specimen. In these cases the nurse can collect urine through a urinary catheter. The nurse can introduce a straight catheter (see Chapter 29) to collect a specimen, or a specimen can be collected from an indwelling catheter. Either method requires strict aseptic technique to ensure sterility and to avoid introducing infection into the urinary tract.

A urine specimen should not be collected for culture tests from a urine drainage bag unless it is the first urine to drain into a new sterile bag. Bacteria grow rapidly in drainage bags and can give a false measurement of bacteria in the urine.

Before beginning this procedure, the nurse should know the normal characteristics of urine and how to maintain an indwelling urinary catheter (Chapter 29).

### Purposes

1. Obtain a sterile specimen with the least risk of contamination.
2. Collect a specimen from a client unable to void voluntarily.

## *Procedure 45-4*

| Steps | Rationale |
|---|---|
| **Assessment** | |
| 1. Assess client or family members' understanding of need for collection of urine from indwelling catheter. | Reveals knowledge of procedure and willingness to cooperate. |
| 2. Assess for signs and symptoms of urinary tract infection: hematuria, flank pain, fever, cloudy urine with sediment. | Suggest bacteria in urine. |

| Steps | Rationale |
| --- | --- |
| 3. Assess indwelling catheter for built-in sampling port and type of material from which it is made. | Provides appropriate place for removal of urine from catheter. Port prevents leakage of urine from catheter. It is safe to insert needle directly into self-sealing rubber catheter. Silastic, silicone, or plastic catheters are not self-sealing and thus should not be punctured with needle for aspiration of urine. |

## Nursing Diagnosis

| Steps | Rationale |
| --- | --- |
| 1. Cluster data to reveal actual or potential nursing diagnoses: | |
| a. Pain: related to urinary catheter placement. | Urinary catheter irritates urethra. Urinary tract infection can cause considerable discomfort. |
| b. Anxiety: related to specimen collection method. | Certain clients, especially children, may become anxious about how specimen is to be removed from catheter. |
| c. Potential for infection: related to indwelling catheter. | Nosocomial infection is commonly caused by catheter placement. |

## Planning

| Steps | Rationale |
| --- | --- |
| 1. Develop individualized goals based on nursing diagnoses: | |
| a. Obtain uncontaminated urine specimen. | Nurse collects only urine that accumulates in catheter tubing. |
| b. Prevent anxiety or discomfort during procedure. | Procedure is painless. |
| 2. Prepare necessary equipment and supplies: | |
| a. 3 ml syringe with 1 in needle (21 to 25 gauge) for culture, or 20 ml syringe with 1 in needle (21 to 25 gauge) for routine urinalysis | Used to aspirate urine from catheter. Small gauge minimizes chance of creating permanent hole in catheter tubing. |
| b. Metal clamp or rubber band | |
| c. Alcohol, povidone-iodine, or other disinfectant swab | Used to cleanse catheter before inserting needle. |
| d. Specimen container: nonsterile for routine urinalysis, sterile for culture | Used to transport specimens to laboratory. |
| e. Completed specimen identification label | Completion of these items before collecting specimens prevents confusion with other specimens and allows more rapid transport to laboratory. |
| f. Completed laboratory requisition with client's name, date, and time of collection | |
| g. Clean, disposable gloves | Prevents urine from coming into contact with hands. |
| 3. Prepare client: | |
| a. Explain that urine specimen is needed and purpose. | Alleviates anxiety when nurse manipulates catheter. |
| b. Explain that urine will be removed from indwelling catheter with syringe and needle, but it will not cause client any discomfort. | Prevents anxiety. |
| c. Explain that catheter will be clamped for 30 min before specimen is collected. | Prevents client from developing anxiety about catheter being clamped. |

## Implementation

| Steps | Rationale |
| --- | --- |
| 1. Wash hands. | Reduces transfer of microorganisms. |
| 2. Clamp drainage tubing with clamp or rubberband for 30 min (Fig. 45-4). | Permits collection of fresh sterile urine in catheter tubing rather than draining into bag. |
| 3. Return to room and inform client that the procedure to collect a specimen from a catheter will begin. | Allows client to anticipate manipulation of urinary catheter, and cope more effectively with discomfort that may occur when catheter is moved. |
| 4. Wash hands and put on gloves. | Reduces transfer of microorganisms. |
| 5. Position client so catheter is easily accessible. | Allows for easy collection of specimen. |
| 6. Cleanse entry port for needle with disinfectant swab. | Prevents entry of microorganisms into catheter. |
| 7. Insert needle at 30-degree angle just above where catheter is attached to drainage tube or at built-in sampling port (Fig. 45-5). | Ensures entrance of needle into catheter lumen and prevents accidental puncture of lumen leading to balloon that holds catheter in place in bladder. Aspiration of water from lumen can result in catheter falling out of bladder. |
| 8. Draw urine into 3 ml syringe for culture or draw urine into 20 ml syringe for routine urinalysis. | Allows collection of urine without contamination. Proper volume is needed to perform test. |
| 9. Transfer urine from syringe into nonsterile urine container for routine urinalysis or transfer urine from syringe into sterile urine container for culture. | Prevents contamination of urine during transfer procedure. |
| 10. Place lid tightly on container. | Prevents contamination of specimen by air and loss by spillage. |
| 11. Unclamp catheter and allow urine to flow into drainage bag. | Allows urine to drain by gravity and prevents stasis of urine in bladder, which can cause much discomfort and potential damage to kidneys. |

| Steps | Rationale |
|---|---|
| 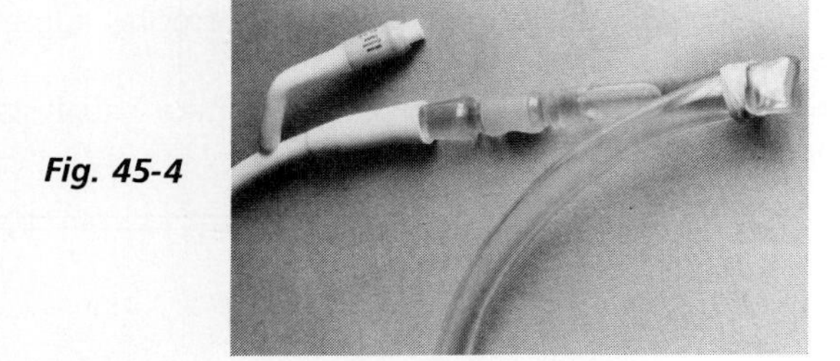 *Fig. 45-4* | *Fig. 45-5* |
| 12. Securely attach properly completed identification label and laboratory requisition to specimen. | Incorrect identification of specimen could result in diagnostic or therapeutic errors. |
| 13. Send specimen to laboratory immediately or place in specimen refrigerator. | Bacteria grow quickly in urine; therefore it should be analyzed or refrigerated immediately. |
| 14. Dispose of soiled supplies; wash hands. | Reduces transmission of microorganisms. |

## Evaluation

| | |
|---|---|
| 1. Check laboratory report for results of tests. | Determines bacteria or other abnormal constituents. May indicate need for nursing interventions. |
| 2. Observe client for signs of infection or discomfort. | |

***Expected outcomes***

| | |
|---|---|
| 1. Urine specimen is obtained from catheter without contamination. | |
| 2. Urine has normal characteristics and no bacterial growth. | Client is free of abnormality. |

***Unexpected outcomes***

| | |
|---|---|
| 1. Urine specimen is contaminated during procedure. | Cannot be evaluated unless nurse obviously contaminates equipment. |
| 2. Lumen that leads to balloon that holds catheter in bladder is punctured. | Will require reinsertion of catheter. |
| 3. Urine has abnormal constituents. | Indicates infection or other alteration. |

## Recording and Reporting

| | |
|---|---|
| 1. Record collection of specimen in nurses' notes; note time and date, appearance, odor. | Verifies collection of specimen if report is slow to return to laboratory. |
| 2. Notify physician of any significant differences in urine. | Allows physician to begin therapeutic action if needed. |

## Special Considerations

- See Procedure 45-1.

# *SKILL 45-5 Measuring Specific Gravity of Urine*

A simple test for the nurse to perform in any clinical setting is the measurement of urine specific gravity. Specific gravity is the concentration of dissolved substances in water. The nurse places a urinometer with a mercury bulb in a cylinder containing urine. The density or concentration of urine determines the level at which the urinometer suspends within the cylinder. If the urine is diluted, the urinometer tends to sink. Concentrated solutes in urine will cause the urinometer to float. The test takes only a few seconds and can often provide useful information about kidney function and the need to regulate fluid intake.

Before beginning this procedure, the nurse should know how to collect a random or catheterized urine specimen (Skills 45-2 and 45-4).

### Purposes

1. Assess the extent to which urine is concentrated in the kidneys.
2. Monitor the client's response to select therapies (e.g., fluid volume infusion, antidiuretic hormone administration).
3. Eliminate the need for expensive laboratory analysis of specimen.

## *Procedure 45-5*

| Steps | Rationale |
|---|---|
| **Assessment** | |
| 1. Assess client or family members' understanding of need to test specific gravity and how test is performed. | Provides nurse with information on which to base teaching. |
| 2. Determine client's ability to collect specimen. | Determines level of assistance required from nurse. |
| 3. Assess client's hydration status: skin turgor, condition of mucous membranes, I & O, integrity of fontanels (infants). | Specific gravity measures concentration of urine solutes and is affected by state of hydration. |
| 4. Assess client's medical history for evidence of renal disease. | Renal tubular disease results in loss of capacity of kidney to concentrate urine. |
| **Nursing Diagnosis** | |
| 1. Cluster data to reveal actual or potential nursing diagnoses: | |
| a. Fluid volume excess: related to renal impairment. | Hypervolemia can cause reduced urine concentration. |
| b. Fluid volume deficit: related to diuresis. | Reduction in fluid volume can cause increase in specific gravity. |
| **Planning** | |
| 1. Develop individualized goals based on nursing diagnoses: | |
| a. Accurately measure specific gravity. | Incorrect measurement may result in inappropriate therapies being instituted. |
| b. Obtain urine specimen free of feces or toilet tissue. | Materials increase solutes in urine and interfere with test results. |
| 2. Prepare necessary equipment and supplies: | |
| a. At least 20 ml of fresh urine. Urine need not be sterile. Random specimen is adequate if client can void. Otherwise obtain specimen from catheter. | Enough urine is needed to fill glass cylinder ⅔ full to float urinometer. |
| b. Urinometer (Validate accuracy of calibration by filling cylinder ⅔ full with water.) | Calibrated hydrometer, with scale at top and mercury bulb at bottom should read 1.000 as it floats in water. Since urine specific gravity is determined by comparing weight of urine with water. If tap water is heavier than 1.000, use distilled water. |
| c. Clean, dry, glass cylinder | Used to hold urine and float urinometer. |
| d. Clean, disposable gloves | Used to prevent contact of urine with skin. |
| 3. Explain purpose of test and how specimen can be obtained. | Relieves anxiety and promotes cooperation. |
| **Implementation** | |
| 1. Wash hands and put on clean, disposable gloves. | Reduces transmission of microorganisms. |
| 2. Carefully pour fresh urine specimen into glass cylinder until it is ⅔ to ¾ full. | Cylinder must be at least ⅔ full to cause urinometer to float. |
| 3. Place urinometer in cylinder of urine and gently twirl top of stem. | Prevents urinometer from adhering to sides of cylinder. |
| 4. Wait until urinometer stops bobbing, then with urinometer scale at eye level, read point where urine level touches calibrated scale. Read scale at lowest point of meniscus for best accuracy (Fig. 45-6). | Concentration of dissolved solutes in urine influences depth at which urinometer floats. Point at which urine reaches scale is specific gravity. |
| 5. Discard urine and wash cylinder and urinometer in cool water. | Warm water coagulates proteins in urine and causes them to stick to glass surfaces. |
| 6. Remove gloves and wash hands. | Reduces transfer of microorganisms. |

| Steps | Rationale |
| --- | --- |

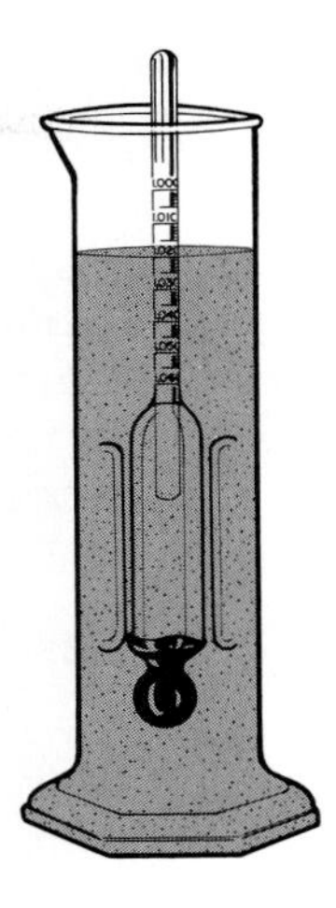

*Fig. 45-6*

## Evaluation

| Steps | Rationale |
| --- | --- |
| 1. Compare results with normal findings for specific gravity. | Determines relative concentration of urine. |
| ***Expected outcomes*** | |
| 1. Specific gravity is between 1.010 and 1.025.<br>2. Urine specimen is free of contaminants. | Normal range of values. |
| ***Unexpected outcomes*** | |
| 1. Specific gravity is less than 1.010 or greater than 1.025. | Dilute urine is less than 1.010; concentrated urine is greater than 1.025. |
| 2. Urine contains feces. | Causes elevated specific gravity reading. |

## Recording and Reporting

| Steps | Rationale |
| --- | --- |
| 1. Record specific gravity reading and note character of urine in nurses' notes. | Allows for early treatment intervention. |
| 2. If client on I & O record urine volume on flow sheet. | All urine must be measured to obtain accurate 24 hr output. |
| 3. Report abnormal values to nurse in charge or physician. | Results may indicate need for further therapy. |

## Follow-up Activity

| Steps | Rationale |
| --- | --- |
| 1. Check physician's orders to determine if specific nursing care is required for given reading (e.g., regulate IV rate, administer pitressin, regulate oral intake of fluids). | Control of fluid intake or reduction in urinary water excretion can regulate specific gravity. In cases of diabetes insipidus, most frequently resulting from tumor or postoperative swelling near pituitary gland, pitressin is given to decrease water excretion. |

## Special Considerations

- Urine should be at room temperature for testing because the urinometer is calibrated at room temperature.
- Special flow sheets should be placed in chart for recording readings when clients require frequent measurements of specific gravity.
- Diluted, watery urine results in low specific gravity readings and dark yellow, concentrated urine results in high specific gravity readings.
- The refractometer, a small telescope-like instrument, is newer technique for measuring specific gravity. One drop of urine is placed on slide and viewed through refractometer, which allows visualization of density of urine on calibrated scale.

## Teaching Considerations

- Instruct client on proper method for collecting random urine specimen.
- Explain reason for measuring specific gravity.
- Discuss significance of test if client shows interest.

# SKILL 45-6 Measuring Urine Glucose and Ketones

Another laboratory test a nurse may perform is measurement of urine glucose and ketones. There are clients with diabetes who learn to perform the test so they can monitor blood glucose regulation. Abnormal test results help these clients to adjust dietary intake, exercise levels, and insulin dosages. Normally glucose and ketones are not present in urine. Either element appearing in urine generally indicates that glucose is not effectively reaching the body's cells. A more accurate way to monitor blood glucose levels is by use of reflectance meters (Skill 45-15).

Testing urine can be performed by immersing a special chemically prepared strip of paper into a clean urine specimen or by adding drops of urine onto chemically prepared tablets. The change in color of the strip or tablet will indicate whether glucose or ketones are in urine.

Before beginning this procedure, the nurse should know the physiology of diabetes mellitus and how to collect a random or catheterized urine specimen (Skills 45-1 and 45-4).

### Purposes

1. Detect glucose or ketones in urine.
2. Monitor glucose and ketone levels to determine need for change in diabetic therapy.

## Procedure 45-6

| Steps | Rationale |
|---|---|
| **Assessment** | |
| 1. Assess if client or family member performs urine testing at home or if there is need for client to learn skill. | Client accustomed to testing own urine may prefer continuing to do so. |
| 2. Determine if physician has recommended specific type of reagent test for client to use. | Variety of reagent strips and tablets permit fast, accurate monitoring of urine glucose and ketones. |
| 3. Assess whether client, if diabetic, is familiar with double-voided specimens and uses technique regularly. | Double-voided specimen is essential for accuracy of glucose test. Clients often do not perceive importance of procedure. |
| 4. Assess type of medications client receives; check drug literature for effects on reagent strips and tablets. | Certain drug components create false-positive glucose readings. Some drugs that can alter reagents include cephalothin sodium (Keflin), ascorbic acid, chloral hydrate, sulfonamides, tetracyclines, and Levodopa. |
| 5. Assess client for signs and symptoms of diabetes mellitus: increased thirst, polyuria, polyphagia, recent loss of weight, pruritus of skin, fatigue. | Presence of these symptoms is often accompanied by glucose in urine (glucosuria). |
| 6. If diabetic, assess client's ability to perform urine test. | Determines level of instruction or assistance required from nurse. Diabetics may suffer from visual alterations or peripheral nerve damage that prevents them from performing test. |
| **Nursing Diagnosis** | |
| 1. Cluster data to reveal actual or potential nursing diagnoses: | |
| a. Fluid volume deficit: related to elevated blood sugar. | When high concentration of glucose is in blood, kidney excretes glucose. Glucose has diuretic effect of pulling water with it. Blood and protein may occur in urine when genitourinary tract is inflamed or damaged. |
| b. Altered nutrition: less than body requirements. | If glucose fails to reach body's cells, protein is broken down for energy. |
| c. Knowledge deficit regarding urine testing: related to inexperience. | Client's knowledge may not be sufficient to test urine correcty. |
| d. Noncompliance with urine testing: related to lack of interest. | May result from lack of understanding, lack of interest, or inability to perform test regularly. Client needs to understand implications of poor blood sugar control. |
| **Planning** | |
| 1. Develop individualized goals based on nursing diagnoses: | |
| a. Accurately detect amount of glucose and ketones in urine. | Amount in urine dictates dietary intake, exercise level, insulin dosage. |
| b. Regulate diet, exercise, medication at appropriate levels. | Keeping urine glucose between trace levels and negative and ketones at negative ensures glucose regulation. |
| c. Provide client with knowledge and skills to measure own urine. | Chronic diabetics must learn to monitor glucose levels in urine at home. |

| Steps | Rationale |
|---|---|
| 2. Prepare equipment and supplies: | |
| a. Bedpan or urinal (optional) | |
| b. Specimen container | |
| c. Watch with second hand or digital counter | Tablets must be exposed to urine for precise length of time. |
| d. *Reagent tablet testing:* | |
| ▪ 10 ml test tube | |
| ▪ Test tube holder | |
| ▪ Medicine dropper | |
| ▪ Clean container with 10 ml water | |
| ▪ Clinitest or Acetest tablets | |
| ▪ Tablet color chart | Color changes indicate amount of glucose/ketones in urine. |
| ▪ Facial tissue | |
| e. *Reagent strip testing:* | |
| ▪ Reagent test strip | Many different companies manufacture reagent strips. |
| ▪ Test strip color chart | Color changes indicate amount of glucose/ketones, blood and protein in urine. |
| f. Clean, disposable gloves (if person other than client tests urine.) | Universal precautions advocated by CDC. |
| 3. Explain reason for collecting double-voided specimen and how it is obtained. | Client must understand importance of precise glucose measurement for monitoring status of condition. Knowledge improves compliance. |
| 4. Explain why urine is tested. | Clients with diabetes should understand effects of disease and need for control of blood glucose. |

## Implementation

| Steps | Rationale |
|---|---|
| 1. Obtain double-voided specimen: | |
| a. Ask client to collect random urine specimen and discard. | Stagnant urine stored in bladder overnight or for long periods does not reveal amount of glucose and ketones excreted by kidney at time of testing. |
| b. Have client drink at least 8 oz water or preferred liquid. | Facilitates ability to void again within short time period. |
| c. 30 to 45 min later, have client collect another random specimen. | Fresh specimen will provide accurate test measurements. If client is catheterized, single, fresh specimen from catheter is adequate. |
| 2. Don gloves. | Universal precautions advocated by CDC. |
| 3. Perform glucose reagent tablet test, 5-drop test: | Measures 0% to 2% glucose. |
| a. Use medicine dropper to transfer 5 drops of well-mixed urine from container to test tube. Use 2-drop or 1-drop test with young children: 2-drop test = 2 drops urine and 10 drops water; 1-drop test = 1 drop urine and 11 drops water. | Proper volume of urine needed to ensure proper reaction of urine to agents in tablet. |
| b. Rinse dropper. | Prevents excess urine from being added to tube. |
| c. Add 10 drops of water to test tube. | Reagent tablet contains sodium hydroxide, which boils in water. |
| d. Add reagent tablet to test tube without touching to bare skin. | Combination of tablet and solution results in boiling effect. If fingers are moist, tablet will be caustic. |
| e. Place tube in holder or hold tube near top. | Chemical reacton produces heat that can cause burn. |
| f. Observe color change occurring as tablet boils. | Heat of reaction causes reduction of chemicals in tablet if glucose is present. Concentration of glucose determines color of urine solution. |
| g. 15 sec after boiling stops, shake tube gently and compare color of solution with color chart. | Comparison of color in test tube with standardized color chart indicates glucose concentration in urine. Delay in reading causes inaccuracy that can cause serious problems if treatments are initiated because of results. |
| h. Rinse test tube and drain. | Tube should be dry and free of chemicals for next test. |
| 4. Perform glucose/ketone reagent test strip test: | Strip test is often preferred over tablet test (3 above). |
| a. Immerse end of strip impregnated with chemical reagent into urine specimen (Fig. 45-7). | Immersion exposes reagent to urine constituents. Although Diastix, Clinistix, and Testape all measure quantity of glucose in urine, measurement scales are not interchangeable. |
| b. Remove strip immediately from container and tap it gently against container's side. | Excess urine can dilute reagents. |
| c. Hold strip in horizontal position. | Prevents possible mixing of chemical reagents. |
| d. Time for specified number of seconds and compare color of strip with color chart (Fig. 45-8). | Accurate interpretation of results depends on precise timing. Keto Stix, 15 sec; Clinistix, 10 sec; Diastix, 30 sec; Testape, 60 sec; Compare darkest part of tape with color chart. If results exceed 0.5%, wait another 60 sec and read (Table 45-1). |
| e. Dispose of reagent strip in trash. | Maintains neat environment and reduces spread of infection. |

**Steps** | **Rationale**

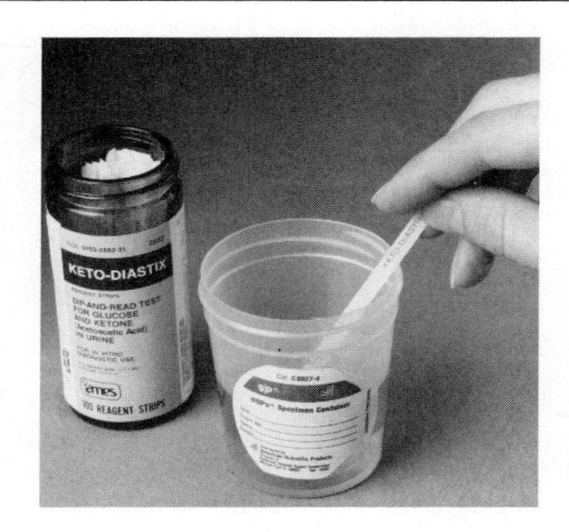

*Fig. 45-7*

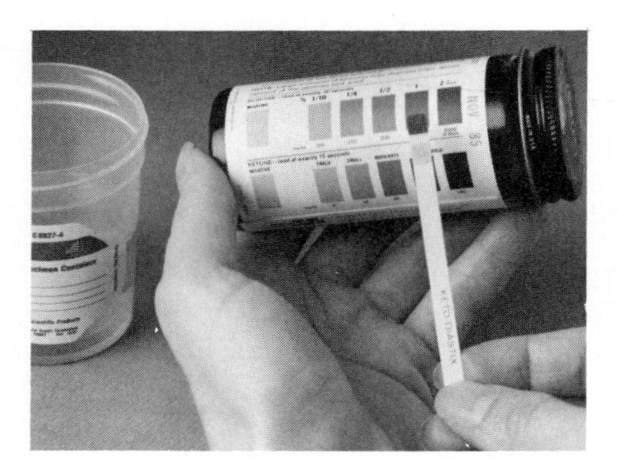
*Fig. 45-8*

***TABLE 45-1*** Multistix

| Test | When to Read | Range of Results |
|---|---|---|
| pH | Anytime | 5 to 9 |
| Protein | Anytime | (−) to +4 (72000 mg/d) |
| Glucose | 10 sec (qualitative) | (−) to +4 |
| | 30 sec (quantitative) | (−) to +4 (270) |
| Ketones | 15 sec | (−) to +3 (large) |
| Blood | 25 sec | (−) to +3 (large) |

5. Perform ketone (Acetest) tablet test. — Unnecessary if Ketostix, Multistix, and Diastix reagent test strips are used.
   a. Place Acetest tablet on white tissue. — Color of tablet changes to shades of tan or gray that can be seen more easily on white background.
   b. Add one drop of urine to tablet. — Begins chemical reaction.
   c. Time for 30 sec and compare tablet's color with Acetest color chart. — Time required for reagent to indicate ketone bodies.
   d. Discard tablet and tissue in trash. — Reduces transmission of microorganisms.
6. Wash hands after removing and discarding gloves. — Reduces transmission of microorganisms.
7. Discuss test results with client. — Client should participate in care to improve understanding and compliance.

## Evaluation

1. Note concentration of glucose or ketones in urine and compare with normal findings. — Determines if blood glucose is regulated.
2. Have client demonstrate testing and reading of results. — Reveals knowledge and understanding of procedure. Return demonstration is best form of feedback.

### *Expected outcomes*

1. Client is able to perform urine test. — Demonstrates learning.
2. Test results are negative for glucose and ketones. — Urine glucose is normally negligible and is reported as none, trace, 1+, 2+, 3+, or 4+. Acetones are reported as negative or positive.
3. Urine is not contaminated with feces.

### *Unexpected outcomes*

1. Client is unable to perform urine test. — Client may require further teaching or family member may need to learn skill.

| Steps | Rationale |
|---|---|
| 2. Test results reveal glucose, ketones, blood, and protein in urine. | Renal threshold for glucose is 180 mg/ml. Ketones appear as waste products in urine when fatty acids are used as energy. Ketones may appear in clients who are fasting, clients on low carbohydrate diets, clients with diabetes. Blood and protein may occur in urine when genitourinary tract is inflamed or damaged. |
| 3. Urine contaminated with feces. | |

## Recording and Reporting

| | |
|---|---|
| 1. Record results immediately in nurses' notes or glucose testing flow sheet. | Timely documentation ensures accurate therapeutic intervention. |
| 2. Have client in home setting record results of test on flow sheet. | Allows client to see variations in testing over several days. Provides record of testing between visits to physician. |
| 3. Report abnormal results to physician. | Physician usually sets guidelines as to what levels of glucose require insulin administration. Client should be informed when to call physician. |

## Follow-up Activity

| | |
|---|---|
| 1. Based on test results, nurse should check physician's orders to determine if insulin should be administered. | Physicians may order sliding scale of insulin dosage. For each concentration of glucose, different dosage of insulin is ordered. |

## Special Considerations

- Carefully read directions on bottles of test tablets and strips.
- Clarify with other health team member that Clinitest is to be done with one drop, two drops, or five drops of urine.
- School-age children can learn to test urine accurately; parents should learn to provide backup for the child.
- Other clients who undergo glucose testing are those receiving high concentrations of intravenous glucose (Chapter 29).
- Flow sheet may also require charting of any medication given and amount of urine.
- If client has difficulty complying with double-void specimen, first check voided specimen for sugar and acetone; however, this is not an accurate assessment of current blood glucose level.
- Urine testing for glucose and acetone has been used for many years to monitor glucose control by diet and insulin. Test is acceptable to clients because it is easily performed and causes no pain; however, it is being replaced by testing capillary blood, which is obtained by skin puncture of fingertip (Skill 45-15). This change is being made because capillary blood monitoring directly reflects current serum glucose levels and is not affected by renal threshold for glucose or fluid volume. Hypoglycemia, which cannot be detected by urine testing, may be identified by sampling of serum glucose.

## Teaching Considerations

- Instruct client on proper method for collecting random urine sample.
- If reagent tablets are used, keep them away from small children. Tablets contain caustic soda that can burn mouth and oral mucosa.
- Teach clients to check expiration date on bottle.
- Teach clients to store tablets in clean, dry area. Moisture can alter chemical makeup of tablets.
- Clients should be taught to tightly close bottles after removing reagent strips to prevent them from absorbing moisture and altering future results.
- Explain rationale for double-voided specimen and seek appropriate client feedback.
- Discuss the drugs that alter effect of urine on reagent.
- Explain relationship of urinary findings of glucose with blood glucose.
- Discuss possible reasons for finding acetone, blood, and protein in urine.
- Discuss relationship of urinary pH to urinary tract infection and formation of renal calculi when appropriate.
- Discuss reason for special precautions for Clinitest tablets.
- Have client return demonstrations on urine testing until they are correct.
- Discuss client's plans for testing urine at home, if indicated.

## Home Care Considerations

- Most kits sold in drug stores contain all equipment necessary for testing urine except specimen container.
- Clients at home may prefer to use large clock with second hand for timing urine tests.

# SKILL 45-7 Collecting a Stool Specimen

Laboratory examination and analysis of stool contains useful information about the nature of elimination. Stool specimens are collected to determine pathologic conditions such as tumors, hemorrhage, infection, and malabsorption problems. These conditions are detected by blood, bile, urobilinogen, fat, nitrogen content, ova, parasites, protozoa, and bacteria. Single stool specimens are most frequently collected but occasionally stool is collected for a timed period such as 72 hr.

Medical aseptic technique should be followed during collection of any stool specimen. Feces contain a variety of microorganisms that can easily be transmitted if specimens are handled incorrectly. Often, clients are capable of collecting their own specimens; thus it is important for them to know about aseptic technique. Because of the relative infrequency of defecation clients should also receive careful instructions about the purpose and technique of stool collection to ensure specimens are not accidentally discarded or mixed with urine or water.

Before beginning this procedure, the nurse should know how to assist a client with a bedpan (Chapter 30).

### Purposes

1. Screen for abnormal constituents in stool.
2. Measure the volume of fecal contents to determine intestinal absorption problems.

## Procedure 45-7

| Steps | Rationale |
|---|---|
| **Assessment** | |
| 1. Determine purpose of stool specimen and correct method of obtaining and handling specimen. | Prevents collection of specimen at time when laboratory cannot test it. |
| 2. Determine if client should have dietary modifications or restrictions before test. | Prevents invalid test results on stool specimen. |
| 3. Assess understanding of reason for collection of stool specimen. | Reveals client's ability and willingness to cooperate in collection of specimen. |
| 4. Ask client when next bowel movement is anticipated. Determine normal defecation pattern. | Allows for more effective planning. If client has bowel movement only once every 3 to 5 days it may be best to give client suppository or enema or have client obtain specimen at home. |
| 5. Assess ability to assist in collection of stool specimen:<br>a. Ability to use toilet facilities.<br>b. Ability to handle specimen container. | Because defecation is private matter, most clients prefer to be as independent in collection as possible. |
| 6. Assess client for discomfort associated with defecation. | Particular type of discomfort might suggest specific elimination problem such as hemorrhoids. |
| 7. Assess client for gastrointestinal dysfunction, such as abdominal pain, nausea, vomiting, excessive flatus, diarrhea. | May indicate specific physical problem. |
| **Nursing Diagnosis** | |
| 1. Cluster data to reveal actual or potential nursing diagnoses: | |
| a. Constipation: related to dietary habits. | Nurse will observe stool specimen closely for blood. |
| b. Fluid volume deficit: related to dehydration. | Chronic diarrheal stools can lead to dehydration. |
| c. Knowledge deficit regarding test procedure: related to inexperience. | Client may require instruction about purpose and importance of test. |
| d. Anxiety: related to specimen collection. | Client may suffer embarrassment about test procedure. |
| e. Toileting self-care deficit: related to physical weakness. | Client will often require assistance to collect specimen. |
| **Planning** | |
| 1. Develop individualized goals based on nursing diagnoses: | |
| a. Obtain fecal specimen uncontaminated by urine, water, or toilet tissue. | Ensures accurate test results. |
| b. Protect client's privacy. | Allows client to relax during defecation so specimen can more easily be obtained. |
| c. Promote client's understanding of elimination alterations. | Client may require information as to significance of test and its relationship to physical condition. |

| Steps | Rationale |
|---|---|
| 2. Prepare equipment and supplies: | |
| a. Waxed cardboard container with lid or sterile test tube with swab | |
| b. Two tongue blades | Used to transfer feces into cardboard container. |
| c. Paper towel | Used to wrap tongue blades before disposal. |
| d. Clean or sterile bedpan, bedside commode, specimen hat, potty chair | Feces should not be mixed with water or urine. Clean, dry receptacle should be used. |
| e. Clean, disposable gloves | Prevents contact of hands with feces, reducing risk of transfer of infection. |
| f. Completed specimen identification label<br>g. Completed laboratory requisition | Completion of label and requisition before collecting specimen prevents confusing it with other specimens and allows more rapid transport to laboratory. |
| h. Signs to remind client and staff of timed specimen (optional) | Prevents accidental disposal of specimens. |
| 3. Prepare client or family member for procedure: | |
| a. Explain reason stool specimen is needed and how client can assist with collection. | Understanding promotes cooperation. Client will more likely be able to collect specimen independently. |
| b. Explain that specimen should be free of urine, water, toilet tissue. | Urine changes character of feces. Water can dilute constituents of stool. |
| c. Ask client to notify nurse immediately after defecating. | Nurse can contain specimen before odor permeates client's room. |
| 4. Refer to agency procedures for proper way to collect or handle specimens. | Agencies may vary as to specimen collection procedures. |

## Implementation

| Steps | Rationale |
|---|---|
| 1. If client unable to use bathroom, close room door or bedside curtains. | Allows client to relax, promoting defecation. |
| 2. Wash hands. | Reduces spread of infection. |
| 3. Assist client as needed into bathroom or onto commode bedpan. | Client's physical mobility and level of fatigue will influence amount of assistance needed. |
| 4. Instruct client to void into toilet before defecating (discard urine before collecting specimen in bedpan or potty chair container). | Feces should not be mixed with urine or toilet tissue. Urine inhibits fecal bacterial growth. Toilet tissue contains bismuth, which interferes with test results. |
| 5. Provide client with clean, dry bedpan, specimen hat, potty chair in which to defecate. | Feces should not be mixed with urine or water. |
| 6. If needed, assist client in washing after toileting and leave in safe, comfortable position after defecation. | Promotes comfort and sense of well-being. |
| 7. Take covered bedpan or other container with stool to bathroom or utility room. | Covering bedpan and removing it from client's room reduces odor and client's embarrassment. |
| 8. Put on clean, disposable gloves (optional). | Provide extra barrier between nurse and stool and prevents transfer of bacteria to skin; however, they do not substitute for good handwashing technique. |
| 9. Obtain specimen: | |
| a. *For culture:* Remove swab from sterile test tube, gather bean-size piece of stool, return swab to tube. If stool is liquid, soak cotton swab in it and return to tube. | Stool is touched only by sterile swab to prevent introduction of extraneous bacteria. |
| b. *For other tests:* Obtain specimen by using tongue blades to transfer representative portion of stool to container. (An inch of formed stool or 15 ml liquid stool). | Use of tongue blades prevents transfer of bacteria to hands or other objects. |
| c. *For timed stool specimen:* All of each stool is placed in waxed cardboard containers for specific time ordered and kept in specimen refrigerator. | Tests for dietary products and digestive enzymes such as fat content or bile require analysis of all feces over time. |
| 10. For timed tests, place signs stating, "Save all stool" over client's bed, on bathroom door, above toilet. | Helps prevent accidental disposal of stool. |
| 11. Immediately place lid on container tightly. | Prevents spread of microorganisms by air or contact with other articles. |
| 12. Wrap used tongue blades in paper towels and dispose in trash. Remove disposable gloves and discard. | Reduces spread of microorganisms. |
| 13. Empty and clean bedpan or other container used to collect specimen and return it to its place. | Makes them ready for use when needed. |
| 14. Wash hands. | Reduces spread of microorganisms. |
| 15. Attach specimen identification label and laboratory requisition with date, time, test name on it. | Inappropriate identification of specimen can lead to errors in diagnosis and therapy. |
| 16. Send specimen to laboratory immediately or place in specimen refrigerator. (See Special Considerations.) | Fresh specimen provides most accurate results. |

| Steps | Rationale |
|---|---|
| **Evaluation** | |
| 1. Check laboratory test results and compare with normal stool test values. | Determines abnormal amounts or types of contituents. |
| 2. Note character of stool during collection. | Certain abnormal constituents such as blood, mucus, pus may be seen by naked eye. |
| 3. Ask client to describe how to obtain specimen. | Reveals knowledge or understanding of procedure. |
| ***Expected outcomes*** | |
| 1. Stool specimen is not contaminated with urine. | Ensures test results will be accurate. |
| 2. Stool does not have any abnormal constituents. | Documents absence of specific gastrointestinal problems. |
| ***Unexpected outcomes*** | |
| 1. Stool specimen is discarded. | Client may have very infrequent bowel routine or be constipated. Instructions were insufficient. |
| 2. Stool contains abnormal constituents. | Indicates some type of medical problem. |
| **Reporting and Recording** | |
| 1. Record time and date specimen collected and disposition in nurses' notes. | Documents collection of specimen. |
| 2. Record appearance and odor of stool and if client had any discomfort during defecation. | Data may help confirm some specific medical problem. |
| 3. Discuss significant test results with physician. | Allows for more prompt interventions when needed. |
| **Follow-up Activity** | |
| 1. If diet was modified because of specimen collection, arrange for client to receive ordered diet. | Maintains normal dietary intake. |

## Special Considerations

- Check institutional policy for types of specimen containers; some tests may require preservatives.
- If a question exists about when and how specimen should be collected, consult institutional policy or procedural manual or consult laboratory.
- With infant or non-toilet-trained child, specimen of stool can be taken from diaper. If stool is liquid, plastic liner inside diaper eases collection.
- Children are often unable to predict next bowel movement; however, defecation tends to occur more frequently. Parents can often assist.
- Children will be more cooperative if able to use familiar toileting facilities.
- If client does not have bowel movement within 24 hrs after specimen is requested, physician may desire insertion of cotton swab into rectum for specimen, particularly if it is for culture *and* if the client is infant or young child.
- Commercially available culture tubes contain ampule of medium that can be crushed within tube. Moisture permits bacteria to remain viable until they reach laboratory.
- If feces contains blood, pus, mucus, sample should be included in specimen.
- Specimen for ova and parasites should be sent to the lab while it is still warm and examined within 30 min. Three random, normally passed stools are needed to ensure accurate test results.
- If client is in isolation, specimen is placed in paper bag for transport.

## Teaching Considerations

- Clients collecting their own specimens at home should be instructed when and how to collect specimen.
- Clients should be instructed to properly store specimen before bringing it to the laboratory for analysis.
- Discuss purpose of collecting stool specimen.
- Discuss client's role in collecting specimen.
- Instruct client about procedure to use to keep stool free from urine and paper.

# SKILL 45-8 Measuring Occult Blood in Stool

A common fecal laboratory test is the guaiac test for occult blood. The test measures microscopic amounts of blood in the feces. Normally a person loses small amounts of blood daily in the feces as a result of minor abrasions of the nasopharyngeal or oral mucosa. If greater than 50 ml of blood enters the feces from the upper gastrointestinal tract, the blood can be visualized as melena. The guaiac test helps to reveal blood visually undetectable. The test is a useful diagnostic tool for conditions such as colon cancer, upper gastrointestinal ulcers, and localized gastric or intestinal irritation.

The test is easy to perform. Clients are often instructed on how to collect fecal specimens for the test in the home. Only a small amount of stool is needed to perform the test successfully. The most common guaiac tests are the Hemoccult slides and the Hematest tablets.

Before beginning this procedure, the nurse should know how to collect a stool specimen (Skill 45-7).

### Purposes

1. Screen clients at known risk for developing gastrointestinal bleeding.
2. Detect colon cancer at an early stage.

## Procedure 45-8

| Steps | Rationale |
|---|---|
| **Assessment** | |
| 1. Assess client's or family members' understanding of need for stool test. | Provides nurse with data base on which to provide necessary health teaching. |
| 2. Assess client's ability to cooperate with procedure and collect specimen. | To avoid embarrassment, clients often prefer to collect own stool specimen. Some clients will require assistance. |
| 3. Assess client's medical history for bleeding or gastrointestinal disorder. | Routine screening can be instituted by nurse. |
| 4. Assess type of medications client receives. Note drugs that can cause gastrointestinal mucosal bleeding. | Anticoagulants will increase risk of bleeding in gastrointestinal tract, even from minor trauma to mucosa. Long-term use of steroids and acetylsalicylic acid can irritate mucosa. |
| 5. Refer to physician's orders for medication or dietary modifications or restrictions before test. | Certain medications such as iron supplement and bismuth compounds can cause stools to resemble melena. Rare meats can cause same results. |
| **Nursing Diagnosis** | |
| 1. Cluster data to reveal actual or potential nursing diagnoses: | |
| a. Anxiety related to:<br>▪ Possible gastrointestinal bleeding.<br>▪ Knowledge deficit regarding testing or risk for bleeding. | When client undergoes screening tests, there can be much apprehension over possible findings. Nurse's instructions may include steps and purpose of procedure and why certain conditions or medications cause risk of bleeding. |
| **Planning** | |
| 1. Develop individualized goals based on nursing diagnoses: | |
| a. Accurately determine microscopic presence of blood in stool. | Detection of gastrointestinal bleeding is important for diagnosis and treatment intervention. |
| b. Obtain specimen free of urine. | Ensures accurate test results. |
| c. Instruct client on importance of occult blood screening. | Explanation of purpose of procedure clarifies importance of health promotion. |
| 2. Prepare equipment and supplies:<br>a. Paper towel<br>b. Disposable gloves<br>c. Wooden applicator<br>d. *Hemoccult test* (Fig. 45-9):<br>▪ Cardboard Hemoccult slide<br>▪ Hemoccult developing solution | |

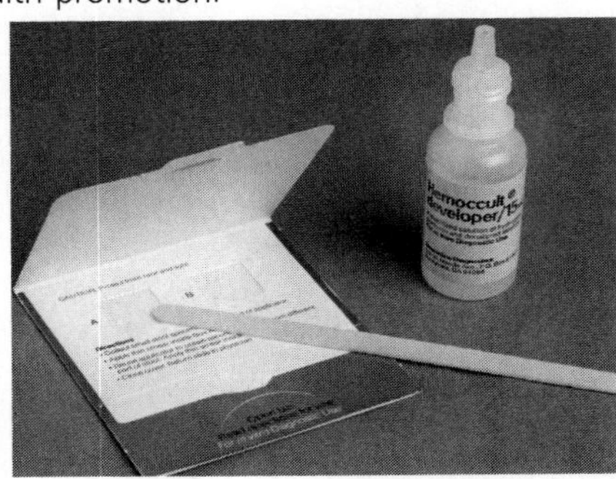


*Fig. 45-9*

| Steps | Rationale |
|---|---|

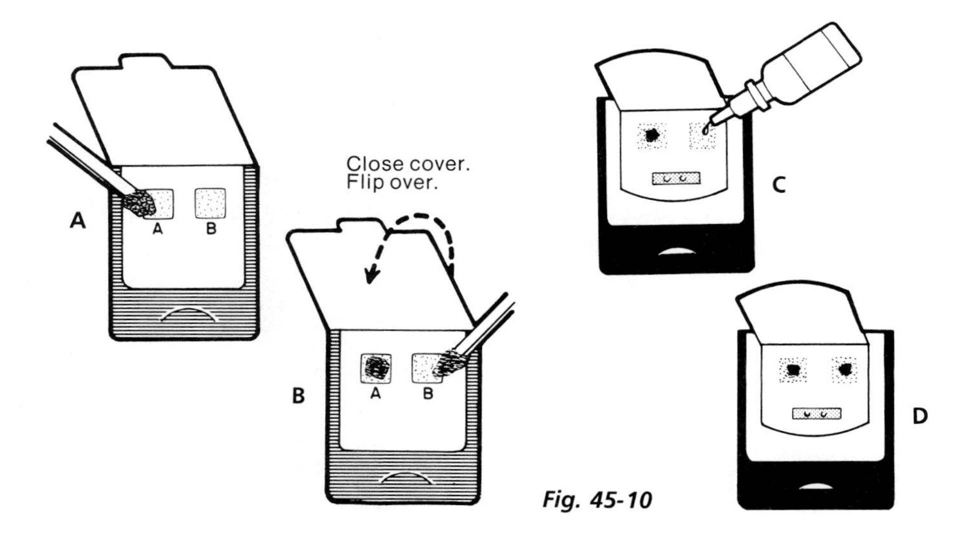

*Fig. 45-10*

| Steps | Rationale |
|---|---|
| e. *Hematest:* | |
| ▪ Hematest tablets | Tablets must be protected from moisture, heat, and light. |
| ▪ Guaiac paper | Reagent tablet produces blue reaction on guaiac paper if fecal smear contains blood. |
| ▪ Sink with running water | |
| 3. Explain purpose of test and how client can assist. | Client's understanding of test's purpose provides cooperation and minimizes anxiety. |
| 4. Be sure dietary or medication restrictions were followed. | Ensures accurate test results. |

## Implementation

| Steps | Rationale |
|---|---|
| 1. Wash hands and apply clean, disposable gloves. | Reduces transmission of microorganisms from fecal specimen to nurse's hands. |
| 2. Obtain uncontaminated stool specimen (Skill 45-7). | Specimen is obtained in clean, dry container and not contaminated with urine, water, toilet tissue. |
| 3. Use tip of wooden applicator to obtain small portion of feces. | Small specimen is sufficient for measuring blood content. |
| 4. Perform Hemoccult slide test: | |
| a. Open flap of slide and apply thin smear of stool on paper in first box (Fig. 45-10, *A*). | Guaiac paper inside box is sensitive to fecal blood content. Occult blood from upper gastrointestinal tract is not always equally dispersed through stool. |
| b. Obtain second fecal specimen from different portion of stool and apply thinly to slide's second box (Fig. 45-10, *B*). | Findings of occult blood are more conclusive for gastrointestinal bleeding when entire specimen is found to contain blood. |
| c. Close slide cover and turn slide over to reverse side. Open cardboard flap and apply 2 drops of Hemoccult developing solution on each box of guaiac paper (Fig. 45-10, *C*). | Developing solution penetrates underlying fecal specimen. Blood is indicated by change in color of guaiac paper. |
| d. Read results of test after 30 to 60 sec (Fig. 45-10, *D*). Note color changes. | Bluish discoloration indicates occult blood (guaiac positive). No change in color of guaiac paper indicates negative results. |
| e. Dispose of test slide in proper receptacle. | Reduces transfer of microorganisms. |
| 5. Perform test using Hematest tablets: | |
| a. Place small amount of fecal specimen on guaiac paper. | Guaiac paper is sensitive in detecting fecal blood content. |
| b. Place Hematest tablet on top of stool specimen. | Tablet contains solid form of developing solution. |
| c. Apply 2 to 3 drops of tap water on tablet, allowing water to flow onto guaiac paper. | Tap water dissolves Hematest tablet and thus dispenses developing solution over specimen and guaiac paper. |
| d. Observe color of guaiac paper within 2 min. | Bluish discoloration is guaiac positive. Do not read color after 2 min. False findings may occur. |
| e. Dispose of tablet and paper in proper receptacle. | Reduces transmission of microorganisms. |
| 6. Wrap wooden applicator in paper towel and dispose in proper receptacle. | Reduces risk of microorganisms. |
| 7. Wash hands after removing and discarding gloves. | Reduces spread of infection. |

| Steps | Rationale |
|---|---|
| **Evaluation** | |
| 1. Note color changes in guaiac paper. | Reveals blood in feces. |
| 2. Note character of stool specimen. | Certain abnormal constituents of stool may be visible. |
| 3. Ask client to explain collection procedure. | Documents level of learning. |
| ***Expected outcome*** | |
| 1. Test for occult blood is negative. | Client only has small amount of blood in feces due to normal nasopharyngeal and oral mucosa abrasions. |
| ***Unexpected outcome*** | |
| 1. Test for occult blood is positive. | Client has quantity of blood greater than 50 ml arising from upper gastrointestinal tract. |
| **Recording and Reporting** | |
| 1. Record results of test in nurses' notes. | All specimen test results should be documented. |
| 2. Record any unusual characteristics of stool in nurses' notes. | Findings may indicate need for further diagnosis. |
| 3. Report positive test results to nurse in charge or physician. | Indication of bleeding may change therapy. |
| **Follow-up Activity** | |
| 1. After tests are completed, confer with physician for renewal of medications or diet. | Findings may result in change of medications and diet. Further testing may be ordered if results are positive. |

## Special Considerations

- Note that hemorrhoids can cause bleeding that may be misinterpreted as upper gastrointestinal bleeding.
- Some physicians order a meat-free diet 3 days before test or restrict clients from taking following medications for 48 hr before test: iron preparations, bromides, iodides, rauwolfia derivatives, indomethacin, salicylates, colchicine, bismuth comounds, ascorbic acid, phenylbutazone, steroids (if client can tolerate).
- Single positive test result does not confirm bleeding or indicate colorectal cancer. For confirmed positive results, test must be repeated at least 3 times while client is on meat-free, high-residue diet. More in-depth diagnosis is needed with positive results.
- Children of school age and over may be curious and ask several questions about test.

## Teaching Considerations

- See Skill 45-7.
- Clients should obtain specimens from two different areas of stool specimen.
- If client has been on long-term steroid or anticoagulant drug therapy, explain how these drugs may result in occult blood in stools.
- If physician orders meat-free diet before test, explain its significance to test results; red meats can cause false positive results.
- Discuss reason for multiple testing of stool for occult blood. Clients are usually requested to obtain specimen every day for 3 days.

## Home Care Considerations

- Many clients are instructed to collect specimens at home and return them to clinic or physician's office.
- Clients who collect specimen at home are asked to prepare slide with feces, close cardboard slide, and return to office or clinic for specimen developing.

# *SKILL 45-9 Collecting Nose and Throat Specimens for Culture*

Clients frequently have signs or symptoms of upper respiratory or sinus infections. A nose or throat culture specimen is a simple diagnostic tool for determining the nature of the client's problem. The laboratory places the specimen on a culture medium to determine if pathogenic organisms will grow.

This specimen collection can cause discomfort to sensitive mucosal membranes. Likewise, collection of a throat culture may cause gagging. Clients should clearly understand how each specimen is to be collected to minimize anxiety or discomfort.

### Purposes

1. Detect pathogenic microorganisms in the nose and throat.
2. Determine which antibiotics are resistant to or effective against the microorganisms discovered.
3. Screen for microorganisms that can colonize in the nose.

## Procedure 45-9

| Steps | Rationale |
|---|---|
| **Assessment** | |
| 1. Assess understanding of purpose of procedure and ability to cooperate. | Provides basis to determine need for health teaching. |
| 2. Assess condition of and drainage from nasal mucosa and sinuses. | Reveals physical signs that may indicate infection or allergic irritation. Clear drainage usually indicates allergy. Yellow, green, brown drainage usually indicates infection. |
| 3. Determine if client has experienced postnasal drip, sinus headache or tenderness, nasal congestion, sore throat. | Symptoms help reveal nature of problem. |
| 4. Assess condition of posterior pharynx. Pay particular attention to areas of inflammation or purulent drainage. | Identification of inflamed or purulent areas allows nurse to swab those sites quickly. |
| 5. Assess client for systemic signs of infection: fever, chills, fatigue. | Infection originating within nasopharynx can become systemic, requiring antibiotic therapy. |
| 6. Review physician's orders to determine if nose, throat, or both cultures are needed. | Prevents exposing client to unnecessary discomfort of repeated cultures. |
| **Diagnosis** | |
| 1. Cluster data to reveal actual or potential nursing diagnoses: | |
| a. Anxiety: related to nature of procedure. | Procedure can be threatening. There is slight discomfort. |
| b. Pain: related to mucosal inflammation. | Nasal, pharyngeal sinus membranes become very sensitive when inflamed. |
| c. Knowledge deficit regarding specimen collection: related to inexperience. | Client requires instructions about procedure and purpose. |
| d. Ineffective breathing pattern: related to nasal or sinus congestion. | Client may experience shortness of breath and have elevated respiratory rate. |
| **Planning** | |
| 1. Develop individualized goals for client based on nursing diagnoses: | |
| a. Obtain specimen not contaminated by saliva. | Allows correct identification of pathogens in nose and throat. |
| b. Minimize trauma to client. | Procedure can cause anxiety and discomfort. |
| 2. Prepare equipment and supplies: | |
| a. 2 sterile swabs in sterile culture tubes (Flexible wire swab with cotton tip may be used for nose cultures.) | Used to collect specimen. |
| b. Nasal speculum (optional) | |
| c. Emesis basin or clean container (optional) | Used to hold speculum. |
| d. Tongue blades | Used to depress tongue to visualize pharynx. |
| e. Penlight | |
| f. Completed identification labels | Label and requisition facilitates correct identification of specimen and ensure prompt delivery to laboratory. |
| g. Completed laboratory requisition (date, time, name of test, source of culture) | |
| h. Facial tissues | |
| i. Clean, disposable gloves | |
| 3. Explain reason nose, throat culture is needed and how client can assist. | Eases anxiety and promotes cooperation. |
| 4. Explain that client may have tickling sensation or gag during swabbing of throat. Nasal swab may create urge to sneeze. Both procedures take only few seconds. | Allows client to be prepared for sensations and thus cooperate more fully. |
| 5. Refer to agency procedures for collection of specimen. | Agency policies may vary. |

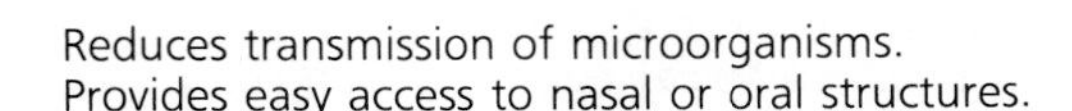

| Steps | Rationale |
|---|---|
| **Implementation** | |
| 1. Wash hands and put on gloves. | Reduces transmission of microorganisms. |
| 2. Ask client to sit erect in bed or chair facing nurse. Acutely ill client or young child may lie back against bed with head of bed raised to 45-degree angle. | Provides easy access to nasal or oral structures. |
| 3. Have swab in tube ready for use. Nurse may wish to loosen top so swab can easily be removed. | Nurse should be able to grasp swab easily without danger of contaminating it. Most commercially prepared tubes have top that fits securely over end of swab, which allows nurse to touch outer top without contaminating swab stick. |
| 4. Collect throat culture: | |
| a. Instruct client to tilt head backward. For clients in bed, place pillow behind shoulders. | Facilitates visualization of pharynx. |
| b. Ask client to open mouth and say "ah." | Permits exposure of pharynx, relaxes throat muscles, minimizes gag reflex. |
| c. If pharynx not visualized, depress tongue with tongue blade and note inflamed areas of pharynx or tonsils. Depress anterior ⅓ of tongue only. (Illuminate with penlight as needed.) | Area to be swabbed should be clearly visualized. Placement of tongue blade along back of tongue more likely initiates gag reflex. |
| d. Insert swab without touching lips, teeth, tongue, cheeks. | Touching lips or oral mucosal structures can contaminate swab with resident bacteria. |
| e. Gently but quickly swab tonsillar area side to side, making contact with inflamed or purulent sites (Fig. 45-11). | These areas contain most microorganisms. |
| f. Carefully withdraw swab without striking oral structures. Immediately place swab in culture tube and crush ampule at bottom of tube. Push tip of swab into liquid medium. | Retains microorganisms within culture tube. Mixing swab tip with culture medium ensures life of bacteria for testing. |
| g. Place top on culture tube securely. | Prevents contamination from microorganisms. |
| h. Discard tongue depressor into trash. | Reduces transmission of microorganisms. |
| i. Remove gloves and discard. | |

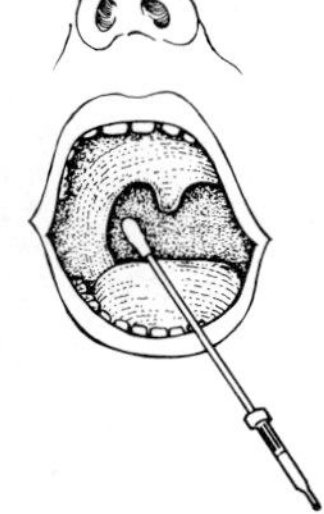

***Fig. 45-11***

| Steps | Rationale |
|---|---|
| 5. Collect nose culture: | |
| a. Encourage client to blow nose and check nostrils for patency with penlight. | Clears nasal passages of mucus containing resident bacteria. |
| b. Ask client to alternatively occlude each nostril and exhale. | Determines nostril with greater patency, from which specimen will be collected. |
| c. Ask client to tilt head back. Clients in bed should have pillow behind shoulders. | Facilitates visualization of nasal septum and sinuses. |
| d. Gently insert nasal speculum in one nostril. | Allows retraction of mucosa for easier swab insertion. |
| e. Carefully pass swab through center of speculum into nostril until it reaches that portion of mucosa that is inflamed or containing exudate. Rotate swab quickly. | Swab should remain sterile until it reaches area to be cultured. Rotating swab covers all surfaces with exudate. |
| f. Remove swab without touching sides of speculum. | Prevents contamination of swab by resident bacteria. |
| g. Carefully remove nasal speculum and place in basin. Offer client facial tissue. | Minimizes period of time client will experience discomfort. |
| h. Insert swab into culture tube. Crush ampule at bottom of tube and push tip of swab into liquid medium. | Retains microorganisms within culture tube. Mixing swab tip with culture medium ensures life of bacteria for testing. |
| i. Place top on tube securely. | Prevents contamination from microorganisms. |
| j. Remove gloves and discard. | |
| 6. Wash hands. | Reduces transmission of microorganisms. |
| 7. Securely attach properly completed identification label and laboratory requisition to culture tube. | Incorrect identification of specimen could result in diagnostic or therapeutic errors. |
| 8. Send specimen immediately to laboratory or refrigerate. | Fresh specimen provides most accurate test results. |
| **Evaluation** | |
| 1. Check laboratory record for results of culture test. | Results reveal type of organisms in nose or pharynx and antibiotics most likely to be effective. |
| 2. Inspect client's nose for evidence of bleeding. | Speculum and swab can traumatize sensitive, fragile mucosa. |

| Steps | Rationale |
|---|---|
| ***Expected outcomes*** | |
| 1. There is no bacterial growth in specimens. | Proves absence of infection. |
| 2. Client does not experience bleeding of nasal mucosa. | Procedure is atraumatic. |
| 3. Specimen is not contaminated. | Evidenced by results of laboratory analysis. |
| ***Unexpected outcomes*** | |
| 1. Nose, throat cultures reveal bacterial growth. | Evidence of upper respiratory or sinus infection. |
| 2. Client experiences minor nasal bleeding. | Trauma to sensitive mucosa causes bleeding, which should disappear with mild pressure over bridge of nose or application of ice. |
| 3. Specimen is contaminated. | Result of abundant number of resident bacteria on swab. |
| **Recording and Reporting** | |
| 1. Record specimen collection, date, time in nurses' notes. | All specimens should be documented to verify procedure performed. |
| 2. Describe appearance of nasal and oral mucosal structures in nurses' notes. | Physical signs may add to diagnostic data base. |
| 3. Report unusual test results to physician or nurse in charge. | Findings may indicate need for therapy (e.g., antibiotic administration). |

### Special Considerations

- The nurse often needs assistance to obtain throat cultures from confused, combative, unconscious, very young clients.
- Immobilization of child's head and arms is important when obtaining nose or throat culture and should be done in firm, gentle, kind manner. Ask parents if they wish to assist or if they prefer another nurse to do it.
- Showing the tongue blade and penlight to child and demonstrating how to say "ah" helps to decrease anxiety.
- School-age child will be more cooperative if given the opportunity to ask questions about procedure and results.
- If client gags, remove tongue blade and allow to relax before reinserting.
- Most agencies use commercially available culture tubes containing special transport medium.
- Agency policy may dictate type of information to place on label. Note on laboratory requisition if client is taking antibiotic or if specific organism is suspected (e.g., *Bordetella pertussis*).

### Teaching Considerations

- Allowing young children to visualize and examine speculum decreases their fear of it.
- Clients should be instructed that procedure is painless but gagging is common.
- Explain how and why specimen is being obtained.
- Discuss relationship between culture results and medication.
- Discuss client's role in collecting specimen.
- Discuss reason for time delay in receiving culture results.

## *SKILL 45-10 Obtaining Vaginal or Urethral Discharge Specimens*

Normally there is minimal discharge from the vagina or urethra. Poor hygiene practices may cause an accumulation of discharge. However, if a client develops an increased amount or change in character of discharge from the vagina or urethra, medical follow-up is necessary. Drainage from the vagina or urethra is normally thin, nonpurulent, whitish or clear, and small in amount. A woman will have bloody discharge during menstruation. A newborn infant may have bloody discharge from the vagina for 2 to 4 weeks after birth due to the abrupt decrease in maternal hormones at birth.

The most common types of clients requiring cultures of vaginal or urethral discharge have signs and symptoms of sexually transmitted disease or urinary tract infection. Clients suspected of having a sexually transmitted disease may be embarrassed by their condition. The nurse must show respect and understanding toward the client. If the client undergoes a complete diagnostic work-up, the many questions can be exhausting and cause anxiety. When collecting vaginal or urethral specimens the nurse should work quickly and calmly, maintaining the client's privacy at all times.

Before beginning this procedure, the nurse should know the communicable nature of sexually transmitted disease and the principles of human sexuality.

**Purposes**

1. Detect pathogenic microorganisms in vaginal or urethral discharge.
2. Determine which antibiotics are effective against or resistant to microorganisms discovered.

## Procedure 45-10

| Steps | Rationale |
|---|---|
| **Assessment** | |
| 1. Assess understanding of need for culture and ability to cooperate with procedure. | Provides data on which nurse develops teaching plan. |
| 2. Assess condition of external genitalia. Observe urethra, meatus, vaginal orifice for redness, swelling, tenderness, discharge that is whitish, mucoid, purulent. | Assessment findings and specimen test results reveal nature of problem. |
| 3. Ask client if dysuria, localized pruritus of genitalia, lower abdominal pain have been experienced. | Symptoms of urinary tract or vaginal infection. |
| 4. If symptoms suggest sexually transmitted disease, collect sexual history of client. | It is important to know nature of client's disease and to what extent sexual partners have been exposed to infection. |
| 5. Refer to physician's order for type of culture. | Client may require one or both types of cultures. |
| **Nursing Diagnosis** | |
| 1. Cluster data to reveal actual or potential nursing diagnoses: | |
| a. Anxiety: related to nature of specimen collection. | Nurse must use caution to protect client's privacy. |
| b. Alteration in comfort: related to vaginal/urethral inflammation. | Pruritus, abdominal pain, and dysuria can be very uncomfortable. |
| c. Potential sexual dysfunction. | Client may have actual or perceived limitations resulting from any discomforts associated with genitalia. |
| d. Alter patterns of urinary elimination: related to dysuria caused from inflamed tissues. | Normal voiding patterns are altered due to client's discomfort. |
| **Planning** | |
| 1. Develop individualized goals based on nursing diagnoses: | |
| a. Collect uncontaminated specimen of urethra or vagina. | Culture should not contain cells of skin or mucous membranes. Exact identification of pathogens in vagina or urethra is necessary for proper treatment. |
| b. Maintain client's privacy. | Need to have culture of urethra or vagina can be very embarrassing. |
| c. Maintain client's self-esteem. | Nurse must not act judgmentally or negatively toward client during specimen collection. |
| 2. Prepare equipment and supplies: | |
| a. Sterile swab in sterile culture tube (Commercially available culture tubes have swab and tube with ampule containing special transport medium.) | Used to collect specimen. |
| b. Sheet, blanket, paper drape | Prevents unnecessary exposure of genitalia. |
| c. Clean, disposable gloves | |
| d. Penlight or gooseneck lamp | |
| e. Completed identification labels | Label and requisition facilitate correct identification of specimen and ensure prompt delivery to lab. |
| f. Completed laboratory requisition (date, time, name of test, type of culture) | |
| 3. Prepare client for procedure: | |
| a. Instruct female client not to douche before specimen collection. | Irrigation of vaginal canal removes discharge containing microorganisms. |
| b. Explain reason vaginal or urethral culture is needed and how client can assist with procedure. | Promotes understanding and cooperation. |
| c. Assure client that procedure will be done in room where privacy can be maintained. | Decreases embarrassment. |
| d. Describe steps of procedure and ensure that it is painless. | Minimizes fear. |

| Steps | Rationale |
|---|---|

## Implementation

1. Wash hands. — Reduces transmission of microorganisms.
2. Draw bedside curtains or close room door. Place "do not enter" sign on door (if available). — Provides privacy for client and demonstrates nurse's respect for client's well-being.
3. Assist client to proper position, raise gown, and drape body parts to be exposed: — Provides easy access to perineal area. Draping minimizes exposure of body parts, minimizing anxiety.
   a. *Female:* Dorsal recumbent position (Fig. 45-12) with sheet draped over each leg and genitalia.
   b. *Male:* Sit on chair or bed or lie supine with sheet draped across lower trunk and genitalia.

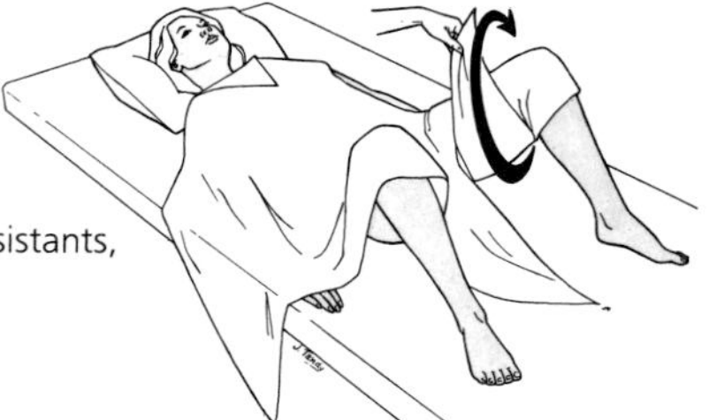

***Fig. 45-12***

From Sorrentino SA: Mosby's textbook for nursing assistants, ed 2, St. Louis, 1987, The CV Mosby Co.

4. Apply clean, disposable gloves. — Prevents contamination of nurse's hands from discharge.
5. Direct light source onto perineum (May not be needed for male client). — Allows better visualization or urethral or vaginal structures.
6. Open culture tube and hold swab in dominant hand. — Provides for easier manipulation of swab during culture collection.
7. Instruct client to slowly deep breathe. — Helps client to relax. Tensing of muscles around pelvic floor may cause discomfort during swabbing.
8. Obtain necessary specimens:
   a. *Female:*
      - With nondominant hand, fully separate labia to expose vaginal orifice. — Exposes perineum and ensures specimen is of vaginal discharge.
      - Touch tip of swab into discharge pool, being careful not to touch skin or mucosa along perineum or vaginal canal. If no discharge is visible, gently insert swabs 1 to 2.5 cm (½ to 1 in) into vaginal orifice and rotate before removal. — Discharge contains the greatest concentration of microorganisms.
      - To expose urethral meatus, use nondominant hand to pull gently on labia minora upward and back. — Labia are often retracted over urethral orifice.
      - Use clean swab and gently apply to tip of meatus where discharge is visible. Avoid touching labia. — Discharge contains greatest concentration of microorganisms.
   b. *Male:*
      - Hold penis near tip with nondominant hand; if male is uncircumcised, gently retract foreskin. — Provides clear exposure of urethral meatus.
      - Use dominant hand to hold swab. Apply gently to area of discharge at urinary meatus. If no discharge is apparent, physician may order swab to be introduced into urinary meatus. — Discharge contains greatest number of microorganisms.
      - Return foreskin to natural position. — Tightening of foreskin around shaft of penis can cause localized discomfort and edema.
9. Return each swab to culture tube and secure top. — Retains microorganisms within tube.
10. Remove and discard gloves. — Reduces spread of microorganisms. Gloves should not be worn while handling outer portion of tube.
11. If using commercial culture tube, immediately squeeze end of tube to crush ampule (Fig. 45-13). Push tip of swab into fluid medium. — Medium supports life of microorganisms until culture is obtained.

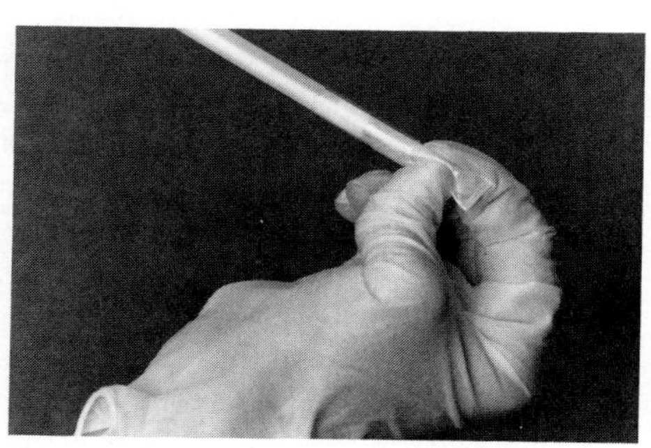

***Fig. 45-13***

| Steps | Rationale |
|---|---|
| 12. Label each culture tube with identification label and affix completed requisition. | Incorrect specimen identification could lead to diagnostic or therapeutic error. |
| 13. Send specimen immediately to laboratory or refrigerate. | Bacteria multiply quickly; specimen should be analyzed quickly for accurate results. |
| 14. Assist client to comfortable position, replace gown, remove drape. | Provides client with sense of self-esteem. |
| 15. Wash hands. | Reduces transmission of microorganisms. |

## Evaluation

| | |
|---|---|
| 1. Check laboratory results for indication of bacterial growth. | Results will reveal type of organisms present. Certain organisms are common to vaginal tract. Urethra should be free of microorganisms. |
| 2. If discharge present, note color and amount. | Characteristics of discharge can indicate specific type of infection. |

### *Expected outcomes*

| | |
|---|---|
| 1. Vaginal, urethral cultures do not reveal growth of microorganisms. | Evidence of absence of infection. |
| 2. Specimen is not contaminated. | Results on laboratory test can reveal whether skin cells or mucosal cells contaminated specimen. |

### *Unexpected outcomes*

| | |
|---|---|
| 1. Vaginal or urethral cultures reveal growth of pathogenic microorganisms. | Indication of infection. |
| 2. Specimen is contaminated with epidermal cells. | Laboratory test results reveal type of cells cultured. |

## Recording and Reporting

| | |
|---|---|
| 1. Record types of cultures obtained and date and time sent to laboratory in nurses' notes. | Documents cultures were obtained. |
| 2. Describe character of discharge and appearance of vaginal orifice or urethral meatus. | Data document infection. |
| 3. Report laboratory results to nurse in charge or physician. | Results may indicate specific therapies such as antibiotic administration. |

## Follow-up Activity

| | |
|---|---|
| 1. Develop care plan for client with sexually transmitted disease. | Treats problem in holistic, humane manner rather than as simple infection. |

## Special Considerations

- Intrusiveness of procedure can arouse anxiety and fear in clients.
- Most clients wish to discuss reason for vaginal or urethral culture privately, and many fear possible results of test.
- Collection of sexual history must be performed nonjudgmentally. Nurse should be comfortable with own sexuality before attempting to collect history.
- Young child will most likely desire parents' presence, whereas adolescent usually will not.
- Parent can assist with specimen collection from infant or young child by gently holding child's legs apart in froglike position.
- Parents should understand that obtaining specimen will not affect virginity of child.
- Hold male genitalia gently. Excess manipulation can cause erection.
- Some institutions have special bags for specimens. If client is in isolation, specimen container must be placed in bag.

## Teaching Considerations

- Clients with urethral or vaginal discharge may require instruction about perineal hygiene measures.
- If topical treatments (e.g., suppositories) are ordered, instruct client in proper administration of medication (Chapter 20).
- Explain how and why specimen is being obtained.
- Discuss client's role in collecting specimen.
- Discuss symptoms of vaginal or urethral infection with client as appropriate.
- Explain relationship between genital discomfort and infection of vaginal or urinary tract.
- Explain time required to obtain results of culture.
- Discuss sexuality and safe sexual practices with client if appropriate.

# SKILL 45-11 Collecting Sputum Specimens

Sputum is produced by cells lining the respiratory tract. Although production is minimal in the healthy state, disease states can increase the amount or change the character of sputum. Examination of sputum may aid in the diagnosis and treatment of several conditions ranging from simple bronchitis to lung cancer.

Three major types of sputum specimens are sputum for cytology, culture and sensitivity, and acid-fast bacilli (AFB). Sputum collected for culture and sensitivity testing can identify specific microorganisms and determine antibiotics to which they are most sensitive. Acid-fast bacilli in sputum indicates tuberculosis. Cytologic or cellular examination of sputum may identify aberrant cells or cancer.

Before beginning this procedure, the nurse should know how to instruct the client in proper coughing exercises (Chapter 15), don sterile gloves by the open method (Chapter 38), and suction the tracheobronchial tree (Chapter 16).

## Purposes

1. Identify pathogenic microorganisms in the tracheobronchial tree.
2. Identify cancerous cells in the tracheobronchial tree.
3. Determine sensitivity of bacterial cells to antibiotics.

## Procedure 45-11

| Steps | Rationale |
|---|---|
| **Assessment** | |
| 1. Check physician's orders for type of sputum analysis and specifications (e.g., amount of sputum, number of specimens, time of collection). | Specific test to be performed may dictate when or how frequently specimens are collected. Ideal time to collect sputum is early AM because bronchial secretions tend to accumulate during night. Bacteria also accumulate as secretions pool. |
| 2. Assess level of understanding of procedure and its purpose. | Provides baseline for nurse to establish teaching plan. |
| 3. Assess client's ability to cough and expectorate specimens. | Adequate cough is essential in production of mucus from tracheobronchial tree. Client may have nonproductive cough due to abdominal or chest pain. Simple clearing of throat is unacceptable. |
| 4. Determine type of assistance needed by client to obtain specimen. | Positioning, postural drainage, deep breathing and coughing exercises may improve ability to cough productively. Suctioning may be indicated if client is unable to cough and expectorate. |
| 5. Assess client's respiratory status, including respiratory rate, depth, pattern, skin color. | Active coughing may alter respiratory status. Respiratory status can depend on amount of sputum in tracheobronchial tree. |
| **Nursing Diagnosis** | |
| 1. Cluster data to reveal actual or potential nursing diagnoses: | |
| a. Ineffective breathing pattern: related to increased mucus secretion. | Increased sputum production may alter breathing patterns. |
| b. Pain: related to postoperative incision site. | Problem can diminish client's effectiveness with coughing. |
| c. Ineffective airway clearance: related to inability to cough. | Client unable to clear airway of mucus may be because of fatigue, positioning, pain. |
| d. Knowledge deficit regarding procedure's purpose: related to inexperience. | Client may require considerable instruction. |
| e. Anxiety: related to impending results of test. | Test results can indicate serious respiratory disease. |
| **Planning** | |
| 1. Develop individualized goals based on nursing diagnoses: | |
| a. Collect specimen uncontaminated by saliva. | Sputum must originate from tracheobronchial tree to ensure accurate test results. |
| b. Minimize client's anxiety. | The need to obtain specimen by suctioning causes anxiety. |
| c. Promote optimal oxygenation during suctioning (if required). | Prolonged suctioning can diminish oxygen supply. |
| d. Minimize discomfort of procedure. | Suctioning or coughing with painful condition can make procedure uncomfortable. |

| Steps | Rationale |
|---|---|
| 2. Prepare equipment and supplies: | |
| a. *Expectorated specimen:* | |
| ▪ Sterile specimen container with cover | Specimen needs to be collected in proper container as described by institution's policy and procedure. |
| ▪ Disposable gloves | Reduces risk of exposure to pathogens in bodily secretions. |
| ▪ Facial tissues | |
| ▪ Emesis basin (optional) | Used to dispose of soiled tissues at bedside. |
| ▪ Toothbrush (optional) | |
| ▪ Completed identification labels | Facilitate correct identification of specimen and ensure prompt delivery to laboratory. |
| ▪ Completed laboratory requisition (date, time, name of test, source of culture) | |
| b. *Suctioned specimen:* | |
| ▪ Suction device (wall or portable) | |
| ▪ Sterile suction catheter (size 14, 16, or 18 Fr) Catheter should not be large enough to cause trauma to nasal mucosa. | |
| ▪ Sterile gloves | |
| ▪ Sterile saline in container | Used to flush suction catheter. |
| ▪ In-line specimen container (sputum trap or Lukino trap (Fig. 45-14) | Connects with suction tubing. |
| ▪ Oxygen therapy equipment if indicated | May be required if client becomes hypoxic. |

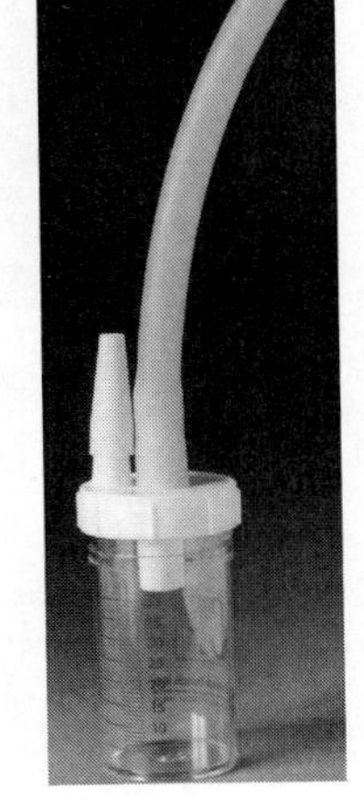

***Fig. 45-14***

| Steps | Rationale |
|---|---|
| 3. Explain steps of procedure and purpose. When client is expectorating sputum, stress importance of deep coughing and need to avoid clearing of throat. If client is to be suctioned, stress importance of relaxing and breathing at normal rate. | Promotes understanding and cooperation. Specimen should not contain saliva. Secretions from oropharynx contain numerous bacteria that will contaminate sputum. Client who is to be suctioned should breathe normally to prevent hyperventilation. |
| 4. For expectorated specimen, have client rinse mouth or brush teeth with water. | Reduces number of oral contaminants that can alter test results. Water is used rather than mouthwash or toothpaste because these substances may decrease viability of microorganisms. |

## Implementation

| Steps | Rationale |
|---|---|
| 1. Wash hands. | Reduces transmission of microorganisms. |
| 2. Provide privacy by closing bedside curtains or room door. | Procedure may be embarrassing or offensive to client and others. |
| 3. Position client in: semi-Fowler's position, sitting on side of bed or chair, standing for coughing and expectorating specimen; high or semi-Fowler's position for suctioning | Promotes full lung expansion and facilitates ability to cough. |
| 4. If client has incision or localized area of discomfort, have client place hands firmly over affected area or place pillow over area. | Splinting or support of painful area minimizes muscular stretching and discomfort during coughing and thus makes cough productive. |
| 5. Collect specimen: | |
| a. *Coughing and expectoration:* | |
| ▪ Provide client with specimen container and instruct not to touch inside. | Prevents risk of contamination. |
| ▪ Instruct client to take 3 to 4 slow deep breaths. | Helps open airways, loosen secretions, and stimulate cough reflex. |
| ▪ Instruct client to emphasize slow, full exhalation. | Moves secretions into larger airways. |
| ▪ After series of deep breaths, ask client to cough after full inhalation. | Full inhalation provides force to move secretions out of airways up to pharynx. |
| ▪ Instruct client to expectorate sputum directly into specimen container. | Retains microorganisms in sterile container. Young children often swallow secretions instead of expectorating. |
| ▪ Have client repeat coughing until adequate amount of sputum has been collected. | Usually 2 to 10 ml (1 to 2 tsp) is required to ensure accurate analysis of specimen. |
| ▪ Apply disposable gloves before accepting specimen from client. | Reduces risk of exposure to pathogens in body secretions. |

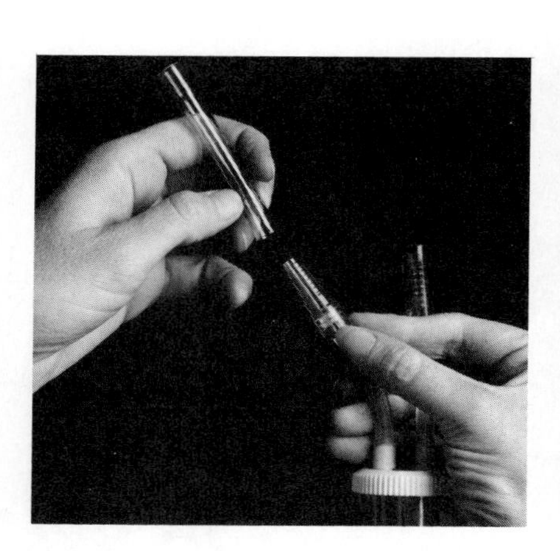

*Fig. 45-15*

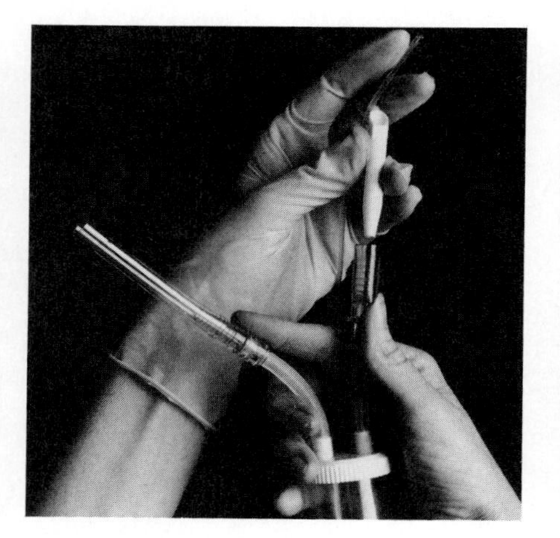

*Fig. 45-16*

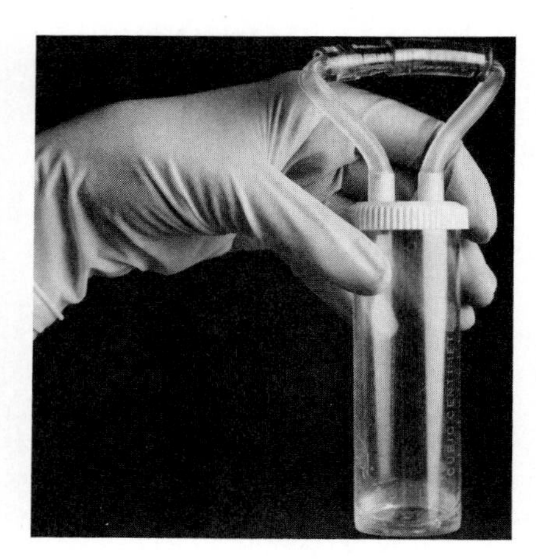

*Fig. 45-17*

| Steps | Rationale |
|---|---|
| b. *Suctioning:* | |
| ▪ Prepare suction machine or device and determine if it functions properly. | Adequate amount of suction is necessary to aspirate sputum. |
| ▪ Connect suction tube to adapter on sputum trap (Fig. 45-15). | Establishes suction that passes through sputum trap to aspirate specimen. |
| ▪ Apply sterile gloves (only dominant hand required). | Tracheobronchial tree is sterile body cavity. Allows nurse to manipulate suction catheter without contamination. |
| ▪ With gloved hand, connect sterile suction catheter to rubber tubing on sputum trap (Fig. 45-16). | Aspirated sputum will go directly to trap instead of suction tubing. |
| ▪ Gently insert tip of suction catheter through nasopharynx, endotracheal tube, tracheostomy without applying suction (Chapter 16). | Minimizes trauma to airway as catheter is inserted. |
| ▪ Advance catheter into trachea. | Entrance of catheter into larynx and trachea triggers cough reflex. |
| ▪ As client coughs, apply suction for 5 to 10 sec, collecting 2 to 10 ml sputum. | Ensures collection of sputum from deep within tracheobronchial tree. Suctioning longer than 15 sec can cause hypoxia. |
| ▪ Remove catheter without applying suction, then turn off suction. | Suction can damage mucosa if applied during withdrawal. |
| ▪ Detach catheter from specimen trap, gather catheter into gloved hand, pull glove off over catheter and dispose. | Decreases risk of spreading microorganisms. |
| 6. Secure top on specimen container tightly. For sputum trap, detach suction tubing, connect rubber tubing on sputum trap to plastic adapter (Fig. 45-17). | Contains microorganisms within container, preventing exposure to personnel handling specimen. |
| 7. If any sputum is on outside of container, wash off with disinfectant. | Prevents spread of infection to persons handling specimen. |
| 8. Offer client tissues after expectorating. Dispose in emesis basin or trash container. | Maintains cleanliness and comfort. |
| 9. Offer client mouth care, if desired. | Promotes comfort. |
| 10. Wash hands. | Reduces spread of microorganisms. |
| 11. Label specimen with identification label and affix requisition. | Incorrect identification could lead to diagnostic or therapeutic error. |
| 12. Send specimen immediately to laboratory or refrigerate. | Bacteria multiply quickly. Specimen should be analyzed promptly for accurate results. |

## Evaluation

| Steps | Rationale |
|---|---|
| 1. Observe client's respiratory status throughout procedure, especially during suctioning. | Excessive coughing or prolonged suctioning can alter respiratory pattern and cause hypoxia. |
| 2. Note anxiety or discomfort in client. | Procedure can be uncomfortable. If client becomes short of breath, anxiety will develop. |
| 3. Observe character of sputum: color, consistency, odor. | Characteristics may indicate disease entities. |
| 4. Refer to laboratory reports for test results. | Determines abnormal cells or microorganisms in sputum. |

| Steps | Rationale |
|---|---|
| ***Expected outcomes*** | |
| 1. Client's respirations are same rate and character as before procedure. | Specimen collection did not alter respiratory status. |
| 2. Client is relaxed, able to answer questions (if no artificial airway present). | Suctioning tends to cause anxiety. |
| 3. Laboratory tests fail to reveal abnormal cells or microorganisms. | Absence of infection or abnormal cells. |
| ***Unexpected outcomes*** | |
| 1. Client becomes hypoxic during procedure; increased respiratory rate and effort are necessary; client feels short of breath. | Most common after suctioning. Clients known to have respiratory alterations may be short of breath or dyspneic and may be anxious. |
| 2. Client remains anxious or complains of discomfort from suction catheter. | Anxiety or discomfort may remain for several minutes until client able to breathe normally. |
| 3. Specimen appears to contain saliva. | Saliva is watery and clear. Requires specimen collection be repeated. |
| 4. Inadequate amount of sputum is collected. | Client may be unable to expectorate or sputum may be very thick or reduced in amount. |
| 5. Specimen contains pathogenic organisms or abnormal cells. | Diagnostic of infection or disorders such as malignancy. |
| **Reporting and Recording** | |
| 1. Record method used to obtain specimen, date and time collected, type of test ordered, laboratory receiving specimen in nurses' notes. | Documents specimens were obtained. |
| 2. Describe characteristics of sputum specimen. | Data can be help in diagnosis of alterations and serve as baseline to detect changes. |
| 3. Describe client's tolerance of procedure. | Provides data to measure respiratory status. |
| 4. Report unusual sputum characteristics and client response to head nurse or physician. | Findings may require specific intervention. |
| 5. When laboratory reports are available, report abnormal findings. | May require new or revised therapies. |
| **Follow-up Activities** | |
| 1. If sputum is positive for AFB, initiate respiratory isolation (Chapter 38). | Tuberculosis organisms are transmitted by air droplet. |
| 2. If specimen could not be obtained under normal procedures, obtain order to induce specimen (e.g., with use of humidification, aerosol therapy, postural drainage, suction). | Procedures can promote loosening and production of sputum. |

## Special Considerations

- Postoperative client benefits from splinting surgical wound to cough deeply (Chapter 39). Parent may assist child in splinting site.
- Clients able to cough effectively may prefer to take specimen container to bathroom.
- Aerosol treatment may be necessary to induce sputum collection.
- Evidence of bright red blood should be immediately reported.
- Children need very clear instructions or demonstration for deep breathing. Infants and young children will be unable to cooperate; aerosol treatment or suctioning may be indicated.
- Parent or another nurse can assist nurse in restraining young child's head and arms during suctioning.
- If client is undergoing oxygen therapy through tracheostomy or endotracheal tube, nurse can insert catheter without removing oxygen tubing.
- If client appears hypoxic or in distress during suctioning, discontinue procedure and provide oxygen therapy as needed.
- Specimens for AFB require three consecutive morning samples; cultures can take up to 8 weeks.
- Refer to institution's policy and procedure for type of specimen container. Some tests require glass instead of plastic containers. Some specimens require additives. Sputum collections over 24 hr require special containers.
- Some agencies have special bags in which to transport specimens.
- Many agencies require nurse to note if client is receiving antibiotics on specimen requisition.

## Teaching Considerations

- Nurse may demonstrate effective coughing techniques vs. clearing of throat.
- Nurse can demonstrate proper splinting technique for postoperative clients.

- If aerosol treatment is indicated, teach client purpose of procedure, explaining that it will stimulate coughing and sputum expectoration.
- Explain purpose of obtaining specimen before breakfast because it is the most concentrated and will be free of food particles.
- Explain purpose of avoiding use of mouthwashes and toothpaste before sputum expectoration, which may decrease viability of microorganisms.

# SKILL 45-12 Obtaining Gastric Specimens

Analysis of gastric contents can aid physicians in diagnosing and treating a number of conditions such as gastric acid irregularities and gastrointestinal bleeding from ulcers or tumors. Gastric pH level determines the acidity of gastrointestinal secretions. Measuring gastric occult blood, which reveals bleeding in the esophagus, stomach, or duodenum, is similar to measuring stool for occult blood.

The testing of gastric specimens for occult blood and pH is relatively easy. The nurse can perform the tests on emesis or on drainage collected from an existing nasogastric tube. Inserting a nasogastric tube solely to collect gastric secretions is very unusual.

Before beginning this procedure, the nurse should know the effect of pH level on gastric contents and how to properly care for nasogastric tubes (Chapter 39).

### Purposes

1. Assess for the presence of blood.
2. Assess the pH level of gastric contents.
3. Determine the need for administering antacid therapy.

## Procedure 45-12

| Steps | Rationale |
|---|---|
| **Assessment** | |
| 1. Review physician's order to determine test and source of specimen. | Provides order when regularly testing specimen. |
| 2. Assess level of understanding of procedure and purpose. | Provides baseline for nurse to establish teaching plan. |
| 3. Review medications client is receiving and foods recently eaten. | Some medications and foods can cause false positive readings for occult blood. |
| 4. Check with laboratory and physician to determine if dietary restrictions or temporary discontinuation of medications is necessary before test. | Gastric analysis for occult blood requires fasting because results depend on peroxidase activity of hemoglobin in red blood cells. Some foods contain peroxidases and cause false results. |
| 5. Assess client for symptoms of abdominal cramping, pain, nausea, vomiting. | Symptoms are characteristic of gastrointestinal alteration. |
| **Nursing Diagnosis** | |
| 1. Cluster data to reveal actual or potential nursing diagnoses: | |
| a. Potential for injury: related to gastrointestinal alteration. | Indication of occult blood can lead to therapies to prevent more serious blood loss. Monitoring of gastric pH level can prevent serious electrolyte alterations. |
| b. Pain: related to gastrointestinal disturbance. | Increased acidity and conditions causing bleeding can result in discomfort. |
| c. Knowledge deficit regarding test procedure and purpose: related to inexperience. | Client requires instruction. |
| d. Anxiety: related to impending test results. | Clients unfamiliar with procedure may fear procedure and findings. |
| **Planning** | |
| 1. Develop individualized goals for client based on nursing diagnoses: | |
| a. Obtain appropriate specimen for analysis. | Specimen should come from stomach to ensure accurate analysis of results. |
| b. Minimize client's anxiety. | Test is painless, unless need exists to insert nasogastric tube, which is rare. |

| Steps | Rationale |
|---|---|
| 2. Prepare equipment and supplies: | |
| a. Disposable gloves | Prevents risk of exposure to pathogens in bodily secretions. |
| b. Facial tissues | |
| c. Emesis basin | |
| d. Wooden applicator or 1 ml syringe | Used to apply sample to pH and guaiac test paper. |
| e. Commercial kit with test paper for pH level and occult blood | Test paper changes color to indicate level of gastric acidity or occult blood. Gastrooccult kit contains paper for both tests. |
| f. Developing solution | Application to test paper causes chemical reaction necessary to measure results. |
| g. 60 ml bulb or catheter tip syringe | Used to aspirate gastric secretions from nasogastric tube. |
| h. Nasogastric tube and supplies for insertion | Used if necessary to insert tube (Chapter 39). |
| 3. Institute dietary or medication restrictions as needed. | Ensures accurate test results. |
| 4. Explain steps of procedure to client. Emphasize that test is painless (unless nasogastric tube insertion is required). | Reduces anxiety and promotes cooperation. |

## Implementation

| Steps | Rationale |
|---|---|
| 1. Wash hands before procedure. | Reduces transfer of microorganisms. |
| 2. Apply disposable gloves. | Prevents risk of exposure to pathogens in bodily secretions. |
| 3. Position client in high Fowler's position in bed or chair. | Minimizes aspiration of gastric contents. Position relieves pressure on abdominal organs. If client is nauseated, flat position in bed or one in which client cannot sit straight may cause abdominal discomfort. |
| 4. Close bedside curtains or door to room. | Maintains privacy. Client who has vomited can become embarrassed. In a semiprivate room, roommate may find vomiting offensive. |
| 5. Insert nasogastric tube, if indicated (Chapter 39). | Allows aspiration of gastric contents. |
| 6. Obtain specimen of gastric contents by attaching bulb syringe to nasogastric tube and aspirating 5 to 10 ml; obtaining sample of emesis with 1 ml syringe or wooden applicator. | Only small amount of specimen is needed for pH and occult blood testing. |
| 7. Using applicator or syringe, apply 1 drop of gastric sample to pH test paper. Be sure drop covers paper completely. | Paper should be completely exposed to secretions to ensure full color change. |
| 8. Read color of pH test paper within 30 sec and compare with pH color guide. | Results range from 1 to 7. Acidic solutions are 4 or less. Basic solutions are 5 or more. |
| 9. Apply 1 drop of gastric sample to Gastrooccult blood test paper. | Sample must cover guaiac paper for test reaction to occur. |
| 10. Apply 2 drops of commercial developer solution over sample and 1 drop between positive and negative performance monitors (Fig. 45-18). | Developer initiates chemical reaction of solution with guaiac paper. |
| 11. After 60 sec, compare color of gastric sample to that of performance monitors. | Positive performance monitor turns blue in 30 sec, and negative monitor remains white or beige. If sample turns blue, test is positive for occult blood. If sample turns green, test is negative. |

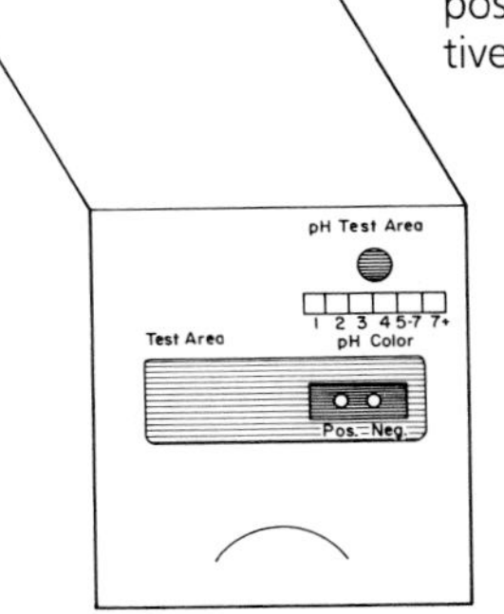


***Fig. 45-18***

| Steps | Rationale |
|---|---|
| 12. Explain results to client. | Immediate results are obtained. Makes client participant in care. |
| 13. Dispose of test slide paper, wooden applicator, and 1 ml syringe in proper receptacle. | Reduces spread of infection and keeps environment clean. |
| 14. Reconnect nasogastric tube to drainage system or clamp as ordered. (Remove tube if only inserted for specimen collection.) | Nasogastric tube serves to decompress abdomen by promoting drainage. Clamping may be ordered to determine tolerance to stomach filling. |
| 15. Remove disposable gloves and dispose. | |
| 16. Assist client to comfortable position and offer oral hygiene. | After vomiting or removal of tube, oral hygiene promotes comfort and helps to reduce nausea. |
| 17. Wash hands. | Reduces transmission of microorganisms. |

| Steps | Rationale |
|---|---|
| **Evaluation** | |
| 1. Assess quantity and character of emesis or gastric secretions. | Characteristics can reveal abnormal status. |
| 2. Compare test findings with normal expected results. | Determines if gastric contents are abnormally acidic or basic. |
| ***Expected outcomes*** | |
| 1. Gastric secretions are greenish to clear, with no evidence of bleeding or clots. | Greenish color results from bile secreted in duodenum. |
| 2. pH level is 1.5 to 3.0. | Gastric secretions are highly acidic. If secretions are collected from lower gastrointestinal tract, results are more basic. |
| 3. Test is negative for occult blood. | Indicates absence of bleeding in gastrointestinal tract. |
| ***Unexpected outcomes*** | |
| 1. Gastric secretions may contain clots or be bloody. Emesis may have "coffee grounds" appearance. | Indicate gastrointestinal bleeding. Bright red blood indicates active bleeding. "Coffee grounds" emesis indicates slow, less active bleeding. |
| 2. pH level is above or below desired range. | Each physician may set guidelines on level at which pH should be maintained. |
| 3. Test is positive for occult blood. | Indicates gastrointestinal bleeding. |
| **Recording and Reporting** | |
| 1. Record test performed, source of specimen, and results in nurses' notes. | Documents specimen obtained and tested. |
| 2. Describe characteristics of gastric contents. | Provides baseline to determine change in client's condition. |
| 3. Report abnormal results to nurse in charge or physician. | May indicate need for additional therapy. |
| **Follow-up Activity** | |
| 1. If results are positive for blood, continue to monitor client for gastrointestinal bleeding. Perform guaiac test on all stools. | Screening helps to indicate location of bleeding. |

## Special Considerations

- Nurses caring for clients at risk for gastrointestinal bleeding, such as critically ill clients prone to stress ulcers, may periodically screen specimen for occult blood or pH level.
- Foods that cause false positive results for occult blood include turnips, horseradish, and red meats. Medications that can cause false positive results include vitamin C in large doses, aspirin, cimetidine (Tagamet), and iron pills.
- Dietary restrictions may be necessary 2 or 3 days before testing.
- Some agencies require gastric test slides be sent to laboratories for application of developer solutions.
- Gastric secretions vary in color if collected from emesis.
- Test may be repeated to confirm results, especially if client did not fast or if indications causing false results were not withheld.

## Teaching Considerations

- Instruct client on foods and medications that may give false test results for occult blood.
- If antacids are ordered, instruct client on proper use.
- If nasogastric tube needs to be inserted, explain procedure to client.

# SKILL 45-13 Obtaining Wound Drainage Specimens

When caring for a client with a wound, the nurse assesses the wound's condition and observes for the development of infection. Localized inflammation, tenderness, and warmth at the wound site, in addition to purulent drainage, usually signify wound infection. Infection cannot be confirmed accurately unless the causative organism is identified. A specimen of wound drainage is analyzed to determine the type and number of pathogenic microorganisms.

The nurse should never collect a wound culture sample from old drainage. Resident colonies of bacteria on the skin grow in wound exudate and may not be the true causative organisms of infection. Separate techniques are used to collect specimens for measuring aerobic vs. anaerobic microorganisms. Aerobic organisms grow in superficial wounds exposed to the air. Anaerobic organisms grow deep within body cavities, where oxygen is normally not present.

Before beginning this procedure, the nurse should know the nature of wound healing and how to apply sterile gloves by the open method (Chapter 38), apply a wound dressing (Chapter 41), and open a sterile package (Chapter 38).

## Purposes

1. Detect pathogenic microorganisms within a wound.
2. Determine type of antibiotics resistant to or effective against identified microorganisms.

## Procedure 45-13

| Steps | Rationale |
|---|---|
| **Assessment** | |
| 1. Assess client's understanding of need for wound culture and ability to cooperate with procedure. | Nurse uses data to develop teaching plan. Wound is painful site. Collection of specimen may arouse anxiety or fear. |
| 2. With disposable gloves, remove any soiled dressings covering wound. Apply sterile gloves and assess condition of wound carefully. Observe for swelling, opening of wound edges, inflammation, drainage. Palpate gently along wound edges and note tenderness or drainage. | Surface of open wound is considered sterile. Sterile gloves allow nurse to palpate area without contamination. Signs indicate wound infection. Gloves needed when contacting bodily secretions to prevent exposure to pathogens. |
| 3. Assess client for signs of fever, chills, thirst, note in laboratory results if white blood cell count is elevated. | Signs and symptoms indicate systemic infection. |
| 4. Ask client about extent and type of pain at wound site. | Pain at wound site often increases with infection. |
| 5. Review physician's orders for aerobic or anaerobic culture. | Specimens are taken from different sites and placed in different containers, depending on type of culture. |
| **Nursing Diagnosis** | |
| 1. Cluster data to reveal actual or potential nursing diagnoses: | |
| a. Potential for injury: related to infectious process. | Client with localized wound infection can develop more serious systemic infection. |
| b. Altered comfort—pain: related to incision. | Localized inflammation and buildup of drainage cause irritation to pain fibers. |
| c. Anxiety: related to fear of specimen collection. | If wound is already painful, client may be apprehensive about how specimen will be obtained. |
| d. Knowledge deficit regarding purpose for procedure: related to misinformation. | Client may be unaware of purpose of procedure or risk of infection. |
| **Planning** | |
| 1. Develop individualized goals for client based on nursing diagnoses: | |
| a. Obtain aerobic specimen uncontaminated by bacteria from skin. | Ensures correct identification of pathogens from wound. |
| b. Obtain anaerobic specimen not exposed to oxygen or contaminated by skin bacteria. | Anaerobes grow only in oxygen-free environment. |
| c. Minimize client's discomfort. | Nurse provides support through thorough explanations and timely nursing care. |
| 2. Prepare equipment and supplies: | |
| a. Culture tube with cotton-tipped swab and transport medium | Used to collect aerobic specimen. |

| Steps | Rationale |
|---|---|
| b. Anaerobic culture tube with swab | Special tubes contain $CO_2$ or nitrogen gas to maintain viability of anaerobes. |
| c. 5 to 10 ml syringe and 21-gauge needle | Used to aspirate anaerobic specimen. |
| d. Disposable gloves | Used to remove soiled dressings. |
| e. Sterile gloves | Used to reapply clean dressing. |
| f. Antiseptic swab | Used to cleanse outer edges of wound of exudate. |
| g. Sterile dressing materials (determined by type of dressing) | Used to cover open wound. |
| h. Paper or plastic disposable bag | Used to contain soiled dressings. |
| i. Completed specimen identification label (according to institutional policy) | Facilitates correct identification of specimen. |
| j. Completed laboratory requisition (date, time, name of test) | Ensures prompt delivery to laboratory. |
| 3. Determine if client may receive analgesic before dressing change or specimen collection. Administer as ordered. | Minimizes discomfort during procedure. |
| 4. Explain reason for wound culture and how it will be collected. | Promotes understanding and cooperation and eases anxiety. |
| 5. Ask parents if they wish to help hold child or if they prefer nurse to do so. | Allows parents to choose. Some prefer to offer child support rather than appear as source of child's discomfort. |
| 6. Explain that client may feel tickling sensation when wound is swabbed. | Anticipation of expected sensations minimizes anxiety. |

## Implementation

| Steps | Rationale |
|---|---|
| 1. Wash hands. | Reduces transfer of microorganisms. |
| 2. Close bedside curtains or door to room. | Avoids embarrassment. |
| 3. Apply disposable gloves and remove old dressing. Observe drainage. Fold soiled sides of dressing together and then dispose of in bag. | Protects hands from contact with drainage. |
| 4. Cleanse area around wound edges with antiseptic swab. Remove old exudate. | Removes skin flora, preventing possible contamination of specimen. |
| 5. Discard swab and dispose of soiled gloves in bag. | Reduces spread of infection. |
| 6. Open packages containing sterile culture tube and dressing supplies. | Provides sterile field from which nurse can pick up and handle sterile supplies. |
| 7. Apply sterile gloves. | Allows nurse to maintain sterility of items while collecting specimen. |
| 8. Collect cultures: | |
| a. *Aerobic culture:* Take cotton-tipped swab from culture tube, insert tip into wound in area of drainage, rotate swab gently. Remove swab and return to culture tube. Crush ampule of medium and push swab into fluid. | Swab should be coated with fresh secretions from within wound. Medium keeps bacteria alive until analysis is complete. |
| b. *Anaerobic culture:* Take cotton-tipped swab from special anaerobic culture tube, swab deeply into draining body cavity, rotate gently. Remove swab and return to culture tube<br>or | Specimen is taken from deep cavity where oxygen is not present. $CO_2$ or nitrogen gas keeps organisms alive until analysis is complete. |
| Insert tip of syringe (without needle) into wound and aspirate 5 to 10 ml of exudate. Attach 21-gauge needle, expel all air, and inject drainage into special culture tube. | Air injected into tube would cause organisms to die. |
| 9. Place each culture tube on correct specimen label. | Maintains sterility of gloves worn. Prevents confusion over aerobic and anaerobic cultures. |
| 10. Ask another nurse to attach labels and proper requisitions to each tube and to send specimens immediately to laboratory. | Bacteria grow rapidly. Cultures should be prepared quickly for accurate results. |
| 11. Clean wound as ordered and apply new sterile dressing. | Protects wound from further contamination and aids in absorbing drainage and debriding wound. |
| 12. Remove gloves by pulling inside out and dispose in trash. Dispose of soiled supplies. | Reduces spread of infection. |
| 13. Secure dressings with tape or ties. | Keeps dressing securely in place over wound. |
| 14. Assist client to comfortable position. | Promotes client's ability to relax. |
| 15. Wash hands after procedure. | Reduces transmission of microorganisms. |

## Evaluation

| Steps | Rationale |
|---|---|
| 1. Refer to laboratory report for results of cultures. | Report indicates if pathogenic organisms are identified. |

| Steps | Rationale |
|---|---|
| ***Expected outcomes*** | |
| 1. Wound culture does not reveal bacterial growth. | Wound remains free of pathogenic microorganisms. |
| 2. Culture swab is not contaminated by bacteria from skin. | Test results indicate type of cells present. Specific cells usually originate from skin. |
| ***Unexpected outcomes*** | |
| 1. Wound cultures reveal heavy bacterial growth. | Wound contaminated by pathogenic microorganisms. |
| 2. Wound culture is contaminated from superficial skin cells. | Inaccurate results require repeat specimen. |
| **Recording and Reporting** | |
| 1. Record types of specimens obtained, source, time and date sent to laboratory in nurses' notes. | Documents that cultures were obtained. |
| 2. Describe appearance of wound and characteristics of drainage in nurses' notes. | Data support evidence of infection and provide baseline to determine change in condition of wound. |
| 3. Report any evidence of infection to nurse in charge or physician. | Findings may indicate need for further therapy, (e.g., antibiotics or wound irrigation). |

## Special Considerations

- Never collect exudate from skin unless it is separate culture and labeled as such.
- Wound cultures are often obtained during dressing change (Chapter 41); thus this step may be performed as part of procedure.
- Commercially prepared culture kits are available.
- If client requires analgesic before dressing changes, medication is ideally given 30 min before to reach peak effect.
- If procedure is to be performed on a child and is anticipated to be painful, some agencies prefer performing procedure in area other than child's room, thus maintaining feeling that child's room is safe place.
- While doing dressing change, client may prefer not to see soiled portion of dressing.
- Some agencies require culture tubes to be transported in bags.

## Teaching Considerations

- Notify client before possible discomfort during procedure.
- Instruct client to inform nurse if procedure causes pain.
- Teach client to assess status of wound for changes.
- Discuss signs and symptoms of infection.

## Home Care Considerations

- When applicable, discuss ways to prevent infection.
- Discuss signs and symptoms of infections and what to report.

# *SKILL 45-14 Collecting Blood Specimens by Venipuncture*

Blood tests are probably the most commonly used diagnostic aid in the care and evaluation of clients. In any health care setting, blood tests can yield valuable information about nutritional, hematologic, metabolic, immune, and biochemical status. Tests allow physicians to screen clients carefully for early signs of physical alterations, plot the course of existing disease, and monitor responses to therapies.

The nurse is often responsible for collecting blood specimens; however, many institutions have specially trained technicians whose sole responsibility is to draw blood. Nurses must be familiar with their institutions' policies and procedures as well as their states' nurse practice act regarding guidelines for drawing blood samples.

The three primary methods of obtaining blood specimens are venipuncture, skin puncture, and arterial stick. Venipuncture, the most common method, involves inserting a hollow bore needle into the lumen of a large vein to obtain a specimen. The nurse may use a needle and syringe or a special vacutainer that allows the drawing of multiple blood samples. Because veins are major sources of blood for laboratory testing and routes for IV fluid or blood replacement, maintaining their integrity is essential. The nurse should be skilled in venipuncture to avoid unnecessary injury to veins.

Skin puncture is the least traumatic method of obtaining a blood specimen. A sterile lancet or needle is used to puncture a vascular area on a finger, toe, or heel. A drop of blood is placed on a test slide or collected within a thin glass, capillary tube for laboratory analysis.

The most traumatic form of obtaining blood specimens is arterial stick. A small-gauge needle is inserted directly into the lumen of an artery to collect a specimen. Of all methods for obtaining blood specimens, arterial stick poses the greatest risks.

Regardless of the method used to obtain a blood specimen, the nurse must anticipate the client's anxiety. The procedures can be painful, and often just the appearance of a needle is frightening, especially to children. The nurse's calm approach and skilled technique helps to limit anxiety.

Before beginning this procedure, the nurse should know the proper technique in using a syringe and needle (Chapter 20).

### Purposes

1. Measure specific constituents or elements within the blood (red blood cells, electrolytes, drug levels, bacteria).
2. Monitor the response to specific therapies.
3. Determine blood type.

## *Procedure 45-13*

| Steps | Rationale |
|---|---|
| **Assessment** | |
| 1. Determine understanding of purpose of procedure and method to be used. | Provides data for nurse to establish teaching plan and provide emotional support. Many clients may have past experiences that increase anxiety. |
| 2. Determine if special conditions need to be met before specimen collection (i.e., client to be NPO, specific time for collection after medication or meal). | Some tests require meeting specific conditions to obtain accurate measurement of blood elements (e.g., fasting blood sugar, drug peak and trough level, and timed endocrine hormone levels). |
| 3. Assess client for possible risk for venipuncture: anticoagulant therapy, low platelet count, bleeding disorders (history of hemophilia or ecchymosis). | Abnormal clotting abilities caused by low platelet count, hemophilia, medications increase risk for bleeding and hematoma formation. |
| 4. Determine ability to cooperate with procedure. | Some clients may need to be restrained, requiring assistance of another nurse. Procedure can appear threatening to client. |
| 5. Assess client for contraindicated sites for venipuncture: presence of IV fluids, hematoma at potential site, history of mastectomy, hemodialysis recipient. | Drawing specimens from such sites can result in false test results or may injure client. |
| 6. Review physician's orders for type of tests. | Multiple samples may be needed; physician's order is required. |
| **Nursing Diagnosis** | |
| 1. Cluster data to reveal actual or potential nursing diagnoses: | |
| a. Anxiety or fear: related to impending venipuncture. | Clients may express anxiety or fear in many ways. Nurse must be aware of client's feelings to perform venipuncture safely. |
| b. Potential for injury: related to venipuncture. | Client is at risk for infection because procedure is invasive and for changes in skin integrity. |
| c. Knowledge deficit regarding procedure and purpose: related to inexperience. | Client often lacks understanding of need for tests. |
| d. Anxiety: related to impending test results. | Blood tests can confirm specific disease states. |
| e. Pain: related to venipuncture. | Insertion of needle causes localized discomfort. Pain thresholds will differ. |
| **Planning** | |
| 1. Develop individualized goals for client based on nursing diagnoses: | |
| a. Obtain appropriate specimen under required conditions (according to agency laboratory policy). | Nurse must collect proper amount of blood under correct conditions to ensure accurate results. |
| b. Minimize discomfort at venipuncture site. | Anxiety heightens pain perception. |
| c. Minimize trauma at needle insertion site. | Nurse uses techniques to avoid hematoma formation. |
| d. Prevent infection at venipuncture site. | Nurse uses aseptic technique to prepare skin and handle sterile items. |
| e. Minimize client's anxiety. | Precise explanations, calm tone of voice, skillful technique help to control anxiety. |
| 2. Prepare equipment and supplies: | |
| a. Alcohol or antiseptic swab | Used to cleanse skin of resident microorganisms. |

| Steps | Rationale |
|---|---|
| b. Disposable gloves | Reduces risk of exposure to HIV, hepatitis, other blood-borne pathogens. |
| c. Small pillow or folded towel | |
| d. Sterile gauze pads (2 × 2) | |
| e. Rubber tourniquet | Applied to extremity to create vein distension. |
| f. Band-Aid or adhesive tape | |
| g. *Syringe method:* | |
| ▪ Sterile needles (20 to 21 gauge for adults, 23 to 25 gauge for children) | Smaller-gauge needle reduces trauma to vein wall. Gauge should be large enough to allow free flow of blood. |
| ▪ Sterile syringe of appropriate size | |
| h. *Vacutainer method:* | |
| ▪ Vacutainer tube with needle holder | Needles designed to attach several blood tubes in succession. |
| ▪ Sterile, double-ended needles (20 to 21 gauge for adults, 23 to 25 gauge for children) (Some nurses prefer to use butterfly or scalp vein needles.) | |
| i. Appropriate blood tubes | Ensures correct testing of specimen. Some tests are performed on clotted blood or unclotted blood and serum. Certain containers contain anticoagulants. |
| j. Completed identification labels according to agency policy | Facilitates correct identification of specimen. |
| k. Completed laboratory requisition (date, time, type of test) | Ensures prompt delivery to laboratory. |
| 3. Explain procedure to client: describe purpose of tests; explain how sensation of tourniquet, alcohol swab, needle stick feel. | Anticipatory guidance helps to reduce anxiety. |

## Implementation

| Steps | Rationale |
|---|---|
| 1. Wash hands. | Reduces transfer of microorganisms. |
| 2. Bring equipment to bedside. | Ensures organized procedure. |
| 3. Close bedside curtain or room door. | Provides for privacy. |
| 4. Raise or lower bed to comfortable working height. | Reduces strain on nurse's back muscles and improves access to body part. |
| 5. Assist client to supine or semi-Fowler's position with arms extended to form straight line from shoulders to wrists. Place small pillow or towel under upper arm. | Helps to stabilize extremity because arms are most common sites of venipuncture. Supported position in bed reduces chance of injury to client if fainting occurs. |
| 6. Ask staff member or parent to restrain child so venipuncture site is immobilized (Fig. 45-19). | Prevents sudden movement, which can cause serious injury to vessel wall or soft tissues. |
| 7. Apply disposable gloves. | Reduces risk of exposure to HIV, Hepatitis other blood-borne bacteria. |

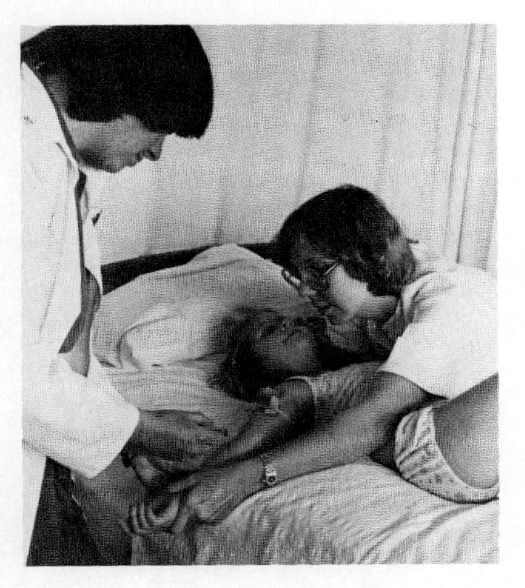

***Fig. 45-19***

From Whaley LF, Wong DL: Nursing care of infants and children, ed 3, St Louis, 1987, The CV Mosby Co.

| Steps | Rationale |
|---|---|
| 8. Apply tourniquet 5 to 15 cm (2 to 6 in) above venipuncture site selected (antecubital fossa site is most often used). Encircle extremity and pull one end of tourniquet tightly over other, looping one end under other (Fig. 45-20). Apply tourniquet so it can be removed by pulling end with single motion. | Tourniquet blocks venous return to heart from extremity, causing veins to dilate for easier visibility. |

***Fig. 45-20***

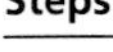

| Steps | Rationale |
|---|---|

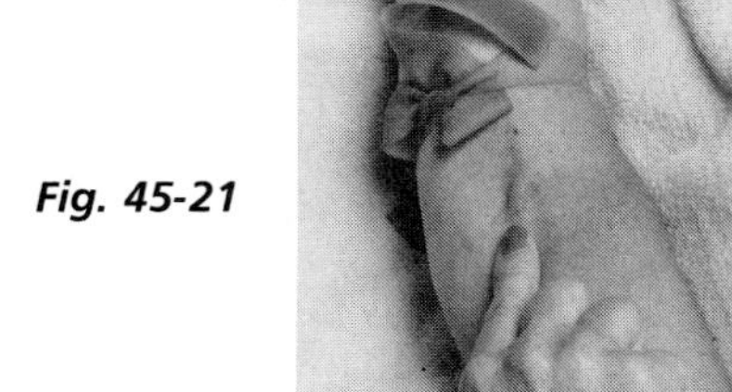

*Fig. 45-21*

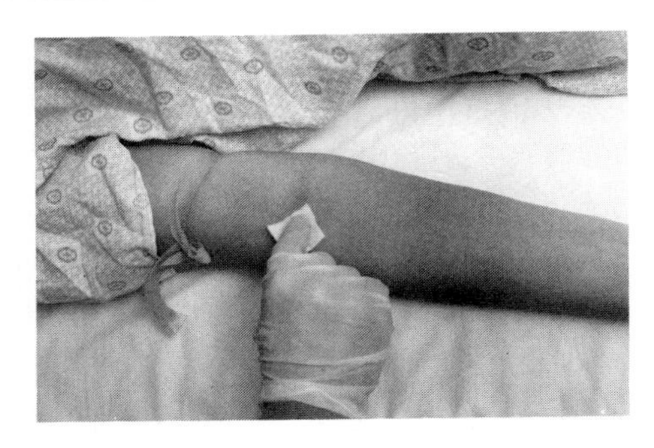

*Fig. 45-22*

| Steps | Rationale |
|---|---|
| 9. Palpate distal pulse (e.g., radial) below tourniquet. If pulse not palpable, reapply tourniquet more loosely. | If tourniquet is too tight, pressure will impede arterial blood flow. |
| 10. Keep tourniquet on no longer than 1 to 2 min. | Prolonged time may alter test results and cause pain and venous stasis (e.g., falsely elevated serum potassium level). |
| 11. Ask client to open and close fist several times, finally leaving fist clenched. | Facilitates distention of veins by forcing blood up from distal veins. |
| 12. Quickly inspect extremity for best venipuncture site, looking for straight, prominent vein without swelling or hematoma. | Straight and intact veins are easier to puncture. |
| 13. Palpate selected vein with index finger. Note if vein is firm and rebounds when palpated or if vein feels rigid and cordlike and rolls when palpated (Fig. 45-21). | Patent, healthy vein is elastic and rebounds on palpation. Thrombosed vein is rigid, rolls easily, is difficult to puncture. |
| 14. Select venipuncture site. (If tourniquet on arm is too long, remove, and assess other extremity or wait 60 sec before reapplying). | Prevents discomfort to client and inaccurate test results. |
| 15. Obtain blood sample: | |
| a. *Syringe method:* | |
| ▪ Have syringe with appropriate needle securely attached. | Needle should not dislodge from syringe during venipuncture. |
| ▪ Cleanse venipuncture site with alcohol swab, moving in circular motion from site for approximately 5 cm (2 in) (Fig. 45-22). Allow to dry. | Antimicrobial agent cleans skin surface of resident bacteria so organisms do not enter puncture site. Allowing alcohol to dry reduces "sting" of venipuncture. |
| ▪ Remove needle cover and inform client "stick" lasting only few seconds will be felt. | Client has better control over anxiety when knows what to expect. |
| ▪ Place thumb or forefinger of nondominant hand 2.5 cm (1 in) above or below site and pull skin taut. | Stabilizes vein and prevents rolling during needle insertion. |
| ▪ Hold syringe and needle at 15- to 30-degree angle from client's arm with bevel up. | Reduces chance of penetrating both sides of vein during insertion. Bevel up reduces vein trauma. |
| ▪ Slowly insert needle into vein (Fig. 45-23). | Prevents puncture on opposite side. |
| ▪ Hold syringe securely and pull back gently on plunger (Fig. 45-24). | Syringe held securely prevents needle from advancing. Pulling on plunger creates vacuum needed to draw blood into syringe. |
| ▪ Look for blood return. | If blood flow fails to appear, indicates needle not in vein. |

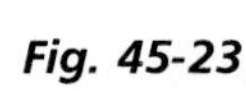

*Fig. 45-23*

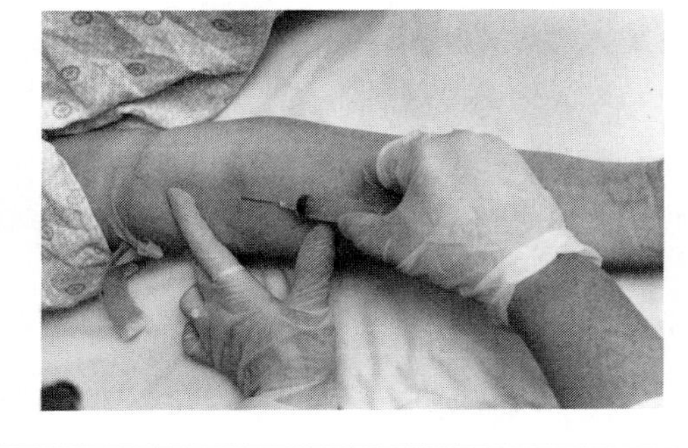

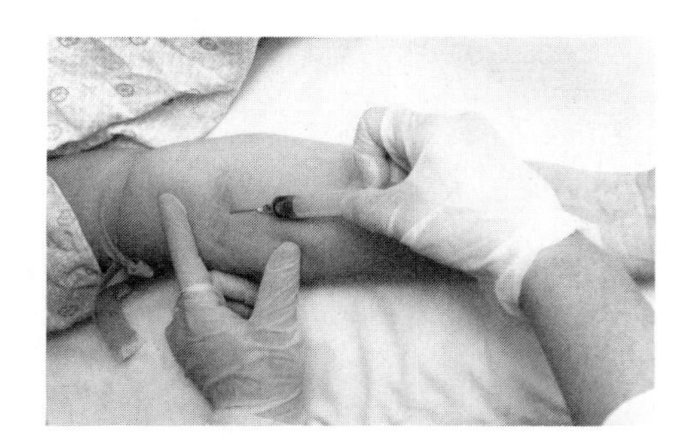

*Fig. 45-24*

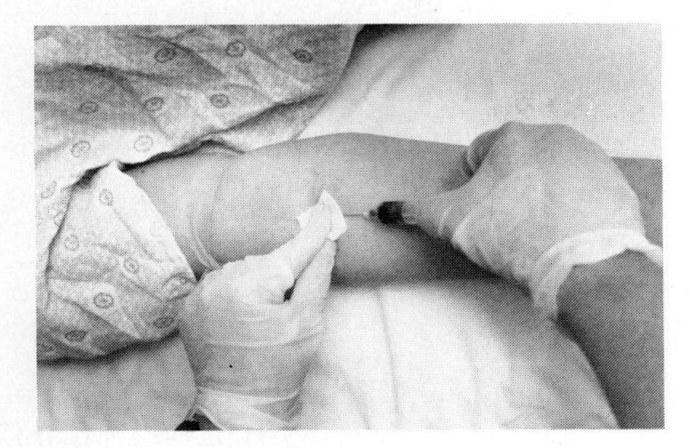
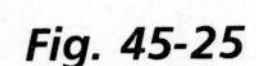

*Fig. 45-25*

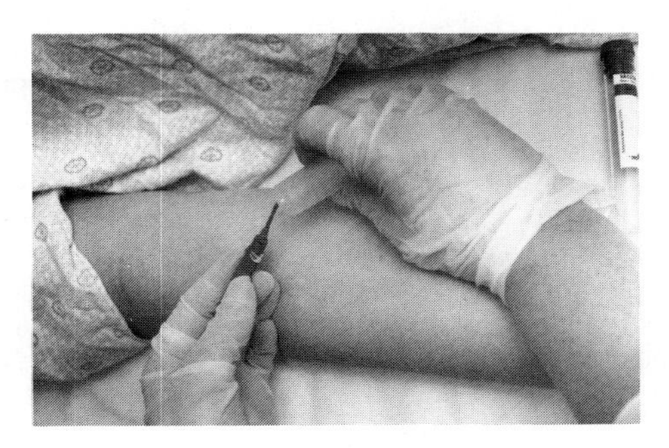

*Fig. 45-26*

| Steps | Rationale |
| --- | --- |
| ▪ Obtain desired amount of blood, keeping needle stabilized. | Test results are more accurate when required amount of blood is obtained. Some tests cannot be performed without minimal blood requirement. Movement of needle increases discomfort. |
| ▪ After specimen is obtained, release tourniquet. | Reduces bleeding at site when needle is withdrawn. |
| ▪ Apply 2 × 2 gauze pad or antiseptic swab over puncture site without applying pressure and quickly but carefully withdraw needle from vein (Fig. 45-25). | Pressure over needle can cause discomfort. Careful removal of needle minimizes discomfort and vein trauma. |
| b. *Vacutainer method:* | |
| ▪ Attach double-ended needle to Vacutainer tube (Fig. 45-26). | Long end of needle used to puncture vein. Short end fits into blood tubes. |
| ▪ Have proper blood specimen tube resting inside Vacutainer but do not puncture rubber stopper. | Causes loss of tube's vacuum. |
| ▪ Cleanse venipuncture site with alcohol swab, moving in circular motion out from site for approximately 5 cm (2 in). | Cleans skin surface of resident bacteria so organisms do not enter puncture site. |
| ▪ Remove needle cover and inform client that "stick" lasting only few seconds will be felt. | Client has better control over anxiety when knows what to expect. |
| ▪ Place thumb or forefinger of nondominant hand 2.5 cm (1 in) above or below site and pull skin taut. Stretch skin down until vein is stabilized. | Helps to stabilize vein and prevent rolling during needle insertion. |
| ▪ Hold Vacutainer at 15- to 30-degree angle from arm with bevel up. | Reduces chance of penetrating both sides of vein during insertion. Bevel up causes less trauma to vein. |
| ▪ Slowly insert needle into vein. | Prevents puncture on opposite side. |
| ▪ Grasp Vacutainer securely and advance specimen tube into needle of holder (do not advance needle in vein) (Fig. 45-27). | Pushing needle through stopper breaks vacuum and causes flow of blood into tube. If needle in vein advances, vein may become punctured on other side. |
| ▪ Note flow of blood into tube (should be fairly rapid). | Failure of blood to appear indicates vacuum in tube lost or needle not in vein. |
| ▪ After specimen tube is filled, grasp vacutainer firmly and remove tube. Insert additional specimen tubes as needed. | Prevents needle from advancing or dislodging. Tube should fill completely because additives in certain tubes are measured in proportion to filled tube. |
| ▪ After last tube is filled, release tourniquet. | Reduces bleeding at site when needle is withdrawn. |
| ▪ Apply 2 × 2 gauze pad over puncture site without applying pressure and quickly but carefully withdraw needle from vein. | Pressure over needle can cause discomfort. Careful removal of needle minimizes discomfort and vein trauma. |

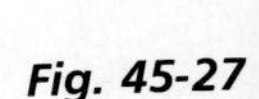
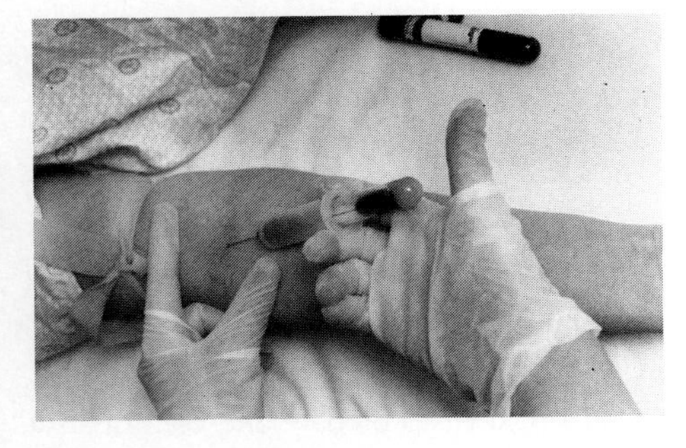

*Fig. 45-27*

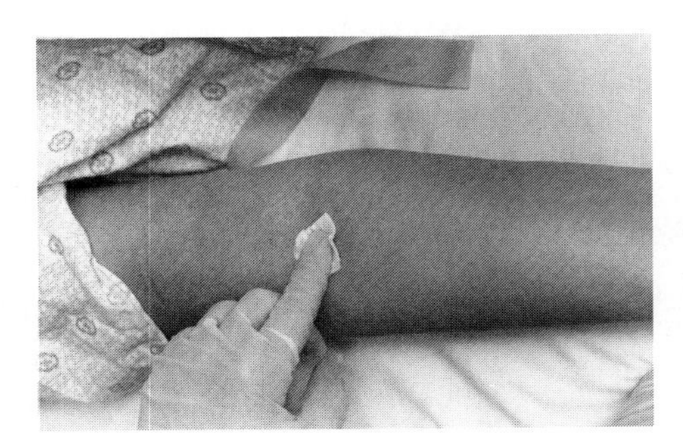

*Fig. 45-28*

| Steps | Rationale |
|---|---|
| 16. Immediately apply pressure over venipuncture site with gauze or antiseptic pad for 2 to 3 min or until bleeding stops (Fig. 45-28). OPTION: apply pressure over site and tape gauze dressing securely. | Direct pressure minimizes bleeding and prevents hematoma formation. Pressure dressing controls bleeding. |
| 17. For blood obtained by syringe, transfer specimen to tubes. Insert needle through stopper of blood tube and allow vacuum to fill tube (Fig. 45-29). Do not force blood into tube. | Blood should not be forced into tube; prevents hemolysis of red blood cells. |
| *or* Remove needle from syringe and stopper to each test tube. Gently inject required amount of blood into each tube. Reapply stopper. | Blood injected too quickly may cause frothing or hemolysis of red blood cells. Stopper maintains sterility of specimen. |
| 18. Take blood tubes containing additives and gently rotate back and forth 8 to 10 times. | Additives should be mixed with blood to prevent clotting. Shaking can cause hemolysis of red blood cells, producing inaccurate test results. |
| 19. Inspect puncture site for bleeding and apply adhesive tape with gauze. | Keeps puncture site clean and controls any final oozing. |
| 20. Check tubes for any sign of external contamination with blood. Decontaminate with 70% alcohol if necessary. | Prevents cross contamination. Reduces risk of exposure to pathogens present in blood. |
| 21. Remove disposable gloves after specimen obtained and any spillage cleaned. | Reduces risk of exposure to HIV, hepatitis, other blood-borne pathogens. |
| 22. Assist client to comfortable position. | |
| 23. Securely attach properly completed identification label to each tube and affix proper requisition. | Incorrect identification of specimen could result in diagnostic or therapeutic errors. |
| 24. Dispose of needles, syringe, soiled equipment in proper container. Do not cap needles. | Prevents cross-contamination through needle sticks and contact with blood. |
| 25. Wash hands after procedure. | Reduces transfer of microorganisms. |
| 26. Send specimens immediately to laboratory. | Fresh specimen ensures accurate results. |

Fig. 45-29

## Evaluation

| | |
|---|---|
| 1. Reinspect venipuncture site. | Determines if bleeding has stopped or hematoma has formed. |
| 2. Determine if client remains anxious or fearful. | Client may require more blood tests in future. Anxiety or concerns should be expressed. |
| 3. Check laboratory report for test results. | Reveals constituents of blood specimen. |

### *Expected outcomes*

| | |
|---|---|
| 1. Venipuncture site shows no evidence of continued bleeding or hematoma. | Indicates hemostasis achieved. |
| 2. Client feels no anxiety or discomfort. | Removal of painful stimulus lessens anxiety. Some clients are not anxious over procedure. |
| 3. Laboratory tests show normal findings. | No abnormalities found in blood elements. |

### *Unexpected outcomes*

| | |
|---|---|
| 1. Hematoma forms at venipuncture site. | Blood has escaped from vein and entered surrounding tissues. |
| 2. Bleeding at site continues. | Clotting mechanisms may be altered. |
| 3. Client continues to be anxious or fearful. | Level of discomfort experienced can heighten anxiety. |
| 4. Laboratory tests reveal abnormal blood constituents. | Tests reveal alterations in physiologic mechanisms. |

## Recording and Reporting

| | |
|---|---|
| 1. Record date and time of venipuncture and test samples obtained in nurses' notes. | Documents samples obtained. |
| 2. Describe venipuncture site after specimen collection and response in nurses' notes. | Documents response to diagnostic therapy. Description of site provides baseline to monitor change. |
| 3. Report any "stat" test results to physician. | Certain tests are ordered stat to determine condition immediately so proper therapies can be selected. |
| 4. Report abnormal test results to physician. | |

## Follow-up Activities

| | |
|---|---|
| 1. If hematoma develops, obtain order from physician to apply cold compress. After bleeding subsides, order for hot compress can be obtained. | Helps to stop bleeding, reduce pain, prevent swelling. After bleeding has stopped, hot compress can improve circulation to area and reduce swelling and discomfort. |
| 2. Inform clients who are to receive further venipunctures about reasons for tests. | Some tests require sequence of specimens over time. Explanations help client to prepare and control anxiety. |

### Special Considerations

- Check with institutional policy regarding designated container for disposal of contaminated needles and syringes.
- If gloves become contaminated with blood, replace with clean pair after proper disposal of contaminated ones. Touch nothing and do not handle supplies with contaminated gloves.
- Infants and young children need to be restrained, as do restless, confused, or combative clients. Check institutional policy on need for physician's order if restraint is necessary. Parent may hold child to facilitate cooperation and decrease anxiety.
- Samples taken from vein near IV infusion may be diluted or contain concentrations of IV fluids. Postmastectomy client may have reduced lymphatic drainage in arm on operative side increasing risk of infection from needle sticks. Arteriovenous shunt should never be used to obtain specimens because of risks of clotting and bleeding. Hematoma indicates existing injury to vessel's wall.
- If drawing sample for blood alcohol level, use only antiseptic swab to ensure accurate test results.
- At times, it is advantageous to draw children's blood specimens in treatment room instead of in bed or room to maintain feeling that room is safe place.
- Clients receiving anticoagulants require pressure over site for at least 5 min.
- If child needs to be restrained during procedure, let parents choose if they want to assist. Person restraining client should speak in calm, reassuring tone. By leaning across child, nurse maintains body and eye contact, which can help to reduce fear.
- In clinics or physician's offices, chair with special arm extension may be used when obtaining blood specimens.
- If client has large distended veins, tourniquet may not be needed.
- Clients undergoing frequent venipunctures may have preferred or undesirable site. Most commonly used vein is median cubital in antecubital fossa. In children, use veins on dorsal aspect of foot or scalp veins. Avoid vessels that pulsate; this indicates artery.
- If vein cannot be palpated or viewed easily, remove tourniquet and apply warm, wet compress over extremity for 10 to 20 min. Heat causes local vasodilation.
- With experience nurse will feel "pop" as needle enters vein. If plunger pulled back too quickly, pressure may cause vein to collapse.

### Teaching Considerations

- Instruct client to briefly apply pressure to venipuncture site. Clients with bleeding disorders or on anticoagulant therapy should apply pressure for at least 5 min.
- Instruct client to notify nurse or physician if persistent or recurrent bleeding or expanding hematoma occurs at venipuncture site.

## *SKILL 45-15 Measuring Blood Glucose Level after Skin Puncture*

Obtaining capillary blood by skin puncture is an alternative when venipuncture cannot be performed or when reducing the frequency of needle sticks is desirable. The procedure is also less painful than venipuncture and is frequently used for routine screening in tests for anemia and blood cell counts. Capillary blood specimens are the primary method of blood collection in children and especially in neonates, for whom venipuncture is technically very difficult.

The ease of skin puncture method in obtaining blood samples makes it possible for clients to perform this procedure. This, along with the development of reagent strips and home glucose monitors, has revoluntionized home management care of clients with diabetes. Although not all blood tests can be performed on capillary samples, it is a viable alternative to venipuncture in many situations.

Self-testing of blood glucose can be performed by two methods. Both methods require obtaining a large drop of blood by skin puncture. The blood is applied to a specially prepared chemical reagent strip.

The first method involves visually reading the reagent strip by comparing it to the color chart on the container. Examples of such strips include Visidex, Dextrostix, Chemstrip BG. If the color on the strip falls between two reference blocks on the chart, the results may need to be estimated. Thus, accurate results of blood glucose may not always be obtained.

The second type of blood glucose monitoring is done by the use of reflectance meters. A variety of meters are on the market, including the Glucometer (Ames), Accu-Check BG (Bio-Dynamics), and the Glucoscan II (LifeScan). After applying a drop of blood from skin puncture onto the reagent strip, the client inserts the strip into the meter. In less than 5 minutes, an accurate measure of blood glucose can be obtained.

The meters use a wet-wash or dry-wipe method of testing. To perform a wet wash, the user flushes the blood-coated reagent strip with water before inserting the strip into the glucose meter. The dry wipe method is somewhat simpler, requiring the user to wipe off the blood-coated reagent strip with a dry cotton ball before making a reading. Both methods allow for measurement of blood glucose between 20 and 800 mg/100 ml, thus providing a sensitive measure of blood glucose.

The glucose meters are rapidly replacing urine glucose testing in the management of clients with diabetes. This skill describes the techniques used to measure blood glucose with a glucose meter using the dry wipe method. Figures 45-34 through 45-36 depict self-testing of blood glucose. When a nurse measures blood glucose, gloves are worn per CDC's universal blood or body fluid precautions (1987).

Before beginning this procedure, the nurse should know normal metabolism and regulation of blood glucose levels.

### Purposes

1. Monitor blood glucose levels of clients at risk for hypoglycemia and hyperglycemia.
2. Provide a method for evaluating the effectiveness of insulin administration.
3. Improve diabetic clients ability to control blood glucose levels independently.

## *Procedure 45-15*

| Steps | Rationale |
|---|---|
| **Assessment** | |
| 1. Assess understanding of procedure and purpose. Determine if clients with diabetes understand how to perform test and realize importance of glucose monitoring. | Data set guidelines for nurse to develop teaching plan. |
| 2. Determine if specific conditions need to be met before sample collection (e.g., with fasting, after meals, or after certain medications). | Dietary intake of carbohydrates and ingestion of concentrated glucose preparations alter blood glucose levels. |
| 3. Determine if risks exist for performing skin puncture (e.g., low platelet count, anticoagulant therapy, bleeding disorders). | Abnormal clotting mechanisms increase risk for local ecchymosis and bleeding. |
| 4. Assess area of skin to be used as puncture site. Inspect fingers, toes, heel. Avoid areas of bruising and open lesions. | Sides of fingers, toes, heels are commonly selected because they have fewer nerve endings and are quite vascular. Area should be free of lesions or abnormalities. |
| 5. Review physician's order for time of frequency of measurement. | Physician determines test schedule on basis of client's physiologic status and risk for glucose imbalance. |
| 6. For diabetic client who performs test at home, assess ability to handle skin puncturing device. | Client's physical health may change (e.g., from fatigue, pain, disease state), preventing client from performing test. |
| **Nursing Diagnosis** | |
| 1. Cluster data to reveal actual or potential nursing diagnoses: | |
| a. Knowledge deficit regarding testing procedure: related to inexperience. | Extent of teaching depends on client's experience with test. |
| b. Altered health maintenance: related to need for continual glucose monitoring. | Results from inability of client to monitor glucose. |
| c. Anxiety: related to discomfort of skin puncture. | Children in particular can be apprehensive about procedure. |
| d. Potential for infection: related to skin puncture. | Potential exists for infection because of break in skin. |
| **Planning** | |
| 1. Develop individualized goals for client: | |
| a. Prevent injury to tissues and vessels. | Correct selection of puncture site and proper use of puncture device can minimize injury to client. |
| b. Obtain appropriate specimen. | Vascular area must be punctured to produce adequate drop of blood. |
| c. Improve client's understanding of glucose monitoring techniques. | Nurse can provide explanations and opportunity for client to practice technique. |
| d. Minimize client's anxiety. | Skin can be punctured quickly with little discomfort. |
| 2. Prepare equipment and supplies (Fig. 45-30): | |
| a. Antiseptic swab | Used to cleanse skin before puncture. |
| b. Cotton ball | Used to wipe glucose reagent strip. |
| c. Sterile lancet or blood-letting device (Autolet) | Used to puncture skin. |
| d. Heel-warming device | Used with infants to increase circulation to heel before puncture. |
| e. Paper towel | |
| f. Glucose testing meter | |
| g. Blood glucose reagent strip | Brand determined by meter used. |
| h. Disposable gloves | Reduces risk of contamination by blood. |
| 3. Explain procedure and purpose to client or family. | Promotes cooperation. |

| **Steps** | **Rationale** |
|---|---|

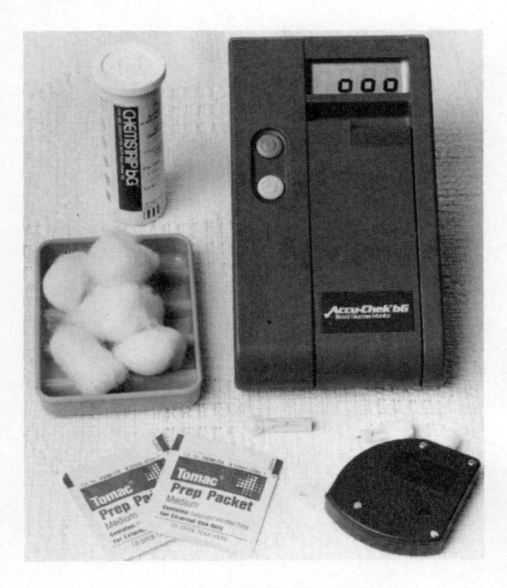


*Fig. 45-30*

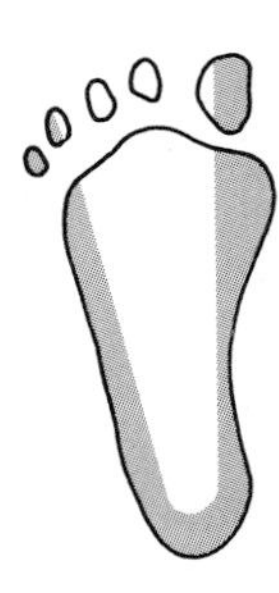

*Fig. 45-31*

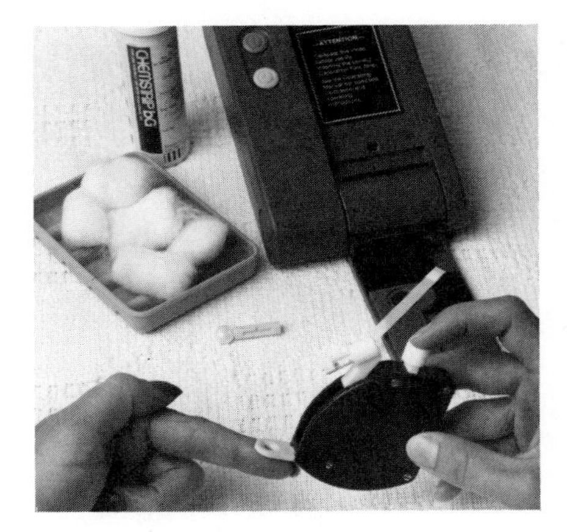

*Fig. 45-32*

## Implementation

| Steps | Rationale |
|---|---|
| 1. Wash hands before procedure. | |
| 2. Instruct adult to wash hands with soap and warm water, if able. | Reduces transfer of microorganisms. Promotes skin cleansing and vasodilation at selected puncture site. Handwashing establishes practice for client when test is performed at home. |
| 3. Position client comfortably in chair or semi-Fowler's position in bed. | Ensures easy accessibility to puncture site. Client will assume position when self-testing. |
| 4. Remove reagent strip from container and tightly seal caps. | Protects strips from accidental discoloration. |
| 5. Insert strip into glucose meter (see manufacturer's directions) and make necessary adjustments. | Some machines must be calibrated; others require zeroing of timer. Each meter is adjusted differently. |
| 6. Remove unused reagent strip from meter and place on paper towel or clean, dry surface with test pad facing up. | Moisture on strip can change its color, altering reading of final test results. |
| 7. Apply disposable gloves. | Reduces risk of contamination by blood. |
| 8. Choose puncture site; side of finger (adult) or outer aspect of heel (infant) (Fig. 45-31). | Puncture site should be vascular. Heel site avoids possible penetration of underlying calcaneus bone. |
| 9. Hold finger to be punctured in dependent position while gently massaging finger toward puncture site. | Increases blood flow to area before puncture. |
| 10. Clean site with antiseptic swab and allow to dry completely. | Alcohol can cause blood to hemolyze. |
| 11. Remove cover of lancet or blood-letting device. | Cover keeps tip of lancet/needle sterile. |
| 12. Place blood-letting device firmly against side of finger and push release button, causing needle to pierce skin (Fig. 45-32). Hold lancet perpendicular to puncture site and pierce finger or heel quickly in one continuous motion (do not force lancet). | Blood-letting devices are designed to pierce skin for specific depth, ensuring adequate blood flow. Perpendicular position ensures proper skin penetration. |
| 13. Wipe away first droplet of blood with cotton ball. | First drop of blood generally contains large portion of serous fluid, which can dilute specimen and cause false results. |
| 14. Lightly squeeze puncture site until large droplet of blood has formed (Fig. 45-33). | Ensure proper coverage of test pad on reagent strip. |
| 15. Hold reagent strip test pad close to drop of blood and lightly transfer droplet to test pad. Do not smear blood. | Droplet must be absorbed by test pad to ensure proper chemical reaction. Smearing causes inaccurate test results. |
| 16. Immediately press timer on glucose meter and place reagent strip on paper towel or on side of timer. | Blood must be exposed to test strip for prescribed time to ensure proper results. Strip should lay flat so blood does not pool on only one part of pad. |
| 17. Apply pressure to skin puncture site. | Promotes hemostasis. |
| 18. When timer displays 60 sec (for Accu-Chek model), use moderate pressure to wipe blood from test pad with cotton ball. No blood should remain on test pad (Fig. 45-34). | In order for meter to read glucose levels, strip must be dry. Refer to product directions for timing used with each type of meter. |

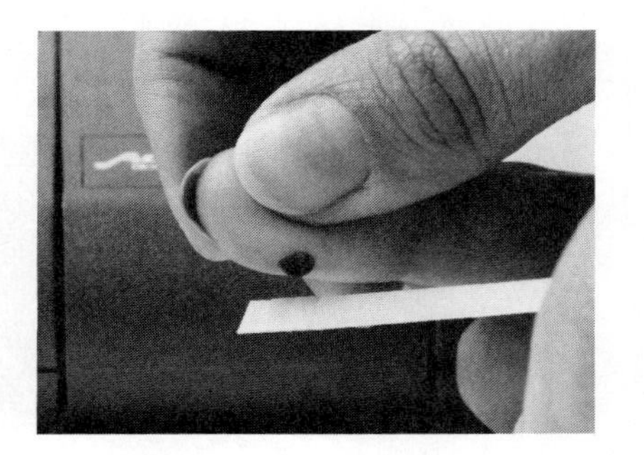

*Fig. 45-33*

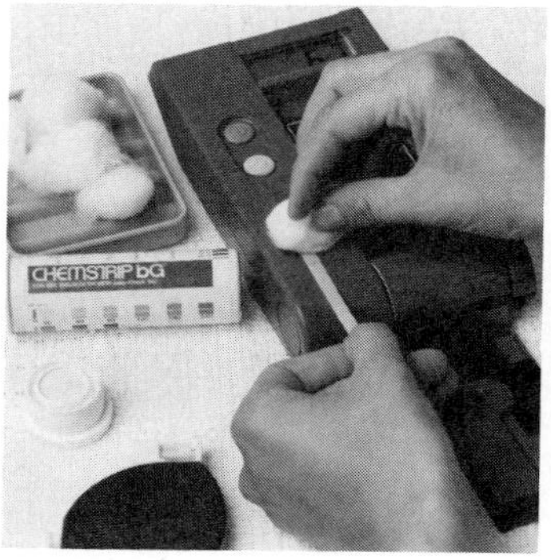

*Fig. 45-34*

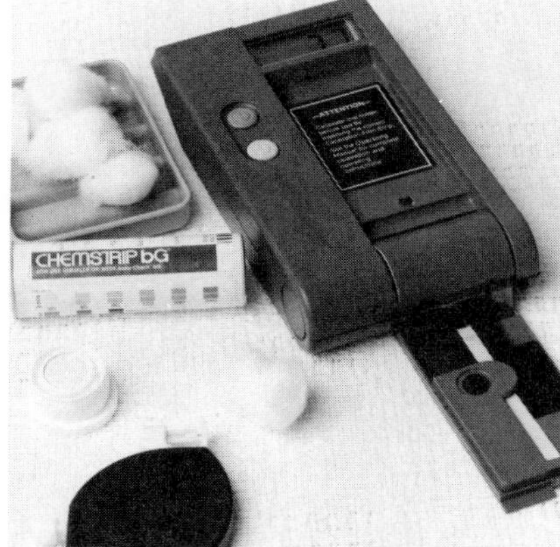

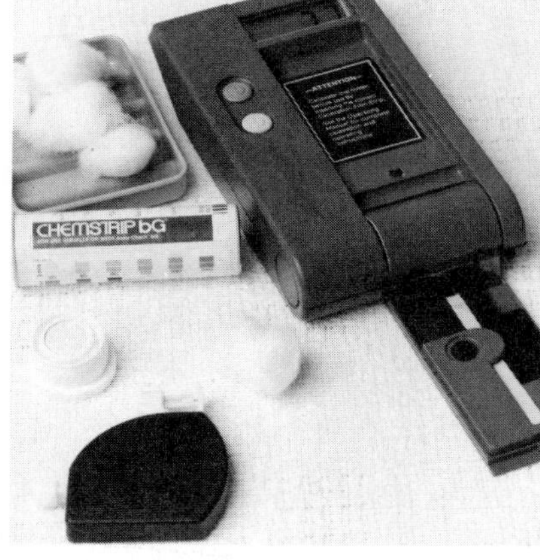



*Fig. 45-35*

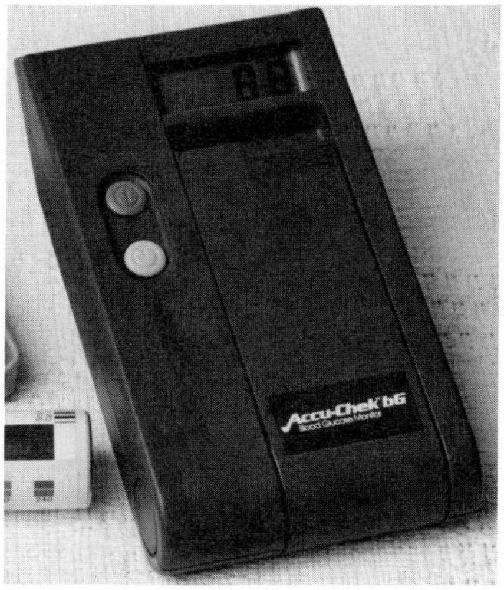

*Fig. 45-36*

| Steps | Rationale |
|---|---|
| 19. While timer continues to count, place reagent strip into meter (Fig. 45-35). | Strip must be inserted correctly to obtain accurate reading. |
| 20. At 2 min, activate meter to display glucose reading. Note reading on display (Fig. 45-36). | Correct timing ensures proper reading of glucose level. |
| 21. Turn meter off and dispose of test strip and cotton balls in proper receptacle. | Meter is battery-powered. Proper disposal reduces spread of microorganisms. |
| 22. Remove disposable gloves. | |
| 23. Wash hands. | Reduces transmission of infection. |
| 24. Share test results with client. | Promotes participation and compliance with therapy. |

## Evaluation

| | |
|---|---|
| 1. Compare glucose meter reading with normal blood glucose levels. | Determines if glucose level is normal. |
| 2. Reinspect puncture site for bleeding or tissue injury. | Can be source of discomfort. |
| 3. Determine if client has any questions or concerns. | Results of test may cause anxiety. Client may misunderstand specific step of procedure. |

### *Expected outcomes*

| | |
|---|---|
| 1. Puncture site shows no evidence of bleeding or tissue damage. | Hemostasis achieved. Lancet or needle did not puncture skin too deeply. |
| 2. Blood glucose level is normal. | Normal fasting glucose is 70 to 120 mg/100 ml, indicating good metabolic control. |
| 3. Client expresses understanding of procedure and test results. | Shows success of nurse's instructions and demonstration. |

### *Unexpected outcomes*

| | |
|---|---|
| 1. Puncture site is bruised or continues to bleed. | Adequate pressure may not have been applied to site, or clotting mechanisms may be altered. |

| Steps | Rationale |
|---|---|
| 2. Blood glucose level above or below normal range. | Client is hypoglycemic or hyperglycemic. |
| 3. Glucose meter malfunctions. | Technique not properly followed as directed; battery may be low; instrument may not be clean. |
| 4. Client expresses misunderstanding of procedure and results. | Attention span or interest in subject may be lessened. Nurse may not have explained steps clearly. |
| **Recording and Reporting** | |
| 1. Record procedure and glucose level in nurses' notes or special flow sheet. | Documents testing. |
| 2. Describe response, including appearance of puncture site, in nurses' notes. | Documents response to therapy. |
| 3. Describe explanations or teaching provided in nurses' notes. | Ensures continuity of health education. |
| 4. Report abnormal blood glucose levels to physician. | Findings may indicate need for new therapy. |
| **Follow-up Activities** | |
| 1. Administer insulin or carbohydrate source as ordered, depending on glucose level. | Diabetic client's insulin dosage is often regulated by blood glucose levels. Clients who are hypoglycemic require increase in carbohydrates. |
| 2. Offer client and family opportunity to practice testing procedures. | Provides for health maintenance in home setting. |
| 3. Provide information on where diabetic client can obtain testing supplies. | Compliance with testing improves when supplies are readily available. |

### Special Considerations

- Some clients with diabetes may already routinely monitor blood glucose at home and wish to continue doing so in hospital.
- Blood glucose levels are frequently assessed before meals to help to determine required insulin dosages.
- Heel is frequently punctured in infants. Clients who undergo frequent skin punctures may develop callous at finger sites they prefer to use.
- Heel punctures should not exceed 2.5 mm because of risk of penetrating calcaneus. Puncture of bone can cause serious osteochordritis.
- Repuncturing skin may be necessary if large enough droplet of blood does not form to ensure accurate test results.
- Diabetic clients frequently have peripheral vascular disease, making it difficult to produce a large droplet of blood after a finger stick. Be sure finger is held in a dependent position prior to stick to improve blood flow to area.

### Teaching Considerations

- Instruct client on correct performance of glucose monitoring procedure.
- Instruct client to to keep accurate records of results.
- Instruct client on how to interpret test results.
- Have client return demonstration of procedure.
- Instruct client about interpretation and correction of erroneous results.
- Instruct client about various alternative sample sites.

## *SKILL 45-16 Measuring Arterial Blood Gases*

Assessment of oxygenation and ventilation can be accomplished by measuring arterial blood gases. The parameters measured include arterial blood pH, partial pressure of oxygen, partial pressure of carbon dioxide, and arterial oxygen saturation. The arterial blood gas sample is easily obtained and can be quickly analyzed to provide the nurse with a clear picture of acid-base balance, oxygenation, and to some extent, ventilation. Alterations from normal show the nurse how the client is adapting to the disease process.

Measuring arterial blood gases aids the nurse in assessment. A decision to draw arterial blood gases may be frequently a direct result of the nurse's physical assessment (Chapter 13). Nursing diagnosis and interventions can be determined based on the clinical picture and laboratory data.

Obtaining arterial blood gases is an invasive procedure. A complete assessment, as well as a medical order, must be completed before obtaining the sample.

Before beginning this procedure, the nurse should know how to prepare a syringe from a vial or ampule (Chapter 20).

## Purposes

1. Assess oxygenation status.
2. Assess effectiveness of current oxygen therapy or ventilatory support.
3. Assess ventilatory status.
4. Assess acid-base balance.

## Procedure 45-16

| Steps | Rationale |
|---|---|
| **Assessment** | |
| 1. Determine need to obtain arterial blood gas sample. Signs and symptoms of alteration in respiratory status requiring sampling may include dyspnea, sudden change in respiratory rate or pattern, unequal breath sounds, unequal chest expansion, cyanosis, change in level of consciousness, self-extubation without need for immediate reintubation, increased work of breathing. | Some situations and medical conditions place clients at risk for alteration in acid-base balance and ventilation status. |
| 2. Assess for factors that influence arterial blood gas measurements: a. From client just awakened. b. immediately after suctioning. c. less than 20 to 30 min after oxygen therapy or ventilator setting change. d. from client whose oxygen has not been in place continually for at least 20 to 30 min. | Allows nurse to eliminate factors that cause inaccurate results. |
| 3. Perform physical assessment of thorax and lungs. | Physical signs and symptoms may indicate need for arterial blood gas sample. |
| 4. Review criteria for choosing site for arterial blood gas sample: | |
| a. Collateral blood flow. | Arterial puncture may result in spasm of artery, clotting, hematoma; any of these factors may result in reduced or obstructed blood flow to tissues supplied by vessel. Collateral blood flow availability is essential if complications occur. |
| ▪ Perform Allen's test: | Determines adequate collateral flow for radial artery. |
| ▫ Have client make tight fist. | Removes as much blood from hand as possible. |
| ▫ Apply direct pressure to both radial and ulnar arteries (Fig. 45-37). | Obstructs arterial blood flow to hand. |
| ▫ Have client open hand (Fig. 45-38). | Fingers and hand should be pale and blanched, indicating lack of arterial blood flow. |
| ▫ Release pressure over ulnar artery; observe color of fingers, thumbs, and hand (Fig. 45-39). Fingers and hand should flush within 15 sec. Flushing is positive Allen's test. If test is negative (no flushing), radial artery should be avoided. Check other hand. | If collateral circulation is present through ulnar artery, hand and fingers flush. Ulnar artery is capable of supplying blood flow to hand if radial artery is damaged or becomes occluded during procedure. |
| b. Accessibility of vessel. | Palpating, stabilizing and performing venipuncture of superficial artery is easier. Superficial arteries are located at distal ends of extremities. |
| c. Tissue surrounding artery. | Muscle, tendon, fat have decreased sensation to pain. Bony periosteum and nerves are very sensitive to pain. |
| d. Arteries surrounded by relatively insensitive tissues. | These are preferred sites; reduces discomfort to client. |
| e. Arteries not directly adjacent to veins. | Help reduce chance of venous puncture and possibility of inaccurate samples. |

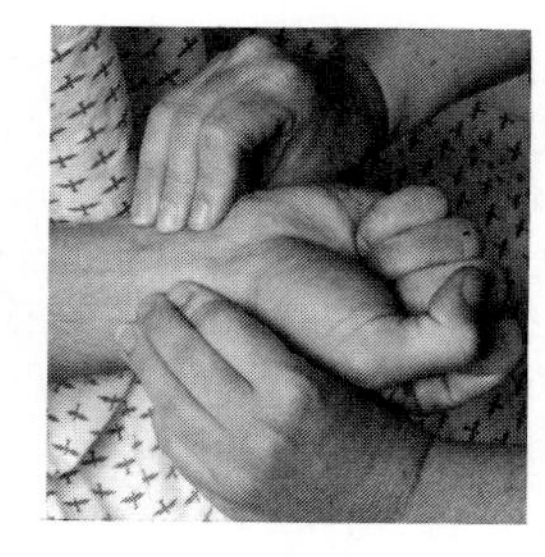

*Fig. 45-37*

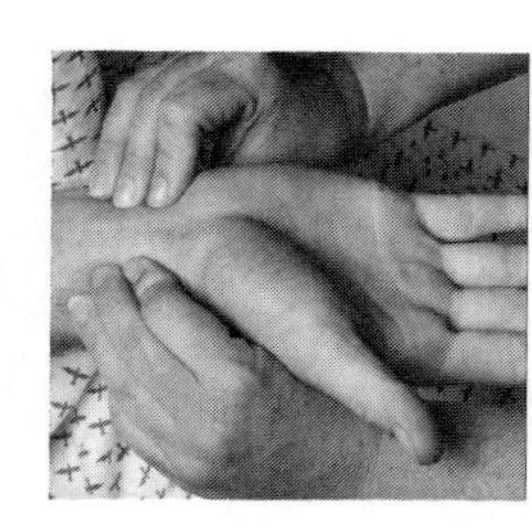

*Fig. 45-38*

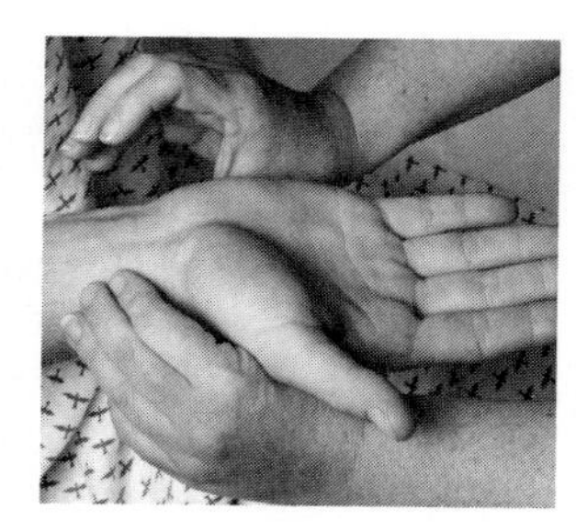

*Fig. 45-39*

| Steps | Rationale |
|---|---|
| 5. Assess arterial sites for use in obtaining specimen: | Previous punctures or preexisting conditions may eliminate potential sites. Artery should be easily accessible. |
| a. Radial artery. | Safest, most accessible site for puncture. Is superficial, is not adjacent to large veins, usually has adequate collateral circulation by ulnar artery, is relatively painless if periosteum is avoided, is used when Allen's test is positive. |
| b. Brachial artery. | Has reasonable collateral blood flow, is less superficial, is more difficult to palpate and stabilize, carries increased risk of venous puncture, results in increased discomfort for client if brachial nerve punctured, is used when radial artery is inaccessible or Allen's test is negative. |
| c. Femoral artery. | Should not be used by nurses without specialized training. Has no adequate collateral flow if obstructed below inguinal ligament, is difficult to stabilize, is deep, is directly adjacent to femoral vein. Is best artery to use in emergency (e.g., cardiac arrest or hypovolemic shock when pulses difficult to palpate). |
| 6. Determine baseline arterial blood gases for client. | Provides basis for comparison and evaluation of therapies. |

## Nursing Diagnosis

| | |
|---|---|
| 1. Cluster data to reveal actual or potential nursing diagnoses: | |
| a. Impaired gas exchange: related to altered oxygen supply. | Blood gas results can assist nurse in confirming diagnoses. |
| b. Ineffective breathing pattern: related to pain. | |
| c. Altered peripheral tissue perfusion: related to poor arterial flow. | Nurse uses precautions to prevent altering arterial blood flow. |
| d. Pain: related to arterial puncture. | Radial artery punctures are painful. |

## Planning

| | |
|---|---|
| 1. Develop individualized goals for client: | |
| a. Minimize client's discomfort. | Arterial puncture is painful; smooth, efficient maneuvers minimize discomfort. |
| b. Ensure accuracy of specimen values. | Techniques for collection and transport of specimen are important in preventing inaccurate results. |
| c. Maintain arterial blood flow. | Nurse uses precautions to prevent arterial obstruction or damage. |
| 2. Prepare equipment and supplies (Commercial blood gas kits are available): | |
| a. 3 ml heparinized syringe | 2 ml blood sample is adequate for most laboratories. |
| b. 23- or 25-gauge needle (scalp vein needle optional) | Smaller-gauge needle reduces risk of hematoma and minimizes damage to arterial wall. |
| c. Syringe cap | Used to seal syringe after sample is collected. |
| d. Two alcohol swabs | |
| e. 2 × 2 gauze pad | |
| f. Heparin (1:1000 solution) | Higher concentration over-dilutes sample and causes inaccurate results. |
| g. Cup or plastic bag with crushed ice | Ice reduces metabolism of red blood cells to prevent reduction in oxygen pressure ($Po_2$) level. Cup or bag is used to transport specimen. |
| h. Label with client identification | Need to label blood sample properly so results reported for correct client. |
| i. Laboratory requisition | Ensures laboratory will run sample for correct test and report results. |
| j. Disposable gloves | |
| 3. Prepare heparinized syringe (if heparinized syringes are unavailable): | |
| a. Aspirate 0.5 ml sodium heparin, 1000 units/ml, into syringe from vial or ampule. | Prevents blood sample from clotting before reaching laboratory. Excessive heparin can affect pH of arterial sample. |
| b. Withdraw plunger entire length of syringe and maintain asepsis. | Coats barrel of syringe with heparin. |
| c. Eject all heparin in barrel out of syringe. | 0.15 to 0.25 ml of sodium heparin remains in hub of syringe. 0.05 ml of sodium heparin adequately anticoagulates 1 ml of blood; 0.15 ml adequately anticoagulates 3 ml without affecting pH level. |
| 4. Explain steps and purpose of procedure to client. | Reduces anxiety and promotes understanding and cooperation. |

| Steps | Rationale |
|---|---|
| **Implementation** | |
| 1. Wash hands and apply gloves. | Reduces transmission of infection. |
| 2. Palpate selected radial site with fingertips. | Determines area of maximal impulse for puncture site. |
| 3. Stabilize artery by hyperextending wrist slightly. | Reduces mobility of artery and makes insertion of needle easier. |
| 4. Clean over area of maximal impulse with alcohol swab, wiping in circular motion. | Reduces number of resident bacteria on skin's surface. |
| 5. Hold alcohol swab with same fingers used to palpate artery. | Keeps swab accessible when covering of puncture site becomes necessary. |
| 6. Keep fingertip on artery, just above chosen puncture site. | Maintaining location of artery improves likelihood of successful puncture because multiple sticks are painful. |
| 7. Hold needle bevel up and insert at 45-degree angle into artery, with bevel directed proximally. | Angle allows for better arterial flow into needle. Oblique hole in artery seals more easily. |
| 8. Stop advancing needle when blood is noted returning into hub of needle, into syringe, into plastic tube of scalp vein needle. | Quick return of blood indicates arterial flow obtained. Prevents completely transversing needle through artery. |
| 9. If using open needle, attach syringe securely. | Prevents air bubbles from entering sample. |
| 10. Use 2 × 2 gauze or antiseptic swab to catch blood that may spill when syringe is attached. | Maintains cleanliness. |
| 11. Draw 2 to 3 ml of arterial blood into heparinized syringe slowly (Fig. 45-40). | Rapidly withdrawing blood creates turbulence and contaminates sample with air bubbles. Bubbles can alter blood gas results. |
| 12. When sampling is complete, hold alcohol swab over puncture site and withdraw needle. | Swab minimizes pulling of skin as needle is withdrawn. |
| 13. Apply pressure over and just proximal to puncture site with swab (Fig. 45-41). | Insertion of needle into artery is just proximal to insertion site through skin. Gauze absorbs any blood that might ooze from site. |
| 14. Maintain continuous pressure over and proximal to site for 5 min, or 10 min if client is on anticoagulant therapy or has bleeding disorder. | Ensures adequate coagulation of arterial puncture site. |
| 15. Visually inspect site for signs of bleeding. | Determines if continued need exists to exert pressure. |
| 16. Palpate artery below or distal to puncture site. | Determines if pulse quality has changed, indicating alteration in arterial flow. |
| 17. Remove gloves and wash hands. | Reduces transmission of microorganisms. |
| 18. Expel air bubbles from syringe. | Air bubbles can falsely elevate arterial oxygen pressure ($Pa_{O_2}$) and lower arterial carbon dioxide pressure ($Pa_{CO_2}$). |
| 19. Prepare syringe for laboratory analysis according to agency policy. Common principles include: | |
| a. Place client identification label on syringe. | Permits proper identification of sample for laboratory. |
| b. Place syringe in cup of crushed ice. | Reduces blood cell metabolism (e.g., oxygen consumption and carbon dioxide ($CO_2$ production) within sample. |
| c. Attach properly labeled requisition to blood gas sample. | Prevents mislabeled specimens in laboratory. Ensures correct results received for correct client. |
| d. Indicate client's fractional inspired oxygen concentration ($Fi_{O_2}$) on requisition. | Essential for proper identification of sample. |
| e. Send sample to laboratory immediately. | Prevents changes in sample resulting from delay in procedure. Provides more timely return of results to nurse. |

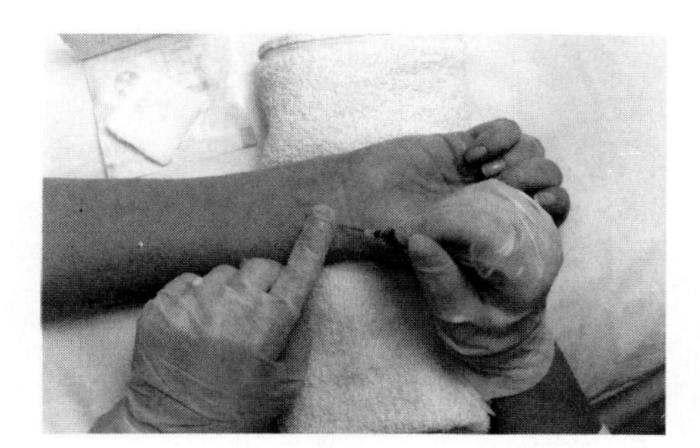

*Fig. 45-40*

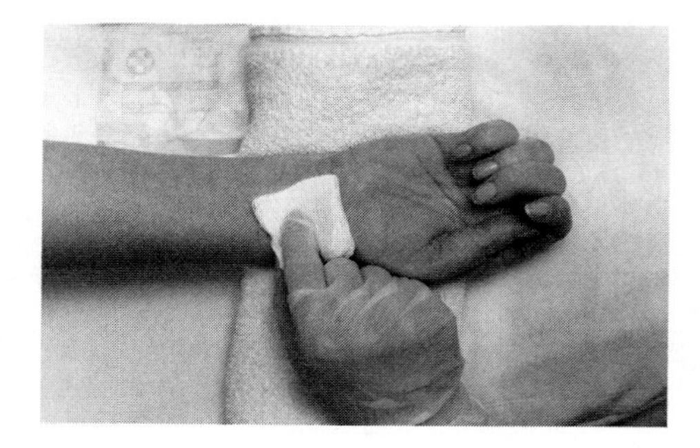

*Fig. 45-41*

| Steps | Rationale |
|---|---|
| **Evaluation** | |
| 1. Inspect area distal to puncture site for complications. | Obstruction of artery can develop from hematoma or damage to vessel wall, reducing arterial flow. |
| 2. Review results of sample as soon as possible. | Identifies any abnormality. |
| ***Expected outcomes*** | |
| 1. Client has normal arterial blood gas values within following ranges: pH—7.35 to 7.45; $Paco_2$—35 to 45; $Pao_2$—80 to 100; $Sao_2$—94% to 98% | Determining normal values is essential for accurate interpretation. |
| ***Unexpected outcomes*** | |
| 1. Client has elevated pH and lowered $Paco_2$. | Indicates respiratory alkalosis. |
| 2. Client has lowered pH and elevated $Paco_2$. | Indicates respiratory acidosis. |
| 3. Client has elevated $Pao_2$. | Indicates possible contamination of sample. |
| 4. Client has lowered $Pao_2$. | Indicates inadequate $Fio_2$; client unable to oxygenate efficiently. |
| **Reporting and Recording** | |
| 1. Report arterial blood gas results to physician as soon as available. | Timely assessment of results and reporting enable physician to make decisions regarding care. |
| 2. Be sure to include client's $Fio_2$ and any ventilator settings (e.g., $V_T$, respiratory frequency [$R_F$] mode of ventilation). | Necessary to interpret $Pao_2$ and $Paco_2$ accurately. |
| 3. Record results of test and condition of puncture site in nurses' notes. | Documents test results and indicates proper evaluation of puncture site. |
| **Follow-up Activities** | |
| 1. Continue to observe puncture site and assess pulse. | Hematoma can form from gradual oozing of blood around vessel. |
| 2. If client's oxygenation status is poor, indicated by low $Pao_2$, lower pH, elevated $Paco_2$ (respiratory acidosis): | |
| a. Encourage coughing and deep breathing. | Removes retained secretions that interfere with gas exchange. |
| b. Perform tracheal suctioning. | |
| c. Elevate head of bed. | Position maximizes chest and lung expansion. |
| d. Administer oxygen therapy. | Increases $Fio_2$ to improve diffusion. |
| e. Hold pain medication administration if possible. | Prevents further depression of respirations. |
| 3. If oxygenation status is poor, indicated by elevated pH, and low $Paco_2$ (respiratory alkalosis): | |
| a. Encourage slow, deep breaths or have client breathe into paper bag. | Prevents further exhalation of $CO_2$. Allows $Paco_2$ to return to normal level. |
| b. Administer pain medication. | Reduces pain sensation that led to hyperventilation. |
| c. Talk with client about fears or concerns. | Relieves anxiety that led to hyperventilation. |
| d. Initiate tepid sponging, control room temperature, or administer antipyretics as ordered. | Reduces body temperature. |

## Special Considerations

- Venous sample has low $Po_2$ and high $Pco_2$ compared to arterial sample.
- Factors that contraindicate use of arterial site include amputation, contractures, dressing or cast.
- Check with laboratory to verify quantity of sample required. Blood should return easily into syringe because of arterial pressure.
- If hyperventilated, client may feel dizzy and confused and may require coaching to slow breathing.

## Teaching Considerations

- Prepare client for needle stick because radial sticks are painful. Prepared client will not reflexively withdraw arm.
- Instruct client to breathe normally.
- Client is taught to report numbness, burning, and/or tingling in hand that had radial artery puncture.

# SKILL 45-17 Pulse Oximetry

Pulse oximetry is the noninvasive measurement of arterial oxygen saturation ($Sao_2$) first developed in Japan. The pulse oximeter uses fiberoptics to measure the amount of oxygenated hemoglobin in arterial blood (Fig. 45-42). The oximeter probe can be applied to the ear, finger, or bridge of the nose.

Pulse oximetry is clinically indicated in clients in whom constant monitoring of $Sao_2$ is desirable. The noninvasive measurement is perferable to frequent arterial blood gas samples or continuous arterial catheters. Clients who are being weaned from mechanical ventilators, have recently been extubated, or are weaning from oxygen therapy are candidates for oximetric measurement.

Before beginning this procedure, the nurse should know oxygen content and saturation, the oxyhemoglobin dissociation curve, and oxygen transport and consumption.

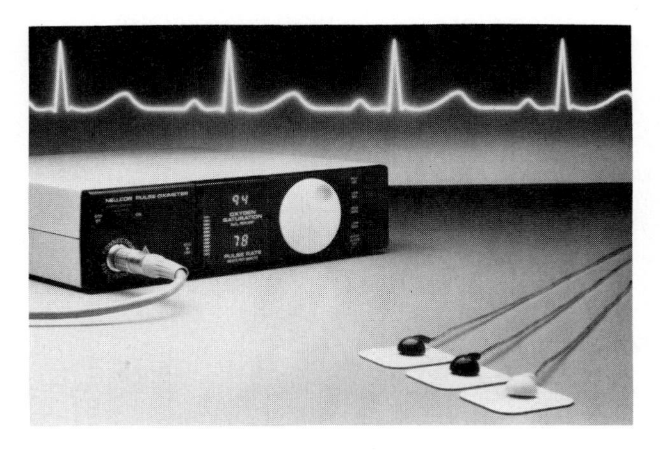


*Fig. 45-42*

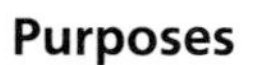

## Purposes

1. Monitor oxygen therapy.
2. Assess withdrawal of oxygen therapy.
3. Monitor oxygenation.

## Procedure 45-17

| Steps | Rationale |
|---|---|
| **Assessment** | |
| 1. Identify clients who would benefit from pulse oximetry. | Alerts health personnel to clients with respiratory alterations who could be monitored. |
| 2. Assess client's respiratory status: oxygen therapy, hemoglobin level. | Indicates factors important in oxygenation assessment. |
| 3. Review client's medical record for physician's order for pulse oximetry. | Medical order is required to administer pulse oximetry. |
| **Nursing Diagnosis** | |
| 1. Cluster data to reveal actual or potential nursing diagnoses: | |
| a. Impaired gas exchange: related to alveolar hypoventilation. | Airway and alveolar collapse result in decreased surface area for gas exchange. |
| b. Impaired gas exchange: related to retained secretions. | |
| **Planning** | |
| 1. Develop individualized goals for client based on nursing diagnoses: | |
| a. Monitor exercise tolerance. | $Sao_2$ indicates client's tolerance to increasing levels of exercise. |
| b. Assess oxygenation status. | Determines pulmonary perfusion or ventilation problems. |
| 2. Obtain equipment and place at bedside: | |
| a. Pulse oximeter | |
| b. Senser probe | |
| c. Continuous printout (optional) | |
| 3. Explain purpose of procedure to client and family. | Assures client and family and increases compliance. |

| Steps | Rationale |
|---|---|
| **Implementation** | |
| 1. Wash hands. | Reduces transmission of microorganisms. |
| 2. Position client comfortably and support dependent extremity to be used for monitoring. | Ensures probe positioning and decreases motion interferences with signal. |
| 3. Instruct client to breath normally. | Prevents large fluctuations in minute ventilation and possible changes in $Sao_2$. |
| 4. Remove finger nail polish (if finger is to be used). | Polish can falsely alter saturation. |
| 5. Attach sensor probe to finger or bridge of nose. | Select sensor site based on peripheral circulation and extremity temperature. Peripheral vasoconstriction alter $Sao_2$. |
| 6. Watch pulse bar for pulse sensing. | Amplitude of pulse bar sensor indicates how well oximeter monitors pulse. |
| 7. Determine that client's radial pulse on arm sensor is in place. | Ensures accuracy of oximeter; double-checks pulse against machine. |
| 8. Read saturation and chart as appropriate. | Documents $Sao_2$ level. |
| ***Expected outcomes*** | |
| 1. Client's $Sao_2$ remains between 90% and 100%. | Indicates adequate oxygenation. |
| 2. Client's oxygenation therapies can be adjusted without invasive measures. | |
| ***Unexpected outcome*** | |
| 1. Client's $Sao_2$ is less than 80%. | Client may demonstrate signs and symptoms of hypoxemia |
| **Recording and Reporting** | |
| 1. Record in nurses' notes client's use of continuous pulse oximetry. | Documents use of equipment for third-party payers. |
| 2. Record $Sao_2$ in nurse's notes. | Documents $Sao_2$. |
| 3. Correlate with arterial blood gas measurements if available. | Documents reliability of oximeter. |
| 4. Report $Sao_2$ and response to changes in therapy to oncoming shift. | Provides oncoming nurse with baseline information and response to therapy. |
| **Follow-up Activity** | |
| 1. Ensure oximeter sensor is functioning properly. | Sensors need to be changed every 48 to 72 hours. |

## Special Considerations

- Clients who smoke cigarettes or who are use nicotine gum may have reduced peripheral circulation, which can make monitoring difficult and reduce accuracy of arterial saturation monitor.
- Clients who have peripheral vascular disease or Reynaud's syndrome or who simply have cold hands may have difficulty in obtaining readings.
- Decreased pH, increased temperature, and increased $Paco_2$ cause oxyhemoglobin curve to shift to right, resulting in lower saturation for the same $Pao_2$. Conversely, elevated pH, low temperature, decreased 2,3-diphosphogycerate (DPG) and decreased $Paco_2$ shift curve to left, resulting in higher saturation at lower $Pao_2$.

## Teaching Considerations

- Teach significance of monitoring arterial saturation.
- Teach signs and symptoms of hypoxemia: headache, somulence, confusion, dusky color, shortness of breath.

## Home Care Consideration

- Pulse oximetry is used in home care to monitor oxygen therapy or changes in oxygen therapy noninvasively.

## BIBLIOGRAPHY

Beare PG: Nursing implications of diagnostic tests, ed 2, Philadelphia, 1985, JB Lippincott Co.

Burton GE, Hodgkin JE: Respiratory care: a guide to clinical practice, ed 2, Philadelphia, JB Lippincott Co.

Centers for Disease Control: Recommendations for prevention of HIV transmission in health care settings, MMWR 36(suppl. 25):35, 1987.

Cherniack RM, Cherniack L: Respiration in health and disease, ed 3, Philadelphia, 1983, WB Saunders Co.

Corbett JV: Laboratory tests in nursing practice, Norwalk, Conn, 1982, Appleton-Century-Crofts.

Gabrielczyk MR, Burst RJ: Pulse oximetry and postoperative hypothermia, Anaesthesia 43:402, 1988.

Kersten L: Philadelphia, 1989, WB Saunders Co.

King T, Simon RH: Pulse oximetry for tapering supplemental oxygen in hospitalized patients, Chest 92:713, 1987.

Lamb JO: Laboratory tests for clinical nursing, Englewood Cliffs, NJ, 1984, Prentice-Hall.

Mihm FG, Halperin BD: Noninvasive detection of profound arterial desaturations using a pulse oximeter device, Anesthesiology 62(1):85, 1985.

Milliam DA: Getting into an artery, Am J Nurs 88(9):1214, 1988.

Nellcor, Inc: Principles of pulse oximetry: clinical education, Nellcor, Inc. 1988.

Nurses Reference Library, Nursing '83, Horsham, Penn, 1983, Intermed Communications, Inc, Springhouse Publishers.

Pagana KD, Pagana TJ: Diagnostic testing and nursing implications, ed 3, St Louis, 1986, The CV Mosby Co.

Pendergraph GE: Handbook of phlebotomy, Philadelphia, 1984, Lea & Febiger.

Shapiro BA, Harrison RA, Walton JR: Clinical application of blood gases, ed 2, Chicago, 1977, Yearbook Medical Publishers, Inc.

Surr CW: New blood-glucose monitoring products. I. Nurs '83 13:42, 1983.

Surr CW: New blood-glucose monitoring products. II. Nurs '83 13:58, 1983.

Taylor MB, Whitwam A: The current status of pulse oximetry, Anaesthesia 41:943, 1986.

Whaley LF, Wong DL: Nursing care of infants and children, ed 3, St Louis, 1987, The CV Mosby Co.

Yelderman M, New W: Evaluation of pulse oximetry, Anesthesiology 59(4):349, 1983.

# 46

# DIAGNOSTIC PROCEDURES

### OBJECTIVES

*Mastery of content in this chapter will enable the nurse to:*

- Define key terms.
- Identify physiologic factors related to diagnostic procedures.
- Perform physical and psychologic assessment related to procedures.
- Demonstrate organizational skills in planning procedures.
- Effectively assist the physician with abdominal paracentesis, bone marrow aspiration, bronchoscopy, CT scanning, chest x-ray examination, electrocardiogram, endoscopy, lumbar puncture, proctoscopy, sigmoidoscopy, and thoracentesis.
- Demonstrate understanding of expected and unexpected outcomes and follow-up activities of procedures.
- Apply knowledge of proper recording and reporting procedures.
- Demonstrate understanding of the physician's and nurse's responsibilities relating to procedure.

### KEY TERMS

*Abdominal girth*
*Antiseptic*
*Anus*
*Ascites*
*Aspiration*
*Biopsy*
*Bone marrow*
*Cannula*
*Cerebrospinal fluid*
*Circulatory fluid*
*Coagulopathy*
*Cytologic*
*Exploratory laparotomy*
*Fiberoptic*
*Foramen magnum*
*Hematopoiesis*
*Hemodynamics*
*Herniation*
*Homeostasis*
*Intercostal space*
*Intraabdominal pressure*
*Intracranial pressure*
*Lavage*
*Lumen*
*Manometer*
*Opening pressure*
*Peritoneal fluid*
*Pleural cavity*
*Pleural fluid*
*Rectum*
*Sigmoid colon*
*Stopcock*
*Subarachnoid space*
*Tracheobronchial tree*
*Trocar*

### SKILLS



Diagnostic tests may be performed by a physician at the client's bedside or in a specially equipped room for therapeutic or diagnostic purposes. The nurse is responsible for assessing the client's knowledge of and preparing the client for the procedure, assisting the physician with the procedure, and caring for the client after tests are completed. The nurse's knowledge of and organization in carrying out the procedure can be the keys to success in performing the procedure. In the implementation phase of each test described (except for Skills 47-5 and 47-6, which are not routinely performed by a physician), the physician's responsibility is outlined separately from the nurse's responsibility. There are two main reasons for this separation of duties in the skills. First, the nurse anticipates the needs of the physician to have supplies ready. Second and most important, the nurse keeps the client adequately informed of procedural details that could cause discomfort.

The nurse must think about legal considerations when dealing with diagnostic procedures. Most invasive diagnostic tests require a signed informed consent. The physician is responsible for it, but the nurse must be aware of institutional policies regarding consent forms and ensure that informed consent is obtained before the procedure. The nurse must also record and report the client's status before and after the procedure.

The nurse assists the client through a procedure. Most of these procedures cause moderate discomfort. The client may tolerate the procedure better if a well-informed nurse stays at the bedside and communicates each step to the client.

### GUIDELINES

1. Know the client's baseline vital signs. Some of the diagnostic tests are invasive procedures and have associated complications. Changes from the baseline vital signs can provide early physiologic data about potential complications.
2. Know the client's level of education. Diagnostic tests require the nurse to teach the client about the test. Knowing the educational background enables the nurse to develop an individualized teaching plan.
3. Determine the client's awareness of actual or potential medical diagnoses. This determination provides the nurse with data about the client's knowledge and perception of medical diagnoses.
4. Through nursing assessment, determine abnormal findings, which can indicate or contraindicate a diagnostic test.
5. Determine the client's previous experience with diagnostic testing. Clients who have had smooth, uncomplicated diagnostic tests are usually less anxious about a test. If a client has had a complication from a diagnostic test, the client may require more preprocedure education and support.

### PREREQUISITE KNOWLEDGE

1. Principles of medical and surgical aepsis.
2. Principles of fluid balance.
3. Normal anatomy and physiology of body systems.
4. Principles of infection control.
5. Normal conduction of a heartbeat (Skill 46-6).

### PREREQUISITE SKILLS

1. Proper handwashing techniques (Chapter 37).
2. Proper positioning techniques (Chapter 33).
3. Physical assessment (Chapter 13).
4. Assessment of vital signs (Chapter 12).
5. Client communication techniques (Chapter 3).
6. Techniques of surgical asepsis (Chapter 38).
7. Transfer techniques (Chapter 33).

## *SKILL 46-1 Assisting with Abdominal Paracentesis*

Abdominal paracentesis is a sterile procedure performed to obtain peritoneal fluid for observation, laboratory tests, or for therapeutic reasons such as reducing intraabdominal pressure. There are two types of abdominal paracentesis: (1) peritoneal lavage, and (2) abdominal aspiration. The two most common medical diagnoses requiring abdominal paracentesis are (1) blunt abdominal trauma with possible perforation of organs and (2) ascites or excess peritoneal fluid.

Peritoneal fluid is obtained to check for blood, which may indicate the need for an exploratory laparotomy following trauma. It is also obtained to determine protein levels and cell types because ascitic fluid is usually high in protein. The client with ascites may experience increased intraabdominal pressure, which can hinder intestinal and respiratory function; therefore ascites may be relieved by paracentesis.

### Purposes

1. Obtain peritoneal fluid for examination to rule out intraabdominal bleeding.
2. Obtain peritoneal fluid to relieve intraabdominal pressure caused by ascites.
3. Obtain ascitic fluid for laboratory examination.

## *Procedure 46-1*

| Steps | Rationale |
|---|---|
| **Assessment** | |
| 1. Assess stability of vital signs, especially blood pressure. | Baseline vital signs are essential so comparisons are available in case of potential complications caused by drainage of large fluid volumes. |
| 2. Assess client's mobility status. | Client may be asked to assume lateral position on either side, and/or semi-Fowler's position is used to circulate fluid instilled into peritoneum during peritoneal lavage. |

| Steps | Rationale |
|---|---|
| 3. Assess client's bladder for distention or time of last void. | Chances of puncture of bladder are greater if bladder is full or distended. |
| 4. Determine whether client is allergic to local anesthetic or antiseptic solutions that may be used. | Common allergic reactions to anesthetic agents are central nervous system depression, respiratory difficulties, hypotension. Allergic reactions to antiseptic solutions are usually skin irritations. |
| 5. Assess client's abdomen for general appearance and degree of ascites if present: | Prenursing and postnursing observations are important in evaluation of amount of fluid aspirated or lavaged. |
| a. Note skin turgor. | |
| b. With ascites, measure abdominal girth in centimeters at largest point of abdomen. Use ink pen to mark where measuring tape lies. | Abdominal girth is measured in same place to accurately note abdominal size before and after paracentesis. |
| 6. Assess client's knowledge regarding procedure. | Client must be informed of impending procedure and its purpose. |
| 7. Assess client's diagnosis or query physician about purpose of procedure. | Enables nurse to anticipate position to be used and type of paracentesis to be performed. |
| 8. Check institution's policy and procedure manual regarding possible requirement of written informed consent. | Some institutions may require written permission for procedure. |

## Nursing Diagnoses

| Steps | Rationale |
|---|---|
| 1. Cluster data to reveal actual or potential nursing diagnoses: | |
| a. Decreased cardiac output: related to drainage or excessive amount of fluid. | Drainage of large amount of ascitic fluid (≈ 1500 ml maximum) could cause hypovolemic shock symptoms and tachycardia. |
| b. Pain: related to needle and position(s) used. | Depending on reason for procedure, client may or may not receive pain medication or local anesthetic. Procedure is painful because of large needle and catheter used and position(s) client assumes to facilitate proper drainage of peritoneal fluid. |
| c. Knowledge deficit regarding purpose and steps of procedure: related to inexperience. | Client will require instruction before and during procedure. |

## Planning

| Steps | Rationale |
|---|---|
| 1. Develop individualized goals based on nursing diagnoses: | |
| a. Promote relaxation and comfort of client before, during, after procedure | Relaxation techniques may help to reduce discomfort. |
| b. Reassure client that you will be assisting during procedure. | Helps client to relax. |
| c. Monitor vital signs carefully. | Vital signs should be obtained before, during, after procedure at frequent intervals because of possibility of complications. |
| 2. Prepare equipment and supplies: | |
| a. Antiseptic solution for handwashing (e.g., povidone-iodine scrub) | |
| b. Paracentesis tray, if available from central supply, which may include: | |
| ▪ Antiseptic solution (e.g., povidone-iodine solution) | Used for skin disinfection. |
| ▪ Sterile gauze sponges (4 × 4) | |
| ▪ Four sterile towels | Used for draping over abdomen to isolate sterile area. |
| ▪ Local anesthetic solution for injection (e.g., lidocaine 1%) | |
| ▪ Sterile syringes: two 3 ml, 23- to 25-gauze needles for anesthetic; four 10 to 30 ml 19- 21-gauge needles | Larger syringes are used if abdominal aspiration is to be performed. |
| ▪ Small, sterile knife blade | Used for small skin incision. |
| ▪ Two sterile cannula needles with inner trocar (CAPD catheter is usually used if available) for lavage | Trocar is sharp-pointed instrument that fits inside large, long needle called *cannula.* After insertion, trocar is removed and plastic tubing is attached for abdominal fluid instillation and drainage. CAPD catheter is supplied with plastic tubing. |
| c. 2 to 3 L IV fluids as ordered | For peritoneal lavage with abdominal trauma, fluid may be instilled to irrigate peritoneum. |
| d. IV tubing, usually macrodrip size or 10 gtt/ml | |
| e. Sterile cups and receptacle for rest of fluid not sent for tests | |
| f. Two packages of sterile gloves: (check physician's preferred size) | |
| g. Masks for physician and nurse (check institution's policy) | |

| Steps | Rationale |
|---|---|
| h. Sterile gauze sponges (2 × 2), tape, antiseptic ointment for dressing of insertion site | |
| i. Pain medication if ordered (given 30 min before procedure) | Reduces client's pain threshold. |
| j. Laboratory requisitions and labels | |
| 3. Organize equipment on bedside table. | Ensures ease and success of procedure. |
| 4. Prepare client: | |
| a. Explain procedure. | Ensures knowledge of procedure; ensures cooperation; promotes relaxation. |
| b. Have client void or check patency of bladder catheter. | Full or distended bladder increases possibility of puncturing bladder. |
| c. Assist client in assuming position desired by physician. | Semi-Fowler's position is used to drain ascites because of effect of gravity on fluid in peritoneal cavity. Fluid accumulates in lower abdomen and may be drained easier in this position (Fig. 46-1). |

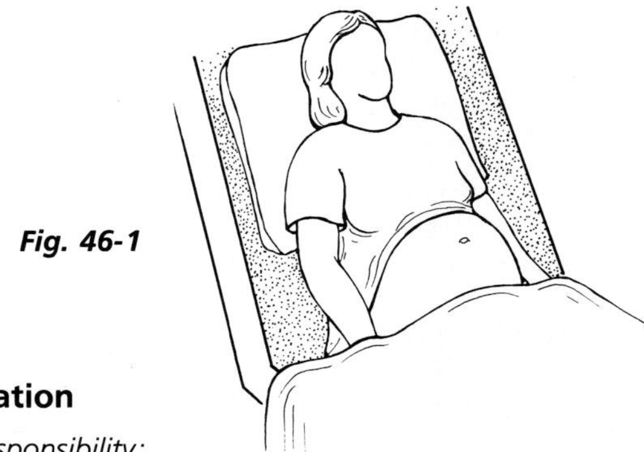

***Fig. 46-1***

## Implementation

| Steps | Rationale |
|---|---|
| *Physician's responsibility:* | |
| 1. Cleanse abdomen with antiseptic solution and 4 × 4 sponges. | Reduces transmission of microorganisms. |
| 2. Don mask. | |
| 3. Don sterile gloves. | Maintains surgical asepsis. |
| 4. Drape client with sterile towels. | |
| 5. Inject local anesthetic and allow to take effect. | Provides local anesthetic to abdomen. |
| 6. Insert 10-gauge needle attached to 10 ml syringe through abdominal wall. Aspirate peritoneal fluid or blood from each quadrant. Use new syringe and needle for each quadrant. | Peritoneal fluid is normally small amount and clear. Blood-tinged fluid needs to be evaluated because blood may be from trauma of needle insertion or from intraabdominal bleed. |
| 7. For lavage, make small incision with knife blade and insert cannula with trocar into lower abdomen between umbilicus and symphysis pubis. Remove trocar and insert CAPD or plastic catheter for fluid instillation or drainage. | Facilitates placement of catheter into abdominal cavity for instillation and drainage of fluid. |
| 8. Remove plastic catheter, cannula, needle. | Prevents further drainage of fluid from peritoneum. |
| 9. Place manual pressure over insertion site until drainage ceases. | Prevents excessive drainage from puncture site. |
| 10. Place antiseptic ointment with 2 × 2 gauze sponge over insertion site. | Prevents growth of bacteria at puncture site. |
| *Nurse's responsibility:* | |
| 1. Set up sterile tray or open sterile supplies and make accessible for physician. | |
| 2. Prepare fluid to be used for lavage; attach to IV tubing. | If fluid instillation is to be performed, as with blunt abdominal trauma. Fluid is ready to attach to plastic tubing after cannula is in place in abdomen. |
| 3. Hold anesthetic solution bottle upside down. | Allows physician to withdraw solution properly while maintaining surgical asepsis. |
| 4. Assist client through procedure: | |
| a. Hold hands tightly. | Allows client opportunity to reciprocate squeeze if pain is experienced. |
| b. Reassure client in coaching manner. | Assists client in estimating when procedure is completed. |
| 5. Implement fluid instillation: | |
| a. After plastic catheter is in place inside cannula, deliver extension tubing to physician while maintaining surgical asepsis. | Provides route for administering fluid for lavage. Allows client mobility for changing position if extension and IV tubing are of sufficient length. |
| b. Attach IV tubing to distal end of extension tubing. | |
| c. Administer physician-ordered amount of fluid at ordered rate. | Promotes infusion of prescribed fluid into peritoneum. |

| Steps | Rationale |
|---|---|
| d. Clamp IV tubing after fluid is instilled. | Prevents accidental infusion of fluid into peritoneum. |
| e. If physician ordered, assist client in changing positions. | Promotes irrigation of all areas of peritoneal cavity. |
| f. Place tubing below client's abdominal level. | Promotes gravitational drainage of fluid from peritoneal cavity. |
| 6. Place sterile specimen cup for laboratory examination under tip of drainage tubing. | Provides sterile container for laboratory specimen. |
| 7. Open tubing clamp to allow drainage of peritoneal lavage fluid. Maximum amount of ascitic fluid usually allowed to drain is 1500 ml. | Permits gravitational flow of solution from abdomen. |
| 8. Assess client's vital signs during procedure. | Enables nurse to detect signs of possible hypovolemic shock. |
| 9. Assess client's toleration of procedure. | Nurse should keep physician informed of client's condition: vital signs, sensorium. |
| 10. Assist client through removal of cannula by holding hands tightly. | Promotes cooperation. |
| 11. Dispose of equipment and wash hands. | Reduces transmission of microorganisms. |

## Evaluation

| Steps | Rationale |
|---|---|
| 1. Evaluate client's status: | |
| a. Take vital signs q 15 min for 1 hr and then q 30 min for 2 hr; check for stability by comparing with preprocedure signs. | Verifies client's physiologic status. |
| b. Check dressing over insertion site for bleeding or drainage. | Provides for continued observation of puncture site. May indicate buildup of blood or fluid in abdominal cavity. |
| c. Measure abdominal girth and skin turgor. | Determines change after fluid drainage. |
| 2. Observe client for signs of discomfort. | Verifies discomfort after procedure. |
| ***Expected outcomes*** | |
| 1. Client can assume positions without problems, has little pain, has few changes in vital signs, has no complications. | Client tolerates procedure well. |
| 2. For peritoneal lavage and abdominal aspiration, aspirate is clear or slightly blood tinged. | Slight amount of blood-tinged drainage may be caused by irritation to tissue by needle. Amount needs to be confirmed by laboratory test. |
| 3. For therapeutic treatment of ascites by peritoneal lavage, amount of fluid drained is sufficient to allow: | |
| a. Decreased size of abdominal girth. | Related to therapeutic ascitic fluid loss. |
| b. Decreased abdominal skin tightness. | Related to therapeutic ascitic fluid loss. |
| c. Increased comfort. | Related to relief of pressure on abdominal contents. |
| d. Improved respiratory status. | Related to relief of pressure on diaphragm. |
| ***Unexpected outcomes*** | |
| 1. Client does not assume lateral positions well. | Increased abdominal pressure resulting from ascites prevents client from assuming lateral position. |
| 2. Changes in vital signs are not within normal limits. | Hypotension may indicate impending hypovolemic shock. Slight hypertension and tachycardia may be caused by anxiety. |
| 3. In client who has experienced blunt abdominal trauma that may have perforated or injured abdominal contents: | Injured or perforated contents may bleed into peritoneal cavity, result of which may be observed through this procedure. |
| a. Aspirate or drained fluid is bloody—bright or dark red. | Indicates blood in peritoneal cavity. |
| 4. Paracentesis complications include: | |
| a. Infection. | Contaminated techniques may cause peritonitis. Also, accidental perforation of organs cause peritonitis. |
| b. Bleeding. | Results from irritation and breakage of blood vessels during procedure. |
| c. Hypovolemic shock. | When excessive peritoneal fluid is drained, fluid shifts occur in circulation and intravascular fluid may enter abdominal cavity where ascites was present. This shift decreases intravascular volume, causing hypovolemia and possible hypovolemic shock. |
| 5. Laboratory test results, including cell counts, protein levels, specific gravity, are not within normal limits. | Indicates abnormal process such as infection, cancer, fluid retention. |

| Steps | Rationale |
| --- | --- |
| **Recording and Reporting** | |
| 1. Record in nurses' notes or on client's chart: type of procedure (aspiration or lavage), client's toleration of procedure (pain level, vital signs and changes), type of dressing over insertion and whether drainage is present. | Documents client's response to invasive procedure. |
| 2. Report to physician immediately: | |
| a. Changes in vital signs beyond normal limits for client. | May indicate hypovolemic shock or peritonitis. |
| b. Severe abdominal pain. | May indicate perforation of abdomen. |
| c. Excessive bloody drainage from insertion site. | May indicate irritation and clotting problem of skin artery. Place manual pressure over insertion site. |
| 3. Report to nurses on next shift all data that have been recorded in nurses' notes and to physician. | Ensures continuity of care. |
| **Follow-up Activities** | |
| 1. Monitor vital signs: q 15 min if change is noted; then q 1 h × 2 if client stabilizes. | Provides for continual assessment of physiologic status. |
| 2. Assist client in assuming comfortable position in bed. | Promotes comfort. |
| 3. Explain to client that procedure is completed. | |
| 4. Label specimens to be sent to laboratory and attach proper requisitions. Send to appropriate laboratory. | Provides for proper disposition of specimens to correct laboratory. |
| 5. Clean up area and send supplies to proper sterilization department. | Prevents transmission of microorganisms. |
| 6. Monitor abdominal dressing for drainage. | |
| 7. Obtain laboratory data for interpretation by nurse and physician. | Reveals cause of ascites or other pathology. |

## Special Considerations

- Client with blunt abdominal trauma or large amount of ascites may experience problems in assuming different positions, especially semi-Fowler's.
- Client with a large amount of ascites may prefer the Fowler's or semi-Fowler's position to increase respiratory function.
- If in doubt as to whether laboratory specimen will be needed, collect sterile specimen. Specimen can easily be discarded, at no cost to the client, if it is not needed.
- If large amount of fluid is expected to be drained, it is drained slowly to prevent great fluid shifts, which may cause hypovolemic shock. IV fluids or albumin may be given to prevent hypotension.
- In addition to signing consent for procedure, clients who have experienced blunt abdominal trauma should also sign consent for emergency abdominal surgery.
- Blood aspirate is called "plus (or positive) tap" or "plus (positive) lavage."
- Client with plus (or positive) tap or lavage is usually sent to operating room (OR) for exploratory laporotomy. OR personnel need to be notified of pending emergency surgery before tap takes place.

## Teaching Considerations

- Explain to client that procedure will be more safely performed if bladder is empty. This decreases chance of bladder perforation.
- Tell client with ascites that comfort will probably increase and respiration will be easier after paracentesis.

# *SKILL 46-2 Assisting with Bone Marrow Aspiration*

Bone marrow aspiration is the removal of a small amount of liquid organic material inside selected bones to evaluate hematopoiesis. The marrow is examined in a laboratory to reveal the number, size, shape, and development of red blood cells (RBCs), white blood cells (WBCs), and megakaryocytes (platelet precursors). The sterile procedure is usually performed by a physician assisted by a nurse, usually in the client's room. A bone marrow biopsy is performed in the operating room, with the client under general anesthesia, to remove a larger sample of marrow. Complications of bone marrow aspiration are bleeding, especially if a coagulopathy is present, infection, and less commonly, organ puncture. The nurse should know normal hematologic laboratory values before assisting with the procedure.

## Purposes

1. Aspirate bone marrow for laboratory examination of RBCs, WBCs, and megakaryocytes.
2. Examine bone marrow for fibrotic tissue or neoplasm.
3. Remove bone marrow for treatment and readministration intravenously as a bone marrow transplant.

# *Procedure 46-2*

| Steps | Rationale |
|---|---|
| **Assessment** | |
| 1. Assess client's knowledge of procedure. | Procedure may need to be explained to relieve client's anxiety. |
| 2. Assess client's ability to assume position required for procedure. | Required position depends on site that is used for bone marrow aspiration (e.g., sternum or anterior iliac spine = supine position; posterior iliac spine or iliac crest = prone or lateral position). |
| 3. Assess vital signs to obtain baseline data. | Ensures stability of hemodynamic status and provides for comparison with postprocedure vital signs. |
| 4. Assess client's coagulation status: use of anticoagulants, platelet count, prothrombin time. | Factors can increase risk of bleeding. |
| 5. Determine purpose of procedure. | Allows nurse to determine whether aspiration or biopsy will be performed to anticipate laboratory requisitions. |
| 6. Check record for signed consent form, (check institution's policy). | Provides written documentation that client has consented to procedure. |
| 7. Determine whether client is allergic to antiseptic or anesthetic solutions. | Decreases chance of complications from anesthetic. |
| 8. Assess need for preprocedure pain medication. | Procedure can be painful, and it is important that client remain motionless to avoid complications. |
| **Nursing Diagnosis** | |
| 1. Cluster data to reveal actual or potential nursing diagnoses: | |
| a. Pain: related to procedure. | Procedure is painful; client may receive preprocedure medication to reduce anxiety and pain perception. |
| b. Decreased cardiac output: related to possible complications from procedure. | Severe blood loss can occur in client whose blood coagulation is deficient or in whom organ is punctured. |
| c. Anxiety: related to impending procedure. | Nurse's calm approach helps to relieve apprehension. |
| d. Knowledge deficit regarding procedural techniques: related to inexperience. | Nurse provides thorough explanation of procedure. |
| **Planning** | |
| 1. Develop individualized goals based on nursing diagnoses: | |
| a. Promote client's comfort. | Helps to maintain cooperation during procedure. |
| b. Prevent client from moving. | Client must remain in selected position until aspiration is complete. Failure to do so can result in incomplete tissue sampling or complications. |
| c. Ensure client's understanding of purpose of procedure. | Increases client cooperation. |
| 2. Prepare equipment and supplies: | |
| a. Antiseptic solution for handwashing | Prevents transmission of microorganisms. |
| b. Bone marrow aspiration tray, if available from central supply, which may include: | |
| ▪ Antiseptic solution (e.g., povidone-iodine) | Used for cleansing puncture site before obtaining specimen. |
| ▪ Gauze sponges (4 × 4) | |
| ▪ Sterile towels | Used to drape and isolate sterile area. |
| ▪ Local anesthetic solution for injection (e.g., lidocaine 1%) | Provides local anesthesia at puncture site. |
| ▪ Sterile syringes: two 3 ml, 23- to 25-gauge needles for anesthetic; two 50 ml for marrow aspiration | Marrow aspiration is performed to obtain marrow sample to be analyzed in laboratory. |
| ▪ Two bone marrow needles with inner stylus | |
| c. Sterile gloves of proper size for physician | Maintains surgical asepsis. |
| d. Masks for physician and nurse (check institution's policy) | Used to prevent transmission of microorganisms to client when client is severely immunocompromised. |
| e. Gauze 2 × 2 tape and antiseptic ointment | Used for dressing or needle insertion site. |
| f. Pain medication if ordered (given 30 min before procedure) | Helps client relax and reduces client's pain threshold. |

| Steps | Rationale |
|---|---|
| 3. Organize equipment on bedside table. | Ensures ease and success of procedure. |
| 4. Explain steps of skin preparation, anesthetic injection, needle insertion. | Anticipation or expected sensation reduces anxiety. |

## Implementation

*Physician's responsibility:*

| Steps | Rationale |
|---|---|
| 1. Select site to be used for bone marrow aspiration. | Sites are chosen for direct access to area of spongy bone. These sites include anterior and posterior iliac spines, iliac crest, body of sternum, tibia. |
| 2. Disinfect skin with antiseptic solution and 4 × 4 gauze sponges. | Removes surface bacteria from skin at area of puncture site. |
| 3. Don sterile mask. | Maintains surgical asepsis. |
| 4. Don sterile gloves. | Maintains surgical asepsis. |
| 5. Drape client with sterile towels. | Maintains surgical asepsis. |
| 6. Inject local anesthetic and allow to take effect. | Provides optimal effect of anesthesia at time of bone marrow aspiration. |
| 7. Insert bone marrow needle with inner stylus into bone. | Stylus is stiff and has longer bevel to enter bone with more ease. |
| 8. Advance needle until it reaches area of spongy bone and remove stylus. | Spongy bone is location of bone marrow (Fig. 46-2). |

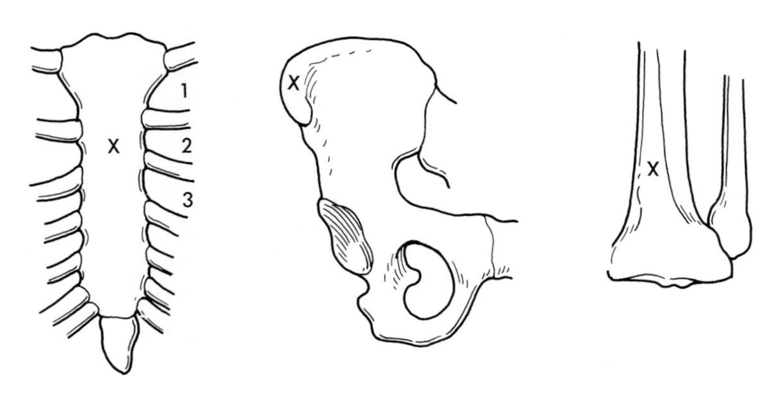


***Fig. 46-2***

From Phipps WJ, Long BC, and Woods NF: Medical-surgical nursing: concepts and clinical practice, ed 3, St Louis, 1987, The CV Mosby Co.

| Steps | Rationale |
|---|---|
| 9. Attach 50 ml syringe to needle and aspirate bone marrow. | Amount aspirated is determined by purpose of procedure: small amount (approximately 5 to 10 ml) for laboratory testings; moderate amount (approximately 50 to 100 ml) for aspiration and treatment to readminister for bone marrow transplant. |
| 10. Remove needle and apply pressure to puncture site. | Prevents bleeding from puncture site. |
| 11. Place antiseptic ointment, 2 × 2 gauze, tape on site for dressing. | Reduces bacterial growth at site of puncture. |

*Nurse's responsibility:*

| Steps | Rationale |
|---|---|
| 1. Set up sterile tray or open supplies to make accessible for physician. | Reduces risk of contamination of sterile field and promotes prompt completion of procedure. |
| 2. Assist client in maintaining correct position. | Decreases chance of complications occurring during procedure. |
| 3. Assist client through procedure by holding hands tightly and reassuring client in coaching manner. | Promotes reassurance, relaxation, and comfort of client and increases cooperation. |
| 4. Hold anesthetic vial upside down for physician to withdraw solution properly. | Allows physician to aspirate anesthesia into syringe while maintaining sterility. |
| 5. Assess client's condition during procedure: respiratory status, vital signs if indicated. | Identifies any changes that may indicate complication. |
| 6. Note characteristics of bone marrow aspirate (e.g., amount, color). | Characteristics are used for observation, reporting, recording. |

| Steps | Rationale |
|---|---|
| **Evaluation** | |
| 1. Monitor vital signs. Check hospital policy; may be as often as every 15 minutes for 2 hours. | Verifies client's physiologic status in response to potential blood loss. |
| 2. Inspect dressing over puncture site. | Determines further blood loss from puncture site. |
| 3. Observe client's level of comfort. | Client may require postprocedure analgesia. |
| ***Expected outcomes*** | |
| 1. Client can assume position without problems, has little pain and few complications. | Client tolerates procedure well. |
| 2. Amount of aspirate is sufficient to perform laboratory testing or for other purpose. | Insufficient aspirate necessitates another bone marrow aspiration. |
| ***Unexpected outcomes*** | |
| 1. Client moves during procedure. | Position changes could cause needle movement, predisposing client to complications. |
| 2. Other complications such as bleeding or infection occur. | Bleeding is common complication if client has coagulopathy. Check coagulation studies before procedure to anticipate possible bleeding side effects. |
| **Recording and Reporting** | |
| 1. Record in nurse's notes or on client's chart: | Accurate recording of procedure is legal necessity. |
| a. Name of procedure. | |
| b. Location of puncture site. | |
| c. Amount and color of marrow aspirated. | |
| d. Duration of procedure. | |
| e. Client's toleration of procedure (e.g., vital signs, pain, complications). | Provides ongoing assessment of physical assessment status. |
| f. Laboratory tests ordered and sent. | Documents that specimen was obtained and to which laboratory it was delivered. |
| g. Type of dressing over puncture site and drainage. | Provides baseline data for monitoring amount of blood loss and drainage from puncture site. |
| 2. Report to physician immediately: | |
| a. Change in vital signs beyond client's normal limits. | Could indicate possible complications such as organ puncture or bleeding. |
| b. Excessive drainage from dressing over puncture site. | Could indicate postprocedure bleeding or localized infection at puncture site. |
| 3. Report results of procedure to nurses on the next shift. | Ensures continuity of care. |
| **Follow-up Activities** | |
| 1. Explain to client that procedure is completed. | |
| 2. Assist client in assuming comfortable position in bed. | Client should avoid lying directly on puncture site until drainage is stopped. |
| 3. Clean up area and send supplies to proper sterilization department. | Reduces transmission of microorganisms. |
| 4. Obtain laboratory data for interpretation. | Receipt of laboratory results in medical record assists in accurate diagnosis of pathologic condition. |

## Special Considerations

- A written informed consent usually must be obtained (check agency policy).
- If client experiences respiratory distress when supine or prone, physician may elect to perform aspiration in semi-Fowler's position.
- When client is uncooperative, procedure may need to be performed in OR with more extensive anesthesia.
- Masks are used with immunocompromised clients including those receiving cancer chemotherapy or high-dose steroid therapy and those in reverse isolation.
- Complications are rare but include sternal puncture, heart and lung puncture, iliac crest or spine puncture, and bowel puncture.

## Teaching Considerations

- After explaining this procedure, encourage client to verbalize concerns. Many clients are anxious about procedure.
- Emphasize importance of remaining still during procedure. Movement can cause needle to accidently puncture vital organ.

# SKILL 46-3 Assisting with Bronchoscopy

Bronchoscopy is the examination of the tracheobronchial tree through a lighted tube containing mirrors. The tube, or bronchoscope, most commonly used is a fiberoptic bronchoscope. A rigid bronchoscope was used before the invention of the flexible type and may still be used in operating rooms. The fiberoptic bronchoscope has lumens for visualization and for obtaining sputum, foreign bodies, and biopsy specimens.

Bronchoscopy may be an emergency or elective procedure and is performed for diagnostic or therapeutic reasons. The main purposes of this procedure are to aspirate excessive sputum that cannot be sufficiently suctioned nasotracheally and to visualize the tracheobronchial tree for assessment of abnormalities of the mucosa. Complications may include hypoxemia, laryngospasm, bronchospasm, pneumothorax, and hemorrhage. The nurse should be able to perform nasotracheal and orotracheal suctioning before assisting with the procedure.

### Purposes

1. Directly visualize the tracheobronchial tree.
2. Remove biopsy specimens.
3. Aspirate sputum.
4. Remove small aspirated objects.

## Procedure 46-3

| Steps | Rationale |
|---|---|
| **Assessment** | |
| 1. Assess client's knowledge of procedure. | Procedure may need to be explained in detail. |
| 2. Assess vital signs to obtain baseline data. | Provides for comparison with findings during and after procedure. |
| 3. Assess respiratory function: type of cough, sputum produced, lung sounds. | Provides for comparison with respiratory status during and after procedure. |
| 4. Determine purpose of procedure: for sputum aspiration, for observation, for tissue biopsy. | Enables nurse to anticipate needs. |
| 5. Assess need for signed consent form (check institution's policy). | Usually requires signed consent form. |
| 6. Determine whether client is allergic to local anesthetic used for spraying throat. | Allergy could cause laryngeal edema or laryngospasm. |
| 7. Assess need for preprocedure medication. | If procedure is performed in OR, preoperative medication is usually given. If procedure is performed in treatment room or at bedside, preoperative medication may not be given. |
| 8. Assess time client last ingested food. Client should have been NPO for 8 hours before procedure. | Reduces risk of aspiration. |
| **Nursing Diagnosis** | |
| 1. Cluster data to reveal actual or potential nursing diagnoses: | |
| a. Impaired gas exchange: related to bronchopulmonary secretions. | Excessive sputum in airways can decrease transfer of oxygen and carbon dioxide from blood to lungs. |
| b. Potential ineffective breathing pattern: related to post-procedure complications. | Client may demonstrate asymmetrical chest wall movement as result of procedure-induced pneumothorax, bronchospasm, laryngospasm. |
| c. Pain: related to procedure. | Procedure can cause discomfort; client will need comfort measures during and after (Chapter 5). |
| d. Anxiety: related to impending procedure. | Nurse's calm approach helps to relieve apprehension. |
| e. Knowledge deficit regarding procedure: related to inexperience. | Nurse's explanation of procedure will clarify client's concerns and fears. |
| **Planning** | |
| 1. Develop individualized goals based on nursing diagnoses: | |
| a. Promote client comfort. | Invasive nature of procedure causes discomfort in some clients. In addition, preprocedure anxiety also causes discomfort. |

*Fig. 46-3*

From Phipps WJ, Long BC, Woods NF: Medical-surgical nursing: concepts and clinical practice, ed 2, St Louis, 1983, The CV Mosby Co; courtesy American Cystoscope Makers, Inc, Pelham, NY.

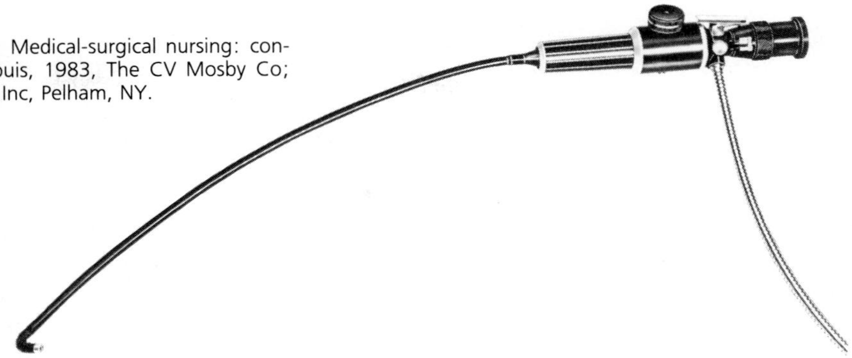

| Steps | Rationale |
|---|---|
| b. Promote optimal respiratory function during and after procedure. | Airway is partially occluded with bronchoscope; client may have sensation of suffocation. |
| 2. Assemble equipment and supplies: | |
| a. Antiseptic solution for handwashing | Reduces transmission of microorganisms. |
| b. Bronchoscopy tray, if available from central supply, which may include: | |
| ▪ Flexible fiberoptic bronchoscope (Fig. 46-3) | Physician or OR will supply machine to attach to bronchoscope for electric light source. |
| ▪ Gauze sponges (4 × 4) | |
| ▪ Local anesthetic spray | Inactivates gag reflex. |
| ▪ Sterile tracheal suction equipment (Chapter 16) | Used for suctioning sputum. |
| ▪ Sterile gloves (proper size for physician) | Used to maintain surgical asepsis. |
| ▪ Sterile water-soluble lubricating jelly | Used to lubricate bronchoscope for ease in intubation of client. |
| ▪ Emesis basin | Used for expectoration of local anesthetic or vomitus. |
| 3. Prepare client: | |
| a. Explain steps of procedure. | Relieves anxiety and promotes cooperation. |
| b. Administer pain or preprocedure medication if ordered. | Promotes relaxation and reduces anxiety. |

## Implementation

| Steps | Rationale |
|---|---|
| *Physician's responsibility:* | |
| 1. Spray nasopharynx and oropharynx with topical anesthetic. | Throat is sprayed early for anesthesia to take effect. |
| 2. Attach bronchoscope to machine for light source. | Another physician, OR personnel, or nurse attaches machine cable to bronchoscope. |
| 3. Don sterile gloves. | Reduces transmission of infection. |
| 4. Introduce bronchoscope into nose to pharynx, and pass through glottis. May use more anesthetic spray at glottis to prevent cough reflex. | Bronchoscope must be passed through upper airway structures to promote visualization of lower airways. |
| 5. Pass tube into trachea and bronchi for observation. | |
| 6. Obtain cytological specimens with wire brush or curette. | Cytological specimens are obtained to determine carcinoma. |
| 7. Suction both bronchi if needed. | Suctioning causes removal of mucus plugs in lower airways. |
| *Nurse's responsibility:* | |
| 1. Assist client in maintaining position desired by physician: semi-Fowler's, supine, or lateral. | Provides maximal visualization of lower airways and adequate lung expansion. |
| 2. Remove and safely store client's dentures and eyeglasses. | Dentures may complicate intubation. Glasses may hinder tube manipulation. |
| 3. Assist client through procedure by holding hands tightly and reassuring in coaching manner. | Although premedicated and drowsy, clients need to be reminded not to change position and to cooperate. |
| 4. Assess client's respiratory status during procedure: observe degree of restlessness and respiratory rate; observe capillary refill and color of nail beds. | Bronchoscope may cause feelings of suffocation; In addition, because airway is partially occluded, client may become hypoxic during procedure. |
| 5. Note characteristics of suctioned material. | Information used to record and report and to make further client observations. |
| 6. At opportune time, ask physician to describe what was seen or to allow you to observe in bronchoscope. | Information is needed for nurse to stay up-to-date on condition and to learn appearance of pathologic conditions. |
| 7. Wipe client's nose to remove lubricant after bronchoscope is removed. | Promotes hygiene and comfort. |
| 8. Do not allow client to eat or drink until the tracheobronchial anesthesia has worn off. | Prevents aspiration of food or fluid, which could cause pneumonia. |

| Steps | Rationale |
|---|---|
| **Evaluation** | |
| 1. Monitor vital signs. | Verifies physiologic response. |
| 2. Observe character and amount of sputum. | Sputum may be blood tinged, which indicates superficial tissue damage. Severe hemoptysis is emergency. |
| 3. Observe respiratory status closely. | May provide evidence of laryngeal bronchospasm. |
| 4. Assess for return of gag reflex. | Reflex return allows client to resume eating and drinking. |
| ***Expected outcomes*** | |
| 1. Client has little pain and few complications and respiratory complications. | Client tolerates procedure well. |
| 2. Physician is able to observe, suction, and obtain specimens from tracheobronchial tree. | Indicates that purpose of procedure was achieved. |
| ***Unexpected outcomes*** | |
| 1. Laryngospasm and bronchospasm indicated by sudden, severe shortness of breath. | Constriction of large airways is response to laryngeal or bronchial irritation from bronchoscope or topical anesthetic. |
| 2. Hypoxemia indicated by gradual shortness of breath and decreasing level of consciousness. | Hypoxemia is caused by occlusions of airways resulting from mucous plug or bronchoscope. |
| 3. Hemorrhage occurs. | Results from trauma to major vessels in airways. |
| **Recording and Reporting** | |
| 1. Record in nurses' notes or client's chart: name of procedure (include biopsy if performed), duration of procedure, client's tolerance of procedure and complications, collection and disposition of specimen. | Accurate recording of procedure is legal necessity. |
| 2. Report to physician immediately: | |
| a. Excessive bleeding after procedure. | May indicate tracheal perforation. |
| b. Changes in vital signs beyond client's normal limits. | May indicate signs of hypoxia. |
| 3. Report results of procedure to nurses on the next shift. | Ensures continuity of care. |
| **Follow-up Activities** | |
| 1. Clean up area and send supplies to proper sterilization area. | Prevents transmission of microorganisms. |
| 2. Assist client in assuming comfortable position in bed. | |
| 3. Obtain laboratory data for interpretation. | Receipt of laboratory results in medical record assists in accurate diagnosis of pathologic condition. |

## Special Considerations

- Cetacaine and lidocaine are commonly used for throat spraying.
- Anesthetic spray is not needed with intubated client.
- For intubated client, bronchoscope is passed through endotracheal tube. Adaptor accompanies bronchoscope and may be used for Ambu bag or ventilator use.
- Meperidine (Demerol) or diazepam and atropine are usual drugs of choice for preoperative medication.
- To reduce risk of aspiration, following restrictions apply:
  *OR:* Client to be npo after midnight.
  *Bedside:* Client NPO for at least 8 hr.
- Petroleum-based lubricants should not be used because of hazard of aspiration and subsequent pneumonia.
- Clients with thick, tenacious sputum may receive bronchoscopy to remove secretions from airways.
- If needed, oxygen, may be administered through bronchoscope. Small amount of bleeding in suctioned material is expected because of tissue trauma.
- Complications are rare with fiberoptic, flexible bronchoscope; they are more common with rigid bronchoscope. Possible complications include extreme shortness of breath, excessive bleeding, damage to glottis, tracheal, or bronchial tissues.
- After bronchoscopy, physician may order serial sputum collections for 24 hr for cytological examination.

## Teaching Considerations

- After thoroughly explaining procedure, assure client that client will be able to breath during procedure.
- Make sure client knows not to eat or drink until gag reflex returns. Before return of reflex, client could aspirate food or fluids.

# *SKILL 46-4 Assisting with CT Scanning*

Computed tomography (CT) scanning consists of a computerized analysis of multiple tomographic x-ray films taken of specific body organs and tissues. The CT scan looks at multiple layers of tissues to provide a three-dimensional view of organs. This particular skill will describe a CT scan of the brain (Fig. 46-4). This remarkable study can be performed with or without a dye injection. CT scanning is performed by trained technologists in a special x-ray room in approximately 1 hour. This equipment is not routinely available to all hospitals. Transportation arrangements may need to be made for clients from smaller hospitals.

### Purposes

1. Visualize structures of the brain and surrounding structures.
2. Identify cranial neoplasms, cerebral infarctions and aneurysms, ventricular displacement and enlargement, and intracranial hemorrhage.
3. Monitor the progress of disease.
4. Monitor the healing process.

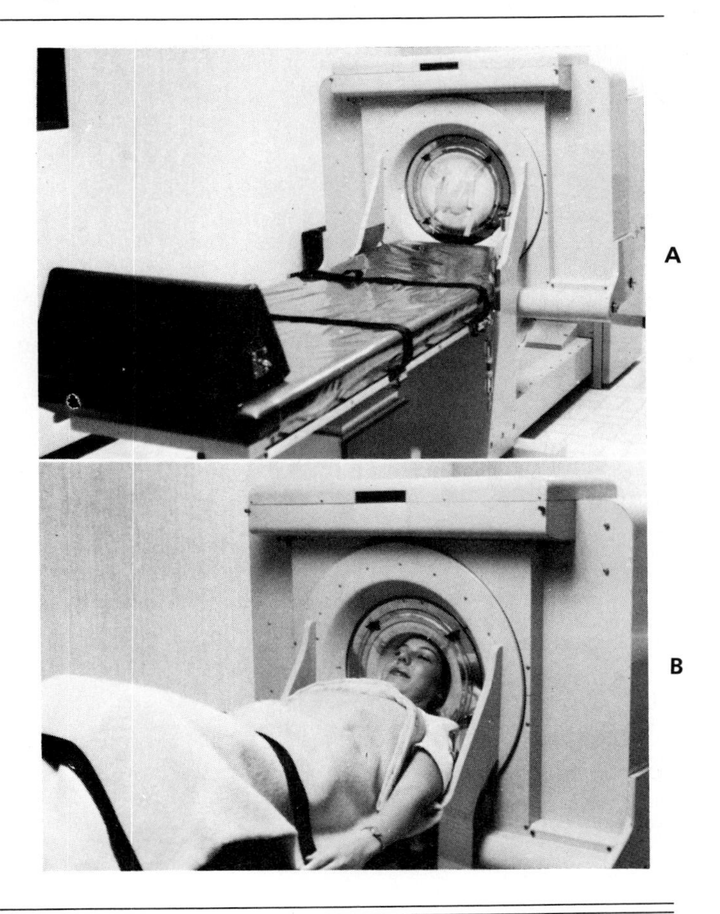


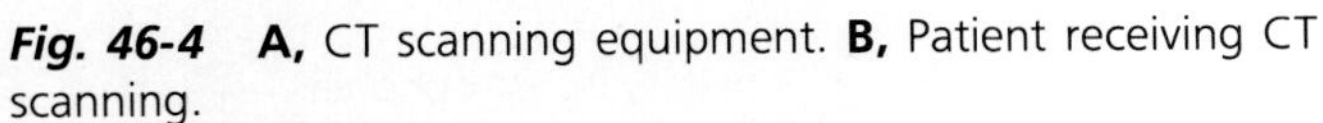

***Fig. 46-4*** **A,** CT scanning equipment. **B,** Patient receiving CT scanning.

From Conway-Rutkowski BL: Carini and Owens' neurologic and neurosurgical nursing, ed 8, St. Louis, 1982, The CV Mosby Co.

## *Procedure 46-4*

| Steps | Rationale |
|---|---|
| **Assessment** | |
| 1. Assess client's knowledge of procedure. | Determines what education may be necessary. |
| 2. Determine if client is allergic to iodine dye. | Detects allergic reaction if contrast dye is used. |
| 3. Assess if client has tendency to be claustrophobic. | Some clients become claustrophobic due to positioning in scanner during procedure. |
| **Nursing Diagnosis** | |
| 1. Cluster data to reveal actual or potential nursing diagnoses: | |
| a. Pain: related to positioning. | Lying still on hard table can be uncomfortable. |
| b. Anxiety: related to impending procedure. | Positioning during scanning and unknown sensations of procedure can cause anxiety. |
| c. Knowledge deficit regarding procedural steps: related to lack of information or inexperience. | |
| **Planning** | |
| 1. Develop individualized goals based on nursing diagnoses. | |
| a. Promote client's comfort. | |
| b. Increase client's understanding of role during procedure. | |

| Steps | Rationale |
|---|---|
| 2. Arrange for transportation of clients to x-ray department. | Transportation in ambulance to another facility may be necessary if the institution does not have a CT scanning device. |
| 3. Inform client that metal objects such as hair clips must be removed. | Metal objects block bony structures and will show up on x-ray film. |
| 4. Keep the client npo for 4 hours before study. | Iodine dye may induce nausea. |
| 5. Explain time frame for procedure. | Promotes client's cooperation. |
| **Implementation** | |
| 1. Assist client into supine position on examining table with head resting in snug-fitting rubber cap. | Position is necessary to obtain good films. |
| 2. Instruct client not to move head, talk, or sigh during procedure. | Movement causes computer-generated artifacts on image produced. |
| 3. X-ray beams pass through the brain from one side to other through 180-degree arc. | Multiple tomographic x-rays taken in successive layers provides three dimensional view of cranial contents. |
| 4. Iodinated dye is administered through peripheral IV line usually started in arm. | Dye enhances contrast and provides improved visualization. |
| 5. Observe client for signs of anaphylaxis. | Signs include respiratory distress, palpitations, itching, diaphoresis. |
| 6. X-ray procedure is repeated. | |
| **Evaluation** | |
| 1. Determine if client feels back pain. | Common post-procedure complaint results from lying on hard examining table. |
| ***Expected outcomes*** | |
| 1. Client tolerates procedure well. Client can maintain position without moving. | Indicates absence of complications. |
| 2. Client has no reaction to iodinated dye. | |
| 3. Satisfactory x-ray films were obtained. | Purpose of procedure was accomplished. |
| ***Unexpected outcomes*** | |
| 1. Client is unable to maintain desired position. | Results from discomfort, anxiety, claustrophobia. |
| 2. Anaphylactic reaction to contrast media occurs. | Results from allergy to iodine. |
| **Recording and Reporting** | |
| 1. Record in the nurses note: date, time, place scan was performed; if contrast dye was administered; client's tolerance of procedure. | Provides documentation of procedure in record. |
| 2. Report duration of procedure and client's tolerance to nurse in charge. | Assures prompt follow-up for unexpected outcomes. |
| **Follow-up Activities** | |
| 1. Assist client in assuming comfortable position after scan. | Client may complain of back discomfort from lying on hard table. |
| 2. Provide meal for client. | After study is completed, npo status is terminated. |
| 3. Check with physician regarding test results. | Ensures that nurses' knowledge of physical condition is current. |

## Special Considerations

- Hospitalization is not required for this procedure. Street clothes can be worn.
- Sedation is restricted to client who cannot lie still during procedure.

## Teaching Considerations

- Assure client that scan is safe and painless.
- If possible, show client a picture of machine to minimize signs of claustrophobia.
- Tell client "clicking" noise will be heard as scanner moves around head. Client will not be able to feel scanner rotating.
- After procedure, encourage fluids for client who received dye injection. Dye is excreted through kidneys and causes diuresis.

# SKILL 46-5 Assisting with Chest X-ray Examination

Several types of x-ray procedures are performed on clients in an inpatient or outpatient setting. Chest x-ray examination is performed to visualize the lungs and surrounding structures. This procedure is often part of the general admission workup or complete physical examination of the adult client.

### Purposes

1. Visualize structures of the lungs and surrounding structures.
2. Identify tumors, inflammation, or fluid in the lung.
3. Identify air in the pleura.
4. Identify fractures of the bones of the thorax.

## Procedure 46-5

| Steps | Rationale |
|---|---|
| **Assessment** | |
| 1. Assess client's knowledge of procedure. | Determines what education may be necessary. |
| 2. Determine if female client is pregnant. | X-ray procedures are contraindicated in pregnant client because of potential risk of causing congenital deformities in the fetus. |
| 3. Determine client's smoking history. | Clients with history of smoking have radiographic changes on chest x-ray films. |
| **Nursing Diagnosis** | |
| 1. Cluster data to reveal actual or potential nursing diagnoses. All nursing diagnoses are possible. | |
| **Planning** | |
| 1. Arrange for transportation of client to x-ray department. | Better quality chest x-ray films are taken with client standing 6 ft from machine. Portable x-rays at bedside are not of high quality. |
| 2. Inform client that metal objects such as necklaces must be removed. | Metal objects block bony structures and will appear on film. |
| **Implementation** | |
| 1. Instruct client to face x-ray film. | Obtains posteroanterior (PA) angle for chest film. |
| 2. Position client's chin on chin rest and shoulders against film. | Optimal position for chest film. |
| 3. Instruct client to take deep breath and hold. | Provides maximal inspiration for PA chest film. |
| 4. Position client with side perpendicular to second film. | Proper position for obtaining lateral film. |
| 5. Instruct client to take deep breath and hold. | Provides maximal inspiration for lateral chest film. |
| **Evaluation** | |
| 1. Reassess client to determine response to chest x-ray examination. | Is noninvasive procedure and does not have any side effects. |
| **Recording and Reporting** | |
| 1. Record in nurses' notes: date and time chest x-ray film was taken. | Documents that x-ray film was taken. Operative procedures require that preoperative chest x-ray film be taken; documentation in nurses' notes verifies film in institution's radiology department. |
| 2. Report status of client's chest x-ray film to oncoming nursing personnel. | Informs personnel of future need to transport client to or from radiology department. |
| **Follow-up Activity** | |
| 1. Review chest x-ray film to determine tumor, inflammation, fluid, fractured bones. | Enables prompt treatment of medical conditions. |

### Special Considerations

- Occasionally, inspiratory and expiratory films are ordered. If so, client remains in same position, fully exhales, and holds breath.
- Clients frequently have order for PA and lateral chest x-ray films.
- If chest x-ray examination is absolutely essential in pregnant client, lead apron should be placed over uterus.
- Men should cover testes and women should cover ovaries with lead shields to prevent radiation-induced abnormalities that could cause congenital abnormalities in future offspring.
- Severely ill client may have portable film taken at bedside; however, x-ray film is not as clear as standing film.
- If portable x-ray is performed at bedside, nurse should leave room or wear lead apron when x-ray is taken.

### Teaching Considerations

- Tell client that to take a deep breath and hold it while x-ray film is being taken. Movement blurs x-ray film.
- Explain necessary shielding to prevent radiation-induced abnormalities that could cause congenital abnormalities in future offspring.

## *SKILL 46-6 Assisting with Electrocardiogram*

An electrocardiogram (ECG or EKG) is a graphic representation of the electrical impulses generated by the heart during the cardiac cycle. The electrical impulses are conducted to the body's surface, where they are detected by electrodes placed on limbs and chest. The electrodes carry the electrical impulses to a continuously running graph that plots the EKG wave pattern. The appearance of the EKG pattern helps diagnose whether there are any abnormalities interfering with electrical conduction through the heart. The 12-lead ECG is composed of five electrodes. One electrode is placed on each of the four extremities, and one is successively placed at varying sites on the chest.

If a continuous ECG recording is needed over an extended period of time, a Holter monitor is used. A Holter monitor is a small, portable device that records electrical activity of the heart for up to 24 hr. The ECG is recorded on magnetic tape and monitors cardiac rhythm during activity, rest, and sleep.

### Purposes

1. Identify abnormal cardiac rhythm.
2. Measure cardiac electrical activity.
3. Diagnose acute myocardial infarction.

## *Procedure 46-6*

| Steps | Rationale |
|---|---|
| **Assessment** | |
| 1. Assess client's knowledge of procedure. | Identifies need for further client education. |
| 2. Obtain baseline vital signs. | Provides for comparison with vital sign data at later date. |
| 3. Obtain previous ECG tracings on file. | Used as comparison with ECG to be taken. |
| **Nursing Diagnosis** | |
| 1. Cluster data to reveal actual or potential nursing diagnoses: | |
| a. Decreased cardiac output: related to electrocardiac disturbances. | Electrocardiac disturbances can decrease frequency and strength of each cardiac contraction, which can cause decrease in cardiac output. |
| b. Anxiety: related to diagnostic test. | Unfamiliarity with test can cause anxiety, which can cause alterations in cardiac rate and rhythm. |
| c. Knowledge deficit regarding ECG procedure: related to lack of information or inexperience. | |
| **Planning** | |
| 1. Develop individualized goals based on nursing diagnoses: | |
| a. Promote client's comfort. | Attachment of leads can cause temporary discomfort and skin irritation, which is relieved once leads are removed. |

| Steps | Rationale |
|---|---|
| b. Reduce anxiety related to procedure. | Reduction in anxiety improves client's participation. |
| 2. Assemble equipment: | |
| a. ECG machine | |
| b. Electrode paste | Ensures electrical conduction between skin and electrodes. |
| c. ECG leads or electrodes | Are attached to client's chest or extremities to monitor ECG tracings. |
| d. Alcohol wipes | Used to remove oil and dirt from skin at site of lead attachment. |
| e. Fine-grade sandpaper | Sometimes used to slightly abrade skin for secure attachment of leads. |
| f. Razor | Used to remove excess chest hair to facilitate attachment of leads. |
| 3. Prepare client for procedure: | |
| a. Remove clothing from waist up. | Facilitates correct placement of cardiac leads. |
| b. Place client in supine position. | Exposes client for lead placement. |
| c. Instruct client to lie still without talking (12-lead ECG only). | Prevents recording of electrical artifacts caused by motion of chest wall. |

## Implementation

| Steps | Rationale |
|---|---|
| 1. Wash hands. | Reduces transmission of microorganisms. |
| 2. Close room door or bedside curtains. | Provides privacy. |
| 3. Cleanse and prepare skin; wipe sites with alcohol and abrade with fine sandpaper. | Promotes adherence of leads (electrodes) to chest or extremity. |
| 4. Apply electrode paste and attach leads. For 12-lead ECG:<br>a. Chest:<br>▪ $V_1$—Fourth intercostal space (ICS) at right sternal border.<br>▪ $V_2$—Fourth ICS at left sternal border.<br>▪ $V_3$—Midway between $V_2$ and $V_4$.<br>▪ $V_4$—Fifth ICS at midclavicular line.<br>▪ $V_5$—Left anterior axillary line at level of $V_4$ horizontally.<br>▪ $V_6$—Left midaxillary line at level of $V_4$ horizontally.<br>b. Extremities: one on each extremity. | Position of leads promotes proper display of ECG on paper. |
| 5. Obtain tracing; 12-lead ECG may be obtained without removing precordial leads. | Transfers electrocardiac conduction on ECG tracing paper for subsequent analysis by cardiologist. |
| 6. Disconnect leads and wipe excess electrode paste from chest. | Promotes comfort and hygiene. |
| 7. Wash hands. | Provides for review of ECG by cardiologist. |
| 8. Deliver ECG tracing to appropriate laboratory or heart station. | Reduces transmission of microorganisms. |

## Evaluation

| Steps | Rationale |
|---|---|
| 1. Determine if client has chest pain. | Determines worsening of condition. |
| 2. Measure vital signs. | Electrocardiac changes may result in vital sign alterations. |

### *Expected outcome*

| Steps | Rationale |
|---|---|
| 1. Client tolerates procedure without anxiety, pain, cardiac abnormalities. | Procedure is noninvasive and does not result in procedure-related complications. |

### *Unexpected outcome*

| Steps | Rationale |
|---|---|
| 1. Unexpected outcomes are not related to test but to underlying condition of client. | |
| a. Client experiences chest pain. | May be related to myocardial ischemia or anxiety. |
| b. Client experiences anxiety. | Anxiety may be result of fears regarding test results. |

## Recording and Reporting

| Steps | Rationale |
|---|---|
| 1. Record in nurse's notes: when ECG was obtained and where tracing was sent, pain or discomfort, baseline vital signs. | Documents completion of test and complications. |
| 2. Report any unexpected outcomes immediately. | Indicates whether there is need for prompt medical follow-up. |

| Steps | Rationale |
|---|---|
| **Follow-up Activity** | |
| 1. If client experiences severe chest pain, notify physician, continue to monitor cardiac activity with ECG, obtain vital signs, remain with client. | Prompt assessment, monitoring of ECG, medical treatment can assist in reducing myocardial damage if chest pain is caused by myocardial infarction. |

### Special Considerations

- Crushing substernal chest pain that radiates to jaw or arm may indicate angina or myocardial infarction. Chest pain should be brought to immediate attention of physician.
- If Holter monitoring is selected, client may require further explanation of how cardiac cycle is monitored.

### Teaching Consideration

- After explaining procedure, assure client that flow of electric current is from him to machine. Client will not feel anything during procedure.

# *SKILL 46-7 Assisting with Endoscopy*

Endoscopy enables direct visualization of the upper and lower gastrointestinal (GI) tract by means of a long, fiberoptic, flexible scope. The procedure is indicated for the diagnosis of gastric ulcers with atypical radiologic features, to locate the source of upper GI bleeding, to establish the presence and extent of varices in the lower esophagus and stomach in clients with liver disease, and to detect abnormalities of the lower colon. For examination of the upper GI tract, the throat is sprayed with a topical anesthetic and the client is positioned on the side. Before examination of the lower colon, fecal material is removed by enema, laxative, or suppository, and the client is placed in the knee-chest position. This procedure is usually performed in a specially equipped endoscopy unit.

### Purposes

1. Examine the esophagus, stomach, duodenum, and colon for tumors, varices, inflammations, polyps, ulcers, and obstructions.
2. Remove tissues for biopsy for suspected conditions.
3. Coagulate sources of active GI bleeding.

## *Procedure 46-7*

| Steps | Rationale |
|---|---|
| **Assessment** | |
| 1. Assess client's knowledge of procedure. | To ensure cooperation, procedure may need to be explained in detail. |
| 2. Assess vital signs. | Provides baseline data for comparison with postprocedure measurements. |
| 3. Determine GI bleeding. Observe character of emesis, stool, nasogastric tube drainage. | Test is contraindicated in clients with severe upper GI bleeding because viewing lens may get covered with blood clots, preventing visualization. |
| 4. Determine purpose of procedure: biopsy, examination, coagulation of bleeding sites. | Enables nurse to anticipate needs. |
| 5. Assess need for signed consent form (check institution's policy). | Invasive procedures require consent form. |
| 6. Verify that client has been npo for at least 8 hr for endoscopy of upper GI tract. | Introduction of endoscope can induce vomiting. Empty stomach reduces risk of aspiration of stomach contents. |
| 7. Verify that client does not have esophageal diverticulum. | Esophageal diverticulum is contraindication to endoscopy because scope can easily fall into diverticulum and perforate its wall. |
| 8. Review physician's orders for preprocedure medication: | |
| a. Diazepam. | Decreases anxiety and promotes muscle relaxation. |
| b. Atropine. | Decreases oral secretions. |

| Steps | Rationale |
|---|---|
| **Nursing Diagnosis** | |
| 1. Cluster data to reveal actual or potential nursing diagnoses: | |
| a. Anxiety: related to procedure. | Unfamiliarity with procedure increases anxiety. |
| b. Pain: related to procedure. | Introduction of endoscope causes discomfort; client will need comfort measures during and after procedure (Chapter 5). |
| c. Decreased cardiac output: related to postprocedure bleeding. | |
| d. Knowledge deficit regarding purpose and steps of procedure: related to inexperience. | Nurse provides thorough explanation to relieve client's anxiety. |
| **Planning** | |
| 1. Develop individualized goals based on nursing diagnoses: | |
| a. Reduce anxiety. | Insertion of endoscope into mouth and throat partially occludes airway; client may have sensations of fear and suffocation. |
| b. Promote comfort. | Can decrease anxiety. |
| 2. Assemble supplies and equipment: | |
| a. Antiseptic solution for handwashing | Reduces transmission of microorganisms. |
| b. Endoscopy tray: | |
| ▪ Fiberoptic endoscope (Fig. 46-5) | Physician or OR supplies machine to attach to endoscope for electric light source. |

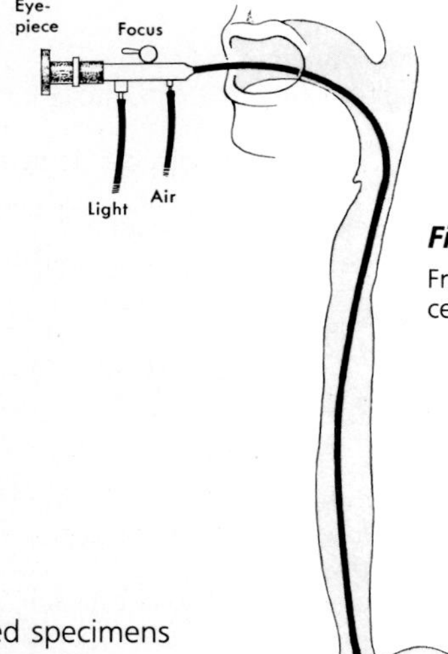


***Fig. 46-5***

From Phipps WJ, Long BC, Woods NF: Medical-surgical nursing: concepts and clinical practice, ed 3, St Louis, 1989, The CV Mosby Co.

| Steps | Rationale |
|---|---|
| ▪ Camera | Physician may elect to photograph unusual or abnormal lesion. Physician may provide own camera. |
| ▪ Solutions for biopsied specimens | Used to preserve specimen for microscopic examination. |
| c. Local anesthetic spray | Inactivates gag reflex. |
| d. Tracheal suction equipment (Chapter 16) | Used for removal of aspirated gastric secretions or sputum from airways. |
| e. Sterile water-soluble jelly | Provides for smooth intubation of client with endoscope. |
| f. Sterile gloves for physician | Maintains surgical asepsis. |
| g. Emesis basin | |
| 3. Prepare client: | |
| a. Explain steps of procedure, including sensations to expect. | Nurse can relieve anxiety and answer clients questions. |
| b. Administer pain or preprocedure medication. | Promotes relaxation and reduces anxiety. |
| **Implementation** | |
| *Physician's responsibility:* | |
| 1. Spray nasopharynx and oropharynx with local anesthetic. | Early application of anesthetic allows for optimal effect of anesthesia. |
| 2. Attach distal end of endoscope to light source. | Provides for direct visualization of upper GI tract. |
| 3. With nursing assistance, position client in left lateral (Sim's) position. | Provides for airway clearance if client gags and vomits gastric contents. |
| 4. Slowly pass endoscope into mouth, esophagus, stomach, duodenum. | Provides visualization of gastric structures. |
| 5. Insufflate air into endoscope. | Maintains patency of endoscopic lumen. |
| 6. Examine or perform biopsy of gastric structures. | Provides data from which physician makes diagnosis. |

| Steps | Rationale |
|---|---|
| *Nurse's responsibility:* | |
| 1. Wash hands. | |
| 2. Remove dentures and partial bridges. | Prevents dislodgment of dental structures during intubation phase. |
| 3. Assist client in maintaining left lateral position. | Unexpected change of position can cause accidental perforation of esophagus, stomach, duodenum. |
| 4. Assist client through procedure: | |
| a. Anticipate needs. | Client is unable to speak after tube is passed into throat. |
| b. Promote comfort. | |
| c. Tell client what is happening. | Reassures client about procedure and how long it will last. |
| d. Hold client's hand. | |
| 5. Place tissue specimens in proper laboratory containers. | Ensures proper labeling and preparation of specimens for microscopic examination. |
| 6. Suction if client begins to vomit. | Prevents aspiration of gastric contents. |
| 7. Maintain client's npo status until gag reflex returns. | Full effects of local anesthetic take 2 to 4 hr to wear off. Ingestion of food before return of gag reflex can increase risk of pulmonary aspiration. |
| 8. Provide oral hygiene when gag reflex returns. | Refreshens mouth after passage of tube. |
| 9. Assist client to comfortable position. | Promotes rest and relaxation. |
| 10. Wash hands. | Reduces transmission of microorganisms. |

## Evaluation

| | |
|---|---|
| 1. Reassess client to determine response to endoscopy. | Identifies unexpected events. |
| a. Monitor vital signs according to hospital policy. May be as often as every 15 min for 2 hrs. | Change in vital signs can indicate new bleeding in abdomen. |
| b. Observe for pain. | Sudden abdominal pain can indicate rupture of abdominal organs. |
| c. Evaluate emesis or aspirate for occult blood (Chapter 45). | Indicates abdominal bleeding. |
| d. Assess for return of gag reflex. | Determines when effects of anesthetic have disappeared. |

### *Expected outcome*

| | |
|---|---|
| 1. Client tolerates procedure. Client has little pain or discomfort, does not aspirate, has no postprocedure bleeding. | Indicates absence of complications. |

### *Unexpected outcomes*

| | |
|---|---|
| 1. Client has abdominal pain. | Occurs with perforation of abdominal structures; pain is accompanied by abdominal distention or bleeding. |
| 2. Client develops aspiration pneumonia. | Caused by aspiration of gastric contents into lungs; may be accompanied by fever, chest pain, productive cough. |
| 3. Client has bleeding. | Results from trauma to biopsy site or reinitiation of upper GI bleeding. |
| 4. Vital signs indicate deterioration of condition. | Results from loss of blood volume related to bleeding or perforation of abdominal structures. |

## Recording and Reporting

| | |
|---|---|
| 1. Record in nurses' notes: procedure, duration, client's tolerance, collection and disposition of specimen. | Provides documentation of procedure in client's record. |
| 2. Report onset of bleeding, abdominal pain, and vital sign changes to physician. | May require emergent treatment. |
| 3. Report to nurse in charge: duration of procedure, client's tolerance, changes in vital signs. | Enables prompt medical follow-up for unexpected outcomes. |

## Follow-up Activities

| | |
|---|---|
| 1. Do not allow the client to eat or drink anything until the tracheobronchial anesthesia has worn off. | Prevents aspiration of food or fluid which could cause pneumonia. |

### Special Considerations

- Procedure may be contraindicated in clients unable to fully cooperate.
- Vital signs are especially crucial in clients who have had GI bleeding.
- If client is actively bleeding, stomach should be lavaged and aspirated clear of clots before procedure is attempted.
- Lidocaine is frequently used to inactivate gag reflex.
- If endoscopy of the upper GI tract is emergency and client has had something to eat or drink, be sure physician is informed first.
- Meperidine may also be used as relaxation agent. Decision to use diazepam or meperidine is usually physician's preference.
- Know in advance if specimens are to be immediately delivered to laboratory and have person available to transport specimen.
- Initially, client may experience internal bleeding without visible signs of blood loss after procedure.

### Teaching Considerations

- Inform client of preprocedure medication and anticipated effects.
- Explain method for endoscope insertion.
- Explain that client will be unable to speak when the endoscope is positioned in GI tract.
- Make sure client knows not to eat or drink until gag reflex returns. Before return of gag reflex, client could aspirate and develop pneumonia.

## *SKILL 46-8 Assisting with Lumbar Puncture*

A lumbar puncture, also called spinal puncture or spinal tap, involves the introduction of a spinal needle into the subarachnoid space of the spinal column. The actual procedure is performed by a physician, but a well-prepared nurse is required to assist in most aspects of it.

The purposes of a lumbar puncture are to measure cerebrospinal fluid (CSF) pressure in the subarachnoid space and to obtain CSF for visual and laboratory examination.

This procedure is contraindicated if there is evidence of greatly increased intracranial pressure because the sudden release of pressure may cause herniation of the brain structures through the foramen magnum. This herniation places pressure on the medulla oblongata, which houses the respiratory center, possibly causing severe respiratory distress.

Lumbar punctures are considered uncomfortable by most clients. A well-prepared nurse can help the client undergo the procedure smoothly and successfully. The nurse explains the entire procedure to the client, reassuring that assistance will be provided throughout. The nurse's knowledge of the procedural details and preparation for the lumbar puncture also helps the physician to complete the procedure in a timely manner.

### Purposes

1. Measure pressure of the subarachnoid space in the spinal column.
2. Obtain CSF for examination.
3. Administer diagnostic agents, spinal anesthetics, or chemotherapeutic agents.

### *Procedure 46-8*

| Steps | Rationale |
|---|---|
| **Assessment** | |
| 1. Assess client's ability to understand and follow directions. | Procedure requires client to follow directions closely and attain proper position. Clients with neurologic problems may have reduced level of consciousness. |
| 2. Assess musculoskeletal flexibility of client to assume lateral decubitus (fetal) position. | Lateral decubitus position is important to place spinal needle in proper position. |
| 3. Assess degree of cooperativeness of client to remain in position without excessive movement. | Movement can cause injury from spinal needle. |
| 4. Examine medical record for contraindications of increased intracranial pressure or degenerative joint disease. | Excessive intracranial pressure may cause brain herniation. Degenerative joint disease may prevent client from attaining proper position or physician from easily entering subarachnoid space for procedure. |

| Steps | Rationale |
|---|---|
| 5. Determine whether client is allergic to medication to be used as local anesthetic agent (e.g., lidocaine). | Previous allergies to anesthetic agents should be noted so these agents may be avoided by physician. |
| 6. Check signed consent form (ascertain institution's policy). | Consent forms are required for most invasive diagnostic testing procedures. |
| 7. Assess client's knowledge regarding procedure. | Procedure needs to be explained to client. |
| 8. Assess vital signs and neurologic status. | Provides baseline data for comparison with postprocedural measurements. |

## Nursing Diagnosis

| Steps | Rationale |
|---|---|
| 1. Cluster data to reveal actual or potential nursing diagnoses: | |
| a. Pain: related to needle insertion and/or related to positioning. | Postprocedure headache and position required for lumbar puncture can cause physical discomfort. |
| b. Anxiety: related to test procedure and findings. | Depending on reason for test, client may exhibit anxiety related to procedure and findings. |
| c. Altered thought processes: related to neurologic impairment. | Client may be disoriented or unable to follow directions. |
| d. Knowledge deficit regarding procedural steps: related to inexperience. | Thorough explanation promotes client's cooperation during procedure. |

## Planning

| Steps | Rationale |
|---|---|
| 1. Develop individualized goals for client based on nursing diagnoses: | |
| a. Promote client comfort. | Client may experience discomfort at puncture site or headache for 6 to 12 hr that may be relieved by bedrest and analgesics. |
| b. Allay client anxieties about procedure and test findings. | Explanation of procedure and results can help to reduce anxiety. |
| c. Ensure client safety. | Proper positioning and restraining prevents injury to spinal cord. |
| 2. Prepare equipment and supplies: | |
| a. Lumbar puncture tray, including: | |
| ■ Antiseptic solution (e.g., povidone-iodine) | Used for topical cleansing of skin. |
| ■ Ten gauze sponges (4 × 4) | |
| ■ Sterile towels | Used to isolate area on back required for lumbar puncture. |
| ■ Three spinal needles (various sizes) with inner obturators | Size depends on size of client. Inner obturators are used to introduce needle into spinal column. |
| ■ Alcohol swabs | |
| ■ Anesthetic agent (e.g., lidocaine 1%) | Provides local anesthetic at puncture site. |
| ■ Syringes (3 to 5 ml) | Used to deliver anesthesia to superficial and deep tissues. |
| ■ Two rolled bath towels | Used to place under client's side for spinal positioning. |
| ■ Needles (5/8 in, 25 g to 1½ in, 21 g) | |
| ■ Sterile gloves (check physician's size) | Obtain several pairs of gloves in more than one size for physician preference and to replace if contaminated. |
| ■ Glass or plastic manometer with three-way stopcock | Used to measure opening and closing pressure of CSF in spinal column. |
| ■ Four test tubes | |
| ■ Antiseptic ointment | |
| ■ Band-Aid | |
| ■ Straight chair for physician | Physician needs to sit at side of bed to work with spine at eye level. Physician needs to be comfortable because of difficulty of procedure. |
| 3. Explain procedure to client. | Physician may have already done this, but nurse should tell client in understandable terms about potential discomfort associated with procedure and length of procedure. |
| 4. Have client empty bladder and bowels before procedure begins. | Avoids interruption of test. |
| 5. Position client in lateral decubitus (fetal) position with head and neck flexed (Fig. 46-6). | Flexion of lumbar spine allows for easy access to CSF in spinal column. |
| a. Bring both arms and knees toward center of body. | Gives spinal column full curvature. Spinal column should be flexed as much as possible to allow maximal space between vertebrae. |
| b. May place pillow between knees. | Prevents discomfort and possibility of upper leg rolling forward. |

| Steps | Rationale |
|---|---|

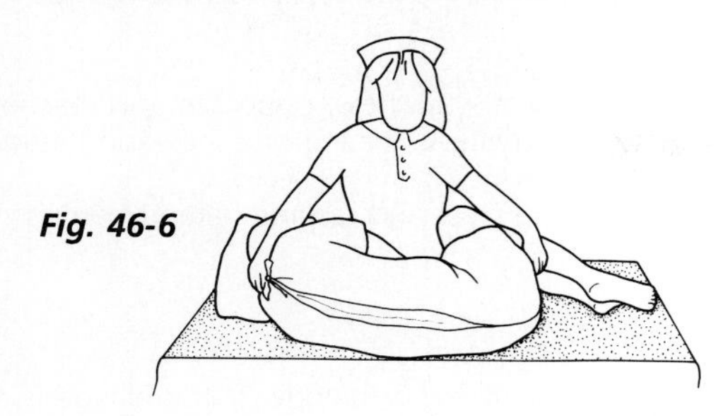
Fig. 46-6

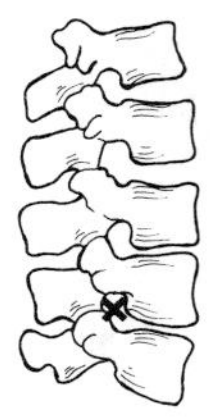
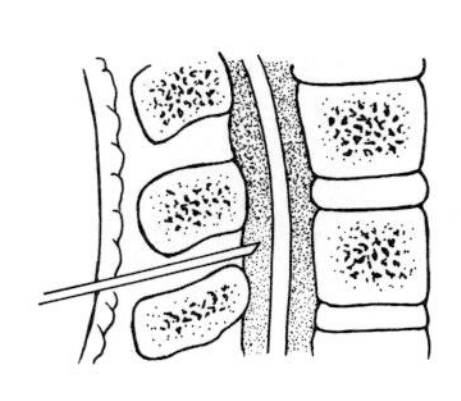
Fig. 46-7

## Implementation

*Physician's responsibility:*

| Steps | Rationale |
|---|---|
| 1. Set up sterile field of equipment. | Provides sterile work area. |
| 2. Don sterile gloves. | |
| 3. Prepare area with antiseptic solution and gauze sponges. | Prevents entry of microorganisms from skin to CSF in spinal cord. |
| 4. Drape with sterile towels. | |
| 5. Inject topical anesthetic agent. | Provides local anesthetic to skin surrounding puncture site. |
| 6. Insert spinal needle with inner obturator into spinal column between L5 and S1 (Fig. 46-7). | This area is chosen because spinal cord ends approximately at L2, which decreases chance of trauma to spinal nerves. |
| 7. After entering subarachnoid space, obturator is removed. | Allows flow of CSF from subarachnoid space. |
| 8. Attach manometer with stopcock and read manometer for "opening pressure." | Manometer is calibrated in centimeters (millimeters of water). "Opening" or "initial" pressure is read by watching CSF fill manometer to stable level. |
| 9. Turn stopcock to allow CSF drainage to drip into test tubes to send for appropriate testing. Each test tube is filled with 2 to 3 ml of CSF. | Maintains patent conduit from CSF to test tube. |
| 10. Remove spinal needle. | |
| 11. Place direct pressure on insertion site. | Decreases or stops CSF leakage from spinal column and blood from subcutaneous tissue track of needle. |
| 12. Place adhesive gauze or Band-Aid over insertion site. | Ensures sterility of insertion site. |

*Nurse's responsibility:*

| Steps | Rationale |
|---|---|
| 1. Explain that client must lie in flexed position for entire procedure. | Client must remain still throughout procedure to ensure no movement of spinal needle within spinal column. |
| 2. Hold arms and legs in position for clients who are restless. | Prevents sudden movement on part of client. |
| 3. Hold client's hands tightly and encourage client to squeeze hands when he feels uncomfortable. | May prevent client from moving in bed in response to discomfort. |
| 4. Explain each step that may give discomfort (e.g., injection of anesthesia): "The medication that numbs the skin is going to be given now. You will feel a burning sensation. It will last just a few seconds and then go away." | Client should know exactly what is occurring so that discomfort can be anticipated and surprises eliminated. |
| 5. Assist physician in holding manometer straight. If not wearing sterile gloves, hold very top of manometer. Manometer is hooked directly to spinal needle. | Prevents movement of needle and contamination of sterile field. |
| 6. Note "opening pressure" and color of CSF. | Remember this pressure for documentation. Normal CSF is colorless; note color for documentation. |
| 7. Assist physician in filling test tubes with CSF. | Physician will have one hand on stopcock and only one hand free and usually needs assistance in filling tubes. |
| 8. Properly label tubes with client information and name of test desired. | Nurse is responsible for labeling tubes with client's name and test desired. Test tubes are numbered in sequence of collection (e.g., Nos. 1-4). Physician orders certain tests on each tube for specific reasons. |
| 9. Assist with placement of direct pressure and gauze bandage. | Pressure helps minimize CSF loss and bleeding. |
| 10. Wash hands thoroughly after procedure, especially if tubes with CSF have been handled. | Tubes might contain virulent organisms. |
| 11. Assist client in assuming comfortable position. | |
| 12. Ask client to maintain reclining position (bedrest), usually 4 to 12 hr. | Reclining position reduces risk of spinal headache, which may result if client sits upright. |
| 13. Provide for client's comfort with medication if ordered, desirable, and not contraindicated. | Procedure is usually described as painful by client. |

| Steps | Rationale |
|---|---|
| 14. During and after procedure, observe client for;<br>a. Changes in level of consciousness.<br>b. Pupil size and reaction.<br>c. Respiratory status.<br>d. Vital signs. | Changes in level of consciousness, pupil size and reaction, respiratory status, and vital signs indicate increasing intracranial pressure. |
| 15. Encourage client to force fluids by mouth if not contraindicated. | Needed to replace CSF loss and resume hemodynamics. |

## Evaluation

| Steps | Rationale |
|---|---|
| 1. Assess needle insertion site for drainage. | Small amount of CSF (clear) or bloody (red) drainage is considered normal. (Small amount would be 1 to 2 cm stain on 4 × 4 gauze.) CSF may leak minimally through insertion site, but leakage usually decreases within short period. |
| 2. Assess level of consciousness, vital signs, pupils, respiratory status. | May indicate complications of brain herniation. |

### *Expected outcomes*

| Steps | Rationale |
|---|---|
| 1. Small amount (1 to 2 cm circle) of clear or red drainage is present. | Small amount of CSF or bloody drainage is considered normal and expected. |
| 2. Client does not experience postpuncture headache or other complications. | Without CSF leakage through subcutaneous track, postpuncture headache does not occur. |
| 3. Test results of CSF are normal: | |
| a. Opening pressure is 80 to 180 mm $H_2O$. | Pressures over 200 mm $H_2O$ are considered abnormal. |
| b. CSF is clear and colorless. | Color and opacity may indicate presence of RBCs or organisms. |
| c. Blood: none present. | |
| d. Cells: no RBCs present; lymphocytes fewer than 5/mm$^3$. | |
| e. Culture and sensitivity: no organisms present. | |
| f. Protein: 15 to 45 mg/100 ml CSF. | |
| g. Glucose: 50 to 75 mg/100 ml CSF or greater than 40% serum glucose level. | |
| h. LDH (lactic dehydrogenase): less than 2 to 7.2 $\mu$/ml. | |
| i. Cytology: no malignant cells present. | |
| j. Serology for syphilis: negative. | |

### *Unexpected outcomes*

| Steps | Rationale |
|---|---|
| 1. Client has excessive drainage from insertion site. | Indicates CSF or blood leakage through subcutaneous track. |
| 2. Client has postpuncture headache. | Precise cause of postpuncture headache is unknown, although CSF leak is theorized cause. Also called spinal headache; is typically bifrontal and suboccipital and appears a few hours to several days after procedure. Is characteristically relieved when client is supine but resumes on sitting. |
| 3. Pain or tingling sensation in lower extremities. | Could be caused by nerve root irritation related to needle trauma to spinal nerves. |

## Recording and Reporting

| Steps | Rationale |
|---|---|
| 1. Record in nurses' notes: procedure performed, including time, physician's name, client's toleration (e.g., opening pressure, color of CSF, amount of drainage on dressing, whether headache and leg tingling are present). | Accurate documentation of procedure is important for legal reasons. |
| 2. Record and report pertinent findings to nurse in charge and physician: changes in vital signs, nausea, vomiting, changes in level of consciousness. | May dictate medical emergency. |

## Follow-up Activities

| Steps | Rationale |
|---|---|
| 1. Provide for client's comfort through positioning, relaxation techniques, and analgesics if indicated. | Promotes sense of well-being. |
| 2. Initiate client teaching for usual post–lumbar puncture care, including activity and forcing fluids. | Promotes cooperation. |

### Special Considerations

- Consider which side of bed physician will need to sit on to perform procedure. Position client so spine (dorsal side) is against proper side of bed.
- Even though physician performs procedure, nurse needs to understand details of procedure to assist and anticipate needs of physician and client. Nurse may set up or help to set up sterile field while physician is disinfecting skin with 4 × 4 sponges and povidone-iodine.
- "Opening" pressure may be compared with "closing" pressure for interest. "Closing" pressure is not as significant a number.
- Client's feelings of discomfort may vary depending on toleration of pain, degree of difficulty in obtaining CSF, and extent of CSF leakage after end of procedure.
- After procedure, some say to place client in prone position with pillow under abdomen to increase intraabdominal pressure, increase pressure on tissues surrounding spinal column, decrease drainage.
- Some physicians order bed rest after lumbar puncture; some do not. Treatment for headache is bed rest, icepack applied to head, and analgesia. Forcing fluids may also help reestablish CSF level.
- Cerebral or cerebellar herniation may occur in client with increased intracranial pressure as result of dramatic decreases in pressure.
- Report any excessive drainage (e.g., saturation of gauze dressing). If excessive drainage occurs, place pressure dressing on site and place client in prone position.
- Excessive drainage from insertion site may predispose client to postpuncture headache and infection because moisture may function as growth medium for bacteria.
- Duration of lumbar puncture is 15 to 60 min, and ease of attaining CSF depends on position held.

### Teaching Considerations

- Thoroughly explain procedure and postprocedure routine to client. Many clients have misconceptions regarding procedure.
- Assure client that insertion of needle into spine will not cause paralysis because needle is inserted into area below spinal cord.
- Make sure clients understands importance of remaining still during procedure. Movement could cause traumatic injury.

# *SKILL 46-9 Assisting with Proctoscopy*

Proctoscopy is a lighted examination of the rectum. It is a form of endoscopy of the lower GI tract. Other forms include anoscopy and sigmoidoscopy, which are examinations of the anus and sigmoid colon, respectively. Proctoscopy, a procedure performed by a physician assisted by a nurse, usually takes place in a treatment room of the nursing division. Direct visualization of the anal and rectal walls is preferable to radiography because this procedure is less traumatic and less expensive for the client. A proctoscopy is performed to visualize anatomy for pathophysiology conditions (e.g., tumors, polyps, or ulcerations). A biopsy may be performed to obtain tissue specimens for microscopic examination.

### Purposes

1. Visualize anal and rectal walls for pathophysiologic conditions.
2. Obtain tissue specimens for microscopic examination.

## *Procedure 46-9*

| Steps | Rationale |
|---|---|
| **Assessment** | |
| 1. Assess client's knowledge of procedure. | Procedure may need to be explained to client. |
| 2. Assess client's ability to assume position required for procedure. | Preferred position for proctoscopy in noncritical client is genupectoral, or knee-chest, position (Fig. 46-8). |
| 3. Assess vital signs to obtain baseline data. | Ensures stability of hemodynamic status and provides for comparison with postprocedure vital signs. |
| 4. Determine purpose of procedure. | Enables nurse to anticipate needed supplies. |
| 5. Assess need for signed consent form (check institution's policy). | Provides written documentation of consent and understanding of procedure. |
| 6. Assess need for preprocedure pain medication. | Procedure may be painful, but need for pain medication should be carefully assessed because it may affect ability to maintain knee-chest position. |

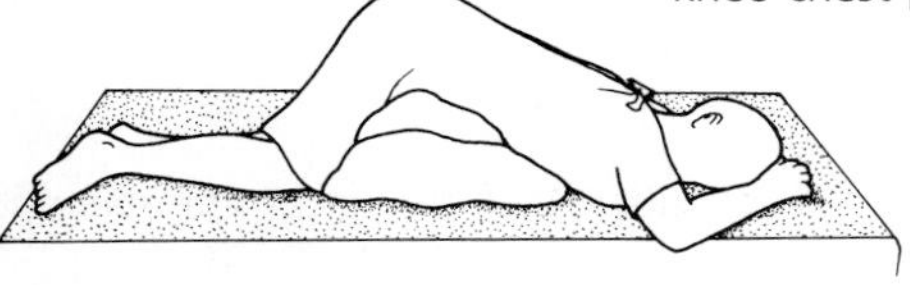

*Fig. 46-8*

| Steps | Rationale |
|---|---|
| 7. Assess client's feces if possible (e.g., color, odor, consistency, abnormalities if present). | Provides for postprocedure comparison. |
| 8. Determine possible order and administration of preprocedure bowel preparation. | Lower bowel preparation may be ordered (e.g., cleansing enema). |

## Nursing Diagnosis

| Steps | Rationale |
|---|---|
| 1. Cluster data to reveal actual or potential nursing diagnoses: | |
| a. Pain: related to procedure. | Client's position required for test and insertion of lighted proctoscope into anus causes physical and emotional discomfort. |
| b. Anxiety: related to procedure. | Position can be embarrassing. |
| c. Knowledge deficit regarding procedural steps: related to inexperience. | Nurse's explanation of procedure will relieve client's anxiety. |

## Planning

| Steps | Rationale |
|---|---|
| 1. Develop individualized goals based on nursing diagnoses: | |
| a. Promote client's comfort. | Relieves client anxiety. |
| b. Promote ease of procedure by coaching client in relaxation techniques. | Allow relaxation of perineal muscles and increase ease of insertion of proctoscope. |
| 2. Prepare equipment and supplies: | |
| a. Proctoscopy tray, if available from central supply, which may include: | |
| ▪ Large sterile drape or halfsheet | Maintains surgical asepsis. |
| ▪ Proctoscope (for proctoscopy) and biopsy forceps (for other procedures: anoscope for anoscopy; sigmoidoscope for sigmoidoscopy) | |
| ▪ Gauze sponges (4 × 4) | Used for cleansing proctoscope tube and anus after procedure. |
| ▪ Lubricant for proctoscope | Promotes ease of insertion of proctoscope. |
| ▪ Long cotton-tipped applicators | Used for removal of fecal contents at distal end of colon. |
| b. Sterile and clean gloves for physician | Clean gloves are used for digital examination; sterile gloves are to be used for procedure. |
| c. Suction machine | Attaches to some models of proctoscopes for suction of fecal matter. |
| d. Air insufflator | Sometimes used to force air into colon to separate mucosal folds. |
| e. Specimen container | |
| f. Guaiac testing card and proper solution | Used for testing for occult blood in stool. |
| g. Small stool for physician | Physician will most likely need to perform procedure in sitting position. |
| h. Portable bright light | Used to illuminate anal region for proper visualization. |
| i. Bedsheet or blanket | Provides adequate privacy during procedure. |
| 3. Arrange equipment in organized manner on bedside table. | Promotes organized and rapid completion of procedure. |

## Implementation

| Steps | Rationale |
|---|---|
| *Physician's responsibility:* | |
| 1. Attach suction machine tubing to outlet on proctoscope. | Allows physician to remove feces from colon. |
| 2. Check proctoscopic light source for functioning. | Proctoscope is tubular instrument with appropriate illumination for rectal inspection. |
| 3. Don clean gloves and lubricate fingers with lubricant. | Physician may examine rectum digitally to ensure patent rectum and dilate anal sphincter. |
| 4. Don sterile gloves. | Maintains sterile asepsis after digital examination of anus. |
| 5. Lubricate proctoscope. | Provides for ease of insertion. |
| 6. Insert proctoscope into rectum and turn on proctoscopic light source. | Observation of rectal walls is performed as proctoscope is advanced. |
| 7. Suction fecal material as needed. | Provides for proper visualization and keeps colon free of fecal material. |
| 8. Insert long cotton-tipped applicators into proctoscope. | Applicators obtain fecal specimen for guaiac or other laboratory testing. |
| 9. If needed, insert air from insufflator. | Air expands bowel wall for proper visualization. |
| *Nurse's responsibility:* | |
| 1. Set up proctoscopy set or open supplies to make accessible for physician. | |
| 2. Assist client in maintaining genupectoral, knee-chest, left lateral position. | This is uncomfortable procedure; client must be encouraged to assume position. |

| Steps | Rationale |
| --- | --- |
| 3. Drape sheet over client's body, exposing only anal area. | Provides privacy and prevents chilling. |
| 4. Assist client through procedure by holding hands tightly and reassuring client in coaching manner. | Promotes comfort and cooperation on part of client. |
| 5. Explain procedure to client as it occurs. | Will help client to anticipate changes before they occur. |
| 6. Assess client's condition during procedure: ability to maintain position, color of face, respiratory rate. | Rectal stimulation may elicit vagal response, which could cause client to experience facial flushing or pallor, faintness, and nausea. |
| 7. After procedure is completed, assist client to comfortable position in bed. | Assists client in relaxing. |

## Evaluation

| Steps | Rationale |
| --- | --- |
| 1. Reassess client to determine response to procedure: | Identifies complication or need to modify care plan. |
| a. Assess bowel sounds. | Indicates peristalsis. |
| b. Monitor vital signs. | Verifies physiologic response to procedure. |
| c. Determine level of comfort. | Sharp pain may indicate bowel perforation. |
| ***Expected outcomes*** | |
| 1. Client tolerates procedure well. Client can assume position without problems, and has little discomfort; vital signs are stable. | Indicates absence of complications. |
| 2. Rectum is patent without obstruction or excessive fecal material. | Indicates that preprocedure bowel preparation was satisfactory. |
| 3. Physician is able to observe and obtain specimens from rectal wall. | Documents that purpose of procedure was accomplished. |
| ***Unexpected outcomes*** | |
| 1. Client is unable to maintain desired position. | Results from musculoskeletal alterations, fatigue, discomfort. |
| 2. Complications occur: | |
| a. Small amount of bleeding from rectum. | Result of rectal wall irritation. Bleeding usually stops within short period of time. |
| b. Profuse amount of bleeding from rectum. | Result of rectal wall perforation. |
| c. Vagal response causing hypotension or fainting. | Stimulation of vagus nerve decreases heart rate and cardiac output. |

## Recording and Reporting

| Steps | Rationale |
| --- | --- |
| 1. Record in nurses' notes or on client's chart: name of procedure (include biopsy if performed), duration of procedure, toleration of procedure, any complications. | Accurate recording of procedure is legal necessity. |
| 2. Report to physician immediately: | |
| a. Bleeding after procedure. | Could indicate bowel perforation. |
| b. Changes in vital signs beyond normal limit. | |

## Follow-up Activities

| Steps | Rationale |
| --- | --- |
| 1. Note presence and characteristics of drainage from anus and perform guaiac test for occult blood. | |
| 2. Check with physician for interpretation of proctoscopic examination. | Nurse's knowledge of physicial condition is current. |
| 3. Clean up area and send supplies to proper sterilization department. | Reduces transmission of microorganisms. |

## Special Considerations

- For more seriously ill client, lateral (preferably, left lateral), side-lying position is used for proctoscopy.
- Proctoscopy trays are usually prepared with biopsy equipment in case unanticipated biopsy is needed.
- Clients taking antihypertensive or other cardiac medication may be susceptible to fainting from rectal stimulation.
- If rectum or colon is occluded with stool, procedure may need to be postponed until adequate bowel preparation has been accomplished.
- Client is encouraged to maintain genupectoral position for as long as possible during procedure. If not possible, left lateral position is assumed.

- Vagal response is common complication, causing slowed heart rate. Remove proctoscope and administer treatment symptomatically as ordered by physician.

**Teaching Considerations**

- Explain procedure to client. Warn that discomfort and urge to defecate may be felt as proctoscope is inserted.
- Tell client that "gas pain" may be experienced as air is insufflated during procedure.

# *SKILL 46-10 Assisting with Sigmoidoscopy*

Sigmoidoscopy is the most commonly performed endoscopic procedure of the lower GI tract. Through the use of a fiber-optic flexible endoscope, sigmoidoscopy allows direct visualization and examination of the anus, rectum, and sigmoid colon. Direct visualization of the lower GI tract is very desirable because the lower GI tract is difficult to visualize radiographically. During this procedure, polyps can be removed and sources of GI bleeding can be coagulated. Microscopic review of biopsy specimens obtained during this procedure can provide a diagnosis for many lower bowel disorders. Sigmoidoscopy, a procedure performed by a physician and assisted by a nurse, usually takes place in a specially equipped endoscopy room.

## Purposes

1. Visualize the anus, rectum, and sigmoid colon for pathophysiologic conditions.
2. Obtain tissue specimens for microscopic examination.
3. Coagulate sources of GI bleeding.

## *Procedure 46-10*

| Steps | Rationale |
|---|---|
| **Assessment** | |
| 1. Assess client's knowledge of procedure. | Procedure may need to be explained to the client. |
| 2. Assess client's ability to assume position required for procedure. | Preferred position for sigmoidoscopy is knee-chest position. |
| 3. Assess vital signs to obtain baseline data. | Ensures stability of hemodynamic status and provides comparison with post-procedure vital signs. |
| 4. Determine purpose of procedure. | Enables nurse to anticipate supplies. |
| 5. Check institutions' policy regarding the need for signed consent. | Most institutions require written permission for procedure. |
| 6. Assess client's feces if possible for color, odor, consistency, other abnormalities. | Provides for postprocedure comparison. |
| 7. Obtain order for preprocedure bowel preparation. | Fleet enema is usually given night before and on morning of procedure. |
| **Nursing Diagnosis** | |
| 1. Cluster data to reveal actual or potential nursing diagnoses: | |
| a. Pain: related to procedure. | Client's position during sigmoidoscopy and insertion of lighted sigmoidoscope causes discomfort. |
| b. Anxiety: related to procedure. | Position client assumes and unknown sensations of procedure cause anxiety. |
| c. Knowledge deficit regarding procedure: related to inexperience. | Nurse's explanation of procedure promotes client's cooperation. |
| **Planning** | |
| 1. Develop individualized goals based on nursing diagnoses: | |
| a. Promote client comfort. | Relaxation techniques may help to reduce discomfort. |
| b. Allay client's anxieties. | Explanation of procedure and sensations can reduce anxiety. |
| 2. Administer enemas as ordered evening before and on day of procedure. | Ensures optimal visualization of lower GI tract. |
| 3. Prepare equipment and supplies: | |
| a. Sigmoidoscopy tray, if available from central supply, which may contain: | |
| ▪ Sterile drape | Used to maintain surgical asepsis. |
| ▪ Sigmoidoscope | |

| Steps | Rationale |
|---|---|
| ▪ Gauze sponges (4 × 4) | Used for cleaning sigmoidoscopy and anus after procedure. |
| ▪ Lubricant for sigmoidoscope | Fosters ease of insertion of sigmoidoscope. |
| ▪ Long cotton-tipped applicator | Used for removal of fecal contents. |
| b. Sterile and clean gloves for physician | Clean gloves are worn for digital examination; sterile gloves are used during procedure. |
| c. Suction machine | Used for removal of fecal matter. |
| d. Air insufflator | Used to instill air to distend bowel, allowing better visualization. |
| e. Specimen container | |
| f. Guaiac testing card and proper solution | Used to detect occult blood in feces. |
| g. Small stool for physician | Physicians usually performs procedure in sitting position. |
| h. Portable bright light | Used to illuminate anal area for better visualization. |
| i. Bedsheet or blanket | Provides privacy during procedure. |
| 4. Arrange equipment in organized manner on bedside table. | Promotes organized and rapid completion of procedure. |

## Implementation

| Steps | Rationale |
|---|---|
| *Physician's responsibility:* | |
| 1. Attach suction machine tubing to outlet on sigmoidoscope. | Allows physician to remove feces from colon. |
| 2. Check sigmoidoscopic light source. | Appropriate illumination is needed for inspection of anus, rectum, sigmoid colon. |
| 3. Don clean gloves and lubricate fingers with lubricant. | Physician performs digital examination of rectum, which slowly dilates anal sphincter. |
| 4. Don sterile gloves. | Maintains asepsis after digital examination of the anus. |
| 5. Lubricate sigmoidoscope. | Fosters ease of insertion. |
| 6. Insert sigmoidoscope into anus, rectum, sigmoid colon. | Observation of anus, rectum, sigmoid colon is performed as scope is slowly advanced. |
| 7. Suction fecal material as necessary. | Provides for proper visualization and maintains colon free of fecal material. |
| 8. Insert long, cotton-tipped applicator into sigmoidoscope. | Used to obtain fecal specimens for lab testing. |
| 9. Insert air from insufflator. | Air expands bowel wall for proper visualization. |
| *Nurse's responsibility:* | |
| 1. Set up sigmoidoscopy set or open supplies to make accessible for physician. | |
| 2. Assist client in maintaining knee-chest position. | Procedure is uncomfortable; client needs to be encouraged to remain still in assumed position. |
| 3. Drape sheet over client's body, exposing only anal area. | Provides privacy and prevents chilling. |
| 4. Assist client through procedure by holding hand and reassuring client in coaching manner. | Promotes comfort and cooperation. |
| 5. Explain procedure to client as it occurs. | Step-by-step explanation helps client to anticipate changes before they occur. |
| 6. Assess client's condition during procedure, ability to maintain position, color of face, respiratory sounds. | Rectal stimulation may elicit vagal response, which could cause facial flushing or palor, faintness, nausea. |
| 7. After procedure is completed, assist client to comfortable position in bed. | Helps client relax. |

## Evaluation

| Steps | Rationale |
|---|---|
| 1. Reassess client to determine response to procedure: | Identifies complication or need to modify care plan. |
| a. Assess bowel sounds. | Indicates presence or absence of peristalsis. |
| b. Monitor vital signs. | Verifies physiologic response to procedure. |
| c. Determine client's level of comfort. | Sharp pain may indicate bowel perforation. |
| ***Expected outcomes*** | |
| 1. Client tolerates procedure well, can maintain position without problem, and has little discomfort; vital signs are stable. | Indicates absence of complications. |
| 2. Rectum is patent without excessive fecal material. | Indicates that preprocedure bowel preparation was adequate. |
| 3. Physician is able to observe and obtain desired specimens from rectum or sigmoid colon. | Purpose of procedure was accomplished. |
| ***Unexpected outcomes*** | |
| 1. Client is unable to maintain desired position. | Result of musculoskeletal alteration, fatigue, discomfort, vagal response. |
| 2. Complications occur: | |
| a. Small amount of bleeding from rectum. | Results from rectal wall irritation. Bleeding usually stops within short time. |

| Steps | Rationale |
|---|---|
| b. Profuse amount of bleeding from rectum. | Result of bowel perforation. |
| c. Vagal response causing hypotension or fainting. | Stimulation of vagus nerve decreases heart rate and cardiac output. |

### Recording and Reporting

| Steps | Rationale |
|---|---|
| 1. Record in nurses' note or in client's chart: type of procedure (include biopsy if performed), duration, tolerance, complications. | Accurate recording of procedure is legal necessity. |
| 2. Report to physician immediately: | |
| a. Bleeding after procedure. | Could indicate bowel perforation. |
| b. Changes in vital signs beyond normal limit. | |
| c. Client complaints of severe abdominal pain. | |

### Follow-up Activities

| Steps | Rationale |
|---|---|
| 1. Note presence and characteristics of drainage from anus. | |
| 2. Check with physician for interpretation of sigmoidoscopy examination. | Knowledge of client's condition is current. |
| 3. Clean up area and send supplies for proper sterilization. | Reduces transmission of microorganisms. |

### Special Considerations

- If client cannot tolerate knee-chest position, lateral or Sims' position is used with buttocks positioned 10 to 12 cm over edge of bed to facilitate complete rotation of sigmoidoscope. Maximum convenience is provided by sigmodoscopy table, which tilts client into desired position.

### Teaching Considerations

- Explain procedure to client. Warn that discomfort and urge to defecate will be felt as sigmoidoscope is passed.
- Explain to client that enemas are administered evening before and morning of test to ensure optimal visualization of lower GI tract.
- Tell client that because air is insufflated into bowel during procedure, "gas pains" may be experienced during sigmoidoscopy.

# SKILL 46-11 Assisting with Thoracentesis

Thoracentesis is a sterile procedure performed by a physician and assisted by a nurse, in which a needle is passed into the pleural cavity to remove excess fluid. The excess pleural fluid can be the result of injury, infection, or disease, (e.g., pulmonary contusion, empyema, or pleural effusion, respectively). The primary purpose of thoracentesis is to reduce difficulty in breathing. Other reasons for removing the fluid are to obtain specimens of fluid or lung tissue for diagnostic purposes and to introduce chemotherapeutic drugs intrapleurally. This procedure is not difficult to perform, but the nurse's role in helping the client to refrain from coughing or moving is extremely important because surrounding organs could be punctured.

### Purposes

1. Aspirate excess pleural fluid for improvement of respiratory status.
2. Obtain pleural fluid for laboratory testing.

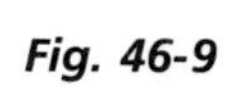
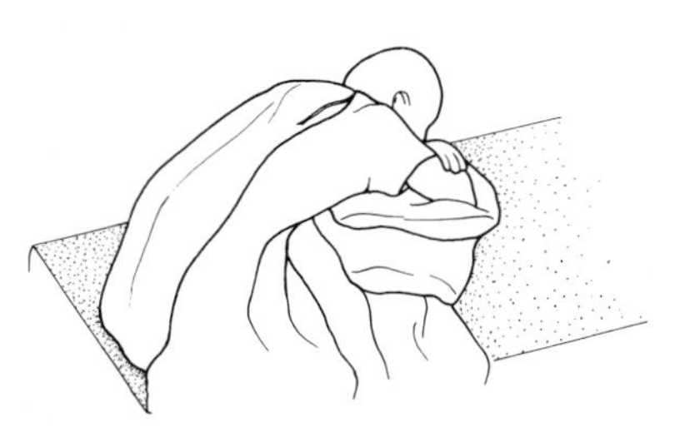

*Fig. 46-9*

## *Procedure 46-11*

| Steps | Rationale |
|---|---|
| **Assessment** | |
| 1. Assess client's knowledge of procedure. | Determines level of health teaching required. |
| 2. Assess client's ability to assume position required for procedure (Fig. 46-9). | Clients with musculoskeletal or respiratory alterations may be unable to sit on side of bed with arms draped over high bedside table. |
| 3. Assess vital signs. | Provides for comparison with vital signs during and after procedure. |
| 4. Assess respiratory function: symmetry of chest on inspiration and expiration, respiratory difficulty, type of cough and sputum produced. | Provides for comparison with respiratory status during and after procedure. |
| 5. Determine purpose of procedure. | Enables nurse to anticipate needed supplies and laboratory requisitions. |
| 6. Assess need for signed consent form (check institution's policy). | |
| 7. Determine whether client is allergic to antiseptic or anesthetic solutions. | Decreases chances of complications. |
| 8. Assess need for preprocedure pain medication. | Procedure can be painful, and client must remain still throughout it because of potential complications. |
| **Nursing Diagnosis** | |
| 1. Cluster data to reveal actual or potential nursing diagnoses: | |
| a. Ineffective breathing pattern: related to excess fluid in pleural cavity. | Fluid decreases ability of lungs to expand with each inspiration. |
| b. Pain: related to procedure. | Frequently, procedure and conditions requiring procedure are painful. |
| c. Knowledge deficit regarding procedure: related to inexperience. | Explanation of procedure promotes client's cooperation. |
| **Planning** | |
| 1. Develop individualized goals based on nursing diagnoses: | |
| a. Promote client's comfort.<br>b. Prevent client from moving to decrease chances of complications. | Placing client in proper position maximizes comfort and respirations and ultimately reduces risk of movement during procedure. |
| c. Promote optimal respiratory function during and after procedure. | |
| 2. Prepare equipment and supplies: | |
| a. Antiseptic solution for handwashing | |
| b. Thoracentesis tray, if available from central supply, which may include: | |
| ▪ Antiseptic solution (e.g., povidone-iodine) | Used to disinfect skin. |
| ▪ Gauze sponges (4 × 4) | |
| ▪ Sterile towels | Used to isolate sterile area. |
| ▪ Local anesthetic solution for injection (e.g., lidocaine 1%) | Provides topical anesthesia. |
| ▪ Sterile syringes: two 3 ml, 23- 25-gauge needles for anesthetic; two 50 ml, 14- 17-gauge needles, 5 to 7 cm long (or 2 to 3 in), for drainage of pleural fluid | |
| ▪ Receptacle for fluid | |
| ▪ Three-way stopcock | Attaches to end of 16-gauge needle so air does not enter pleural space. |
| ▪ Two-way stopcock with extension tubing | Used for drainage of pleural fluid into receptacle. |
| ▪ Test tubes | Used for laboratory tests. |
| c. Sterile gloves of proper size for physician | |
| d. Masks for physician and nurse (check institution's policy) | |
| e. Gauze (2 × 2), tape, and antiseptic ointment for dressing on insertion site | |
| f. Cough or pain medication if ordered | |
| 3. Organize equipment on bedside table. | Ensures ease and success of procedure. |

| Steps | Rationale |
|---|---|
| 4. Prepare client: | |
| a. Explain procedure. | Ensures knowledge of procedure, thus promoting cooperation and relaxation. |
| b. Assist in assuming position desired by physician. | Position in high-Fowler's position: sitting on side of bed, leaning over bedside table. Arms are draped over one or two pillows on table to slightly spread intercostal spaces. |

## Implementation

| Steps | Rationale |
|---|---|
| *Physician's responsibility:* | |
| 1. Disinfect skin with antiseptic solution and 4 × 4 gauze sponges. | Removes surface bacteria on skin. |
| 2. Don mask. | |
| 3. Don sterile gloves. | Maintains surgical asepsis. |
| 4. Drape client with sterile towels. | |
| 5. Inject anesthetic and allow time for it to take effect. | Provides local anesthesia at needle insertion site. |
| 6. Palpate exact site needed for thoracentesis (most often just below angle of scapula at seventh intercostal space). | If needle is inserted too low, liver or spleen may be punctured, causing serious complications. |
| 7. Attach thoracentesis needle to three-way stopcock, which is turned off to needle lumen. | Ensures that no air enters pleural space when needle is introduced. |
| 8. Ready two-way stopcock extension tubing and receptacle for fluid. | Ensures drainage of pleural fluid into proper receptacle. |
| 9. Insert needle into determined site slowly until pleural space is reached. | Places needle in pleural space to facilitate removal of pleural fluid. |
| 10. Slowly and gently aspirate fluid. | Fluid is aspirated slowly to decrease complications of drawing lung tissue into needle. |
| 11. Remove needle and apply pressure to puncture site. | Pressure assists in sealing puncture site. |
| 12. If desired, order chest x-ray film and blood work (e.g., hematocrit and hemoglobin, serum electrolytes). | Chest x-ray may show decreased fluid level in pleural space. Blood work is performed to check cell count and electrolytes in case replacement is needed. |
| 13. Place antiseptic ointment, 2 × 2 gauze, and tape on site for dressing. | Prevents possible air leak and entrance of infection. |
| *Nurse's responsibility:* | |
| 1. Set up sterile tray or open supplies to make them accessible for physician. | |
| 2. Assist client in maintaining correct position. | Prevents sudden movement on part of client. |
| 3. Assist client through procedure by holding shoulders or sides and reassuring in coaching manner. | |
| 4. Hold anesthetic vial upside down for physician to withdraw solution properly. | Allows physician to withdraw solution properly while maintaining surgical asepsis. |
| 5. Assess client's respiratory status during procedure: rate, difficulty, color of mucous membranes and nail beds. | Enables nurse to detect toleration of procedure. |
| 6. Assist client through removal of needle and placement of dressing. | May be painful. |
| 7. Assist client in assuming comfortable position in bed. | If leakage into pleural space is suspected, client is positioned recumbent with punctured chest side up. |

## Evaluation

| Steps | Rationale |
|---|---|
| 1. Note characteristics of pleural fluid (e.g., amount and color). | Characteristics are used for observation, reporting, recording. |
| 2. Monitor vital signs according to hospital policy. | Monitors physiologic status. |
| 3. Note drainage on chest dressing. | Documents leakage of fluid from puncture site. |

### *Expected outcomes*

| Steps | Rationale |
|---|---|
| 1. Client tolerates procedure well. Client can assume position without problems; has little discomfort; has no depression of respiratory function or complications. | |
| 2. Improved respiratory status as evidenced by nonlabored respirations, improvement in arterial blood gases, improved comfort. | Removal of pleural fluid permits optimal expansion of lungs and improves respiration. |

### *Unexpected outcomes*

| Steps | Rationale |
|---|---|
| 1. Client does not assume position well. | May be result of anxiety, pain, musculoskeletal alteration, respiratory distress. |

| Steps | Rationale |
|---|---|
| 2. Client moves abruptly or coughs during procedure. | May be result of underlying pathologic condition of lungs. |
| 3. Other complications, (e.g., liver or spleen perforation) occur. | Result of improper needle placement or abrupt movement. |

### Recording and Reporting

| Steps | Rationale |
|---|---|
| 1. Record in nurses' notes or on client's chart: name of procedure, location of puncture site, amount and color of fluid drained, duration, toleration (e.g., vital signs, pain, respiratory status, complications), laboratory tests ordered and sent, type of dressing over puncture site, drainage. | Accurate recording of any procedure is legal necessity in nursing. |
| 2. Report to physician immediately: | |
| a. Decreased respiratory function. | Could indicate lung perforation with resultant pneumothorax or hemothorax. |
| b. Changes in vital signs beyond normal limits. | |
| c. Changes in postprocedure hemoglobin, hematocrit, serum electrolyte values. | |
| d. If chest x-ray film is obtained after procedure, notify physician if any complications were detected. | |
| 3. Report to nurses on next shift all data that have been recorded in chart and reported to physician. | Allows for continuity of care. |

### Follow-up Activities

| Steps | Rationale |
|---|---|
| 1. Explain to client that procedure is completed. | |
| 2. Label specimens to be sent to laboratory and attach proper requisitions. Send to appropriate laboratory. | |
| 3. Clean up area and send supplies to proper sterilization department. | Prevents transmission of microorganisms. |
| 4. Obtain laboratory data for interpretation by nurse and physician. | |

## Special Considerations

- Nurse may need to obtain sterile jar for collection of large amount of fluid.
- Client must not move or cough during procedure because it could cause displacement of needle into lung.
- If client cannot assume high-Fowler's position sitting on side of bed, lateral high-Fowler's position is used. Affected lung is on top with arm from that side placed up over head.
- If high-Fowler's leaning-forward position cannot be assumed or maintained, accessibility of intrathoracic spaces is decreased, making it more difficult to find intrapleural space.
- During procedure, nurse remains in front of client, ensuring little or no movement. If physician requires something not in room, another nurse should be called to help.
- Determining exact site for needle insertion is performed by examining chest x-ray film and noting level of fluid in pleural space.
- Not more than 1200 ml of pleural fluid is aspirated at a time to decrease complications of circulatory fluid shift and pulmonary edema.
- Movement or coughing during procedure can cause needle displacement and puncture of lung. If lung becomes punctured and air escapes into pleural space, chest tube will need to be inserted as soon as possible.
- The complications of liver and spleen perforation are less common than lung perforation. Symptoms are subtle and may not be noted for several days. Symptoms include decreasing hemoglobin and hematocrit values and possibly abdominal pain.
- If thoracentesis was traumatic, client is positioned recumbent with punctured chest side up because this position minimizes fluid seepage into pleural space and allows puncture site to heal.

## Teaching Considerations

- After explaining procedure, make certain client knows that movement or coughing could cause damage to lung or pleura. Cough suppressant may be administered before test if client has cough.
- Explain to client that chest x-ray is often ordered after procedure to check for adequate lung expansion.

## BIBLIOGRAPHY

Beck ML: Three more gastrointestinal tests—and how to help your patient through each, Nurs 81 8:22, 1981.

Braunwald E, et al., editors: Harrison's principles of internal medicine, ed 11, New York, 1988, McGraw-Hill, Inc.

Felson B, Weinstein AS, Spitz HB: Principles of chest roentgenology: a programmed text, Philadelphia, 1965, WB Saunders Co.

Gibb SP, et al.: Use of fiberoptic endoscopy in diagnosis and therapy of upper gastrointestinal disorders, Med Clin North Am 70(6):1307, 1986.

LeMay M: CT changes in dementing diseases, AJR, 147(5):963, 1986.

Markus S: Taking the fear out of bone marrow examinations, Nurs 81 11:64, 1981.

Pagana KD, Pagana TJ: Diagnostic testing and nursing implications: a case study approach, St. Louis, 1986, The CV Mosby Co.

Pagana KD, Pagana TJ: Pocket nurse guide to laboratory and diagnostic tests, St Louis, 1986, The CV Mosby Co.

Potter PA, Perry AG: Fundamentals of nursing: concepts, process, and practice, St Louis, ed 2, 1989, The CV Mosby Co.

Rakel RE, editor: Conn's current therapy, Philadelphia, 1988, WB Saunders Co.

Sabiston DC, editor: Textbook of surgery, ed 13, Philadelphia, 1986, WB Saunders Co.

# 47

# CARE AFTER DEATH

### OBJECTIVES

*Mastery of content in this chapter will enable the nurse to:*

- Define key terms.
- Describe and compare the phases of grieving from Engle, Kubler-Ross, and Martocchio.
- Explain principles to follow when making organ or tissue donation requests.
- Describe postmortem care techniques.
- Describe the physiologic changes after death.
- Correctly prepare a client's body after death.

### KEY TERMS

*Algor mortis*
*Anorexia*
*Antiemetics*
*Autopsy*
*Epidemiology*
*Grief*
*Hope*
*Loss*
*Livor mortis*
*Morgue*
*Rigor mortis*

### SKILLS

**47-1** Care of the Body After Death

Death is an overwhelming experience that affects the dying person, as well as family, friends, and care givers. Feelings, values, and experiences influence the extent to which nurses can support clients and families during a loss or death. The nurse may be the best person to care for the client's body after death because of the therapeutic nurse-client relationship previously established. A nurse can be sensitive to the need of caring for the body with dignity and sensitivity.

It is important for the nurse to recognize that proper care of the dying and dead has social, religious, cultural, and legal implications. Each client and family member must be cared for in a unique way on the basis of their reaction to the loss. The nurse may find it easy and nonthreatening to relieve physical symptoms associated with illness and death, but becoming involved in meaningful interpersonal relationships to support a dying client is difficult.

## STAGES OF GRIEVING AND DYING

Behaviors and feelings associated with the grieving process occur in individuals suffering losses such as death of a relative or close friend. They also occur in individuals facing their own death. Both the person undergoing loss and the significant others in that person's life experience grief. The nurse uses the theories regarding stages of grieving and dying to anticipate emotional needs of clients and families and to plan interventions to help them understand their grief and deal with it. The nurse's role is to assess grieving behaviors, recognize how grief is influencing behavior, and provide empathetic support. A number of theories exist to describe the grieving process. They also can be applied to support of the dying person (Table 47-1).

## ENGLE'S THEORY

The classic work of Engle (1964) proposes that the grieving process has three phases: shock and disbelief, developing awareness, and reorganization and restitution. In phase one the person denies reality of the loss and may withdraw. It may seem to observers that the full impact has not hit the person. Physical reactions include fainting, diaphoresis, nausea, diarrhea, rapid heart rate, restlessness, insomnia, and fatigue.

In phase two, the person feels the loss acutely and may experience desperation. Anger, guilt, frustration, and depression occur. During phase three, the inevitability of the loss is acknowledged. The loss is accepted and the person begins to reorganize life.

## KUBLER-ROSS' STAGES OF DYING

The framework provided by Kubler-Ross (1969) includes five stages: denial, anger, bargaining, depression, and acceptance (Table 47-2). A person may waver back

***TABLE 47-1*** Comparison of Three Theories of the Grieving Process

| Engle (1964) | Kubler-Ross (1969) | Martocchio (1985) |
|---|---|---|
| Shock and disbelief | Denial | Shock and disbelief |
| | Anger | Yearning and protest |
| Developing awareness | Bargaining | Anguish, disorganization, despair |
| | Depression | |
| Reorganization and restitution | Acceptance | Identification in bereavement |
| | | Reorganization and restitution |

***TABLE 47-2*** Behaviors Representative of Kübler-Ross' Stages of Dying

| Stage | Behaviors |
|---|---|
| Denial | Avoids reality, cannot deal with decisions about treatment; may attempt activities of which one is no longer physically capable; isolates self from sources of accurate information; fails to comply with medical therapy; uses considerable emotional energy to deny truth; may appear artificially happy. |
| Anger | May retaliate against family members, nursing staff, or physicians; becomes demanding and accusing; anger may arouse guilt because client is aware of dependence on care givers; guilt may foster feelings of anxiety and low self-esteem. |
| Bargaining | Is fearful of losing body functions, experiencing uncontrollable pain, and losing control; is willing to do anything to change prognosis or fate; accepts new forms of therapies. |
| Depression | Recognizes potential loss of loved ones; may withdraw from important relationships to avoid painful feelings; may become quiet and noncommunicative when feeling loss of control; may express feelings of loneliness; does little to maintain appearance; may become suicidal when unrealistic hopes of a cure fade. |
| Acceptance | Accepts terms of death; begins to make plans for death (e.g., writes a will, completes financial arrangements for the family, gives up personal possessions); is able to discuss feelings about death; reminisces about the past. |

and forth through the stages of dying until acceptance finally occurs. There is no set time frame in which a person works through grief. It may take one to two years or longer.

## MARTOCCHIO'S PHASES OF GRIEVING

Although the grieving process has a predictable course and distinctive symptoms, no two persons react or progress through it in the same way. Martocchio (1985) describes five phases of grief that have overlapping boundaries and no expected order (Table 47-3). Remember that while a client is passing through phases of grief, family and friends also experience grief in their way at their pace.

Clients and their families facing terminal illness also experience hope during the grieving process. Hope is characterized by a confident yet uncertain expectation of achieving a future goal (Dufault and Martocchio, 1985). Hope is a complex series of thoughts, feelings, and actions that change often (see box 1, p. 1024). Awareness of the dimensions of hope helps the nurse support a client's hope. This can help relieve the grieving associated with terminal illness (see box 2, p. 1024).

## PHYSICAL CARE FOR THE DYING CLIENT

Nursing care of the terminally ill can be demanding and stressful. A client may experience many symptoms for months before death occurs. A dying client must be cared for with respect and concern. Promoting comfort in the terminally ill is important so that the dying person retains energy to maintain quality life activities.

### Pain Control

1. Research suggests that only 50% of cancer patients experience pain. Pain affecting the terminally ill may be acute or chronic. Any source of physical irritation can worsen a client's pain.
2. As death approaches, a person's mouth remains open, the tongue becomes dry and swollen, and the lips become dry and cracked.
3. The blinking reflex diminishes near death, causing drying of the cornea.

#### Nursing Implications

1. Administer narcotic analgesics on a regular schedule and not PRN.
2. Relaxation, guided imagery, distraction, and peripheral nerve stimulators offer relief.

**TABLE 47-3** Martocchio's Phases of Grief

| Stage | Client Behaviors | Nursing Implications |
|---|---|---|
| Shock and disbelief | A person's immediate response after death or serious loss. | Do not share client's denial. |
| | Physiologic responses may include muscular weakness, tremors, deep sighs, diaphoresis, flushed or cold and clammy sensations, anorexia, discomfort. | Be accepting. |
| | Mood swings are common. | Do not discuss reasons for client's behavior or the need to cope. |
| | Offers of comfort and support are often rejected. | |
| | Person disbelieves and searches for evidence that death or loss has not occurred. | |
| Yearning and protest | Bereaved person experiences anger toward the deceased for dying. | Assure client that anger is normal. |
| | Anger expressed toward God and care givers. | Do not take anger personally. |
| | Bereaved person may feel jealous or resentful of others who still have loved one. | Meet those needs that cause the angry response. |
| | Bereaved person may be reluctant to share thoughts and feelings with others. | |
| Anguish, disorganization, and despair | Reality and permanence of loss becomes recognized. | Be empathetic. |
| | Bereaved person becomes confused, unmotivated, disinterested, and indecisive. | |
| | Crying is common | Show support and understanding during crying episode. |
| | Withdrawal from activities and social relationships. | Use touch to communicate caring. |
| | Reminiscent about lost loved one. | Listen attentively. |
| | Gains new awareness of value of life, but may cope by following unhealthy behaviors such as excess drinking. | |
| Identification in bereavement | The bereaved takes on the behavior, qualities, habits and goals of the lost loved one. | Carefully assess symptoms to rule out presence of physical illness. |
| | May experience symptoms of the same illness the deceased suffered. | Do not ignore client's complaints. |
| Reorganization and restitution | Process begins about 6 months after the loss and lasts 1 or more years. | Offer person opportunity to discuss feelings about loss. |
| | Recurring episodes of depression mixed with periods of well-being. | Show acceptance during episodes of depression. |
| | Life begins to stabilize. | Assist client in discussing plans for the future. |

3. Use combinations of analgesics.
4. Position the client comfortably or employ other therapies as client's needs change.
5. Thorough skin care including daily baths, skin lubrication, massage to pressure sites, and dry and clean bed linens minimize irritants.
6. Give frequent oral care, at least every 2 to 4 hours, using a soft toothbrush or foam swab. Apply a light film of petroleum jelly to the lips and tongue.
7. Eye care removes crusts from eyelid margins.
8. Artificial tears reduce corneal drying.

## Relief of Nausea and Vomiting

The terminal disease process, complications of the disease, and therapeutic medications can cause nausea and vomiting.

### Nursing Implications

1. Administer antiemetics before meals.
2. Confer with physician about changing medications when possible.
3. Bowel decompression with insertion of a nasogastric tube may provide relief from obstruction.
4. Provide mouth care and promptly clean up emesis.

## Energy Conservation

The metabolic demands created by cancerous tumors and systemic chronic disease cause weakness and fatigue.

### Nursing Implications

1. Set mutual goals with client after identifying valued or desired tasks, then conserve energy for only those tasks.
2. Offer frequent rest periods in a quiet environment.
3. Time and pace nursing care activities to conserve client's energy.

## Maintenance of Bowel Function

Frequently the terminally ill receive narcotic medications that slow peristalsis. Immobility resulting from illness adds to this problem. Lack of bulk in the diet or a reduced fluid intake may result from appetite changes predisposing clients to constipation. Diarrhea may result from the disease process itself or complications of medical therapies.

### Nursing Implications

1. Prevention of constipation is achieved by increasing fluid intake; providing bran, whole grain products, and fresh vegetables in the diet; and encouraging exercise.
2. Prophylactic stool softeners prevent constipation.
3. A low residue diet is indicated for diarrhea.
4. Confer with physician to change medications causing diarrhea or constipation if possible.

## Treating Urinary Incontinence

Progressive disease can cause incontinence as a result of reduced levels of consciousness or spinal cord involvement (from cancer).

### Nursing Implications

1. Protect skin from irritation or breakdown using absorbent pads and clean linen.
2. Indwelling urinary catheter or condom catheters may be used.

## Promoting Nutrition

Nausea and vomiting resulting from disease or medications can decrease appetite. Depression from grieving may also cause anorexia.

### *DIMENSIONS OF HOPE*

**Affective**

- Sensations and emotions (i.e., feelings of confidence or an attraction to the desirable outcome) that are part of hoping.

**Cognitive**

- Processes by which persons wish, imagine, perceive, think, learn, or judge in relation to hope.

**Behavioral**

- Actions a person takes to directly achieve hope. Actions may be physiologic, psychosocial, cultural, or spiritual.

**Affiliative**

- A person's sense of involvement beyond self. Social interaction, mutuality, attachment, and intimacy compose affiliation. There is a relationship with others.

**Temporal**

- The person's experience of time (past, present, and future) in relation to hoping.

**Contextual**

- Hope is perceived within the context of life as interpreted by the person. Life situations influence and are a part of hope. An actual or potential loss may be the context in which hope arises.

### *NURSING IMPLICATIONS FOR PROMOTING HOPE*

**Affective dimension**

- Convey an empathetic understanding of client's worries, fears, and doubts. Reduce degree to which client becomes immobilized by concerns; build on client and family strengths of patience and courage.

**Cognitive dimension**

- Clarify or modify the hoping person's reality perceptions: offer information about illness or treatment, correct misinformation, share experiences of others as a basis of comparison.

**Behavioral dimension**

- Assist client to use own resources and those of others in relation to hope. Balance levels of independence, interdependence, and dependence when planning care.
- Enhance person's self-esteem and capabilities; give praise and encouragement appropriately.

**Affiliative dimension**

- Strengthen or foster the relationships with others that are consistent with hope.
- Help clients know they are loved, cared for, and important to others.

**Temporal dimension**

- Attend to a client's experience of time. Apply client's insights from past experiences to the present.

**Contextual dimension**

- Provide opportunity to communicate about life situations that have an influence on hope.
- Encourage discussion of desired goals, reminiscing, reviewing values, and reflecting on the meaning of suffering, life, or death.

#### Nursing Implications

1. Smaller portions and bland foods may be more palatable.
2. Home cooked meals may be preferred by client and gives the family a chance to participate.
3. Have food available on nursing unit at all times.
4. Offer fluids with nutritive value.

### Preventing Dehydration

As terminal disease progresses a client is less willing or unable to maintain oral fluid intake. Certain cancers may obstruct the gastrointestinal tract.

#### Nursing Implications

1. Relieve thirst by offering ice chips, sips of fluids, or a moist cloth to the lips.
2. Provide frequent mouth care.
3. Monitor and maintain intravenous fluid infusions.

### Promoting Oxygenation

A client may suffer ineffective breathing patterns if the disease involves lung tissue capacity, pneumonia, or pulmonary edema. Clients may become severely anemic, causing reduced oxygen carrying capacity.

#### Nursing Implications

1. Position client semi-Fowler's or high Fowler's to improve lung expansion.
2. Administer bronchodilators as ordered.
3. Narcotics can suppress cough and ease breathing and apprehension.
4. Suction accumulated secretions from the mouth and throat.

## SIGNS OF DEATH

When death occurs the traditional clinical signs are cessation of the apical pulse, respirations, and blood pressure. Many clients, however, are maintained on mechanical ventilators, artificial pacemakers, and supportive intravenous medications that maintain respiration and blood circulation. Thus, identifying clinical death is often difficult. Institutions have brain death protocols to determine death. Brain death is an irreversible form of unconsciousness that is characterized by complete loss of brain function while the heart continues to beat. The legal definition of brain death varies from state to state and the provinces of Canada. The usual clinical criteria for brain death include the absence of reflex activity, movements, and respiration, with the pupils dilated and fixed. Before brain death is formally determined a client usually undergoes two to three electroencephalograms (EEGs) which measure electrical brain activity, over 12 to 24 hours. A cerebral arteriogram, which measures circulation to the brain, may also be performed. The EEGs must show no electrical impulses in order to confirm death. A physician pronounces death and then stops all life support systems.

There are times when the decision is made either by a client or his family to not initiate CPR measures after the client's heart fails. Do not resuscitate (DNR) or no-code orders are required to prevent resuscitation from being initiated. The nurse is required to initiate and maintain CPR for all other clients (see Chapter 18) until the client recovers or the physician pronounces the client's death.

## PHYSIOLOGIC CHANGES AFTER DEATH

When death occurs cellular and circulatory changes create alterations in the body's tissues (Table 47-4). These changes influence the manner in which the nurse cares for the body after death. It is important for the nurse to prepare the body for family viewing as quickly as possible. Because the body undergoes changes after death the longer a nurse waits to care for the body the more difficult it is to make the body appear natural.

## PREREQUISITE KNOWLEDGE

1. The grieving process.
2. Principles of medical asepsis.

## PREREQUISITE SKILLS

1. Basic handwashing techniques (Chapter 37).

***TABLE 47-4*** Physiologic Changes After Death

| Change | Related Interventions |
|---|---|
| Stiffening of body (rigor mortis), developing in 2-4 hr after death; involves contraction of skeletal and smooth muscle owing to lack of adenosine 5′-triphosphate (ATP). | Before rigor mortis develops, position body in normal anatomic alignment, close eyelids and mouth, insert dentures in mouth. |
| Reduction in body temperature with loss of skin elasticity (algor mortis). | Gently remove tape and dressings to avoid tissue breakdown. Avoid pulling on skin or body parts. |
| Purple discoloration of skin (livor mortis) in dependent areas owing to breakdown of red blood cells. | Elevate head to prevent discoloration. |
| Body tissues soften and liquify by bacterial fermentation. | Store body in cool place in hospital morgue or other designated area. |

# *SKILL 47-1 Care of the Body After Death*

When a client's death is pronounced the physician certifies the death in the medical record and records the time of death and a description of therapies or actions taken. The physician may request permission from the family for an autopsy. An autopsy or postmortem examination is performed to confirm or determine the cause of death, gather data regarding the nature and progress of a disease, study the effects of therapies on body tissues, and provide statistical data for epidemiology and research purposes. A consent form must be signed by the most immediate family member and the physician or designated requestor. Autopsies are required in circumstances of unusual death (for example, violent trauma or unexpected death in the home) as well as death occuring within a set time frame following hospitalization. Each state has guidelines for when autopsies are requested. Autopsies normally do not delay burial of the deceased.

A trained nursing staff member or a physician is required in most states to ask the family or client's guardian for organ or tissue donation (see box). The client must be a suitable donor as determined by age and preexisting medical condition. Families must be properly informed of their right to donate as well as to decline. State laws govern the procedure for documenting organ and tissue requests. Institutional policies for required request procedures must encourage discretion and sensitivity in dealing with potential donor families. Nurses may feel uncomfortable making donation requests, since families of deceased clients often undergo considerable grief. However, research has shown that families are willing to donate if they are asked and if the requester feels comfortable making the request (Malecki and Hoffman, 1986).

***TISSUES AND ORGANS USED FOR TRANSPLANT***

**Nonvital tissues**
- Corneas, skin, long bones, middle ear bones.

**Vital organs**
- Heart, liver, lung, kidney, pancreas (recovered after a client is pronounced clinically dead or brain dead; circulatory and ventilatory support is maintained to perfuse the organs before removal).

After all requests are made it becomes the responsibility of the nurse to care for the client's body. Often family wish to view the body before final preparations are made. The nurse should give family members the time needed to say goodbye to the deceased before the body is transferred to the morgue.

### Purposes

1. Make the body presentable in appearance to family members.
2. Expedite timely transfer of the body for tissue retrieval.
3. Maintain dignity of the deceased.

## *Procedure 47-1*

| Steps | Rationale |
|---|---|
| **Assessment** | |
| 1. Assess for presence of family or significant others and whether they have been informed of the client's death. Ask if they wish to view the body. Observe their response. | It is the physician's responsibility to notify family of the client's death. Nurse provides emotional support and properly prepares body for viewing. |
| 2. Assess client's religious preference or cultural heritage. Determine if family wishes to have a minister or priest at the bedside. | Specific religions dictate ceremonies at time of death. |
| 3. Determine if client was on isolation precautions for an infectious disease. | Precautions must be taken to prevent spread of infection to others. |
| 4. Review agency policy for method of preparing the body including: removal of equipment, care of dentures or hairpieces, wrapping of the body. | Each agency may differ. Procedure incorporates legal guidelines, especially if an autopsy is scheduled. |
| **Nursing Diagnosis** | |
| 1. Cluster data to reveal actual or potential nursing diagnoses as they apply to the family: | |

| Steps | Rationale |
|---|---|
| a. Ineffective individual coping: related to loss of spouse or friend. | Family member or significant other faces grief related to death of client. |
| b. Altered family processes: related to death of parent. | Family system is faced with loss and individual members may be unable to support one another. |
| c. Dysfunctional grieving: related to death of significant other. | Person is actively grieving and is unable to accept loss. |

## Planning

| Steps | Rationale |
|---|---|
| 1. Develop individualized goals for client and family based on nursing diagnoses: | |
| a. Family member or significant other will have opportunity to verbalize grief. | Nurse provides empathetic support after preparing the body. |
| b. Body prepared without skin damage or discoloration. | Tissues become fragile, requiring extra care during tape or tube removal. |
| 2. Prepare needed equipment and supplies: | |
| a. Body bag or shroud kit (contains plastic or paper sheet, gauze ties, and two identification tags) | Used to enclose or wrap the body. |
| b. Wash basin, water, washcloth, and bath towel | Used to clean soiled body parts. |
| c. Clean gown (optional, depending on agency policy) | |
| d. Absorbent pads | Used to place under anal area. |
| e. Adhesive or masking tape | Used if shroud is applied. |
| f. Small pillow or towel | |
| g. Paper bag | To transfer client's belongings. |
| h. Disposable gloves | Protects nurse's hands from contacting body secretions. |
| i. Valuables list and envelopes | Documents valuables brought to agency by client. Must be safely returned to family. |
| j. Gauze dressings (optional) | Used to change soiled dressings. |
| 3. Explain to family that it will take a short time to prepare the body for viewing (do this in a private place). | Family requires privacy to ease expression of grief. |
| 4. If another client is in the room, explain what has happened and offer them the opportunity to leave room until procedure is completed. | Serves to relieve client's anxiety. |

## Implementation

| Steps | Rationale |
|---|---|
| 1. Wash hands. | Reduces transmission of microorganisms. |
| 2. Apply disposable gloves. | Body excretions may harbor infectious microorganisms. Withdrawal of IVs or other tubing may cause temporary bleeding. |
| 3. Close room door or draw bedside curtain. | Provides privacy for the deceased and family. |
| 4. Identify the body according to agency policy. | Ensures proper name used in labeling and completion of forms. |
| 5. Position client supine with arms at sides, palms down, or arms across the abdomen. Do not place hands on top of one another because bottom hand will become discolored. | Client appears natural and comfortable. |
| 6. Place small pillow or folded towel under the head. | Prevents pooling of blood in the face and subsequent discoloration. |
| 7. Gently place your fingers over the client's closed eyelids for a few sec. (optional: place moistened cotton balls over closed eyelids.) | Holds eyelids in place to create a natural appearance. |
| 8. Insert client's dentures into the client's mouth. If mouth fails to close, place a rolled up towel under the chin. | It is difficult to insert dentures after rigor mortis. Dentures maintain natural facial expression. |
| 9. Remove all bottles, bags, or receptacles from urinary catheters, nasogastric tubes, IV lines, or drainage tubes. | Collection devices and contents are not needed for autopsy exams. |
| 10. For tubes remaining in the body either remove, clamp, or cut to within 1 in (2.5 cm) of the skin and tape in place. | Agency policy dictates tube care. Specific guidelines apply if an autopsy is to be performed. |
| 11. Remove soiled dressings and replace with clean gauze dressings. | Controls odor caused by microorganisms. |
| 12. Wash body parts soiled by blood, urine, feces, or other drainage. (A mortician will provide a complete bath.) | Prepares body for viewing and reduces odors. |
| 13. Place an absorbent pad under the client's buttocks. | Relaxation of sphincter muscles after death may cause release of urine or feces. |
| 14. Brush and comb client's hair. Remove any clips, hairpins, or rubber bands. | During viewing the client should appear well-groomed. Hard objects such as pins can damage or discolor the face and scalp. |

| Steps | Rationale |
|---|---|
| 15. Remove all jewelry. *Exception:* family may request wedding band be left in place. Place a small strip of tape around client's finger. | Prevents loss of client's valuables. |
| 16. Place a clean gown on the client (agency policy may require removal before body is wrapped). | Prepares body for viewing. |
| 17. Account for all valuables remaining in the client's room. Label each. Use valuables list to inventory all items. Return valuables to immediate family members when they arrive or store in locked container. | Nurse is responsible for safekeeping of client's personal valuables, e.g., jewelry, wallet, eyeglasses, or religious medals. |
| 18. Place client's clothing and shoes in a labeled bag and return to family members. | Keeps items safely secured. |
| 19. Complete identification tags and attach one to the client's ankle. The remaining tag should be attached to the outside of the shroud. The identification bracelet on the client's wrist remains in place. | Ensures proper identification of the body for eventual transfer to the morgue and mortician. |
| 20. If the family requests viewing, place a sheet or light blanket over the body with only the head and upper shoulders exposed. Provide soft lighting and offer chairs to the family. | Maintains dignity and respect for the client and family. Prevents exposure of body parts. |
| 21. Remain at bedside with the family, then allow them time to view the body privately. Do not rush the family. | Families need time to express their grief and say goodbye to their loved one. |
| 22. After the family has left remove all linen and the client's gown (refer to agency policy). Then place body in body bag or apply the shroud. Be sure the shroud completely encircles all body parts (Fig. 47-1). | Prevents injury to skin and extremities, avoids unnecessary exposure of body parts. |

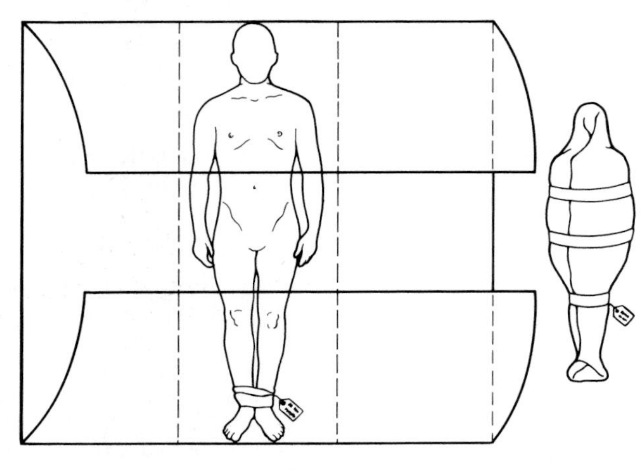

***Fig. 47-1***

| Steps | Rationale |
|---|---|
| 23. Secure shroud with tape wrapped over the shoulders, waist, and legs. | Keeps shroud secure, protects body during transfer. |
| 24. Attach second completed label to outside of the body bag or shroud (check agency policy for location). | Ensures proper identification of the body. |
| 25. If client had a transmissable infection, special labeling may be used. | Alerts health care workers who transport and store the body. |
| 26. Arrange transportation of the body to the morgue or mortuary. | If delay is anticipated before the mortician arrives, the body should be cooled in the morgue to prevent further tissue damage. |
| 27. Carefully transfer the body to a regular or false bottom stretcher. Keep body aligned. Cover with a clean sheet. | Prevents damage to body tissues. False bottom stretcher makes it appear there is no body lying on stretcher. |
| 28. Close other clients' room doors, arrange for an elevator to arrive on the floor and transport the body as inconspicuously as possible. | Appearance of a body can be emotionally upsetting to other clients. |
| 29. Remove remaining items and linen from the client's room. Wash hands. | Prevents transfer of microorganisms. |

## Evaluation

| | |
|---|---|
| 1. Observe family's response to loss of loved one. | Nonverbal expressions reveal level of family's grief. |

| Steps | Rationale |
|---|---|
| 2. Offer family the opportunity to ask questions or express feelings. | Family members often seek opportunity to express feelings with someone other than an immediate family member. If client's death is sudden, many questions may be asked. |
| 3. Note appearance and condition of client's skin during preparation of body. | Determines if damage to tissues occurs after preparation. |
| ***Expected outcomes*** | |
| 1. Family members express grief verbally and nonverbally. | Family acknowledges loss of loved one. |
| 2. Skin of deceased is clear of bruises, lacerations, or abrasions. | No additional injury to tissues as a result of care. |
| ***Unexpected outcomes*** | |
| 1. Family members fail to express grief. | Family members are unwilling or unable to express grief during this initial phase. |
| 2. Lacerations, bruises, or abrasions noted on skin surfaces. | Positioning or preparation of the body results in skin injury. |
| **Recording and Reporting** | |
| 1. Record date and time of death, time physician notified, name of physician pronouncing death, disposition of valuables and belongings, family member accepting valuables, care delivered to body, identification of body, consent form signed by family, disposition of the body, and information provided to family members. | Ensures that client's death is accurately and legally recorded. |

## Special Considerations

- At time of death last rites are performed by Eastern Orthodox Christians and Roman Catholics. Members of Islamic religion believe only family should touch and wash body.
- Members of the Jewish faith do not favor autopsy and cremation.
- If a client is an eye donor, place small ice packs over closed eyelids to help preserve corneal tissues.
- Do not use safety pins to secure shroud; damage may occur to skin.
- When a person dies, law requires completion of death certificate. This is usually prepared by the medical records department and signed by physician. Certificate is filed by local health or government office and family receives copy.
- Endotracheal tubes should be removed to avoid disfigurement of client's face. (Confer with agency policy.)

## Home Care Consideration

- In hospice programs, clients are often able to experience a peaceful, dignified death at home. The nurse assists the family in care of the body.

## BIBLIOGRAPHY

Anthony M: No code, helping the family understands what it means, Nursing '86 16(8):55, 1986.

Beland JA: Grief responses to long-term illness and disability, Reston, Va, 1981 Reston Publishing, Prentice-Hall Co.

Dufault K, Martocchio BC: Hope: its spheres and dimensions, Nurs Clin North Am 20:379, 1985.

Engle GL: Grief and grieving, Am J Nurs 64:93, 1964.

Golden S: Nursing a loved one at home, Philadelphia, 1988, Running Press.

Hogstel M: Home nursing care for the elderly, Bowie, Md, 1985, Brady Communications Co, Inc.

Kemp B, Pillitteri A: Fundamentals of nursing, Boston, 1984, Little, Brown & Co.

Kubler-Ross E: On death and dying, New York, 1969, Macmillan Inc.

Malecki M, Hoffman M: Personal level of discomfort among nurses and its effect on obtaining consent for organ and tissue donation, It's News (Illinois Transplant Society), vol. 3, Summer, 1986.

Martocchio BC: Grief and bereavement: healing through hurt, Nurs Clin North Am 20:327, 1985.

Potter P: Making required request work, Nursing Management 19:50, 1988.

Potter P, Perry A: Fundamentals of nursing, ed. 2, St. Louis, 1989, The CV Mosby Co.

Stoddard S: The hospice movement, New York, 1978, Vintage Books.

The Gallup Organization: Attitudes and opinions of the American public towards kidney donation, The National Kidney Foundation, February, 1983.

Ufema J: How to talk to a dying patient, Nursing '87 17(8):43, 1987.

Ufema J: Insights on death and dying, Nursing '88 18(10):97, 1988.

# GLOSSARY

**abdominal girth** The measurement of the abdomen's circumference, taken at the same place with each measurement.

**abduction** Movement of an extremity away from the midline of the body.

**accommodation reflex** Adjustment of the eyes for near vision, composed of pupillary constriction, convergence of the visual axes, and increased convexity of the lens.

**accurate empathy** Communication technique used by nurse to show understanding of client's feelings and experiences.

**Acetest** A test that measures the presence of ketone (acetone) bodies in the urine. A large quantity of acetone causes rapid change in the color of the Acetest tablet.

**activity tolerance** Kind and amount of exercise or work that a person is able to perform.

**adduction** Movement of an extremity toward midline of the body.

**adrenergic drug** A medication that mimics the effects of sympathetic nerve stimulation of the autonomic nervous system.

**aerobe** A microorganism that lives and grows in the presence of free oxygen.

**air embolus** A quantity of air that circulates in the bloodstream to eventually lodge in a blood vessel.

**air fluidization** The process of blowing warm air through a collection of microspheres to create a fluid-like environment; used in special mattresses designed to reduce pressure against a person's skin.

**airway obstruction** An abnormal condition of the respiratory system characterized by a mechanical impediment to the delivery or the absorption of oxygen in the lungs.

**aldosterone** A steroid hormone produced by the adrenal cortex that causes the kidney tubules to excrete potassium and reabsorb sodium and water.

**allergen** A substance that can produce a hypersensitive reaction in the body but that is not necessarily intrinsically harmful.

**alopecia** Partial or complete lack of hair.

**AMBU bag** Portable resuscitation device that provides manual inflation of the lungs. An AMBU bag is usually used with supplemental oxygen.

**The American Society of Parenteral and Enteral Nutrition (ASPEN)** An organization that provides education, support, and accreditation to individuals in the nutritional support field.

**amino acid** An organic compound composed of one or more basic amino groups and one or more carboxyl groups. Amino acids are the building blocks that construct proteins and the end products of protein digestion.

**ampule** Small sterile glass or plastic container that usually contains a single dose of solution to be administered parenterally.

**anaerobic** Pertaining to absence of air or oxygen.

**anaphylactic reaction** Exaggerated hypersensitivity reaction to a previously encountered antigen. It is a severe and sometimes fatal systemic reaction characterized by itching, hyperemia, angioedema, and in severe cases vascular collapse, bronchospasm, and shock.

**anaphylaxis** An exaggerated hypersensitivity reaction to a previously encountered antigen. The reaction may be localized or generalized.

**anergy** Lack of activity.

**anesthesia** The absence of normal sensation, especially sensitivity to pain.

**anions** Negatively charged ions.

**anorexia** The loss of appetite or the loss of the physiologic desire to eat.

**anoxia** An abnormal condition characterized by a lack of oxygen.

**anthropometry** Measurements of various body parts to determine nutritional and caloric status, muscular development, brain growth, and other parameters.

**antianginal drug** A medication that dilates coronary arteries, improving blood flow to the myocardium to prevent angina.

**antiarrhythmic** A class of medications that possesses properties for controlling abnormal cardiac rhythms, e.g., quinidine and propranolol (Inderal).

**antibody** Protein substance made by the body after exposure to a foreign substance or antigen. Antibodies provide the body with immunity.

**antigens** Substances, usually protein, which cause the formation of an antibody and which react specifically with that antibody.

**antipyretic** Pertaining to a substance, such as a medication, that reduces fever.

**antiseptic** A substance that will inhibit the growth and reproduction of microorganisms.

**anus** The distal or terminal orifice of the alimentary canal.

**apical pulse** Measurement of the heartbeat as taken with the stethoscope placed over the apex of the heart.

**apnea** An absence of spontaneous respirations.

**approximate** To come together, as in the edges of a wound.

**aqueous** Watery or waterlike; referring to a medication prepared with water.

**artificial airway** Plastic or rubber device inserted into the upper or lower respiratory tract to facilitate ventilation or secretion removal.

**ascites** Effusion and accumulation of serous fluid in the abdominal cavity.

**asepsis** Absence of germs or microorganisms.

**aseptic technique** Method by which contamination with microorganisms is prevented.

**aspirant** Fluid or particulate that is aspirated.

**aspirate** Withdrawal of fluid or air into the barrel of a syringe or suction device.

**aspiration** The removal of fluids such as mucus, serum, or gases from the body by the application of suction.

**aspiration (of medication), drug abuse** The inhalation of liquid or solid drug preparations into the pulmonary system; use of a chemical substance for nontherapeutic purposes that do not comply with cultural or social standards.

**astigmatism** Abnormal condition of the eye in which the light rays cannot be focused clearly in a point on the retina because the spherical curve of the cornea is not equal in all meridians. Vision is blurred and use of the eyes causes discomfort.

**astringent** A topical substance that causes constriction of tissues upon application; commonly used for cleansing the skin.

**atelectasis** An abnormal condition characterized by the collapse of lung tissue, preventing the respiratory exchange of carbon dioxide and oxygen.

**atrophy** Wasting or diminution of size or physiologic activity of a part of the body caused by disease or other influences.

**atmospheric pressure** Pressure exerted by the atmosphere. (Atmospheric pressure at sea level is 760 mm Hg.)

**autoclave** An instrument used to sterilize objects. Consists of a vault or chamber that produces steam under pressure.

**autolet** A small instrument with a lancet used to obtain a capillary blood specimen.

**autologous transfusion** Procedure in which blood removed from a donor is subsequently returned to the donor's circulation after a variable period of storage.

**autotransfusion** The collection, anticoagulation, filtration, and reinfusion of blood from an active bleeding site.

**axillary** Pertaining to the pyramid-shaped space that forms the underside of the shoulder between the upper part of the arm and the side of the chest.

**bacteremia** Presence of bacteria in the blood.

**bacteriostatic** Inhibits development of bacteria.

**basal metabolism** Energy needed to maintain the body's basic processes such as respiration, circulation, and temperature.

**base of support** Surface area on which an object rests.

**bed rest** Placement of the client in bed for therapeutic reasons for a prescribed period.

**belt restraints** Type of restraint used to secure a client on a stretcher.

**bile** A digestive juice secreted by the liver, stored in the gallbladder, and secreted in the small intestine to digest fat. Bile causes brown color of feces.

**binder** Bandage made of a large piece of material to fit and support a specific body part.

**biopsy** The removal and microscopic examination of tissue, performed to establish precise diagnosis.

**blood group** Classification of blood based on the presence or absence of genetically determined antigens on the surface of the red cell.

**blood plasma** The liquid portion of the blood, free of its formed elements and particles.

**blood pump** Device placed externally over a unit of blood that regulates the flow of blood into the blood vessel during transfusion.

**blood transfusion** Administration of whole blood or a blood component as cells to replace blood lost through trauma, surgery, or disease.

**blood typing** Identification of genetically determined antigens on the surface of the red blood cell, used to determine a person's blood group.

**blood warming coil** Device constructed of coiled plastic tubing used to warm reserve blood before massive transfusion.

**body alignment** Refers to the condition of joints, tendons, ligaments, and muscles in various body positions.

**body mechanics** The coordinated efforts of the musculoskeletal and nervous systems as the person moves, lifts, bends, assumes a standing, sitting, or lying posture, and completes activities of daily living.

**bolus** A dose of a medication injected all at once intravenously.

**bone marrow** Specialized, soft tissue filling the spaces in cancellous bone of the epiphyses, responsible for red blood cell production.

**borborygmus** Audible abdominal sound produced by hyperactive intestinal peristalsis.

**bradycardia** An abnormality in heart rate in which the heart contracts steadily at a rate less than 60 contractions per minute.

**broad-spectrum antibiotic** Refers to a group of antibiotics that are effective against a large variety of infectious microorganisms.

**bronchospasm** Abnormal contraction of the smooth muscles of the bronchi.

**bronchus** One of several large air passages in the lungs through which pass inspired air and exhaled gases.

**bruit** Abnormal sound or murmur created by turbulent blood flow heard while auscultating an organ, gland, or artery.

**buccal** Of or pertaining to the inside of the cheek; surface of a tooth or gum next to the cheek.

**cachexia** General ill health and malnutrition marked by weakness and emaciation.

**calipers** Instrument used to measure skinfold thickness.

**calorie (Kcal)** A calorie is the amount of heat required to raise the temperature of 1 g of water 1° C at atmospheric pressure.

**cannula** A hollow tube for insertion into a duct or cavity. During its insertion its lumen is usually occluded by a trocar.

**caput medusa** A spidery varicose appearance around a stoma caused by portal hypertension.

**carcinoma** Malignant epithelial neoplasm that tends to invade surrounding tissue and spread to distant regions of the body.

**cardiopulmonary arrest** Sudden cessation of respirations, pulse, and circulation.

**cardiopulmonary resuscitation (CPR)** Basic emergency procedure for life support, consisting of artificial respiration and manual external cardiac massage.

**cardiotonic** A class of medications that possesses properties for increasing the force of myocardial contractions, e.g., digitalis.

**caries** Decay of a tooth; progressive decalcification of enamel and dentin of a tooth.

**cast** Rigid plaster or fiberglass application molded over skin tissues to hold musculoskeletal tissues to permit healing of injuries.

**cast brace** Combination of a brace within a cast at a joint.

**cast saw** Saw used to cut through plaster to remove cast.

**cast shoe** Shoe worn over the foot encased in plaster.

**cast stabilization** Use of rods, pins, broom handles, or sticks to lend stability to a particular cast.

**cast syndrome** A series of client signs indicative of an untoward (claustrophobic) reaction to being in a cast.

**casting tape** Rolls of adhesive or resin-impregnated tape for use as lightweight casts.

**cathartic** Drug that acts to promote bowel evacuation.

**catheter hub** Plastic threaded connection at end of an intravenous catheter.

**catheterization** Introduction of a rubber or plastic tube through the urethra and into the bladder.

**cations** Positively charged ions.

**center of gravity** Midpoint or center of body weight. In the adult it is the midpelvic cavity between the symphysis pubis and the umbilicus.

**central venous catheter** Catheter placed into a large vein, usually with the tip resting in the superior vena cava or right atrium.

**cephalic vein** One of the four superficial veins of the upper limb.

**cerebrospinal fluid** Substance contained within the four ventricles of the brain, the subarachnoid space, and the central canal of the spinal cord.

**cerumen** Earwax; a waxy secretion produced by apocrine sweat glands in the external ear canal.

**chart** A client's record; or, to note data in a client's record, usually at prescribed intervals.

**cheilosis** Disorder of the lips and mouth characterized by scales and fissures.

**chemical indicator** Commercially prepared device that monitors all or part of the physical conditions of the sterilization cycle; it usually consists of a sensitive ink dye that changes colors under certain conditions.

**chemotherapeutic agent** A medication used to treat cancer, which alters the growth of a cancer cell.

**chemotherapy** Use of drugs to prevent cancer cells from multiplying, invading adjacent tissue, and metastasizing.

**chest physiotherapy** Physical maneuvers, including postural drainage, chest percussion, vibration, rib shaking, and cough, to improve airway mucus clearance in clients with retained tracheobronchial secretions.

**chest tube** Catheter inserted through the chest wall into the intrapleural space by the physician.

**circulatory fluid** Pertaining to the blood pumped by the heart through the arteries, veins, and capillaries.

**circumduction** The circular movement of a limb; the motion of the head of a bone within an articulating cavity, such as the hip joint.

**class II biologic safety cabinet** A vertical containment or biologic safety cabinet that recirculates air through a high-efficiency air (HEPA) filter.

**clean-voided specimen** A technique used to collect a urine specimen as free from bacterial contamination as possible without catheterizing the client.

**cleansing enema** An enema, usually soap suds, administered repeatedly until the colon is free of all formed fecal material.

**client-centered air leak** The entry of air, which originates from the client, into a closed chest drainage system, as opposed to the entry of air originating from the chest drainage system itself.

**Clinitest** A test that measures the amount of glucose and acetone in a urine specimen.

**Clinitron bed** A special bed containing an air-fluidization mattress that conforms to the shape of a person's body to reduce pressure exerted against skin and soft tissues.

**colon** Portion of large intestine from the cecum to the rectum.

**colostomy** Surgical formation of an opening of the colon onto the surface of the abdomen through which fecal matter is emptied.

**compartment syndrome** Insufficient arterial perfusion to an extremity caused by trauma or stasis; leads to ischemia and tissue necrosis if not reversed.

**compliance** Fulfillment by the client of the caregiver's prescribed course of treatment.

**compound** A substance composed of two or more different elements, chemically combined, that cannot be separated by physical means.

**compress** Soft pad of gauze or cloth used to apply heat, cold, or medications to the surface of a body part.

**concreteness** Communication that includes specific feelings, behaviors, and experiences or situations; communication that is not vague.

**conduction** Mechanism of heat transfer involving flow of heat from one object to another with which it is in contact.

**conduit** An artificially created channel for drainage of urine, e.g., ileoloop.

**congruent** Harmonious and consistent; the verbal and nonverbal message is congruent when the nonverbal message is the same or consistent with the verbal message.

**conjunctiva** Mucous membrane lining the inner surfaces of the eyelids and anterior part of the sclera.

**consensual light reflex** Constriction of the pupil of one eye when the other eye is illuminated.

**constipation** Condition characterized by difficulty in passing stool, or an infrequent passage of hard stool.

**contact lens** A small, transparent, curved glass or plastic lens shaped to fit over a person's cornea; the lens floats on a precorneal tear film.

**contamination** The existence of an infectious agent on the body, a piece of equipment, or surface area.

**contracture** Abnormal condition of a joint, characterized by flexion and fixation and caused by atrophy and shortening of muscle fibers or by loss of normal elasticity of the skin.

**coronary bypass surgery** Open heart surgery in which a section of a blood vessel or an artificial vessel is grafted onto one or more of the coronary arteries and connected to the ascending aorta, bypassing narrowing or blockage of the coronary arteries.

**cough** Forced exhalation following in order after these normal series of events: (a) partial or full inhalation; (b) closure of the glottis; (c) active contraction of expiratory muscles; and (d) rapid glottic opening.

**countertraction** Use of client's body weight or other weights, ropes, and pulleys to counter the pull of the traction weight.

**crackle** Fine bubbling sound heard on auscultation of the lung.

**croupette** A device that provides cool humidification with controlled oxygen concentration to an infant or toddler.

**crutch gait** Gait assumed by a person on crutches by alternately bearing weight on one or both legs and on the crutches.

**crutch palsy** Temporary or permanent loss of sensation or movement resulting from pressure on axilla from crutch.

**culture** Laboratory test involving the cultivation of microorganisms or cells in a special growth medium.

**cycloplegic** Pertaining to a drug that paralyzes ciliary muscles of the eye causing pupillary dilation for ophthalmologic examination or surgery.

**Dacron cuff** Dacron sheath, 1 cm wide, surrounding an atrial catheter to prevent ascending infections and accidental displacement of catheter.

**debride** To remove dead or damaged tissue from a wound; to remove dirt, foreign objects, damaged tissue, and cellular debris from a wound or burn in order to prevent infection and promote healing.

**debridement** Removal of dead tissue in a wound.

**decompression** Removal of pressure as from gas and fluid in the stomach and intestinal tract.

**defecation** Passage of feces from the digestive tract through the rectum.

**dehiscence** Partial or total separation of wound layers resulting from improper wound healing.

**dentifrice** A pharmaceutic compound used with a toothbrush for cleaning and polishing teeth.

**dermatitis** An inflammatory condition of the skin, characterized by erythema and pain or pruritis.

**dextrose** The hydrated form of glucose.

**diastolic pressure** The lower blood pressure measurement that reflects pressure within the arterial system during the period of ventricular relaxation—diastole.

**diluent** Agent that makes a solution or mixture thinner or more liquid by admixture.

**discharge planning** The process by which the nurse plans for a client's eventual release from a health care agency; the process begins upon a client's admission to the agency.

**don** To put on.

**dorsal** Pertaining to the back or posterior.

**dorsiflexion** Flexion of the foot at the ankle (or flexion of other joints).

**double-void** A procedure of discarding the first urine specimen and testing the second urine specimen that was obtained 30-45 minutes later; this procedure gives a more accurate amount of glucose being spilled into the urine at that particular time.

**drawsheet** A special sheet placed over the regular sheet on a bed and used to move a person in bed.

**drug abuse** Use of a drug to obtain effects for which it is not prescribed. May lead to physical, social, and psychologic harm.

**drug addiction** Inability to control a drive or craving for a chemical substance.

**drug dependence** Psychologic or physiologic reliance on a chemical substance.

**drug plateau** Blood serum concentration reached and maintained after repeated, fixed doses of a medication.

**duration** A characteristic used in assessing a symptom; the length of time a symptom lasts.

**dyspnea** Difficulty in breathing.

**dysrhythmia** An irregularity or deviation from the normal pattern of a heartbeat.

**ecchymosis** Discoloration of an area of the skin or mucous membrane resulting from extravasation of blood into the subcutaneous tissues as a result of trauma to the underlying blood vessels or to fragility of the vessel walls.

**eczema** Superficial dermatitis of unknown cause.

**edema** Abnormal accumulation of fluid in interstitial spaces of tissues.

**effluent** Drainage from a stoma such as urine, liquid stool, or formed stool.

**elastic bandage** Bandage of elasticized fabric that provides support and allows movement.

**elbow restraints** Restraints used to maintain elbow joint rigidity; made of fabric with slots for tongue blades.

**electrolyte** An element or compound that, when melted or dissolved in water or another solvent, dissociates into ions and is able to carry an electric current.

**emaciation** Excessive leanness caused by disease or malnutrition.

**embolus** A solid, liquid, or gaseous mass that either arises within or is introduced into circulation. The embolus obstructs the blood vessel, halting flow of blood to a particular body part.

**empathy** Ability to recognize and to some extent share the emotions and state of mind of another and to understand the meaning and significance of that person's behavior.

**endotracheal tube** Artificial airway inserted through the mouth into the trachea.

**enema** Procedure involving introduction of a solution into the rectum for cleansing or therapeutic purposes.

**enteral nutrition** The administration of nutrition via the gastrointestinal tract (i.e., by mouth, tube feeding, or oral supplement).

**enteric-coated** Tablets coated with a substance that does not dissolve until reaching the intestine. Drug constituents are irritating to oral and gastric mucosa.

**enterostomy** Surgical procedure that produces an artificial anus or fistula in the intestine by incision through the abdominal wall.

**enucleation** Removal of the eyeball, performed in cases of malignancy, severe infection, extensive trauma, or to control pain in glaucoma.

**episiotomy** A surgical procedure in which an incision is made in a woman's perineum to enlarge her vaginal opening for delivery of a newborn infant; procedure prevents tearing of perineum.

**erythema** An area of diffuse redness.

**erythroblastosis fetalis** A type of hemolytic anemia that occurs in newborns as a result of maternal-fetal blood group incompatibility, specifically involving the Rh factor and the ABO blood groups.

**evaporation** Mechanism of heat loss whereby moisture from the body's surface changes to vapor and transfers heat to the surrounding air.

**eversion** Turning the foot outward at the ankle.

**excoriation** An epidermal abrasion caused by trauma, chemicals, or burns.

**excretion** The process of eliminating, shedding, or getting rid of substances by body organs or tissues.

**exercise** Performance of any physical activity for the purpose of conditioning the body, improving health, maintaining fitness, or as a therapeutic measure.

**exit site** Site at which catheter exits to outside of body from subcutaneous tunnel.

**exophthalmos** Abnormal protrusion of one or both eyeballs caused by trauma, intracranial lesions, intraorbital disorders, or systemic disease, most commonly hyperthyroidism.

**expectorant** An agent that facilitates removal of bronchopulmonary secretions.

**expectoration** Expulsion of mucus or sputum from the mouth or lungs.

**exploratory laparotomy** The surgical exploration or examination of an abdominal organ or part.

**extended care facility** An institution that provides medical, nursing, and/or custodial care for an individual over a prolonged period of time, as during the course of a chronic disease or during the rehabilitation phase after an acute illness.

**extension** Movement increasing angle between two adjoining bones.

**external air leak** The presence of air originating from outside of the closed chest drainage system.

**external jugular vein** One of a pair of large vessels in the neck that receive most of the blood from the exterior of the cranium and the deep tissues of the face.

**external rotation** Rotation of a joint outward.

**extravasation** The inadvertent infiltration of intravenous fluids or medications into the subcutaneous tissues surrounding the infusion site.

**extremity restraints** Restraint used to immobilize one or all extremities.

**exudate** Fluid, cells, or other substances that have slowly discharged from cells or blood vessels through breaks in cell membranes. May accumulate in a cavity, as in a wound.

**fascia** Fibrous connective tissue.

**febrile** Pertaining to or characterized by fever or an elevation in body temperature.

**feces** The waste material excreted by the rectum after digestion; stool.

**fenestrated drape** A drape with a round or slitlike opening in the center.

**fever** An abnormal elevation of body temperature.

**fiberoptic** Pertaining to fiberoptics; referring to the transmission of an image along flexible bundles of coated glass or plastic fibers having special optical properties.

**flatulence** Condition characterized by the accumulation of gas within the lumen of the intestines.

**flexion** Movement decreasing the angle between two adjoining bones; bending of a limb.

**flotation device** A foam mattress with a gel-like pad located in its center, designed to protect bony prominences and distribute pressure more evenly against the skin's surface.

**flora** Microorganisms that reside on and within the body to compete with disease producing microorganisms to provide a natural immunity against certain infections.

**flossing** Mechanical cleansing of tooth surfaces with the use of stringlike waxed or unwaxed dental floss.

**flow sheet** A graphic summary of several changing factors, especially the client's vital signs or weight, and the treatments and medications given.

**fontanel** A space covered by tough membranes between the bones of an infant's cranium.

**foramen magnum** The large opening in the anterior and inferior part of the occipital bone, interconnecting the vertebral canal and cranial cavity.

**foreign body airway maneuver** One of three methods used to remove a foreign object which is obstructing the airway.

**footboard** Board placed perpendicular to the mattress, parallel to and touching the plantar surface of the client's foot and used to maintain dorsiflexion of the feet.

**footdrop** A falling or dragging of the foot from paralysis of the flexors of the ankle.

**four-poster cast** Cast placed over shoulders; contains four vertical posts or poles on the anterior and posterior lateral sides of the head to immobilize the cervical vertebrae.

**Fowler's position** Posture assumed by a client when the head of the bed is raised approximately 45 to 90 degrees, as though the client is sitting upright.

**frequency** Symptom of urinary disorder involving repetitive voidings over a fixed time period.

**friction** Effect of rubbing, or the resistance that a moving body meets from the surface on which it moves; a force that occurs in a direction to oppose movement; in massage, technique in which deeper tissues are stroked or rubbed, usually through strong circular movements of the hand.

**friction rub** Dry grating sound heard during auscultation, caused by rubbing of tissue surfaces.

**gag reflex** A normal neural reflex elicited by touching the soft palate or posterior pharynx.

**gait** Manner or style of walking, including rhythm, cadence, and speed.

**gastrostomy feeding tube** Long, hollow, flexible tube inserted into the stomach through a stab wound in the upper left abdominal quadrant.

**genuineness** Communication of authenticity or sincerity.

**gingiva** The gum of the mouth.

**gingivitis** Inflammatory condition in which the gums are red, swollen, and bleeding.

**glaucoma** An abnormal condition of elevated pressure within the anterior chamber of an eye due to obstruction of outflow of aqueous humor.

**granulation** The presence of red, granular, moist tissue that appears during the healing of open wounds; type of tissue containing new blood vessels that bleed readily.

**granulation tissue** Soft, pink, fleshy projection of tissue that forms during the healing process in a wound not healing by primary intention.

**gravity** Heaviness of an object resulting from the universal effect of the attraction of a planetary body.

**guided imagery** Technique in which client focuses on an image, becoming less aware of pain.

**gurgle** Abnormal coarse sound heard during auscultation of the lung; produced by air entering large mucus-containing airways.

**gypsum** Plaster of Paris; material used for casts as it becomes hard and rigid.

**halitosis** Offensive breath resulting from poor oral hygiene, dental or oral infections, ingestion of certain foods, or systemic diseases.

**hand roll** Cylindric roll of cloth or gauze placed against the palmar surface of a client's hand to maintain hand, thumb, and fingers in a functional position.

**Harris splint** Expandable splint that supports the thigh in skeletal traction.

**head halter** Support for the head, made of cotton material, used for traction.

**hematemesis** Vomiting of blood.

**hematology** The study of blood cells.

**hematoma** Collection of extravasated blood trapped in the tissues of the skin or in an organ; results from trauma or incomplete coagulation.

**hematopoiesis** The formation and development of blood cells in bone marrow.

**hemiplegia** Paralysis of one side of the body.

**hemoconcentration** The concentration of red blood cells in one area.

**hemodialysis** A procedure in which impurities or wastes are removed from the blood; used in treating renal insufficiency and various toxic conditions.

**hemodynamics** The study of movements of the blood and of the forces concerned therein.

**hemolysis** The destruction of red blood cells.

**hemoptysis** Coughing up of blood from the respiratory tract.

**hemostasis** Termination of bleeding by mechanical or chemical means or by the coagulation process of the body.

**hemothorax** An accumulation of blood in the intrapleural space caused by a pulmonary infarction, tissue damage due to lung cancer or other chest trauma, or a complication of anticoagulant therapy after chest surgery. This condition is characterized by tachycardia, hypotension, diaphoresis, chest pain, dyspnea, asymmetric chest movements, decreased breath sounds on the affected side, and dullness on percussion on the affected side.

**hemopneumothorax** An accumulation of both air and blood in the intrapleural space. This condition is characterized by the signs and symptoms listed with pneumothorax and hemothorax.

**heparin lock** An intravenous needle connected to a small "well" that allows for the intermittent injection of medication without the need for repeated venipuncture.

**herniation** The abnormal protrusion of an organ or other body structure through a defect or natural opening in a covering, membrane, muscle, or bone.

**hirsutism** Excessive body hair in a masculine distribution, caused by heredity, hormonal dysfunction, or medication.

**homeostasis** The state of equilibrium (balance between opposing pressures) in the internal environment of the body, naturally maintained by adaptive responses that promote healthy survival.

**Hoyer lift** Mechanical device that uses a canvas sling to easily lift dependent clients for transferring.

**Huber needle** Special needle with a deflected point designed to prevent damage to the silicone septum of implanted infusion ports.

**hyperemia** Increased blood in part of the body, caused by increased blood flow, as in the inflammatory response, local relaxation of arterioles, or obstruction of the outflow of blood from an area.

**hyperextension** Movement of a body part beyond its normal resting extended position.

**hyperkalemia** Elevated concentration of potassium in the blood serum.

**hypernatremia** Greater-than-normal concentration of sodium in the blood, caused by excessive loss of water and electrolytes owing to polyuria, diarrhea, excessive sweating, or inadequate water intake.

**hyperopia** A refractive error of the eye in which parallel rays of light focus behind the retina; the person has difficulty seeing near objects.

**hyperpigmentation** Unusual darkening of the skin.

**hypokalemia** Decreased concentration of potassium in blood serum.

**hyponatremia** Lower-than-normal concentration of sodium in the blood, caused by inadequate excretion of water or by excessive water in the circulating bloodstream.

**hypothermia** An abnormal lowering of body temperature; usually due to prolonged exposure to cold.

**hypovolemic shock** State of physical collapse caused by massive blood loss, circulatory dysfunction, and inadequate tissue perfusion.

**hypoxemia** Abnormal deficiency of oxygen in arterial blood.

**hypoxia** Insufficient oxygen available to meet the metabolic needs of tissues and cells.

**idiosyncratic reaction** A response to a medication or therapy that is unique to an individual.

**ileal conduit** A method of urinary diversion through intestinal tissue. Ureters are implanted in a section of dissected ileum that is then sewed to an ostomy in the abdominal wall.

**ileostomy** Surgical formation of an opening of the ileum onto the surface of the abdomen, through which fecal matter is emptied.

**immobility** Pertaining to the inability of a body part or limb to be moved.

**immunosuppressive** Pertaining to a substance or procedure that lessens or prevents a normal immune response.

**impaction** Presence of large or hard fecal mass in the rectum or colon.

**implanted infusion port** Self-sealing silicone septum encased in a metal or plastic case with an attached silicone catheter.

**incentive spirometry** Method of encouraging voluntary deep breathing by providing visual feedback to clients concerning their inspiratory volume.

**incident report** Confidential document that describes any client accident while the person is on the premises of a health care agency.

**incompatibility** Inability to coexist; describes two medications of different chemical makeups that cannot be mixed together.

**incontinence** Inability to control urination or defecation.

**induration** Hardening of a tissue, particularly the skin.

**infection** Invasion of the body by pathogenic microorganisms that reproduce and multiply, causing disease by local cellular injury, secretion of a toxin, or antigen-antibody reaction in the host.

**infiltration** Presence of intravenous fluids within the subcutaneous space surrounding a venipuncture site.

**infusate** Volume parenteral fluid infused into a client over an established period of time.

**infusion** Introduction of a substance such as a fluid, drug, electrolyte, or nutrient, directly into a vein by means of gravity flow.

**infusion pump** Device designed to deliver a measured amount of fluid over a period of time.

**injection** Act of forcing a liquid into the body by means of a syringe.

**injection cap** Rubber diaphragm covering a plastic cap; permits needle insertion into a catheter.

**insertion site** Site of large vein into which a catheter is threaded.

**insulation** (1) The act of insulating; (2) a nonconducting substance that offers a barrier to the passage of heat or electricity.

**intake** Measurement of the ingestion or infusion of liquids into the body, including all liquids and semiliquids, liquid medications, enteral tube feedings, intravenous therapy, blood components, and total parenteral nutrition.

**integument** Skin and its appendages: hair, nails, and sweat and sebaceous glands.

**intercostal space** Area between any two ribs.

**intermittent positive pressure breathing (IPPB)** A form of assisted or controlled respiration produced by a ventilatory apparatus in which compressed gas is delivered under positive pressure into the person's airways until a preset pressure is reached.

**internal rotation** Rotation of a joint inward.

**intraabdominal pressure** Amount of tension within abdominal cavity.

**intracavitary** Within a body cavity.

**intracellular fluid** Liquid within the cell membrane.

**intraclavicular fossa** Small pocket area or indentation just below the clavicle on both sides of the neck.

**intracranial pressure** Pressure exerted by cerebrospinal fluid within the subarachnoid space surrounding the brain and spinal cord.

**intradermal injection** Form of injection in which a solution is introduced into the dermal skin layer.

**intramuscular (IM) injection** Form of injection in which a solution is introduced into the body of a muscle.

**intrapleural** Pertaining to, or affecting, the potential space between the parietal and visceral pleura.

**intrapulmonic** Pertaining to, or affecting, the spaces within the lungs.

**intrathecal** Of or pertaining to a structure, process, or substance within a sheath, as within the spinal canal.

**intravenous (IV) injection** Form of injection in which a solution is introduced into a vein.

**intubation** The process of passing a flexible plastic tube through the upper respiratory tract into the trachea.

**invasive** Referring to procedures that involve puncture, incision, or insertion of a foreign object into the body.

**irrigate** To flush with fluid using slow, steady pressure on a syringe plunger. Done to clear tubing or cleanse a wound.

**irrigation** Gentle washing of an area with a stream of solution.

**isolation** The separation of a person or persons with an infectious process or with the potential to develop an infection process from others.

**isometric contraction** Increased muscle tension without muscle shortening.

**iso-osmotic solution** A solution with electrolytes that will exert the same osmotic pressure as the solution it is being compared with, e.g., peripheral vein solution and RBC's.

**isotonic (solution)** Having the same concentration of solute as another solution, hence exerting the same amount of osmotic pressure as the solution.

**isotonic contraction** Increased muscle tension resulting in muscle contraction and muscle shortening.

**jacket restraint** Vestlike restraint that usually crosses in the back of the client but may also cross in the front.

**jejunal feeding tube** A hollow tube inserted into the jejunum through the abdominal wall for administration of liquefied foods.

**joint** Portion of body where two or more bones join.

**kilogram** The metric conversion for a pound; weight (lbs.) × 2.2 = kilograms.

**kinesthetic** Related to the ability to perceive the existence or direction of weight or movement.

**knee exercise** Mechanical apparatus for passive exercises of the knee joint.

**knee sling** Support in sling form used under the knee for Russel's traction.

**lavage** The irrigation or washing out of an organ or cavity.

**leukopenia** A decrease in circulating white blood cells.

**ligaments** White, shiny, flexible bonds of fibrous tissues that bind joints together and connect various bones and cartilage.

**line of gravity** An imaginary line that goes from the center of gravity to the base of support.

**lipodystrophy** Any abnormality in metabolism and deposition of fat.

**lotion** Liquid preparation applied externally to protect the skin or treat a dermatologic disorder.

**lower airway respiratory system** All respiratory structures below the epiglottis, including trachea, bronchi, and alveoli.

**lumen** The hollow channel within a tube.

**MAC** Mid-upper arm circumference. Measurement midpoint between tip of acromial process of scapula and olecranon process of ulna. Measurement value denotes muscle wasting.

**macerate** To soften, usually by soaking in water.

**maceration** Softening of the skin from soaking or exposure to moisture.

**malabsorption** The inability to absorb nutrients via the gastrointestinal system.

**malnutrition** Any nutritional disorder, such as unbalanced, insufficient, or excessive diet, or impaired absorption, assimilation, or utilization of food.

**MAMC** Mid-arm muscle circumference (MAC). Calculation obtained by subtracting the triceps skin fold (TSF) from the mid-upper arm circumference measurement. Value assists in denoting muscle wasting.

**manometer** An instrument for measuring pressure or tension of liquids or gases.

**mastication** Chewing, tearing, or grinding food with the teeth while it mixes with saliva.

**meatus** Any opening or tunnel through any part of the body, e.g., the point at which the urethra opens onto the skin.

**medical asepsis** Technique used to reduce the number of surface microorganisms and help prevent or reduce their spread.

**mediastinal shift** A condition in which the mediastinal contents move toward the unaffected side in the presence of a pneumothorax, hemothorax, or pneumothorax. The mediastinal shift causes compression of the organs and it is a life-threatening situation. This condition is characterized by deviation of the trachea from the midline toward the unaffected side, cardiac dysrhythmias, hypotension, and distended neck veins.

**medicated enema** Administration of a medication via an enema. Usually used preoperatively with clients scheduled for bowel surgery.

**melanin** Black or dark brown pigment that occurs naturally in the skin, hair, and iris.

**melanocyte** A body cell capable of producing melanin, the pigment of the skin.

**melena** Darkening of the feces by blood pigments.

**metastasis** Process by which tumor cells are spread to the distant parts of the body.

**microorganism** Any microscopic entity capable of sustaining living processes, such as bacteria, virus, and fungi.

**microvasculature** The portion of the circulatory system composed of the capillary network.

**micturition** Urination; act of passing or expelling urine voluntarily through the urethra.

**midstream** Procedure in which the client initiates a stream of urine, inserts a sterile collection cup into the stream, and then withdraws the cup before the stream of urine stops.

**milliequivalent per liter (mEg/L)** Number of grams of a specific electrolyte dissolved in 1 liter of plasma.

**minerva jacket** Cast encasing the head (with face and ears uncasted), continuing over the thorax and back to the iliac crests.

**mitered corner** A triangular folded corner of a bed sheet, used to prevent the sheet from pulling out from the mattress.

**mitten restraints** Thumbless mitten devices used to restrain a client's hands.

**moleskin** Adhesive-backed tape used for some forms of skin traction.

**mucociliary transport** Process in which cilia lining the tracheobronchial tree sweep mucus upward toward the esophagus to keep airways clear of inhaled particulate.

**mummy restraint** Blanket or sheet folded in such a manner as to restrain a small child or infant.

**muscle tone** Normal state of balanced muscle tension.

**mydriasis** Dilation of the pupil of the eye caused by contraction of dilator muscles of the iris.

**myelosuppression** A decrease in the cellular components of the bone marrow.

**myocardial infarction** An occlusion of a coronary artery, caused by atherosclerosis or an embolus that necroses an area in the artery.

**myopia** A refractive error of the eye in which parallel rays of light focus in front of the retina; the person has difficulty seeing far objects clearly.

**nares** The pairs of anterior and posterior openings in the nose that allow for passage of air to the pharynx and lungs.

**nasal** Of or pertaining to the nose and nasal cavity.

**nasal airway** Flexible, curved piece of rubber or plastic, with one wide or trumpet-like end and one narrow end that is inserted through the nose into the pharynx.

**nasal cannula** A device for delivering oxygen by way of two small tubes that are inserted into the nares.

**nasal catheter** A flexible, small-bore tube inserted into the oropharynx by way of the nose.

**nasogastric feeding tube** A small tube that is passed via the nares into the stomach.

**naso-intestinal feeding tube** Tungsten-weighted tube inserted through the naris to allow natural peristaltic movement of the tube through the pyloric sphincter into the duodenum or jejunum.

**nebulization** Vaporization or dispersion of a liquid in a fine spray.

**necrotic** Related to death of a portion of tissue.

**negative pressure** Pressure, measured in mm Hg, which is less than atmospheric pressure.

**neurologic** Pertaining to the study and treatment of the nervous system.

**neuropathy** An abnormal condition characterized by inflammation and degeneration of the peripheral nerves.

**neurovascular checks** Series of eight observations (checks) required to measure neurologic and circulatory status of a client's peripheral tissues.

**neutropenia** An abnormal decrease in the number of neutrophils in the blood.

**nitroglycerin** Medication that causes dilation of coronary arteries.

**nosocomial infection** Infection acquired during hospitalization or stay in a health care facility.

**noxious** Harmful, injurious, or detrimental to health.

**NPO** Abbreviation for nothing-per-mouth; client is restricted from taking food or fluids orally.

**nursing home** Type of extended-care facility that is licensed to provide nursing and custodial care for persons over a prolonged period of time. Some nursing homes have living quarters that allow residents to continue normal living routines under staff supervision.

**objective data** Data obtained by an observer (nurse) through direct physical examination, including observation, palpation, and auscultation, and by laboratory analyses and radiologic and other studies.

**occult blood** A minute or hidden quantity of blood that can be detected only by means of a chemical test or by microscopic or spectroscopic examination.

**O.D.** Abbreviation for *oculus dexter,* Latin phrase meaning "right eye."

**oil retention enema** An enema containing a small volume (200-250 ml) of an oil-based solution; used to soften fecal mass.

**ointment** A semisolid externally applied preparation, usually containing a drug.

**oncology** A branch of medicine regarding the study of tumors.

**onset of action** Period of time after a drug is administered for it to produce a response.

**opening pressure** The amount of tension measured in a manometer following insertion of a spinal needle into the subarachnoid space.

**ophthalmic** Of or pertaining to the eye.

**ophthalmologist** A medical doctor whose practice is limited to diseases, conditions, and trauma to the eyes. An ophthalmologist also prescribes corrective lenses for clients whose visual acuity is impaired.

**optometrist** A person who practices optometry, tests the eyes for visual acuity, prescribes corrective lenses, and recommends eye exercises.

**oral airway** Minimally flexible curved piece of plastic extending from the exterior of the lips over the tongue to the pharynx.

**orthopedics** Branch of medicine devoted to the study and treatment of the skeletal system, its joints, muscles, and associated structures.

**orthopnea** An abnormal condition in which a person must sit or stand in order to breathe deeply or comfortably.

**O.S.** Abbreviation for *oculus sinister,* a Latin phrase meaning "left eye."

**osmolality** The characteristics of a solution determined by the ionic concentration of the solvent.

**otic** Of or pertaining to the ear.

**O.U.** Abbreviation for *oculus uterque,* a Latin phrase meaning "each eye."

**output** Includes all liquids excreted, such as urine, vomitus, and diarrhea, and drainage from wounds, fistulas, and suction equipment.

**overdose** Oral or parenteral ingestion of an excessive quantity of a medication or drug.

**over-the-counter drug** Drug available to a consumer without a prescription.

**oxygen hood** Used with pediatric clients to deliver high concentrations of oxygen.

**oxygen mask** A flexible mask that fits snugly and securely over the client's nose and mouth for delivery of oxygen.

**oxygen therapy** Administration of oxygen by any route to a client, to prevent or relieve hypoxia.

**pain** Subjective, unpleasant sensation caused by noxious stimulation of sensory nerve endings.

**pain tolerance** Point at which a person is not willing to accept pain of greater severity or duration.

**pallor** Unnatural paleness or absence of color in the skin.

**palpate** To feel with the hand.

**palpebra** Portion of the conjunctiva that lines the inner surface of the eyelids; it is thick, opaque, and highly vascular.

**paralysis** An abnormal condition characterized by loss of muscle function or the loss of sensation.

**paralytic ileus** A decrease in or absence of intestinal paralysis that may occur after abdominal surgery, illness, or trauma.

**parenteral** Not in or through the digestive system; typically refers to administering medications by injection.

**parenteral nutrition** The administration of nutrition into the vascular system.

**paresis** Slight or partial paralysis related to some cases to local neuritis.

**parietal pleura** Serous membrane lining the pleural wall of the thoracic cavity.

**patency** Absence of clots within an intravenous needle, or kinks within an intravenous tubing.

**pathogen** Any microorganism capable of producing disease.

**Patient's Bill of Rights** A list of patient's rights promulgated by the American Hospital Association; it offers some guidance and protection to clients by stating the responsibilities that a hospital and its staff have toward clients and families during hospitalization; it is not a legally binding document.

**peak action** Time it takes for a drug to reach its highest effective concentration.

**Pearson's attachment** The support used under the leg in balanced suspension skeletal traction.

**pediculosis** Infestation of the integument with blood-sucking lice.

**pelvic belt** Girdle-shaped cotton belt or support that fits around the hips, lumbosacral area, and abdomen for attaching ropes and weights in pelvic belt traction.

**pelvic sling** A hammock-like sling that fits under the client's lumbosacral area and hips and is then connected to ropes and weights; it suspends the pelvis off the bed as treatment for fractures of pelvic bones.

**perception** The conscious recognition and interpretation of sensory stimuli through unconscious associations, especially memory, that serve as a basis for understanding, learning, and knowing or for the motivation of a particular action or reaction.

**percutaneous** A procedure performed through the skin, like the aspiration of fluid from a space below the skin, using a needle, catheter, or syringe.

**perfusion** Effect of pulmonary circulation in moving blood to and from the blood-gas barrier so gas exchange can occur.

**periodontal** Referring to tissues surrounding the teeth, such as the gums and buccal mucosa.

**peristomal** Referring to the area of skin surrounding a surgically created stoma.

**peritoneal fluid** Substance in the abdominal cavity for lubrication of peritoneal membrane and internal organs.

**peritonitis** Inflammation of peritoneum produced by bacteria or irritating substances introduced into the abdominal cavity by a penetrating wound or perforation of an organ in the gastrointestinal or reproductive tract.

**PERRLA** Acronym for "pupils equal, round, reactive to light, accommodative"; the acronym is recorded in the physical examination if pupil assessment is normal.

**PEH** Acronym for pseudoepitheliomatous hyperplasia; maceration of skin surrounding the stoma.

**petaling** Finishing the raw or ragged edges of a plastic cast to prevent skin irritation or pressure.

**pétrissage** A massage technique in which the skin is gently lifted and squeezed.

**pH** Reflection of the hydrogen ion concentration of a liquid.

**pharmacologic agents** Oral, parenteral, or topical substances used to alleviate symptoms and treat or control illness.

**phlebitis** Inflammation of a vein.

**phlebotomy** The incision of a vein for the letting of blood, as in collecting blood from a donor.

**Physician's Desk Reference (PDR)** A compendium, compiled annually, containing information about drugs supplied by a manufacturer.

**PIE** An acronym for Problem, Intervention, and Evaluation, used as an organizing framework for narrative nurses' notes.

**piggyback infusion** Method for administering intravenous medications intermittently; a piggyback IV set is a supplementary set that connects with the primary IV tubing.

**piloerection** Erection of the hairs of the skin in response to a chilly environment, emotional stimulus, or irritation of the skin.

**plantar flexion** Flexion of the foot and toes toward the sole.

**plasmaphoresis** Laboratory procedure in which the plasma proteins are separated by electrophoresis for identification and evaluation of the proportions of the various proteins.

**plaque (dental)** A thin film on teeth made up of mucin and colloidal material found in saliva and often secondarily invaded by bacteria.

**platelet** Formed particle found in blood that relates directly to the ability of the blood to clot.

**pleura** Delicate serous membrane enclosing the lung.

**pleural cavity** Space between visceral and parietal pleura; pressure within the cavity is negative when compared to atmospheric pressure.

**pleural fluid** Substance contained between visceral and parietal pleurae for lubrication of the membranes.

**pneumonitis** Inflammation of the lung; may be caused by a virus, or may be a hypersensitivity reaction due to allergy to chemical or organic dusts.

**pneumothorax** An accumulation of air in the intrapleural space caused by a severe blow to the chest, extremely forceful cough, chest trauma, or open chest surgery. This condition is characterized by sudden sharp pain in the chest or referred pain across the chest to the shoulder or abdomen, dyspnea, dry cough, asymmetric hyperresonance on percussion on the affected side, decreased breath sounds on the affected side, and possible subcutaneous emphysema around the neck. A pneumothorax causes air to enter the intrapleural space with each inspiration.

**podiatrist** A health professional trained to diagnose and treat diseases and disorders of the feet.

**point of maximal impulse (PMI)** Point at which the heartbeat can most easily be palpated through the chest wall, usually along the left-midclavicular line at the fourth or fifth intercostal space.

**poison** Any substance that impairs health or destroys life when ingested, inhaled, or absorbed by the body in relatively small amounts.

**poison control center** One of a network of facilities that provides information regarding all aspects of poisoning or intoxication, maintains records of their occurrence, and refers clients to treatment centers.

**POMR** An acronym for Problem Oriented Medical Record, used as an organizing framework for a client's complete medical record.

**positive pressure** Pressure, measured in mm Hg, that is greater than atmospheric pressure.

**postcast care** Nursing interventions performed for and with clients in casts or after cast removal.

**postoperative** Period of time after completion of a surgical procedure wherein the nurse monitors the client's recovery.

**postural drainage** Gravitational clearance of airway secretions by assumption of one or more of 10 different body positions for 5 to 15 minutes each; each posture corresponds to specific segments of bronchi in the lung.

**posture** Position of the body in relation to the surrounding space.

**premature ventricular contraction (PVC)** A cardiac dysrhythmia characterized by a ventricular contraction preceding the expected contraction; it appears on an electrocardiogram as an early, wide QRS complex without a preceding P wave.

**preoperative** The period of time preceding induction of anesthesia and the beginning of a surgical procedure.

**pressure ulcer** Inflammation, sore, or ulcer in the skin usually over a bony prominence, caused by a compromise in circulation to the skin.

**primary intention** Primary union of the edges of a wound, progressing to complete scar formation with granulation.

**problem-oriented record (POR)** Method of recording data about the health status of a client that fosters a collaborative problem-solving approach by all members of the health care team.

**pronation** Movement of a body part so the front or ventral surface faces downward.

**proprioception** Sensation achieved through stimuli originating from within the body regarding spatial position and muscular activity.

**prospective reimbursement** A method of payment to an agency for health care services to be delivered based on predictions of what the agency's costs will be for the coming year.

**prosthesis** An artificial replacement for a missing part of the body.

**pruritus** The symptom of itching, an uncomfortable sensation leading to the urge to scratch.

***pseudomonas*** A genus of gram-negative bacteria that includes several free-living species of soil and water and some opportunistic pathogens, isolated from wounds and sputum; may produce blue and yellow pigments.

**pulley** Mechanical round, grooved disks over which ropes can move freely for traction pull.

**quality assurance** In health care, any evaluation of services provided and of the results achieved as compared with accepted standards.

**random voided specimen** A specimen obtained at any point of a 24-hour period.

**reagent** Chemical used to indicate the presence of a particular substance.

**rectal tube** Flexible tube inserted into the rectum to assist in relief of flatus.

**rectum** Portion of the large intestine, about 12 cm long, continuous with the descending sigmoid colon, just proximal to the anal canal.

**refractive error** Condition in which parallel rays of light are not brought to focus upon the retina.

**relaxation exercise** Pain relief treatment in which clients perform controlled breathing and relaxation exercises and concentrate on a pleasant situation when a noxious stimulus is applied.

**remission** The partial or complete disappearance of the clinical and subjective characteristics of a chronic or malignant disease.

**renal** Pertaining to the kidney.

**residual urine** Volume of urine remaining in the bladder after a normal voiding; the bladder normally is almost completely empty after micturition.

**respect** Communication of esteem, honor, or consideration of another.

**respiratory arrest** Cessation of respirations.

**restraint** Device used to immobilize a client or an extremity.

**reverse Trendelenburg** Position in which the lower extremities are low and the body and head are elevated on an inclined plane.

**rib shaking** Step in chest physiotherapy involving constant downward pressure with an intermittent shaking motion of the hands on the rib cage over the area being drained; it is done with the flat part of the palm of the hand during 4 to 12 prolonged exhalations through pursed lips.

**rib vibration** Step in chest physiotherapy involving a downward vibrating pressure done only during exhalation by the flat part of the palm of the hand over the lung segment being drained; usually done during 4 to 12 prolonged exhalations through pursed lips over each segment drained.

**right atrial catheter** An indwelling intravenous catheter inserted centrally or peripherally and threaded into the superior vena cava and right atrium.

**rigidity** Condition of hardness, stiffness, or inflexibility.

**Rotokinetic treatment table** A special bed equipped with an automatic turning device that completely immobilizes clients while rotating them from 90 to 270 degrees along a horizontal axis.

**$S_1$** Symbol for the first heart sound in the cardiac cycle occurring with ventricular systole; it is associated with the closure of the mitral and tricuspid valves.

**$S_2$** Symbol for the second heart sound in the cardiac cycle; it is associated with closure of the aortic and pulmonary valves just before ventricular diastole.

**saliva** A digestive secretion emitted from the salivary glands in the mouth.

**sclerosis** Condition characterized by hardening of tissue resulting from any of several causes, including inflammation, the deposit of mineral salts, and infiltration of connective tissue cells.

**scrubbed team members** Includes the surgeon and scrub nurse or technician and assisting physicians who are scrubbed.

**scultetus binder** Many-tailed binder with an attached central piece.

**sebaceous gland** One of the small glands in the dermis that secretes an oily substance (sebum) on the skin's surface and in the hair.

**seborrheic dermatitis** A common chronic, inflammatory skin disease characterized by dry or moist greasy scales and yellow crusts.

**secondary intention** Wound closure in which the edges are separated, granulation tissue develops to fill the gap, and, finally, epithelium grows in over the granulation, producing a larger scar than results with primary intention.

**secretion** A product produced by a gland of the body.

**semi-Fowler's position** Placement of client in an inclined position, with the upper half of the body raised by elevating the head of the bed approximately 30 to 45 degrees.

**sensitivity** Laboratory test used in conjunction with culture; it measures the response of microorganisms to antibiotics that have been placed on a culture plate.

**sepsis** Infection, contamination.

**serology** Branch of medicine dealing with serum and blood products.

**shearing** Pressure exerted against the surface and layers of the skin as tissues slide underneath the body as it moves against a surface.

**sheet wadding** Stretchable sheets of cotton padding used to cover skin before a cast is applied; the stretching allows for some extremity edema without the cast becoming too tight.

**side effect** An effect caused by a drug that is different from the therapeutic (desired) action; the effect may be harmless or injurious.

**sigmoid colon** The part of the large intestine that extends from the descending colon to the rectum.

**sign** Objective finding perceived by an examiner, such as a fever, rash, abnormal reflex, or abnormal breath sound.

**silicone septum** Silicone partition that covers the port chamber housed in the metal or plastic body of the implanted infusion port.

**sitz bath** Special bath in which only the hips and buttocks are immersed in fluid.

**skin barrier** An artificial layer of skin, made of plastic or vinyl-like material, applied to skin before application of tape or ostomy drainage bags. Protects skin from chronic irritation.

**sling** Used to support, limit movement, enhance circulation, and prevent edema of the arm, hand, or wrist.

**SOAP** Acronym for subjective, objective, assessment, and plan, the four parts of the written account of a client's health problem in a problem-oriented record.

**solvent** Any liquid in which another substance can be dissolved.

**spasm** Involuntary muscle contraction.

**specific gravity** The ratio between the density of a solution and that of water.

**speculum** A retractor used to separate the walls of a cavity, e.g., the vaginal cavity.

**spica cast** An orthopedic cast applied to immobilize part or all of the trunk of the body and part or all of one or more extremities.

**sponge** Gauze dressing used to absorb blood in a surgical wound.

**spore** An inactive but viable state of microorganisms; certain bacteria and fungi will sustain themselves in this form until the environment is favorable for vegetative growth; while in this stage, the microorganism is highly resistant to heat, toxic chemicals, and other methods of destruction.

**spreader bar** A metal bar with curved hoop areas for attaching hooks or pins for traction.

**sputum** Lung mucus; normally thin, watery, and white or clear and watery.

**standardized care plan** A written care plan to be used for groups of clients that have similar health problems.

**staples** Stainless steel wire used to close a surgical wound.

**sterile** Free of microorganisms, including all spores.

**sterile field** Area immediately around the client that has been prepared for a surgical procedure; this area includes personnel who are properly attired and all furniture covered with sterile drapes.

**sterilization** Process by which microorganisms, including spores, are killed.

**stockinette** Stretchable cotton materials of various sizes and widths used immediately over the skin to protect tissues from the irritation of felt or plaster.

**stoma** Surgically created opening between a body cavity and the body's surface, such as a colostomy.

**stomatitis** Any inflammatory condition of the mouth. It may result from infection by bacteria, viruses, or fungi; from exposure to certain chemicals or drugs; from vitamin deficiency; or from a systemic inflammatory disease.

**stopcock** A valve that controls the flow of fluid or air through a tube.

**stroke volume** The volume of blood ejected from the left ventricle with each ventricular contraction.

**subarachnoid space** Situated or occurring between the arachnoid and the pia mater membranes, which cover the brain and spinal cord.

**subcutaneous (SQ or SC) injection** Form of injection in which a solution is introduced into subcutaneous tissues.

**subjective data** Data collected from a client.

**sublingual** Route for administering a drug beneath the tongue.

**suction** The act of sucking up a substance by reducing air pressure over its surface.

**suction catheter** Thin plastic or rubber tubing used to remove secretions.

**supination** Movement of a body part so the front or ventral surface faces upward.

**suppository** A solid form of medication inserted into a body cavity, e.g., the rectum or vagina. The drug is absorbed after it dissolves in the cavity.

**surgical asepsis** Techniques used to eliminate microorganisms from an area.

**surgical scrub** Process of removing as many microorganisms as possible from the hands and arms by mechanical washing and chemical antisepsis.

**suspension** A liquid in which small particles of a solid are dispersed, but not dissolved, and in which the dispersal is maintained by stirring or shaking the mixture.

**sympathomimetic** A pharmacologic agent that mimics the effects of stimulation of organs and structures by the sympathetic nervous system.

**syrup of ipecac** An emetic used with certain types of poisoning and drug overdoses.

**systemic** Of or pertaining to the whole body rather than to a localized area.

**systolic pressure** The higher blood pressure measurement; reflects pressure within the arterial system during the period of ventricular contraction (systole).

**T binder** Bandage in the shape of a letter T; used to support perineal dressing for delivery of humidified air.

**T tube** A T-shaped device that is attached to an endotracheal or tracheostomy tube.

**tachycardia** An abnormality in heart rate in which the myocardium contracts regularly, but at a rate over 100 beats per minute.

**tartar** A hard, gritty deposit composed of organic matter, phosphates, and carbonates that collects on teeth and gums.

**tension pneumothorax** An accumulation of air in the intrapleural space that with each inspiration becomes trapped and causes pressure to rise. This condition can result from mechanical ventilation delivering positive end-expiratory pressure (PEEP), faulty water-seal chest tube drainage systems, or prolonged clamping of the chest tube. As symptoms become increasingly severe the client develops a mediastinal shift to the unaffected side, as well as the symptoms noted with a pneumothorax.

**tepid** Moderately warm to the touch.

**terminal disinfection and sterilization** Procedures carried out at the completion of a surgical procedure to destroy pathogens.

**therapeutic silence** The use of silence that encourages verbal description and reflection; avoidance of premature verbal communication that may be due to the nurse's anxiety.

**thermoregulation** Internal control of body temperature.

**Thomas splint** A long splint with a half or full ring at one end; covered with towels and lined with felt or other soft material, it is used to suspend the thigh in skeletal traction.

**thrombocytopenia** A decrease in circulating platelets.

**thrombophlebitis** Inflammation of a vein.

**thrombus** Accumulation of platelets, fibrin, clotting factors, and the cellular elements of the blood attached to the interior wall of a vein or artery, sometimes occluding the lumen of the vessel.

**timed collection** The collection of a substance such as urine or stool for a specific period of time.

**tinnitus** Ringing heard in one or both ears.

**tissue ischemia** Decreased blood supply to body tissues.

**topical** Of or pertaining to a drug or treatment applied to the surface of a body part.

**tourniquet** An item used for the compression of blood vessels.

**tracheal malacia** An abnormal softening or sponginess of the tracheal tissue.

**tracheobronchial tree** Anatomical divisions of the respiratory tract, including the combination of trachea, bifurcations into the right and left mainstem bronchi, and subsequent bifurcations into smaller bronchi and bronchioles.

**tracheostomy** Opening through the neck into the trachea with an indwelling tube inserted; created surgically to produce an airway.

**tracheostomy collar** Curved oxygen delivery device with an adjustable neck strap that fits around the tracheostomy.

**traction** Force or pull applied to limbs, bones, or other tissues to pull the tissues apart.

**traction boot** A foam rubber boot shaped to fit a forearm or leg, used for a type of skin traction.

**transdermal** Refers to a form of medication that is applied to the skin's surface and is absorbed across the dermal or outer skin layer.

**transfusion reaction** Systemic response by the body to the administration of blood incompatible with that of the recipient.

**transilluminate** To pass light through body tissues to examine a structure interposed between the observer and the light source.

**Trendelenburg position** Position in which the head is low and the body and legs are elevated.

**trocar** Sharp, pointed rod that fits inside a tube; used to pierce the skin and the wall of a cavity or canal in the body in order to aspirate fluids, to instill a medication or solution, or to guide placement of a soft catheter.

**TSF** Triceps skin fold. Measurement determining the mass of the triceps muscle. Useful in denoting muscle wasting.

**unit dose system** System of drug distribution in which a portable cart containing a drawer for each client's medications is prepared by the pharmacy with a 24-hour supply of medications.

**unscrubbed team members** Includes the anesthesiologist or anesthetist and the circulating nurse, who wear surgical attire but are not gowned or gloved.

**upper airway respiratory system** All respiratory structures above the epiglottis, including nose, sinuses, mouth, and pharynx.

**uretheral sphincter** Voluntary muscle at the neck of the bladder that relaxes to allow micturition.

**urgency** The need to void immediately.

**urinal** Plastic or metal receptacle for urine.

**urinary retention** Inability to empty the bladder, resulting in accumulation of urine in the bladder.

**urinary tract infection** Inflammation of any structure of the urinary tract caused by an entrance of bacteria into the urinary tract.

**urine** Fluid secreted by the kidneys, transported by the ureters, stored in the bladder, and voided through the urethra.

**urine specific gravity** Measurement of the degree of concentration of the urine.

**urinometer** Device used for determining specific gravity of urine.

**urostomy** Diversion of urine away from a diseased or defective bladder through a surgically created opening (stoma) in the skin.

**uterostomy** An ostomy site in which one or both ureters are surgically brought to the abdominal surface for the excretion of urine.

**Vacu-tainer tube** A glass tube with a rubber stopper; air has been removed to create a vacuum.

**vascular access device (VAD)** Indwelling catheter, cannula, or other instrumentation used to obtain venous or arterial access.

**vein lumen** Central opening through which blood flows in a vein.

**vellus** Soft, fine hair covering all parts of the body except the palms, soles, and areas where other types of hair are normally found.

**venipuncture** Technique in which a vein is punctured transcutaneously by a sharp rigid stylet (such as a butterfly needle), a cannula (such as an angiocatheter that contains a flexible plastic catheter), or a needle attached to a syringe.

**ventilation** Respiratory process by which gases are moved into and out of the lungs.

**ventral** Of or pertaining to an anterior position, toward the abdomen.

**vertigo** A sensation of faintness or an inability to maintain normal balance in a standing or seated position, sometimes associated with giddiness, mental confusion, nausea, and weakness.

**vesicant** A drug capable of causing tissue necrosis when extravasated.

**vial** Glass container with a metal-enclosed rubber seal.

**visceral pleura** A serous membrane lining both lungs.

**visceral protein status** The amount of protein that pertains to the internal organs (e.g., abdominal).

**void** The process of emptying the bladder of urine; urinate; micturate.

**walking belt** Leather device with handles that enables the nurse to help a client walk.

**walking heel** Plastic or rubber heel placed in the sole of a leg cast to allow weight-bearing.

**webril** Stretchable cotton material applied over the skin to protect from plaster irritation.

**weight** Force exerted on a body by the gravity of the earth.

**weight holder** A metal, T-shaped bar that holds weights for traction.

**weights** Filled bags or metal disks of varying poundage used for traction.

**windowing** Cutting a small area of a cast to permit inspection of the tissues below.

**Z-track** Method for injecting irritating preparations into muscle without tracking residual medication through sensitive tissues.

# INDEX

## C

**N**



**O**

## Q



## R

# ALSO AVAILABLE!

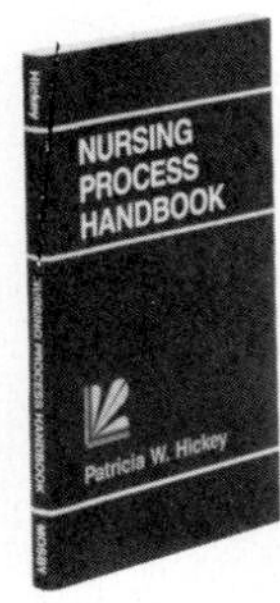


**NEW!**
**NURSING PROCESS HANDBOOK**
**Patricia W. Hickey, R.N., M.N.**
**1990. ISBN 0-8016-6041-6**

This definitive new text emphasizes the practical application of the nursing process in the clinical setting. Each step of the process is explained as well as the relationships between steps, reinforcing the logic of the problem-solving approach to planning and delivering care. Pertinent and commonly encountered examples illustrate each concept, enabling the nurse to plan and document care easily and effectively.

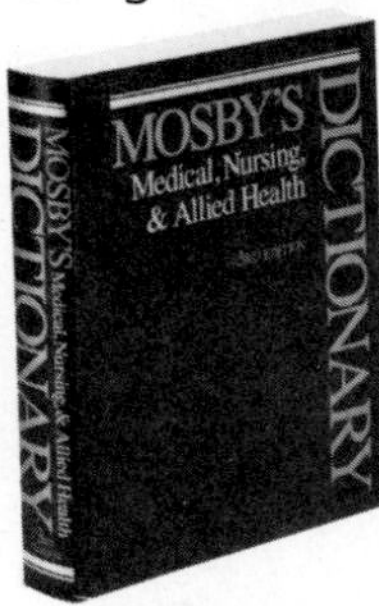


**MOSBY'S MEDICAL, NURSING,**
**AND ALLIED HEALTH DICTIONARY**
**3rd Edition**
**Kenneth N. Anderson**
**Lois Anderson**
**Walter D. Glanze**
**1990. ISBN 0-8016-3227-7**

The third edition of this respected and widely used dictionary offers in-depth definitions of specialized terms currently used by physicians, nurses, and allied health professionals. Featuring comprehensive and easy-to-read definitions, this dictionary is an indispensable reference for all nurses.

**POCKET GUIDE TO PHYSICAL ASSESSMENT**
**2nd Edition**
**Patricia A. Potter, R.N., M.S.N.**
**March 1990. ISBN 0-8016-3377-X**

This practical, pocket-sized handbook succinctly outlines the purpose, skills, and nursing considerations of physical assessment including rationales, normal findings (including deviations from normal), and appropriate pediatric and geriatric considerations for each assessment.

**POCKET GUIDE TO BASIC SKILLS AND PROCEDURES**
**2nd Edition**
**Anne G. Perry, R.N., M.S.N., A.N.P.**
**March 1990. ISBN 0-8016-5527-7**

This portable, quick-reference handbook features over 100 basic nursing skills and has been thoroughly updated to include the latest CDC guidelines and nursing diagnoses from the 8th NANDA Conference.

---

**To order, ask your bookstore manager or call toll-free 1-800-426-4545.**
**We look forward to hearing from you.**

NMA-028